ARCHIVES OF SURGERY

JANUARY 1999

PULMONARY FUNCTION FOLLOWING LAPAROSCOPIC OR CONVENTIONAL COLORECTAL RESECTION

DOES THE FACE PROTECT THE BRAIN? A CASE-CONTROL STUDY OF TRAUMATIC BRAIN INJURY AND FACIAL FRACTURES

IMPAIRMENT OF CARDIAC PERFORMANCE BY LAPAROSCOPY IN PATIENTS RECEIVING POSITIVE END-EXPIRATORY PRESSURE

PRIMARY COMMON BILE DUCT CLOSURE

PERFORATION OF THE SIGMOID COLON DUE TO GEOPHAGIA

CHANGES IN RESPIRATORY MECHANICS AFTER TRACHEOSTOMY

TRANSECTION OF THE APPENDIX: A SEAT BELT INJURY

COMPLETE TABLE OF CONTENTS INSIDE

American Medical Association
Physicians dedicated to the health of America
www.ama-assn.org/surgery

Once-daily dosing for a wide range of patients

Indication	Loading dose	Daily therapy
Oropharyngeal candidiasis	**200 mg**	100 mg
Esophageal candidiasis	**200 mg**	100 mg*
Candidal UTI and peritonitis	†	50 to 200 mg‡
Systemic candidal Infections†	†	up to 400 mg
Cryptococcal meningitis (acute)§	**400 mg**	200 mg*
Cryptococcal meningitis (maintenance to prevent relapse)		200 mg
Bone marrow transplant prophylaxis‖		400 mg

*Doses up to 400 mg/day may be used, based on medical judgment of the patient's response to therapy.

†In general, a loading dose of twice the daily dose is recommended on the first day of therapy to result in plasma concentrations close to steady-state by the second day of therapy.

‡Including candidemia, disseminated candidiasis, and pneumonia.

§Three risk factors that may predict a negative outcome for AIDS patients with cryptococcal meningitis are abnormal mental status, CSF with antigen titer >1:1024, and CSF WBC <20 cells per cubic millimeter.

‖Therapy should be continued for 7 days after neutrophil count rises above 1000 cells/mm^3. Patients who are anticipated to have severe granulocytopenia (<500 neutrophils/mm^3) should start Diflucan prophylaxis several days before the anticipated onset of neutropenia and continue for 7 days after the neutrophil count rises above 1000 cells per cubic millimeter.

Pediatric patient dose conversion

Pediatric patients	Adults
3 mg/kg	100 mg
6 mg/kg	200 mg
12 mg/kg‖	400 mg

‖Some older children may have clearances similar to that of adults. Absolute doses exceeding 600 mg/day are not recommended.

References: 1. Data available on request from Roerig. **2.** Laine L, Dretler RH, Conteas CN, et al. Fluconazole compared with ketoconazole for the treatment of candida esophagitis in AIDS: a randomized trial. *Ann Intern Med.* 1992;117:655-660. **3.** Powderly WG, Saag MS, Cloud GA, et al. A controlled trial of fluconazole or amphotericin B to prevent relapse of cryptococcal meningitis in patients with the acquired immunodeficiency syndrome. *N Engl J Med.* 1992;326:793-798. **4.** Saag MS, Powderly WG, Cloud GA, et al. Comparison of amphotericin B with fluconazole in the treatment of acute AIDS-associated cryptococcal meningitis. *N Engl J Med.* 1992;326:83-89.

Diflucan® (fluconazole)

100/150/200 mg Tablets, 10/40 mg/mL Oral Suspension, 200/400 mg IV Injection

BRIEF SUMMARY

INDICATIONS AND USAGE

DIFLUCAN (fluconazole) is indicated for the treatment of:
1. Vaginal candidiasis (vaginal yeast infections due to *Candida*).
2. Oropharyngeal and esophageal candidiasis. In open noncomparative studies of relatively small numbers of patients, DIFLUCAN was also effective for the treatment of *Candida* urinary tract infections, peritonitis, and systemic *Candida* infections including candidemia, disseminated candidiasis, and pneumonia.
3. Cryptococcal meningitis. Before prescribing DIFLUCAN for AIDS patients with cryptococcal meningitis, please see CLINICAL STUDIES section (in full prescribing information). Studies comparing DIFLUCAN to amphotericin B in non-HIV infected patients have not been conducted.

Prophylaxis. DIFLUCAN is also indicated to decrease the incidence of candidiasis in patients undergoing bone marrow transplantation who receive cytotoxic chemotherapy and/or radiation therapy.

Specimens for fungal culture and other relevant laboratory studies (serology, histopathology) should be obtained prior to therapy to isolate and identify causative organisms. Therapy may be instituted before the results of the cultures and other laboratory studies are known; however, once these results become available, anti-infective therapy should be adjusted accordingly.

CONTRAINDICATIONS

DIFLUCAN is contraindicated in patients who have shown hypersensitivity to fluconazole or to any of its excipients. There is no information regarding cross-hypersensitivity between fluconazole and other azole antifungal agents. Caution should be used in prescribing DIFLUCAN to patients with hypersensitivity to other azoles. Coadministration of terfenadine is contraindicated in patients receiving DIFLUCAN at multiple doses of 400 mg or higher based upon results of a multiple dose interaction study. Coadministration of cisapride is contraindicated in patients receiving DIFLUCAN. (See PRECAUTIONS below.)

WARNINGS

(1) Hepatic injury: DIFLUCAN has been associated with rare cases of serious hepatic toxicity, including fatalities primarily in patients with serious underlying medical conditions. In cases of DIFLUCAN-associated hepatotoxicity, no obvious relationship to total daily dose, duration of therapy, sex or age of the patient has been observed. DIFLUCAN hepatotoxicity has usually, but not always, been reversible on discontinuation of therapy. Patients who develop abnormal liver function tests during DIFLUCAN therapy should be monitored for the development of more severe hepatic injury. DIFLUCAN should be discontinued if clinical signs and symptoms consistent with liver disease develop that may be attributable to DIFLUCAN.

(2) Anaphylaxis: In rare cases, anaphylaxis has been reported.

(3) Dermatologic: Patients have rarely developed exfoliative skin disorders during treatment with DIFLUCAN. In patients with serious underlying diseases (predominantly AIDS and malignancy) these have rarely resulted in a fatal outcome. Patients who develop rashes during treatment with DIFLUCAN should be monitored closely and the drug discontinued if lesions progress.

PRECAUTIONS

General: Single Dose. The convenience and efficacy of the single dose oral tablet of fluconazole regimen for the treatment of vaginal yeast infections should be weighed against the acceptability of a higher incidence of drug related adverse events with DIFLUCAN (26%) versus intravaginal agents (16%) in U.S. comparative clinical studies. (See ADVERSE REACTIONS.)

Drug Interactions: Clinically or potentially significant drug interactions between DIFLUCAN and the following agents/classes have been observed. These are described in greater detail below: Oral hypoglycemics, coumarin-type anticoagulants, phenytoin, cyclosporine, rifampin, theophylline, terfenadine, cisapride, astemizole, rifabutin, tacrolimus.

Oral hypoglycemics: Clinically significant hypoglycemia may be precipitated by the use of DIFLUCAN with oral hypoglycemic agents; one fatality has been reported from hypoglycemia in association with combined DIFLUCAN and glyburide use. DIFLUCAN reduces the metabolism of tolbutamide, glyburide, and glipizide and increases the plasma concentration of these agents. When DIFLUCAN is used concomitantly with these or other sulfonylurea oral hypoglycemic agents, blood glucose concentrations should be carefully monitored and the dose of the sulfonylurea should be adjusted as necessary.

Coumarin-type anticoagulants: Prothrombin time may be increased in patients receiving concomitant DIFLUCAN and coumarin-type anticoagulants. Careful monitoring of prothrombin time in patients receiving DIFLUCAN and coumarin-type anticoagulants is recommended.

Phenytoin: DIFLUCAN increases the plasma concentrations of phenytoin. Careful monitoring of phenytoin concentrations in patients receiving DIFLUCAN and phenytoin is recommended.

Cyclosporine: DIFLUCAN may significantly increase cyclosporine levels in renal transplant patients with or without renal impairment. Careful monitoring of cyclosporine concentrations and serum creatinine is recommended in patients receiving DIFLUCAN and cyclosporine.

Rifampin: Rifampin enhances the metabolism of concurrently administered DIFLUCAN. Depending on clinical circumstances, consideration should be given to increasing the dose of DIFLUCAN when it is administered with rifampin.

Theophylline: DIFLUCAN increases the serum concentrations of theophylline. Careful monitoring of serum theophylline concentrations in patients receiving DIFLUCAN and theophylline is recommended.

Terfenadine: Because of the occurrence of serious cardiac dysrhythmias secondary to prolongation of the QTc interval in patients receiving azole antifungals in conjunction with terfenadine, interaction studies have been performed. One study at a 200-mg daily dose of fluconazole failed to demonstrate a prolongation of QTc interval. Another study at a 400-mg and 800-mg daily dose of fluconazole demonstrated that DIFLUCAN taken in doses of 400 mg per day or greater significantly increases plasma levels of terfenadine when taken concomitantly. The combined use of fluconazole at doses of 400 mg or greater with terfenadine is contraindicated. (See CONTRAINDICATIONS.) The coadministration of fluconazole at doses lower than 400 mg/day with terfenadine should be carefully monitored.

Cisapride: There have been reports of cardiac events, including torsade de pointes in patients to whom fluconazole and cisapride were coadministered. The combined use of fluconazole and cisapride is contraindicated. (See CONTRAINDICATIONS.)

Astemizole: The use of fluconazole in patients concurrently taking astemizole or other drugs metabolized by the cytochrome P450 system may be associated with elevations in serum levels of these drugs. In the absence of definitive information, caution should be used when coadministering fluconazole. Patients should be carefully monitored.

Rifabutin: There have been reports of uveitis in patients to whom fluconazole and rifabutin were coadministered. Patients receiving rifabutin and fluconazole concomitantly should be carefully monitored.

Tacrolimus: There have been reports of nephrotoxicity in patients to whom fluconazole and tacrolimus were coadministered. Patients receiving tacrolimus and fluconazole concomitantly should be carefully monitored.

Fluconazole tablets coadministered with ethinyl estradiol-and levonorgestrel-containing oral contraceptives produced an overall mean increase in ethinyl estradiol and levonorgestrel levels; however, in some patients there were decreases up to 47% and 33% of ethinyl estradiol and levonorgestrel levels. The data presently available indicate that the decreases in some individual ethinyl estradiol and levonorgestrel AUC values with fluconazole treatment are likely the result of random variation. While there is evidence that fluconazole can inhibit the metabolism of ethinyl estradiol and levonorgestrel, there is no evidence that fluconazole is a net inducer of ethinyl estradiol or levonorgestrel metabolism. The clinical significance of these effects is presently unknown.

Physicians should be aware that interaction studies with medications other than those listed in the CLINICAL PHARMACOLOGY section (in full prescribing information) have not been conducted, but such interactions may occur.

Carcinogenesis, Mutagenesis and Impairment of Fertility: Fluconazole showed no evidence of carcinogenic potential in mice and rats treated orally for 24 months at doses of 2.5, 5 or 10 mg/kg/day (approximately 2-7x the recommended human dose). Male rats treated with 5 and 10 mg/kg/day had an increased incidence of hepatocellular adenomas.

Fluconazole, with or without metabolic activation, was negative in tests for mutagenicity in 4 strains of *S. typhimurium*, and in the mouse lymphoma L5178Y system. Cytogenetic studies *in vivo* (murine bone marrow cells, following oral administration of fluconazole) and *in vitro* (human lymphocytes exposed to fluconazole at 1000 µg/mL) showed no evidence of chromosomal mutations.

Fluconazole did not affect the fertility of male or female rats treated orally with daily doses of 5, 10 or 20 mg/kg or with parenteral doses of 5, 25 or 75 mg/kg, although the onset of parturition was slightly delayed at 20 mg/kg PO. In an intravenous perinatal study in rats at 5, 20 and 40 mg/kg, dystocia and prolongation of parturition were observed in a few dams at 20 mg/kg (approximately 5-15x the recommended human dose) and 40 mg/kg, but not at 5 mg/kg. The disturbances in parturition were reflected by a slight increase in the number of still-born pups and decrease of neonatal survival at these dose levels. The effects on parturition in rats are consistent with the species specific estrogen-lowering property produced by high doses of fluconazole. Such a hormone change has not been observed in women treated with fluconazole.

Pregnancy: Teratogenic Effects. Pregnancy Category C: Fluconazole was administered orally to pregnant rabbits during organogenesis in two studies, at 5, 10 and 20 mg/kg, and at 5, 25, and 75 mg/kg respectively. Maternal weight gain was impaired at all dose levels, and abortions occurred at 75 mg/kg (approximately 20-60x the recommended human dose); no adverse fetal effects were detected. In several studies in which pregnant rats were treated orally with fluconazole during organogenesis, maternal weight gain was impaired and placental weights were increased at 25 mg/kg. There were no fetal effects at 5 or 10 mg/kg; increases in fetal anatomical variants (supernumerary ribs, renal pelvis dilation) and delays in ossification were observed at 25 and 50 mg/kg and higher doses. At doses ranging from 80 mg/kg (approximately 20-60x the recommended human dose) to 320 mg/kg embryolethality in rats was increased and fetal abnormalities included wavy ribs, cleft palate and abnormal cranio-facial ossification. These effects are consistent with the inhibition of estrogen synthesis in rats and may be a result of known effects of lowered estrogen on pregnancy, organogenesis and parturition.

There are no adequate and well controlled studies in pregnant women. There have been reports of multiple congenital abnormalities in infants whose mothers were being treated for 3 or more months with high dose (400-800 mg/day) fluconazole therapy for coccidioidomycosis (an unindicated use). The relationship between fluconazole use and these events is unclear. DIFLUCAN® (fluconazole) should be used in pregnancy only if the potential benefit justifies the possible risk to the fetus.

Nursing Mothers: Fluconazole is secreted in human milk at concentrations similar to plasma. Therefore, the use of DIFLUCAN in nursing mothers is not recommended.

Pediatric Use: An open-label, randomized, controlled trial has shown DIFLUCAN to be effective in the treatment of oropharyngeal candidiasis in children 6 months to 13 years of age.

The use of DIFLUCAN in children with cryptococcal meningitis, *Candida* esophagitis, or systemic *Candida* infections is supported by the efficacy shown for these indications in adults and by the results from several small noncomparative pediatric clinical studies. In addition, pharmacokinetic studies in children have established a dose proportionality between children and adults. (See DOSING.)

In a noncomparative study of children with serious systemic fungal infections, most of which were candidemia, the effectiveness of DIFLUCAN was similar to that reported for the treatment of candidemia in adults. Of 17 subjects with culture-confirmed candidemia, 11 of 14 (79%) with baseline symptoms (3 were asymptomatic) had a clinical cure; 13/15 (87%) of evaluable patients had a mycologic cure at the end of treatment but two of these patients relapsed at 10 and 18 days, respectively, following cessation of therapy.

The efficacy of DIFLUCAN for the suppression of cryptococcal meningitis was successful in 4 of 5 children treated in a compassionate-use study of fluconazole for the treatment of life-threatening or serious mycosis. There is no information regarding the efficacy of fluconazole for primary treatment of cryptococcal meningitis in children.

The safety profile of DIFLUCAN in children has been studied in 577 children ages 1 day to 17 years who received doses ranging from 1 to 15 mg/kg/day for 1 to 1,616 days. (See ADVERSE REACTIONS.)

Efficacy of DIFLUCAN has not been established in infants less than 6 months of age. A small number of patients (29) ranging in age from 1 day to 6 months have been treated safely with DIFLUCAN.

ADVERSE REACTIONS

In Patients Receiving a Single Dose for Vaginal Candidiasis: During comparative clinical studies conducted in the United States, 448 patients with vaginal candidiasis were treated with DIFLUCAN, 150 mg single dose. The overall incidence of side effects possibly related to DIFLUCAN was 26%. In 422 patients receiving active comparative agents, the incidence was 16%. The most common treatment-related adverse events reported in the patients who received 150 mg single dose fluconazole for vaginitis were headache (13%), nausea (7%), and abdominal pain (6%). Other side effects reported with an incidence equal to or greater than 1% included diarrhea (3%), dyspepsia (1%), dizziness (1%), and taste perversion (1%). Most of the reported side effects were mild to moderate in severity. Rarely, angioedema and anaphylactic reaction have been reported in marketing experience.

In Patients receiving multiple doses for other infections: Sixteen percent of over 4000 patients treated with DIFLUCAN in clinical trials of 7 days or more experienced adverse events. Treatment was discontinued in 1.5% of patients due to adverse clinical events and in 1.3% of patients due to laboratory test abnormalities.

Clinical adverse events were reported more frequently in HIV infected patients (21%) than in non-HIV infected patients (13%); however, the patterns in HIV infected and non-HIV infected patients were similar. The proportions of patients discontinuing therapy due to clinical adverse events were similar in the two groups (1.5%).

The following treatment-related clinical adverse events occurred at an incidence of 1% or greater in 4048 patients receiving DIFLUCAN for 7 or more days in clinical trials: nausea 3.7%, headache 1.9%, skin rash 1.8%, vomiting 1.7%, abdominal pain 1.7%, and diarrhea, 1.5%.

The following adverse events have occurred under conditions where a causal association is probable: *Hepatobiliary:* In combined clinical trials and marketing experience, there have been rare cases of serious hepatic reactions during treatment with DIFLUCAN. (See WARNINGS.) The spectrum of these hepatic reactions has ranged from mild transient elevations in transaminases to clinical hepatitis, cholestasis and fulminant hepatic failure, including fatalities. Instances of fatal hepatic reactions were noted to occur primarily in patients with serious underlying medical conditions (predominantly AIDS or malignancy) and often while taking multiple concomitant medications. Transient hepatic reactions, including hepatitis and jaundice have occurred among patients with no other identifiable risk factors. In each of these cases, liver function returned to baseline on discontinuation of DIFLUCAN.

In two comparative trials evaluating the efficacy of DIFLUCAN for the suppression of relapse of cryptococcal meningitis, a statistically significant increase was observed in median AST (SGOT) levels from a baseline value of 30 IU/L to 41 IU/L in one trial and 34 IU/L to 66 IU/L in the other. The overall rate of serum transaminase elevations of more than 8 times the upper limit of normal was approximately 1% in fluconazole-treated patients in clinical trials. These elevations occurred in patients with severe underlying disease, predominantly AIDS or malignancies, most of whom were receiving multiple concomitant medications, including many known to be hepatotoxic. The incidence of abnormally elevated serum transaminases was greater in patients taking DIFLUCAN concomitantly with one or more of the following medications: rifampin, phenytoin, isoniazid, valproic acid, or oral sulfonylurea hypoglycemic agents.

Immunologic: In rare cases, anaphylaxis has been reported.

The following adverse events have occurred under conditions where a causal association is uncertain: *Central Nervous System:* seizures. *Dermatologic:* Exfoliative skin disorders including Stevens-Johnson Syndrome and toxic epidermal necrolysis (see WARNINGS), alopecia. *Hematopoietic and Lymphatic:* leukopenia, including neutropenia and agranulocytosis, thrombocytopenia. *Metabolic:* hypercholesterolemia, hypertriglyceridemia, hypokalemia.

Adverse Reactions in Children: In Phase II/III clinical trials conducted in the United States and in Europe, 577 pediatric patients, ages 1 day to 17 years were treated with DIFLUCAN at doses of up to 15 mg/kg/day for up to 1,616 days. Thirteen percent of children experienced treatment-related adverse events. The most commonly reported events were vomiting (5%), abdominal pain (3%), nausea (2%), and diarrhea (2%). Treatment was discontinued in 2.3% of patients due to adverse clinical events and in 1.4% of patients due to laboratory test abnormalities. The majority of treatment-related laboratory abnormalities were elevations of transaminases or alkaline phosphatase.

Percentage of Patients With Treatment-Related Side Effects

	Fluconazole (N=577)	Comparative Agents (N=451)
With any side effect	13.0	9.3
Vomiting	5.4	5.1
Abdominal pain	2.8	1.6
Nausea	2.3	1.6
Diarrhea	2.1	2.2

Pfizer U.S. Pharmaceuticals

FC255A98

Rev. October 1998

OVERWHELMING ANTIFUNGAL SUCCESS

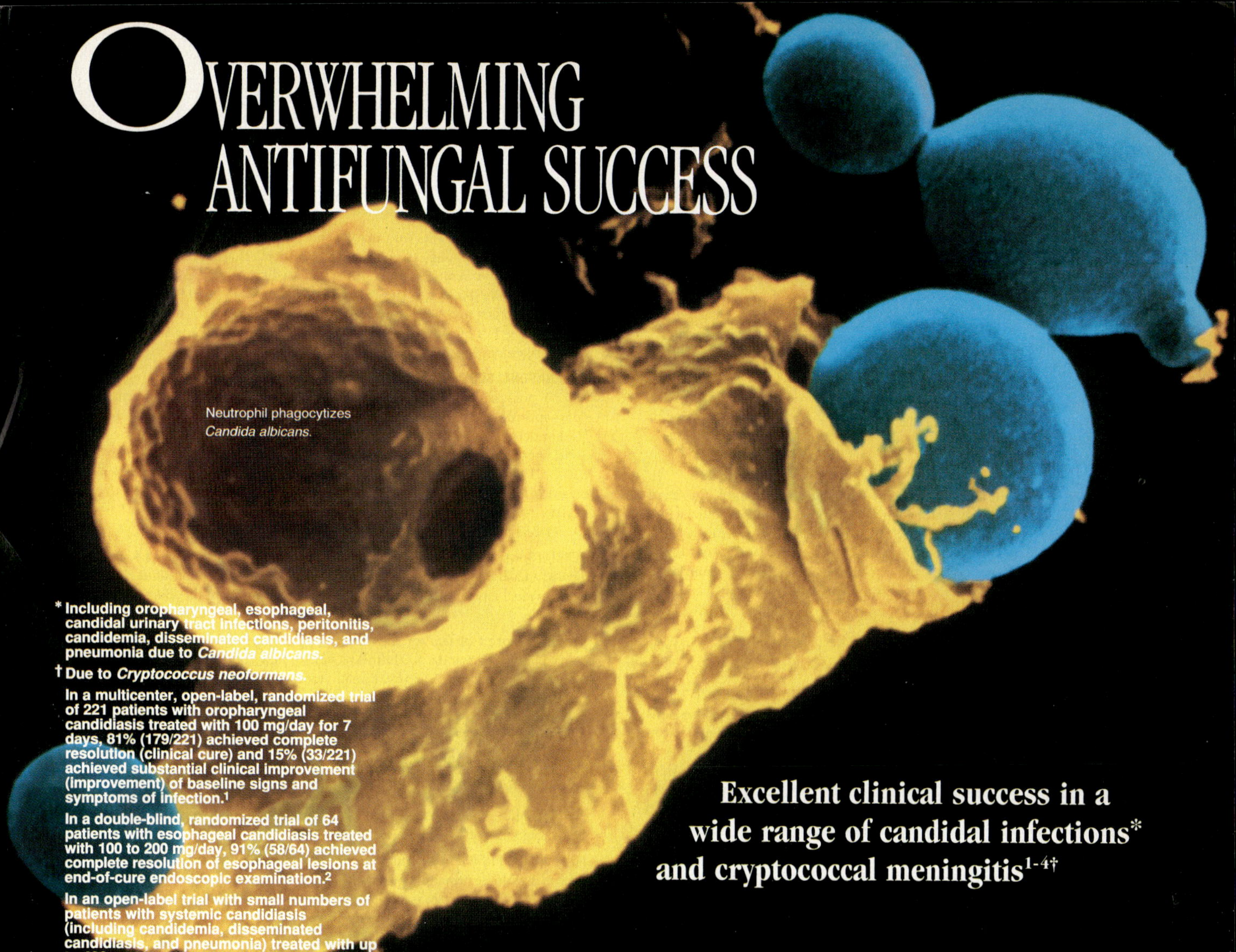

Neutrophil phagocytizes *Candida albicans.*

* Including oropharyngeal, esophageal, candidal urinary tract infections, peritonitis, candidemia, disseminated candidiasis, and pneumonia due to *Candida albicans.*

† Due to *Cryptococcus neoformans.*

In a multicenter, open-label, randomized trial of 221 patients with oropharyngeal candidiasis treated with 100 mg/day for 7 days, 81% (179/221) achieved complete resolution (clinical cure) and 15% (33/221) achieved substantial clinical improvement (improvement) of baseline signs and symptoms of infection.[1]

In a double-blind, randomized trial of 64 patients with esophageal candidiasis treated with 100 to 200 mg/day, 91% (58/64) achieved complete resolution of esophageal lesions at end-of-cure endoscopic examination.[2]

In an open-label trial with small numbers of patients with systemic candidiasis (including candidemia, disseminated candidiasis, and pneumonia) treated with up to 400 mg/day, 69% (22/32) of candidemia patients achieved complete resolution (clinical cure), and 22% (7/32) achieved substantial clinical improvement (improvement) of baseline signs and symptoms of infection. In patients with disseminated candidiasis, 52% (16/31) achieved complete resolution (clinical cure), and 19% (6/31) achieved substantial clinical improvement (improvement) of baseline signs and symptoms of infection. In patients with pneumonia, 58% (11/19) achieved complete resolution (clinical cure), and 37% (7/19) achieved substantial clinical improvement (improvement) of baseline signs and symptoms of infection.

In an open-label trial with small numbers of patients with candidal urinary tract infections (UTI) and peritonitis treated with doses of 50 mg to 200 mg/day, 53% (20/38) of those with candidal UTI achieved complete resolution (clinical cure), and 26% (10/38) achieved substantial clinical improvement (improvement) of baseline signs and symptoms of infection. In peritonitis patients, 66% (23/35) achieved complete resolution (clinical cure), and 25% (9/35) achieved substantial clinical improvement (improvement) of baseline signs and symptoms of infection.

In a multicenter comparative study of 111 patients treated with 200 mg/day for suppression of relapse of cryptococcal meningitis, 93% (103/111) achieved successful maintenance without culture-confirmed relapse and without toxicity necessitating discontinuance. Three risk factors which may predict a negative outcome for AIDS patients with cryptococcal meningitis are: abnormal mental status, CSF with antigen titer>1:1024, and CSF WBC<20 cells per cubic millimeter.[3]

In a multicenter, open-label, 10-week trial of 131 AIDS patients treated with 200 mg/day for culture-confirmed acute cryptococcal meningitis, an overall response rate (cure and quiescent disease) of 60% (78/131) was achieved.[4]

Excellent clinical success in a wide range of candidal infections* and cryptococcal meningitis[1-4†]

Excellent clinical safety

In more than 4,000 patients who received Diflucan for at least 7 days, the most common adverse events were nausea (3.7%), headache (1.9%), skin rash (1.8%), vomiting (1.7%), abdominal pain (1.7%), and diarrhea (1.5%).[1]

Diflucan has been associated with rare cases of serious hepatotoxicity. Patients have rarely developed exfoliative skin disorders during treatment with Diflucan.

ONCE-A-DAY **Diflucan**® ORAL IV (fluconazole)

100/200 mg Tablets, 10/40 mg/mL Oral Suspension, 200/400 mg IV Injection

Overwhelming antifungal success

Please see brief summary of prescribing information on adjacent page of this advertisement.

ARCHIVES OF SURGERY

The ARCHIVES OF SURGERY is a member of the consortium of AMA journals listed below. The complete text of all AMA journals is available online from Dialog Information Services and Information Access Company.

The Journal of the American Medical Association (JAMA)
Archives of Dermatology
Archives of Family Medicine
Archives of General Psychiatry
Archives of Internal Medicine
Archives of Neurology
Archives of Ophthalmology
Archives of Otolaryngology–Head & Neck Surgery
Archives of Pathology & Laboratory Medicine
Archives of Pediatrics & Adolescent Medicine
Archives of Surgery

The ARCHIVES OF SURGERY (ISSN 0004-0010) is published monthly by the American Medical Association, 515 N State St, Chicago, IL 60610, and is an official publication of the Association. The ARCHIVES OF SURGERY reaches more than 19 000 readers in over 69 countries each month. Periodicals postage paid at Chicago, IL, and at additional mailing offices. GST registration number 12622 5556 RT. Canada Post International Publications Mail (Canadian Distribution) Sales Agreement No. 319309.

Printed in the USA.

Official Publication of the New England Surgical Society, Pacific Coast Surgical Association, Surgical Infection Society, Western Surgical Association.

SUBSCRIPTION RATES—The personal subscription rates for the ARCHIVES OF SURGERY are $145 for 1 year (12 issues) in the United States and US possessions; $195 in the Americas; £125 outside the Americas. The institution rates for 1 year are $245 in the US; $345 in the Americas; £195 outside the Americas. Special rates for residents and medical students are available. Address all subscription communications to: Subscriber Services Center, American Medical Association, PO Box 10946, Chicago, IL 60610-0946. Phone: (800) 262-2350. Fax: (312) 464-5831. E-mail: ama-subs@ama-assn.org. For mailing addresses outside the United States and US possessions, see International Subscription Information.

CHANGE OF ADDRESS—POSTMASTER, send all address changes to ARCHIVES OF SURGERY, c/o Subscriber Services, American Medical Association, 515 N State St, Chicago, IL 60610. Please notify us of address change at least 6 weeks in advance to ensure uninterrupted service. Include both old and new addresses, a recent mailing label, and new ZIP code. For mailing addresses outside the United States and US possessions, see International Subscription Information.

SUBSCRIBER SERVICES—For information about subscribing to any of the AMA publications, change of address, missing issues, or purchasing back issues, please contact Subscriber Services Center, American Medical Association, PO Box 10946, Chicago, IL 60610-0946, or call (800) 262-2350 or (312) 670-SUBS (670-7827) between 8:30 AM and 4:30 PM CST. Fax: (312) 464-5831. E-mail: ama-subs@ama-assn.org. For mailing addresses outside the United States and US possessions, see International Subscription Information.

INTERNATIONAL SUBSCRIPTION INFORMATION—Subscriptions outside the United States and US possessions are served according to geographic region. Please address correspondence to the following 2 offices based on delivery address: (1) For delivery in North America, Central America, and South America, contact Subscriber Services, AMA, PO Box 10946, Chicago, IL 60610-0946. Phone: (312) 670-7827. Fax: (312) 464-5831. E-mail: ama-subs@ama-assn.org. (2) For delivery outside the Americas contact JAMA & Archives Journals, Reader Services Centre, PO Box 299, London WC1H 9TD, England. Phone: +44 (0)171-383-6270. Fax: +44 (0)171-383-6402. E-mail: jama-archives@dial.pipex.com.

REPRINTS—Authors place their reprint order at the time the edited typescript is reviewed and should allow 4 to 6 weeks for delivery following publication. Requests for individual reprints should be sent directly to the author at the address shown in the article.

For bulk reprint orders for distribution by commercial organizations, please contact Wanda Bartolotta, 500 Fifth Ave, #2210, New York, NY 10110. Phone: (212) 354-0050. Fax: (212) 354-1169. E-mail: wanda_bartolotta@ama-assn.org. For reprint orders in limited quantities for distribution by educational organizations and for author reprints, please contact Joseph R. Rekash, 515 N State St, Chicago, IL 60610. Phone: (312) 464-4594. Fax: (312) 464-4849.

WORLD WIDE WEB ADDRESS—http://www.ama-assn.org.

SURGERY HOME PAGE—http://www.ama-assn.org/surgery.

PERMISSIONS—Contact Ada Jimenez-Walker, Permissions Assistant, 515 N State St, Chicago, IL 60610. Phone: (312) 464-2513.

ADVERTISING PRINCIPLES—Each advertisement in this issue has been reviewed and complies with the principles governing advertising in AMA scientific publications. A copy of these principles is available on request. The appearance of advertising in AMA publications is not an AMA guarantee or endorsement of the product or the claims made for the product by the manufacturer.

ARCHIVES OF SURGERY

www.ama-assn.org/surgery

VOL 134 NO. 1, JANUARY 1999

MISSION STATEMENT

To promote the art and science of surgery by publishing relevant peer-reviewed clinical and basic science information to assist the surgeon in optimizing patient care. The *Archives of Surgery* will also serve as a forum for the discussion of issues that involve ethics, teaching, surgical history, and socioeconomic concerns.

*Approved by the Editorial Board, *Archives of Surgery*, July 19, 1996.

ORIGINAL ARTICLES

Pulmonary Function Following Laparoscopic or Conventional Colorectal Resection: A Randomized Controlled Evaluation 6
Wolfgang Schwenk, MD; Bartolomäus Böhm, MD, PhD; Christoph Witt, MD; Tido Junghans, MD; Kerstin Gründel, MD; Jochen M. Müller, MD

Invited Critique 13
Andrew A. Shelton, MD; Robert D. Madoff, MD

Does the Face Protect the Brain? A Case-Control Study of Traumatic Brain Injury and Facial Fractures 14
Heather T. Keenan, MD; Susan I. Brundage, MD; Diane C. Thompson, MS; Ronald V. Maier, MD; Frederick P. Rivara, MD, MPH

Antireflux Surgery Enhances Gastric Emptying 18
Mikko Viljakka, MD; Keijo Saali, MSc; Matti Koskinen, PhD; Lauri Karhumäki, MD; Jyrki Kössi, MD; Markku Luostarinen, MD; Ossi Teerenhovi, MD; Jouko Isolauri, MD

Primary Common Bile Duct Closure 22
A. Kent Seale, MD; Walter P. Ledet, Jr, MD

Effect of Intraoperative Blood Transfusion on Patient Outcome in Hepatic Transplantation 25
Thomas V. Cacciarelli, MD; Emmet B. Keeffe, MD; Dan H. Moore, PhD; Washington Burns, MD; Stephan Busque, MD; Waldo Concepcion, MD; Samuel K. S. So, MD; Carlos O. Esquivel, MD, PhD

The Relationship Between Hospital Volume and Outcomes of Hepatic Resection for Hepatocellular Carcinoma 30
Robert E. Glasgow, MD; Jonathan A. Showstack, PhD, MPH; Patricia P. Katz, PhD; Carlos U. Corvera, MD; Robert S. Warren, MD; Sean J. Mulvihill, MD

Invited Critique 35
Christian Herfarth, MD; Peter Kienle, MD

Preoperative Serum Albumin Level as a Predictor of Operative Mortality and Morbidity: Results From the National VA Surgical Risk Study 36
James Gibbs, PhD; William Cull, PhD; William Henderson, PhD; Jennifer Daley, MD; Kwan Hur, MS; Shukri F. Khuri, MD

Comparison of Blue Dye and Probe-Assisted Intraoperative Lymphatic Mapping in Melanoma to Identify Sentinel Nodes in 100 Lymphatic Basins 43
Peter Bostick, MD; Richard Essner, MD; Edwin Glass, MD; Mark Kelley, MD; Terry Sarantou, MD; Leland J. Foshag, MD; Karen Qi, MS; Donald Morton, MD

Prognostic Factors in T1 and T2 Squamous Cell Carcinoma of the Thoracic Esophagus 50
Mitsuo Tachibana, MD; Shoichi Kinugasa, MD; Dipok Kumar Dhar, MD; Hideki Tabara, MD; Reiko Masunaga, MD; Tsukasa Kotoh, MD; Hirofumi Kubota, MD; Naofumi Nagasue, MD

Lower Esophageal Sphincter Dysfunction Often Precludes Safe Gastric Feeding in Stroke Patients 55
Charles E. Lucas, MD; Pingyang Yu, MD; Angie Vlahos, MS; Anna M. Ledgerwood, MD

Changes in Respiratory Mechanics After Tracheostomy 59
Kenneth Davis, Jr, MD; Robert S. Campbell, RRT; Jay A. Johannigman, MD; John F. Valente, MD; Richard D. Branson, BA, RRT

Resection With External Beam and Intraoperative Radiotherapy for Recurrent Colon Cancer 63
Richard D. Pezner, MD; David Z. J. Chu, MD; Lawrence D. Wagman, MD; Nayana Vora, MD; Jeffrey Y. C. Wong, MD; Stephen I. Shibata, MD

Invited Critique 67
Raj M. Nambiar, MD

ARCHIVES OF SURGERY

Prospective Evaluation of Total Parathyroidectomy and Autotransplantation for the Treatment of Secondary Hyperparathyroidism 68
Francesco Zaraca, MD; Sandro Mazzaferro, MD; Marco Catarci, MD; Alessandra Saputelli, MD; Piero Alò, MD; Manlio Carboni, MD

Invited Critique 72
James Norman, MD

The Value of Acute-Phase Protein Measurements After Curative Gastric Cancer Surgery 73
Tetsuji Fujita, MD; Akihiko Hara, MD; Yoji Yamazaki, MD

Impairment of Cardiac Performance by Laparoscopy in Patients Receiving Positive End-Expiratory Pressure 76
Eric J. Kraut, MD; John T. Anderson, MD; Amira Safwat, MD; Ronald Barbosa, BS; Bruce M. Wolfe, MD

Relationship of Systemic Inflammatory Response Syndrome to Organ Dysfunction, Length of Stay, and Mortality in Critical Surgical Illness: Effect of Intensive Care Unit Resuscitation 81
Mia Talmor, MD; Lynn Hydo, BS; Philip S. Barie, MD, FCCM

CLINICAL OBSERVATIONS

Perforation of the Sigmoid Colon Due to Geophagia 88
Alexander Woywodt, MD; Akos Kiss, MD, FCSSA

Transection of the Appendix: A Seat Belt Injury 90
Robert A. Edwards, DO; Douglas B. Paul, DO; Gary L. Anderson, DO; Mary C. McCarthy, MD

SPECIAL ARTICLE

Surgery in the Netherlands 92
H. Jaap Bonjer, MD, PhD; Hajo A. Bruining, MD, PhD

SURGICAL TECHNIQUE

Laparoscopic Splenectomy 99
Richard T. Schlinkert, MD; Sumeet S. Teotia, MD

Invited Critique 103
Vafa Shayani, MD

SURGICAL REMINISCENCES

Necessity Is the Mother of Invention 104
Roger T. Sherman, MD

MOMENTS IN SURGICAL HISTORY

Henry H. Smith's *A System of Operative Surgery* 105
Ira M. Rutkow, MD, MPH, DrPH

DEPARTMENTS

Surgical Anatomy 24

Products & Services 106

Instructions for Authors 107

Classified Advertising 116

Index to Advertisers 119

Pulmonary Function Following Laparoscopic or Conventional Colorectal Resection

A Randomized Controlled Evaluation

Wolfgang Schwenk, MD; Bartolomäus Böhm, MD, PhD; Christoph Witt, MD; Tido Junghans, MD; Kerstin Gründel, MD; Jochen M. Müller, MD

Background: Laparotomy causes a significant reduction of pulmonary function, and atelectasis and pneumonia occur after elective conventional colorectal resections.

Objective: To evaluate the hypothesis that pulmonary function is less restricted after laparoscopic than after conventional colorectal resection.

Design: A randomized clinical trial.

Setting: The surgical department of an academic medical center.

Patients: Sixty patients underwent laparoscopic (n = 30) or conventional (n = 30) resection of colorectal tumors. The 2 groups did not differ significantly in age, sex, localization or stage of tumor, or preoperative pulmonary function.

Main Outcome Measures: Forced vital capacity, forced expiratory volume in 1 second, peak expiratory flow, midexpiratory phase of forced expiratory flow, and oxygen saturation of arterial blood.

Results: The forced vital capacity (mean ± SD values: conventional resection group, 1.73 ± 0.60 L; laparoscopic surgery group, 2.59 ± 1.11 L; $P<.01$) and the forced expiratory volume in 1 second (conventional resection group, 1.19 ± 0.51 L/s; laparoscopic surgery group, 1.80 ± 0.80 L/s; $P<.01$) were more profoundly suppressed in the patients having conventional resection than in those having laparoscopic surgery. Similar results were found for the peak expiratory flow (conventional resection group, 2.51 ± 1.37 L/s; laparoscopic resection group, 3.60 ± 2.22 L/s; $P<.05$) and the midexpiratory phase of forced expiratory flow (conventional resection group, 1.87 ± 1.12 L/s; laparoscopic surgery group, 2.67 ± 1.76 L/s; $P<.05$). The oxygen saturation of arterial blood, measured while the patients were breathing room air, was lower after conventional than after laparoscopic resections ($P<.01$). The recovery of the forced vital capacity and forced expiratory volume in 1 second to 80% of the preoperative value took longer in patients having conventional resection than in those having laparoscopic resection ($P<.01$). Pneumonia developed in 2 patients having conventional resection, but no pulmonary infection occurred in the laparoscopic resection group ($P>.05$).

Conclusions: Pulmonary function is better preserved after laparoscopic than after conventional colorectal resection. Pulmonary complications may be reduced after laparoscopic resections because of the better postoperative pulmonary function.

Arch Surg. 1999;134:6-12

From the Department of General, Visceral, Vascular, and Thoracic Surgery (Drs Schwenk, Böhm, Junghans, Gründel, and Müller), and the First Department of Internal Medicine (Dr Witt), Medical Faculty of the Humboldt–University of Berlin, Charité, Berlin, Germany.

The suppression of pulmonary function is a well-known sequela of abdominal surgery and was first described in 1933 by Beecher.[1] Following upper abdominal incisions, forced vital capacity (FVC) and forced expiratory volume in 1 second (FEV_1) are reduced by almost 60%[2-4] because of a reflectory dysfunction of the diaphragm. Because the functional residual capacity is decreased postoperatively, small airways collapse[5] and atelectasis occurs in most patients.[6] Regardless of the anesthetic technique, pulmonary function does not recover to preoperative values within the first postoperative week after conventional abdominal surgery, and intensive physiotherapy does not prevent pulmonary dysfunction.[1,7-10] Pneumonia is clinically apparent in more than 5% of all patients undergoing elective conventional colorectal resection and constitutes the most common general postoperative complication after conventional colorectal resection.[11-13]

See Invited Critique at end of article

Pulmonary function is better after simple laparoscopic procedures than after conventional surgery. Arterial oxygen saturation (SaO_2) is less impaired and at-

PATIENTS AND METHODS

HYPOTHESIS, END POINTS, AND SAMPLE SIZE CALCULATION

We hypothesized that pulmonary function is less suppressed and recovers faster following laparoscopic than conventional colorectal resections. To test this hypothesis, we recorded postoperative changes in FVC, FEV_1, peak expiratory flow (PEF), the midexpiratory phase of forced expiratory flow ($FEF_{25\%-75\%}$), the relation of the FEV_1 to the FVC (FEV_1/FVC ratio), and Sa_{O_2}. The sample size needed to test the hypothesis was calculated according to the methods described by Altman.[19] The FVC and FEV_1 were chosen as major criteria for calculating the sample size. It was assumed that FVC and FEV_1 values decrease by 50% ± 20% (±SD) following conventional colorectal resections.[6] A difference of 15% in the postoperative FVC and FEV_1 values between the laparoscopic and conventional resection groups can be detected by a 2-tailed test with an α level of .05, a β level of .20 (power, 80%), and 30 patients in each group.

STUDY POPULATION

All patients with the diagnosis of a colorectal tumor who were scheduled for elective ascending colectomy, sigmoidectomy, proctosigmoidectomy, or abdominoperineal resection were included in the study. Patients who were scheduled for a sphincter-preserving anterior resection with total mesorectal excision of carcinoma of the middle or lower rectum (<12 cm from the anal verge) were excluded. Further exclusion criteria were intestinal obstruction, intraabdominal abscess or sepsis, infiltration of tumor into adjacent organs or a tumor of more than 8 cm in diameter on computed tomographic scan, severe obesity (body mass index [or Quetelet index], calculated as weight in kilograms divided by the square of the height in meters, >32), operative risk greater than the American Society of Anesthesiologists' class III, and uncorrectable coagulopathy or thrombocytopenia.

STUDY DESIGN

The study was approved by the local ethics committee. Concomitant cardiopulmonary diseases of all patients were recorded, and medical treatment was optimized before surgery. An informed consent was obtained from every patient. Mechanical bowel preparation and the perioperative administration of antibiotics were the same in the 2 groups. Anesthesia with endotracheal intubation was performed in a standardized manner by the same anesthesiological team using sufentanil, propofol, and atracurium besylate. Intraoperative sufentanil doses in micrograms per kilogram of body weight per minute were comparable in both groups.

OPERATIVE TECHNIQUE AND INTRAOPERATIVE RANDOMIZATION

All patients underwent a diagnostic laparoscopy. When the surgeon decided during the diagnostic laparoscopy that laparoscopic resection of the tumor was feasible, intraoperative randomization was accomplished, and a laparoscopic or conventional resection was carried out. If the surgeon decided that laparoscopic resection could not be performed, the patient was excluded from further evaluation and underwent a conventional resection. All laparoscopic procedures were performed by an experienced laparoscopic team using a standardized 5-trocar technique (infraumbilical and middle and lower abdomen bilaterally) that has been described in detail elsewhere.[20] During proctosigmoidectomy and abdominoperineal resection, high ligation of the inferior mesenteric artery was accomplished with a linear endoscopic stapling device (EndoGIA 30; Autosuture Germany,

Continued on next page

electasis occurs less often after laparoscopic than after conventional cholecystectomy.[3,14-16] Although the laparoscopic approach to colorectal diseases has been reported by some authors[11,17] to be beneficial, it is still questionable whether laparoscopic colorectal resection actually results in better postoperative pulmonary function.[18] A randomized study was conducted to determine whether postoperative pulmonary function is better following laparoscopic than conventional colorectal resections.

RESULTS

From April 19, 1995, to October 24, 1996, 60 patients were randomly assigned to laparoscopic (n = 30) or conventional (n = 30) resection of colorectal tumors. An 86-year-old patient in the laparoscopic resection group was switched to a laparoscopic-assisted sigmoidectomy because of tumor infiltration of the left ovary and was included in the laparoscopic group for an intent-to-treat analysis. After conventional sigmoidectomy, 1 patient required a second laparotomy because of hemorrhage from the greater omentum at the splenic flexure. The patient received mechanical ventilation for 24 hours after primary surgery.

Patient demographics are shown in **Table 1**. There were no significant differences in these characteristics between the groups. Preoperatively, the FVC and FEV_1 values, the FEV_1/FVC ratio, and the PEF, $FEF_{25\%-75\%}$, and Sa_{O_2} values were comparable between the groups (**Table 2**). None of the patients had pulmonary function values below 70% of expected for their age. Preoperative results of the spirometric tests were correlated to the results of body plethysmography (FVC, $r = 0.93$, $P < .001$; and FEV_1, $r = 0.89$, $P < .001$).

The operating time was 219 ± 64 minutes for the laparoscopic resection group and 146 ± 41 minutes for the conventional resection group ($P < .01$). Postoperative morbidity and the number of deaths are shown in **Table 3**. The mean length of postoperative hospital stays was 10.1 ± 3.0 days in the laparoscopic resection group and 11.6 ± 2.0 days in the conventional resection group ($P < .05$). One patient with sigmoid carcinoma and diffuse liver metastases was discharged 9 days after conventional surgery but died 14 days later of hepatic failure.

The postoperative suppression of pulmonary function (FVC, FEV_1, PEF, and $FEF_{25\%-75\%}$) was more severe after conventional than after laparoscopic resection

Toenisvorst, Germany). During ascending colectomies, the ileocolic and right colic arteries were dissected with a stapler close to their origin from the superior mesenteric artery. In all resections with curative intent, a systematic regional lymphadenectomy was performed. After resection, the specimen was retrieved through a minilaparotomy of 3 to 4 cm in the left lower abdomen (proctosigmoidectomy) or the infraumbilical region (ascending colectomy). During ascending colectomy, a functional end-to-end ileotransversostomy was performed extracorporeally with a linear stapling device (GIA80; Autosuture Germany). For a proctosigmoidectomy, the anvil of a circular stapling device (Premium Plus CEEA; Autosuture Germany) was inserted into the descending colon extracorporeally. Then the minilaparotomy was closed, the pneumoperitoneum was reestablished, and the anastomosis between the descending colon and rectum was performed using the "double-stapling" technique. The anatomical extent of resection and the anastomotic technique were similar in the conventional surgery, but the resection was accomplished through a wide midline laparotomy.

POSTOPERATIVE ANALGESIA, PULMONARY FUNCTION, AND Sa_{O_2}

All patients received patient-controlled analgesia with morphine sulfate until the morning of the fourth postoperative day and, from then on, tramadol hydrochloride orally until discharge. Pain was assessed using a visual analog scale during rest and during coughing. The patient-controlled anesthesia bolus was increased when the visual analog scale score at rest was higher than 50. All patients received supplemental oxygen (2-6 L/min) until the morning of the first postoperative day. Patients were discharged from the surgical intensive care unit to the regular nursing floor on the first postoperative day. Bedside spirometry (Renaissance Spirometer; Firma Puritan Bennett Hoyer, Gräfeling, Germany) was carried out with the patients lying in bed and the upper body elevated by 45°. Each test was repeated 3 times, and the best of the 3 results for FVC, FEV_1, PEF, and $FEF_{25\%-75\%}$ were chosen for further analysis.[21] The FEV_1/FVC ratio (in percentage) was calculated from these values. Spirometry was performed preoperatively, 3 times per day from the first to the third day, twice a day from the fourth to the sixth day, and once a day from the seventh day until discharge. At the same time, Sa_{O_2} was measured by pulse oximetry (Oxyshuttle+2; Critikon, Norderstedt, Germany) while the patients were breathing room air. Body plethysmography was performed preoperatively and on the fifth postoperative day in the Department of Pulmonology to validate the results of the spirometric tests.

All patients received patient-controlled analgesia with morphine sulfate immediately after surgery until the eighth postoperative day. The doses were adjusted according to the patients' subjective pain perception, which was assessed every 8 hours by visual analog scale. All intraoperative and postoperative complications and mortality were recorded until 30 days after surgery. Pneumonia was diagnosed when patients had a temperature higher than 38°C, a productive cough, and radiological evidence of infection. To complete the measurements of the first postoperative week, patients were not discharged before the seventh postoperative day.

DATA COLLECTION AND STATISTICAL ANALYSIS

Normally distributed continuous data are given as mean ± SD and were compared between the groups using the Student *t* test. If appropriate, the Wilcoxon rank sum test was performed. Categorical data were compared using the Fisher exact test. Correlations between continuous values were calculated using the Spearman rank test. A *P* value of .05 was considered significant. Statistical analysis of all data was performed using commercial software (SAS for Windows; SAS Institute Inc, Cary, NC).

(**Table 4**). The results of spirometric tests and body plethysmography in the postoperative period were also highly correlated (FVC, $r = 0.96$, $P < .001$; and FEV_1, $r = 0.94$, $P < .001$). Improvement of pulmonary function had the same slope in both groups (**Figure 1** through **Figure 3**). Recovery to 80% of the preoperative FVC value was achieved after 2.9 ± 2.0 days in the laparoscopic resection group and after 5.2 ± 2.6 days in the conventional resection group ($P < .01$) (Figure 1). Recovery of 80% of the preoperative FEV_1 value took 3.0 ± 2.2 days in the laparoscopic resection group and 5.7 ± 3.2 days in the conventional resection group ($P < .01$) (Figure 2). The postoperative values of the PEF reached 80% of the preoperative level within 3.9 ± 3.3 days in the laparoscopic resection group and 5.7 ± 3.7 days in the conventional resection group (Figure 3). The $FEF_{25\%-75\%}$ reached 80% of the preoperative value within 3.2 ± 2.9 days after laparoscopic resection and 4.9 ± 3.2 days after conventional resection ($P < .05$). There were no differences in the FEV_1/FVC ratio between the groups.

Preoperative Sa_{O_2} values were comparable between the groups (Table 2). From the morning of the first postoperative day, the Sa_{O_2} value was lower after conventional resection than after laparoscopic surgery (**Figure 4**). Although the Sa_{O_2} value remained almost unchanged in the laparoscopic resection group, it continuously decreased in the conventional resection group until 2 PM of the second day after surgery (Figure 4). The Sa_{O_2} value at least once was lower than 90% in 22 patients (73%) having conventional resection but in only 14 patients (47%) having laparoscopic resection ($P = .06$).

COMMENT

Postoperative pneumonia occurs in more than 5% of all patients after elective conventional colorectal resection.[11-13] The reason for this incidence of postoperative pneumonia is a prolonged impairment of pulmonary function induced by laparotomy.[3-7,23] After a midline laparotomy, pulmonary function is depressed to about 50% of the preoperative value,[3,5,6,23] and complete recovery of pulmonary function after abdominal surgery usually takes 7 or more days.[3,4] Pulmonary function is more depressed after incisions in the upper abdomen than after lower abdominal laparotomy.[3,5,7] Colorectal carcinoma, inflammatory bowel disease, or diverticular disease require the resection of larger bowel segments.[24] Mobili-

Table 1. Characteristics of Patients Undergoing Laparoscopic or Conventional Resection of Colorectal Tumors*

Characteristic	Patient Group: Laparoscopic Resection (n = 30)	Conventional Resection (n = 30)	*P*†
Age, mean ± SD, y	63.3 ± 12.2	64.8 ± 14.7	.67
BMI, mean ± SD, kg/m²	24.7 ± 2.9	24.7 ± 2.4	>.99
Sex			
Male	14 (47)	16 (53)	.80
Female	16 (53)	14 (47)	
Concomitant diseases‡			
Cardiac	6 (20)	10 (33)	.38
Arterial hypertension	7 (23)	4 (13)	.51
Diabetes mellitus	2 (7)	4 (13)	.67
Pulmonary	1 (3)	3 (10)	.61
Hepatic	0	1 (3)	>.99
None	20 (67)	13 (43)	.12
ASA class			
I	14 (47)	9 (30)	
II	14 (47)	19 (63)	.29
III	2 (7)	2 (7)	
Type of resection			
Ascending colectomy	4 (13)	3 (10)	
Proctosigmoidectomy	22 (73)	24 (80)	.83
Abdominoperineal resection	4 (13)	3 (10)	
Tumor stage§			
0 (adenoma)	1 (3)	3 (10)	
I	9 (30)	8 (27)	
II	12 (40)	5 (17)	.19
III	6 (20)	8 (27)	
IV	2 (7)	6 (20)	

*Values are number (percentage) unless otherwise indicated.
†For age and BMI, the Student *t* test was used; for all other variables, the Fisher exact test.
‡Some patients had more than 1 concomitant disease.
§From the Union Internationale Contre le Cancer.[22]

Table 2. Preoperative Values of Pulmonary Function Tests and Pulse Oximetry in Patients Undergoing Laparoscopic or Conventional Resection of Colorectal Tumors*

Test	Patient Group: Laparoscopic Resection (n = 30)	Conventional Resection (n = 30)	*P*†
FVC, L	3.62 ± 1.26	3.38 ± 1.07	.44
FEV_1, L/s	2.57 ± 0.90	2.36 ± 0.95	.39
FEV/FVC ratio, %	81.2 ± 4.6	78.9 ± 10.8	.30
PEF, L/min	5.83 ± 2.64	5.57 ± 2.89	.71
$FEF_{25\%-75\%}$, L/min	4.11 ± 2.19	4.07 ± 2.58	.94
$Sa{O_2}$, %	95.76 ± 1.24	95.77 ± 1.52	.98

*Data are given as mean ± SD. FVC indicates forced vital capacity; FEV_1, forced expiratory volume in 1 second; PEF, peak expiratory flow; $FEF_{25\%-75\%}$, midexpiratory phase of forced expiratory flow; and SaO_2, arterial oxygen saturation.
†Student *t* test.

zation of the splenic or hepatic flexure is necessary in many cases, and exploration of the upper abdomen and the liver is mandatory in patients with malignant neoplasms. Therefore, the midline laparotomy is extended to the upper abdomen in most colorectal resections.

Table 3. Postoperative Morbidity and Death After Laparoscopic and Conventional Resection of Colorectal Tumors*

Variable	Patient Group: Laparoscopic Resection (n = 30)	Conventional Resection (n = 30)	*P*†
Major complications‡			
Hemorrhage on day of primary surgery	0	1	>.99
Intraperitoneal abscess§	0	1	>.99
Minor complications‖			
Pneumonia	0	2	.49
Perineal wound healing impairment	0	1	>.99
Symptomatic hyperglycemia	0	1	>.99
Central venous (CV) line infection	0	1	>.99
Brachial plexus lesion (CV line)	0	1	>.99
Urinary tract infection	2	0	.49
Surgical morbidity	0	3	.20
Total morbidity	2	8	.08
Death			
In hospital	0	0	>.99
<30 d	0	1	>.99

*Data are the number of patients.
†Fisher exact test.
‡Requiring a laparotomy.
§On 17th postoperative day.
‖Requiring medical treatment.

Table 4. Pulmonary Function at 2 PM on the First Day After Laparoscopic or Conventional Resection of Colorectal Tumors*

Test	Patient Group: Laparoscopic Resection (n = 30)	Conventional Resection (n = 30)	*P*†
FVC, L	2.59 ± 1.11	1.73 ± 0.60	<.01
FEV_1, L/s	1.80 ± 0.80	1.19 ± 0.51	<.01
PEF, L/s	3.60 ± 2.22	2.51 ± 1.37	<.05
FEV_1/FVC ratio, %	69.6 ± 11.0	67.7 ± 9.8	.51
$FEF_{25\%-75\%}$, L/s	2.67 ± 1.76	1.87 ± 1.12	<.05
SaO_2, %	93.8 ± 1.9	92.1 ± 3.3	<.05

*Data are given as mean ± SD of actual values and percentage of preoperative values. The abbreviations are the same as explained in the first footnote of Table 2.
†Student *t* test.

The main reason for the suppression of pulmonary function after laparotomy is a decreased or even a paradoxical upward movement of the diaphragm during inspiration.[25-27] Because of this diaphragmatic malfunction, a postoperative shift from abdominal (ie, diaphragmatic) to thoracic (ie, rib cage) breathing occurs, tidal volume is markedly decreased, and respiratory frequency is increased.[28] The small airways of the lung (<1.0 mm in diameter) are not supported by cartilage and are influenced by transmitted intrapleural pressures. Normally, pleural pressures are less than atmospheric pressure, producing a positive transpulmonary pressure that

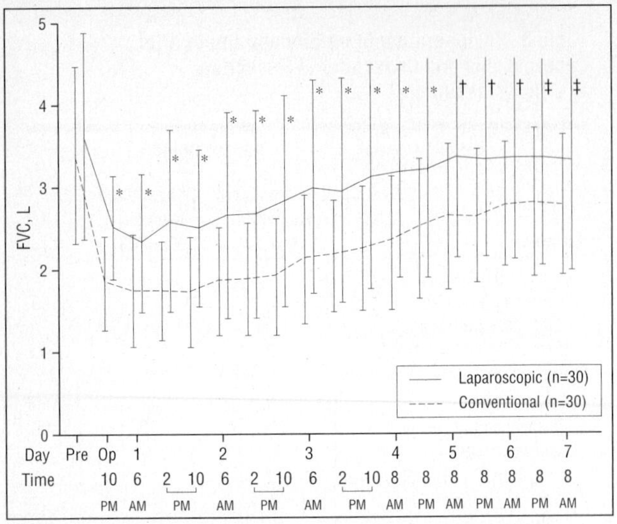

Figure 1. *Postoperative changes in forced vital capacity (FVC) following laparoscopic or conventional resection of colorectal tumors. Pre indicates preoperative measurement; Op, day of surgery; asterisk,* P = *.01; dagger,* P<*.05; and double dagger,* P = *.06.*

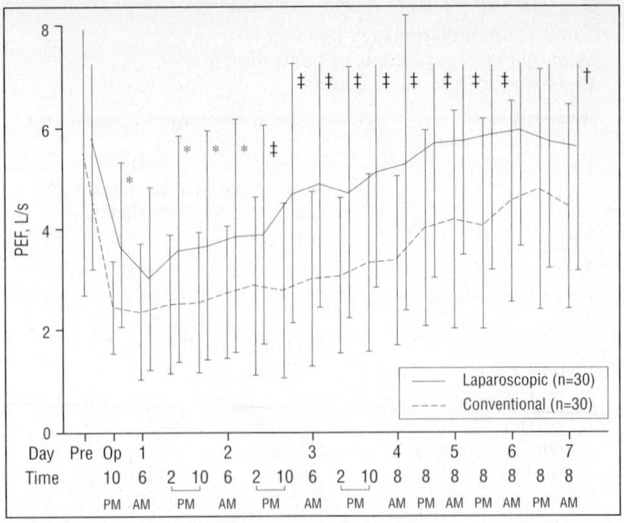

Figure 3. *Postoperative changes in peak expiratory flow (PEF) following laparoscopic or conventional resection of colorectal tumors. Pre indicates preoperative measurement; Op, day of surgery; asterisk,* P<*.05; dagger,* P = *.06; and double dagger,* P<*.01.*

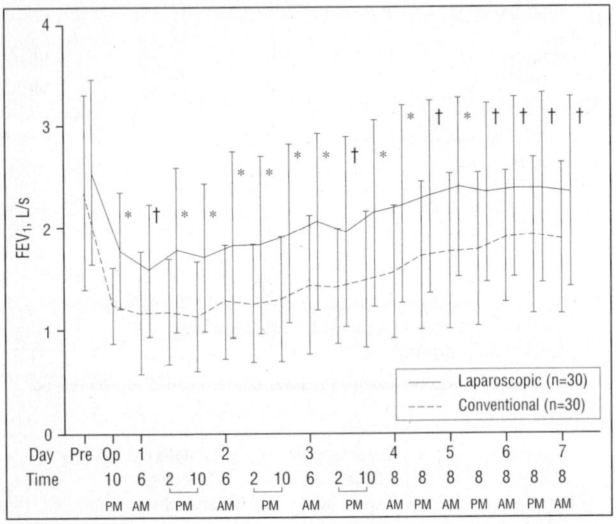

Figure 2. *Postoperative changes in forced expiratory volume in 1 second (FEV_1) following laparoscopic or conventional resection of colorectal tumors. Pre indicates preoperative measurement; Op, day of surgery; asterisk,* P<*.01; and dagger,* P<*.05.*

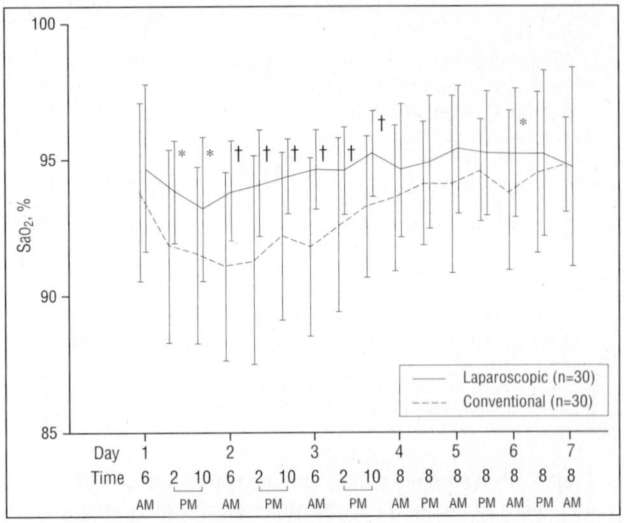

Figure 4. *Postoperative changes in oxygen saturation of the arterial blood (Sao_2), measured while patients are breathing room air, following laparoscopic or conventional resection of colorectal tumors. Asterisk indicates* P<*.05; dagger,* P<*.01.*

distends these small airways.[4] Because of the postoperative diaphragmatic malfunction, the intrapleural pressure rises and a negative transpulmonary pressure develops. This negative transpulmonary pressure causes the small airways to collapse.[4] Collapse or narrowing of small airways will result in a reduction of ventilation to affected lung regions and produce a low ventilation-perfusion relationship. The lung volume at which a small airway begins to close is called the closing capacity of the lung. If the functional residual capacity (ie, volume of air remaining in the lungs at the end of a normal expiration) is decreased below the closing capacity of the lung, regions with a low ventilation-perfusion ratio will develop, which leads to impaired gas exchange. The failure of closed airways to reopen leads to a total collapse of the lung unit served by the airway, producing atelectasis and a reduced Sao_2 value.[4-6,28]

The influence of modern anesthesiological,[8,29] analgesic,[5,30] and physiotherapeutic techniques[14] on postoperative pulmonary function after conventional abdominal surgery has been evaluated to reduce the high incidence of pulmonary complications after gastrointestinal tract resections. Pain relief or intensive physiotherapy has improved the postoperative recovery of pulmonary function only marginally.[5,10,30-32] A reduction of the functional residual capacity by 25%[30] and the FVC or FEV_1 by about 50% appears to be inevitable because the degree of diaphragmatic dysfunction after upper abdominal laparotomy cannot be substantially influenced. This reduction of the pulmonary function will cause atelectasis in more than 50% of patients,[3,4,6,23,25] and pneumonia will develop in up to 7% of patients after conventional colorectal resection, regardless of supportive therapy.[11-13]

LAPAROSCOPIC SURGERY, however, may reduce the degree of diaphragmatic dysfunction and the incidence of pulmonary complications.[14,16] Residual pneumoperitoneum does not influence pulmonary function after diagnostic laparoscopy,[33] but changes in diaphragmatic function have been found after laparoscopic cholecystectomy.[34] After laparoscopic cholecystectomy, the FVC decreases to 54% to 79%, the FEV_1 to 54% to 80%, the PEF to 49% to 76%, and the $FEF_{25\%-75\%}$ to 68% to 88% of the preoperative value.[14,16,35,36] Furthermore, the total lung capacity is suppressed to 92% and the maximum minute ventilation to 78% of the preoperative values.[14]

Several randomized trials have proved that FVC, FEV_1, and $FEF_{25\%-75\%}$ values are suppressed by almost 50% after conventional cholecystectomy, whereas they are reduced by only 19% to 27% after laparoscopic gallbladder surgery.[14,16,35,37] The postoperative SaO_2 decreased one third less in a laparoscopic resection group than in a conventional resection group,[14,16] and there were significant differences in postoperative pulmonary function between the 2 groups, even when conventional cholecystectomy was performed by minilaparotomy.[16,35] Furthermore, the SaO_2, measured while patients were breathing room air, was significantly lower after conventional than after laparoscopic cholecystectomy.[14,16]

Few data have been available regarding postoperative pulmonary function after laparoscopic and conventional colectomy. Franklin et al[17] compared 84 laparoscopic and 110 conventional colorectal resections and found that "pulmonary toilet" was promoted after laparoscopic surgery. Senagore et al[11] described 5 cases of pneumonia (19%) after 26 laparoscopic colectomies and 11 cases of pneumonia (10%) after 110 conventional colorectal resections. All cases of pneumonia were diagnosed early in this series after surgery with a pneumoperitoneum of 15 mm Hg. Later, all resections were performed with an intra-abdominal pressure of 10 mm Hg, and no further patients with pulmonary infection were observed.[11] In our department, laparoscopic colorectal resections are performed with a maximum intra-abdominal pressure of 12 mm Hg, and after more than 100 laparoscopic colorectal procedures, no cases of pneumonia have developed.

Only 2 clinical trials[18,38] addressing pulmonary function after laparoscopic and conventional colorectal resection have been published. Azagra et al[18] performed laparoscopic proctosigmoidectomies in 7 patients using trocar positions comparable to those used in our technique. Postoperative changes in FVC, FEV_1, and PEF values after laparoscopic surgery were compared with those of laparoscopic-assisted (n = 7) and conventional (n = 7) proctosigmoidectomies. The authors did not find any significant difference in postoperative pulmonary function between the 2 groups. On the first postoperative day, the difference in PEF values between both groups was about 15%. This difference is almost identical to the difference in PEF values 24 hours after surgery in our trial (18.8%). To detect a 15% difference in PEF values between laparoscopic and conventional resections with a power of 80%, a sample size of 30 patients in each group would have been necessary.[19] Therefore, it can be assumed that Azagra et al[18] were not able to detect significant differences in pulmonary function after laparoscopic, laparoscopic-assisted, and conventional proctosigmoidectomy because of the small sample size of their study.

Stage et al[38] randomly assigned 29 patients from 3 different departments to laparoscopic (n = 15) or conventional (n = 14) colectomy and did not find any significant differences in pulmonary function between the groups. There are, however, some important differences between this study and our own trial. All patients investigated by these authors underwent perioperative thoracic epidural analgesia, which was not used in our trial. Almost 50% of their patients (n = 14) underwent an ascending colectomy, whereas 46 of our patients (77%) underwent proctosigmoidectomy, which is the most common laparoscopic and conventional colorectal cancer resection. Although no exact data for mean preoperative pulmonary function are given by Stage et al, and no SD is shown in the figures given, the preoperative pulmonary function seemed to be much worse in their study (FVC, 2.3-2.5 L; and FEV_1, about 1.8 L/s) than in our patients (preoperative FVC, 3.6 ± 1.3 L and 3.4 ± 1.0 L; and preoperative FEV_1, 2.6 ± 0.9 L/s and 2.4 ± 1.0 L/s). Although the mean patient age was about 10 years lower in our study, other factors might be responsible for this considerable difference in preoperative pulmonary function between the groups, and these may explain the different postoperative findings.

Our randomized study supports 3 theses reported by other authors: First, a wide midline laparotomy causes a postoperative depression of pulmonary function by 50% to 60%[3,5,6,23]; second, complete recovery of pulmonary function takes more than 7 days[3,4]; and third, significant decreases in SaO_2 values may occur several days after laparotomy, despite an uneventful course, suggesting the formation of atelectatic areas in the lung.[6] In contrast to the conventional resection group, pulmonary function was reduced by only 35% after laparoscopic colorectal resection. Furthermore, it recovered within 3 days, and the postoperative SaO_2 was almost unchanged in the laparoscopic resection group. However, although a greater initial diminution of pulmonary function occurred in patients undergoing conventional colorectal resection compared with those having laparoscopic surgery, the daily amount of pulmonary recovery was comparable in both groups. The previously suggested pathogenesis may explain why the SaO_2 was more severely reduced from day 1 to day 4 after conventional colorectal resection in our study. Lindberg et al[6] have shown a significant correlation between pulmonary function, atelectatic areas, and the PaO_2 value after conventional colorectal resection. Therefore, the differences in SaO_2 values between the groups in our study (Figure 4) indicate a greater impairment of functional residual capacity[14] and a higher incidence of atelectasis.[6,14] Furthermore, the lower levels of SaO_2 may indicate an increased risk for postoperative complications[16,23] after conventional than after laparoscopic surgery.

Clinical data from randomized trials[14,16] regarding pulmonary function after conventional and laparoscopic cholecystectomy support the assumption that the incidence of pneumonia may be reduced by laparoscopic surgery because radiological evidence of atelectasis occurred less often (40%) after laparoscopic than after conventional (90%) surgery, and the incidence of chest infection was higher after minilaparotomy (8%) than after laparoscopic cholecystectomies (1%). In our study, pneumonia developed in 2 patients (7%) after conventional colorectal resection, but not after laparoscopic surgery; this difference was not significant. Further randomized multicenter trials will need to evaluate whether the incidence of pneumonia is lower after laparoscopic colorectal resections than after conventional procedures.

The data of our randomized trial demonstrate that pulmonary function is 30% to 35% less suppressed and recovers 40% to 45% faster after laparoscopic surgery than after conventional colorectal resection. No other change in surgical, anesthesiological, or physiotherapeutic technique has resulted in such an improvement of postoperative pulmonary function after colorectal resection. Because of these major advantages, the use of the laparoscopic approach may decrease the incidence of postoperative pulmonary complications after elective colorectal resections. Therefore, laparoscopic resection should be considered in every patient scheduled for an elective segmental resection of benign colorectal disease. Laparoscopic procedures, however, cannot be recommended for the curative treatment of malignant disease, unless randomized multicenter studies have determined the long-term results of the new technique.

Corresponding author: Wolfgang Schwenk, MD, Universitätsklinik für Allgemein, Viszeral Gefäss und Thoraxchirurgie, Medizinische Fakultät der Humboldt–Universität zu Berlin, Charité, Schumannstr 20/21, 10117 Berlin, Germany (e-mail: schwenk@charite.de).

REFERENCES

1. Beecher HK. The measured effect of laparotomy on the respiration. *J Clin Invest.* 1933;12:639-650.
2. Williams CD, Brenowitz JB. Ventilatory patterns after vertical and tranverse upper abdominal incisions. *Am J Surg.* 1975;130:725-728.
3. Latimer RG, Dickmann M, Day EC. Ventilatory pattern and pulmonary complications after upper abdominal surgery determined by preoperative and postoperative computerized spirometry and blood gas analysis. *Am J Surg.* 1971;122:622-632.
4. Craig DB. Postoperative recovery of pulmonary function. *Anesth Analg.* 1981; 60:46-52.
5. Hedenstierna G. Mechanisms of postoperative pulmonary dysfunction. *Acta Chir Scand Suppl.* 1989;550:152-158.
6. Lindberg P, Gunnarsson L, Tokics L, et al. Atelectasis and lung function in the postoperative period. *Acta Anaesthesiol Scand.* 1992;36:546-553.
7. Marshall BE, Wyche MQ Jr. Hypoxemia during and after anesthesia. *Anesthesiology.* 1972;37:178-209.
8. Hendolin H, Lahtinen J, Lansimies E, Tuppurainen T, Partanen K. The effect of thoracic epidural analgesia on respiratory function after cholecystectomy. *Acta Anaesthesiol Scand.* 1987;31:645-651.
9. Bartlett RH, Brennan ML, Gazzaniga AL, Hanson EL. Studies on the pathogenesis and prevention of postoperative pulmonary complications. *Surg Gynecol Obstet.* 1973;137:925-933.
10. Christensen EF, Schultz P, Jensen OV. Postoperative pulmonary complications and lung function in high-risk patients: a comparison of three physiotherapy regimens after upper abdominal surgery in general anesthesia. *Acta Anaesthesiol Scand.* 1991;35:97-104.
11. Senagore AJ, Luchtefeld MA, Mackeigan JM, Mazier PW. Open colectomy versus laparoscopic colectomy: are there differences? *Am Surg.* 1993;59:549-553.
12. Hansen O, Schwenk W, Hucke HP, Stock W. Colorectal stapled anastomoses: experiences and results. *Dis Colon Rectum.* 1996;39:30-36.
13. Böhm B, Nouchirvani K, Hucke HP, Stock W. Morbidity and mortality after elective resections of colorectal cancers [in German]. *Langenbecks Arch Chir.* 1991; 376:93-101.
14. Schauer PR, Luna J, Ghiatas AA, Glen ME, Warren JM, Sirinek KR. Pulmonary function after laparoscopic cholecystectomy. *Surgery.* 1993;114:389-399.
15. Gunnarsson L, Tokics L, Gustavsson H, Hedenstierna G. Influence of age on atelectasis formation and gas exchange impairment during general anaesthesia. *Br J Anaesth.* 1991;66:423-432.
16. McMahon AJ, Baxter JN, Kenney G, O'Dwyer PJ. Ventilatory and blood gas changes during laparoscopic and open cholecystectomy. *Br J Surg.* 1993;80:1252-1254.
17. Franklin ME, Rosenthal D, Norem RF. Prospective evaluation of laparoscopic colon resection versus open colon resection for adenocarcinoma. *Surg Endosc.* 1995;9:811-816.
18. Azagra JS, Goergen M, Gilbart E, Jacobs D, Lejeune P, Carlier E. Anterior resection: the total laparoscopic approach. In: Monson JRT, Darzi A, eds. *Laparoscopic Colorectal Surgery.* Oxford, England: Isis Medical Media; 1995:38-55.
19. Altman DG. *Practical Statistics for Medical Research.* London, England: Chapman & Hall; 1991.
20. Milsom JW, Böhm B. *Laparoscopic Colorectal Surgery.* New York, NY: Springer-Verlag NY Inc; 1996.
21. American Thoracic Society. Standardization of spirometry: 1987 update. *Am Rev Respir Dis.* 1987;136:1285-1298.
22. Union Internationale Contre le Cancer. *TNM Classification of Malignant Tumours.* Berlin, Germany: Springer Publishing Co; 1987.
23. Hansen G, Drablos PA, Steinert R. Pulmonary complications, ventilation and blood gases after upper abdominal surgery. *Acta Anaesthesiol Scand.* 1977;21:211-215.
24. Rinnert-Gongora S, Tartter PI. Multivariate analysis of recurrence after anterior resection for colorectal carcinoma. *Am J Surg.* 1989;157:573-576.
25. Ford GT, Whitelaw WA, Rosenal TW, Cruse PJ, Guenter CA. Diaphragm function after upper abdominal surgery in humans. *Am Rev Respir Dis.* 1983;127: 431-436.
26. Dureuil B, Cantineau JP, Desmonts JM. Effects of upper or lower abdominal surgery on diaphragmatic function. *Br J Anaesthiol.* 1987;59:1230-1235.
27. Dureuil B, Viires N, Cantineau JP, Aubier M, Desmonts JM. Diaphragmatic contractility after upper abdominal surgery. *J Appl Physiol.* 1986;61:1775-1780.
28. Wahba RWM. Perioperative functional residual capacity. *Can J Anaesth.* 1991; 38:384-400.
29. Rademaker BM, Ringers J, Odoom JA, de Wit LT, Kalkman CJ, Oosting J. Pulmonary function and stress response after laparoscopic cholecystectomy: comparison with subcostal incision and influence of thoracic epidural analgesia. *Anesth Analg.* 1992;75:381-385.
30. Bonnet F, Blery C, Zatan M, Simonet O, Brage D, Gaudy J. Effect of epidural morphine on post-operative pulmonary dysfunction. *Acta Anaesthesiol Scand.* 1984; 28:147-151.
31. Simonneau G, Vivien A, Sartene R, et al. Diaphragm dysfunction induced by upper abdominal surgery: role of postoperative pain. *Am Rev Respir Dis.* 1983; 128:899-903.
32. Sprung J, Cheng EY, Nimphius N, Hubmayr RD, Rodarte JR, Kampine JP. Diaphragm dysfunction and respiratory insufficiency after upper abdominal surgery. *Plucne Bolesti.* 1991;43:5-12.
33. Benhamou D, Simonneau G, Poynard T, Goldman M, Chaput JC, Duroux P. Diaphragm function is not impaired by pneumoperitoneum after laparoscopy. *Arch Surg.* 1993;128:430-432.
34. Erice F, Fox GS, Salib YM, Romano E, Meakins JL, Magder SA. Diaphragmatic function before and after laparoscopic cholecystectomy. *Anesthesiology.* 1993; 79:966-975.
35. Kanellos I, Zarogilidis K, Ziogas E, Dadoukis I. Prospektiv-vergleichende Studie der Lungenfunktion nach laparoskopischer, Mini-Lap oder konventioneller Cholezystektomie. *Minim Invasive Chir.* 1995;4:169-171.
36. Kum CK, Eypasch E, Aljaziri A, Troidl H. Randomized comparison of pulmonary function after the "French" and "American" techniques of laparoscopic cholecystectomy. *Br J Surg.* 1996;83:938-941.
37. Frazee RC, Roberts JW, Okeson GC, et al. Open versus laparoscopic cholecystectomy: a comparison of postoperative pulmonary function. *Ann Surg.* 1991; 213:651-654.
38. Stage JG, Schulze S, Moller P, et al. Prospective randomized study of laparoscopic versus open colonic resection for adenocarcinoma. *Br J Surg.* 1997;84: 391-396.

New surgical techniques invariably arrive amid a flurry of claimed advantages, often unsubstantiated. Laparoscopic colectomy is no exception, and surgical journals are replete with claims of an early return of gastrointestinal function, reduced pain, shorter lengths of stay, and decreased morbidity. Advocates of laparoscopic surgery have long argued that decreased postoperative pain leads to better pulmonary function, a finding borne out in comparative trials of open vs laparoscopic cholecystectomy.[1-3] In the preceding article, Schwenk et al address the issue of pulmonary function following large-bowel resection: Is the well-documented impairment of pulmonary function following conventional colectomy ameliorated by a laparoscopic approach?

Alterations in pulmonary function are common following abdominal surgery because of pain, central nervous system–depressant medications, muscle weakness, and elevation of the diaphragm. Reduced functional residual capacity, vital capacity, and forced expiratory volume in 1 second conspire to cause atelectasis, which is reported in varying percentages of patients but accounts for most pulmonary complications. Although atelectasis is usually of little clinical consequence, its presence sets the stage for a progression to pneumonia, which occurs in up to 5% of patients following abdominal surgery. Efforts to improve pulmonary function are ultimately directed at the prevention of pneumonia.

The present study is a well-designed, randomized controlled trial that demonstrates less impairment in pulmonary function following laparoscopic than open colectomy, findings that echo the results of previous cholecystectomy trials. How broadly applicable are the results, and what do they mean practically?

First, it is worth considering whether the patients with open colectomy received optimal management with respect to postoperative pulmonary function. Most patients studied underwent the resection of rectal or rectosigmoid lesions. One assumes that the authors' "wide midline laparotomy" includes extension of the incision into the upper abdomen in the group undergoing conventional resection. At our institution (Division of Colon and Rectal Surgery, University of Minnesota, Minneapolis), most sigmoid colectomies, anterior resections, and abdominoperineal resections are performed through either a transverse infraumbilical or a lower midline incision. Avoiding upper abdominal incisions may limit some of the detrimental effects of laparotomy on pulmonary function. Furthermore, although certainly not a uniform finding, improvement in pulmonary function with the use of epidural analgesia has been shown in several studies.[4-6] The authors note the conflicting results of the study by Stage et al,[7] which showed no significant difference in pulmonary function following laparoscopic or open colectomy, a study that, interestingly, used epidural analgesics for pain control in the group undergoing conventional colectomy. Perhaps a similar approach to pain management in the patients having open surgery in the present study would have mitigated their impaired pulmonary function.

Second, the authors have included few patients in their trial with underlying pulmonary disease, and none of their patients had severely compromised pulmonary function. Thus, those at highest risk for pulmonary complications were not part of the study population. In addition, severe chronic obstructive pulmonary disease can be a relative contraindication to laparoscopy. The Trendelenburg position and positive-pressure pneumoperitoneum can exacerbate the general anesthesia–associated decline in functional residual capacity, particularly in patients with chronic obstructive pulmonary disease, and carbon dioxide absorption can lead to hypercarbia, requiring increased ventilation.[8-10] Because of these issues, extrapolating the present results to high-risk patients must be undertaken with caution.

Most important, although the authors have clearly shown an improvement in pulmonary function test results, they have not demonstrated a significant difference in serious pulmonary morbidity—although, because of the overall low incidence of postoperative pneumonia following colectomy, a large trial would be necessary to demonstrate a significant difference between open and laparoscopic techniques with pneumonia as the primary end point.

The present study convincingly demonstrates less deterioration in pulmonary function following laparoscopic than conventional colectomy. Does this mean, as the authors state, that *every* patient scheduled for elective segmental resection of benign disease should be considered for laparoscopic resection? This far-reaching conclusion remains premature. Schwenk et al have clearly set a benchmark for postoperative pulmonary function using laparoscopic colectomy that optimized conventional surgery must now attempt to match. But whether improvement in this surrogate end point can be translated into a clinically significant improvement in outcome that justifies the additional operative time and cost of laparoscopy and whether the present results are applicable to patients at high risk for pulmonary complications await further study.

Andrew A. Shelton, MD
Robert D. Madoff, MD
St Paul, Minn

1. Hall JC, Tarala RA, Hall JL. A case-control study of postoperative pulmonary complications after laparoscopic and open cholecystectomy. *J Laparoendosc Surg.* 1996;6:87-92.
2. Karayiannakis AJ, Makri GG, Mantzioka A, Karousos D, Karatzas G. Postoperative pulmonary function after laparoscopic and open cholecystectomy. *Br J Anaesth.* 1996;77:448-452.
3. McMahon AJ, Russell IT, Ramsay G, et al. Laparoscopic and minilaparotomy cholecystectomy: a randomized trial comparing postoperative pain and pulmonary function. *Surgery.* 1994;115:533-539.
4. Major CP Jr, Greer MS, Russell WL, Roe SM. Postoperative pulmonary complications and morbidity after abdominal aneurysmectomy: a comparison of postoperative epidural versus parenteral opioid analgesia. *Am Surg.* 1996;62:45-51.
5. Simpson T, Wahl G, DeTraglia M, Speck E, Taylor D. A pilot study of pain, analgesia use, and pulmonary function after colectomy with or without a preoperative bolus of epidural morphine. *Heart Lung.* 1993;22:316-327.
6. Scott NB, James K, Murphy M, Kehlet M. Continuous thoracic epidural analgesia versus combined spinal/thoracic epidural analgesia on pain, pulmonary function, and the metabolic response following colonic resection. *Acta Anaesthesiol Scand.* 1996;40:691-696.
7. Stage JG, Schulze S, Moller P, et al. Prospective randomized study of laparoscopic versus open colonic resection for adenocarcinoma. *Br J Surg.* 1997;84:391-396.
8. Puri GD, Singh H. Ventilatory effects of laparoscopy under general anaesthesia. *Br J Anaesth.* 1992;68:211-213.
9. Wittgen CM, Andrus CH, Fitzgerald SD, Baudendistel LJ, Dahms TE, Kaminski DL. Analysis of the hemodynamic and ventilatory effects of laparoscopic cholecystectomy. *Arch Surg.* 1991;126:997-1001.
10. Williams MD, Murr PC. Laparoscopic insufflation of the abdomen depresses cardiopulmonary function. *Surg Endosc.* 1993;7:12-16.

Does the Face Protect the Brain?

A Case-Control Study of Traumatic Brain Injury and Facial Fractures

Heather T. Keenan, MD; Susan I. Brundage, MD; Diane C. Thompson, MS; Ronald V. Maier, MD; Frederick P. Rivara, MD, MPH

Background: The relationship between facial fractures and traumatic brain injury is controversial. Some studies show an increased risk of brain injury with the presence of facial fractures while others claim that facial fractures protect against brain injury.

Objective: To examine the association between facial fractures and traumatic brain injuries.

Design: Case-control study.

Setting: Subjects were recruited from the emergency departments of 7 hospitals in the Seattle, Wash, area.

Patients: Three thousand eight hundred forty-nine injured bicyclists and 5 scene deaths were identified from March 1, 1992, to August 31, 1994, with complete data available on 3388 bicyclists.

Interventions: None.

Results: The study group was composed of 1602 cases with injuries to the head, face, or brain and 1540 control subjects. There were 203 bicyclists with traumatic brain injuries, of whom 62 had an identifiable intracranial injury and 141 suffered a concussion. A total of 81 patients sustained facial fractures. The odds ratio for the risk of intracranial injury associated with facial fractures after adjustment for significant confounders was 9.9 (95% confidence interval, 5.1-19.3). The effect was less strong but still present when all traumatic brain injuries including concussions were considered (odds ratio, 2; 95% confidence interval, 1.1-3.7). No association was found for concussion only.

Conclusions: This study demonstrates no evidence that facial fractures help prevent traumatic brain injury. Data indicate that facial fractures are markers for increased risk of brain injury.

Arch Surg. 1999;134:14-17

From the Department of Pediatrics, University of North Carolina, Chapel Hill (Dr Keenan); Department of Surgery, Harborview Medical Center (Drs Brundage and Maier), Department of Pediatrics and Epidemiology (Dr Rivara), and the Harborview Injury Prevention and Research Center (Ms Thompson and Dr Rivara), University of Washington, Seattle.

IT HAS BEEN proposed that the face protects the brain from injury the way an airbag protects the chest in a motor vehicle crash. Actual data on this are scant and conflicting. Lee et al[1] reported that facial fractures are associated with a decreased risk of a traumatic brain injury, while Davidoff et al[2] found facial fracture to be highly associated with traumatic brain injury. This question has important clinical implications. Multiple origins and potentially significant confounding variables make accurate assessment of the association between traumatic head injury and facial fractures difficult.

In our study, we used a large database of individuals with injuries from bicycle crashes to examine the association between traumatic brain injury and facial fracture using a case-control design.

RESULTS

Seven hospital EDs treated 3849 injured bicyclists, 5 of whom died at the scene during the 2½-year study. Two bicyclists were excluded because of incomplete data, leaving 3388 injured cyclists for analysis. Of these bicyclists, 1602 had head, face, or brain injury or recounted that they hit their helmet, head, or face. They constitute the study group. There were 203 bicyclists (14.4%) with traumatic brain injuries of whom 62 (3.9%) had intracranial injuries.

Cases (intracranial injuries, n = 62) and controls (all other face or head injured bicyclists, n = 1540) did not differ significantly by age or sex; however, more controls (45.8%) than cases (24.2%) were wearing a helmet (**Table 1**). Characteristics of the crash (**Table 2**), including the bicyclists' self-reported speed and the type of surface (paved vs other) were not different between cases and controls; however, bicyclists whose speed was unknown were at a higher risk of intracranial injury (OR, 10.7; 95% CI, 3.3-33.3), most likely reflecting a recall bias for patients suffering intracranial injury. Col-

MATERIALS AND METHODS

DATA COLLECTION

Our current study data were collected as part of a case-control study examining head injuries caused by bicycle crashes. Methods of data collection are described in detail in a larger study that examined the effectiveness of bicycle safety helmets in preventing head injuries.[3] Our case-control study was conducted at 7 major hospitals in the Seattle, Wash, area: Central and Eastside Hospitals of Group Health Cooperative of Puget Sound, a large health maintenance organization; University of Washington Medical Center; Harborview Medical Center, a regional level I trauma center; Overlake Hospital, a community hospital that cares for a large portion of trauma patients; and Children's Hospital and Medical Center of Seattle and the Mary Bridge Hospital and Medical Center of Tacoma, 2 children's hospitals. The medical examiner's offices of Pierce and King counties (Washington) were visited regularly to identify deaths at the scene that might have eluded the surveillance system.

SUBJECT IDENTIFICATION

Subjects were identified prospectively by regular surveillance (1 to 2 times a week) of the emergency department (ED) logs and records in each of the 7 study hospitals from March 1, 1992, to August 31, 1994. Automated hospital admission records were screened monthly by *International Classification of Diseases, Ninth Revision, Clinical Modification* coding (*ICD-9-CM* E codes 800-802, 805-807, 810-816, 818-823, 825-829) to identify admissions that were not recorded in ED records. Any individual injured on a bicycle was eligible for the study, including child passengers (<6 years) riding in a child carrier, (n = 4), but excluding older bicycle passengers, pedestrians injured by a bicycle, and individuals assaulted while riding a bicycle.

MEDICAL RECORD ABSTRACTION

Trained abstractors reviewed the complete medical record of each patient, recording the following: mental status (nausea, headaches, amnesia, and length of unconsciousness), description of the incident, Glasgow Coma Scale scores, radiological procedures, helmet use, and a detailed description of all injuries. All radiology reports, surgical procedures, and discharge summaries were reviewed. Medical examiners' reports were abstracted for all deaths. A computer software program (TRICODE, TRIANALYTICS, Bel Air, Md) was used to convert text descriptions into *ICD-9-CM* codes and to calculate Abbreviated Injury Scale score and Injury Severity Score.

DEFINITIONS

Patients who sought care for a bicycle-related traumatic brain injury in the ED of a study hospital during the period from March 1, 1992, to August 31, 1994, were enrolled in this study. They were classified by injury into 2 groups: those with intracranial injuries and those with concussions. Intracranial injury included the following: cerebral lacerations, cerebral contusions, and subarachnoid, subdural, and extradural hemorrhages. Patients with loss of consciousness without signs of intracranial hemorrhage were defined as having a concussion. Loss of consciousness was defined by either a transient state of witnessed unresponsiveness or a patient report of temporary loss of awareness. A large group of individuals with traumatic brain injury were defined as having intracranial hemorrhage/contusions and a concussion. Control subjects were defined as bicyclists treated in the same EDs who reported hitting their helmet, head, or face or sustaining an injury to their head or face, without any traumatic brain injury. This control group was chosen to include only those bicyclists at risk of traumatic brain injury and/or facial fracture. Facial injury was defined as any injury to the jaw, lips, cheeks, nose, ears (external), eyes (external), forehead, or mouth (intraoral). Facial fracture was defined as injury to the maxilla, orbits, zygoma, or mandible.

QUESTIONNAIRES

Detailed questionnaires were sent to all injured bicyclists treated in this period regarding the circumstances of the crash, including helmet use, speed, and motor vehicle involvement. Telephone follow-up occurred within 2 weeks of the ED visit. Response rate to the questionnaires was 88%; complete data were available for analysis on 3388 injured bicyclists.

STATISTICAL ANALYSIS

The SAS statistical package was used for all analyses (SAS Institute Inc, Cary, NC). Descriptive information and crude odds ratios (ORs) were generated for all traumatic brain injuries. Unconditional logistic regression modeling was performed for traumatic brain injuries to estimate the OR and 95% confidence intervals (CIs) of traumatic brain injury while controlling for multiple confounders.[4]

To determine whether facial fracture was associated with severity of brain injury, analyses of all cases of traumatic brain injury, as well as the subcategories of intracranial injury and concussions were done.

lision with a motor vehicle occurred in 55% of cases, which significantly increased the odds of intracranial injury (OR, 6.6; 95% CI, 4.2-10.4).

A total of 81 patients had facial fractures distributed between cases (29%) and controls (4.1%), including the following: 31 mandibular fractures or dislocations (28.3%); 6 maxillary fractures (7.4%); 29 nasal fractures (35.8%); and 15 orbital fractures (18.5%). Characteristics of cyclists' injuries are given in **Table 3**. Bicyclists with intracranial injuries were more likely to have concomitant neck injuries (OR, 3.1; 95% CI, 1.3-7.1). Injury Severity Scores ranged from 0 to 75; 24.2 % of the patients and 99.6% of controls had scores lower than 15. Patients with traumatic brain injuries had higher Injury Severity Scores, with 66.1% of the cases having scores of 16 to 40 compared with 0.4% of controls, and 9.7% of the cases having scores of 41 to 75 compared with no controls. The Glasgow Coma Scale scores were higher in the control group, with 98.9% of controls receiving scores from 12 to 15 compared with 56.5% of the cases.

Table 1. Demographic Characteristics of and Helmet Use by Patients and Controls With Intracranial Injury Due to a Bicycle Crash

Characteristic	No. (%) of Intracranial Injury		Unadjusted Odds Ratio (95% CI*)
	Patients	Controls	
Sex			
Male	46 (74.2)	1116 (72.5)	1.1 (0.6-2.0)
Female	16 (25.8)	424 (27.5)	1.0†
Age, y			
<13	32 (51.6)	758 (49.2)	1.0 (0.6-1.7)
13-19	6 (9.7)	238 (15.5)	0.6 (0.2-1.4)
≥20	24 (38.7)	544 (35.3)	1.0†
Helmet use	15 (24.2)	720 (45.8)	0.4 (0.2-0.7)
No helmet use	47 (75.8)	820 (54.2)	1.0†

**CI indicates confidence interval.*
†Reference group.

Table 2. Characteristics Contributing to Crash Severity for Patients Involved in Bicycle Crashes

Characteristic	No. (%) of Intracranial Injury		Unadjusted Odds Ratio (95% CI*)
	Patients	Controls	
Self-reported speed			
Slow (<5 mph)	24 (38.7)	517 (33.6)	1.0†
Moderate (5-15 mph)	17 (27.4)	657 (42.6)	0.6 (0.3-1.1)
Fast (>15 mph)	16 (25.8)	356 (23.1)	1.0 (0.5-2.0)
Unknown	5 (8.1)	10 (0.7)	10.7 (3.3-33.3)
Paved surface	54 (87.1)	1259 (81.8)	1.5 (0.7-3.2)
Other surface	8 (12.9)	281 (18.2)	1.0†
Motor vehicle collision	34 (54.8)	240 (15.6)	6.6 (4.2-10.4)
Other collisions	28 (45.2)	1300 (84.4)	1.0†

**CI indicates confidence interval.*
†Reference group.

The OR for the effect of facial fracture on the risk of intracranial injury was adjusted for significant confounders including helmet use, motor vehicle involvement, and speed. Further adjustment for other variables including sex, age, and surface type had almost no effect on the OR. The adjusted OR for the risk of intracranial injury (n = 62) associated with facial fracture was 9.9 (95% CI, 5.1-19.3). The effect was weakened, but still present, when all traumatic brain injuries (n = 203), including concussions, were considered (OR, 2; 95% CI, 1.1-3.7); when only concussions (n = 141) were considered, no association was found (OR, 0.6; 95% CI, 0.2-1.6).

COMMENT

This study demonstrates no evidence that facial fractures help prevent traumatic brain injury. In fact, the risk of intracranial injury in those bicyclists with facial injury was increased almost 10-fold, and the risk for all brain injuries including concussion was doubled. This does not imply that facial fractures cause traumatic brain injury, but suggests that blunt impact with enough force to break facial bones could also produce

Table 3. Characteristics of Injuries Sustained From Bicycle Crashes for Patients Seen in an Emergency Department

Characteristic	No. (%) of Intracranial Injury		Unadjusted Odds Ratio (95% CI*)
	Patients	Controls	
All facial fractures	18 (29.0)	63 (4.1)	9.6 (5.8-15.9)
Orbit	7 (11.3)	8 (0.5)	24.4 (7.6-77.3)
Maxilla	5 (8.1)	1 (0.07)	135 (14.6-6388)
Nose	2 (3.2)	27 (1.8)	1.9 (0.2-7.7)
Mandible	4 (6.4)	27 (1.8)	3.9 (0.95-11.6)
Neck injury	6 (9.7)	52 (3.4)	3.1 (1.3-7.1)
Injury Severity Score			
0-15	15 (24.2)	1534 (99.6)	1.0†
16-40	41 (66.1)	6 (0.4)	698.8 (238-2179)
41-75	6 (9.7)	0 (0)	. . .‡
Glasgow Coma Scale scores			
<7-9	22 (35.5)	6 (0.4)	160 (57-502)
10-12	5 (8.0)	10 (0.7)	21.8 (5.5-73.9)
12-15	35 (56.5)	1524 (98.9)	1.0†

**CI indicates confidence interval.*
†Reference group.
‡Odds ratio not calculated due to no injuries in the control group.

brain injury. Patients with intracranial injuries were more likely to have been involved in a crash involving a motor vehicle, to have had a higher Injury Severity Scale score, and to have coexisting neck injuries than bicyclists who had an injury to the head or face that suggested a more severe crash. Importantly, no protective effect of facial fracture was found, even in bicyclists with less severe brain injury such as concussion. In the group who had concussions, no association with facial fracture was observed.

These results disagree with the previously reported decreased risk of traumatic brain injury in patients with facial fracture. Lee et al[1] theorized that the facial bones act as a protective cushion for the brain to explain why injuries that crush the facial bones frequently caused no apparent brain damage. Our results are more in agreement with Davidoff et al[2] who reported a 55% incidence of concomitant facial fracture and brain injury (defined as loss of consciousness or posttraumatic amnesia) and a 6% incidence of intracranial injury in a retrospective case series of 156 patients admitted to an ED with facial fractures from a variety of causes; however, the Davidoff study lacked a control group.

There are some limitations to our study. The controls were limited to patients who fell and hit their head or face and sought care for a bicycle-related injury. Those patients who fell, but were not badly injured, and did not seek medical care were excluded from this study. This could underestimate the association of facial fracture with brain injury.

Our study only examined 1 population, bicyclists who crashed, so we cannot comment on other mechanisms of injury that are reported as causes of facial fractures such as motor vehicle crashes or assaults.[5,6] While our choice of patient population limits generalizability, it is a homogeneous data set from which to draw associations.

CONCLUSIONS

Our study shows no evidence that facial fractures are protective of traumatic brain injury. In fact, the risk of intracranial hemorrhage in bicyclists with a facial injury was increased by almost 10-fold, and the risk of any traumatic brain injury including a concussion was doubled. This suggests that the presence of enough force to cause facial fractures is likely to produce brain damage. Facial fractures are a marker for an increased risk of injury to the brain rather than protection against traumatic brain injury. Patients with facial fractures seen in the ED need to be evaluated for potentially serious brain injury.

Reprints: Frederick P. Rivara, MD, MPH, Department of Pediatrics and Epidemiology, Harborview Injury Prevention and Research Center, Box 359960, 325 Ninth Ave, University of Washington, Seattle, WA 98104-2499 (e-mail: fpr@u.washington.edu).

REFERENCES

1. Lee KF, Wagner LK, Lee YE, Suh JH, Lee SR. The impact-absorbing effects of facial fractures in closed-head injuries. *J Neurosurg.* 1987;66:542-547.
2. Davidoff G, Jakubowski M, Thomas D, Alpert M. The spectrum of closed-head injuries in facial trauma victims: incidence and impact. *Ann Emerg Med.* 1988; 17:6-9.
3. Thompson DC, Rivara FP, Thompson RS. Effectiveness of bicycle safety helmets in preventing head injuries: a case-control study. *JAMA.* 1996;276:1968-1973.
4. Breslow NE, Day NE. Statistical methods in cancer research. In: Breslow NE, Day NE, eds. *The Analysis of Case-Control Studies.* Vol 1. Lyon, France: International Agency for Research on Cancer; 1980. International Agency for Research on Cancer Series, No. 32.
5. Turvey TA. Midfacial fractures: a retrospective analysis of 593 cases. *J Oral Surg.* 1977;35:887-891.
6. Cannell H, King JB, Wich RD. Head and facial injuries after low speed motorcycle accidents. *Br J Oral Surg.* 1982;20:183-191.

IN OTHER AMA JOURNALS

JAMA

Molecular Staging of Malignant Melanoma: Correlation With Clinical Outcome

Steven C. Shivers, PhD; Xiangning Wang, MD; Weiguo Li, MD; Emmanuella Joseph, MD; Jane Messina, MD; L. Frank Glass, MD; Ronald DeConti, MD; C. Wayne Cruse, MD; Claudia Berman, MD; Neil A. Fenske, MD; Gary H. Lyman, MD, MPH; Douglas S. Reintgen, MD

Context: For most solid tumors, the metastatic status of regional lymph nodes is the strongest predictor of relapse and survival. However, routine pathological examination of lymph nodes may underestimate the number of patients with melanoma who have nodal metastases.
Objective: To determine the clinical significance of a highly sensitive molecular assay for occult nodal metastases for the staging of patients with melanoma.
Design: A prospective cohort study of consecutive patients in which lymphatic mapping and sentinel lymph node (SLN) biopsy were performed on 114 melanoma patients with clinical stage I and stage II disease. The SLNs were bivalved, and half of each specimen was submitted for routine pathological examination. The other half was submitted for molecular detection of submicroscopic metastases using a reverse transcriptase–polymerase chain reaction (RT-PCR) assay for tyrosinase messenger RNA as a marker for the presence of melanoma cells. Patient follow-up averaged 28 months.
Setting: A major university-based melanoma referral center at a National Cancer Institute–designated cancer center.
Patients: A total of 114 patients with newly diagnosed cutaneous malignant melanoma who were at risk for regional nodal metastases.
Main Outcome Measure: Melanoma recurrence and overall survival.
Results: Twenty-three patients (20%) had pathologically positive SLNs, and all of these patients were also RT-PCR positive. Of the 91 pathologically negative patients, 44 were RT-PCR negative and 47 were RT-PCR positive. There was a recurrence rate among 14 (61%) of the 23 patients who were both pathologically and RT-PCR positive and a recurrence rate among 1 (2%) of 44 patients who were both pathologically and RT-PCR negative. For patients who were upstaged by the molecular assay (pathologically negative, RT-PCR positive), there was a recurrence rate among 6 (13%) of 47 patients. The differences in recurrence rates and overall survival between the pathologically negative, RT-PCR–negative and pathologically negative, RT-PCR–positive patient groups were statistically significant ($P = .02$ for disease-free survival and for overall survival). In both univariate and multivariate regression analyses, the histological and RT-PCR status of the SLNs were the best predictors of disease-free survival.
Conclusions: The use of an RT-PCR assay for detection of submicroscopic melanoma metastases in SLNs improved the prediction of melanoma recurrence and overall survival over routine pathological examination. *(1998;280:1410-1415)*

Reprints: Douglas S. Reintgen, MD, Cutaneous Oncology Program, H. Lee Moffitt Cancer Center and Research Institute at the University of South Florida, 12902 Magnolia Dr, Tampa, FL 33612 (e-mail: doug@moffitt.usf.edu).

Antireflux Surgery Enhances Gastric Emptying

Mikko Viljakka, MD; Keijo Saali, MSc; Matti Koskinen, PhD; Lauri Karhumäki, MD; Jyrki Kössi, MD; Markku Luostarinen, MD; Ossi Teerenhovi, MD; Jouko Isolauri, MD

Objective: To evaluate the influence of antireflux surgery on gastric emptying.

Design: Nonrandomized controlled trial 3 months before and after surgical intervention.

Setting: Secondary and tertiary referral center.

Patients and Control Subjects: Twenty consecutive patients (7 women, 13 men), mean age 49.2 years, with symptomatic, objectively confirmed gastroesophageal reflux disease and 10 healthy control subjects (3 women, 7 men), mean age 37.3 years.

Intervention: Laparoscopic or open Nissen fundoplication (in 1 case Toupet 180° posterior hemifundoplication).

Main Outcome Measures: Gastric emptying scintigraphy, using solid food, in control subjects and patients 3 months before and 3 months after the operation; time to halving of the maximal activity and the activity remaining at 60, 100, and 120 minutes.

Results: Preoperative symptoms included pyrosis in 19 of 20 patients and regurgitation in 18. Three months postoperatively, 19 patients were symptom-free. The mean time to halving of the maximal activity decreased from 113 to 78 minutes ($P = .001$). Delayed gastric emptying was found postoperatively in 3 patients, compared with preoperative values, using activity at 60, 100, 120 minutes and the mean time to halving of the maximal activity as the variables. Compared with control subjects, gastric emptying was slower in patients preoperatively and faster postoperatively, but the difference was not statistically significant.

Conclusion: Gastric emptying is enhanced after antireflux surgery, along with cessation of symptoms and healing of esophagitis.

Arch Surg. 1999;134:18-21

From the Department of Surgery, the Medical School, University of Tampere, Tampere (Dr Viljakka); the Departments of Clinical Physiology and Surgery, Kanta-Häme Central Hospital, Hämeenlinna (Mr Saali and Dr Karhumäki); the Departments of Clinical Physiology and Surgery, Tampere University Central Hospital, Tampere (Drs Koskinen, Luostarinen, and Teerenhovi); the Department of Surgery, Loimaa District Hospital, Loimaa (Dr Kössi); and Department of Surgery, Turku University Central Hospital, Turku (Dr Isolauri), Finland.

THE PATHOGENESIS of gastroesophageal reflux disease is multifactorial.[1] In surgical management, Nissen fundoplication is the favored method, with success rates of 91% to 95%.[2,3] Multiple mechanisms of action have been suggested for Nissen fundoplication.[4-9] Restoration of the normal lower esophageal sphincter pressure with reduced frequency of transient lower esophageal relaxation is documented,[4,5] but its role in curing the esophagitis has been questioned.[6,7] Esophageal motor activity was found to improve after fundoplication.[8,9]

The role of gastric emptying in the pathogenesis of gastroesophageal reflux disease is controversial. Some investigators reported delayed gastric emptying in about 40% of patients with reflux[10,11] and esophagitis,[11,12] whereas others found no correlation between reflux and delayed gastric emptying,[13,14] and such delay was associated with normal rather than inflamed esophageal mucosa.[15] Accelerated gastric emptying could be demonstrated after Nissen fundoplication,[16,17] but not after the Hill operation.[18] The failure of antireflux operations has been associated with delayed gastric emptying.[19] The aim of the present study was to evaluate the influence of antireflux surgery on gastric emptying.

RESULTS

CLINICAL EXAMINATIONS

All patients had received medication for reflux symptoms; 14 had used proton pump inhibitors, and 8 had used histamine$_2$ blocking agents (some patients had used both types of medications). Cisapride, antacids, and sucralfate also were used. Preoperatively, 19 patients had pyrosis, 18 had regurgitation, and 5 had ex-

PATIENTS, CONTROL SUBJECTS, AND METHODS

PATIENTS, CLINICAL EXAMINATIONS, AND SUBJECTS

Twenty patients (7 women, 13 men), mean age 49 years (range, 28-70 years), underwent surgery for the treatment of symptomatic gastroesophageal reflux disease at the Kanta-Häme Central Hospital, Hämeenlinna, Finland, between October 1, 1995, and August 31, 1996. The diagnosis was based preoperatively on the presence and duration of pyrosis, regurgitation, and dysphagia and the use of medication to treat reflux symptoms. Preoperative examinations included esophagogastroduodenoscopy, esophageal manometry, and 24-hour pH monitoring. Pathological reflux was found by the 24-hour pH recording (pH $<$4.00 for $>$4.2% of the recording time) in 18 of 20 patients (mean, 23.3% of the total monitoring time). The other 2 patients had erosive esophagitis and had experienced symptoms for many years. The clinical assessment was repeated 1 month and 3 months after the operation, and at 3 months, a control esophagogastroduodenoscopy was performed to observe the healing of esophagitis and the location and competence of the fundic wrap.

Ten healthy volunteers (3 women, 7 men; mean age, 37 years; age range, 25-52 years) served as control subjects. The control subjects were using no medications.

OPERATION

Nissen fundoplication was performed on 16 patients by using a laparoscopic procedure and on 3 patients by using an open procedure (2 of these owing to previous abdominal surgery). A wrap 2 cm in length was constructed with a 50F Maloney bougie inside the esophagus. The short gastric vessels were not divided. One of the open operations was begun as a laparoscopic procedure but was converted to an open procedure owing to technical problems. For 1 patient with propulsive, low-amplitude peristalsis, the Toupet hemifundoplication was preferred.

GASTRIC EMPTYING SCINTIGRAPHY

The patients fasted from midnight before the test. The test meal was taken with a glass of water. The test steak consisted of technetium Tc 99m colloid–labeled egg (20 MBq), 50 g of minced meat, and 1 to 2 spoons of bread crumbs cooked in a microwave oven. Immediately after the meal, imaging with a gamma camera was begun with the patient in a semisitting position. Two cobalt 57 (^{57}Co) markers were attached on the skin. The dynamic stage of imaging lasted 30 minutes. Acquisition, at 1 frame per 20 seconds, was performed in an anteroposterior direction. Thereafter, static images for 5-minute periods were collected at 15- to 30-minute intervals, during which the patients were permitted to get up. The camera and seat positions were kept constant, and minor shifts were corrected with the aid of the ^{57}Co marker. Imaging was continued until the activity of gastric contents had decreased to less than half of the maximal value, or for a maximum of 240 minutes. The 10 control subjects underwent the same gastric emptying scintigraphy.

ANALYSIS OF GAMMA IMAGING

The dynamic imaging and the 5-minute static images were linked in a file in temporal order. At this stage, if necessary, the static images were adjusted with the spots of the ^{57}Co markers. Dynamic images were added as 5-minute periods to obtain dynamic stage activity values at 5, 10, 15, 20, 25, and 30 minutes. Half-time correction of technetium Tc 99m was performed. By using dynamic and static values, an activity curve was plotted, with background activity subtracted, expressing the activity as a percentage of the first time point. Activities (as percentages of the maximal activity) at 60, 100, and 120 minutes (A_{60}, A_{100}, and A_{120}) were interpolated from the 2 nearest measurement points, and the time required for the activity to decrease to half of the maximal activity was defined ($T_{1/2}$).

STATISTICAL ANALYSIS

We used the *t* test for paired samples to compare preoperative and postoperative data and the *t* test for unpaired samples to compare data for the patients and control subjects, with $P<.05$ considered significant. The mean differences with 95% confidence limits were calculated. Correlation coefficients were calculated for age and emptying data ($T_{1/2}$ and A_{60}). The study was approved by the ethics committees of Kanta-Häme Central Hospital and Tampere University Hospital, Tampere.

perienced dysphagia at some time. The respective numbers of patients experiencing these symptoms at 1 month after the operation were 0, 1, and 9, and at 3 months, they were 1, 1, and 2, respectively. The preoperative esophagogastroduodenoscopy grades for esophagitis (using Savary-Miller grading [grade 1, linear, nonconfluent erosions; grade 2, longitudinal, confluent, noncircumferential erosions; grade 3, longitudinal, confluent, circumferential erosions bleeding readily; and grade 4, ulcer]) were as follows: grade 0, 7 patients; grade 1, 7 patients; grade 2, 4 patients; grade 3, 1 patient; and grade 4, 1 patient. Two patients had Barrett esophagus, that was histologically confirmed (gastric-type epithelium $>$3 cm above the most cranial fold of gastric mucosa). Postoperative esophagogastroduodenoscopy showed no esophagitis (grade 0) in 18 patients and grade 1 in 1 patient; 1 patient refused to undergo esophagogastroduodenoscopy.

GASTRIC EMPTYING

In the preoperative imaging, the activity had fallen below 50% of the maximal before 100 minutes in 2 patients and before 120 minutes in 3 patients. In the postoperative imaging, the respective numbers of patients were 7 and 13. For these patients, the values at respective times were linearly extrapolated for statistical comparison. The means for all variables (**Table**) indicated enhanced gastric emptying 3 months after the operation. All changes were significant. For 3 patients, gastric emptying at 60, 100, or 120 minutes was slower or the $T_{1/2}$ was longer than

Comparison of Preoperative vs Postoperative Gastric Emptying Data for Patients and Data for Patients vs Control Subjects*

	Preoperative	Mean Difference† (95% Confidence Interval)	Postoperative	*P*†	Control Subjects‡
$T_{1/2}$, min	113.1 (40.5)	−35 (−54 to −17)	77.6 (26.6)	.001	93.3 (40.8)
A_{60}, %	83.1 (13.3)	−20 (−31 to −9)	63.2 (20.4)	.001	76.9 (28.5)
A_{100}, %	56.4 (16.7)	−28 (−40 to −16)	28.5 (24.4)	<.001	40.7 (31.6)
A_{120},%	42.9 (20.0)	−26 (−38 to −15)	16.5 (22.1)	<.001	29.3 (29.3)

**Unless otherwise indicated, data are given as mean (SD). $T_{1/2}$ indicates time until half of the radioactivity leaves the stomach; A_{60}, A_{100}, and A_{120}, activity remaining after 60, 100, and 120 minutes, respectively.*

†Preoperative vs postoperative data.

‡Comparisons of preoperative and postoperative data for patients vs control subjects were not significant.

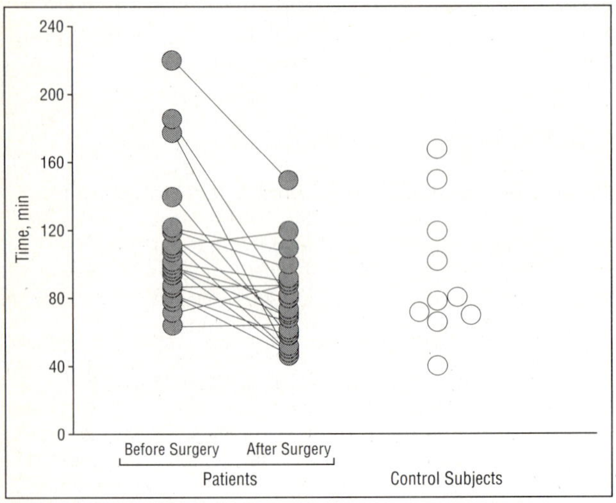

Figure 1. *The time required for half of the gastric contents to leave the stomach in patients before and after the operation and in control subjects.*

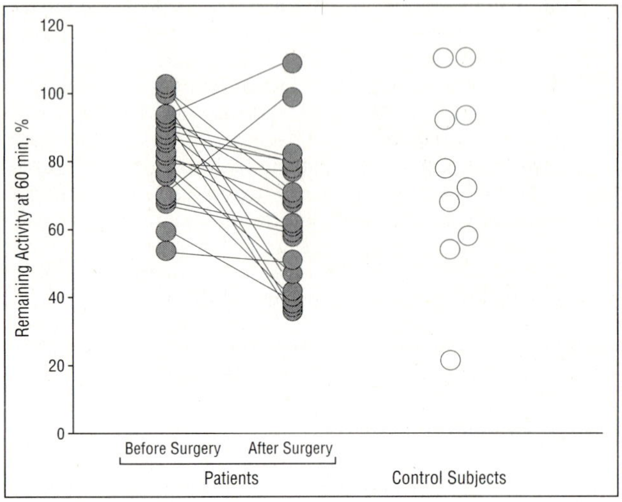

Figure 2. *The percentage of solid food retained at 60 minutes in patients before and after the operation and in control subjects.*

in the preoperative examinations. Compared with control subjects, the preoperative gastric emptying was slower in patients (Table), but no statistical difference was noted between the patients for preoperative or postoperative examinations and the control subjects. The variation in the gastric emptying rate was wide for the patients and the control subjects (**Figure 1** and **Figure 2**). No significant correlation was found between age and $T_{1/2}$ or A_{60} in the preoperative and postoperative examination results for patients or between age and $T_{1/2}$ or A_{60} for the patients and the control subjects.

COMMENT

Three months after antireflux surgery, gastric emptying was enhanced in most patients. By using $T_{1/2}$ or activity at 60 minutes as the variables, gastric emptying was enhanced in 18 of 20 patients. Simultaneously, there was total abolition of symptoms and esophagitis in 18 patients (90%). Although these findings may not be mutually explanatory,[18] they agree with the findings of previous studies[16,17] and could suggest a role for accelerated gastric emptying in the action mechanism of antireflux procedures.

For 3 of the patients in the present study, gastric emptying was slower after fundoplication than before, but for 2 of them, the preoperative rate was faster than the average of the patients. Delayed gastric emptying has been associated with the failure of antireflux procedures to abolish symptoms of reflux,[19] but these 3 patients were totally asymptomatic 3 months after the operation. These cases suggest that enhanced gastric emptying is not essential to the effectiveness of antireflux surgery. All patients with postoperative symptoms at 3 months had improved gastric emptying. Furthermore, no statistical difference in gastric emptying was found between preoperative and postoperative examination results for patients or between patients and control subjects.

Although the preoperative gastric emptying was slower in patients, we could not demonstrate as clear a distinction between patients with gastroesophageal reflux disease and control subjects as was demonstrated in previous studies,[10-12] because there was considerable overlap between and variation within the present study groups.

The enhancement of gastric emptying could have resulted from the reduction in gastric volume related to the use of the fundus for plication. Similar enhancement was not found with the Angelchik prosthesis.[20] Functional studies showed that the proximal stomach initially stores the solid component of food before its redistribution and emptying from the stomach,[21] and removal of this reservoir may lead to accelerated emptying. It also has been suggested that delayed proximal rather than total gastric emptying could be important in the induction of transient lower esophageal sphincter relaxation.[22] With simultaneous restoration of the lower esophageal sphincter pressure,[4] enhanced gastric emptying can promote the progress of gastric contents into the intestine, thus inhibiting reflux into the esophagus.

Esophageal transit times tend to normalize after Nissen fundoplication when the fundus is not mobilized,[23] as in the present study. The improvement of esophageal transit[23] and gastric emptying together may reflect improved upper gastrointestinal tract motility after antireflux surgery. Optimum esophageal motor function is desirable, since impairment is associated with esophagitis and reflux disease,[24,25] although the significance of this finding has been questioned.[26]

After fundoplication, some patients complain of postprandial fullness,[27] which may be related to delayed gastric emptying.[28] Postoperatively, the increased gastric wall tension together with the reduced gastric volume also may account for the fullness.[29] Heightened gastric tone can, in turn, enhance emptying. Flatulence also increases after fundoplication in some patients,[30] but it is not accompanied by an increase of the intra-abdominal gas volume,[30] which likewise may be explained by accelerated gastric emptying and possibly by normal, instead of abnormal, esophageal motility.[31]

To study gastric emptying, we used solid food, which seems to be preferable to liquids for detecting delayed emptying in patients with gastroesophageal reflux disease[18] or esophagitis.[11] Furthermore, solid food (with a glass of water) more closely mimics the postprandial state, when some patients experience excessive reflux.[32] In postoperative tests, the percentage of retention of solid food at 100 minutes was similar to the findings in previous studies,[16,17,19,28] as was the $T_{1/2}$.[33] The ages of the control subjects (mean, 37 years) and patients (mean, 49 years) differed, but there was no correlation between the age and gastric emptying, and gastric emptying was not influenced by age in previous studies.[10,13]

The symptoms of gastroesophageal reflux disease were relieved by antireflux surgery. At the 3-month postoperative follow-up, scintigraphy showed significantly enhanced gastric emptying. The preoperative gastric emptying for the patients was slower than for the control subjects, but in the small groups in the present study, no significant difference was found.

This study was supported by grants from the Finnish Foundation for Gastroenterological Research, Helsinki, and the Medical Research Fund of Tampere University Hospital, Tampere; and Medical Research Fund of Kanta-Häme Central Hospital, Hämeelinna.

Reprints: Jouko Isolauri, MD, Turku University Central Hospital, Kiinamyllynkatu 4-8, 20520 Turku, Finland (e-mail: jouko.isolauri@tyks.fi).

REFERENCES

1. Katz PO. Pathogenesis and management of gastroesophageal reflux disease. *J Clin Gastroenterol.* 1991;13(suppl 2):S6-S15.
2. DeMeester TR, Bonavina L, Albertucci M. Nissen fundoplication for gastroesophageal reflux disease: evaluation of primary repair in 100 consecutive patients. *Ann Surg.* 1986;204:9-20.
3. Shirazi S, Schulze K, Soper R. Long-term follow-up for treatment of complicated chronic reflux esophagitis. *Arch Surg.* 1987;122:548-551.
4. Ellis FH, Crozier RE. Reflux control by fundoplication: a clinical and manometric assessment of the Nissen fundoplication. *Ann Thorac Surg.* 1984;38:387-392.
5. Ireland AC, Holloway RH, Toouli J, Dent J. Mechanisms underlying the antireflux action of fundoplication. *Gut.* 1993;34:303-308.
6. Bancewicz J, Mughal M, Marples M. The lower oesophageal sphincter after floppy Nissen fundoplication. *Br J Surg.* 1987;74:162-164.
7. Fisher RS, Malmud LS, Lobis IF, Maier WP. Antireflux surgery for symptomatic gastroesophageal reflux. *Dig Dis.* 1978;23:152-160.
8. Gill RC, Bowes KL, Murphy PD, Kingma YJ. Esophageal motor abnormalities in gastroesophageal reflux and the effects of fundoplication. *Gastroenterology.* 1986; 91:364-369.
9. Grande L, Lacima G, Ros E, et al. Dysphagia and esophageal motor dysfunction in gastroesophageal reflux are corrected by fundoplication. *J Clin Gastroenterol.* 1991;13:11-16.
10. McCallum RW, Berkowitz DM, Lerner E. Gastric emptying in patients with gastroesophageal reflux. *Gastroenterology.* 1981;80:285-291.
11. Maddern GJ, Chatterton BE, Collins PJ, Horowitz M, Shearman DJC, Jamieson GG. Solid and liquid gastric emptying in patients with gastro-oesophageal reflux. *Br J Surg.* 1985;72:344-347.
12. Little AG, DeMeester TR, Kirchner PT, O'Sullivan GC, Skinner DB. Pathogenesis of esophagitis in patients with gastroesophageal reflux. *Surgery.* 1980;80:101-107.
13. Shay SS, Eggli D, McDonald C, Johnson LF. Gastric emptying of solid food in patients with gastroesophageal reflux. *Gastroenterology.* 1987;92:459-465.
14. Keshavarzian A, Bushnell DL, Sontag S, Yegelwel EJ, Smid K. Gastric emptying in patients with severe reflux esophagitis. *Am J Gastroenterol.* 1991;86: 738-742.
15. Schwizer W, Hinder RA, DeMeester TR. Does delayed gastric emptying contribute to gastroesophageal reflux disease? *Am J Surg.* 1989;157:74-80.
16. Maddern GJ, Jamieson GG. Fundoplication enhances gastric emptying. *Ann Surg.* 1985;201:296-299.
17. Jamieson GG, Maddern GJ, Myers JC. Gastric emptying after fundoplication with and without proximal gastric vagotomy. *Arch Surg.* 1991;126:1414-1417.
18. Velasco N, Hill LD, Gannan RM, Pope CE II. Gastric emptying and gastroesophageal reflux. *Am J Surg.* 1982;144:58-62.
19. Maddern GJ, Jamieson GG, Chatterton BE. Is there an association between failed antireflux procedures and delayed gastric emptying? *Ann Surg.* 1985;202:162-165.
20. Maddern GJ, Myers JC, McIntosh N, Bridgewater FHG, Jamieson GG. The effect of the Angelchik prosthesis on esophageal and gastric function. *Arch Surg.* 1991; 126:1418-1422.
21. Collins PJ, Houghton LA, Read NW, et al. Role of proximal and distal stomach in mixed solid and liquid meal emptying. *Gut.* 1991;32:615-619.
22. Lundell L, Anvari M, Collins PJ, Myers JC, Jamieson GG. The association between gastric emptying, gastric distension and transient lower esophageal sphincter relaxations in patients with gastroesophageal reflux disease. *Gastroenterology.* 1992;102:A478.
23. Luostarinen MES, Koskinen MO, Isolauri JO. Effect of fundal mobilisation in Nissen-Rossetti fundoplication on oesophageal transit and dysphagia. *Eur J Surg.* 1996; 162:37-42.
24. Singh P, Adamopoulos A, Taylor RH, Colin-Jones DG. Oesophageal motor function before and after healing of esophagitis. *Gut.* 1992;33:1590-1596.
25. Lin S, Ke M, Xu J, Kahrilas PJ. Impaired esophageal emptying in reflux disease. *Am J Gastroenterol.* 1994;89:1003-1006.
26. Timmer R, Breumelhof R, Nadorp JHSM, Smout AJPM. Ambulatory esophageal pressure and pH monitoring in patients with high-grade reflux esophagitis. *Dig Dis Sci.* 1994;39:2084-2089.
27. Negre JB. Post-fundoplication symptoms: do they restrict the success of Nissen fundoplication? *Ann Surg.* 1983;198:698-700.
28. Lundell LR, Myers JC, Jamieson GG. Delayed gastric emptying and its relationship to symptoms of "gas-bloat" after antireflux surgery. *Eur J Surg.* 1994;160: 161-166.
29. Holloway RH, Hongo M, Berger K, McCallum RW. Gastric distension: a mechanism for postprandial gastroesophageal reflux. *Gastroenterology.* 1985;89: 779-784.
30. Luostarinen M, Koskinen M, Reinikainen P, Karvonen J, Isolauri J. Two antireflux operations: floppy versus standard Nissen fundoplication. *Ann Med.* 1995; 27:199-205.
31. Bremner RM, DeMeester TR, Crookes PF, et al. The effect of symptoms and nonspecific motility abnormalities on outcomes of surgical therapy for gastroesophageal reflux disease. *J Thorac Cardiovasc Surg.* 1994;107:1244-1250.
32. DeMeester TR, Johnson LF, Joseph GJ, Toscano MS, Hall AW, Skinner DB. Patterns of gastroesophageal reflux in health and disease. *Ann Surg.* 1976;184: 459-469.
33. Vassilakis JS, Xynos E, Kasapidis P, Chrysos E, Mantides A. The effect of floppy Nissen fundoplication on esophageal and gastric motility in gastroesophageal reflux. *Surg Gynecol Obstet.* 1993;177:608-616.

Primary Common Bile Duct Closure

A. Kent Seale, MD; Walter P. Ledet, Jr, MD

Objective: To show that primary closure of the common bile duct following minicholecystectomy is safe and effective.

Design: Eighty-nine primary common bile duct closures done over 13 years.

Setting: General community hospital.

Patients: Patients with cholangiographic evidence of stones in the common bile duct.

Interventions: Minicholecystectomy followed by a primary common bile duct closure or common bile duct closure over a T tube.

Main Outcome Measures: Successful clinical result of primary common bile duct closure following minicholecystectomy.

Results: Eighty-nine primary closures of the common bile duct between 1983 and 1986, resulting in successful clinical outcomes.

Conclusion: Primary closure of the common bile duct following minicholecystectomy is safe, effective, and inexpensive.

Arch Surg. 1999;134:22-24

OBSTRUCTION of the common bile duct as a result of the presence of stones has historically been corrected by opening the common bile duct and removing the stones. The duct is then closed around a T tube. Unfortunately, the use of T tubes carries a significant morbidity. The tube can be dislodged before a tract has developed and reoperation becomes necessary. A T tube must be left in place from 3 to 4 weeks before removal. There is a large amount of pain associated with the presence of the T tube over such a long period. In addition, a drain must also be positioned, and postoperative x-ray films are necessary before removal. Patients are reluctant to return to work with a T tube in place and can lose from 3 to 4 weeks of work.

We believe that primary common bile duct closure using modern operative techniques can be as safe as primary common bile duct closure using a T tube. The patient returns home with 1 drain instead of 2 and the drain remains in place an average of 3 to 5 days. Early dislodgment of the drain does not always require reoperation and postdischarge x-ray films are not required. The patient has a smoother postoperative course, with less pain and an earlier return to work.

Recently, common bile duct stones found during laparoscopic cholecystectomy have been handled by laparoscopic transcystic duct exploration or endoscopic sphincterotomy. Liberman and Phillips[1] reviewed a group of 76 patients, 59 of whom had a laparoscopic cholecystectomy and laparoscopic transcystic duct exploration and 17 of whom had laparoscopic cholecystectomy and endoscopic sphincterotomy. Their length of hospital stay of 6 to 7 days and their cost of $15 000 to $20 000 was considerably higher than a common bile duct exploration with primary closure.

As early as 1917, Halstead[2] described primary closure of the common bile duct that was drained using a tube through the cystic duct stump. Later closures were done using only a Penrose drain in the hepatorenal recess. Mayo,[3] Kirschner,[4] Mirrizzi,[5] Edwards and Herrington,[6] and Herrington et al[7] have written articles supportive of primary closure of the

This article is also available on our Web site: www.ama-assn.org/surgery.

From the Sulphur Surgical Clinic, Sulphur, La.

MATERIALS AND METHODS

Methods for primary bile duct closure were developed in 1983. After a minicholecystectomy, a cholangiogram is done on the patients with laboratory and visual indications of an obstructed common bile duct. The ducts with stones are opened longitudinally in a convenient area. The relationship of the cystic duct to the incision in the common bile duct is not proven to be of consequence. The incision should not be extended within 1 cm of the bifurcation of the common bile duct. The stones in the common bile duct are removed either blind or using a choledochoscope, as well as Fogarty catheters, grasping forceps, irrigation, or stone baskets. The absence of stones in the common bile duct is verified using the choledochoscope. Using a headlight and ×2 magnification, the common bile duct is closed primarily using a 3-0 chromic running stitch (**Figure**). It is imperative that only small bites of the common bile duct are taken. A cystic duct cholangiogram is repeated after the bile duct has been primarily closed. A closed suction drain is always positioned.

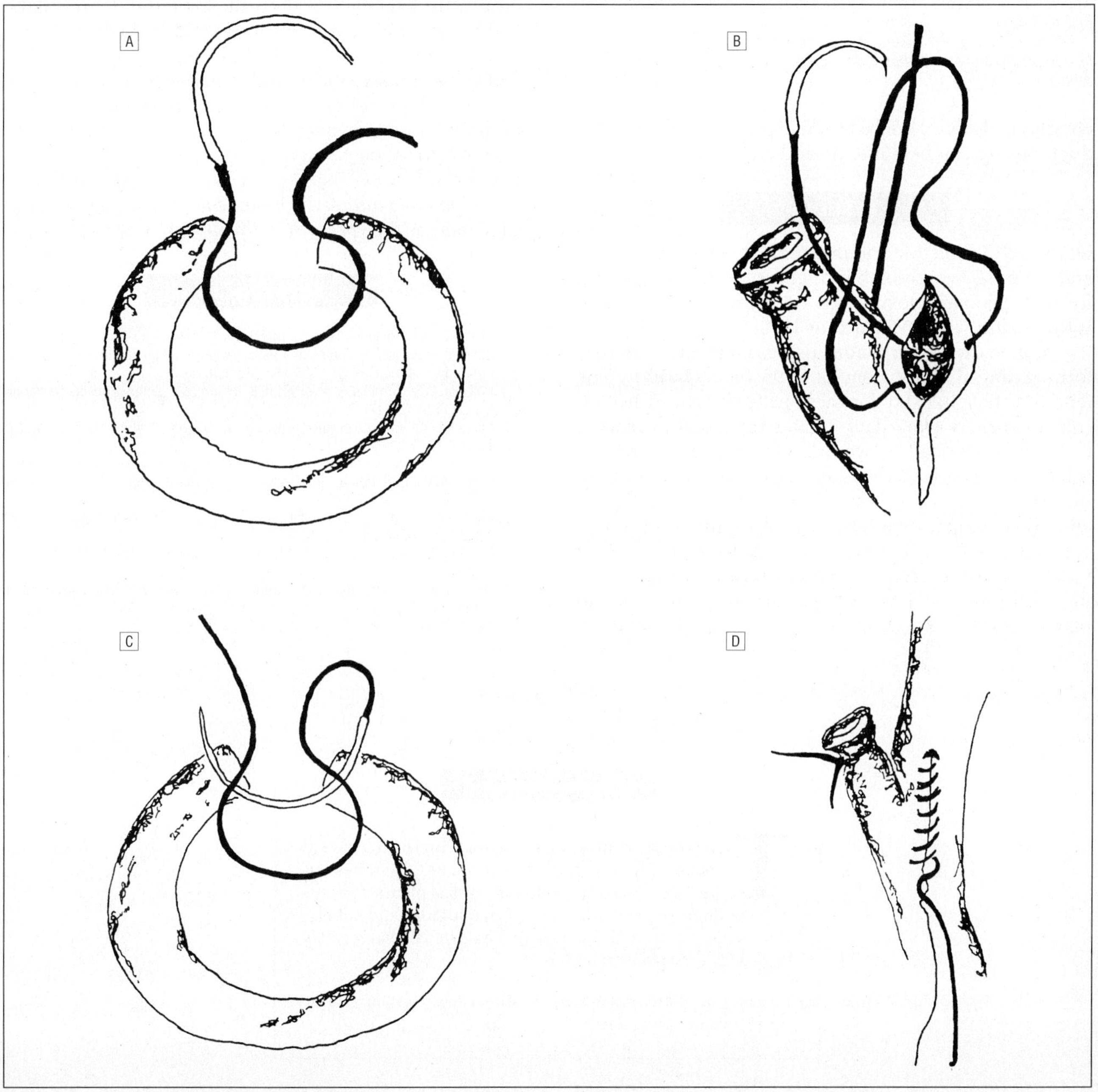

A, The initial stitch approximating only muscularis and mucosa is positioned at the proximal apex. B, The tail of the stitch is held and not tied. C, The suture proceeds distally to the apex, holding tension behind the running stitch. D, After reaching the apex, the suture line proceeds proximally approximating only the serosal layer. On reaching the proximal apex, the suture is tied.

Characteristics of Patients Who Underwent Primary Common Duct Closure

Patient Age Group, y	Primary Closure	Average Stay, d	T Tube†
20-30	7	2.5	1
30-40	7	2.1	1
40-50	5	3.8	2
50-60	9	2.1	0
60-70	16	3.1	4
70-80	27	4.1	10
80-90	15	4.5	0
90-100	3	6.0	0
Total	**89**	**3.6**	**18**

**The duration of hospital stay is an average of the length of stay for each designated age group. In calculating the average, there were some patients who stayed as short as 0 days (day of surgery) and some who stayed as long as 7 days.*

†A comparison of the average stay of patients with a T tube is inappropriate as this procedure is done on sicker patients with multiple problems.

common bile duct. We believe that primary common bile duct closure can be both safe and effective.

RESULTS

Of the 1882 cholecystectomies performed between 1983 and 1996, 107 common bile duct explorations were performed: primary closure was performed in 89 and T-tube closure was performed in 18.

Our patients for whom primary closure was performed ranged in age from 22 to 90 years (**Table**). The length of hospital stay for these patients ranged from 0 (day of surgery) to 7 days. Drains remained in place 3 to 10 days. We had no wound infections or drain tract infections. There were no associated intra-abdominal infections or abscesses and no phlebitis or pulmonary emboli. Postoperative bile leakage in all patients was controlled with the closed suction drainage; no reoperations were necessary. No patient returned with common bile duct strictures or retained stones and no patient who underwent primary common bile duct closure died postoperatively or within 90 days of discharge from the hospital.

CONCLUSIONS

Primary closure of the common bile duct offers improved patient care and should be considered a primary option. The average hospital costs for a minicholecystectomy, common bile duct exploration, and primary closure of the common bile duct was $5000 and the average length of hospital stay was 3.6 days. As opposed to T-tube drainage, the patient remained in the hospital for a shorter period and was not burdened over a 3- to 6-week interval by the T tube. Compared with laparoscopic transcystic exploration or endoscopic sphincterotomy, the average stay in the hospital was 2.6 less days, and the average cost was approximately $10 000 less.

Closure of the common bile duct is a safe, effective, and less expensive means of handling stones in the common bile duct. It requires a shorter hospital stay and is notably less expensive. Many patients return to work within 5 to 10 days.

Corresponding author: A. Kent Seale, MD, Sulphur Surgical Clinic, 914 Cypress St, Sulphur, LA 70663.

REFERENCES

1. Liberman MA, Phillips EH. Cost-effective management of complicated choledocholithiasis: laparoscopic transcystic duct exploration or endoscopic sphincterotomy. *J Am Coll Surg.* 1996;182:488-494.
2. Halstead WS. *Surgical Papers.* Vol 2. Baltimore, Md: Johns Hopkins University Press. 1924:427-472.
3. Mayo WI. An address on the surgery of the hepactic and common bile ducts. *Lancet.* 1923;1:1299-1302.
4. Kirschner M, ed. Operations on the gall bladder and the bile passage. In: Radvin IS, trans. Vol 2. *Abdomen and Rectum.* In: *Operative Surgery.* Philadelphia, Pa: JB Lippincott; 1933:460-517.
5. Mirrizzi PL. Primary suture of the common bile duct in choledocholithiasis. *Arch Surg.* 1942;44:44-54.
6. Edwards LW, Herrington JL Jr. Closure of the common bile duct following its exploration. *Am Surg.* 1953;137:189.
7. Herrington JL Jr, Dawson RE, Edwards WH, Edwards LW. Further consideration in the evaluation of primary closure of the common bile duct following its exploration. *Am Surg.* 1957;145:153-161.

Surgical Anatomy

The thoracic duct enters the neck on the left side of the esophagus, and, at the level of C7, arches laterally and forward on to the cervical pleura. It opens into the angle between the left internal jugular and subclavian veins. Its last half inch (ie, beyond its last valve) may be distended with venous blood.

1. Grant JCB. *A Method of Anatomy: Descriptive and Deductive.* 5th ed. Baltimore, Md: Williams & Wilkins; 1952:682-683.

ORIGINAL ARTICLE

Effect of Intraoperative Blood Transfusion on Patient Outcome in Hepatic Transplantation

Thomas V. Cacciarelli, MD; Emmet B. Keeffe, MD; Dan H. Moore, PhD; Washington Burns, MD; Stephan Busque, MD; Waldo Concepcion, MD; Samuel K. S. So, MD; Carlos O. Esquivel, MD, PhD

Objective: To evaluate the effect of intraoperative transfusion of red blood cells (RBCs) on patient and graft survival.

Design: A retrospective study.

Setting: A tertiary care referral center.

Patients: Between January 1, 1992, and December 31, 1994, medical records from 225 adult patients who underwent primary liver transplantations were analyzed.

Results: Overall patient survival was 90% at 1 year and 86% at 3 years, while graft survival was 89% at 1 year and 85% at 3 years. The following factors were associated with patient and graft survival: age, sex, medical condition at the time of transplantation, and intraoperative transfusion of RBCs. When these factors were subjected to a multivariate analysis, all were independently associated with survival. Fifty-four recipients (24%) underwent transplantation without intraoperative transfusion of RBCs, while 171 recipients (76%) received at least 1 U of RBCs intraoperatively. Recipients who did not receive transfusion of RBCs had higher patient and graft survival rates than patients who did receive RBCs. By multivariate analysis, transplantation without intraoperative transfusion of RBCs no longer remained statistically significant, and only sex and the patient's medical condition were independently associated with patient and graft survival. Patient and graft survival decreased if 5 or more U were transfused, but transfusion of 5 or more U was not independently associated with survival by multivariate analysis.

Conclusions: Increased transfusion requirement for RBCs was independently associated with patient and graft survival. While transplantation without transfusion of intraoperative RBCs was associated with superior patient and graft survival, these effects were overridden by patient sex and medical condition at the time of transplantation.

Arch Surg. 1999;134:25-29

From the Department of Surgery, Stanford University Medical Center, Stanford, Calif (Drs Cacciarelli, Keeffe, Busque, Concepcion, So, and Esquivel); and the Research Institute (Dr Moore) and Department of Pathology (Dr Burns), California Pacific Medical Center, San Francisco.

IMPROVEMENTS IN patient selection, surgical techniques, postoperative management, and immunosuppression for orthotopic liver transplantation (OLT) have led to patient survival approaching 80% at 1 year.[1] While attempts have been made to identify factors affecting patient and graft survival, no set of uniform predictive variables has been described.[2-5] The effect of intraoperative blood loss and transfusions on survival after liver transplantation has been assessed by several different centers, with most data showing a correlation between blood use and postoperative morbidity and mortality rates.[2,3,6-8] During a 3-year period, a substantial proportion of our adult patients underwent OLT without intraoperative transfusion of red blood cells (RBCs). These patients were compared with recipients who received at least 1 U of RBCs intraoperatively to determine the effect of not giving patients RBC transfusions on patient and graft survival rates after OLT.

RESULTS

In the present study, the overall patient survival rates were 90% at 1 year and 86% at 3 years, and graft survival rates were 89% at 1 year and 85% at 3 years. Patient and graft survival for patients undergoing OLT with and without intraoperative transfusion of RBCs are shown in **Figure 1**. Transplant recipients who did not receive RBCs intraoperatively had significantly higher patient and graft survival compared with transfused recipients ($P = .01$ and $P = .03$, respectively). However, the following factors were also associated with patient survival: age ($P = .04$), sex ($P = .005$), and the patient's medical condition ($P = .002$). When these factors, along with whether a patient was trans-

PATIENTS AND METHODS

Between January 1, 1992, and December 31, 1994, a total of 334 OLTs were performed at California Pacific Medical Center, San Francisco. Pediatric recipients (82 transplants) and retransplantations (27 transplants) were excluded from this study, leaving a total of 225 adult primary OLT patients for analysis. There were 105 female and 120 male patients, respectively. The mean age for the entire group was 49.5 years, 47.4 years for those patients who did not receive RBC transfusions, and 50.2 years for those who did receive RBC transfusions. Techniques for procuring and transplanting the donor liver have been described elsewhere.[9-11] The mean (±SD) cold ischemia preservation times in the transfused and nontransfused groups were 11.6 ± 0.2 and 10.7 ± 0.4, respectively. The difference was not statistically significant. The 225 OLTs were performed by the following techniques: 169 piggyback (75%), 36 standard with venovenous bypass (16%), and 20 standard without venovenous bypass (9%). Recipients were divided into 2 groups based on intraoperative RBC transfusion requirement. The transfused group included 171 recipients (76%) who received at least 1 U of RBCs intraoperatively, while 54 recipients (24%) received no RBCs (either packed cells or salvaged blood) intraoperatively (nontransfused group). Cell saver was not used in patients requiring less than 30 U of blood. For the effect of RBC transfusion on patient and graft survival, the groups were arbitrarily divided into 3 groups: intraoperative transfusion of 0 (54 patients), 1 to 4 (64 patients), and 5 or more (107 patients) U of RBCs, respectively. The transfused group included 171 recipients (76%) who received at least 1 U of RBCs intraoperatively.

STATISTICAL ANALYSIS

The influence of the following variables on patient and graft survival after OLT were determined by univariate analysis: age, sex, primary diagnosis, medical condition at the time of transplantation, previous abdominal surgery, transjugular intrahepatic portosystemic shunts, preoperative prothrombin time, intraoperative RBC requirement, cold ischemia time, and operative time. The patient's condition at the time of transplantation was based on Child's classification and United Network for Organ Sharing (UNOS) status. Patient and graft survival were also calculated for the transfused and nontransfused groups. Variables that had a substantial effect on patient and graft survival by univariate analysis were entered into a proportional hazards regression analysis along with transfused and nontransfused recipients to determine whether transfusion of packed RBCs was independently associated with survival or whether confounding variables were present.

Univariate analysis was performed by the Mann-Whitney nonparametric test. Patient and graft survival were determined using a log rank (Mantel-Cox) test and Kaplan-Meier cumulative survival plot. A proportional hazards model was used to control for any intergroup differences based on the aforementioned variables found to have a substantial effect on survival. Factors that were significant in univariate (Mann-Whitney) tests ($P < .05$) were considered in a multivariate proportional hazards regression model. Backward stepwise selection was used to find a group of factors that best influenced outcome. In the first step, all factors that had a significant effect on outcome as determined by univariate analysis were considered. At each step, the factor with the largest P value for significance was removed until only those factors with $P < .05$ remained. These remaining factors were then considered to be those that were statistically significant in predicting outcome. Statistical software (S-PLUS, Version 3.2, StatSci, Division of MathSoft Inc, Seattle, Wash) was used to perform the logistic regression analysis.

fused intraoperatively, were subjected to stepwise multivariate analysis, intraoperative transfusion of RBCs was not significant and only age ($P = .03$), sex ($P = .004$), and patient's medical condition ($P = .003$) remained significant (**Table 1**). The results of similar univariate and multivariate analyses for graft survival are given in Table 1. Men had poorer survival than women and survival was worse for critically ill patients (status 1 and 2a based on current UNOS classification).

When survival rates were examined, patient and graft survival decreased if 5 U or more were transfused ($P = .006$ and $P = .01$, respectively) (**Figure 2**). When subjected to multivariate analysis along with age, sex, and patient's medical condition, transfusion of 5 U or more was not independently associated with patient or graft survival (**Table 2**).

Transfusion of packed RBCs, when examined as a continuous variable, was found to influence patient and graft survival by univariate analysis ($P < .001$). When subjected to multivariate analysis, blood transfusion as a continuous variable remained significant for both patient ($P = .008$) and graft ($P = .03$) survival, along with age, sex, and the patient's medical condition (**Table 3**). **Figure 3** shows relative survival as a function of amount of RBC transfusion and demonstrates decreasing survival with increasing transfusion requirement.

When causes of patient and graft loss were examined, only 1 patient died (primary nonfunction) and 1 patient lost a graft (hepatic artery thrombosis) in the nontransfused group. Twenty-nine recipients in the transfused group died, and 45% (13 patients) died of septic complications, including generalized sepsis, endocarditis, aspergillosis, and bacterial pneumonia. The remaining causes of death were cancer (5 patients), cardiovascular disease (3 patients), trauma (3 patients), intraoperative cardiac arrest (2 patients), primary graft nonfunction (2 patients), natural causes (2 patients), and recurrent disease (1 patient). Causes of graft loss in the group included biliary strictures, hepatic artery thrombosis, and primary graft nonfunction, 1 patient each.

COMMENT

Several centers have examined factors that influence patient and graft survival after OLT, but no consensus exists as to which variables accurately predict outcome after OLT.[2-7] According to these studies, factors that have increased the risk of death or graft loss for patients

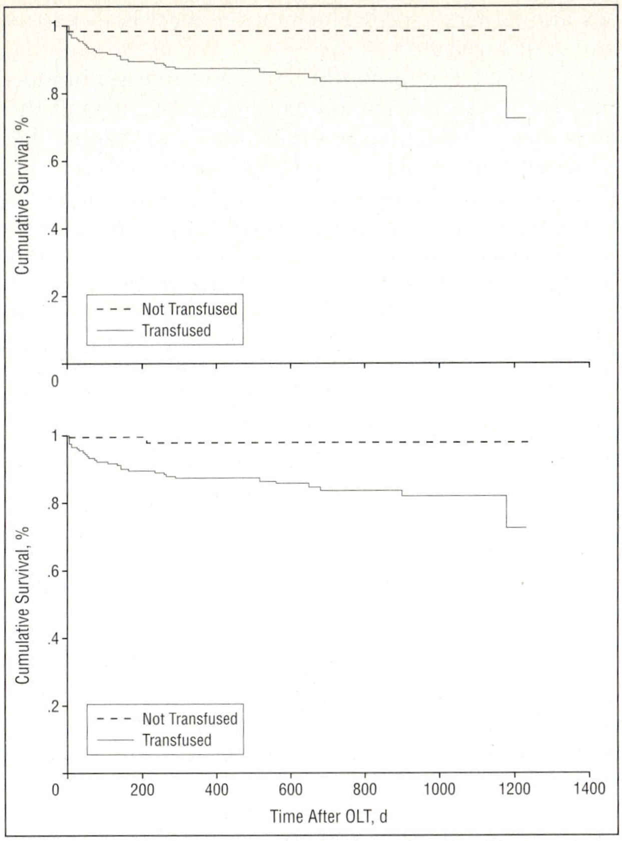

Figure 1. *Patient survival (top) and graft survival (bottom) by intraoperative transfusion of red blood cells in 225 orthotopic liver transplantations (OLTs). The differences in patient survival (P = .01) and graft survival (P = .3) between recipients transfused and not transfused intraoperatively were statistically significant.*

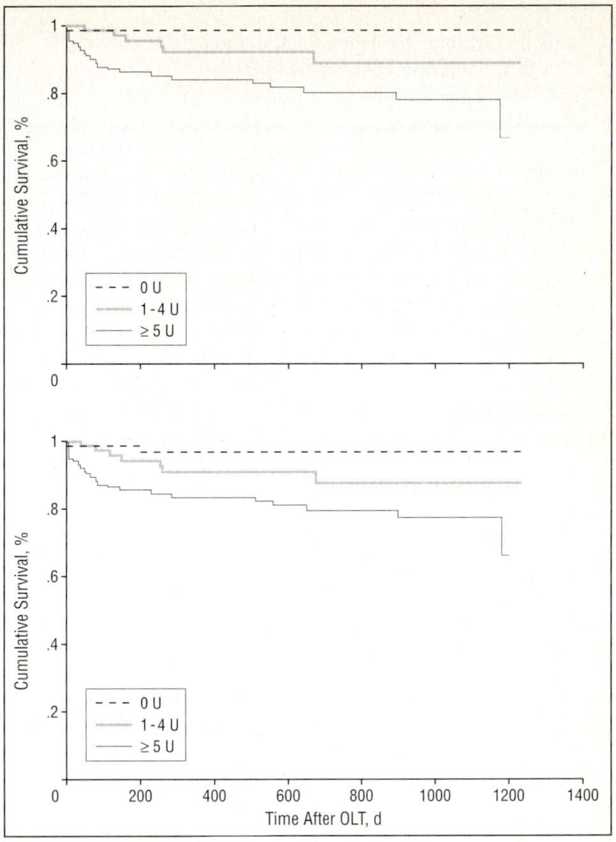

Figure 2. *Patient survival (top) and graft survival (bottom) by intraoperative transfusion of red blood cells (RBCs) in 225 orthotopic liver transplantation (OLT) recipients. The differences in patient survival (P = .006) and graft survival (P = .01) between recipients transfused 0 U and 5 or more U of RBCs intraoperatively was statistically significant.*

Table 1. Variables Influencing Patient and Graft Survival After OLT in Recipients Receiving No RBCs vs 1 Unit or More of RBCs Intraoperatively*

Variable	Univariate Analysis	Multivariate Analysis
Patient survival		
0 vs ≥1 U RBCs	.01	.17
Age	.04	.03
Sex	.005	.004
Patient's medical condition	.002	.003
Graft survival		
0 vs ≥1 U RBCs	.03	.30
Sex	.008	.005
Patient's medical condition	.002	.002

**OLT indicates orthotopic liver transplantation; RBCs, red blood cells. P values were calculated using proportional hazards regression analysis.*

Table 2. Variables Influencing Patient and Graft Survival After OLT in Recipients Receiving Less Than 5 vs 5 Units or More of RBCs Intraoperatively*

Variable	Univariate Analysis	Multivariate Analysis
Patient survival		
<5 vs ≥ 5 U RBCs	.004	.12
Age	.04	.02
Sex	.005	.005
Patient's medical condition	.002	.006
Graft survival		
<5 vs ≥5 U RBCs	.01	.20
Sex	.008	.006
Patient's medical condition	.002	.01

**OLT indicates orthotopic liver transplantation; RBCs, red blood cells. P values were calculated using proportional hazards regression analysis.*

undergoing OLT vary and include UNOS status, Child's classification, fulminant hepatic failure, ABO incompatibility, compromised renal function, and infection before transplantation. In addition, some studies have reported a detrimental effect of intraoperative blood loss and massive transfusion requirements after liver transplantation.[2,3,7,8] In a previous study, we conducted an analysis of several factors on the need for blood transfusion.[12] These factors were recipient's age at the time of transplantation, sex, Child's classification, UNOS status, preoperative hematocrit, prothrombin time, partial thromboplastin time, platelet count, and fibrinogen level. In addition, other factors examined were primary liver disease, year of transplantation, history of abdominal surgery, transjugular intrahepatic portosystemic shunt placed prior to transplantation, use of venovenous bypass technique for transplantation, cold ischemia time, and operative time. The univariate

Table 3. Variables Influencing Patient and Graft Survival After OLT, Analyzing Transfusion of RBCs as a Continuous Variable*

Variable	Univariate Analysis	Multivariate Analysis
Patient survival		
RBC transfusion	.0001	.39
Age	.04	.02
Sex	.005	.003
Patient's medical condition	.002	.003
Graft survival		
RBC transfusion	.0001	.61
Sex	.008	.004
Patient's medical condition	.002	.005

**OLT indicates orthotopic liver transplantation; RBCs, red blood cells. P values were calculated using proportional hazards regression analysis.*

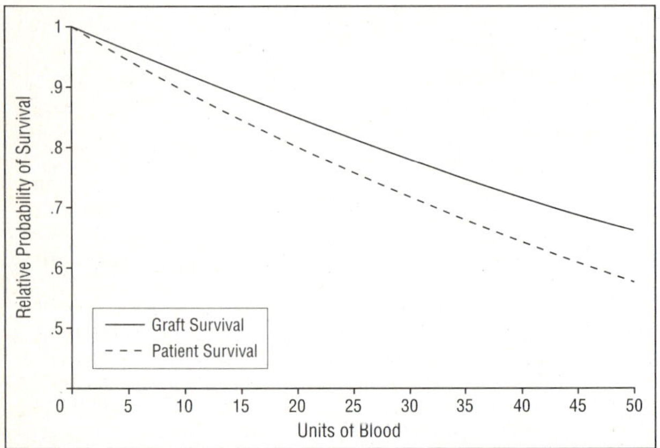

Figure 3. *Relative probability of patient and graft survival based on transfusion requirements when analyzed as a continuous variable.*

analysis showed the following factors to be associated with OLT without blood transfusions: Child's classification, UNOS status, lack of previous right upper quadrant surgery, preoperative hematocrit, prothrombin time, activated partial thromboplastin time, piggyback technique, operative time, adult recipient status, and year of transplantation. A regression analysis showed that UNOS status (healthier patients required less blood), preoperative hematocrit, piggyback technique, operative time, and year of transplantation remained independently associated with OLT without transfusion of RBCs.[12] Unfortunately, donor information was not available for the analysis.

The present study examined the effect of OLT without transfusion of any RBCs on patient and graft outcome. A significant improvement was noted in both patient and graft survival when recipients underwent OLT without intraoperative transfusion of RBCs. However, other factors, rather than the presence or absence of intraoperative blood transfusions, appear to have a more substantial effect on outcome. Male sex and severity of the patient's medical condition (patients in an intensive care unit) had a negative influence on patient and graft survival. This finding is in agreement with UNOS scientific registry data, which have shown that sex and patient's medical condition affect both patient and graft survival.[1,12]

Why OLT without RBCs transfusion was not independently associated with superior patient and graft survival may be related to several factors. Previous studies demonstrating an adverse effect of transfusion requirements on outcome were conducted during an earlier era of OLT and examined the effects of massive intraoperative transfusion of blood and blood products.[2,3,8] A more recent study also divided patients into a group of "bleeders" who received 10 U or more of RBCs.[7] The present study compared patients receiving no RBCs with a group who received at least 1 U of RBC intraoperatively, and the study population did not contain a large proportion of bleeders. In fact, 50 patients (29%) in the transfused group received 3 U of packed RBCs or less intraoperatively (mean 5.7 U, median 4.0 U, range 1-67 U). The small number of RBCs required intraoperatively in the present study is probably due to technical improvements in performing OLT. Even when a group of recipients who received 5 U or more of RBCs was examined, an independent association with survival was not seen. Because many patients in the transfused group received few RBCs, the detrimental effect of massive transfusions in the few patients who required it were most likely masked by the remaining patients receiving only a few units of RBCs.

When cutoff points were not employed and blood transfusion was examined as a continuous variable, it did have an independent association with survival. The concept that increased blood loss, and hence, a greater transfusion requirement during the transplantation, affects survival agrees with other data.[2,3,7] Although blood loss is not the only factor that influences survival, it does point to the need for attention to detail during the procedure.

Previous studies have reported a high mortality rate secondary to infectious complications in general,[13,14] and particularly in patients who have received blood transfusions.[7] Almost half the deaths in the present study involved septic complications, similar to the previous studies. In addition, all deaths due to sepsis occurred in the group that received transfusions, and the mean intraoperative RBC transfusion requirement for these patients was 13 U.

The present study demonstrates that recipients who undergo OLT without transfusion of RBCs have superior patient and graft survival when compared with transfusion recipients, but other factors have a substantial effect on outcome after OLT, namely, age, male sex, and medical condition at the time of transplantation. When the effect of intraoperative blood transfusion on survival was examined as a continuous variable, an independent association with survival was noted, suggesting that blood loss should be kept to a minimum during the transplantation.

We thank Katie Allen for the skillful preparation of the manuscript.

Corresponding author: Carlos O. Esquivel, MD, PhD, Professor of Surgery, Stanford University Medical Center, 750 Welch Rd, Suite 319, Palo Alto, CA 94304-1510.

REFERENCES

1. *1995 Annual Report of the US Scientific Registry of Transplant Recipients and the Organ Procurement and Transplantation Network-Transplant Data: 1988-1994.* Bethesda, MD: Division of Organ Transplantation, Bureau of Health Resources Development, Health Resources and Services Administration, US Dept of Health and Human Services; 1995. No. 1076-8874.
2. Shaw BW Jr, Wood RP, Gordon RD, Iwatsuki S, Gillquist WP, Starzl TE. Influence of selected patient variables and operative blood loss on six-month survival following liver transplantation. *Semin Liver Dis.* 1985;5:385-393.
3. Brems JJ, Hiatt JR, Colonna JO, et al. Variables influencing the outcome following orthotopic liver transplantation. *Arch Surg.* 1987;122:1109-1111.
4. Beliga P, Merion RM, Turcotte JG, et al. Preoperative risk factor assessment in liver transplantation. *Surgery.* 1992;112:704-711.
5. Cuervas-Mons V, Millan I, Gavaler JS, Starzl TE, Van Thiel DH. Prognostic value of preoperatively obtained clinical and laboratory data in predicting survival following orthotopic liver transplantation. *Hepatology.* 1986;6:922-927.
6. Motschman TL, Taswell HF, Brecher ME, Rakela J, Grambsch PM, Larson-Keller JJ. Transplantation: their relationship to clinical and laboratory data. *Mayo Clin Proc.* 1989;64:346-355.
7. Mor E, Jennings L, Gonwa TA, et al. The impact of operative bleeding on outcome in transplantation of the liver. *Surg Gynecol Obstet.* 1993;176: 219-227.
8. Rouch DA, Thistlethwaite JR, Lichtor L, et al. Effect of massive transfusion during liver transplantation on rejection and infection. *Transplant Proc.* 1988;20: 1135-1137.
9. Nakazato P, Concepcion W, Bry W, et al. Total abdominal evisceration: an en-bloc technique for abdominal organ harvesting. *Surgery.* 1992;111:37.
10. Starzl TE, Iwatsuki S, Shaw BW Jr. Technique of liver transplantation. In: Blumgart CH, ed. *Surgery of the Liver and Biliary Tract.* Edinburgh, Scotland: Churchill Livingstone Inc; 1987:1537.
11. Tzakis A, Todo S, Starzl TE. Orthotopic liver transplantation with preservation of the inferior vena cava. *Ann Surg.* 1989;210:649-652.
12. Cacciarelli TV, Keeffe EB, Moore DH, et al. Primary liver transplantation without transfusion of red blood cells. *Surgery.* 1996;120:698-705.
13. Cuervas-Mons V, Martinez AJ, Dekker A, et al. Adult liver transplantation: an analysis of the cause of death in 40 consecutive cases. *Hepatology.* 1986;6: 495-501.
14. Shaw BW Jr, Wood RP, Stratta RJ, Pillen TJ, Langnas AN. Stratifying the causes of death in liver transplant recipients: an approach to improving survival. *Arch Surg.* 1989;124:895-900.

IN OTHER AMA JOURNALS

JAMA

Acupuncture

NIN Consensus Development Panel on Acupuncture

Objective: To provide clinicians, patients, and the general public with a responsible assessment of the use and effectiveness of acupuncture to treat a variety of conditions.

Participants: A nonfederal, nonadvocate, 12-member panel representing the fields of acupuncture, pain, psychology, psychiatry, physical medicine and rehabilitation, drug abuse, family practice, internal medicine, health policy, epidemiology, statistics, physiology, biophysics, and the representatives of the public. In addition, 25 experts from these same fields presented data to the panel and a conference audience of 1200. Presentations and discussions were divided into 3 phases over 2½ days: (1) presentations by investigators working in areas relevant to the consensus questions during a 2-day public session; (2) questions and statements from conference attendees during open discussion periods that were part of the public session; and (3) closed deliberations by the panel during the remainder of the second day and morning of the third. The conference was organized and supported by the Office of Alternative Medicine and the Office of Medical Applications of Research, National Institutes of Health, Bethesda, Md.

Evidence: The literature, produced from January 1970 to October 1997, was searched through MEDLINE, Allied and Alternative Medicine, EMBASE, and MANTIS, as well as through a hand search of 9 journals that were not indexed by the National Library of Medicine. An extensive bibliography of 2302 references was provided to the panel and the conference audience. Expert speakers prepared abstracts of their own conference presentations with relevant citations from the literature. Scientific evidence was given precedence over clinical anecdotal experience.

Consensus Process: The panel, answering predefined questions, developed their conclusions based on the scientific evidence presented in the open forum and scientific literature. The panel composed a draft statement, which was read in its entirety and circulated to the experts and the audience for comment. Thereafter, the panel resolved conflicting recommendations and released a revised statement at the end of the conference. The panel finalized the revisions within a few weeks after the conference. The draft statement was made available on the World Wide Web immediately following its release at the conference and was updated with the panel's final revisions within a few weeks of the conference. The statement is available at http://consensus.nih.gov.

Conclusions: Acupuncture as a therapeutic intervention is widely practiced in the United States. Although there have been many studies of its potential usefulness, many of these studies provide equivocal results because of design, sample size, and other factors. The issue is further complicated by inherent difficulties in the use of appropriate controls, such as placebos and sham acupuncture groups. However, promising results have emerged, for example, showing efficacy of acupuncture in adult postoperative and chemotherapy nausea and vomiting and in postoperative dental pain. There are other situations, such as addiction, stroke rehabilitation, headache, menstrual cramps, tennis elbow, fibromyalgia, myofascial pain, osteoarthritis, low back pain, carpal tunnel syndrome, and asthma, in which acupuncture may be useful as an adjunct treatment or an acceptable alternative or be included in a comprehensive management program. Further research is likely to uncover additional areas where acupuncture interventions will be useful. *(1998;280:1518-1524)*

NIH Consensus Statements, NIH Technology Assessment Statements, and related materials are available by writing to the NIH Consensus Program Information Center, PO Box 2577, Kensington, MD 20891, by calling toll free 1 (888) 644-2667, or by visiting the NIH Consensus Development Program home page at http://consensus.nih.gov.

ARTICLE

The Relationship Between Hospital Volume and Outcomes of Hepatic Resection for Hepatocellular Carcinoma

Robert E. Glasgow, MD; Jonathan A. Showstack, PhD, MPH; Patricia P. Katz, PhD; Carlos U. Corvera, MD; Robert S. Warren, MD; Sean J. Mulvihill, MD

Background: Volume-outcome relations have been established for several complex therapies. However, few studies have examined volume-outcome relations for high-risk procedures in general surgery, such as hepatectomy for hepatocellular carcinoma (HCC).

Objective: To evaluate the relation between hospital volume and outcome for patients undergoing hepatectomy for HCC.

Design: Retrospective cohort study.

Setting: All acute-care hospitals in California.

Patients: Hospital discharge data were analyzed for each patient in California who underwent major hepatic resection for HCC from January 1, 1990, through December 31, 1994. Hospitals were grouped according to number of hepatectomies performed at each center during the 5-year study.

Main Outcome Measures: Outcome measures included operative mortality and length of hospital stay. Regression analyses were used to adjust for differences in patient mix.

Results: Five hundred seven patients underwent hepatectomy for HCC during the study. Hepatic resections were performed in 138 hospitals, with an overall in-hospital mortality rate of 14.8%. Three quarters of patients were treated at hospitals that average 3 or fewer hepatic resections for HCC per year. These low-volume providers represent 97.1% of all hospitals treating patients with HCC statewide. Significant reductions in risk-adjusted operative mortality rates (22.7%-9.4%; $P = .002$, multiple logistic regression) and risk-adjusted length of stay (14.3-11.3 days; $P = .03$, multiple linear regression) were observed as hospital volume increased.

Conclusions: Low operative mortality and length of stay were associated with high-volume centers. These data support regionalization of high-risk procedures in general surgery, such as hepatectomy for HCC.

Arch Surg. 1999;134:30-35

TODAY'S CHANGING health care environment is being driven, in part, by external pressures on providers to deliver economical, high-quality care. For some medical therapies, quality of care varies little among providers, making cost a primary focus.[1,2] For other treatments, however, quality of care is not uniform. Such is the case with coronary angioplasty, coronary surgery, and bone marrow and solid organ transplantation. For these complex therapies, a volume-outcome relationship exists where poor patient outcome, such as in-hospital mortality, is related to low provider volume and inexperience.[1,3-6] These volume-outcome relations serve as the basis for the argument that high-risk procedures should be regionalized to centers of excellence.[3,7,8]

In the case of coronary angioplasty, coronary surgery, and transplantation, regionalization is beginning to occur as payers selectively contract with providers for these services. However, this is not the case with other complex therapies. In general surgical practice, standards for the minimum of experience necessary to perform highly complex and risky procedures, ie, major hepatic, pancreatic, or esophageal resection for neoplasia, do not exist. The number of these complex operations performed each year is insufficient for all surgeons and hospitals to have experience. Most of these operations are performed on an elective rather than emergent basis. Thus, if centers with superior patient outcomes could be identified, these procedures could be regionalized as a means of providing the most efficacious and cost-effective care.

See Invited Critique at end of article

From the Departments of Surgery (Drs Glasgow, Corvera, Warren, and Mulvihill) and Medicine (Drs Showstack and Katz) and the Institute for Health Policy Studies (Drs Showstack and Katz), University of California, San Francisco.

MATERIALS AND METHODS

DATA SOURCES

We retrospectively analyzed standardized patient discharge abstracts obtained from the California Office of Statewide Health Planning and Development (OSHPD), Sacramento. This database contains discharge data abstracts for every patient hospitalization from every acute-care facility in the state of California. Each abstract includes a variety of demographic, clinical, and hospitalization data that characterize a specific hospitalization. Each patient is assigned a principal diagnosis and procedure and up to 16 secondary diagnoses and procedures. The OSHPD database uses diagnostic and procedural codes derived from the *International Classification of Diseases, Ninth Revision, Clinical Modification* (4th ed) (*ICD-9-CM*), issued by the US Department of Health and Human Services.[9]

All discharge abstracts from January 1, 1990, through December 31, 1994, were included in the initial search of the OSHPD database. From these abstracts, all patients who underwent hepatic lobectomy (*ICD-9-CM* code 50.3) or partial hepatectomy (*ICD-9-CM* code 50.22) were examined. From this group, a subset of patients undergoing hepatic resection for HCC was selected (*ICD-9-CM* code 155.0). Hospitals were characterized with regard to the number of acute and intensive care beds, discharges and patient hospital days per year, yearly overall surgical volume and number of hepatic resections for benign and malignant neoplasia, presence of a liver transplantation program and general surgery residency program, university affiliation, and capability for other complex surgery, as determined by the presence of cardiac surgery services. These data were derived, in part, from the *Licensed Services and Utilization Profiles: Annual Report of Hospitals* for January 11, 1991, through December 31, 1991.[10] Frequency distributions for the individual patient characteristics within the data set and hospital characteristics listed above were computed.

DATA ANALYSIS

Patients were grouped according to hospital identification number. Hospitals were then classified into quartile groups based on the number of hepatic resections performed in the study period. Crude operative mortality rate and length of hospital stay were calculated for each volume range. Operative mortality in this study was defined as patient death before hospital discharge. Because length of hospital stay is directly related to events within the postoperative course, patients with long hospital stays are most likely patients in whom significant perioperative complications develop. Thus, the percentage of patients with hospital stays longer than the 75th percentile (14 days) was calculated for each volume group. This measure served as a surrogate for postoperative complications, as other reliable objective measures of postoperative complications were not directly available within this database.[4] To characterize a profile of hospitals within each volume group, the distribution of the various hospital characteristics was analyzed.

Regression modeling was used to evaluate the independent associations of patient and hospital characteristics with the primary outcomes of interest (ie, operative mortality and length of hospital stay). The patient was the unit of analysis, with hospital volume group defined as a patient characteristic. This allowed for a volume group effect to be assessed while controlling for the characteristics of individual patients. Multiple logistic regression was used to model the dichotomous outcome, in-hospital mortality, and multiple linear regression was used to model length of hospital stay.

The independent variables in these analyses included hospital volume, age group, sex, year of surgery, source of admission, type of resection (hepatic lobectomy or partial hepatectomy), presence of chronic liver disease, and presence of other preoperative comorbid illnesses. Age was entered into the regression equations as the following sets of dummy variables: 45 to 60 years, 60 to 75 years, and older than 75 years, with younger than 45 years as the reference group. Significant preoperative comorbid illnesses within a given patient abstract were grouped into 1 dichotomous variable to minimize potential colinearities among the various comorbidities. For example, patients with a history of congestive heart failure are likely to also have coronary artery disease. We believed the following comorbidities to have a significant influence on operative risk: coronary artery disease (*ICD-9-CM* codes 412-414), chronic obstructive pulmonary disease (*ICD-9-CM* codes 490-496), diabetes mellitus (*ICD-9-CM* codes 250), congestive heart failure (*ICD-9-CM* code 428), nutritional deficiencies (*ICD-9-CM* codes 260-263), and preoperative intra-abdominal hemorrhage (*ICD-9-CM* code 459). The presence of chronic liver disease, including cirrhosis (*ICD-9-CM* code 571), was treated as a separate dichotomous variable, as it represents an independent factor associated with poor operative risk. The dependent variables for these analyses were operative mortality or death before discharge and length of hospital stay.

Adjusted means for operative mortality rate and length of hospital stay were calculated from regression equations that included all of the independent variables. A complete description of the process of adjustment is provided by Cohen and Cohen.[11] An adjusted mean is an estimate based on the hypothetical situation that all hospital volume groups had the same mean values on each of the independent variables that were entered into the equation. In other words, the adjusted mean represents the estimated operative mortality rate or length of stay if each of the volume groups treated patients with similar patient characteristics. To further evaluate this volume-outcome relation, an additional analysis was performed, where hospital volume was defined by the total number of hepatic resections for benign and malignant neoplasia, including metastatic disease.

A key goal of any reorganization of health care delivery practices in the United States is to preserve or improve quality while reducing costs. Quality of a surgical procedure is measured by operative morbidity and mortality, outcome, effectiveness compared with alternate therapies, and patient satisfaction. It is an open question whether regionalization of high-risk procedures in general surgical practice is desirable or warranted from this standpoint. To help answer this question, we analyzed the relation between hospital volume and postoperative outcome in 1 high-risk, complex general surgical operation, major hepatic resection for hepatocellular carcinoma (HCC). We hypothesized that the risk, as measured by operative mortality, and the cost, as measured by length of hospital stay, are reduced when these patients are cared for in hospitals with greater experience with the procedure.

RESULTS

During the study, 507 patients underwent major hepatic resection for HCC in the state of California. The number of resections performed each year was relatively constant, ranging from 117 in 1990 to 87 in 1993 (**Table 1**). A total of 138 hospitals reported to the database during the 5 years but, because a hepatic resection was not performed at all hospitals in each year, the yearly average number of hospitals in which a hepatic resection for HCC was performed was 53 (Table 1).

Patient ages were distributed as seen in the following tabulation:

Age Range, y	No. (%) of Patients
<45	126 (24.8)
45-59	125 (24.6)
60-74	203 (40.0)
≥75	53 (10.4)

The median age was 60 to 64 years. Men outnumbered women by a ratio of nearly 3:2 (293 [57.8%] vs 214 [42.2%], respectively). The most common race of treated patients was white (263 [51.9%] of the study population), followed by Asian (135 [26.6%]), Hispanic (68 [13.4%]), other (21 [4.1%]), and African American (20 [3.9%]). Payer source is presented in the following tabulation:

Source	No. (%) of Patients
Medicare	160 (31.6)
Medi-Cal	76 (15.0)
Blue Cross/Blue Shield	28 (5.5)
Private insurance	94 (18.5)
Health maintenance or preferred health provider organization	128 (25.2)
Other	21 (4.1)

Source of admission and presence of comorbid medical illnesses were analyzed as indicators of severity of illness. Patients transferred from other acute-care hospitals and those admitted on an elective basis for surgery far outnumbered patients admitted from the emergency department (453 [89.3%] vs 54 [10.6%]). Preoperative comorbidities included diabetes mellitus (46 [9.1%]), coronary artery disease (37 [7.3%]), chronic obstructive pulmonary disease (36 [7.1%]), chronic nutritional deficiencies (17 [3.4%]), congestive heart failure (9 [1.8%]), and chronic renal insufficiency (6 [1.2%]). Eight patients, or 1.6% of the total, presented emergently with a diagnosis of intra-abdominal hemorrhage. Six (11.1%) of the 54 patients admitted through the emergency department had a diagnosis of intra-abdominal hemorrhage, compared with 2 (0.4%) of the 453 patients admitted on a routine basis or transferred from another acute-care facility. The median number of significant comorbidities per patient was 0, with a mean ± SE of 0.70 ± 0.04.

Chronic liver disease, including cirrhosis, was present in 192 (37.9%) of patients overall. For patients with chronic liver disease, the crude operative mortality rate was 27.1% compared with 7.3% in patients without chronic liver disease ($P<.001$ by χ^2 analysis). Likewise, increasing number of comorbidities correlated with increased crude operative mortality. For patients with no comorbidities, the operative mortality was 5.0%. This rate increased significantly with increasing number of secondary diagnoses ($P<.001$ by linear regression analysis). For patients with 4 or more comorbidities, the operative mortality was 50.0%. Partial hepatectomy (*ICD-9-CM* code 50.22) was performed in 299 patients compared with 208 patients who underwent hepatic lobectomy (*ICD-9-CM* code 50.3).

Each of the 4 volume groups included approximately 127 patients (25.0% of the total number of patients). One half of all patients were treated at centers where 6 or fewer resections were performed during the study (**Table 2**). These centers accounted for 88.4% of all reporting hospitals. In contrast, the highest-volume centers averaged 37 patients each during the 5 years and accounted for only 2.9% of the reporting hospitals statewide.

Hospital volume groups varied widely with regard to hospital characteristics (**Table 3**). The highest-volume providers were larger, with more acute and intensive care unit beds and more discharges and patient days per year. They also were more likely to be university hospitals with a general surgery residency training program. In addition to a higher overall surgical volume per year, the highest-volume providers were more likely to perform other complex operations (ie, coronary artery bypass) and to have a higher overall volume of hepatic resections for benign and malignant neoplasia. Three of the 4 highest-volume providers had a liver transplantation program, indicating an institutional interest in hepatology and hepatic surgery. In contrast, none of the lowest-volume providers performed liver transplantation.

The overall mortality rate for the study population was 14.8%. Crude operative mortality rates decreased with increasing hospital volume, from 24.4% in the lowest-volume centers to 6.2% in the highest-volume centers (**Table 4**). This inverse relationship between decreasing operative mortality rate and increasing hospital volume is summarized in the **Figure**. This relationship was highly significant ($P<.001$

Table 1. Distribution of Hospitals and Patients by Year of Surgery

Year	No. of Hospitals*	No. of Patients
1990	59	117
1991	57	95
1992	50	101
1993	45	87
1994	56	107
Total	138†	**507**

Indicates hospitals at which hepatic resection for hepatocellular carcinoma was performed.

†Total number of hospitals reporting during the study period.

Table 2. Hospital Volume Group Assignments

Hospital Volume Group, No. of Operations/5 y	Hospitals, No. (%)*	Patients, No. (%)
1-2	90 (65.2)	115 (22.7)
3-6	32 (23.2)	130 (25.6)
7-16	12 (8.7)	116 (22.9)
≥17	4 (2.9)	146 (28.8)

Indicates hospitals at which hepatic resections for hepatocellular carcinoma were performed.

Table 3. Hospital Characteristics by Hospital Volume Groups

Characteristic	All	Hospital Volume Groups, No. of Operations/5 y: 1-2	3-6	7-16	≥17
University hospital, %*	6.5	0.0	12.5	25.0	50.0
Liver transplantation program, %*	8.0	0.0	12.5	33.3	75.0
Residency training center, %*	18.7	7.0	37.5	33.3	75.0
No. of acute-care beds, mean ± SEM*	302 ± 18	243 ± 20	337 ± 32	493 ± 53	734 ± 92
No. of patient days/y, mean ± SEM*	63 877 ± 4130	47 548 ± 4224	74 753 ± 6884	114 606 ± 11 242	171 701 ± 19 472
No. of discharges/y, mean ± SEM*	11 906 ± 738	9498 ± 789	12 643 ± 0.2	21 273 ± 2099	29 056 ± 3637
No. of intensive care unit beds, mean ± SEM*	21.3 ± 1.7	14.4 ± 1.7	28.2 ± 2.9	39.8 ± 4.7	56.7 ± 8.1
No. of operations/y, mean ± SEM*	7356 ± 482	5808 ± 532	8022 ± 862	13 456 ± 1408	16 245 ± 2439
No. of hepatectomies for neoplasia in 1990 through 1994, mean ± SEM*†	55.1 ± 1.3	6.3 ± 1.0	19.8 ± 0.9	52.4 ± 1.0	139.8 ± 0.92
Cardiac surgery center, %‡	54	45.6	62.5	83.3	100

*$P<.001$ by analysis of variance, linear regression analysis.
†Indicates January 1, 1990, through December 31, 1994.
‡$P<.01$ by analysis of variance, linear regression analysis.

Table 4. Crude and Adjusted Operative Mortality Rates by Hospital Volume Groups

Hospital Volume Group, No. of Operations/5 y	Crude Operative Mortality Rate, Mean %*	Risk-Adjusted Operative Mortality Rate, Mean %†‡
1-2	24.4	22.7
3-6	16.2	13.3
7-16	14.7	15.4
≥17	6.2§	9.4
All	14.8	. . .‖

*$P<.001$, using logistic regression analysis.
†Indicates risk-adjusted using multiple logistic regression analysis for sex, age, year of operation, source of admission, type of resection, presence of chronic liver disease, and presence of significant comorbid illnesses.
‡$P<.05$, hospitals with 17 or more operations vs those with 1 to 2, 3 to 6, and 7 to 16; hospitals with 1 to 2 operations vs those with 3 to 6, 7 to 16, and ≥17; and hospitals with ≥17 operations vs those with 1 to 2, using multiple logistic regression analysis.
§$P<.05$, hospitals with ≥17 operations vs those with 1 to 2, 3 to 6, and 7 to 16, using χ^2 analysis.
‖Not applicable.

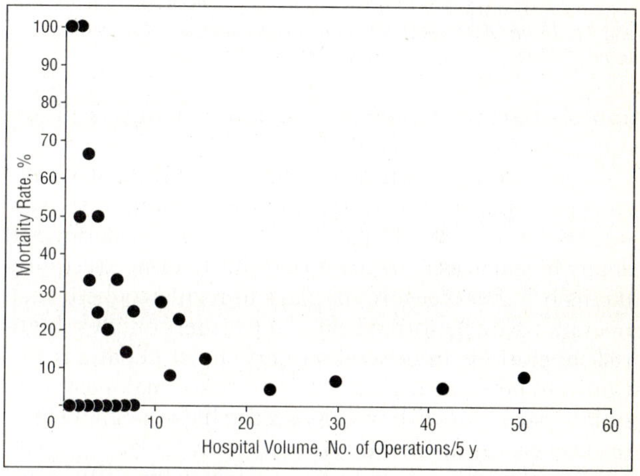

Scatterplot diagram of hospital volume plotted against operative mortality rate.

by logistic regression analysis). When the crude mortality rates for each volume group were adjusted to account for differences in patient characteristics, this highly significant volume-outcome relationship persisted (Table 4).

A similar volume-outcome relationship was observed when length of hospital stay was analyzed. The mean hospital stay was 12.9 days. The lowest-volume providers had a mean length of stay of 14.7 days compared with 10.8 days in the highest-volume providers (**Table 5**). When the length of hospital stay for each volume group was adjusted to account for differences in patient characteristics, this significant volume-outcome relationship persisted (Table 5). In addition, lowest-volume providers were more likely to have patients with hospital stays beyond the 75th percentile (Table 5). This implies that patients treated at lowest-volume providers were twice as likely to have complicated postoperative courses than patients treated at highest-volume providers. The mean (±SEM) length of stay for patients who died was longer than that for patients who survived (18.4 ± 2.24 vs 12.0 ± 0.42 days). When patients who died were excluded from the length-of-stay analysis, a significant volume outcome relationship persisted.

When hospital volume was defined as total number of hepatic resections for benign and malignant neoplasia, these significant volume-outcome relations persisted. In 2004 patients, the overall operative mortality rate was 6.9%, ranging from 9.3% in the lowest-volume providers to 4.1% in the highest-volume providers.

COMMENT

In an era of limited resources, increased attention is being paid in the United States to the most efficient delivery of health care services. The desired goal is to provide the highest quality of care while using the fewest resources. Volume-outcome analyses have shown that for certain complex surgical procedures, including heart transplantation and coronary artery bypass, the results of treatment are directly linked to experience. These observations have led to the suggestion that these complex, high-risk procedures should be regionalized to high-volume centers of excellence. To determine if similar volume-outcome relations exist in general surgical practice, we examined the relation between hospital volume

Table 5. Crude and Adjusted Operative Length of Hospital Stay by Hospital Volume Group

Hospital Volume Group, No. of Operations/5 y	Length of Hospital Stay, Mean ± SEM, d*	Risk-Adjusted Length of Hospital Stay, d†	Length of Stay >75th Percentile, Mean %‡§
1-2	14.7 ± 1.0	14.3	30.4
3-6	13.7 ± 1.0	13.4	28.5
7-16	12.9 ± 1.0	13.1	24.1
≥17	10.8 ± 0.9	11.3‖	15.8
All	12.9 ± 0.5	. . .	24.3

*$P<.05$, using linear regression analysis, hospitals with ≥17 operations vs those with 1 to 2, using Tukey-Kramer honestly significant difference.

†Indicates risk-adjusted using multiple linear regression analysis, adjusting for sex, age, year of operation, source of admission, type of resection, presence of chronic liver disease, and presence of significant comorbid illnesses. Ellipses indicate not applicable.

‡Indicates more than 14 days.

§$P<.05$, using linear regression analysis, hospitals with 17 or more operations vs those with 1 to 2 and 3 to 6, using χ^2 analysis.

‖$P<.05$, hospitals with 17 or more operations vs those with 1 to 2, 3 to 6, and 7 to 16; and hospitals with 17 or more operations vs those with 1 to 2, using multiple linear regression analysis.

and operative outcome in 1 complex, high-risk procedure, hepatic resection for HCC.

Hepatic resection was selected for this analysis because it represents a technically challenging, resource-intensive procedure. Hepatic resection may be performed at any hospital, as there are no certificate-of-need requirements or other measures in place to regulate where such operations are performed. Similar to other complex, high-risk operations in general surgery, most hepatic resections are performed on an elective basis, making it possible for such cases to be regionalized to high-volume centers of excellence. Furthermore, hepatectomy for HCC is an infrequently performed procedure for which the average surgeon or hospital is not likely to have substantial experience. Hepatocellular carcinoma was selected as a model in this study, because it is a diagnosis for which major hepatic resection would be considered and represents a disease entity associated with significantly higher rates of operative morbidity and mortality compared with hepatic resection for other indications.[12-14]

Our main finding was a highly significant relationship between hospital volume and operative outcome for patients undergoing hepatic resection for HCC in California during the 5-year study. The sample size was large, encompassing 507 patients treated at 138 hospitals. The effect of hospital volume on operative mortality was substantial, with a 4-fold difference in mortality between the lowest- and highest-volume groups. In addition to reduced operative mortality rates, high-volume centers were found to have shorter average lengths of hospital stay. These findings suggest that the highest-volume hospitals not only treat patients undergoing hepatic resection for HCC with substantially lower operative mortality, but also accomplish this by using fewer resources.

There are 3 possible explanations for these results. First, the data may have been flawed, and systematic reporting or coding errors may have favored the highest-volume providers. In previous studies of population database reliability, a 10% to 30% error rate in diagnosis and procedure coding has been reported.[15-17] In our study, concordance between diagnosis and procedure codes was required for each patient as part of the inclusion criteria, thereby reducing the number of erroneously coded patient discharge abstracts from further analysis. An error rate of only 1% has been identified in the reporting of the end point of patient mortality when the OSHPD database has been reconciled to primary data from individual patient medical records.[15] This error rate is not sufficiently large to explain the differences in operative mortality found between low- and high-volume hospitals in this study.

Second, differences in patient characteristics could account for the observed variations in patient outcome. We controlled for these differences in 2 ways. First, the data were pooled by hospital volume such that the number of patients in each volume group was sufficiently large to offset small differences in patient mix at any one hospital. Second, we used multivariate statistical techniques to adjust mortality rates and length of hospital stay for differences in patient characteristics. This risk adjustment did not alter the primary finding of a highly significant association between hospital volume and patient outcome. Additional risks may have been present but not identifiable in the OSHPD database, and the distribution of patients with these unknown risk factors may have been skewed toward hospitals with low volume, but this seems unlikely.

Finally, our findings probably represent true differences in outcome related to variations in patient care in hospitals of various volume groups. Supporting evidence suggests that this interpretation of the data is correct. First, the overall operative mortality rate of 14.8% and the rates for the lower-volume hospital groups in this study are comparable with previously reported operative mortality rates for this procedure in other large-population studies, including the nationwide Veterans Administration experience.[14] Second, the operative mortality rates of the highest-volume centers in our study mirror the recently published results of other high-volume centers around the world.[12,18-21] Therefore, the recently cited improvements in operative outcome in patients undergoing hepatectomy for HCC may apply only to high-volume centers and not more generally to the medical community. Finally, when the analysis in our study was extended to hepatic resection for all benign and malignant neoplasia, the volume-outcome relation persisted.

Only a limited insight into potential differences in patient care leading to lower operative mortality in the high-volume centers could be gleaned from the available data. High-volume centers were larger hospitals with higher overall surgical volume and university and residency program affiliation. They were more likely to perform other complex operations, such as cardiac surgery. The highest-volume providers performed a greater overall number of hepatic resections per year, and 3 of 4 had active liver transplantation programs, compared with none of the lowest-volume providers. Furthermore, a greater percentage of patients treated at low-volume providers had extended hospital stays, suggesting complicated postoperative courses. Patients treated at high-volume centers were less likely to have postoperative complications, or these centers have developed the means to better manage these complications should they arise. Thus, the improved in-hospital mortality rates and shorter lengths of hospital stay for patients with HCC at high-volume centers likely represent not only increased volume or experience, but an institutional interest and expertise in the treatment of patients undergoing liver surgery.

In today's health care environment, quality of care is measured not only in terms of patients' clinical outcome, but also cost-effectiveness. In California, most patients undergoing hepatic resection for HCC are treated at hospitals with limited experience. This study demonstrates a strong relationship between hospital volume and outcome in these patients. The standard of patient care for hepatic resection for HCC is not uniform across California. If the adjusted outcomes estimated for the highest-volume hospitals were applied statewide in 1990 through 1994, 44 additional patients would have survived their operation, with a savings of 1067 hospital days. Our results support the regionalization of high-risk general surgical procedures, such as hepatic resection for HCC, as a means of providing the most efficacious and cost-effective care.

Corresponding author: Sean J. Mulvihill, MD, Department of Surgery, Room U-122, University of California–San Francisco Medical Center, San Francisco, CA 94143-0788 (e-mail: sjm@itsa.ucsf.edu).

REFERENCES

1. Hannan EL, O'Donnell JF, Kilburn H Jr, Bernard HR, Yazici A. Investigation of the relationship between volume and mortality for surgical procedures performed in New York State hospitals. *JAMA.* 1989;262:503-510.
2. Rosenthal GE, Harper DL, Quinn LM, Cooper GS. Severity-adjusted mortality and length of stay in teaching and nonteaching hospitals. *JAMA.* 1997;278:485-490.
3. Luft HS, Bunker JP, Enthoven AC. Should operations be regionalized? *N Engl J Med.* 1979;301:1364-1369.
4. Showstack JA, Rosenfeld KE, Garnick DW, Luft HS, Schaffarzick RW, Fowles J. Association of volume with outcome of coronary artery bypass graft surgery: scheduled vs nonscheduled operations. *JAMA.* 1987;257:785-789.
5. Laffel G, Barnett A, Finkelstein S, Kaye M. The relation between experience and outcome in heart transplantation. *N Engl J Med.* 1992;327:1220-1225.
6. Hannan EL, Racz M, Ryan TJ, et al. Coronary angioplasty volume-outcome relationships for hospitals and cardiologists. *JAMA.* 1997;279:892-898.
7. Bunker JP, Luft HS, Enthoven A. Should surgery be regionalized? *Surg Clin North Am.* 1982;62:657-668.
8. Gordon T, Burleyson G, Tielsch J, Cameron J. The effects of regionalization on cost and outcome for one general high-risk surgical procedure. *Ann Surg.* 1995;221:43-49.
9. Jones M, Brouch K, Hall D, Aaron W. *St Anthony's Compact ICD-9-CM: Code Book for Physician Payment, 1995.* Reston, Va: St Anthony's Publishing Inc; 1994:1-2.
10. Office of Statewide Health Planning and Development. *Licensed Services and Utilization Profiles: Annual Report of Hospitals.* Sacramento, Calif: Office of Statewide Health Planning and Development; 1991.
11. Cohen J, Cohen P. *Applied Multiple Regression/Correlation Analysis for the Behavioral Sciences.* 2nd ed. Hillsdale, NJ: Lawrence Eribaum Associates Inc; 1983.
12. Tsao JI, Loftus JP, Nagorney DM, Adson MA, Ilstrup DM. Trends in morbidity and mortality of hepatic resection for malignancy. *Ann Surg.* 1994;220:199-205.
13. Doci R, Gennanri L, Bignami P, et al. Morbidity and mortality after hepatic resection of metastatic colorectal carcinoma. *Br J Surg.* 1995;82:377-381.
14. Nadig DE, Wade TP, Fairchild RB, Virgo KS, Johnson FE. Major hepatic resection: indications and results in a national hospital system from 1988 to 1992. *Arch Surg.* 1997;132:115-119.
15. Chen A, Meux E, Cox G. *Report of the Results From the OSHPD Reabstracting Project: An Evaluation of the Reliability of Selected Patient Discharge Data July Through December 1990.* Sacramento, Calif: Office of Statewide Health Planning and Development; 1993.
16. How good are the data? *Am J Kidney Dis.* 1992;46:675-683.
17. Lloyd SS, Rissing JP. Physician and coding errors in patient records. *JAMA.* 1985;254:1330-1336.
18. Segawa T, Tsuchiya R, Furui J, Isawa K, Tsunoda T, Kanematsu T. Operative results in 143 patients with hepatocellular carcinoma. *World J Surg.* 1993;17:663-668.
19. Vauthey J, Klimstra D, Franceschi D, et al. Factors affecting long-term outcome after hepatic resection for hepatocellular carcinoma. *Am J Surg.* 1995;169:28-35.
20. Bismuth H, Chiche L, Castaing D. Surgical treatment of hepatocellular carcinoma in noncirrhotic liver. *World J Surg.* 1995;19:35-41.
21. Lai EC, Fan S-T, Lo C-M, Chu K-M, Liu C-L, Wong J. Hepatic resection for hepatocellular carcinoma. *Ann Surg.* 1995;221:291-298.

Invited Critique

The article from Glasgow et al for the first time describes the relationship between high volume and outcome after liver resection for HCC. The authors clearly demonstrate lower postoperative mortality rates and a shorter hospital stay for high-volume centers. These results are not surprising, as Gordon et al[1] have already shown lower postoperative morbidity and mortality rates for other intricate oncological operations in visceral surgery: the early results after the Whipple operation were distinctly better in high-volume centers. Similar results have been published for orthopedic and traumatological operations, cardiac and vascular surgery, and gynecological operations. This proves that not only specific surgical technical skills but the combination of a well-equipped center with potent intensive care and experienced anesthesiologists as well as a general training for large operations are important for successful therapy. In conclusion, we merely learn a truism.

In oncological surgery, however, the late results after 5 or 10 years, depending on tumor stage, additional therapies, and the surgeon, are crucial. To our knowledge, only Anderson et al[2] in a prospective study and Hermanek et al[3] in a multicenter observation have proven that the surgeon actually can be a bigger risk factor for the prognosis of the patient than the tumor stage. Recently, similar results for breast cancer have been reported from a multicenter study in Denmark.

The study by Glasgow et al is a step in the right direction; however, further studies for longer observation periods focusing on surgeon and center should be encouraged, as only these can sufficiently prove the success or failure of different surgical oncological concepts. In his programmatic presentation of the future work of the American College of Surgeons, Wells[4] showed perspectives that we must follow. Similar concepts also exist in several centers in Europe; we hope that new focused knowledge will be generated here through the European unification process.

Christian Herfarth, MD
Peter Kienle, MD
Heidelberg, Germany

1. Gordon TA, Burleyson GP, Tielsch JM, Cameron JL. The effects of regionalization on cost and outcome for one general high-risk surgical procedure. *Ann Surg.* 1995;221:43-49.
2. Anderson JH, Hole D, McArdle CS. Elective versus emergency surgery for patients with colorectal cancer. *Br J Surg.* 1992;79:706-709.
3. Hermanek P Jr, Wiebelt H, Riedl S, Staimmer D, Hermanek P. Long-term results of surgical therapy of colon cancer: results of the Cancer Study Group. *Chirurg.* 1994;65:287-297.
4. Wells SA. The American College of Surgeons Oncology Group: its genesis and future directions. *Bull Am Coll Surg.* 1998;83:13-19.

ORIGINAL ARTICLE

Preoperative Serum Albumin Level as a Predictor of Operative Mortality and Morbidity

Results From the National VA Surgical Risk Study

James Gibbs, PhD; William Cull, PhD; William Henderson, PhD; Jennifer Daley, MD; Kwan Hur, MS; Shukri F. Khuri, MD

Objective: To improve the precision and reliability of estimates of the association between preoperative serum albumin concentration and surgical outcomes.

Design: Prospective observational study. Patients were followed up for 30 days postoperatively. Multiple logistic regression models were developed to evaluate serum albumin level as a predictor of operative mortality and morbidity in relation to 61 other preoperative patient risk variables.

Setting: Forty-four tertiary care Veterans Affairs (VA) medical centers.

Patients: A total of 54 215 major noncardiac surgery cases from the National VA Surgical Risk Study.

Main Outcome Measures: Thirty-day operative mortality and morbidity.

Results: A decrease in serum albumin from concentrations greater than 46 g/L to less than 21 g/L was associated with an exponential increase in mortality rates from less than 1% to 29% and in morbidity rates from 10% to 65%. In the regression models, albumin level was the strongest predictor of mortality and morbidity for surgery as a whole and within several subspecialties selected for further analysis. Albumin level was a better predictor of some types of morbidity, particularly sepsis and major infections, than other types.

Conclusions: Serum albumin concentration is a better predictor of surgical outcomes than many other preoperative patient characteristics. It is a relatively low-cost test that should be used more frequently as a prognostic tool to detect malnutrition and risk of adverse surgical outcomes, particularly in populations in whom comorbid conditions are relatively frequent.

Arch Surg. 1999;134:36-42

From the Cooperative Studies Program Coordinating Center, the Edward Hines, Jr, VA Hospital, Hines, Ill (Drs Gibbs, Cull, and Henderson and Mr Hur); Institute for Health Services Research and Policy Studies, Northwestern University, Evanston, Ill (Drs Gibbs, Cull, and Henderson); Brockton/West Roxbury VA Medical Center, West Roxbury, Mass (Drs Daley and Khuri); and Harvard Medical School (Drs Daley and Khuri), Division of General Medicine and Primary Care, Beth Israel Deaconess Medical Center (Dr Daley), and Brigham and Women's Hospital (Dr Khuri), Boston, Mass.

HYPOALBUMINEMIA has been shown to be associated with increased mortality and morbidity rates in both hospitalized patients[1-4] and samples of community-dwelling elderly persons.[5,6] In surgery, an association between hypoalbuminemia and adverse outcome has been recognized for many years. In an early series of 26 patients, most operated on for diseases of the digestive tract, Jones and Eaton[7] found that postoperative edema was associated with low concentrations of serum albumin and serum protein, which they attributed to preoperative and postoperative undernutrition. More recently, Rich et al[4] found that patients undergoing cardiac surgery who had lower serum albumin levels showed a trend toward having higher postoperative mortality rates and had significantly higher rates of several complications than did patients with higher serum albumin levels, while controlling for other risk factors. Albumin also has been found to predict postoperative mortality and morbidity for patients undergoing elective surgery[8] and postoperative morbidity for those undergoing gastrointestinal tract surgery.[9,10]

Although it is well established that hypoalbuminemia, as a marker of malnutrition and disease, is associated with greater risk of adverse surgical outcome, previous studies have been based on relatively small samples and selected types of operations and have failed to adequately separate the predictive ability of albumin level from other risk factors. We used a large database, the National VA Surgical Risk Study,[11-14] which included all major surgical procedures, to improve the precision and reliability of estimates of the association between albumin levels and mortality and morbidity. This database was sufficiently large and detailed to allow separate as well as summary analysis for

MATERIALS AND METHODS

OVERVIEW OF THE NATIONAL VA SURGICAL RISK STUDY

The National VA Surgical Risk Study was initiated in 44 academically affiliated Veterans Affairs (VA) medical centers with the aim of developing and validating risk-adjusted models for the prediction of surgical outcome (30-day mortality and morbidity).[11-14] Clinical nurse reviewers at each site prospectively collected 46 preoperative, 12 operative, and 24 postoperative variables for 87 078 major surgery cases between October 1, 1991, and December 31, 1993. Preoperative variables included health risk behaviors, comorbidities, and 14 laboratory test results. All surgical operations conducted under general, spinal, and epidural anesthesia were eligible for inclusion as the index operation except (1) operations on patients who had been enrolled in the study for an index operation within the previous 30 days, (2) operations with very low mortality rates (eg, ophthalmologic procedures), and (3) organ transplantation, because this is performed at a limited number of VA medical centers. The study protocol is described in detail elsewhere.[11]

ALBUMIN STUDY DATABASE

The analyses presented here were based on 54 215 (62%) of the 87 078 cases from the National VA Surgical Risk Study database for which preoperative serum albumin values were reported. The omitted cases, those not tested for albumin level (38%), were similar in age to those included in the analysis but were somewhat less likely to have comorbid conditions or severe disease. For example, 33% of the omitted cases vs 38% of the included cases had hypertension requiring medication, 12% vs 15% had diabetes mellitus requiring an oral agent or insulin, and 51% vs 64% were assigned an American Society of Anesthesiology (ASA) class of 3 or higher. (An ASA class of 1 indicates a healthy patient; 2, mild systemic disease but no functional limitations; 3, severe systemic disease with definite functional limitations; 4, severe systemic disease that is a constant threat to life; and 5, moribund patient unlikely to survive 24 hours with or without operation.) An analysis using all cases, in which missing albumin values were imputed from scores on the other preoperative variables, yielded very similar results to those reported here for cases tested for albumin level.

INDEPENDENT VARIABLES

Preoperative serum albumin values closest to the day of surgery were used in the analysis. Only those measurements that occurred within 30 days prior to surgery were considered valid. The number of days intervening between the last albumin measurement and surgery (mean=5.03 days, SD=6.15 days) was not found to affect the association between albumin level and mortality as indicated by a lack of statistical interaction between time of measurement and albumin level (χ^2=1.47, *P*=.23). The predictive ability of serum albumin levels was evaluated against 61 other preoperative patient characteristics. These variables are listed in a previous publication.[11] They include age, sex, tobacco use, alcohol use, substance abuse, functional status, weight loss, emergency operation, presence or absence of comorbidities covering all major organ systems, and 14 preoperative laboratory values.

DEPENDENT VARIABLES

Operative mortality was defined as death due to any cause occurring within 30 days of the operation. Operative morbidity

Continued on next page

21 postoperative complications. The availability of comprehensive preoperative risk data permitted comparison of the predictive ability of serum albumin level with many other variables and measurement of the contribution of albumin level to prediction independent of the effects of other risk factors. Our results should better define the usefulness of preoperative albumin levels as a prognostic indicator.

RESULTS

SAMPLE CHARACTERISTICS

Reflecting the composition of all VA hospital patients, 97.1% of the albumin study cases were male, and the mean age was 61.0 years (SD=13.0 years). Seventy-six percent were white, 18% were black, and 6% were of other racial backgrounds (eg, Hispanic, Asian American). The most frequent subspecialty was general surgery (28.3%), followed by orthopedics (18.0%), urology (14.8%), vascular surgery (11.7%), neurosurgery (8.4), thoracic surgery (7.3%), otolaryngology (5.9%), plastic surgery (3.7%), and other (2.0%). The 30-day mortality rate was 3.9%, and the 30-day morbidity rate (1 or more of the 21 complications) was 19.6%. The mean preoperative serum albumin level was 38 g/L (SD=6.5 g/L). Twenty-three percent of the cases had albumin values less than 35 g/L, which is generally considered the lower boundary of the normal range.

UNIVARIATE ANALYSES

Table 1 shows the 10 strongest predictors of 30-day mortality and morbidity, ranked by the *c* index, from the set of 62 preoperative variables. For both outcomes, albumin level was the best predictor, with ASA class and hematocrit ranking second and third, respectively. Albumin level alone correctly discriminated between survivors and nonsurvivors 78% of the time. In general, the *c* values are higher for mortality than morbidity, indicating that the variables predict mortality better than the occurrence of 1 or more complications.

Figure 1 and **Figure 2** display the relationship between serum albumin and mortality and morbidity for all operations and for the 3 selected subspecialties. For all operations, the mortality rate increases from less than included 21 predefined complications recorded in the 30 days after the operation. The summary measure used in this analysis was the presence or absence of 1 or more of the 21 complications. In other analysis of the National VA Surgical Risk Study database, this score was found to be strongly correlated with summary scores based on several weighting schemes, including the total number of morbidities reported (r=0.74), weights based on the regression relationship between postoperative length of stay and the 21 morbidities (r=0.75), weights based on the relative proportion of a morbidity occurring with other morbidities (r=0.96), and the mean ratings by the chiefs of surgery at the 44 participating VA medical centers on a scale of 1 to 5 as to the likelihood that the morbidity could result in death, permanent sequelae, prolonged length of stay, or patient dissatisfaction (r=0.97).

STATISTICAL ANALYSIS

First, the association between preoperative serum albumin levels and mortality and morbidity was assessed univariately. We compared the predictive ability of albumin level with that of each of the 61 other preoperative variables. The predictive ability of each variable was determined by the c index[15] from logistic regressions with 1 independent variable. A c index of 0.5 or less indicates prediction no better than chance, and values from 0.5 to 1.0 (perfect prediction) indicate improvement over chance.

Second, multivariate logistic regression models were developed to assess the predictive ability of albumin level independent of the effects of other variables. The large number of candidate predictor variables was reduced in several steps. First, the variables were screened for significant univariate association (P<.001) with the dependent variables, which eliminated only 10 of the 62 candidate variables for mortality modeling and only 4 for morbidity modeling. Next, we eliminated variables that predicted the dependent variables with a c index less than 0.57, a cutoff level that substantially reduced the number of variables but retained a diverse set of variables. We further reduced the number of remaining variables by developing separate stepwise regression models for the remaining comorbidity and laboratory variables, requiring $P \leq .0001$ (Wald χ^2) to enter the models and $P \leq .0005$ (Wald χ^2) to stay, and then eliminating variables that did not increase the c index for the model by at least 0.01. These steps identified a diverse set of 7 strong predictors of mortality, including serum albumin level, that were forced in a final model to assess their relative predictive ability. Likewise, 6 variables were selected for a final morbidity model. These variables were tested for intercorrelation, and none of the correlations between pairs of predictor variables exceeded r=0.37.

In addition to analysis of all operations in the database, we assessed the predictive ability of albumin levels within 3 subspecialties chosen to represent variation in mortality and morbidity rates as well as different types of surgery—general surgery and noncardiac thoracic surgery, which had the highest subspecialty 30-day mortality rates (6.4% and 6.0%, respectively) and higher than average morbidity rates (26.3% and 23.6%, respectively), and orthopedics, with a mortality rate of 2.5% and a morbidity rate of 13.7%. The model development process described for all operations was also used for the subspecialty analyses except that less stringent screening and model entry criteria were used owing to smaller sample sizes. Split-sample cross-validation of the all operations and subspecialty models showed little degradation of the c values, ranging from no decrease from learning to test samples in 3 of the models to a decrease of 0.03 in the c value for the orthopedic mortality model.

1% for albumin levels of 46 g/L or higher to 28% for albumin levels below 21 g/L. The increase in mortality seems to be exponential as albumin level decreases from a level of approximately 40 g/L. Figure 2 shows that morbidity increases from approximately 10% to 65% as albumin values decline from 46 g/L to less than 21 g/L. The subspecialties show similar trends except that the mortality and morbidity rates are lower for orthopedics than the other subspecialties.

MULTIVARIATE ANALYSES

Table 2 presents the final models developed from the 62 preoperative variables for all operations and for 3 selected subspecialties. The models predict mortality very well for all operations, general surgery, and orthopedics, with c values ranging from 0.86 to 0.91. The c values for the morbidity models are not as high, ranging from 0.67 to 0.76. The predictive variables are listed in Table 2 in order of the magnitude of their Wald χ^2 values, which indicates their relative importance in the models. Albumin level appears in all of the models and is the strongest predictor in both the mortality and morbidity models for all operations and in several of the subspecialty models. The odds ratios for albumin level in the all operations models indicate that a decrease of 10 g/L in albumin value was associated with more than a 2-fold increase in the odds of dying and almost a 2-fold increase in the odds of a complication. The ASA class was also a strong predictor, particularly in the mortality models. Both serum albumin levels and weight loss appear in the mortality model for thoracic surgery, indicating that albumin level detects risk not associated with weight loss of greater than 10% of body weight in the 6 months prior to surgery.

COMPLICATION-SPECIFIC ANALYSIS

In addition to analysis of morbidity using the summary measure of complications, we analyzed the association between preoperative serum albumin and each of the 21 predefined complications. **Table 3** gives the mortality rate, incidence, and regression results for each of the complications, listed in order of the magnitude of the c index for the regression of the complication on serum albumin level. The complications with the higher c values

Table 1. Preoperative Predictors of 30-Day Mortality and Morbidity After Major Surgery, Ranked by *c* Index Magnitude (Albumin Study Database)*

Mortality		Morbidity	
Variable†	*c* Index	Variable	*c* Index
Albumin, g/L	0.78	Albumin, g/L	0.68
ASA class	0.77	ASA class	0.67
Hematocrit, %	0.72	Hematocrit, %	0.66
Serum urea nitrogen, mmol/L	0.69	Functional status	0.60
Functional status	0.67	Age, y	0.60
Prothrombin time, s	0.67	Prothrombin time, s	0.59
Age, y	0.64	Serum urea nitrogen, mmol/L	0.58
Emergency operation	0.64	Alkaline phosphatase, U/L	0.58
WBC, >11 000/μL	0.63	Emergency operation	0.57
Alkaline phosphatase, U/L	0.62	WBC, >11 000/μL	0.57

**ASA indicates American Society of Anesthesiology; WBC, white blood cell count.*

†All variables were examined using single-variable logistic regression models, and all variables were significant at P<.001.

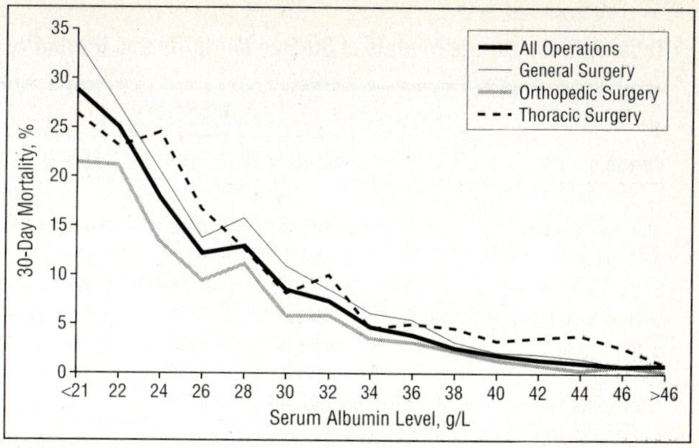

Figure 1. *Thirty-day mortality rate by preoperative serum albumin level for all operations and 3 subspecialties.*

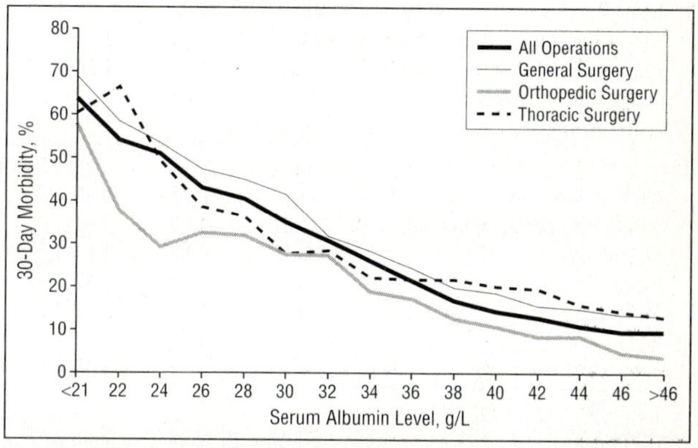

Figure 2. *Thirty-day morbidity rate by preoperative serum albumin level for all operations and 3 subspecialties.*

tend to have higher mortality rates. They also are characterized by incidence rates that are markedly higher for cases with albumin levels below normal (<35 g/L) than for cases in the normal range (≥35 g/L).

The last column of Table 3 shows the entry step of albumin level in stepwise logistic regression using all 62 preoperative variables and an entry criterion of $P<.05$. In these multivariate analyses, albumin level was a relatively strong predictor of most of the complications, entering the models at the first, second, or third step. Albumin level was the first variable to enter for the major infection complications (systemic sepsis, pneumonia, deep wound infection). For several complications, albumin level was not a significant predictor in the regression analyses.

The variation in the predictive ability of albumin level for different complications partially explains why albumin level was not as strong a predictor of operative morbidity for some types of surgery as it was for others in our analysis using a summary measure of morbidity (Table 2). For example, albumin level did not predict morbidity as well in orthopedic surgery as it did for all operations, and we found that most of the complications that were predicted best by albumin level for all operations in Table 3, such as systemic sepsis and failure to wean from ventilation, were proportionately underrepresented in orthopedic surgery, whereas several that were predicted less well by albumin level for all operations, such as pulmonary embolism and deep vein thrombosis/thrombophlebitis, were overrepresented in orthopedic surgery.

Veterans who receive surgical care at VA hospitals are predominantly male and older, with higher rates of comorbid conditions than those undergoing surgery elsewhere. To demonstrate the applicability of the findings beyond VA patients, we performed separate analyses for a lower-risk segment of the sample and for women. All cases were identified in which the patient was younger than 70 years, had an ASA classification of 1 or 2 (healthy patient or mild disease), was independent in functional status, and did not report a weight loss of more than 10% within the last 6 months prior to surgery. There were 15 555 patients in our sample who met these criteria. The 30-day death rate for these low-risk patients was 0.32%. As shown in **Figure 3**, there was a negative association (c=0.72, $P<.001$) between serum albumin level and mortality even within this lower-risk subgroup. Likewise, for the women in the sample (n=1575), there was a strong association between serum albumin level and mortality (c index=0.86, $P<.001$), with a graded increase in mortality rates as albumin values declined, similar to the finding for the total sample.

COMMENT

We used a large national sample of VA patients to determine the association between preoperative serum albumin level and 30-day postoperative mortality and morbidity. We found large, graded increases in mortality and morbidity as albumin level declined from high to low levels. We found that for all major operations combined and for selected surgical subspecialties, serum albumin level was a strong predictor of mortality and morbidity independent of the effects of a large, diverse set of prospectively determined patient risk variables. The association between albumin concentration and operative mortality persisted in a subsample of patients who were classified as low risk on

Table 2. Multivariate Models of 30-Day Mortality and Morbidity After Major Surgery (Albumin Study Database)*

	Mortality				Morbidity		
Variable	Wald χ^2†	OR	95% CI	Variable	Wald χ^2†	OR	95% CI
All Operations‡							
Albumin level, g/L	541.0	0.44	0.41-0.48	Albumin level, g/L	813.9	0.58	0.56-0.60
ASA class	416.1	2.33	2.15-2.53	ASA class	745.8	1.71	1.65-1.78
Emergency operation	212.0	2.26	2.02-2.53	Emergency operation	422.1	2.00	1.87-2.14
Serum urea nitrogen, mmol/L	109.2	1.01	1.01-1.02	Functional status	351.2	1.48	1.42-1.55
Age, y	108.9	1.03	1.02-1.03	Age, y	115.1	1.01	1.01-1.01
Dyspnea	63.8	1.38	1.27-1.49	Serum urea nitrogen, mmol/L	82.2	1.01	1.01-1.01
Functional status	47.4	1.28	1.19-1.37				
General Surgery§							
Albumin level, g/L	162.9	0.49	0.44-0.55	Albumin level, g/L	245.2	0.61	0.57-0.65
ASA class	140.1	2.18	1.91-2.49	ASA class	199.6	1.60	1.50-1.71
Ascites	86.1	4.47	3.23-6.17	Emergency operation	181.8	1.96	1.77-2.16
Age, y	45.7	1.03	1.02-1.03	Functional status	84.7	1.46	1.34-1.58
Serum urea nitrogen, mmol/L	44.1	1.01	1.01-1.02	Age, y	55.2	1.01	1.01-1.02
Functional status	36.6	1.41	1.26-1.57	Transfusions (>4 U preoperatively)	34.4	1.75	1.44-2.11
Emergency operation	34.4	1.68	1.41-2.01	Serum urea nitrogen, mmol/L	25.8	1.01	1.01-1.01
Prothrombin time, s	28.5	1.11	1.07-1.15				
Thoracic Surgery‖							
Albumin level, g/L	40.5	0.51	0.41-0.63	Age, y	29.7	1.02	1.02-1.03
Serum urea nitrogen, mmol/L	13.9	1.02	1.01-1.03	Ventilator use (preoperative)	29.6	4.66	2.64-8.19
Weight loss	12.5	1.86	1.31-2.65	Albumin level, g/L	25.7	0.70	0.61-0.81
Dyspnea	12.0	1.45	1.17-1.79	ASA class	15.6	1.35	1.16-1.58
ASA class	8.5	1.47	1.12-1.92	Functional status	12.0	1.39	1.15-1.69
Age, y	7.7	1.02	1.01-1.04	Prothrombin time, s	6.6	1.08	1.02-1.15
Emergency operation	6.9	1.82	1.15-2.86	Dyspnea	5.4	1.18	1.02-1.36
Orthopedic Surgery¶							
ASA class	70.4	2.95	2.28-3.18	Age, y	36.1	1.02	1.01-1.02
Albumin level, g/L	40.3	0.49	0.39-0.61	Wound infection (preoperative)	28.6	1.71	1.40-2.09
Age, y	27.7	1.04	1.02-1.05	Functional status	27.7	1.38	1.22-1.56
Emergency operation	26.1	2.38	1.70-3.34	ASA class	19.3	1.31	1.16-1.47
Weight loss	24.2	3.14	1.97-5.00	Hematocrit, %	17.0	0.97	0.96-0.99
DNR orders	17.1	2.47	1.60-3.83	COPD	16.0	1.43	1.19-1.70
Functional status	16.2	1.54	1.24-1.90	Alkaline phosphatase, U/L	15.7	1.00	1.00-1.00
Serum urea nitrogen, mmol/L	10.0	1.01	1.01-1.02	Albumin level, g/L	12.5	0.78	0.68-0.90
				Emergency operation	11.8	1.42	1.16-1.74
				WBC, >11 000/μL	11.1	1.32	1.12-1.56
				Impaired senses	9.1	1.38	1.12-1.72
				Serum urea nitrogen, mmol/L	5.9	1.01	1.00-1.01

**OR indicates odds ratio; CI, confidence interval; ASA, American Society of Anesthesiology; DNR, do not resuscitate; COPD, chronic obstructive pulmonary disease; and WBC, white blood cell count. Total sample size is reduced slightly from 54 215, and sample sizes differ between the mortality and morbidity models because of varying numbers of missing values associated with each set of predictor variables. The number of cases for the subspecialty models do not add to the totals for the all operations models because the all operations models also include cases from all other subspecialties in the database.*

†$P \leq .001$ for all variables in the all operations models. $P \leq .05$ for all variables in the subspecialty models.

‡For all operations, mortality data, N = 53 055, with 2076 deaths and a c index of 0.86. For morbidity data, N = 53 136, with 10 358 cases of complications and a c index of 0.73.

§For general surgery, mortality data, N = 13 566, with 864 deaths and a c index of 0.87. For morbidity data, N = 14 782, with 3888 cases of complications and a c index of 0.74.

‖For thoracic surgery, mortality data, N = 3740, with 228 deaths and a c index of 0.74. For morbidity data, N = 3685, with 877 cases of complications and a c index of 0.67.

¶For orthopedic surgery, mortality data, N = 9467, with 235 deaths and a c index of 0.91. For morbidity data, N = 8673, with 1141 cases of complications and a c index of 0.76.

the basis of clinically recognizable risk factors. With regard to operative morbidity, we showed that albumin level was a better predictor of some types of complications than others.

Although serum albumin level may also be affected by acute factors such as trauma and surgical stress, it is predictive of operative outcome because it is a marker of disease and malnutrition as well as possibly conferring a direct protective effect through several biological mechanisms.[16] It is a better prognostic indicator than anthropomorphic markers of nutritional status[8-10,17-19] because of its ability to detect protein-energy malnutrition, which is not necessarily accompanied by lower body weight and may not be clinically recognizable, but is associated with significantly increased risk of morbidity and mortality.[20-22] Protein-energy malnutrition results from increased protein and energy requirements associated with the stress of illness, injury, or infection.[23,24] If the increased needs are not met from dietary or therapeutic sources, visceral protein stores are depleted, leading to

Table 3. Association Between Preoperative Serum Albumin Level and Selected Complications After Major Surgery (Albumin Study Database)*

Complication (Mortality Rate, %†)	Incidence When Albumin Level <35 g/L, %	Incidence When Albumin Level ≥35 g/L, %	*c* Index for Univariate Prediction‡	Entry Step of Albumin Level in Stepwise Logistic Regression
Systemic sepsis (40.0)	8.0	1.3	0.78	1
Acute renal failure (47.8)	2.1	0.4	0.76	2
Coma (64.1)	2.3	0.4	0.76	2
Renal insufficiency (41.3)	3.0	0.6	0.75	3
Failure to wean from ventilation (30.9)	11.2	2.3	0.75	3
Bleeding/transfusions (27.3)	7.1	1.6	0.72	2
Cardiac arrest (77.8)	4.4	1.1	0.72	2
Pneumonia (22.1)	10.6	2.9	0.71	1
Urinary infection (8.1)	8.9	2.6	0.69	2
Pulmonary edema (27.1)	5.9	1.9	0.69	3
Reintubation (35.6)	6.2	2.0	0.68	2
Deep wound infection (10.2)	5.9	2.0	0.66	1
Wound dehiscence (11.3)	2.0	0.8	0.64	3
Prolonged ileus (14.3)	3.9	1.9	0.61	...
Pulmonary embolism (44.0)	0.6	0.3	0.60	1
Myocardial infarction (42.2)	1.1	0.6	0.59	...
Neurological deficits (29.9)	1.7	0.8	0.59	...
Superficial wound infection (3.6)	4.4	2.4	0.59	...
DVT/thrombophlebitis (12.0)	0.9	0.5	0.58	...
CVA (27.6)	0.9	0.5	0.58	...
Graft failure (9.2)	1.0	0.7	0.53	10

**DVT indicates deep vein thrombosis; CVA, cerebrovascular accident; and ellipses, not applicable.*
†Thirty-day mortality associated with occurrence of the complication, occurring by itself or in combination with other complications.
‡All relationships were significant at $P<.001$.

abnormal function in organ systems, including gastrointestinal malabsorption, impaired immunologic response, and impaired production of albumin and other plasma proteins in the liver.[24,25] However, albumin infusion usually is not an effective therapy because the albumin will degrade quickly and infusion does not address the underlying causes of adverse operative outcome.[26]

There was wide variation in the rate of preoperative serum albumin testing among the 44 participating hospitals, ranging from 20% to 98% of cases, with a median testing rate of 60%. Even if the analysis is restricted to cases with an ASA score of 3 or higher (severe systemic disease with functional limitation; 59% of all cases), the variation by hospital in the proportion tested remains large (from 27% to 97% of cases, with a median of 72%). In contrast, the ordering of blood counts and portions of the SMA-7 (eg, serum sodium and potassium) was consistently high (>90%) across hospitals.

These findings suggest that preoperative serum albumin testing is underutilized by some surgeons. The cost of the test ($2-$4, based on cost data from 2 VA hospitals and 1 large community hospital) is low in relation to its prognostic value. In addition to its value as a prognostic tool, serum albumin level is a key element in accurate nutritional assessment,[9,10,17,27] and it has been shown that nutritional therapy is more effective in reducing operative mortality and morbidity when the diagnosis of malnutrition is based on objective nutritional indices that include serum albumin rather than on subjective assessment.[28,29] Particularly in patient populations with high rates of comorbidities, such as VA patients, it would seem that the test should be used more frequently as a prognostic tool and for detecting malnutrition.

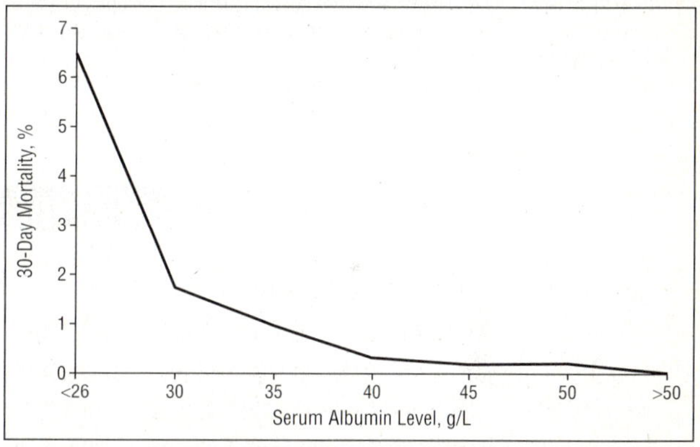

Figure 3. *Thirty-day mortality by preoperative serum albumin for low-risk cases (American Society of Anesthesiology class of 2 or lower, independent functional status, no weight loss of >10% in 6 months prior to surgery, and age younger than 70 years).*

This research was supported by a grant from the American Association for Clinical Chemistry Inc, Washington, DC, to the Institute for Health Services Research and Policy Studies at Northwestern University, Evanston, Ill; and by the Office of Patient Care Services and Cooperative Studies Program, US Department of Veterans Affairs Headquarters, Washington. Dr Daley is a Senior Research Associate in the Health Services Research and Development Program in the Department of Veterans Affairs.

Reprints: James Gibbs, PhD, CSPCC (151K), Edward Hines, Jr, VA Hospital, PO Box 5000, Hines, IL 60141-5151 (e-mail: jgibbs@nwu.edu).

REFERENCES

1. Ferguson RP, O'Connor P, Crabtree B, Batchelor A, Mitchell J, Coppola D. Serum albumin and prealbumin as predictors of clinical outcomes of hospitalized elderly nursing home residents. *J Am Geriatr Soc.* 1993;41:545-549.
2. Herrmann FR, Safran C, Levkoff SE, Minaker KL. Serum albumin level on admission as a predictor of death, length of stay, and readmission. *Arch Intern Med.* 1992;152:125-130.
3. Reinhardt GF, Myscofski JW, Wilkens DB, Dobrin PB, Mangan JE, Stannard RT. Incidence and mortality of hypoalbuminemic patients in hospitalized veterans. *JPEN J Parenter Enter Nutr.* 1980;11:140-143.
4. Rich MW, Keller AJ, Schechtman KB, Marshall WG, Jr, Kouchoukos NT. Increased complications and prolonged hospital stay in elderly cardiac surgical patients with low serum albumin. *Am J Cardiol.* 1989;63:714-718.
5. Corti MC, Guralnik JM, Salive ME, Sorkin JD. Serum albumin level and physical disability as predictors of mortality in older persons. *JAMA.* 1994;272:1036-1042.
6. Klonoff-Cohen H, Barrett-Connor EL, Edelstein SL. Albumin levels as a predictor of mortality in the healthy elderly. *J Clin Epidemiol.* 1992;45:207-212.
7. Jones CM, Eaton FB. Postoperative nutritional edema. *Arch Surg.* 1933;27:159-177.
8. Mullen JL, Gertner MH, Buzby GP, Goodhart GL, Rosato EF. Implications of malnutrition in the surgical patient. *Arch Surg.* 1979;114:121-125.
9. Buzby GP, Mullen JL, Matthews DC, Hobbs CL, Rosato EF. Prognostic nutritional index in gastrointestinal surgery. *Am J Surg.* 1980;139:160-167.
10. Detsky AS, Baker JP, O'Rourke K. Predicting nutrition-associated complications for patients undergoing gastrointestinal surgery. *JPEN J Parenter Enter Nutr.* 1987;11:440-446.
11. Khuri SF, Daley J, Henderson W, et al. The National VA Surgical Risk Study: risk adjustment for the comparative assessment of the quality of surgical care. *J Am Coll Surg.* 1995;180:519-531.
12. Khuri SF, Daley J, Henderson W, et al. Risk adjustment of the postoperative mortality rate for the comparative assessment of the quality of surgical care. *J Am Coll Surg.* 1997;185:315-327.
13. Daley J, Khuri SF, Henderson W, et al. Risk adjustment of the postoperative morbidity rate for the comparative assessment of the quality of surgical care. *J Am Coll Surg.* 1997;185:328-340.
14. Daley J, Forbes MG, Young GJ, et al. Validating risk-adjusted surgical outcomes: site visit assessment of process and structure. *J Am Coll Surg.* 1997;185:341-351.
15. Hanley JA, McNeil BJ. The meaning and use of the area under a receiver operating characteristic (ROC) curve. *Radiology.* 1982;143:29-36.
16. Goldwasser P, Feldman J. Association of serum albumin and mortality risk. *J Clin Epidemiol.* 1997;50:693-703.
17. Mullen JL, Buzby GP, Waldman MT, Gertner MH, Hobbs CL, Rosato EF. Prediction of operative morbidity and mortality by preoperative nutritional assessment. *Surg Forum.* 1979;30:80-82.
18. Agarwal N, Acevedo F, Leighton LS. Predictive ability of various nutritional variables for mortality in elderly people. *Am J Clin Nutr.* 1988;48:1173-1178.
19. Apelgren KN, Rombeau JL, Twomey PL, Miller RA. Comparison of nutritional indices and outcome in critically ill patients. *Crit Care Med.* 1982;10:305-307.
20. Blackburn GL, Harvey KB. Nutritional assessment as a routine in clinical medicine. *Postgrad Med.* 1982;71:46-63.
21. Blackburn GL, Harvey KB. Prognostic strength of nutritional assessment. *Progr Clin Biol Res.* 1981;77:689-697.
22. Lipschitz DA. Protein calorie malnutrition in the hospitalized elderly. *Primary Care.* 1982;9:531-543.
23. Homsy FN, Blackburn GL. Modern parenteral and enteral nutrition in critical care. *J Am Coll Nutr.* 1983;2:75-95.
24. Lipschitz DA. Protein-energy malnutrition. *Hosp Pract.* 1988:87-99.
25. McClave SA, Mitoraj TE, Thielmeier KA, Greenburg RA. Differentiating subtypes (hypoalbuminemic vs marasmic) of protein-calorie malnutrition: incidence and clinical significance in a university hospital setting. *JPEN J Parenter Enter Nutr.* 1992;16:337-342.
26. Rothschild MA, Oratz M, Schreiber SS. Serum albumin. *Hepatology.* 1988;8:385-401.
27. Buzby GP, Williford WO, Peterson OL, et al. A randomized clinical trial of total parenteral nutrition in malnourished surgical patients: the rationale and impact of previous clinical trials and pilot study on protocol design. *Am J Clin Nutr.* 1988;47:357-365.
28. Mullen JL, Buzby GP, Matthews DC, Smale BF, Rosato EF. Reduction of operative morbidity and mortality by combined preoperative and postoperative nutritional support. *Ann Surg.* 1980;192:604-613.
29. Buzby GP, Blouin G, Colling CL, et al. Perioperative total parenteral nutrition in surgical patients. *N Engl J Med.* 1991;325:525-532.

IN OTHER AMA JOURNALS

ARCHIVES OF INTERNAL MEDICINE

Dyspepsia in the Community Is Linked to Smoking and Aspirin Use but Not to *Helicobacter pylori* Infection

Sanjay Nandurkar, FRACP; Nicholas J. Talley, MD, PhD, FRACP; Harry Xia, PhD; Hazel Mitchell, PhD; Stuart Hazel, PhD; Michael Jones, PhD

Background: The relationship between *Helicobacter pylori* infection and symptoms remains controversial. We aimed to determine if an association exists between unexplained dyspepsia (pain or discomfort centered in the upper part of the abdomen) and *H pylori*.

Methods:A validated questionnaire was completed by 592 healthy blood donors. *Helicobacter pylori* serologic values (via enzyme-linked immunosorbent assay), blood group status, and Rh status were measured; 4.9% of subjects who had a history of peptic ulcer disease were excluded from the analyses.

Results: The prevalence of dyspepsia and no ulcer history was 11% (95% confidence interval [CI], 8.6%-13.8%); 15.4% of subjects with dyspepsia had *H pylori* while 14.6% of subjects without dyspepsia were infected ($P = .90$). The mean dyspepsia impact scores (combining frequency and severity) in those with and without *H pylori* were 4.7 and 5.4, respectively ($P = .20$). The median *H pylori* optical density values in dyspepsia vs no dyspepsia were not significantly different ($P = .30$). Independent risk factors for dyspepsia were the use of aspirin (odds ratio [OR], 2.2; 95% CI, 1.3-3.7) and smoking (OR, 2.1; 95% CI, 1.3-3.6) but not age, sex, marital status, educational level, income, or the use of alcohol, coffee, or nonsteroidal anti-inflammatory drugs. Independent risk factors for *H pylori* were increasing age (OR, 1.8 per decade; 95% CI, 1.5-2.3), male sex (OR, 2.1; 95% CI, 1.3-3.4), and net family income (OR, 1.8; 95% CI, 1.2-3.3).

Conclusion: Dyspepsia in the community is linked to smoking and aspirin use, but not to *H pylori* infection. *(1998;158:1427-1433)*

Reprints: Nicholas J. Talley, MD, PhD, Department of Medicine, University of Sydney, Nepean Hospital, Penrith, New South Wales 2751, Australia.

Comparison of Blue Dye and Probe-Assisted Intraoperative Lymphatic Mapping in Melanoma to Identify Sentinel Nodes in 100 Lymphatic Basins

Peter Bostick, MD; Richard Essner, MD; Edwin Glass, MD; Mark Kelley, MD; Terry Sarantou, MD; Leland J. Foshag, MD; Karen Qi, MS; Donald Morton, MD

Objective: To determine whether combining isosulfan blue dye with a radiopharmaceutical agent will increase intraoperative detection of sentinel nodes (SNs) in patients with early-stage melanoma.

Patients and Design: Clinical trial with a consecutive sample. Eighty-seven patients with clinical stage I melanoma underwent preoperative lymphoscintigraphy with 1 of 3 radiopharmaceutical agents to identify the lymphatic basin and the site of the SN. All patients subsequently underwent intraoperative lymphatic mapping and selective lymph node dissection (SLND) with isosulfan blue dye and a radiopharmaceutical agent. A handheld gamma probe determined the radioactive counts over the draining lymph node basins and individual blue-stained lymph nodes before (in vivo) and after (ex vivo) their removal. An irrelevant body site was used as the denominator of a count ratio by which absolute counts were standardized for comparison. Completion lymphadenectomy was undertaken in patients whose SLND specimen had histopathologic evidence of tumor cells.

Setting: Tertiary care cancer center.

Intervention: Lymph node sampling.

Main Outcome Measure: Accuracy of SN detection by blue dye and radiopharmaceutical techniques.

Results: Preoperative lymphoscintigraphic images identified 100 lymph node basins and 135 lymph nodes in 87 patients. All 3 radiopharmaceutical agents were equally effective in imaging the SN before surgery. During SLND, we identified and removed 136 blue-stained and radioactive (hot) SNs and 8 additional non–blue-stained hot nodes from 98 basins (98.0%). Of the 144 excised lymph nodes, 132 nodes (91.7%) from 83 basins had either an in vivo– or an ex vivo–background count ratio of 2:1 or more and 125 nodes (86.8%) from 77 basins had a count ratio of 3:1 or more. Twelve blue-stained SNs had count ratios of less than 2:1. Seventeen SNs (11.8%) from 15 basins contained metastases: 16 were identified with blue dye and probe and 1 was identified with blue dye alone. Four (1.1%) of 377 non-SNs excised during completion lymphadenectomy contained metastases. There have been no lymph node recurrences during mean follow-up of 16.3 months (range, 7-42 months).

Conclusions: The blue dye technique remains the criterion standard for SLND in melanoma. The addition of a radiopharmaceutical tracer serves as a useful adjunct to the visualization of blue-stained SNs.

Arch Surg. 1999;134:43-49

Surgical management of the regional lymph nodes in patients with clinical stage I melanoma remains controversial. More than 100 years ago, elective lymph node dissection (ELND) was proposed as a method to control the permeation of melanoma from the primary site to the regional lymph nodes.[1] Results of multiple retrospective studies[2-5] support this approach by demonstrating a survival advantage for patients who undergo ELND compared with those being treated by delayed (therapeutic) lymph node dissection. Results of 3 prospective randomized trials[6-8] fail to confirm a survival benefit for patients who undergo ELND and raise the question as to the efficacy of this treatment. We suspect that any overall survival advantage for early removal of the tumor-positive regional lymph nodes in these randomized trials was likely obscured because only a few patients were likely to have occult lymph node metastases.

Factors such as the primary melanoma's thickness, Clark level of invasion, ulceration, and anatomic location have clear prognostic significance in clinical stage I melanoma, but they are not adequate criteria on which to base the decision for ELND.[9,10] Even if ELND is reserved for patients in clinical stage I whose primary melanomas meet the criteria for high risk,

From the Roy E. Coats Research Laboratories of the John Wayne Cancer Institute (Drs Bostick, Essner, Kelley, Sarantou, Foshag, and Morton and Ms Qi) and the Department of Nuclear Medicine, Saint John's Health Center (Dr Glass), Santa Monica, Calif.

PATIENTS AND METHODS

Eighty-seven consecutive patients (56 men and 31 women) with American Joint Committee on Cancer stage I and II melanoma underwent preoperative LS followed either immediately or at least 24 hours later by SLND. All primary melanomas were diagnosed by either incisional or excisional biopsy examination, and all were Breslow thickness 0.65 mm or greater and Clark level II or greater or had ominous histological features such as regression or ulceration.[22,23] None of the patients underwent excision of the primary site with margins of 1.5 cm or greater or a previous operative procedure that disrupted lymphatic drainage to the regional nodal basin.

PREOPERATIVE LS

Preoperative dynamic LS was performed with 1 of 3 technetium Tc 99m–labeled radiopharmaceutical agents: Tc 99m HSA (Amersham-Medi-Physics, Arlington Heights, Ill), technetium Tc 99m albumin colloid (Tc 99m AC, CIS-US Inc, Bedford, Mass), or technetium Tc 99m sulfur colloid (Tc 99m SC, Amersham-Medi-Physics). Of 87 patients, 71 underwent LS at least 24 hours before surgery with either Tc 99m HSA ($n = 57$) or Tc 99m AC ($n = 14$) and had SLND performed with concurrent intraoperative injection of isosulfan blue dye and Tc 99m HSA. The remaining 16 patients underwent LS with Tc 99m SC performed no more than 4 hours before surgery.

All radiopharmaceutical agents were prepared and stored according to the instructions of the manufacturers. Both colloids were filtered through 0.20-μm filters to remove larger-sized particles, which tend to migrate slowly from the primary site.[24,25] The primary site was injected with approximately 18.5 to 30 MBq (500-800 μCi) of the radiopharmaceutical agent at 4 circumferential points, and a large-field stationary scintillation camera (Siemens ZLC, Des Plaines, Ill) was used to image the primary site, afferent lymphatics, and regional drainage basins. After injection of the radiopharmaceutical agent, continuous monitoring was performed until the first nodes or SNs were visualized. The SNs were defined as the first lymph nodes visualized on LS images. Occasionally, 1 or more lymph nodes would be identified simultaneously, and in some cases 2 or more afferent lymphatic channels would lead to different lymph nodes. Each of these lymph nodes were considered SNs. The transit times of the radiopharmaceutical agents were measured from the injection time until the first regional lymph node was visualized. The sites of the afferent lymphatic channels and the SN were marked on the skin with indelible ink and the body image was outlined to create the radiograph.

SURGICAL PROTOCOL

After induction of general or local anesthesia, we injected patients intradermally with isosulfan blue dye (Lymphazurin 1%, Hirsch Industries Inc, Richmond, Va), 1 to 1.5 cm^3, at the primary site. The 71 patients who underwent preoperative LS more than 24 hours before SLND received the dye in a 3:1 ratio with Tc 99m HSA (11-55 MBq); the 16 patients who underwent LS on the day of surgery received blue dye alone. Gentle massage facilitated the passage of the injectate into the lymphatics. Five to 10 minutes after injection, an incision was made at the site marked

up to 60% of patients will not have histopathologic evidence of metastases in the regional lymph nodes and are therefore unlikely to benefit from ELND.[10] On the other hand, although only a small fraction of low-risk patients will ever develop lymph node metastases, excluding them from ELND may ultimately prevent them from obtaining the survival benefit of this procedure.

In 1992, Morton et al[11] reported a minimally invasive operative procedure to determine the presence of occult regional lymph node metastases in patients with clinical stage I melanoma. Intraoperative lymphatic mapping and selective lymph node dissection (SLND) was devised as an alternative to ELND. Morton et al[11] and Wong et al[12] demonstrated that the lymphatic drainage patterns of cutaneous melanoma were predictable by preoperative lymphoscintigraphy (LS) and that the first tumor-draining lymph node could be identified intraoperatively with a single injection of isosulfan blue dye at the primary site. Excision and histopathologic analysis of the sentinel node (SN) was used to determine the tumor status of the regional lymph node basin. Only patients with demonstrated SN metastases would be subject to a complete lymphadenectomy (LND). In their initial experience, Morton et al[11,13] identified the SN in 194 (81.8%) of 237 predicted lymph node basins. By performing LND in all patients, they found that the frequency of false-negative, tumor-positive SNs was less than 1%. Several other investigators[14-16] subsequently validated the SN technique and proved its strength as a staging procedure.

Because the success of the technique is limited by the surgeon's ability to identify blue-stained SNs, we modified the procedure by using isosulfan blue dye in conjunction with technetium Tc 99m human serum albumin (Tc 99m HSA). The radiopharmaceutical agent was tracked with a handheld gamma probe into the regional nodes, where higher radioactive counts were found in SNs than in non-SNs.[17,18] Although other investigators[19-21] published their results with intraoperative probe-directed mapping, none of these early studies clearly defined the radioactive SN using the blue-stained SN as a standard. In this study, we evaluate the utility of several radiopharmaceutical agents for LS and SLND to improve the accuracy of SN detection.

RESULTS

Preoperative LS demonstrated 28 cervical, 44 axillary, and 28 inguinal lymph node basins from the 17 head and neck, 32 torso, and 38 extremity primary sites. Of 87 patients, 13 (15%) had dual pathways of lymphatic drainage, but no patient had more than 2 drainage basins or an ambiguous drainage pattern. Lymphoscintigraphy imaged 135 SNs (mean, 1.35 per basin) within the first hour of injection of the radiopharmaceutical agent. There was no difference ($P = .35$) among the 3 agents in the interval (minutes) between injection and identification of the SN: 9.8 ± 9.8 minutes (range, 1-36 minutes) for Tc 99m HSA; 10.4 ± 7.2 minutes (range, 1-30 minutes) for Tc 99m AC;

by preoperative LS; the exact time of this incision depended on the radiopharmaceutical agent used.[24] The lymphatics at the edge of the basin nearest the primary melanoma were identified and were followed by meticulous dissection to the first blue-stained node in the basin. Sentinel nodes were defined as the first blue-stained lymph nodes or radioactive and non-blue lymph nodes. The site and number of lymph nodes identified as SNs was usually closely correlated to the LS findings. The area several centimeters around the SN was carefully explored for additional blue-stained nodes. Injection was repeated every 20 minutes as necessary to identify an SN. If more than 1 lymph node basin was demonstrated by LS (n = 13) we explored the basins in the order they were found by LS.

A handheld gamma particle probe (Neoprobe 1000, Neoprobe Corp, Dublin, Ohio) was used to determine the radioactivity (counts per second) over the regional lymph node basin at the site marked during LS and over each blue-stained SN before (in vivo) and after (ex vivo) its excision. If a blue-stained lymph node was not identified, the nodes with the highest radioactivity were excised until the counts approached measured background levels. Background counts were obtained from 3 neutral body sites (10-20 cm from the primary injection site and lymph node basin) to avoid confusion with either the primary site or the lymph node basin. In cases in which the primary site was adjacent to the dissected basin, the probe crystal was positioned to diminish the artifact from the primary site. In these cases, radioactivity did not reach the neutral background levels. Triplicate counts were recorded from all sites.

While excised SNs were examined for evidence of metastases, the primary melanoma was excised with radial margins of 1 to 3 cm (depending on the thickness and site of the primary lesion). If results of pathologic examination of the SN were positive for metastases either by frozen or permanent section, LND was performed in the standard fashion.

PATHOLOGIC EXAMINATION

The techniques of pathologic examination have been described previously.[12,26] Briefly, each SN was bisected from the hilum to the periphery. Each face of the cross section of the specimen was processed by frozen-section examination using conventional hematoxylin-eosin staining; the remaining portion of the lymph node was embedded in paraffin and sectioned for reexamination by hematoxylin-eosin and immunohistochemical staining with antibodies for S-100 and the melanoma-specific protein HMB45.[26] Additional lymph nodes removed during LND were examined by hematoxylin-eosin staining alone.

STATISTICS

Preoperative LS transit times of the radiopharmaceutical agents and the first identification of the SN were compared using analysis of variance, and significance was based on $P<.05$. Mean ± SD radioactivity counts were calculated, and count-background ratios were determined from the preincision lymph node basin, the in vivo and ex vivo lymph nodes, and the postexcision lymph node basin. The difference in mean count ratios associated with immediate (≤4 hours after preoperative LS) vs delayed (≥24 hours after LS) SLND was assessed using a 2-sample *t* test with pooled variance.[27]

and 14 ± 15.1 minutes (range, 2-60 minutes) for Tc 99m SC. There was also no difference ($P = .26$) in the number of nodes identified (1.29 ± 0.49 for Tc 99m HSA, 1.53 ± 0.72 for Tc 99m AC, and 1.33 ± 0.49 for Tc 99m SC) per basin by each of the radiopharmaceutical agents, suggesting that the 3 agents were equally effective for preoperative LS.[24]

During SLND, SNs were identified in 98 of 100 regional lymphatic basins. One hundred forty-four SNs (mean, 1.4 per basin) were excised. In one third of the lymph node basins, more than 1 SN was identified (29 basins, 2 SNs; 4 basins, ≥3 SNs). Sentinal nodes were not found in 2 basins. In 1 patient, preoperative LS demonstrated drainage to the inguinal lymph node basin from a proximal calf primary site. The popliteal space was explored first because of concern that lymphatic drainage to this basin may have been obscured by the artifact from the radiopharmaceutical agent injected at the primary site. After injection of isosulfan blue dye, we suspect that the lymphatic channel leading to the inguinal basin may have been transected in the process of our exploration of the popliteal space. In a second patient, the skin overlying the sternocleidomastoid muscle was marked during LS. Lymphoscintigraphic images led us to believe that the SN was located posterior and lateral to the sternocleidomastoid muscle, but we suspect that the SN was likely deep to the muscle and that the lymphatic channel was cut during dissection through the muscle. In both patients, blue dye was injected concurrently with Tc 99m HSA, which prevented us from identifying a radioactive SN. Neither of these 2 patients has had a recurrence after 16 and 17 months of follow-up, respectively.

For the 93 basins in which a blue-stained SN was identified, the mean ± SD absolute radioactivity counts were 104 ± 124 per second (range, 1-690 per second) for the background, 605 ± 834 per second (range, 7-3953 per second) over the basin before incision, 745 ± 1198 per second (range, 5-3136 per second) for the SN in vivo, 551 ± 1104 per second (range, 10-6787 per second) for the SN ex vivo, and 213 ± 440 per second (range, 2-2266 per second) over the basin after excision. The corresponding site-background count ratios (mean ± SD) were as follows (**Figure 1**): preincision basin, 12.9 ± 20.4 (range, 0.7-123.7); in vivo SN, 27.4 ± 100.6 (range, 0.4-963.0); ex vivo SN, 20.1 ± 77.8 (range, 0.2-711.0); and postexcision basin, 2.8 ± 3.8 (range, 0.1-21.0).

There was a wide distribution of in vivo count ratios measured over blue-stained and non–blue-stained SNs (**Figure 2**). Twelve blue-stained SNs (8.3%) had an in vivo count ratio less than 2:1. By increasing the in vivo count ratio to 3:1 or more to improve the specificity of the technique, the number of blue-stained SNs not defined by the gamma probe technique increased to 21 (14.6%). Count ratios varied from less than 1 to 100. We found a similar wide range of count ratios after the SNs were excised. Twenty-two SNs (16.2%) had ex vivo count ratios less than 2 and 37 SNs (27.2%) had ex vivo counts ratios less than 3:1 (data not shown). To account for all

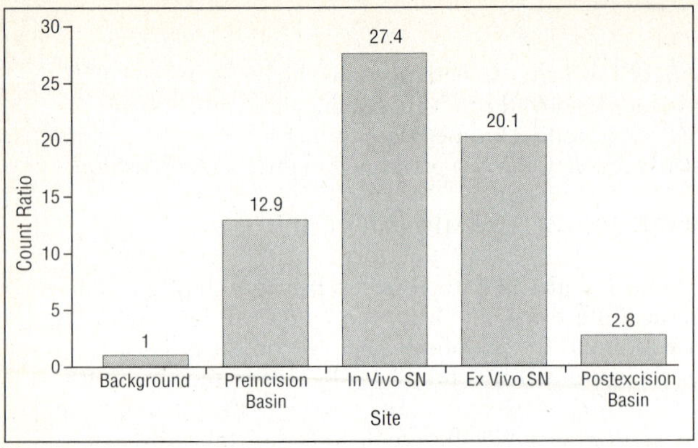

Figure 1. *Relative change in count ratios measured during selective lymph node dissection. Absolute counts were determined over each of the sites using a handheld gamma probe and recorded in triplicate. Count ratios were calculated in each case by comparing site counts with those of an irrelevant background location away from the primary site of the lymph node basin. SN indicates sentinel node.*

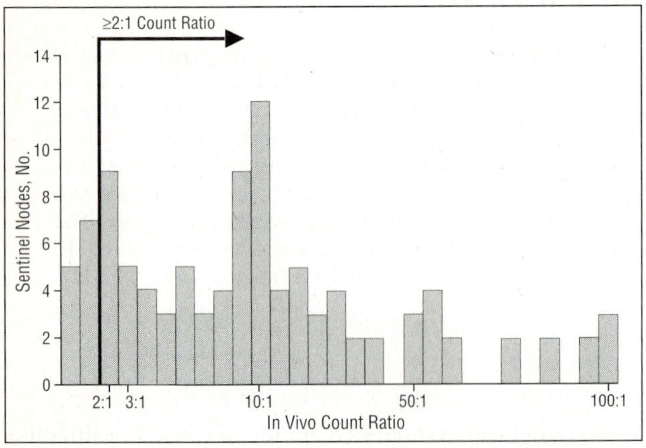

Figure 2. *Distribution of in vivo sentinel node–background count ratios. Blue-stained and non–blue-stained sentinel nodes were assessed for the presence of radioactivity using a handheld gamma probe. Count ratios were calculated by comparing in vivo sentinel node counts with those of an irrelevant body site (background). Twelve blue-stained lymph nodes (8.3%) had count ratios less than 2.*

blue-stained nodes, in vivo and ex vivo count ratios would have to be 1 or less. We found that a count ratio of 1 or less is impractical for routine use of the gamma probe. We therefore defined a radioactive (hot) SN with an in vivo or ex vivo count ratio of 2:1 or more from a blue-stained node because this ratio is sufficiently large for easy detection with the probe.

As shown in **Table 1**, 124 blue-stained lymph nodes (86.1%) from 83 basins (83.0%) met our definition of a hot SN, defined as an in vivo– or ex vivo–background count ratio of 2:1 or more. Whereas 117 lymph nodes (81.2%) from 77 basins (77%) had count ratios of 3:1 or more. Eight non–blue-stained radioactive SNs (count ratios ≥2) were identified in only 5 basins (2 cervical and 3 axillary). None of these lymph nodes contained metastases. The success of the blue dye was 94% and the success of radiopharmaceutical techniques alone was 4%. The combined success rate of the 2 techniques was 98%.

Sixteen patients (18%) underwent LS with Tc 99m SC immediately before surgery (mean time between LS and SLND, 210 minutes; range, 30-240 minutes) and therefore required only a single injection of a radiopharmaceutical agent. In all 16 patients, the SN was successfully identified during surgery. In 15 patients the SN was identified with blue dye and a radiopharmaceutical agent and in 1 patient the SN was identified with blue dye alone (count ratio <2). An SN was identified in all 18 lymphatic basins (100% success), and 27 of 29 SNs (93.1% concordance) were blue stained and hot (in vivo or ex vivo count ratios ≥2). In comparison, in 71 patients who underwent SLND by simultaneous injection of Tc 99m HSA and isosulfan blue dye, the SN was identified in 80 of 82 lymphatic basins (98% success), and 96 of 115 SNs (83.5% concordance) were blue stained and hot. There was no difference in count ratios in vivo (21.6 ± 26 vs 29.5 ± 116.7; $P = .60$) or ex vivo (16.3 ± 19.6 vs 20.7 ± 85.6; $P = .73$) between patients injected with Tc 99m SC vs Tc 99m HSA, respectively.

Table 1. Results of Intraoperative Lymphatic Mapping*

	No. (%)
Lymph nodes, total SN	144 (100.0)
SN blue stained	136 (94.4)
SN hot (ratio ≥2)	132 (91.7)
SN hot (ratio ≥3)	125 (86.8)
SN blue stained only (ratio <2)	12 (8.3)
SN blue stained and ratio ≥2	124 (86.1)
SN blue stained and ratio ≥3	117 (81.2)
SN hot only (ratio ≥2)	8 (5.6)
Lymph node basins, total basins	100 (100.0)
Basins SN identified	98 (98.0)
Basins SN blue stained	93 (93.0)
Basins SN blue stained and hot (ratio ≥2)	83 (83.0)
Basins SN blue stained and hot (ratio ≥3)	77 (77.0)
Basins SN blue stained only (ratio <2)	10 (10.0)
Basins SN hot (ratio ≥2), not blue stained	5 (5.0)
Basins SN hot (ratio ≥3), not blue stained	5 (5.0)

**SN indicates sentinel node.*

Of 87 patients (85 with SNs identified), 14 (16%) had metastases in the SN. Seventeen (11.8%) of 144 SNs removed during SLND were tumor positive. Sixteen (94%) of 17 tumor-containing SNs were blue stained and hot (in vivo or ex vivo ratio ≥2); the remaining SN had an in vivo– and ex vivo–background count ratio less than 2 and was identified with isosulfan blue dye alone. The in vivo and ex vivo count ratios of tumor-containing SNs were 18.2 ± 25.6 (range, 0.4-96.0) and 14.1 ± 26.9 (range, 0.2-91.3), respectively. These count ratios were no different than the in vivo ($P = .82$) or ex vivo ($P = .49$) ratios for SNs that were tumor free (**Figure 3**). Four (1.1%) of 377 lymph nodes removed during completion LND contained metastases. There have been no same-basin recurrences in 87 patients (mean follow-up, 16.3 months).

COMMENT

Intraoperative lymphatic mapping and SLND was introduced by our institution as a means of identifying occult regional lymph node metastases in patients with early-stage melanoma.[12,13] This minimally invasive operative procedure was devised as an alternative to ELND. Results of our initial experience suggest that the blue dye alone was not sufficient. The success of identifying the

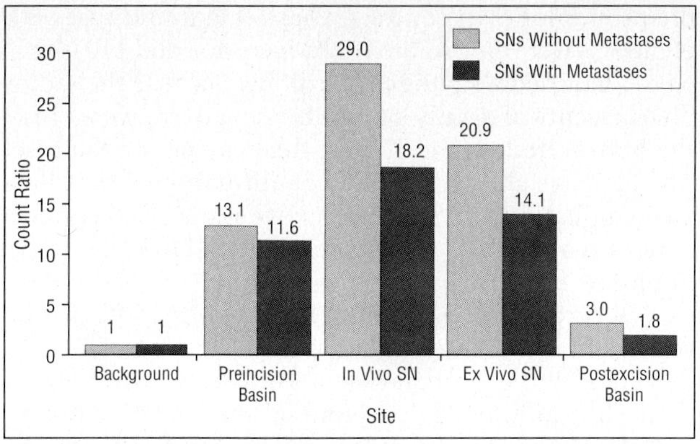

Figure 3. *Relative change in count ratios for sentinel nodes (SNs) with and without metastases. Absolute counts were determined over each site using a handheld gamma probe and recorded in triplicate. Count ratios were calculated in each case by comparing counts with an irrelevant background, away from the primary or lymph basin. Relative count ratios were no different for blue-stained SNs in vivo (*P *= .82) or ex vivo (*P *= .49) with or without metastases.*

SN is dependent on the surgeon locating a blue-stained afferent lymphatic and lymph node. The first improvement in the technique was the addition of preoperative cutaneous LS in all patients so the surgeon would have a landmark for the location of the SN.[28-30]

Preoperative LS has been adapted by most surgeons as an essential component of the SN technique, but there is no standard method or radiopharmaceutical agent used for this procedure. We performed LS with 1 of 3 agents: Tc 99m HSA, Tc 99m AC, or Tc 99m SC. In our series, LS identified the draining lymphatic basin in all patients and demonstrated dual drainage patterns in 13 patients (15% incidence), a rate similar to that reported by other institutions.[24,30,31] Lymphoscintigraphy clearly improves localization of the SN, but the intralymphatic kinetics and retention of the various radiopharmaceutical agents in the lymph nodes have not been well studied. We found that Tc 99m HSA had a slightly faster transit time to the SN than did the 2 filtered particulate agents, Tc 99m AC and Tc 99m SC.[24] The number of SNs identified by LS was similar for all 3 agents when images were obtained within the first hour. We have not seen demonstration of additional lymph node basins later than 1 hour after injection of any of the 3 radiopharmaceutical agents. Yet, with delayed images (3-4 hours), an increasing number of lymph nodes were identified with Tc 99m AC and Tc 99m SC.[24] With longer delay, particulate agents travel from the SN to non-SN, which makes LS unreliable for detecting the site of the SN. Although the concept that particulate agents are trapped in the SN is intriguing, our results suggest that this is not always the case. Transit of the radiopharmaceutical agents in the lymph nodes is time dependent: the longer the imaging period the more nodes that will appear. Our findings indicate that although Tc 99m HSA and particulate agents (Tc 99m AC and Tc 99m SC) have different transit times related to particle size, all 3 are equally effective in identifying the SN by LS if early images are used. The use of a single injection of a radiopharmaceutical agent for both LS and probe-directed SLND would diminish the cost and radiation exposure to patients and may be the most sensible method for this procedure.

Our second goal for this study was to determine the utility of intraoperative probe-directed mapping for identification of the SN. Several institutions have reported that addition of radiopharmaceutical agents to the blue dye improves localization of the SN, but there are discrepancies in the methods in which the radiopharmaceutical agents are used and in the level of radioactivity that defines an SN. Eighteen hours after injecting Tc 99m AC at the primary site, Pijpers et al[32] used a gamma probe to identify the SN but found in most cases high levels of radioactivity in nodes adjacent to the SN. Krag and associates[19] reported successful localization of hot nodes up to 24 hours after injection of unfiltered Tc 99m SC, but they rarely used the blue dye to confirm their findings. Albertini et al[20] recommended waiting 3 to 4 hours after injection of Tc 99m SC to achieve radioactive counts 2-fold higher in SNs than in non-SNs. In these studies, the concordance between blue dye and probe ranged from 60% to 100%. Taylor and associates[33] suggested that Tc 99m HSA was not retained in the lymph nodes long enough for effective intraoperative lymphatic mapping. However, in our 71 patients receiving Tc 99m HSA, we identified the SN in 80 (98%) of 82 lymphatic basins, and 96 of 115 SNs were blue stained and hot (in vivo and ex vivo counts ratios ≥2:1, 83.5% concordance). In 16 patients receiving Tc 99m SC, the SN was identified in all 18 lymphatic basins (100%), and 27 of 29 SNs (93% concordance) were blue stained and hot (in vivo and ex vivo counts ratios ≥2:1). These findings suggest that SLND may be undertaken immediately after injecting Tc 99m HSA or up to 4 hours after injecting filtered Tc 99m SC. We are currently investigating the efficacy of preoperative LS and SLND with filtered Tc 99m SC injected 4 hours or longer before the operative procedure.

An in vivo or ex vivo lymph node count ratio of 2:1 or more identified 132 (91.7%) of 144 lymph nodes excised during SLND (Table 1). Although we are not the first to define an SN by a count ratio, other investigators have used count ratios subject to variability.[19,20,32-38] Albertini et al[20] initially suggested defining the SN by an in vivo count ratio of 3:1 or more and an ex vivo SN–non-SN ratio of 10:1 or more. However, background counts were obtained from the dissected basin and thus would be expected to vary significantly according to the kinetics of the radiopharmaceutical agent and the distance of the gamma probe to the hot SN. More recently, this group of investigators redefined the SN by an in vivo count ratio of 2:1 or more.[39] Only 220 (80.0%) of 275 SNs demonstrated this level of radioactivity. They did not report on the concordance of blue dye and radiopharmaceutical techniques, but because only 165 SNs were blue stained, the concordance between the 2 techniques may have been as low as 60%. Krag et al[19] defined an SN by an absolute count of at least 15 per 10 seconds and a count ratio of 3:1 or more. Sentinel nodes were identified in all 118 patients, but because blue dye was not used in all cases and LND was not performed, the true accuracy of the probe cannot be determined by this approach. Mudun et al[36] defined an SN by an absolute count of 300 to 3000 per 10 seconds and a count ratio of 30:1

Table 2. Results of Probe-Assisted Selective Lymph Node Dissection

	No. (%)	
	Glass et al[39]	Present Study
Total SNs*	275	144
Blue dye success	165 (60.0)	136 (94.4)
Probe success	220 (80.0)	132 (91.7)
SN hot only	110 (40.0)	8 (5.6)
SN blue stained only	55 (20.0)	12 (8.3)
Combined basin success	175/180 (97.2)	98/100 (98.0)

*SNs indicates sentinel nodes.

or more. However, true SNs with ratios less than 30:1 were probably missed, and absolute counts are time dependent and not easily reproducible using the gamma probe. Both Loggie et al[37] and Wong et al[38] defined the SN by the level of radioactivity alone. Using absolute counts for defining the SN may be misleading because the hottest lymph node may vary with the amount of radiopharmaceutical agent injected and the kinetics of the agent.[24,40]

We prefer to use a count ratio as our method of choice for defining the SN, with an irrelevant body site as the background. Before making a skin incision in the lymph node basin (before incision) we found mean count ratios of 12.9 ± 20.4. The count ratio over the blue-stained SN increased approximately 2-fold before (in vivo, 27.4 ± 100.6) and after (ex vivo, 20.1 ± 77.8) its excision. The postexcision ratio (2.8 ± 3.8), determined after excision of all hot blue-stained SNs, was less than the preincision ratio in 96% of patients. In the remaining patients, the postexcision ratio did not drop below preincision levels. We suspect that the elevated counts may relate to the gamma probe detecting counts in the afferent lymphatics or residual non-SNs.

The blue dye technique remains the criterion standard for SN localization, and the gamma probe serves as a useful adjunct. In their initial series, Morton et al[12,13] used blue dye alone to identify the SN in 194 (81.8%) of 237 lymphatic basins. The accuracy of the procedure was determined by performing LND in all cases. After refining the blue dye technique with LS in all cases, Morton et al[29] achieved a 90% success rate in 72 patients. Other institutions[15,16] reported success rates ranging from 90% to 93% using blue dye alone. In this study, the addition of a radiopharmaceutical agent increased our overall basin success to 98%, a rate similar to that reported by others[19,20,32,33] using the combined technique. Although some of our improved success may relate to our experience with SLND, we believe that the use of the gamma probe expedites the SN localization process and diminishes the chance of the surgeon transecting the blue-stained afferent lymphatics.

Although the overall SN detection rates reported by other institutions are similar to ours, one cannot be certain that the SNs removed by the probe alone are true SNs. In comparing our series with the study by Glass and associates[39] (**Table 2**), the overall basin success was similar. In our study, 94.4% of the SNs were blue stained, 91.7% were hot, and only 8 (5.6%) were identified with the probe alone. In contrast, Glass et al found that 60% of the SNs were blue stained, 80% were hot, and 110 (40%) were identified with the probe alone. Because the radiopharmaceutical agents cannot be visualized, we assume the hottest node is the SN, yet this may not be the case. The blue dye allows for visual confirmation of the afferent lymphatics and SN. We believe the lack of concordance between the 2 techniques may lead to higher rates of missed SNs.

Several studies[19,33,39] using blue dye and probe reported an increased incidence of metastases in SNs detected by the probe alone and raise the question of their clinical importance. None of the 17 SNs containing metastases in our study were identified with the probe alone; 16 (94%) of 17 were blue stained and hot and 1 (6%) of 17 was blue stained and did not meet our definition of a radioactive SN. The increased detection of SNs with metastases by the probe alone reported by other investigators[20,39] can be partially explained by their relatively low success rate (60%-70%) with blue dye. We found no difference in the count ratios of SNs with or without metastases (Figure 3). Based on the results of this study, we propose that the following guidelines be used for LS and SLND:

1. Preoperative LS for all patients considered for SLND regardless of the site of the primary melanoma. The radiopharmaceutical agents Tc 99m HSA, Tc 99m AC, and Tc 99m SC are equally effective for localizing the sites of the SN. Dynamic imaging is essential for accurate identification of the SN.
2. Selective LND can be performed by combining blue dye with Tc 99m HSA during surgery or by injecting filtered Tc 99m SC up to 4 hours before administration of blue dye. The SN is identified by a blue-stained afferent lymphatic channel leading into a lymph node. The gamma probe is used as an adjunct for guiding the surgeon to the first and any additional blue-stained SNs.
3. If a blue-stained SN cannot be identified, all lymph nodes with an in vivo or ex vivo count ratio of 2:1 or more are removed until the count ratios in the basin are less than 2:1.

The blue dye and gamma probe techniques are complementary. Probe-directed SLND is a useful adjunct to the blue dye technique and improves the rate of SN detection.[40] Although the radioactivity in the regional lymph nodes is easily detected by the gamma probe technique, the blue dye allows for visual confirmation of the afferent lymphatics leading into the SN. Yet, the blue dye can be difficult to locate, especially in the axilla or when the skin site is not well marked by LS. To improve the rates of SN detection and to standardize the use of the gamma probe technique, further studies are necessary to evaluate the kinetics of the radiopharmaceutical agents through the lymphatics and the retention of these agents in the lymph node basins.

Supported by grant PO NCI CA 29605 from the National Institutes of Health, Bethesda, Md, and by funding from Viasoft Corp, Phoenix, Ariz. Dr Essner is a recipient of an American Cancer Society Career Development Award.

Presented at the 50th Annual Cancer Symposium of the Society of Surgical Oncology, Chicago, Ill, March 23, 1997.

Reprints: Richard Essner, MD, John Wayne Cancer Institute, 2200 Santa Monica Blvd, Santa Monica, CA 90404 (e-mail: essner@jwci.org).

REFERENCES

1. Snow H. Melanotic cancerous disease. *Cancer.* 1892;2:872-875.
2. Milton GW, Shaw HH, McCarthy WJ, et al. Prophylactic lymph node dissection in clinical stage I cutaneous malignant melanoma: results of surgical treatment in 1,319 patients. *Br J Surg.* 1982;69:108-111.
3. Morton DL, Wanek L, Nizze JA, Elashoff RM, Wong JH. Improved long-term survival after lymphadenectomy of melanoma metastatic to regional nodes: analysis of prognostic factors in 1134 patients from the John Wayne Cancer Clinic. *Ann Surg.* 1991;214:491-499.
4. Das Gupta TK. Results of treatment of 265 patients with primary cutaneous melanoma: a five-year prospective study. *Ann Surg.* 1977;186:201-209.
5. Day CL Jr, Mihm MC Jr, Lew RA, et al. Prognostic factors for patients with clinical stage I melanoma of intermediate thickness (1.51-3.99mm): a conceptual model for tumor growth and metastasis. *Ann Surg.* 1982;195:35-43.
6. Sim FH, Taylor WF, Ivins JC, Pritchard DJ, Soule EH. A prospective randomized study of the efficacy of routine elective lymphadenectomy in management of malignant melanoma. *Cancer.* 1978;41:948-956.
7. Veronesi U, Adamus J, Bandiera DC, et al. Inefficacy of immediate node dissection in stage I melanoma of the limbs. *N Engl J Med.* 1977;297:627-630.
8. Balch CM, Soong SJ, Bartolucci AA, et al. Efficacy of an elective regional lymph node dissection of 1 to 4 mm thick melanomas for patients 60 years of age and younger. *Ann Surg.* 1996;224:255-266.
9. Balch CM, Murad TM, Soong SJ, et al. Tumor thickness as a guide to surgical management of clinical stage I melanoma patients. *Cancer.* 1979;43:883-888.
10. Balch CM, Milton GW, Cascinelli N, Sims FH. Elective lymph node dissections: pros and cons. In: Balch CM, Houghton A, Milton GW, Sober AJ, Soongs SJ, eds. *Cutaneous Melanoma.* 2nd ed. Philadelphia, Pa: JB Lippincott; 1992:345-366.
11. Morton DL, Wen DR, Wong JH, et al. Technical details of intraoperative lymphatic mapping for early stage melanoma. *Arch Surg.* 1992;127:392-399.
12. Wong JH, Cagle LA, Morton DL. Lymphatic drainage of skin to a sentinel node in a feline model. *Ann Surg.* 1991;214:637-641.
13. Morton DL, Wen DR, Cochran AJ. Management of early-stage melanoma by intraoperative lymphatic mapping and selective lymphadenectomy: an alternative to routine elective lymphadenectomy or "watch and wait." *Surg Oncol Clin North Am.* 1992;1:247-259.
14. Reintgen D, Cruse CW, Wells K, et al. The orderly progression of melanoma nodal metastases. *Ann Surg.* 1994;220:759-767.
15. Thompson JF, McCarthy WH, Bosch CM, et al. Sentinel lymph node status as an indicator of the presence of metastatic melanoma in regional lymph nodes. *Melanoma Res.* 1995;5:255-260.
16. Karkakousis CP, Velez AF, Spellman JE, et al. The technique of sentinel node biopsy. *Eur J Surg Oncol.* 1996;22:271-275.
17. Essner R, Foshag L, Morton DL. Intraoperative radiolymphoscintigraphy: a useful adjuvant to intraoperative lymphatic mapping and selective lymphadenectomy in patients with clinical stage I melanoma. Paper presented at: Annual Meeting of the Society of Surgical Oncology; March 19, 1994; Houston, Tex.
18. Essner R. The role of lymphoscintigraphy and sentinel node mapping in assessing patient risk in melanoma. *Semin Oncol.* 1997;24:54-60.
19. Krag DN, Meijer SJ, Weaver DL, et al. Minimal-access surgery for staging of malignant melanoma. *Arch Surg.* 1995;130:654-660.
20. Albertini JJ, Cruse CW, Rapaport D, et al. Intraoperative radiolymphoscintigraphy improves sentinel lymph node identification for patients with melanoma. *Ann Surg.* 1996;223:217-224.
21. Leong SPL, Steinmetz I, Habib FA, et al. Optimal selective sentinel lymph node dissection in primary malignant melanoma. *Arch Surg.* 1997;132:666-673.
22. Ronan SG, Eng AM, Briele HA, et al. Thin malignant melanomas with regression and metastasis. *Arch Dermatol.* 1987;123:1326-1330.
23. Soong SJ, Harrison RA, McCarthy WH, et al. Factors affecting survival following local, regional or distant recurrence from localized melanoma. *J Surg Oncol.* 1998; 67:228-233.
24. Glass EC, Essner R, Morton DL. Kinetics of three lymphoscintigraphic agents in patients with cutaneous melanoma. *J Nucl Med.* 1998;39:1185-1190.
25. Hung JC, Wiseman GA, Wahner HW, et al. Filtered technetium-99m-sulfur colloid evaluated for lymphoscintigraphy. *J Nucl Med.* 1995;36:1895-1901.
26. Cochran AJ, Wen DR, Herschman HR. Occult melanoma in lymph nodes detected by antiserum to S-100 protein. *Int J Cancer.* 1984;34:159-163.
27. Campbell MJ, Machin D. *Medical Statistics: A Commonsense Approach.* 2nd ed. New York, NY: John Wiley & Sons Inc; 1995.
28. Fee HJ, Robinson DS, Sample WF, et al. The determination of lymph shed by colloidal gold scanning in patients with malignant melanoma: a preliminary study. *Surgery.* 1978;84:626-632.
29. Morton DL, Wen DR, Foshag LJ, Essner R, Cochran A. Intraoperative lymphatic mapping and selective cervical lymphadenectomy for early-stage melanomas of the head and neck. *J Clin Oncol.* 1993;11:1751-1756.
30. Lamki LM, Logic JR. Defining lymphatic drainage patterns with cutaneous lymphoscintigraphy. In: Balch C, Houghton A, Milton GW, Sober AJ, Soong SJ, eds. *Cutaneous Melanoma.* 2nd ed. Philadelphia, Pa: JB Lippincott; 1992:367-375.
31. Norman J, Cruse CW, Espinosa C, et al. Redefinition of cutaneous lymphatic drainage with the use of lymphoscintigraphy for malignant melanoma. *Am J Surg.* 1991;162:432-437.
32. Pijpers R, Collet GJ, Meijer S, Hoekstra OS. The impact of dynamic lymphoscintigraphy and gamma probe guidance on sentinel node biopsy in melanoma. *Eur J Nucl Med.* 1995;22:1238-1241.
33. Taylor A Jr, Murray D, Herda S, Vansant J, Alazraki N. Dynamic lymphoscintigraphy to identify the sentinel and satellite nodes. *Clin Nucl Med.* 1996;21:755-758.
34. Wong JH, Truelove K, Ko P, Coel MN. Localization and resection of an intransit sentinel lymph node by use of lymphoscintigraphy, intraoperative lymphatic mapping, and a hand-held gamma probe. *Surgery.* 1996;120:114-116.
35. O'Brien CJ, Uren RF, Thompson RF, et al. Prediction of potential metastatic sites in cutaneous head and neck melanoma using lymphoscintigraphy. *Am J Surg.* 1995;170:461-466.
36. Mudun A, Murray DR, Herda SC, et al. Early stage melanoma: lymphoscintigraphy, reproducibility of sentinel node detection, and effectiveness of the intraoperative gamma probe. *Radiology.* 1996;199:171-175.
37. Loggie BW, Hosseinian AA, Watson NE, et al. Prospective evaluation of selective lymph node biopsy for cutaneous malignant melanoma. *Am Surg.* 1997;63: 1051-1056.
38. Wong JH, Terada K, Ko P, et al. Lack of effect of particle size on the identification of the sentinel node in cutaneous malignancies. *Ann Surg Oncol.* 1998;5:77-80.
39. Glass LF, Messina JL, Cruse W, et al. The use of intraoperative radiolymphoscintigraphy for sentinel node biopsy in patients with malignant melanoma. *Dermatol Surg.* 1996;22:715-720.
40. Bostick P, Essner R, Sarantou T, et al. Intraoperative lymphatic mapping for early-stage melanoma of the head and neck. *Am J Surg.* 1997;174:536-539.

ORIGINAL ARTICLE

Prognostic Factors in T1 and T2 Squamous Cell Carcinoma of the Thoracic Esophagus

Mitsuo Tachibana, MD; Shoichi Kinugasa, MD; Dipok Kumar Dhar, MD; Hideki Tabara, MD; Reiko Masunaga, MD; Tsukasa Kotoh, MD; Hirofumi Kubota, MD; Naofumi Nagasue, MD

Background: Prognostic indicators in patients with T2 tumor have not been fully understood.

Objective: To clarify the clinicopathologic characteristics and long-term results of T1 and T2 squamous cell carcinomas of the thoracic esophagus.

Design: Consecutive case series.

Setting: Department of surgery in a university hospital.

Patients: Of 234 patients with primary squamous cell carcinoma of the thoracic esophagus, 142 patients underwent esophagectomy with curative intent: 97 patients had pT1 and pT2 tumors.

Interventions: Investigated were clinicopathologic characteristics of 65 of 97 patients with pT1 and pT2 tumors; excluded were 7 patients who died of postoperative complications and another 25 patients who died of causes other than esophageal cancer.

Main Outcome Measures: Clinicopathologic characteristics and long-term results.

Results: Pathologic tumor stages were pT1 N0 in 23 patients, pT1 N(+) in 7 patients, pT2 N0 in 15 patients, and pT2 N(+) in 20 patients. Fifty patients are alive and free of cancer and 15 patients died of tumor recurrence (1 patient with pT1 N0 tumor, 1 patient with pT1 N[+][+] tumor, 1 patient with pT2 N0 tumor, and 12 patients with pT2 N[+] tumor). The sites of metastatic nodes in 6 survivors with pT1 N(+) tumor were a solitary perigastric node in 4 patients, a solitary mediastinal node in 1 patient, and 2 mediastinal nodes in 1 patient. The 5-year survival rates of patients with pT1 N0, pT1 N(+), and pT2 N0 tumors all exceeded 85%, and the rate of those with pT2 N(+) tumor was 33.9% (pT2 N[+] vs others: pT1 N0, pT1 N[+], and pT2 N0; $P = .003$). The factors affecting survival rate by univariate analysis were Borrmann classification (0, 1 vs 2, 3, 4), tumor size (<4.0 vs ≥4.0 cm), combined T, N factor (pT2 N[+] vs others), time of operation (≤420 vs >420 minutes), estimated blood loss (<1000 vs ≥1000 mL), and lymph vessel invasion (marked vs not marked). Stage pT2 N(+) tumor became a single independent prognostic factor for survival as determined by multivariate analysis (pT2 N[+] vs others; $P = .008$).

Conclusions: Stage pT1 N(+) tumors with a few diseased nodes and pT2 N0 tumors are considered to be a group with an excellent prognosis, similar to pT1 N0 tumors. Patients with pT2 N(+) diseases had worse prognoses and thus should have meticulous lymph node dissection and extensive adjuvant therapy.

Arch Surg. 1999;134:50-54

From the Second Department of Surgery, Shimane Medical University, Shimane, Japan.

ESOPHAGEAL carcinoma is one of the most malignant tumors, with a dismal prognosis. Among several clinicopathologic factors affecting the outcomes of patients with esophageal carcinoma, the depth of penetration is the crucial factor determining the prognosis.[1-3] Patients with superficial (T1) esophageal carcinoma have a significantly favorable clinical course compared with those with advanced cancers. The outcome for patients with T1 cancer is excellent, with a 5-year disease-specific survival rate exceeding 80%.[4-6] Conversely, the prognosis of patients with locally advanced (T3 and T4) tumor is far from satisfactory.[7-9] Prognostic indicators, however, in patients with T2 tumor have not been fully understood.

The operative approach for esophageal cancer varies from conventional transthoracic esophagectomy chiefly for palliation[10] to wide local excision with extensive lymphadenectomy with curative intent[3] to limited excision without thoracotomy.[11] The confusing factors are that adenocarcinomas of the gastric cardia invading the esophagus and those arising from the Barrett esophagus are reviewed in the literature, but their biologic behavior may be different from that of epidermoid cancer. Therefore, such adenocarcinomas of the esophagus were excluded from this study.

To clarify the clinicopathologic characteristics of early-stage squamous cell carcinoma of the thoracic esophagus, data from patients with T1 and T2 tumors were retrospectively investigated. Because these tumors must be evaluated in a series of resected specimens pathologically proven, this study included patients who had undergone surgical intervention.

PATIENTS AND METHODS

Between December 1979 and November 1997, 234 patients with primary squamous cell carcinoma of the thoracic esophagus were admitted to the Second Department of Surgery, Shimane Medical University, Shimane, Japan. Of these, 142 patients (60.7%) underwent esophagectomy with curative intent: 97 patients (68.3%) had pT1 and pT2 esophageal tumors and the remaining 45 patients (31.7%) had pT3 and pT4 tumors. Of these 97 patients with pT1 and pT2 tumors, excluded were 7 patients (7.2%) who died of postoperative complications during the hospital stay and another 25 patients (25.8%) who died of causes other than esophageal cancer, ie, pneumonia or respiratory failure (5 patients), second cancer (5 patients [hepatocellular cancer in 2 patients and gastric tube cancer, sigmoid colon cancer, and pancreas cancer each in 1 patient]), severe emaciation (4 patients), aging (3 patients), cardiac problems (2 patients), cerebrovascular attack (2 patients), and choking accident, gastric tube ulcer perforation, liver failure, and unknown sudden death at home (each in 1 patient). Therefore, 65 patients were enrolled in this analysis.

Most patients underwent a right transthoracic subtotal esophagectomy and dissection of the cervical (bilateral supraclavicular regions), mediastinal (periesophagus and around the trachea), and abdominal (perigastric lesion and around the celiac axis) lymph nodes. Reconstruction was usually carried out with a gastric tube through the retrosternal route, and esophagogastrostomy was done in the neck under the cervical and abdominal incisions.

When the tumor invaded the deeper submucosal layer, 1 or 2 cycles of adjuvant radiochemotherapy was routinely administered. Patients with T2 tumor received 2 cycles of the same schedule of chemotherapy with radiotherapy. One cycle of chemotherapy consisted of bolus administration of cisplatin (50 mg/m^2 per day) on the 1st and 15th days and continuous intravenous infusion of fluorouracil (300 mg/m^2) for 28 days. One cycle of radiotherapy consisted of 1.8 Gy daily directed to the tumor bed. The total dosage was 30.6 Gy.

Clinicopathologic characteristics of these 65 patients were investigated based on the TNM classification of malignant tumors.[12] The outcomes of patients were examined, and those who clearly died of recurrence were regarded as tumor-related deaths. In calculating the 10-year survival rate, those who were alive more than 10 years were counted as being alive at 10 years.

Survival rates were estimated by the Kaplan-Meier method,[13] and statistical analysis was carried out by the log-rank test to test for equality of the survival curves. In multivariate analysis, independent prognostic factors were determined using a Cox proportional hazards model[14] (StatView J4.5, Abacus Concepts Inc, Berkeley, Calif). The level of significance was $P<.05$.

RESULTS

Pathologic tumor stages were pT1 N0 in 23 patients, pT1 N(+) in 7 patients, pT2 N0 in 15 patients, and pT2 N(+) in 20 patients. Fifty patients are alive and free of cancer at the time of this analysis. Fifteen patients died because of recurrence: 1 patient with pT1 N0 tumor, 1 patient with pT1 N(+) tumor, 1 patient with pT2 N0 tumor, and 12 patients with pT2 N(+) tumor. The overall 1-, 3-, 5-, and 10-year survival rates of all 65 patients were 91.3%, 77.4%, 72.1%, and 68.1%, respectively.

SITES OF LYMPH NODE METASTASIS IN pT1 N(+) AND pT2 N(+) TUMORS

In 7 patients with pT1 N(+) tumor, the sites of diseased nodes were a solitary perigastric node in 4 patients, a solitary mediastinal node in 1 patient, 2 mediastinal nodes in 1 patient, and multiple cervical and mediastinal nodes in 1 patient who died of recurrence.

In 20 patients with pT2 N(+) tumor, the sites of metastatic nodes were a solitary perigastric node in 4 patients, mediastinal nodes in 4 patients, mediastinal and perigastric nodes in 3 patients, coeliac nodes (M1a) with mediastinal nodes in 4 patients, and cervical (M1a) and mediastinal nodes in 5 patients.

ADJUVANT TREATMENT

Forty-five patients received adjuvant treatment. Of 23 patients with pT1 N0 tumor, 17 patients did not receive any adjuvant treatment and 6 patients received adjuvant radiochemotherapy. Of 7 patients with pT1 N(+) tumor, 6 patients received radiochemotherapy and 1 patient refused any adjuvant treatment. Of 35 patients with pT2 tumor, 25 patients received adjuvant radiochemotherapy and 8 patients with shallow muscle layer invasion received chemotherapy alone. The remaining 2 patients refused any adjuvant treatment.

CUMULATIVE SURVIVAL RATES OF PATIENTS WITH pT1 AND pT2 TUMORS ACCORDING TO LYMPH NODE METASTASIS

The 5-year survival rates of patients with pT1 N0, pT1 N(+), and pT2 N0 tumors were satisfactory, all exceeding 85% (**Figure 1** and **Figure 2**). Conversely, 12 of 20 patients with pT2 N(+) tumor died of recurrence, and the 5-year survival rate was 33.9% (pT2 N[+] vs others: pT1 N0, pT1 N[+], and pT2 N0; $P=.003$) (**Figure 3**).

CLINICOPATHOLOGIC FACTORS AFFECTING SURVIVAL RATE

Table 1 shows the clinicopathologic variables affecting the cumulative survival rates by univariate analysis.

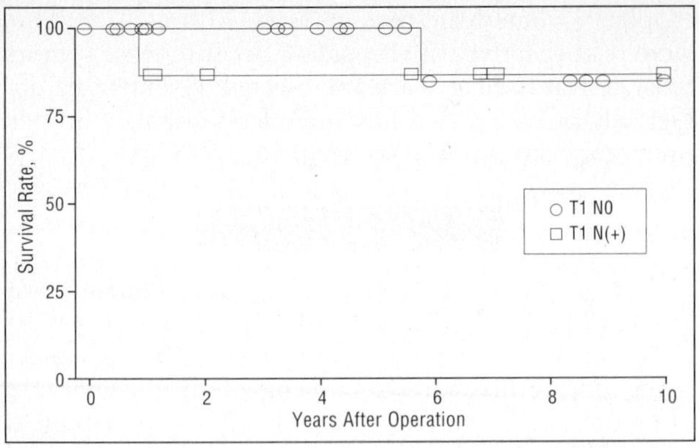

Figure 1. *Cumulative survival curves of patients with pT1 esophageal cancer according to lymph node metastasis. The 3- and 5-year survival rates were 100% for those without lymph node metastasis (n = 23) and 85.7% for those with lymph node metastasis (n = 7) (P = .57, log-rank test).*

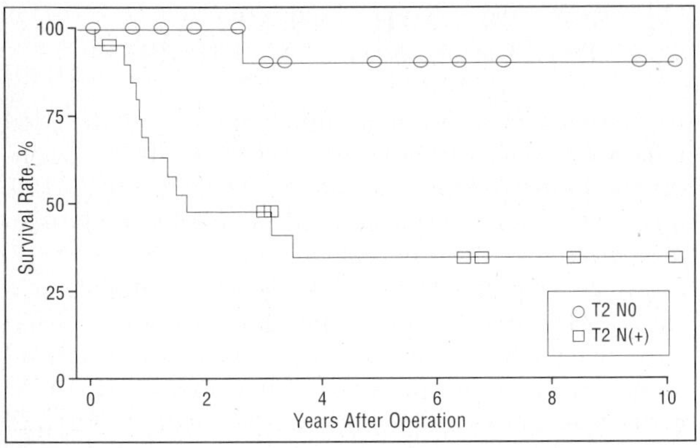

Figure 2. *Cumulative survival curves of patients with pT2 esophageal cancer according to lymph node metastasis. The 3- and 5-year survival rates were 90% for those without lymph node metastasis (n = 15) and 47.5% and 33.9%, respectively, for those with lymph node metastasis (n = 20) (P = .003, log-rank test).*

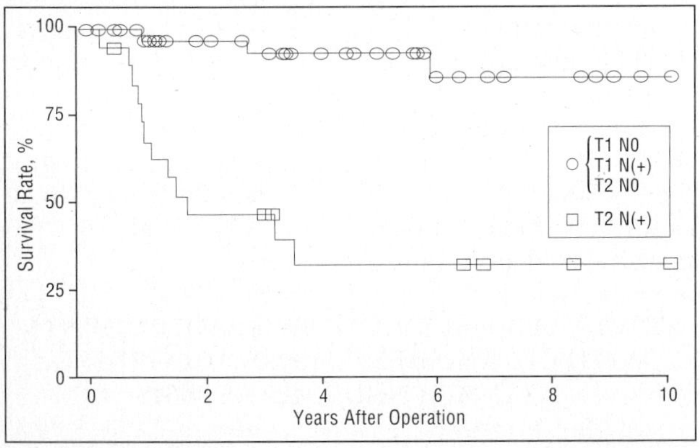

Figure 3. *Cumulative survival curves of patients with pT1 and pT2 esophageal cancers according to combined T, N factor. The 3- and 5-year survival rates were 93.8% for those with pT1 N0, pT1 N(+), and pT2 N0 diseases (n = 45) and 47.5% and 33.9%, respectively, for those with pT2 N(+) disease (n = 20) (P<.001, log-rank test).*

The variables affecting survival rate were Borrmann classification (0,1 vs 2,3,4), tumor size (≤4.0 vs >4.0 cm), combined T, N factor (pT2 N[+] vs others), time of operation (≤420 vs >420 minutes), estimated blood loss (<1000 vs ≥1000 mL), and lymph vessel invasion (marked vs not marked). Sex, histological differentiation, and vessel invasion did not affect the survival rate.

PROGNOSTIC SIGNIFICANCE EVALUATED BY MULTIVARIATE ANALYSIS

Among those 6 significant variables verified by univariate analysis, stage pT2 N(+) tumor was a single independent prognostic factor for survival as determined by multivariate analysis (pT2 N[+] vs others; *P* = .008) (**Table 2**). Therefore, pT1 N(+) and pT2 N0 diseases are considered to be a group with an excellent prognosis, similar to pT1 N0 tumor.

COMMENT

Depth of invasion is a major denominator deciding the prognosis of esophageal cancer. The prognosis of patients with T1 tumor[4-6] is generally good, but the therapeutic result is far from satisfactory for locally advanced (T3 and T4) tumors.[7-9] Although patients with T2 tumor are generally considered to have a favorable prognosis, recurrence of the disease occurs in a certain number of patients. Therefore, it is necessary to identify the high-risk group and to design an appropriate therapy for better survival.

The incidence of T1 and T2 esophageal cancer so far reported varies from 13.1% to 52.2%,[15-18] and the 5-year survival rate of these patients has been reported to be 22.5% to 88.2%.[10,18-20] These data are comparable to the 68.3% incidence of T1 and T2 tumors and 72.1% 5-year survival rate in the present study.

Unlike patients with early gastric carcinoma, the prognosis of patients with esophageal carcinoma is considered to be dismal once the regional lymph nodes are involved.[21-23] However, several European series, including that reported by Hoelscher et al,[24] found no significant difference in survival between the node-positive and node-negative group in T1 tumor and concluded that nodal status was not an independent prognostic factor by multivariate analysis. Similarly, we demonstrated that there was no significant difference in survival between the pT1 N0 and pT1 N(+) groups, and the 5-year survival rates were excellent, exceeding 85% in both groups. This indicates that a certain number of patients with diseased regional lymph nodes might have excellent survival when the primary tumor is pT1. Also, this survival advantage in patients with pT1 N(+) tumor could be associated with the extent and site of involvement of the regional lymph nodes. In these series, only 1 patient with pT1 N(+) tumor died of recurrence and had extensive lymph node involvement at multiple anatomical fields, and all other surviving patients had only a few (<2) metastatic nodes either in the mediastinum or in the perigastric region. Nishimaki et al[25] showed that survival rates of patients with metastases to a single anatomical field were better than those with metastases to 2 fields, similar to another report.[26] Moreover, the number of patients who received adjuvant treatment was high (6 of 7 patients) compared with another study.[22] Therefore, although the number of patients is small in this study, those with a few metastatic nodes confined to a single ana-

Table 1. Clinicopathologic Features and Prognosis of Patients With T1 and T2 Esophageal Cancer

Variable	Patients, No. (%)	Survival Rate, %* 1 y	3 y	5 y	10 y	P
Sex						
Female	4 (6)	100	100	50	. . .	.97
Male	61 (94)	93	76	74	69	
Age, y						
≤65	37 (57)	91	73	64	64	.43
>65	28 (43)	96	84	84	73	
Tumor location						
Nonupper	59 (91)	92	81	76	71	.12
Upper	6 (9)	75	50	50	50	
Borrmann classification						
0, 1	42 (65)	97	87	87	81	.008
2, 3, 4	23 (35)	82	64	50	50	
Size of tumor, cm						
<4.0	31 (48)	100	90	90	81	.03
≥4.0	34 (52)	84	68	59	59	
Combined T, N factor						
pT1, pT2 NO	45 (69)	97	94	94	87	.001
pT2 N(+)	20 (31)	74	48	34	34	
Time of operation, min						
≤420	53 (82)	94	83	80	80	.01
>420	12 (18)	75	50	42	42	
Blood loss, mL						
<1000	49 (75)	95	85	81	76	.03
≥1000	16 (25)	74	60	50	50	
Histological differentiation						
Well	24 (37)	81	70	52	52	.21
Nonwell	41 (63)	97	82	75	75	
Lymph vessel invasion						
Not marked	60 (92)	91	82	77	73	.006
Marked	5 (8)	75	25	. . .	. . .	
Blood vessel invasion						
Not marked	60 (92)	92	79	74	70	.31
Marked	5 (8)	60	60	60	. . .	
Radiotherapy						
Yes	34 (52)	85	70	62	62	.09
No	31 (48)	96	90	90	72	

Ellipses indicate no survivors during this time.

tomical region who undergo proper adjuvant therapy are considered to be a group with an excellent prognosis, similar to those with pT1 N0 diseases.

By TNM classification,[12] pT1 N0 tumor is classified as stage I and pT2 N0 tumor as stage IIa. Stage pT2 N0 tumors, however, yielded an excellent survival rate that was similar to that of pT1 N0 diseases in the present study. Killinger et al[20] compared the survival results in stage II esophageal carcinoma and revealed that survival was not different between T1 N0 and T2 N0 disease (both 50% of 5-year survival rate; $P = .83$). They concluded that the distinction between these subgroups was not warranted. Similarly, Skinner et al[19] grouped submucosal (T1) and T2 tumors in 1 group because without any lymph node metastasis, patients with T1 and T2 tumors have similar survival. There are several possible explanations for such contradictory results. First, most reports included patients with esophageal carcinoma of different pathologic backgrounds, for example, squamous cell carcinoma and adenocarcinomas, making the interpretation difficult.[10,19,20] Second, we considered only disease-specific deaths to evaluate the prognosis, but most others[10,19,20] evaluated the prognosis as overall survival. Last, subtle variations among different institutions, surgeons, or patient characteristics could be another factor. Because our survival data are better than those previously reported, we assume that pT2 N0 disease should be categorized as a group with an excellent prognosis, similar to pT1 N0 tumors.

Table 2. Multivariate Analysis of Prognostic Factors for Survival Using a Cox Proportional Hazards Model

Variables*	Coefficient	P	Hazard Ratio	95% CI†
pT2 N(+)	1.90	.008	6.65	1.64-26.92
Time of operation	1.50	.16	4.50	0.55-37.02
Size of tumor	1.07	.11	2.91	0.78-10.90
Borrmann type	0.88	.13	2.40	0.76-7.55
Lymph vessel invasion	0.79	.28	2.20	0.53-9.10
Blood loss	−0.71	.52	0.49	0.06-4.27

*Variables are categorized as in Table 1.
†CI indicates confidence interval.*

Our results indicate that pT1 N(+) tumors with a few metastatic nodes confined to a single anatomical region and pT2 N0 tumors are considered to be a group with an excellent prognosis, similar to pT1 N0 diseases. However, once the tumor was metastasized to the lymph nodes, the prognosis of pT2 tumor became worse. To improve the prognosis of patients with pT2 N(+) tumors, meticulous lymph node dissection and extensive adjuvant therapy might be important.

Reprints: Mitsuo Tachibana, MD, Second Department of Surgery, Shimane Medical University, Enya-cho 89-1, Izumo 693-8501, Shimane, Japan (e-mail: nigeka33@shimane-med.ac.jp).

REFERENCES

1. Giuli R, Garnier HS. Diagnostic, therapeutic, and prognostic features of cancers of the esophagus: results of the international prospective study conducted by the OESO group (790 patients). *Surgery.* 1986;99:614-622.
2. Ellis FH, Gibb SP, Watkins E. Esophagogastrectomy: a safe, widely applicable, and expeditious form of palliation for patients with carcinoma of the esophagus and cardia. *Ann Surg.* 1983;198:531-540.
3. Skinner DB. En bloc resection for neoplasms of the esophagus and cardia. *J Thorac Cardiovasc Surg.* 1983;85:59-71.
4. Tachibana M, Yoshlmura H, Kinugasa S, et al. Clinicopathological features of superficial squamous cell carcinoma of the esophagus. *Am J Surg.* 1997;174:49-53.
5. Sugimachi K, Ohno S, Matsuda H, Mori M, Matsuoka H, Kuwano H. Clinicopathologic study of early stage esophageal carcinoma. *Surgery.* 1989;105:706-710.
6. Peracchia A, Ruol A, Bonavina L, et al. Early squamous cell carcinoma of the esophagus: diagnosis and management. *Dig Surg.* 1989;6:109-113.
7. Abe S, Tachibana M, Shimokawa T, Shiraishi M, Nakamura T. Surgical treatment of advanced carcinoma of the esophagus. *Surg Gynecol Obstet.* 1989;168:115-120.
8. Daly JM, Karnell LH, Menck HR. National cancer data base report on esophageal carcinoma. *Cancer.* 1996;78:1820-1828.
9. Iizuka T, Isono K, Kakegawa T, Watanabe H. Parameters linked to ten-year survival in Japan of resected esophageal carcinoma. *Chest.* 1989;96:1005-1011.
10. Ellis FH, Heatley GJ, Krasna MJ, Williamson WA, Balogh K. Esophagogastrectomy for carcinoma of the esophagus and cardia: a comparison of findings and results after standard resection in three consecutive eight-year intervals with improved staging criteria. *J Thorac Cardiovasc Surg.* 1997;113:836-848.
11. Orringer MB. Transhiatal esophagectomy without thoracotomy for carcinoma of the thoracic esophagus. *Ann Surg.* 1984;200:282-288.
12. UICC staff. *TNM Classification of Malignant Tumours.* 5th ed. New York, NY: Wiley-Liss Inc; 1997.
13. Kaplan EL, Meier P. Nonparametric estimation for incomplete observations. *J Am Stat Assoc.* 1958;53:457-481.
14. Cox DR. Regression models and life tables. *J R Stat Soc Ser B.* 1972;34:187-220.
15. Fok M, Law SYK, Wong J. Operable esophageal carcinoma: current results from Hong Kong. *World J Surg.* 1994;18:355-360.
16. Kato H, Tachimori Y, Watanabe H, Igaki H, Nakanishi Y, Ochlai A. Recurrent esophageal carcinoma after esophagectomy with three-field lymph node dissection. *J Surg Oncol.* 1996;61:267-272.
17. Junginger T, Dutkowski P. Selective approach to the treatment of oesophageal cancer. *Br J Surg.* 1996;83:1473-1477.
18. Ide H, Nakamura T, Hayashi K, et al. Esophageal squamous cell carcinoma: pathology and prognosis. *World J Surg.* 1994;18:321-330.
19. Skinner DB, Ferguson MK, Soriano A, Little AG, Staszak VM. Selection of operation for esophageal cancer based on staging. *Ann Surg.* 1986;204:391-401.
20. Killinger WA, Rice TW, Adelstein DJ, et al. Stage II esophageal carcinoma: the significance of T and N. *J Thorac Cardiovasc Surg.* 1996;111:935-940.
21. Yoshinaka H, Shimazu H, Fukumoto T, Baba M. Superficial esophageal carcinoma: a clinicopathological review of 59 cases. *Am J Gastroenterol.* 1991;86:1413-1418.
22. Kato H, Tachimori Y, Watanabe H, et al. Superficial esophageal carcinoma: surgical treatment and the results. *Cancer.* 1990;66:2319-2323.
23. Sugimachi K, Ikebe M, Kitamura K, Toh Y, Matsuda H, Kuwano H. Long-term results of esophagectomy for early esophageal carcinoma. *Hepatogastroenterology.* 1993;40:203-206.
24. Hoelscher AH, Bollschweiler E, Schneider PM, Siewert JR. Prognosis of early esophageal cancer: comparison between adeno- and squamous cell carcinoma. *Cancer.* 1995;76:178-186.
25. Nishimaki T, Suzuki T, Suzuki S, Kuwabara S, Hatakeyama K. Outcomes of extended radical esophagectomy for thoracic esophageal cancer. *J Am Coll Surg.* 1998;186:306-312.
26. Yano K, Okamura T, Yoshida Y, Ezaki T, Yasumoto K. The extent and number of metastatic lymph nodes limit the efficacy of lymphadenectomy in patients with oesophageal carcinoma. *Surg Oncol.* 1994;3:187-192.

ORIGINAL ARTICLE

Lower Esophageal Sphincter Dysfunction Often Precludes Safe Gastric Feeding in Stroke Patients

Charles E. Lucas, MD; Pingyang Yu, MD; Angie Vlahos, MS; Anna M. Ledgerwood, MD

Objectives: To determine the relationship between stroke and lower esophageal dysfunction with vomiting and to identify an optimal nutrition protocol based on our findings.

Patients and Methods: The lower and upper esophageal sphincter functions were assessed in 35 patients who had an acute stroke to determine whether gastric or jejunal enteral feeding was the optimal route. Stroke was due to unilateral ischemia in 20 patients, unilateral intracerebral hemorrhage in 8 patients, and global ischemia in 7 patients. Our study consisted of 18 men and 17 women with an average age of 64 years.

Results: Using standard esophageal manometric definitions, the lower esophageal sphincter function was below normal in 24 patients: 3 had global anoxia, 5 had unilateral hemorrhage, and 16 had unilateral ischemia. The upper esophageal sphincter function was low in 30 patients: 6 had global anoxia, 7 had unilateral hemorrhage, and 17 had unilateral ischemia. Based on lower esophageal sphincter pressure, 7 patients underwent tube gastrostomy and 13 patients underwent tube jejunostomy placement. All tolerated enteral alimentation well. Prior to lower esophageal sphincter assessment, 4 patients had percutaneous endoscopy gastrostomy feedings that led to aspiration pneumonitis and consultation for tracheostomy; 2 terminally ill patients were referred to the ethics service, and 2 were converted to feeding via jejunostomy tube at the time of tracheostomy and did well.

Conclusions: Vomiting with aspiration due to lower esophageal sphincter dysfunction is common after acute strokes. Esophageal manometry serves as a guide to find the optimal feeding route.

Arch Surg. 1999;134:55-58

An acute cerebral vascular stroke can lead to multiple problems, both short term and in convalescence. The first challenge is to overcome the life-threatening insults caused by the brain injury and the loss of many central regulatory systems. After surviving the acute phase, the patient enters the recuperative period when many other threats related to independent airway control, nutrition, and mobility must be faced. Success during this phase is strongly influenced by the restitution of an alimental diet.

Following stroke, oral deglutition is often impaired because of central hypopharyngeal dysfunction.[1,2] Attempts at oral feeding are frustrated by aspiration; aspiration pneumonia is a common cause of death following stroke.[3] This hazard may be circumvented by small intragastric feedings through narrow, specifically designed, gastric feeding tubes. The surgeon can be consulted later for placement of a more permanent intragastric feeding tube such as a percutaneous endoscopic gastrostomy.[4-6] Vomiting with aspiration pneumonitis, however, is a frequent complication of intragastric feedings whether given by nasogastric tube or percutaneous endoscopic gastrostomy feedings,[7,8] and is a common cause of death for patients in long-term care facilities.[9]

Prior studies have demonstrated that acute head injury causes a temporary reduction in lower esophageal sphincter (LES) function.[10] Such patients are at high risk for aspiration pneumonitis. Our study was designed to assess esophageal function in patients who had a stroke and were referred to us for feeding tube placement and to identify an optimal nutrition protocol based on our findings. These patients can then be restored to a full alimental diet.

From the Department of Surgery, Wayne State University, Detroit, Mich.

RESULTS

The esophageal manometry was well tolerated by all patients; there were no com-

PATIENTS AND METHODS

Esophageal function was assessed by esophageal manometry in 35 patients who had an acute stroke. All 35 patients were seen in consultation for performance of a tracheostomy for respiratory failure and pneumonia, for placement of a feeding tube for alimental nutrition, or for both. There were 18 men and 17 women with an average age of 64 years (range, 39-100 years). The cause of the acute stroke was unilateral ischemia in 20 patients, unilateral intracerebral hemorrhage in 8 patients, and global ischemia in 7 patients. All 35 patients had severe strokes, with complete unilateral deficits after focal ischemic insults and coma after global ischemia. Although modest neurologic improvement was present at the time of consultation in some patients, all had severe residual deficits. Esophageal manometry was performed during the second week after stroke in 14 patients, during the third week after stroke in 12 patients, and between the third and sixth week after stroke in 9 patients. All patients were receiving histamine$_2$ blocker as prophylaxis for short-term, erosive gastritis. Twenty-six patients received antibiotics (often for aspiration pneumonia), 12 received antihypertensive medicines, and 7 received inotropic support. A detailed history of gastroesophageal reflux disease was difficult to obtain because of the communication impairment but 1 patient was treated for prior symptoms suggestive of reflux esophagitis.

The technique for esophageal manometry has been previously described.[10] Esophageal manometry with direct testing of LES and upper esophageal sphincter (UES) tone was performed with a 3-channel probe connected through appropriate transducers to a computer-based (Sandhill, Sandhill Scientific, Highlands Ranch, Colo) manometric system.[11,12] The esophageal manometric probe is a standard 3-transducer probe with the pressure sensors set at 5-cm intervals near the distal end of the probe. The probe was placed through the nose to a depth of 70 cm and a gastric baseline value was obtained. This measurement was considered the 0 point. The probe was then withdrawn at 5-cm intervals and both continuous and interval manometric measurements were obtained. All ancillary activity during the manometric testing was noted (ie, swallowing, coughing, and suctioning). These events caused a transient artifact in the ongoing measurements and were discounted. The continuous data measurements captured events that did not occur at a set interval,[11,12] and the interval measurements allowed for study of an area to note any changes in tone over time.[10] All 35 patients were given histamine$_2$ blockers as prophylaxis against short-term, erosive gastritis, precluding pH monitoring of reflux from the stomach into the esophagus. All values are expressed as mean±SE.

plications. The LES pressure averaged 15.2+3.01 mm Hg and the UES pressure averaged 23.9±3.75 mm Hg. Both the LES pressure (14 mm Hg) in 24 patients and the UES pressure (40 mm Hg) in 30 patients were below normal (**Table 1**). The 20 patients who had ischemic unilateral strokes had the lowest LES pressure, averaging 12.5±4.5 mm Hg, 4 of whom had an LES pressure above 14 mm Hg. The LES pressure in the 8 patients who had unilateral intracerebral hemorrhagic strokes averaged 17.8±4.6 mm Hg, 5 of whom had an LES pressure below 14 mm Hg (Table 1). The 7 patients who had global ischemia had an average LES pressure of 19.9±6.0 mm Hg, 3 of whom had a low LES pressure (Table 1). The LES and UES pressures were significantly ($P<.05$, unpaired Student t test) below those seen in normal volunteers (LES, 29±2.6; UES, 47±5.6) and in patients with head and neck cancer referred for feeding tube placement (LES, 27.5±5.6).

The UES pressure in the 20 patients who had ischemic strokes averaged 23.6±4.4 mm Hg, 17 of whom had a UES pressure below 40 mm Hg (**Table 2**). The UES pressure in the 8 patients who had unilateral intracerebral hemorrhagic strokes averaged 23.9±11.82; 7 of 8 patients had a UES pressure below 40 mm Hg (Table 2). The UES pressure in the 7 patients who had global ischemia averaged 25±6.04 mm Hg, 6 of whom had a low UES pressure (Table 2). These pressures were significantly lower ($P<.05$) than the UES pressure in normal volunteers.

The decision on the technique for alimental feedings was based on the LES manometric studies. Thirteen patients who had progressive illness died or were referred to the ethics service and never received an operative feeding tube, including 9 patients with low LES pressure and 4 patients with normal LES pressure. Two patients' conditions improved and did not require a feeding tube. The remaining 12 patients with low LES pressure underwent an open feeding jejunostomy; all these patients tolerated their jejunal feedings without aspiration of the liquid diet. Many patients, however, exhibited a syndrome of increased gastric and biliary secretions that were sectioned from the nasogastric tube during the first 1 or 2 weeks of jejunal feedings. This common phenomenon of cryptic origin has been previously described; prevention of aspiration of the gastric and biliary commends requires continued nasogastric suction while the tube feedings are advanced.[13] The addition of blue dye to the tube feedings confirmed that this nasogastric effluent had no blue discoloration and was not tube feeding.[13] The remaining 8 patients with normal LES function were treated by feeding gastrostomy in 7 patients and by a feeding jejunostomy in 1 patient; this latter patient had prior vomiting of nasogastric tube feedings, biasing the surgeon to perform a feeding jejunostomy. The patients with gastrostomy, performed by either the open or percutaneous technique, tolerated the tube feedings without vomiting and aspiration. All 20 patients tolerated tube feeding and were transferred to a rehabilitation hospital or long-term care facility with tube feeding as the sole source of nutrition. Tolerance of the tube feeding persisted until discharge from the rehabilitation institute. Most patients' conditions improved during the rehabilitation care. Four patients regained normal swallowing and had the feeding tube removed; none had a second esophageal manometry at this time. The other patients

Table 1. Lower Esophageal Sphincter (LES) Studies

Characteristics	LES, mm Hg		LES ≥ 14 mm Hg		LES < 14 mm Hg	
	Mean ± SE	Patients, No.	Mean ± SE	Patients, No.	Mean ± SE	Patients, No.
Patients, total No.	15.17 ± 3.01	**35**	32.29 ± 7.26	**11**	7.33 ± 0.75	**24**
Patients with						
Global anoxia	19.89 ± 5.96	7	28.01 ± 8.41	4	9.06 ± 2.13	3
Focal hemorrhage	17.75 ± 4.62	8	32.09 ± 4.48	3	9.15 ± 2.09	5
Focal ischemia	12.45 ± 4.52	20	36.73 ± 19.74	4	6.43 ± 0.80	16

Table 2. Upper Esophageal Sphincter (UES) Studies

Characteristics	UES, mm Hg		UES ≥ 40 mm Hg		UES < 40 mm Hg	
	Mean ± SE	Patients, No.	Mean ± SE	Patients, No.	Mean ± SE	Patients, No.
Patients, total No.	23.90 ± 3.75	**35**	65.23 ± 10.44	**5**	17.06 ± 2.29	**30**
Patients with						
Global anoxia	24.99 ± 6.04	7	44.40 ± 0.00	1	21.75 ± 6.04	6
Focal hemorrhage	23.93 ± 11.82	8	103.10 ± 0.00	1	12.62 ± 3.97	7
Focal ischemia	23.58 ± 4.40	20	59.56 ± 6.01	3	17.23 ± 3.07	17

were lost to follow up after discharge from the rehabilitation hospital.

Four patients were initially consulted for tracheostomy for pneumonitis that developed from aspiration of percutaneous endoscopic gastrostomy feeding. The percutaneous endoscopic gastrostomy, in each instance, had been placed without manometric studies. All 4 patients had low LES tone. The tracheostomy was done in conjunction with percutaneous endoscopic gastrostomy tube removal and placement of an open feeding jejunostomy in 2 patients who rapidly recovered from pneumonitis when they were no longer aspirating intragastric feedings. Both patients tolerated jejunal feedings without vomiting. The other 2 patients had progression of the brain deficit after the onset of aspiration pneumonitis and were transferred to the ethics service.

COMMENT

Many patients who have acute strokes die within 96 hours from the extensive brain injury or associated diseases complicated by the acute stroke. Other patients recover quickly and are able to tolerate a carefully administered and slowly advanced oral diet. The remaining patients require multidisciplinary support as they enter the recuperative phase. A key element in the successful treatment of these patients is the successful institution of alimental nutrition.

During the early poststroke period, when central nervous system dysfunction, adynamic ileus, abdominal distention, and pulmonary distress are paramount, nutrition typically is provided by the intravenous route. Once this acute phase has passed and the adynamic ileus has resolved, the patient should be assessed for hypopharyngeal function and swallowing proficiency. Some patients exhibit adequate swallowing and oral feeding may be carefully started. Presumably, these patients have normal esophageal manometries, although no measurements of LES and UES pressures have been reported in patients who had a stroke and with normal swallowing. Acute stroke often impairs swallowing due to the injurious effects on the cranial nerves that modulate deglutition.[14] When doubt exists about tolerance of oral feedings, a swallowing test can determine if there is evidence of aspiration associated with swallowing.[14] There may also be patients who do not seem to aspirate during a swallowing test but then develop the clinical findings of aspiration pneumonitis.[3] When oral feedings are not tolerated because of hypopharyngeal dysfunction, intragastric feedings should be instituted. Patients who tolerate the intragastric feedings will probably tolerate gastric tube feedings. The benefits of the intragastric route relate both to the maintenance of immunological competence of alimental feedings and the ability to give bolus feedings. Nasogastric tube feedings with monitoring residual volume predicts successful tolerance of gastric tube feedings; however, cryptic vomiting with aspiration may recur and be evidenced by the development of recurrent or worsening pneumonitis. This sequence presages LES dysfunction and can be quickly and safely identified by esophageal manometry. If the LES function is low, the patient requires intrajejunal feedings that can be instituted by an endoscopically placed tube or by open laparotomy. The manometric assessment of LES function, identified herein, seems to accurately define whether a patient should receive a tube gastrostomy or a tube jejunostomy.

These studies identify an interesting but small subgroup of patients who have a normal LES function, but a low UES function. The current level of experience with this subgroup of patients is too small to predict what type of feeding is most desirable. Clearly, more study is needed to identify whether these patients are candidates for intragastric or intrajejunal feeding.

This study was supported by account 4-44966, of the Interstitial Fluid Fund (Dr Lucas).

Reprints: Charles E. Lucas, MD, Department of Surgery, Wayne State University, 420 St Antoine, Room 2V, Detroit, MI 48201.

REFERENCES

1. Logemann J. Swallowing disorders asssociated with neuromuscular disorders. In: *Evaluation and Treatment of Swallowing Disorders.* San Diego, Calif: College-Hill Press; 1983:214-215.
2. Friedman L, Castell D. Esophageal diseases in the elderly. In: Castell D, ed. *The Esophagus.* 2nd ed. Boston, Mass: Little Brown & Co Inc; 1995:778-779.
3. Holas MA, DePippo KL, Reding MJ. Aspiration and relative risk of medical complications following stroke. *Arch Neurol.* 1994;51:1051-1053.
4. Steffes C, Weaver DW, Bouwman DL. Percutaneous endoscopic gastrostomy: new technique—old complications. *Am Surg.* 1989;5:273-277.
5. Larson DE, Burton DD, Schroeder KW, DiMagno EP. Percutaneous endoscopic gastrostomy: indications, success, complications and mortality in 314 consecutive patients. *Gastroenterology.* 1987;93:48-52.
6. Foutch PG, Haynes WC, Bellapravalu S, Sanowski RA. Percutaneous endoscopic gastrostomy: a new procedure comes of age. *J Clin Gastroenterol.* 1986; 8:10-15.
7. Hassett JM, Sunby C, Flint L. No elimination of aspiration in neurologically disabled patients with feeding gastrostomy. *Surg Gynecol Obstet.* 1988;167: 383-388.
8. Olivares L, Segovia A, Revuelta R. Tube feeding and lethal aspiration in neurological patients: a review of 720 autopsy cases. *Stroke.* 1974;5:654-657.
9. Cogen R, Weinry GJ, Pomerantz C, Fenstemacher P. Complications of jejunostomy tube feedings in nursing facility patients. *Am J Gastroenterol.* 1991;86: 1610-1613.
10. Saxe JM, Ledgerwood AM, Lucas CE, Lucas WF. Lower esophageal sphincter dysfunction precludes safe gastric feeding after head injury. *J Trauma.* 1994;37: 581-586.
11. Castell JA, Dalton CB, Castell DO. On-line computer analysis of human lower esophageal sphincter relaxation. *Am J Physiol.* 1988;255:G794.
12. Castell JA, Castell DO. Computer analysis of human esophageal peristalsis and lower esophageal sphincter pressure, II: an interactive system for on-line data collection and analysis. *Dig Dis Sci.* 1986;31:1211.
13. McGonigal MD, Lucas CE, Ledgerwood AM. Feeding jejunostomy in patients who are critically ill. *Surg Gynecol Obstet.* 1989;168:275-277.
14. Gordon C, Hewer RL, Wade DT. Dysphagia in acute stroke. *BMJ.* 1987;295: 411-414.

IN OTHER AMA JOURNALS

JAMA

Finding and Applying Evidence During Clinical Rounds: The "Evidence Cart"

David L. Sackett, MD; Sharon E. Straus, MD; for Firm A of the Nuffield Department of Medicine

Context: Physicians need easy access to evidence for clinical decisions while they care for patients but, to our knowledge, no investigators have assessed use of evidence during rounds with house staff.
Objective: To determine if it was feasible to find and apply evidence during clinical rounds, using an "evidence cart" that contains multiple sources of evidence and the means for projecting and printing them.
Design: Descriptive feasibility study of use of evidence during 1 month (April 1997) and anonymous questionnaire (May 1997).
Setting: General medicine inpatient service.
Patients: Medical students, house staff, fellows, and attending consultant.
Intervention: Evidence cart that included 2 secondary sources developed by the department (critically appraised topics [CATs] and Redbook), *Best Evidence*, *JAMA* Rational Clinical Examination series, the Cochrane Library, MEDLINE, a physical examination textbook, a radiology anatomy textbook, and a Simulscope, which allows several people to listen simultaneously to the same signs on physical examination.
Main Outcome Measures: Number of times sources were used, type of sources searched and success of searches, time needed to search, and whether the search affected patient care.
Results: The evidence cart was used 98 times, but could not be taken on bedside rounds because of its bulk; hard copies of several sources were taken instead. When the evidence cart was used during team rounds and student rounds, some sources could be accessed quickly enough (10.2-25.4 seconds) to be practical on our service. Of 98 searches, 79 (81%) sought evidence that could affect diagnostic and/or treatment decisions. Seventy-one (90%) of 79 searches regarding patient management were successful, and when assessed from the perspective of the most junior team members responsible for each patient's evaluation and management, 37 (52%) of the 71 successful searches confirmed their current or tentative diagnostic or treatment plans, 18 (25%) led to a new diagnostic skill, an additional test, or a new management decision, and 16 (23%) corrected a previous clinical skill, diagnostic test, or treatment. When the cart was removed, the perceived need for evidence rose sharply, but a search for it was carried out only 12% of the time (5 searches performed out of the 41 times evidence was needed).
Conclusions: Making evidence quickly available to clinicians on a busy medical inpatient service using an evidence cart increased the extent to which evidence was sought and incorporated into patient care decisions. *(1998;280:1336-13380)*

Reprints: David L. Sackett, MD, NHS R & D Centre for Evidence-Based Medicine, Level 5, John Radcliffe Hospital, Headington, Oxford OX3 9DU, England (e-mail: sackett@cebm.jr2.ox.ac.uk).

ORIGINAL ARTICLE

Changes in Respiratory Mechanics After Tracheostomy

Kenneth Davis, Jr, MD; Robert S. Campbell, RRT; Jay A. Johannigman, MD; John F. Valente, MD; Richard D. Branson, BA, RRT

Objective: To determine the effects of tracheostomy on respiratory mechanics and work of breathing (WOB).

Design: A before-and-after trial of 20 patients undergoing tracheostomy for repeated extubation failure.

Setting: Surgical intensive care unit at a university teaching hospital and a level I trauma center.

Patients: A consecutive sample of 20 patients who met extubation criteria (PaO_2, >55 mm Hg; pH >7.30; and respiratory rate, <30/min on room air continuous positive airway pressure after 20 minutes) but failed extubation on 2 occasions were eligible for the study.

Interventions: Respiratory mechanics, lung volumes, and WOB were measured before and after tracheostomy.

Main Outcome Measures: Patients in whom extubation fails often progress to unassisted ventilation after tracheostomy. The study hypothesis was that tracheostomy would result in improved pulmonary function through changes in respiratory mechanics.

Results: Data are given as means ± SDs. After tracheostomy, WOB per liter of ventilation (0.97 ± 0.32 vs 0.81 ± 0.46 J/L; $P<.09$), WOB per minute (8.9 ± 2.9 vs 6.6 ± 1.4 J/min; $P<.04$), and airway resistance (9.4 ± 4.1 vs 6.3 ± 4.5 cm H_2O/L per second; $P<.07$) were reduced compared with breathing via an endotracheal tube. These findings, however, do not fully explain the ability of patients to be liberated from mechanical ventilation after tracheostomy. In 4 patients who were extubated before tracheostomy, WOB was significantly greater during extubation than when breathing through an endotracheal or tracheostomy tube (1.2 ± 0.19 vs 0.81 ± 0.24 vs 0.77 ± 0.22 J/L).

Conclusions: We believe that the rigid nature of the tracheostomy tube represents reduced imposed WOB compared with the longer, thermoliable endotracheal tube. The clinical significance of this effect is small, although as respiratory rate increases, the effects are magnified. In patients in whom extubation failed, WOB may be elevated because of incomplete control of the upper airway. Future studies should evaluate the cause of increased WOB after extubation.

Arch Surg. 1999;134:59-62

THE TIMING of tracheostomy during the treatment of respiratory failure remains controversial.[1-3] Results of a recent report[4] suggest that early tracheostomy does not impact intensive care unit length of stay, incidence of pneumonia, or mortality compared with continued translaryngeal intubation. Yet, tracheostomy often results in clinical improvement in respiratory function and liberation from mechanical ventilation. The exact mechanisms for this improvement remain ill-defined.

Differences in work of breathing (WOB) and pressure time product (PTP) between endotracheal and tracheostomy tubes of the same internal diameter in a lung model were previously studied.[5] A slight reduction in WOB with tracheostomy tubes was found owing to a shorter length and more rigid form. Wright et al[6] demonstrated that the in vivo resistance of endotracheal tubes exceeds the in vitro resistance because of thermoliability of materials and the tortuous translaryngeal path. Davis et al[5] also showed that the misconception that tracheostomy significantly reduces dead space is mere myth.

Despite these findings, the mechanism by which tracheostomy allows weaning from mechanical ventilation after failed extubation attempts remains elusive. This study compares the changes in respiratory mechanics before and after tracheostomy in a group of non–head-injured surgical patients in whom extubation failed on 2 occasions.

RESULTS

There were statistically significant reductions in WOB per minute (8.9 ± 2.9 vs 6.6 ± 1.4 J/L per minute; $P = .04$), and PEEP

From the Division of Trauma and Critical Care, Department of Surgery, University of Cincinnati, Cincinnati, Ohio.

PATIENTS, MATERIALS, AND METHODS

Twenty patients (14 men and 6 women) were studied. All patients were recovering from acute lung injury and were intubated orally via a size 7.0 (n = 4) or 8.0 (n = 16) endotracheal tube. Mean ± SD age of the patients was 58 ± 13 years (range, 26-70 years). Mean ± SD duration of ventilatory support before the study was 16 ± 3.3 days (range, 9-23 days). Mean ± SD static compliance for the group was 49 ± 6 mL/cm H_2O (range, 39-61 mL/cm H_2O). All patients had been weaned to a fraction of inspired oxygen (FIO_2) concentration of less than 0.45, a positive end-expiratory pressure (PEEP) of 5 cm H_2O, and a pressure support of less than 10 cm H_2O. Thirteen patients were injured in motor vehicle crashes, 5 patients had undergone repair of abdominal aortic aneurysms, and 2 patients had aspiration pneumonia after major abdominal surgery.

All patients were receiving enteral nutritional support via nasoenteric tubes. Energy (calorie) needs were measured by indirect calorimetry and were adjusted 1 to 2 times per week. Sedation was accomplished with administration of fentanyl citrate or haloperidol lactate as needed.

All patients had resolution of their primary lung injury and were judged ready for extubation by the intensive care unit service. All patients underwent a room air continuous positive airway pressure (CPAP) trial at 5 cm H_2O with no pressure support. After 20 minutes, an arterial blood sample was obtained and was analyzed for pH, $PaCO_2$, PaO_2, and oxygen saturation. If the patient's PaO_2 was greater than 55 mm Hg, spontaneous respiratory rate was less than 30/min, pH was greater than 7.30, and tidal volume was greater than 4 mL/kg, the CPAP trial was considered "passed." Subjective observation of the patient's mental status, ability to control the airway, and ability to handle secretions were made by the intensive care unit physicians and staff. If these were considered adequate, the patient was extubated.

In all study patients, extubation failed on 2 occasions after all the extubation criteria were met. We chose to study these patients based on our previous observations that after repeated extubation failure, many patients are liberated from the ventilator after tracheostomy. By choosing patients with 2 previous extubation failures, we believe our chances of finding differences in measured variables would be enhanced. The reasons for failure included hypoxemia (n = 9), hypercarbia (n = 3), excessive secretions (n = 3), and a combination of the 3 (n = 5). Each patient was scheduled for tracheostomy by the attending physician to aid in weaning from ventilatory support. The protocol was approved by the institutional review board of the University of Cincinnati, Cincinnati, Ohio, and informed consent was obtained.

Six to 10 hours before tracheostomy, patients had an esophageal balloon inserted transnasally (SmartCath, Bicore Monitoring Systems, Irvine, Calif) into the distal third of the esophagus to monitor esophageal pressure (Pes). Patients were placed in the semi-Fowler position with the head elevated a minimum of 30°. Correct placement of the balloon was confirmed using an airway occlusion test, as described by Baydur et al.[7] A variable orifice flow transducer and pressure tap (VariFlex, Bicore Monitoring Systems) was placed on the end of the endotracheal tube to monitor airway flow and pressure. Signals from the flow transducer and esophageal balloon were transmitted to a portable respiratory monitor (Bicore CP-100, Bicore Monitoring Systems). The performance of this device has been validated elsewhere and found to be accurate for clinical measurements.[8] Patients were disconnected from the ventilator and allowed to breathe via a continuous flow of gas at an FIO_2 concentration equal to that set on the ventilator.

After 10 minutes of stabilization, measurements were made. The following variables were measured: tidal volume, respiratory rate, airway pressure, flow, and Pes. These measurements were used to determine all other variables. Work of breathing was expressed in joules per liter and was calculated from the area subtended by the Pes created during inspiration and the relaxation curve of the chest wall (estimated chest wall compliance was 200 mL/cm H_2O). Pressure time product, an estimate of respiratory muscle metabolic work, was measured as the integral Pes and the duration of respiratory muscle contraction and expressed in centimeters of water per second per minute. Intrinsic PEEP was calculated as the difference in Pes from the end of expiration to the initiation of inspiratory flow. Expiratory airway resistance was calculated from the difference in transpulmonary pressure (airway pressure–Pes) divided by the difference in flow. All signals were recorded continuously for 10 minutes and were stored breath by breath in a personal computer for later analysis.

Ten to 12 hours after tracheostomy, the same measurements were repeated. This time was allowed to eliminate the effects of anesthetic agents on respiratory function. As before, the patient was disconnected from the ventilator and allowed to breathe from a continuous flow of gas at the previous FIO_2 concentration. The flow transducer was placed on the proximal end of the tracheostomy tube, and placement of the esophageal catheter was reconfirmed or adjusted as necessary.

Four patients were extubated before tracheostomy and were reintubated. Two patients were extubated at the attending physician's request and 2 patients were self-extubated. In these patients, the same variables were measured while the patients breathed through a mouthpiece.

Data are represented as mean ± SD, and each point represents the average of at least 40 breaths during the 10-minute measurement. Data before and after tracheostomy were compared using a paired t test. A probability of less than .05 was considered significant.

(2.9 ± 1.7 vs 1.6 ± 1.0 cm H_2O; $P = .02$). There was a tendency toward reductions in PTP, expiratory airway resistance, and WOB (joules per liter).

Posttracheostomy tidal volume was reduced slightly (329 ± 104 vs 312 ± 119 mL; $P = .47$), as was respiratory rate (28 ± 5 vs 26 ± 6/min; $P = .51$). **Table 1** depicts the data from the study. All patients were successfully weaned to an FIO_2 concentration of 0.40 delivered via a high-flow aerosol system through a tracheostomy collar within 24 hours of tracheostomy (duration, 8 ± 3 hours; range, 2-15 hours).

In each of the 4 patients who were extubated before tracheostomy, there was a significant increase in WOB (**Figure**) during extubation compared with breathing via an endotracheal or tracheostomy tube. Tidal volume increased, as did respiratory rate and other variables (**Table 2**).

Table 1. Changes in Respiratory Variables Before and After Tracheostomy

Variable	Before Tracheostomy	After Tracheostomy	*P*
Tidal volume, mL/breath	329 ± 104	312 ± 119	.47
Minute volume, L/min	9.2 ± 3.0	8.1 ± 3.1	.26
Respiratory rate, breaths/min	28 ± 5	26 ± 6	.51
Intrinsic positive end-expiratory pressure, cm H_2O	2.9 ± 1.7	1.6 ± 1.0	.02
Pressure time product, cm H_2O/s per minute	236 ± 122	155 ± 101	.09
Work of breathing, J/L	0.97 ± 0.32	0.81 ± 0.46	.09
Work of breathing, J/min	8.9 ± 2.9	6.6 ± 1.4	.04
Expiratory airway resistance, cm H_2O/L per second	9.4 ± 4.1	6.3 ± 4.5	.07

Table 2. Changes in Respiratory Variables in 4 Patients Who Were Extubated Before Tracheostomy

Variable	Endotracheal Tube	Extubated	Tracheostomy
Tidal volume, mL/breath	383 ± 107	429 ± 124	378 ± 81
Minute volume, L/min	11.1 ± 3.1	14.5 ± 4.2	10.6 ± 2.7
Respiratory rate, breaths/min	29 ± 8	34 ± 6	28 ± 5
Pressure time product, cm H_2O/s per minute	277 ± 109	328 ± 132	252 ± 97
Work of breathing, J/L	0.8 ± 0.2	1.2 ± 0.2	0.8 ± 0.2
Work of breathing, J/min	9.0 ± 2.7	17.4 ± 2.8	8.2 ± 2.2

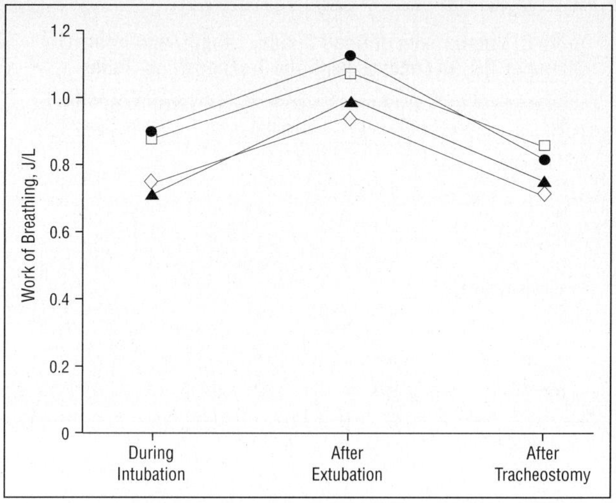

Changes in the work of breathing in 4 patients during endotracheal intubation, after extubation, and after tracheostomy.

COMMENT

The major findings of this study suggest that after tracheostomy, WOB and airway resistance are reduced compared with breathing via an endotracheal tube. These findings agree with laboratory results[5] comparing WOB between endotracheal and tracheostomy tubes in a lung model. These changes are, however, small and in our opinion do not fully explain facilitated weaning often seen after tracheostomy. However, the improvements seen when breathing through a tracheostomy tube are magnified as respiratory rate and tidal volume increase. Another important finding is the statistically and clinically significant increase in WOB after extubation compared with breathing via either a tracheostomy or endotracheal tube.

The imposed WOB caused by the presence of an endotracheal tube has been studied by numerous investigators.[8-12] Decreasing the diameter of the tube and increasing flow (patient demand) through the tube increase the imposed work. Internal diameter is the most important factor, as described by the Poiseuille law, in which pressure drop across the tube is inversely proportional to the fourth power of the radius during laminar flow. In the presence of turbulent flow, pressure drop increases by the fifth power of the radius.

Compared with the number of studies evaluating the untoward effects of the endotracheal tube on respiratory work, the tracheostomy tube has been relatively ignored. Cullen[13] evaluated the effects of tracheostomy in 14 patients with chronic obstructive pulmonary disease. He found that compared with mouth breathing, tracheostomy resulted in a reduction in physiologic dead space, a slight decrease in oxygen consumption, and a slight increase in airway resistance. This work is not immediately applicable to our study because of the difference in patient disease and absence of the endotracheal tube. Cavo et al[14] found that tracheostomy tubes created airway resistance greater than that imposed by the normal upper airway. As expected, decreasing diameter resulted in greater resistance. These authors suggested that the largest diameter tube be used for prolonged tracheostomy. Yung and Snowdon[15] evaluated the resistance of 3 varieties of tracheostomy tubes in the laboratory. They found that design (radius of curvature and roughness of the inner surface) and length of the tube were important in determining resistance.

Results of a previous laboratory study[5] demonstrate that for equivalent inside diameter, endotracheal tubes created greater imposed work than did tracheostomy tubes. We believe that the additional length of the endotracheal tube contributes to the increased resistance but that the major contributor is the tortuous path traveled by the endotracheal tube. In our laboratory study, the endotracheal tube was placed through the upper airway of a resuscitation mannequin. In previous comparisons of endotracheal and tracheostomy tubes, both were placed on the bench top. Comparison of endotracheal and tracheostomy tubes in vivo, as accomplished in this study, seems to support this hypothesis. There were decreases in WOB (joules per liter and joules per minute), PTP, airway resistance, intrinsic PEEP, and minute volume after tracheostomy. These changes represent trends in many instances but seem to suggest that tracheostomy improves the efficiency of breathing compared with breathing via an endotracheal tube. In addition, Wright et al[6] found that the in vivo resistance of endotracheal tubes was significantly greater than anticipated from in vitro studies. They attributed this finding to changes in the shape of the thermolabile endotracheal tubes and adherence of secretions to the inner lumen. Wright et al also demonstrated that flow through endotracheal tubes in vivo was turbulent, causing resistance

Table 3. Comparison of Dead Space, Length, and Internal Diameter (ID) of Endotracheal and Tracheostomy Tubes

Tube	ID, mm	Length, cm	Dead Space, mL
Endotracheal			
No. 6.0	6.0	31.5	11.0
No. 7.0	7.0	34.5	15.0
No. 8.0	8.0	35.5	18.0
No. 8.5	8.5	36.5	24.0
Tracheostomy*			
Size 4	5.0	10.0	3.0
Size 6	7.0	12.0	5.0
Size 8	8.5	12.0	6.0
Size 10	9.0	12.0	8.0

**Note that tracheostomy tube size is not equal to ID.*

to increase with decreasing diameter to the fifth power of the radius.

Our results did not show any difference in tidal volume before and after tracheostomy. It is a misconception that tracheostomy reduces dead space. Compared with mouth breathing, tracheostomy can reduce dead space, as shown by Cullen.[13] However, the added length of the endotracheal tube only results in an increase in dead space of 10 to 18 mL. **Table 3** compares dead space, length, and internal diameter values for endotracheal and tracheostomy tubes used in this study.

The genesis for this study lies in the frequent observation that patients in whom extubation repeatedly fails are quickly weaned from mechanical ventilation after tracheostomy. Results of this study suggest that tracheostomy reduces respiratory work, although this reduction may not be the only explanation. We believe the finding that patients have significant increases in respiratory work after extubation may be the most important finding of our trial. The ability to wean a patient from mechanical ventilation after tracheostomy frequently occurs after failed extubation attempts. In these patients, tracheostomy allows improved secretion clearance, allows simple initiation and discontinuation of ventilatory support, and eliminates the variable of upper airway control. Extubation criteria are frequently quoted with the caveat "ability to control the upper airway." This nebulous definition is subjective and difficult to quantify yet seemingly critically important.

Nathan et al[16] had similar findings during a study designed to use pressure support to overcome the imposed WOB caused by the endotracheal tube. They found that compared with breathing through an endotracheal tube, the WOB and PTP were increased after extubation. The increase in WOB was nearly 30% (0.74 vs 1.04 J/L) and was statistically significant. They also found the presence of "fluttering" in the flow-volume tracings of the patients who were extubated. This finding is often seen in patients with upper airway obstruction, and the authors hypothesized that after extubation, lack of upper airway control causes increased respiratory work. In a follow-up study, Ishaaya et al[17] measured tracheal and glottic diameter after extubation. They confirmed their previous results, finding a consistent increase in WOB after extubation compared with endotracheal tube breathing. However, they did not find evidence of airway narrowing. In fact, the cross-sectional area of the intact upper airway was 3 times that of the endotracheal tube. This finding may suggest that the site of upper airway narrowing is in the oropharynx. If upper airway closure in this instance is similar to that seen during sleep apnea, the use of CPAP by mask or noninvasive ventilation may be helpful. DeHaven et al[18] used CPAP by face mask to treat postextubation hypoxemia successfully.

Results of this study suggest that after tracheostomy, WOB and PTP are reduced compared with breathing through an endotracheal tube. These findings are due to reduced resistance of the tracheostomy tube compared with the thermoliable endotracheal tube, which can become deformed in the upper airway. During extubation, patients with inadequate upper airway control have WOB greater than during spontaneous breathing through either type of artificial airway. Successful discontinuation of mechanical ventilation after tracheostomy represents improved airway control compared with spontaneous breathing via the intact upper airway in select patients. The improvements in respiratory efficiency after tracheostomy compared with endotracheal tube breathing are small and unlikely to fully explain the ability to discontinue mechanical ventilation after tracheostomy.

Reprints: Kenneth Davis, Jr, MD, Division of Trauma and Critical Care, Department of Surgery, University of Cincinnati Medical Center, 231 Bethesda Ave, ML 0558, Cincinnati, OH 45267-0558 (e-mail: Kenneth.Davis@UC.edu).

REFERENCES

1. Lewis RJ. Tracheostomies: indications, timing, and complications. *Clin Chest Med.* 1992;13:137-149.
2. Rodriguez JL, Steinberg SM, Luchette FA, Gibbons KJ, Taheri PA, Flint LM. Early tracheostomy for primary airway management in the surgical care setting. *Surgery.* 1990;108:655-659.
3. Plummer AL, Gracey DR. Consensus conference on artificial airways in patients receiving mechanical ventilation. *Chest.* 1989;96:178-180.
4. Sugerman HJ, Wolfe L, Pasquale MD, et al. Multicenter, randomized, prospective trial of early tracheostomy. *J Trauma Injury Infect Crit Care.* 1997;43:741-747.
5. Davis K Jr, Branson RD, Porembka D. A comparison of the imposed work of breathing with endotracheal and tracheostomy tubes in a lung model. *Respir Care.* 1994; 39:611-616.
6. Wright PE, Marini JJ, Bernard GR. In vitro versus in vivo comparison of endotracheal tube airflow resistance. *Am Rev Respir Dis.* 1989;140:10-16.
7. Baydur A, Behrakis PK, Zin WA, et al. A simple method for assessing the validity of the esophageal balloon technique. *Am Rev Respir Dis.* 1982;126:788-791.
8. Banner MJ, Blanch PB, Kirby RR. Imposed work of breathing and methods of triggering a demand-flow, continuous positive airway pressure system. *Crit Care Med.* 1993;21:183-190.
9. Shapiro M, Wilson RK, Casar G. Work of breathing through different sized endotracheal tubes. *Crit Care Med.* 1986;14:1028-1031.
10. Bersten AD, Rutten AJ, Vadig AE, Skowronski GA. Additional work of breathing imposed by endotracheal tubes, breathing circuits, and intensive care ventilators. *Crit Care Med.* 1989;17:671-677.
11. Bhatt SB, Patel CB, Tan IKS, Vernasco D, Tam YH. Imposed work of breathing during tracheal pressure triggering using a demand valve CPAP system. *Respir Care.* 1996;41:1028-1031.
12. Brochard L, Rua F, Lorino H, et al. Inspiratory pressure support compensates for the additional work of breathing caused by the endotracheal tube. *Anesthesiology.* 1991;75:739-745.
13. Cullen JH. An evaluation of tracheostomy in pulmonary emphysema. *Ann Intern Med.* 1963;58:953-960.
14. Cavo J, Ogura JH, Sessions DG, et al. Flow resistance in tracheostomy tube. *Ann Otolaryngol.* 1973;82:827-830.
15. Yung MW, Snowdon SL. Respiratory resistance of tracheostomy tubes. *Arch Otolaryngol.* 1984;110:591-595.
16. Nathan SD, Ishaaya AM, Koerner SK, Belman MJ. Prediction of minimal pressure support during weaning from mechanical ventilation. *Chest.* 1993;103:1215-1219.
17. Ishaaya AM, Nathan SD, Belman MJ. Work of breathing after extubation. *Chest.* 1995;107:204-209.
18. DeHaven CB, Hurst JM, Branson RD. Post-extubation hypoxemia treated with continuous positive airway pressure by face mask. *Crit Care Med.* 1985;13:46-48.

Resection With External Beam and Intraoperative Radiotherapy for Recurrent Colon Cancer

Richard D. Pezner, MD; David Z. J. Chu, MD; Lawrence D. Wagman, MD; Nayana Vora, MD; Jeffrey Y. C. Wong, MD; Stephen I. Shibata, MD

Objective: To review treatment outcomes for patients with locoregional recurrent colon cancer who underwent resection, intraoperative radiotherapy (IORT), and external beam radiotherapy (EBRT).

Design: Retrospective study of patients treated between January 1990 and June 1994.

Setting: Tertiary care cancer center.

Patients: Eleven patients with bulky recurrent colon cancer extending to adjacent organs or structures signed informed consent forms to receive IORT.

Intervention: Of 10 patients who underwent exploratory laparotomy, 5 had no metastatic disease and underwent resection, IORT, and EBRT. Complete resection was accomplished in 4 patients. Doses of IORT ranged from 13 to 20 Gy depending on residual tumor burden; EBRT was typically delivered postoperatively to a dose of 45 Gy.

Main Outcome Measures: Survival and locoregional tumor control.

Results: All 4 patients who underwent complete resection, IORT, and EBRT are alive without locoregional recurrence 53 to 77 months after treatment. Of these, only 1 patient developed distant metastases. The fifth patient, who had gross residual tumor, developed local recurrence 5 months after IORT. One patient developed an IORT complication—ureteral fibrosis leading to ipsilateral nephrectomy.

Conclusion: Long-term disease-free survival can be achieved in selected patients with bulky regional recurrence of colon cancer with complete tumor resection, IORT, and EBRT.

Arch Surg. 1999;134:63-67

FEW PATIENTS with colon cancer that arises outside the pelvis (ie, not in the rectum or rectosigmoid junction) develop locoregional tumor recurrence after definitive surgical resection. Only 6% to 9% of patients who undergo complete surgical resection develop cancer regrowth in the tumor bed as the first site of recurrence.[1-4] In patients with primary tumors that extend to adjacent organs or structures, 11% to 29% may develop isolated locoregional recurrences.[2,5] Such recurrences are difficult to control. Although some recurrences are limited to the anastomotic site, such that complete resection is possible, most will be bulky tumors that involve adjacent vital structures and produce devastating problems such as bowel obstruction, bleeding, ureteral obstruction, and severe pain from nerve or bone invasion. Selected patients have undergone radical surgical resection, with some having long-term survival benefit.[3,4,6-8] More recently, intraoperative radiotherapy (IORT), usually in combination with external beam radiotherapy (EBRT), has been used at the time of resection.[9,10] The rationale for this approach is that the total radiation dose delivered by the combination of IORT and EBRT would be greater than could be safely delivered by either modality alone, thus offering the possibility of a greater chance of long-term locoregional tumor control.

See Invited Critique at end of article

From the Divisions of Radiation Oncology (Drs Pezner, Vora, and Wong) and Surgery (Drs Chu and Wagman), and Department of Medical Oncology and Therapeutics (Dr Shibata), City of Hope National Medical Center, Duarte, Calif.

RESULTS

Of 4 patients who underwent complete tumor resection, IORT, and EBRT, 3 are alive with no evidence of disease 53, 64, and 66 months after treatment

PATIENTS AND METHODS

Between January 1990—when City of Hope National Medical Center, Duarte, Calif, inaugurated an IORT program—and June 1994, 11 patients with recurrent colon adenocarcinoma signed informed consent forms to receive IORT if indicated at exploratory laparotomy. There were 5 men and 6 women who ranged in age from 31 to 77 years (mean, 60 years). The primary site was the cecum in 2 patients, ascending colon in 1 patient, hepatic flexure in 2 patients, descending colon in 2 patients, and sigmoid in 4 patients. Stage at initial diagnosis was I in 1 patient, II in 4 patients, III in 5 patients, and IV (liver metastases) in 1 patient.[11] Ten patients underwent complete resection on the primary tumor, whereas 1 patient with a T4 primary tumor was left with gross residual tumor. Five patients also received adjuvant 5-fluorouracil chemotherapy with either leucovorin calcium or levamisole hydrochloride.

Recurrent disease, as evaluated by computed tomographic scan, presented as a solitary retroperitoneal, presacral, or psoas mass in 8 patients, liver metastases in 1 patient, tumor bed recurrence and liver metastases in 1 patient, and para-aortic adenopathy in 1 patient. Only 1 of 11 patients had a previous recurrence (ovarian metastasis) before consideration for IORT. Preoperative computed tomographic scan showed ureteral obstruction in 2 patients. Results of cystoscopy showed bladder invasion in another patient. Computed tomographic scan showed tumor sizes ranging from 3 to 8 cm ($\geq$5 cm in 7 patients). Intraoperative radiotherapy was considered for selected patients known to have distant metastases in the event that all sites of disease could be grossly resected.

Six of 11 patients did not receive IORT. One patient did not undergo laparotomy because results of his preoperative radiolabeled anti–carcinoembryonic antigen monoclonal antibody scan led to the discovery of a biopsy-proven nonpalpable supraclavicular nodal metastasis. Five patients underwent laparotomy but did not receive IORT because of the discovery of widespread disease, including peritoneal metastases in 2 patients, liver and peritoneal metastases in 1 patient, porta hepatis nodal and liver metastases in 1 patient, and multiple unresectable para-aortic nodal metastases in 1 patient. Among 6 patients who did not receive IORT, 5 had a history of disease outside the tumor bed before laparotomy (ie, liver metastases in 2 patients and supraclavicular nodal, para-aortic nodal, and previous ovarian metastases in 1 patient each). After documentation of widespread metastases, these 6 patients survived for 6 to 21 months (mean, 11 months).

The other 5 patients had no evidence of metastases found at laparotomy and underwent resection and IORT (**Table 1**). For these 3 men and 2 women, the disease-free interval from initial diagnosis of colon cancer to the date of diagnosis of recurrent cancer ranged from 5 to 31 months (<12 months in 4 patients). All had tumor bed recurrences that extended to adjacent organs or structures (Table 1). Tumors ranged in size from 3 to 8 cm. Complete resection of all gross disease was accomplished in 4 patients. Pathologic margins were clear in 3 patients and were involved by tumor in 1 patient. One patient had gross tumor left on the sacrum despite preoperative EBRT and low anterior resection.

Intraoperative radiotherapy was delivered after resection and before reconstruction. On completion of resection, the surgeon and radiation oncologist evaluated the feasibility of safely and effectively delivering IORT to the tumor bed defined by the surgeon. The patient's wound was closed and covered in sterile drapes. While under anesthesia, the patient was transported to the linear accelerator suite in the radiation oncology department for delivery of IORT. Critical organs such as the bowel, bladder, stomach, and liver were retracted away from the IORT cone applicator placed on the tumor bed. In 1 patient, a ureter that had been encased by tumor was in the IORT field (**Figure 1**). In the other 4 patients, ureters either were not near the tumor bed or were uninvolved and able to be retracted out of the IORT field (**Figure 2**). Fixed critical structures within the IORT field, such as kidney and sciatic nerve, were protected by placement of small sterile lead shields or by limiting dose penetration by selection of appropriate electron beam energy. The cone end protruding out of the wound was then carefully docked to the IORT cone holder, which was attached to the collimator head of the linear accelerator (Clinac 1800, Varian Associates, Palo Alto, Calif). Doses prescribed to the 90% isodose were 13 to 14 Gy for negative margins, 17 Gy for positive margins, and 20 Gy for gross residual tumor (Table 1). Electron beam energies ranged from 9 to 20 MeV, depending on the thickness of the tumor bed. Applicator cone sizes ranged from 5.7 to 9.5 cm. On completion of IORT, the cone was undocked and removed, the wound was closed, and the patient was returned to the operating room to complete the procedure.

External beam radiotherapy was delivered after surgery in 4 patients and before surgery in 1 patient (Table 1). The interval from date of surgery to start of postoperative EBRT ranged from 2 to 11 weeks. The time from the end of preoperative EBRT to surgery was 2 weeks. The EBRT dose was 45 Gy, given in 25 fractions for 5 to 8 weeks. Field sizes were determined so that they encompassed the tumor bed and adjacent nodal sites with generous margins. Survival was estimated from the date of IORT administration.

(**Table 2**). One patient developed lung metastases 30 months after IORT and is alive after 77 months without locoregional recurrence. The patient who had gross residual tumor treated by IORT developed local recurrence 5 months later and died of cancer 1 month afterward.

Complications developed in 3 patients (Table 2). Two were attributed to resection and 1 to IORT. One patient developed an anastomotic bowel leak and fistula that postponed the EBRT start date until 11 weeks after surgery and IORT. Severe diarrhea and the need for long-term total parenteral nutrition developed in the patient who required resection of 126 cm of small bowel with tumor (Table 1). The IORT complication developed in the only patient whose ureter was in the IORT field. Despite prophylactic ureteral stent placement, the patient developed ureteral stenosis leading to loss of ipsilateral kidney function and eventual nephrec-

Table 1. Treatment Details of Patients With Recurrent Colon Cancer Who Received IORT*

Patient No.	Recurrent Tumor Findings	Extent of Resection and IORT	Pathologic Margin Status	EBRT Timing, Dose, Interval Delay†
1	5-cm Mass involving psoas, small bowel, femoral nerve, and abdominal wall	Mass and involved organs; 14-Gy IORT; 9.5-cm cone	Negative	Postoperative, 45 Gy, 15 d
2	3-cm Mass involving psoas	Mass and psoas; 14-Gy IORT; 7.6-cm cone	Negative by 0.7 cm	Postoperative, 45 Gy, 11 wk
3	8-cm Anastomotic mass involving multiple small-bowel loops	Mass with 126-cm small bowel; 13-Gy IORT; 7.6-cm cone	Negative	Postoperative, 45 Gy, 5 wk
4	6-cm Psoas mass encasing ureter	Mass and psoas; 17-Gy IORT; 8.3-cm cone	Microscopic positive	Postoperative, 45 Gy, 21 d
5	6-cm Anastomotic mass fixed to sacrum	Low anterior resection, diverting colostomy; 20-Gy IORT; 5.7-cm cone	Gross residual tumor	Preoperative, 45.3 Gy, 2 wk

**IORT indicates intraoperative radiotherapy; EBRT, external beam radiotherapy.*

†Timing indicates preoperative vs postoperative; dose, 1 Gy = 100 rad; and interval delay, time from date of IORT to first-day postoperative EBRT or time from end preoperative EBRT to date of IORT.

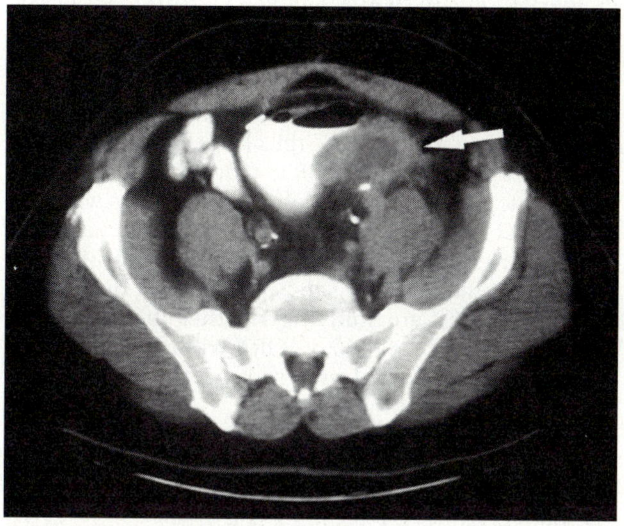

Figure 1. *Computed tomographic scan of patient 4 showing bulky recurrent sigmoid colon cancer encasing the ureter and invading psoas muscle (arrow).*

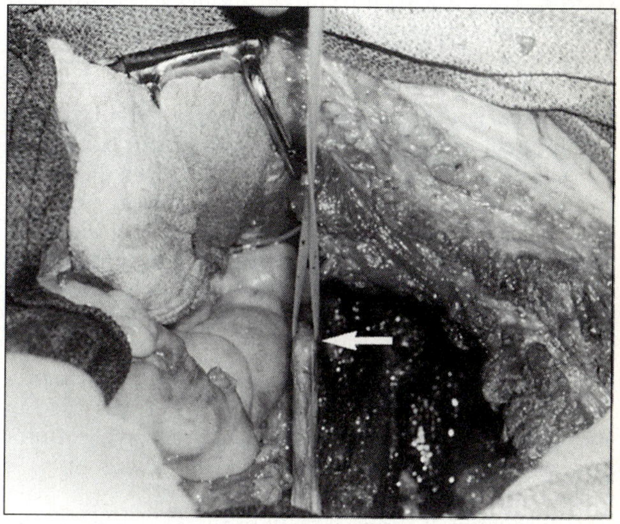

Figure 2. *Ureter retracted out of the resected tumor bed in patient 1 before placement of the intraoperative radiotherapy cone applicator (arrow).*

tomy 15 months after tumor resection and IORT. The patient recuperated well from nephrectomy and never developed pyelonephritis or renal insufficiency.

COMMENT

Complete surgical resection has been the single most effective treatment modality for patients with isolated locoregional recurrence of extrapelvic colon cancer.[3,4,6,7,12,13] Success depends on tumor presentation not involving unresectable structures such as the sciatic nerve and the lumbosacral spine and the ability of the surgeon to perform a procedure that may be as extensive as an exenteration.[7,12-14] A urinary diversion procedure may be performed if a ureter or the bladder must be resected because of tumor involvement.[14] Results of retrospective studies report that up to 40% of selected patients with isolated locoregional tumor bed recurrences, including small-bowel anastomotic site recurrences, may survive at least 5 years after complete surgical resection.[3,4,6,8,12,15] The value of preoperative or postoperative EBRT combined with resection for patients with locoregional recurrent colon cancer has not been well defined.[7] External beam radiotherapy is of palliative value for many patients who have unresect-

Table 2. Outcome for Patients With Locoregional Recurrent Colon Cancer Who Underwent Resection, Intraoperative Radiotherapy, and External Beam Radiotherapy (EBRT)

Patient No.	Complications	Survival
1	None	No evidence of disease, 66 mo; lost to follow-up
2	Postoperative anastomotic leak delaying start of EBRT	Lung metastases, 30 mo; alive without locoregional recurrence, 77 mo
3	Severe short bowel syndrome requiring total parenteral nutrition	No evidence of disease, 64 mo
4	Ureteral stenosis leading to nephrectomy at 15 mo	No evidence of disease, 53 mo
5	None	Local recurrence, 5 mo; died of cancer, 6 mo

able disease, although long-term disease-free survival is rare with EBRT alone.[4,6,8]

Intraoperative radiotherapy is a technique to deliver a large single dose of radiation directly to the tumor bed defined by the surgeon at the time of resection.[9,10] Critical organs such as the small bowel, bladder, and ureters can be moved out of the path of the IORT beam to significantly reduce the risk of late radiation complications. Radiation dose to structures that cannot be easily moved such as the sciatic nerve or kidneys can be limited by placement of small shields at the time of IORT or by choice of electron beam energy to limit the dose of radiation delivered deep to the tumor bed. External beam radiotherapy can be kept to a dose range that is sufficient for microscopic disease beyond the IORT field but below the level of a high risk of bowel complications.[16] Results of retrospective studies[17-22] suggest that IORT may significantly improve control of locoregional recurrent rectal cancer provided that tumor fixation does not prevent resection of all gross disease and previous EBRT does not limit the dose of IORT or EBRT that may be safely delivered.

Locoregional recurrence of cancer originating in the colon outside of the pelvis is not as likely to have limitations such as tumor extension to unresectable structures or a history of previous EBRT. Several institutions have reported use of IORT in some patients with recurrent colon cancers, but the relative benefit of the addition of IORT to surgery has not been analyzed in detail.[12,14,19,21] The largest experience was reported by Gunderson et al.[22] They delivered 10- to 20-Gy IORT to 43 patients with recurrent colon cancer who had no previous history of EBRT. Preoperative EBRT was used in most patients. They reported an actuarial 5-year tumor control rate within the IORT and EBRT region of 80%, with a 5-year disease-free survival of 21%.

In our small series, 4 of 11 evaluable patients, and more important, 4 of 5 patients who received IORT, were long-term survivors. Selection of appropriate candidates may be a factor in our favorable results. Intraoperative radiotherapy was used only in patients who did not have disseminated disease to the liver, peritoneum, or other sites. Resection of all gross disease was accomplished in all of our long-term survivors. None of the patients in our series who underwent IORT had small anastomotic recurrences; all had bulky tumors that extended to adjacent organs or structures. We were also able to deliver both IORT and EBRT, which may yield a higher local control rate than with either radiation modality alone.[17,19,20] A long disease-free interval between initial diagnosis of cancer and diagnosis of recurrence was considered a favorable prognostic factor by others[12] but was not noted in our study.

External beam radiotherapy can be delivered either before or after surgery. Preoperative EBRT may reduce the size of a tumor to make it more likely to be resectable. However, there may be an increased risk of postoperative wound-healing complications. Patients with metastatic disease at laparotomy would not likely have a survival benefit from EBRT. In comparison, EBRT delivered after surgery can be reserved for patients without metastatic disease. The main disadvantage of postoperative EBRT is that a significant delay in treatment start may compromise its effectiveness because of intervening tumor regrowth.

Sciatic neuropathy and ureteral stenosis are the most common complications related to IORT delivered to abdominal and pelvic sites.[9,10,17,22] Although none of our patients had neuropathy, others[17-22] report symptomatic neuropathy in 0% to 17% of patients with recurrent colorectal cancer who received IORT. Intraoperative radiotherapy can produce ureteral stenosis leading to hydronephrosis and possible loss of kidney function.[23] Ureteral stenosis was noted by Gunderson et al[22] in 12 (36%) of 33 patients with recurrent colorectal cancer who received IORT to a ureter. In our patients, the only IORT complication was in the only patient who received treatment to a ureter. Ureters without cancer should be excluded from the IORT field (Figure 2). If the ureter must be in the IORT field, a stent can be placed.[19,22] Alternatively, a urinary diversion procedure can be performed.

Our results demonstrate that selected patients with bulky tumor bed recurrence of colon cancer can be long-term disease-free survivors when treated with a combination of complete surgical resection, IORT, and wide-field postoperative EBRT. Our series is too small to estimate what proportion of treated patients will have a survival benefit. More effective treatment is necessary for patients whose disease cannot be completely resected or who cannot safely receive full-dose IORT and EBRT. We[24] are studying whether the delivery of chemotherapy at the time of IORT will improve locoregional tumor control and reduce the subsequent appearance of distant metastases.

Corresponding author: Richard D. Pezner, MD, Division of Radiation Oncology, City of Hope National Medical Center, 1500 E Duarte Rd, Duarte, CA 91010.

REFERENCES

1. Olson RM, Perencevich NP, Malcolm AW, Chaffey JT, Wilson RE. Patterns of recurrence following curative resection of adenocarcinoma of the colon and rectum. *Cancer.* 1980;45:2969-2974.
2. Willett CG, Tepper JE, Cohen AM, Oklow E, Welch CE. Failure patterns following curative resection of colonic carcinoma. *Ann Surg.* 1984;200:685-690.
3. Michelassi F, Vannucci L, Ayala JJ, Chappel R, Goldberg R, Block GE. Local recurrence after curative resection of colorectal adenocarcinoma. *Surgery.* 1990;108:787-793.
4. Stipa S, Nicolanti W, Botti C, et al. Local recurrence after curative resection for colorectal cancer: frequency, risk factors and treatment. *J Surg Oncol.* 1991;2:155-160.
5. Gunderson LL, Sosin H, Levitt S. Extrapelvic colon: areas of failure in a reoperation series: implications for adjuvant therapy. *Int J Radiat Oncol Biol Phys.* 1985;11:731-741.
6. Welch JP, Donaldson GA. Detection and treatment of recurrent cancer of the colon and rectum. *Am J Surg.* 1978;135:505-511.
7. Schiessel R, Wunderlich M, Herbst F. Local recurrence of colorectal cancer: effect of early detection and aggressive surgery. *Br J Surg.* 1986;73:342-344.
8. Waldron RP, Donovan IA. Clinical follow-up and treatment of locally recurrent colorectal cancer. *Dis Colon Rectum.* 1987;30:428-430.
9. Hoekstra HJ, Sindelar WF, Kinsella TJ, Oldhoff J. History, preliminary results, complications, and future prospects of intraoperative radiotherapy. *J Surg Oncol.* 1987;36:175-182.
10. Calvo FA, Micaily B, Brady LW. Intraoperative radiotherapy: a positive view. *Am J Clin Oncol.* 1993;16:418-423.

11. Beahrs OH, Henson DE, Hutter RVP, Kennedy BJ, eds. *Handbook for Staging of Cancer.* Philadelphia, Pa: JB Lippincott; 1993:95-102.
12. Gwin JL, Hoffman JP, Eisenberg BL. Surgical management of nonhepatic intra-abdominal recurrence of carcinoma of the colon. *Dis Colon Rectum.* 1993;36: 540-544.
13. Yeung RS, Moffat FL, Falk RE. Pelvic exenteration for recurrent and extensive primary colorectal adenocarcinoma. *Cancer.* 1993;72:1853-1858.
14. Steele G, Ravikumar TS, Benotti PN. New surgical treatments for recurrent colorectal cancer. *Cancer.* 1990;65:723-730.
15. Stulc JP, Petrelli NJ, Herrera L, Mittelman A. Anastomotic recurrence of adenocarcinoma of the colon. *Arch Surg.* 1986;121:1077-1080.
16. Coia LR, Myerson RJ, Tepper JE. Late effects of radiation therapy on the gastrointestinal tract. *Int J Radiat Oncol Biol Phys.* 1995;31:1213-1236.
17. Wallace HJ, Willett CG, Shellito PC, Coen JJ, Hoover HC. Intraoperative radiation therapy for locally advanced recurrent rectal or rectosigmoid cancer. *J Surg Oncol.* 1995;60:122-127.
18. Lanciano RM, Calkins AR, Wolkov HB, et al. A phase I/II study of intraoperative radiotherapy in advanced unresectable or recurrent carcinoma of the rectum: a Radiation Therapy Oncology Group (RTOG) study. *J Surg Oncol.* 1993;53: 20-29.
19. Abuchaibe O, Calvo FA, Azinovic I, Aristu J, Pardo F, Alvarez-Cienfuelgos J. Intraoperative radiotherapy in locally advanced recurrent colorectal cancer. *Int J Radiat Oncol Biol Phys.* 1993;26:859-867.
20. Bussieres E, Gilly F-N, Rouanet P, et al. Recurrences of rectal cancers: results of a multimodal approach with intraoperative radiation therapy. *Int J Radiat Oncol Biol Phys.* 1996;34:49-56.
21. Lowy AM, Rich TA, Skibber JM, Dubrow RA, Curley SA. Preoperative infusional chemoradiation, selective intraoperative radiation and resection of locally advanced pelvic recurrence of colorectal adenocarcinoma. *Ann Surg.* 1996;223: 177-185.
22. Gunderson LL, Nelson H, Martenson JA, et al. Intraoperative electron and external beam irradiation with or without 5-fluorouracil and maximum surgical resection for previously unirradiated locally recurrent colorectal cancer. *Dis Colon Rectum.* 1996;39:1379-1395.
23. Sindelar WF, Tepper J, Travis EL, Terrill R. Tolerance of retroperitoneal structures to intraoperative radiation. *Ann Surg.* 1982;196:601-608.
24. Shibata S, Pezner R, Chu D, et al. Pilot study of intraoperative radiation therapy (IORT) with concurrent 5-FU followed by external beam radiation therapy (EBRT) with a prolonged 5-FU infusion in locally advanced gastrointestinal (GI) malignancies. *Proc Am Soc Clin Oncol.* 1997;16:305a. Abstract 1086.

Invited Critique

The role of adjuvant therapy for recurrent colorectal cancer is still evolving. Radical surgical resection alone or combined with external radiotherapy and often with chemotherapy have been commonly used in treating isolated locoregional recurrence of colon cancer. In the past 2 decades, a major advance in this field has been the addition of intraoperative radiotherapy (IORT) to external beam radiotherapy (EBRT).

Using this combination, Pezner and colleagues successfully treated a few patients with bulky recurrent colon tumors and achieved long-term local control and survival. Although small in number, this study has further illustrated important points. Intraoperative radiotherapy has the advantage of delivering a high-energy electron beam in a single dose to a clearly defined residual tumor bed without exposure and damage to adjacent organs and tissues. However, IORT and EBRT cannot eliminate local failures if complete tumor excision is not achieved, as observed in this study and others.[1] Curative resections are often not possible in locally recurrent colon lesions because most recurrent tumors manifest with fixity to adjacent structures.

Intraoperative radiotherapy is not without complications. Radiation injury to nerves, ureter, and bowel may occur when not adequately shielded from the IORT field. This could become an important consideration as more countries embark on this technique.

In recurrent colon cancer, the risk of systemic disease is high. The addition of chemotherapy and radiation modifiers in conjunction with IORT and EBRT seems justifiable. It would be of interest to await the results of controlled studies that are currently in progress of the use of systemic therapy with IORT and EBRT to improve locoregional control and the risk of disseminated disease.

Raj M. Nambiar, MD
Tan Tock Seng Hospital
Singapore, Republic of Singapore

1. Gunderson LL, Nagorney DM, Martenson JA, et al. External beam plus intraoperative irradiation for gastrointestinal cancers. *World J Surg.* 1995;19:191-197.

Prospective Evaluation of Total Parathyroidectomy and Autotransplantation for the Treatment of Secondary Hyperparathyroidism

Francesco Zaraca, MD; Sandro Mazzaferro, MD; Marco Catarci, MD; Alessandra Saputelli, MD; Piero Alò, MD; Manlio Carboni, MD

Objective: To evaluate the clinical effectiveness of total parathyroidectomy with autotransplantation for the treatment of hyperparathyroidism and the recurrence rate of hyperparathyroidism after this procedure.

Design: A prospective study of total parathyroidectomy and autotransplantation in 19 consecutive patients with severe secondary (renal) hyperparathyroidism.

Setting: University hospital department of surgery.

Patients: Nineteen patients operated on for the treatment of secondary hyperparathyroidism between March 1993 and March 1996. Eighteen had been receiving long-term hemodialysis, and 1 had a functioning renal graft.

Intervention: Total parathyroidectomy and autotransplantation of excised parathyroid tissue into the brachioradialis muscle of the arm opposite that in which the arteriovenous fistula had been placed for dialysis.

Main Outcome Measures: Clinical and biochemical improvement, morbidity, mortality, and recurrence rates of hyperparathyroidism after the procedure.

Results: The conditions of 13 (72%) of 18 patients followed up improved, and the clinical and laboratory variables indicating secondary hyperparathyroidism returned to normal. One patient died 50 days after surgery. In 2 patients (10%), mild hypoparathyroidism developed, and in 1 patient (5%), persistent hyperparathyroidism developed and required reoperation. In 2 patients (10%), recurrent hyperparathyroidism developed, and 1 (5%) required reoperation.

Conclusions: Total parathyroidectomy with autotransplantation effectively relieves the symptoms of hyperparathyroidism, and the recurrence rate of hyperparathyroidism is low. Because all procedures used resulted in good control of clinical and biochemical variables, the method used for the surgical treatment of secondary hyperparathyroidism depends on the surgeon's preference.

Arch Surg. 1999;134:68-72

A PROLONGED chronic deficiency of calcitriol secondary to long-standing renal failure is the major cause of increased secretion of parathyroid hormone (PTH) and hypertrophy and hyperplasia of the parathyroid glands. In advanced cases, the treatment of vitamin D deficiency is ineffective for correcting hypersecretion of the parathyroid glands, and surgical removal is warranted.

See Invited Critique at end of article

In 1994, according to the European Dialysis and Transplantation Registry Report, 1.3% of patients with end-stage renal disease who were receiving hemodialysis required parathyroidectomy because of severe secondary hyperparathyroidism that caused bone pain, extraosseous soft tissue calcification, and severe pruritus.[1] Three types of surgical techniques have been proposed for this disease. The first technique was subtotal parathyroidectomy, performed in 1960.[2] Subsequently, total parathyroidectomy was suggested, but a severe form of disabling osteomalacia was reported secondary to this surgical procedure, which then fell out of favor. However, during the following years, it became clear that such a complication was related to a preexisting accumulation of aluminum in the bone and not the surgical procedure, which has been reintroduced. In 1968, Alveryd[3] reported the first experience of total parathyroidectomy with autotransplantation of fresh parathyroid tissue. Since that time, subtotal parathyroidectomy and total parathyroidectomy with autotransplantation have been considered comparable procedures. In 1991, Rothmund et al[4] reported the results of a randomized trial comparing the 2 procedures in 40 patients with secondary hyperparathyroidism. They concluded that total parathyroidectomy with autotransplantation is preferable to subtotal parathy-

From the Second Surgical Clinic (Drs Zaraca, Catarci, Saputelli, and Carboni), the Second Medical Clinic (Dr Mazzaferro), and the Department of Pathology, (Dr Alò), University of Rome "La Sapienza" Medical School, Rome, Italy.

PATIENTS AND METHODS

Between March 1993 and March 1996, 19 consecutive patients were operated on at the University of Rome Department of Surgery, Rome, Italy, for the treatment of secondary hyperparathyroidism. Eighteen had been receiving long-term hemodialysis for a mean of 7.7 years, and 1 had a functioning renal graft. The 9 men and 10 women ranged in age from 30 to 72 years (mean, 50.2 years). Chronic renal failure was caused by glomerulonephritis in 8 patients, polycystic kidney disease in 4, nephrolithiasis in 3, vesicoureteral reflux in 2, diabetic nephropathy in 1, and urate nephropathy in 1.

Preoperative examinations included serial estimations of serum calcium, phosphorus, and alkaline phosphatase concentrations. Serial intact PTH concentrations also were obtained. In all patients, a bone biopsy was performed before surgery to obtain tissue for histological analysis. All patients underwent dialysis the day before operation.

The indications for surgery in the 19 patients are shown in the following tabulation.

Indication	No. (%) of Patients
Bone pain	19 (100)
Hyperparathyroidism	19 (100)
Medical therapy	19 (100)
Pruritus	18 (95)
Muscle weakness	14 (74)
Spontaneous hypercalcemia	8 (42)

All procedures were performed by the chief surgeon (M. C.), and the exploration of the neck was done according to the technique suggested by Rothmund and Wagner.[5] The procedure involved the excision of all identified parathyroid glands and of the thyrothymic ligament. Intraoperatively, all resected specimens were examined microscopically to confirm the diagnosis. Cervical thymectomy was required for 6 patients (32%). For each patient, 20 pieces of tissue ranging from 1 to 2 mm^3 were implanted into the brachioradialis muscle of the arm opposite that in which the arteriovenous fistula had been placed for dialysis, as described by Wells et al.[6] Surplus fragments were sent to the laboratory for cryopreservation, which was performed according to the method of Wagner et al.[7]

We found 4 parathyroid glands in 17 patients and 5 in 1 patient. We found 3 parathyroid glands in the other patient.

Patients were treated and followed up by the referring dialysis centers after discharge. During the first 48 hours, supplemental calcium was given intravenously according to actual serum calcium concentrations. Subsequently, during the first 6 months, calcium and calcitriol supplements were administered orally according to the trends in the serum calcium concentration. The objective effects of surgical treatment on clinical symptoms and the function of the parathyroid glands were evaluated prospectively in all patients by measurement of the serum calcium, phosphorus, alkaline phosphatase, and PTH concentrations. The subjective response to surgical treatment was measured by using a questionnaire completed by the patient and the referring nephrologist during each follow-up examination. The duration of follow-up ranged from 13.6 to 50.6 months (mean ± SE, 27.9 ± 2.9 months). All examinations were performed at 1, 6, and 12 months after surgery and then every year.

All laboratory and clinical data were analyzed by using repeated measures analysis of variance. The level of significance was set at .05.

roidectomy for patients with renal osteodystrophy. Actually, total parathyroidectomy with autotransplantation is a widely accepted surgical treatment for secondary hyperparathyroidism, and a wide range of recurrence rates have been reported.

The aim of the present study was to evaluate the clinical effectiveness of total parathyroidectomy with autotransplantation and the recurrence rate of hyperparathyroidism after this procedure.

RESULTS

Eighteen patients were followed up; 1 (5%) of the 19 patients died 50 days after surgery of a cerebrovascular accident. No perioperative complications occurred. Improvement, defined by a return to normal in the clinical and laboratory variables that indicate secondary hyperparathyroidism, occurred in 13 (72%) of the patients.

The biochemical and clinical data before and after operation are shown in the **Table**. Serum concentrations of intact PTH were normalized on the first postoperative day in all but 1 patient who had persistent hyperparathyroidism. The serum calcium concentration decreased progressively during the first postoperative week, and the clinical symptoms improved. **Figure 1** through **Figure 7** show the time trend for each variable.

There were 2 cases (11%) of postoperative hypoparathyroidism among the 18 patients who survived, which was defined by a serum concentration of intact PTH less than 1.1 pmol/L 12 months after surgery. Both patients are without symptoms, and a low-dose oral calcium and cholecalciferol regimen has resulted in only slight hypocalcemia. Therefore, they are not candidates for reoperation. Of note, 1 of these patients is the only patient in the present series with a functioning renal graft. Of the 19 patients, 1 experienced persistent hyperparathyroidism (5% persistence rate), defined as a reduction of the serum PTH concentration to less than 30% of the preoperative value 1 month after surgery. At the first operation, only 3 parathyroid glands were detected and removed. Postoperatively, the presence of a missed ectopic gland was confirmed by sestamibi scan, and at subsequent reexploration we found the fourth gland in the mediastinum. In 2 of 18 patients, recurrent hyperparathyroidism developed, which was defined as a serum PTH concentration of more than 21.1 pmol/L 1 year after surgery (11% recurrence rate). In one of these patients, further exploration of the neck was successful, with removal of a fifth hyperplastic parathyroid gland from the thymus. The second patient with recurrent disease has not undergone reoperation, but he is undergoing diagnostic evaluation to identify the site of recurrence. The diagnostic procedures (ultrasonography, scintigraphy, and arm-dependent serum PTH concentrations) excluded an autograft-dependent hyperparathyroidism.

Preoperative and Postoperative Data*

	Baseline	Postoperative Interval, mo: 1	6	12	24	36	48	F	*P*
No. of cases	19	19	18	18	17	9	1	. . .	. . .
Laboratory test results									
Calcium, mmol/L	2.60 ± 0.07	2.09 ± 0.08	2.21 ± 0.06	2.35 ± 0.08	2.35 ± 0.05	2.34 ± 0.05	25	0.54	.77
PTH, pmol/L	131.7 ± 12.5	16.8 ± 7.8	16.2 ± 8.2	9.9 ± 2.2	11.8 ± 2.6	9.2 ± 2.1	2.3	26.89	<.001
Phosphorus, mmol/L	1.78 ± 0.12	1.09 ± 0.08	1.49 ± 0.08	1.76 ± 0.09	1.66 ± 0.10	1.74 ± 0.17	1.68	0.27	.93
ALP, U/L	919.5 ± 221.8	762.5 ± 171.8	370.9 ± 67.6	178.5 ± 22.6	237.7 ± 22.6	194.9 ± 29.5	204	1.76	.25
Clinical symptoms									
Bone pain	8.26 ± 0.30	3.05 ± 0.63	2.00 ± 0.64	1.61 ± 0.57	1.05 ± 0.39	0.22 ± 0.14	0.00	4.46	.046
Pruritus	4.57 ± 0.79	1.68 ± 0.67	1.61 ± 0.70	1.38 ± 0.61	1.05 ± 0.39	0.77 ± 0.40	0.00	1.00	.50
Muscle weakness	7.42 ± 0.52	3.21 ± 0.70	1.55 ± 0.62	0.66 ± 0.25	0.50 ± 0.24	0.00 ± 0.00	0.00	8.35	.01

**Data are given as mean ± SE. F and* P *values obtained by repeated measures analysis of variance. PTH indicates parathyroid hormone; ALP, alkaline phosphatase; and ellipses, not applicable. To convert calcium to milligrams per deciliter, divide by 0.25. To convert PTH to picograms per milliliter, divide by 0.1053. To convert phosphorus to milligrams per deciliter, divide by 0.3229.*

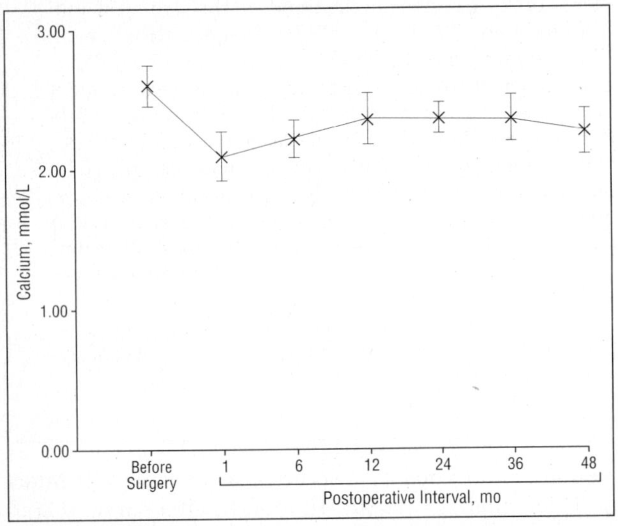

Figure 1. *Time trend of mean preoperative and postoperative serum calcium concentrations. Error bars represent 95% confidence intervals. To convert the calcium concentration from millimoles per liter to milligrams per deciliter, divide by 0.25.*

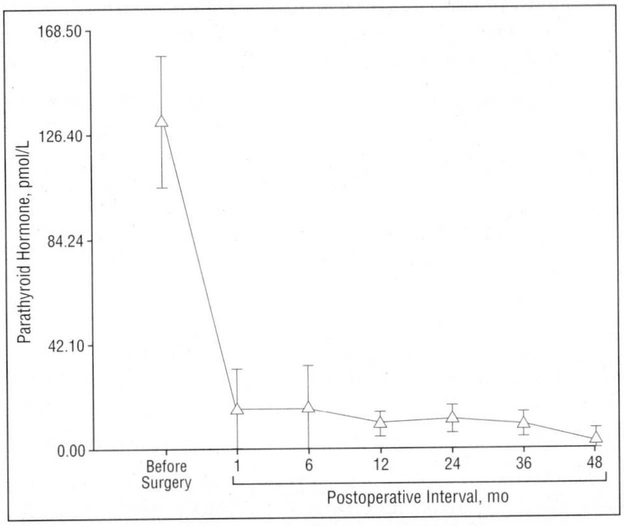

Figure 2. *Time trend of mean preoperative and postoperative serum parathyroid hormone concentrations. Error bars represent 95% confidence intervals. To convert the parathyroid hormone concentration from picomoles per liter to picograms per milliliter, divide by 0.1053.*

COMMENT

Secondary hyperparathyroidism is a classic feature of chronic renal failure. It is controlled in many patients by the use of calcium and vitamin cholecalciferol supplements, but this prophylactic therapy is not always effective. In such cases, we usually perform a total parathyroidectomy with autotransplantation. In all patients, a bone biopsy was performed to determine whether aluminum had accumulated in the bone. When this has occurred, it is important that a parathyroidectomy not be performed because symptoms will not improve, the patient's condition may deteriorate, and increased aluminum deposition may occur on the bone surfaces.[8] In the present series, good subjective improvement of symptoms was noted, similar to that reported in the literature.[4,9-11]

The most appropriate operation for secondary hyperparathyroidism remains a matter of debate. In theory, total parathyroidectomy with autotransplantation is better than subtotal parathyroidectomy, because recurrence in forearm autografts is more easily controlled by excision under local anesthesia. Cervical reoperations for recurrence in the neck are more invasive, require greater surgical expertise, and are associated with a substantial risk of hypoparathyroidism and damage to the recurrent laryngeal nerve. Some authors agree that total parathyroidectomy with autotransplantation complicates the issue when there is a recurrence, because in theory the offending parathyroid tissue may be in the neck, in the mediastinum, or at the site of the graft. On the other hand, when a subtotal parathyroidectomy has been performed, there are only 2 possible sites for the source of PTH. Casanova and coworkers[12] described a new and intriguing technique to solve the aforementioned problem. A complete ischemic blockade of the arm in which the graft was placed quickly reflects acute changes in the PTH concentration in cases of graft-dependent hyperparathyroidism. This finding is based on the short half-life of PTH, and the technique also permits the intraoperative monitoring of the effectiveness of the parathyroidectomy, even for secondary hyperparathyroidism.[13] Concentrations are determined by using a modified immunochemiluminometric assay. In the present series, intraoperative PTH concentrations were determined for the last 3 patients, and results are under evalu-

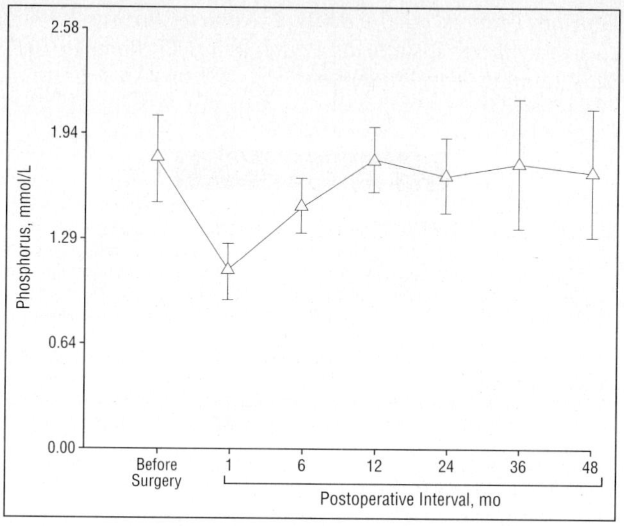

Figure 3. *Time trend of mean preoperative and postoperative serum phosphorus concentrations. Error bars represent 95% confidence intervals. To convert the phosphorus concentration from millimoles per liter to milligrams per deciliter, divide by 0.3229.*

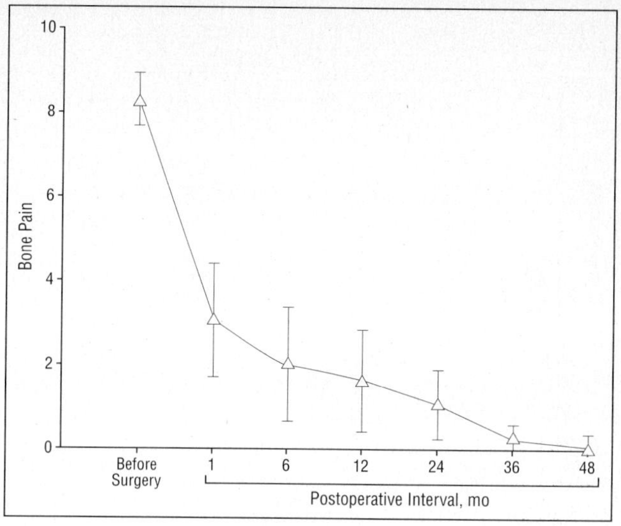

Figure 5. *Time trend of mean subjective intensity of bone pain. Error bars represent 95% confidence intervals. In visual analog scale, 0 indicates no pain; 10, worst pain ever experienced.*

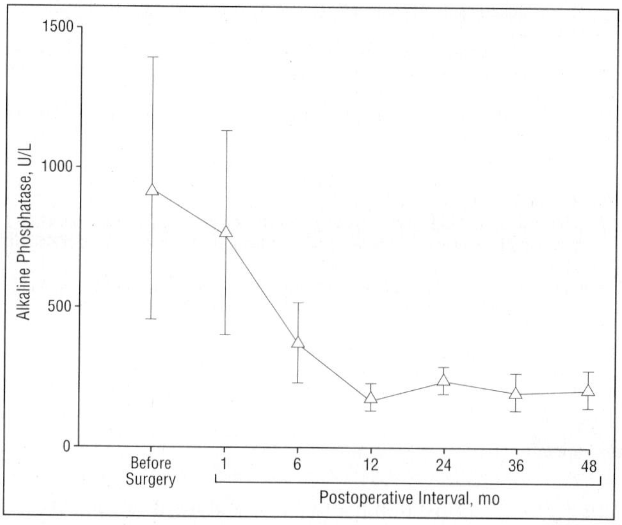

Figure 4. *Time trend of mean preoperative and postoperative serum alkaline phosphatase concentrations. Error bars represent 95% confidence intervals.*

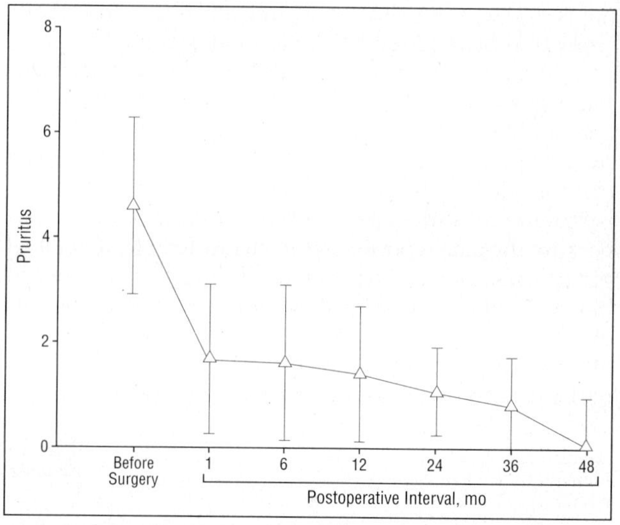

Figure 6. *Time trend of mean subjective intensity of pruritus. Error bars represent 95% confidence intervals. In visual analog scale, 0 indicates no pruritus; 10, worst pruritus ever experienced.*

ation. All 3 patients had substantial decreases in PTH concentrations 10 minutes after total parathyroidectomy (mean, 80% decrease). Long-term follow up and more experience gained by the authors and other groups[13] correlated with standard serum PTH concentration determinations, and results could make the method described helpful during parathyroidectomy for the treatment of secondary hyperparathyroidism.

Furthermore, according to some authors,[9,10] excision of grafted parathyroid tissue in case of graft hyperfunction is not a simple procedure, as the glandular tissue can infiltrate muscle planes, particularly in cases of nodular hyperplasia. Actually, this infiltration also can happen in the neck at the level of the parathyroid remnant. In fact, the capsule is opened, and, therefore, cells can spill and seed in the operative field, although the specimens are macroscopically removed.[14] Therefore, the risk of infiltration should not be used as an argument for one or another procedure, since it can be avoided by an adequate intraoperative histological examination. Intraoperative histological examination of the parathyroid glands is quick and easy to perform, and when performed by a skilled pathologist, it enables selection of the correct gland to be transplanted in the forearm. Hematoxylin-eosin, periodic acid–Schiff, and oil red O are the routine stains used for histological examination of frozen sections of the parathyroid glands. Pathologists determine whether the tissue submitted for intraoperative evaluation is parathyroid tissue, whether the parathyroid tissue is hyperplastic, whether the hyperplasia is nodular or diffuse, and whether the tissue selected is suitable for transplantation. The answers to these questions enable the surgeon to implant the appropriate tissue to avoid recurrent hyperparathyroidism from the graft and iatrogenic hypoparathyroidism. Recent findings enable the evaluation on frozen sections of the proliferative rate of the chief cells of each parathyroid gland. This can be performed by counting the Ki-67–positive cells with a simple 1-step immu-

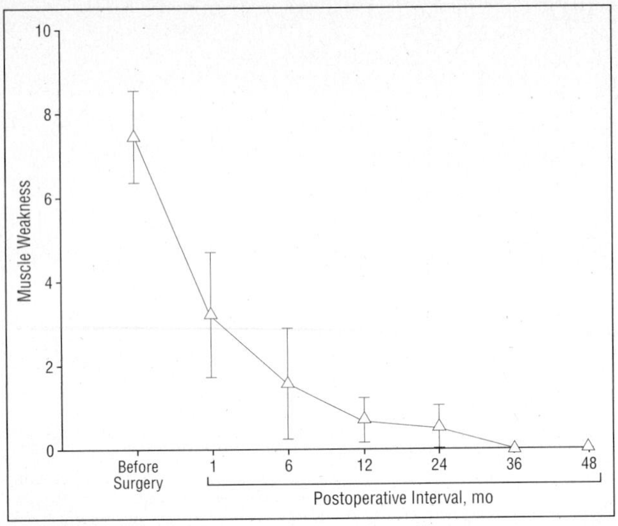

Figure 7. *Time trend of mean subjective intensity of muscle weakness. Error bars represent 95% confidence intervals. In visual analog scale, 0 indicates no muscle weakness; 10, worst muscle weakness ever experienced.*

noperoxidase stain. Studies are directed toward the shortening of time required for the immunostaining.

In our experience, total parathyroidectomy with autotransplantation effectively relieved the symptoms of hyperparathyroidism, and a low rate of recurrence of hyperparathyroidism was associated with this procedure. The method used for the surgical treatment of secondary hyperparathyroidism depends on the surgeon's preference, because the data reported in the literature indicate that all procedures described result in good control of clinical and biochemical variables. Further study is needed of the role of intraoperative monitoring of PTH concentrations and of the evaluation of the proliferative rate of the chief cells of the parathyroid glands on frozen sections.

Reprints: Francesco Zaraca MD, 2° Clinica Chirurgica, Policlinico Umberto I, Viale del Policlinico, 155, Rome 00161, Italy (e-mail: marchir@tin.it).

REFERENCES

1. Valderrabano F, Berthoux FC, Jones EH, Mehls O. Report on management of renal failure in Europe, XXV, 1994 end-stage renal disease and dialysis report: the EDTA-ERA Registry, European Dialysis and Transplant Association–European Renal Association. *Nephrol Dial Transplant.* 1996;11(suppl 1):2-21.
2. Stanbury SW, Lumb GA, Nicholson WF. Elective subtotal parathyroidectomy for renal hyperparathyroidism. *Lancet.* 1960;1:793-798.
3. Alveryd A. Parathyroid glands in thyroid surgery. *Acta Chir Scand Suppl.* 1968; 389:1-2.
4. Rothmund M, Wagner PK, Schark C. Subtotal parathyroidectomy versus total parathyroidectomy and autotransplantation in secondary hyperparathyroidism: a randomized trial. *World J Surg.* 1991;15:745-750.
5. Rothmund M, Wagner PK. Total parathyroidectomy and autotransplantation of parathyroid tissue for renal hyperparathyroidism: a one to six-year follow-up. *Ann Surg.* 1983;197:7-16.
6. Wells SA, Gunnells JC, Shelbourne JD, et al. Transplantation of parathyroid glands in men: clinical indications and results. *Surgery.* 1975;78:34-44.
7. Wagner PK, Rumpelt HJ, Krause U, Rothmund M. The effect of cryopreservation on hormone secretion in vitro and morphology of human parathyroid tissue. *Surgery.* 1986;99:257-264.
8. Andress DL, Ott SM, Maloney NA, Sherrad DJ. Effect of parathyroidectomy on bone aluminum accumulation in chronic renal failure. *N Engl J Med.* 1985;312: 468-473.
9. Neonakis E, Wheeler MH, Krishnan H, Coles GA, Davies F, Woodhead JS. Results of surgical treatment of renal hyperparathyroidism. *Arch Surg.* 1995;130: 643-648.
10. Bessel JR, Proudman WD, Parkyn RF, Disney APS. Parathyroidectomy in the treatment of patients with chronic renal failure: a 10-year review. *Br J Surg.* 1993;80:40-42.
11. Ready AR, Sabharawal T, Barnes AD. Parathyroidectomy in the west Midlands. *Br J Surg.* 1996;83:823-827.
12. Casanova D, Sarfati E, De Francisco A, Amado A, Arias M, Dubost C. Secondary hyperparathyroidism: diagnosis of site of recurrence. *World J Surg.* 1991;15: 546-550.
13. Clary BM, Garner SC, Leight GS. Intraoperative parathyroid hormone monitoring during parathyroidectomy for secondary hyperparathyroidism. *Surgery.* 1997; 122:1034-1038.
14. Rothmund M, Wagner PK. Reoperations for persistent and recurrent secondary hyperparathyroidism. *Ann Surg.* 1988;207:310-314.

Invited Critique

Advanced secondary (renal) hyperparathyroidism (HPT) induced by long-standing chronic renal insufficiency can be a serious complication for patients receiving long-term hemodialysis. As Zaraca and colleagues have pointed out, parathyroidectomy is indicated for patients with advanced secondary HPT that is refractory to medical management; many patients feel dramatically better within days of the operation. The questions that remain, therefore, are when to operate and which operation to perform. Zaraca et al address the second question.

Since 1960, the surgical treatment of secondary HPT has evolved from total parathyroidectomy, to subtotal parathyroidectomy, to total parathyroidectomy with autotransplantation of a portion of 1 gland. The reason that all surgeons are not performing the same operation is that it is unclear which of the latter 2 of these operations has superior long-term results. Although most surgeons have abandoned total parathyroidectomy, numerous reports describe relatively equal short- and long-term clinical success rates for subtotal parathyroidectomy and total parathyroidectomy with autotransplantation (the latter is supported nicely in the article by Zaraca et al).

All patients with secondary HPT will have multigland disease, almost exclusively 4-gland hyperplasia. Because of this, all operations for the treatment of secondary HPT must include bilateral exploration and identification, biopsy, and removal of all 4 (or 3½) glands. There should be little if any use for localizing studies before neck exploration for the treatment of secondary HPT, and in fact, sestamibi scanning should not be used unless it is for reoperation to find a single recurrent gland. This is in stark contrast to patients with primary HPT, which is due to a single adenoma in 87% of patients.[1] Sestamibi scanning is extremely accurate for identifying single adenomas (specificity almost 100%),[1] so minimally invasive parathyroidectomies are now possible. As the newer techniques are embraced, surgeons must realize that secondary HPT has a completely different cause and is not suitable for minimally invasive unilateral operations.

James Norman, MD
University of South Florida
Tampa

1. Denham D, Norman J. Cost-effectiveness of preoperative sestamibi scan for primary hyperparathyroidism is solely dependent upon surgeon's choice of operative procedure. *J Am Coll Surg.* 1998;186:293-304.

ARCHIVES OF SURGERY

SUBSCRIPTION ORDER FORM

☑ **YES!** Enter my personal subscription to ***Archives of Surgery*** at the special money saving rate checked below:

❑ AMA Member rate: One year (12 issues) — $95*.
❑ Individual non-member rate: One year (12 issues) — $145*.
❑ Corporate/Institutional rate: One year (12 issues) — $245.
❑ *My personal check in U.S. $ is enclosed.
(Make check payable to *American Medical Association*).
❑ Charge my personal credit card: ❑ VISA ❑ MASTERCARD ❑ AMEX ❑ OPTIMA

Card No.__________ Exp. Date__________ Signature__________

Name (Please print) __________

Address __________

City__________ State/Province__________ Zip/Postal Code __________

Phone__________ Fax__________ e-mail __________

IMPORTANT: The individual non-member rate is available in the U.S. and Canada only. Payment must accompany order. Corporate/Institutional checks are not accepted for personal subscriptions. Canada residents add 7% GST. GST # (12622 5556 RT).

19X1DZ

ARCHIVES OF SURGERY

SUBSCRIPTION ORDER FORM

☑ **YES!** Enter my personal subscription to ***Archives of Surgery*** at the special money saving rate checked below:

❑ AMA Member rate: One year (12 issues) — $95*.
❑ Individual non-member rate: One year (12 issues) — $145*.
❑ Corporate/Institutional rate: One year (12 issues) — $245.
❑ *My personal check in U.S. $ is enclosed.
(Make check payable to *American Medical Association*).
❑ Charge my personal credit card: ❑ VISA ❑ MASTERCARD ❑ AMEX ❑ OPTIMA

Card No.__________ Exp. Date__________ Signature__________

Name (Please print) __________

Address __________

City__________ State/Province__________ Zip/Postal Code __________

Phone__________ Fax__________ e-mail __________

IMPORTANT: The individual non-member rate is available in the U.S. and Canada only. Payment must accompany order. Corporate/Institutional checks are not accepted for personal subscriptions. Canada residents add 7% GST. GST # (12622 5556 RT).

19X1DZ

BUSINESS REPLY MAIL
FIRST-CLASS MAIL PERMIT NO. 1376 CHICAGO IL

NO POSTAGE NECESSARY IF MAILED IN THE UNITED STATES

POSTAGE WILL BE PAID BY ADDRESSEE

SUBSCRIBER SERVICES CENTER
AMERICAN MEDICAL ASSOCIATION
PO BOX 10945
CHICAGO IL 60610-9902

BUSINESS REPLY MAIL
FIRST-CLASS MAIL PERMIT NO. 1376 CHICAGO IL

NO POSTAGE NECESSARY IF MAILED IN THE UNITED STATES

POSTAGE WILL BE PAID BY ADDRESSEE

SUBSCRIBER SERVICES CENTER
AMERICAN MEDICAL ASSOCIATION
PO BOX 10945
CHICAGO IL 60610-9902

The Value of Acute-Phase Protein Measurements After Curative Gastric Cancer Surgery

Tetsuji Fujita, MD; Akihiko Hara, MD; Yoji Yamazaki, MD

Objective: To determine whether acute-phase protein measurement provides clinically useful information about tumor recurrence.

Patients and Methods: Acute-phase serum protein levels were measured at regular intervals in 43 patients who underwent curative gastrectomy for gastric cancer. At 12 months after surgery, patients were grouped according to the presence or absence of a C-reactive protein response, and were followed up for a minimum of 12 months or until death.

Results: There was a significant difference ($P = .02$) in a recurrence rate between patients with a C-reactive protein response (3 of 4 patients) and those without such a response (4 of 39 patients). Moreover, serum levels of C4 and α_1-antitrypsin 12 months after surgery in patients who eventually recurred were significantly ($P<.05$) higher than those in a group without recurrence.

Conclusion: An acute-phase protein response may be a predictive factor in the early stages of tumor recurrence. Acute-phase protein measurement provided clinically useful information about tumor recurrence after curative gastric cancer surgery.

Arch Surg. 1999;134:73-75

BECAUSE OF the advances in diagnostic methods and the progress of surgical treatment, the 5-year survival rate of patients with gastric cancer has steadily increased, reaching more than 60% in Japan[1,2]; however, approximately a quarter of patients who underwent curative resection of gastric cancer had tumor recurrence.[2] It is known that a proportion of patients develop an acute-phase protein response following tumor recurrence or progression.[3] Although a recent study[4] showed a higher recurrence rate of colorectal cancer for patients with ongoing, acute-phase protein response compared with patients without such a response, there is little evidence that an acute-phase protein response indicates the early phase of tumor recurrence after curative cancer surgery.

We wanted to determine whether acute-phase protein measurement provides clinically useful information about tumor recurrence after curative gastric cancer surgery.

RESULTS

Of the 43 patients studied, 4 had a CRP response at 12 months after gastrectomy. Although radiological examinations did not show definitive evidence of tumor recurrence, peritoneal or lymph node metastases were highly suspected during physical examinations in 2 patients. One had a CRP response and died of massive metastases to the peritoneum 1 month later and another died of metastases to systemic lymph nodes 13 months later. In other 5 patients in whom tumor eventually recurred, a relapse could be detected at 16, 22, 29, 30, and 38 months after surgery. There was a significant difference ($P = .02$) in a recurrence rate between patients with a CRP response (3 of 4 patients) and those without such a response (4 of 39 patients) (**Table 2**). Serum levels of α_1-AT and C4 in patients with subsequent clinical recurrence were significantly higher than those without recurrence (α_1-AT: 2.37 ± 0.49 g/L [236.86 ± 49.01 mg/dL] vs 1.96 ± 0.32 g/L; C4: 0.31 ± 0.01 g/L vs 0.23 ± 0.08 g/L) at 12 months after surgery (**Figure 1** and **Figure 2**). No statistical difference was found between the 2 groups in preoperative and postoperative serum levels of total protein, albumin, prealbumin, transferrin, immunoglobulins, C3, and ceruloplasmin.

From the Department of Surgery, The Jikei University School of Medicine, Tokyo, Japan.

PATIENTS AND METHODS

PATIENTS

Forty-three patients who underwent curative resection of gastric cancer between January 7, 1991 and June 30, 1994 were enrolled in our prospective study after informed consent was obtained. All operations were performed by one of us (T.F.). Curative resections were defined as patients with no residual macroscopic disease after surgery. Distal (subtotal) gastrectomy was carried out in 26 patients, total gastrectomy in 12, and total gastrectomy with splenectomy in 5 (**Table 1**). The new Japanese classification of gastric cancer[5] was used for clinical staging of the tumors. Blood samples were obtained from each patient before surgery to measure serum levels of total protein, albumin, negative acute-phase proteins (prealbumin and transferrin), immunoglobulins, and positive acute-phase proteins (C3 and C4, α_1-antitrypsin [α_1-AT], ceruloplasmin, and C-reactive protein). These protein levels were also measured at 3, 6, and 12 months after surgery. Following an annual computed tomographic scan and ultrasound examination of the upper abdomen, patients were divided into 2 groups according to serum C-reactive protein (CRP) levels at 12 months after surgery (CRP<0.3 mg/dL or CRP ≥ 0.3 mg/dL). At this time, none of the patients showed any evidence of infections or liver dysfunction. They were then followed up once a month for a minimum of 12 months or until death.

PROTEIN ASSAYS

Serum albumin levels were measured using the bromocresol green method.[6] Nephelometric assays[7] were used to determine serum levels of both negative and positive acute-phase proteins. Goat antiserum to human CRP was purchased from the Yatoron Corporation (Tokyo, Japan), rabbit antisera to human prealbumin, transferrin, C3 and C4, α_1-AT, and ceruloplasmin were purchased from Behringwerke Corporation (Marburg, Germany). Light scattering intensity was measured by a nephelometer analyzer (Behring Corporation, Marburg, Germany). The detection limit of CRP concentration in this assay was 0.003 g/L.

STATISTICAL ANALYSIS

Data are presented as mean ±SD, or as means and ranges. Differences in serum protein levels between the 2 groups were statistically analyzed using the Mann-Whitney *U* test. The comparison of a recurrence rate was made with the 2-sided Fisher exact test. Differences were considered significant at $P<.05$.

Table 1. Characteristics of Patients Who Underwent Curative Gastrectomy for Gastric Cancer

Characteristic	No. of Patients
Total No. of patients	**43**
Mean age, y	59
Range	25-82
Sex, M/F	28/15
Stage of tumors*	
1a	27
1b	6
2	5
3a	2
3b	3
Procedures performed	
Distal gastrectomy	26
Total gastrectomy	12
Total gastrectomy with splenectomy	5
Mean follow-up period after surgery, mo	42
Range	13-66

*New Japanese classification of gastric cancer was used for staging of the tumors.[5]

Table 2. Stage, Procedures, and Recurrence Rate by Presence or Absence of C-Reactive Protein (CRP) Response

Characteristic	CRP<0.3 mg/dL	CRP≥0.3 mg/dL
Patients, No.	39	4
Stage of tumors*		
1a	25	2
1b	6	0
2	5	0
3a	2	0
3b	1	2
Procedure performed		
Distal gastrectomy	25	1
Total gastrectomy	9	3
Total gastrectomy with splenectomy	5	0
Recurrence site		
Peritoneum	3	1
Lymph nodes	1	2
Liver	0	0
Rate†	4	3

*New Japanese classification of gastric cancer was used for staging of the tumors.[5]

†The Fisher exact test showed a significant ($P = .02$) difference in a recurrence rate for gastric cancer between patients with a CRP response and those without such a response.

COMMENT

In general, the acute-phase proteins are defined as serum proteins that increase in concentration by 25% or more in the first 7 days following tissue damage.[8] Some serum proteins, however, consistently demonstrate reduction in serum concentration during the acute-phase response, and are often referred to as negative acute-phase proteins.[9] Of these proteins, CRP is the best-studied major acute-phase proteins in human. At 12 months following surgery, a CRP response (CRP level was ≥0.003 g/L) was identified in 4 of 43 patients. This low incidence of a CRP response is in contrast to a high incidence of a CRP response (15 of 36 patients)[4] at 4 months after surgery in patients with colorectal cancer. A difference in a recurrence rate for gastric cancer between patients with a CRP response and those without such a response was noted. This result is in keeping with that of a study[4] showing a higher recurrence rate for colorectal

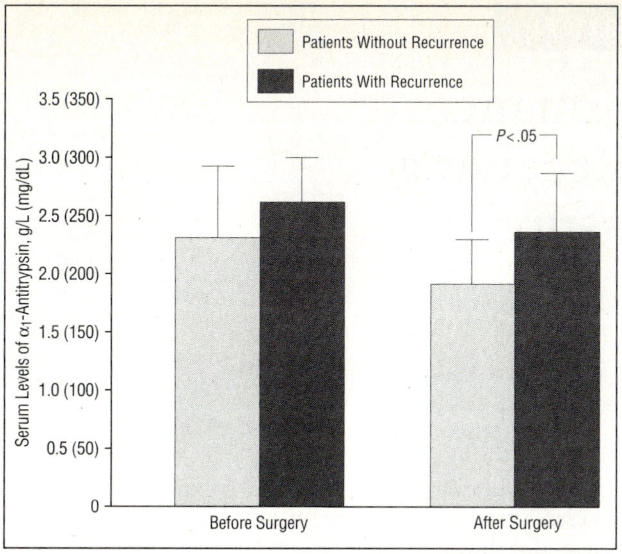

Figure 1. *Serum levels of α_1-antitrypsin in patients with subsequent clinical recurrence were higher than those without recurrence at 12 months after surgery, indicating its possible function as an indicator of malignant tumor recurrence. Error bars indicate SD.*

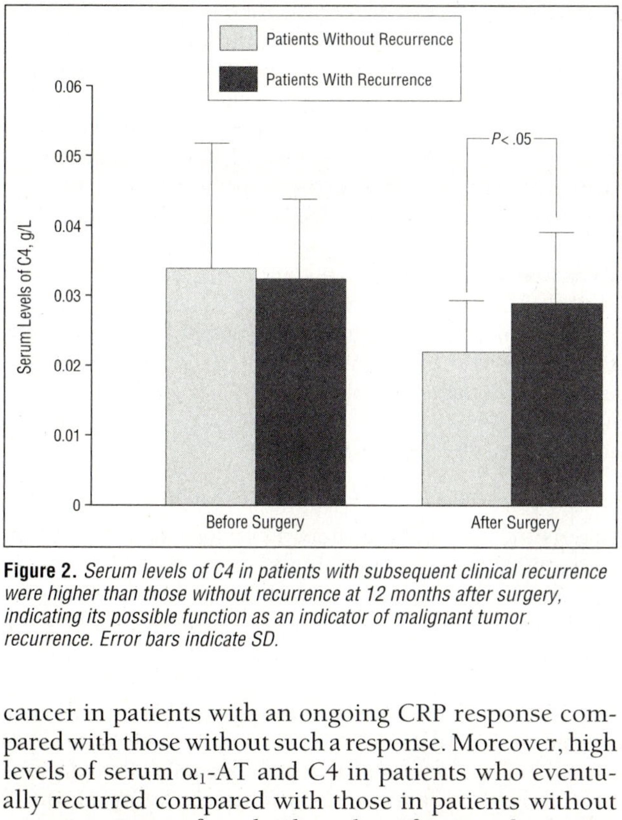

Figure 2. *Serum levels of C4 in patients with subsequent clinical recurrence were higher than those without recurrence at 12 months after surgery, indicating its possible function as an indicator of malignant tumor recurrence. Error bars indicate SD.*

cancer in patients with an ongoing CRP response compared with those without such a response. Moreover, high levels of serum α_1-AT and C4 in patients who eventually recurred compared with those in patients without recurrence were found. The value of acute-phase protein measurement has been studied in patients with malignant diseases. In patients with colorectal cancer, rises of α_1-AT, α_1-acid glycoprotein, and CRP were associated with metastases, and high levels of haptoglobin suggested involvement of the bowel wall by recurrent cancer.[10,11] In gastric cancer, preoperative levels of CRP could help in the identification of the patients with a resectable tumor.[12] Another study of the patients with gastric cancer found an association between postoperative survival time and pretreatment levels of positive acute-phase proteins.[13] These findings indicate that an acute-phase protein response may be sensitive to the early or late phase of tumor growth. The presence of acute-phase protein response may also provide an environment in which tumors are more likely to grow. An inflammatory response with acute-phase protein production may stimulate tumor growth by the increased elaboration of proinflammatory cytokines important in the tissue remodeling.[14]

CONCLUSION

There was a significant difference in the gastric cancer recurrence rate between patients with a CRP response and those without such a response following curative gastric cancer surgery. Higher serum levels of α_1-AT and C4 in patients who eventually recurred were also compared with those in patients without recurrence, and suggest that the presence of an acute-phase protein response is a predictive factor in the early phase of tumor recurrence in patients who undergo curative surgery for gastric cancer.

Corresponding author: Tetsuji Fujita, MD, Department of Surgery, The Jikei University School of Medicine, 3-25-8 Nishishinbashi, Minato-ku, Tokyo 105-0003, Japan.

REFERENCES

1. Noguchi Y, Imada T, Matsumoto A, Coit DG, Brennan MF. Radical surgery for gastric cancer–a review of the Japanese experience. *Cancer.* 1989;64: 2053-2062.
2. Maruyama K, Okabayashi K, Kinoshita T. Progress in gastric cancer surgery in Japan and its limits of radicality. *World J Surg.* 1987;11:418-425.
3. Cooper EH, Stone J. Acute phase reactant proteins in cancer. In: Klein G, Weinhouse S, eds. *Advances in Cancer Research.* 30th ed. Orlando, Fla: Academic Press Inc; 1979:1-44.
4. McMillan DC, Wotherspoon HA, Fearon KCH, et al. A prospective study of tumor recurrence and the acute-phase response after apparently curative colorectal cancer surgery. *Am J Surg.* 1995;170:319-322.
5. Japanese Research Society for Gastric Cancer. *Japanese Classification of Gastric Cancer.* Tokyo, Japan: Kanehara Publishers; 1995.
6. Doumas BT, Watson W, Biggs HG. Albumin standards and the measurement of serum albumin with bromocresol green. *Clin Chim Acta.* 1971;31:87-96.
7. Sternberg JC. A rate nephelometer for measuring specific proteins by immunoprecipitation reactions. *Clin Chem.* 1977;23:1456-1464.
8. Kushner I. The phenomenon of the acute phase response. *Ann N Y Acad Sci.* 1982;389:39-48.
9. Ballou SP, Kushner I. C-reactive protein and the acute phase response. In: Stollerman GH, ed. *Advances in Internal Medicine.* 37th ed. St Louis, Mo: Mosby–Year Book Inc; 1992:313-336.
10. Ward AM, Cooper EH, Turner R, Anderson JA, Neville AM. Acute-phase protein profiles: an aid to monitoring large bowel cancer by CEA and serum enzymes. *Br J Cancer.* 1977;35:170-178.
11. Weinstein PS, Skinner M, Sipe JD, Lokich JJ, Zamcheck N, Cohen AS. Acute-phase proteins or tumour markers: the role of SAA, SAP, CRP and CEA as indicators of metastasis in a broad spectrum of neoplastic diseases. *Scand J Immunol.* 1984;19:193-198.
12. Mello J, Struthers L, Turner R, Cooper EH, Giles GR. Multivariate analyses as aids to diagnosis and assessment of prognosis in gastrointestinal cancer. *Br J Cancer.* 1983;48:341-348.
13. Rashid SA, O'Quigley J, Axon ATR, Cooper EH. Plasma protein profiles and prognosis in gastric cancer. *Br J Cancer.* 1982;45:390-394.
14. Gelin J, Moldawer LL, Lönnroth C, Sherry B, Chizzonite R, Lundholm K. Role of endogenous tumor necrosis factor alpha and interleukin 1 for experimental tumor growth and the development of cancer cachexia. *Cancer Res.* 1991;51: 415-421.

Impairment of Cardiac Performance by Laparoscopy in Patients Receiving Positive End-Expiratory Pressure

Eric J. Kraut, MD; John T. Anderson, MD; Amira Safwat, MD; Ronald Barbosa, BS; Bruce M. Wolfe, MD

Background: The cardiopulmonary effects of the combination of abdominal and thoracic pressures in humans have not been well delineated.

Objective: To study the cardiopulmonary effects of 15 mm Hg of intra-abdominal pressure in the presence and absence of 10 cm H_2O of positive end-expiratory pressure (PEEP).

Design: Prospective.

Setting: University hospital.

Methods: Nine patients undergoing laparoscopic cholecystectomy had pulmonary compliance, cardiac output, exhaled carbon dioxide, and preload (left ventricular end-diastolic volume) determined at 4 points while undergoing ventilation with (1) no PEEP before pneumoperitoneum; (2) 10 cm H_2O of PEEP and no pneumoperitoneum; (3) no PEEP and 15 mm Hg of pneumoperitoneum; and (4) 10 cm H_2O of PEEP and 15 mm Hg of pneumoperitoneum. Preload and cardiac output were determined by means of transesophageal echocardiography. Pulmonary compliance and exhaled carbon dioxide were determined by an attachment to the end of the endotracheal tube.

Main Outcome Measures: Preload, cardiac output, exhaled carbon dioxide, and pulmonary compliance.

Results: There was no significant change from baseline in preload, cardiac output, or pulmonary compliance when either PEEP or pneumoperitoneum was applied separately. However, there was a significant decrease in preload ($P<.01$), cardiac output ($P=.01$), and exhaled carbon dioxide ($P=.04$) when PEEP and pneumoperitoneum were applied together. Pulmonary compliance was not significantly affected at any of these points.

Conclusions: There was a significant reduction in preload and cardiac output when there was intra-abdominal pressure of 15 mm Hg in the presence of 10 cm H_2O of PEEP. This combination of pressures may pose a contraindication to laparoscopic surgery.

Arch Surg. 1999;134:76-80

INTRA-ABDOMINAL hypertension can cause both hemodynamic and pulmonary compromise when there is intra-abdominal bleeding, intra-abdominal packing, intestinal obstruction, or pneumoperitoneum. The pulmonary effects of intra-abdominal hypertension tend to culminate in elevated peak airway pressures when intra-abdominal pressure (IAP) reaches 30 to 40 mm Hg; there is also a fall in pulmonary compliance and vital capacity and an increase in alveolar dead space.[1] The hemodynamic effects of increasing IAP are marked by decreasing cardiac output (CO) thought to be caused by increasing systemic vascular resistance and decreasing venous return.[2,3] In the normovolemic human, an increase in IAP may decrease cardiac output when IAP reaches 40 mm Hg.[4-7] At this point, patient survival may depend on lowering the IAP by decompressing the abdomen.[8,9]

Patients with intra-abdominal hypertension (such as trauma patients with abdominal packing and patients undergoing laparoscopy) frequently receive positive end-expiratory pressure (PEEP) ventilation. An important question to ask is whether the criteria for abdominal decompression in patients receiving elevated PEEP should be the same as for those receiving low PEEP. The answer to this question may clarify the reported discrepancies in the level at which IAP results in hemodynamic consequences. For example, Kashtan et al[2] showed no hemodynamic compromise in dogs until the IAP reached 40 mm Hg, whereas Meldrum et al[9] demonstrated improved CO when the abdomen was decompressed at a mean IAP of 27 mm Hg. This discrepancy in mean

From the Department of Surgery, University of California, Davis Health System, Sacramento.

PATIENTS AND METHODS

Nine patients at the University of California, Davis, who were slated for laparoscopic cholecystectomy gave consent for this study, which was approved by our Human Subjects Committee. A thorough cardiac and pulmonary history was obtained on all patients. Patients were excluded if they had esophageal obstruction, recent upper gastrointestinal tract bleeding, or previous upper gastrointestinal tract surgery. All patients were given an initial bolus of 2 mL of crystalloid per kilogram per hour of preoperative fast. This was followed intraoperatively by 2 mL of crystalloid drip per kilogram per hour as maintenance fluid. A Foley catheter and peripheral intravenous line were placed in all patients. Six patients had a respiratory mechanics workstation (Ventrak, Novametrics Medical Systems Inc, Wallingford, Conn) attached to the end of their endotracheal tubes. Five of these 6 patients had arterial lines placed because of the anesthesiologists' need for blood pressure or blood gas monitoring. A Varess needle or Hassan cannula was placed shortly after induction so that the IAP could be measured before insufflation of the abdomen and not assumed to be 0 mm Hg. Pneumoperitoneum was obtained through either Varess needle or Hassan cannula to 15 mm Hg and maintained through the side port of an 11-mm cannula. A carbon dioxide (CO_2) insufflator (OpPneu 5050E, Wisap GmbH, Munich, Germany) was used.

After induction, a transesophageal echocardiography (TEE) probe (Sonos 2500, Hewlett Packard, Andover, Mass) was placed into the esophagus and advanced to a position 30 to 35 cm from the incisors to obtain a 4-chamber view of the heart. The left ventricular end-diastolic volume (LVEDV), the left ventricular end-systolic volume (LVESV), and the ejection fraction were measured with the probe in the horizontal plane by the method of acoustic quantification.[12] The respiratory mechanics workstation was attached to the end of the endotracheal tube by an in-line adaptor in 6 patients. This machine and arterial blood gases were used to determine the ratio of dead space to tidal volume, pulmonary compliance, autoPEEP (see below), and total exhaled CO_2 per minute ($\dot{V}CO_2$). These values were obtained with the respiratory mechanics workstation by the method of Arnold et al.[13] Data were analyzed off-line with Analysis + respiratory mechanics analysis software (Version 2.0, Novametrics Medical Systems Inc). A CO_2 expirogram was obtained by plotting CO_2 in exhaled breath against exhaled breath volume. The CO_2 was determined with a mainstream capnometer; flow and pressure were determined from a fixed-orifice differential pressure pneumotachograph. Expired CO_2 per breath was calculated as the area under the CO_2 expirogram curve. The CO_2 production was determined as the $\dot{V}CO_2$. The ratio of physiological dead space to tidal volume was determined from the CO_2 expirogram and the arterial CO_2 level by the technique of Fowler[14] and Fletcher et al.[15] Dynamic pulmonary compliance was assessed by the following equation: compliance = tidal volume/(peak inspiratory pressure − PEEP). Total PEEP was determined as the sum of set PEEP and autoPEEP, where set PEEP is the PEEP set on the ventilator. AutoPEEP was measured as the airway pressure in excess of baseline PEEP required to initiate ventilator flow.

The previously mentioned data collected by TEE, the respiratory mechanics workstation, and arterial blood gases were obtained while the patient was placed under 4 conditions within 15 minutes after induction: (1) 0 cm H_2O of PEEP and before pneumoperitoneum, (2) 10 cm H_2O of PEEP and before pneumoperitoneum, (3) 0 cm H_2O of PEEP after pneumoperitoneum at a pressure of 15 mm Hg, and (4) 10 cm H_2O of PEEP after pneumoperitoneum. Data acquisition with each manipulation required approximately 1 to 2 minutes. We waited approximately 1 to 2 minutes between each manipulation and its respective data acquisition. No ventilator changes were made other than PEEP during the data acquisition period.

Stroke volume was determined by the equation LVEDV − LVESV. The CO was determined by the equation heart rate × stroke volume. The ventricular end-systolic elastance (Ees) was used as a measure of myocardial contractility.[16] The equation for Ees is Ees = LVESP/(LVESV − 0.1 × weight [kilograms]). The LVESP was estimated by the equations LVESP = (0.9 × SBP) − 10 mm Hg for patients 50 years or older and LVESP = (0.9 × SBP) − 20 mm Hg for patients younger than 50 years, where SBP is systolic blood pressure.[16]

Data were statistically analyzed by means of a factorial repeated-measures analysis of variance with 2 within factors, IAP and PEEP. The 4 treatment combinations were compared by a repeated-measures model with 1 within factor (treatment) and by pairwise post hoc comparisons among the treatments with the use of the Tukey method.[17] Relationships were considered statistically significant whenever $P < .05$. Variables were transformed logarithmically as necessary to satisfy the assumptions of normality and homoscedasticity. As ventricular volumes and COs were compared within each patient under 4 experimental conditions, the volumes were left unindexed for simplicity.

IAP may have occurred because the patients studied by Meldrum et al had an average of 10 cm H_2O of PEEP, whereas Kashtan et al applied no PEEP. In the context of laparoscopy, 15 mm Hg of IAP may not cause hemodynamic compromise unless the patient is also exposed to 10 cm H_2O of PEEP.

Although both PEEP and IAP are thought to decrease venous return, there is evidence that both 10 cm H_2O of PEEP[10] and mild increases in IAP,[11] when applied separately, are tolerated in the normovolemic state with no decrease in CO. An animal study showed that CO is reduced when intra-abdominal pressures less than 40 mm Hg are applied in conjunction with PEEP.[10] Because elevated intra-abdominal pressures frequently occur in conditions in which PEEP is required in humans, we prospectively studied the cardiopulmonary effects of intra-abdominal pressure in conjunction with PEEP.

RESULTS

Demographic data are given in **Table 1**. One of the patients had acute cholecystitis and severe coronary artery disease with a fractional shortening of 10% and previous congestive heart failure. Another patient had had a myocardial infarction 12 years before our study and had subsequently sustained a cardiac arrest with a previous

Table 1. Demographic Data on 9 Patients Undergoing Laparoscopic Cholecystectomy

Factor	Finding
Age, mean ± SD, y	50.3 ± 16.6
Weight, mean ± SD, kg	87.9 ± 29.7
Height, mean ± SD, cm	162.7 ± 5.1
Diagnoses, No.	
Acute cholecystitis	2
Chronic cholecystitis	7
Sex, No.	
Male	3
Female	6
Heart disease, No.	
Previous myocardial infarctions	2
No cardiac symptoms	7
Pulmonary disease, No.	
Chronic obstructive pulmonary disease	1
No pulmonary symptoms	8

surgery. The other 7 patients had no major cardiac symptoms. One patient had chronic obstructive pulmonary disease but no symptomatic heart disease. The other patients had no pulmonary symptoms.

Nine patients had ventricular volumes determined by TEE under each of the 4 conditions. Pulmonary compliance, autoPEEP, airway pressures, and $V\text{CO}_2$ could be determined in the 6 patients who had respiratory mechanics workstation analysis. The ratio of dead space to tidal volume could be described in only the 5 patients who had arterial lines for an arterial blood gas measurement in each of the 4 conditions. All patients had urine outputs of greater than 50 mL/h during surgery.

Thoracic and abdominal pressures are shown in **Table 2**. The mean autoPEEP was 2.80, 3.40, 0.90, and 3.25 cm H_2O for conditions 1, 2, 3, and 4, respectively. AutoPEEPs were statistically similar in all 4 groups. Total PEEPs were 2.80, 13.40, 0.90, and 13.25 cm H_2O. The average IAP before insufflation was 0.8 mm Hg. After insufflation of the abdomen with CO_2, the average IAP was 15 mm Hg as it was set by the insufflating machine for conditions 3 and 4.

The cardiopulmonary variables evaluated under the 4 conditions are shown in **Table 3**, and the statistical analyses of these variables are shown in **Table 4**. The end-diastolic volume had a significant decrease from baseline only when both PEEP and 15 mm Hg of IAP were applied in condition 4. The end-diastolic volume in condition 4 was also lower than that in conditions 2 and 3. Neither 10 cm H_2O of PEEP (condition 2) nor 15 mm Hg alone (condition 3) had a statistically significant effect on preload because conditions 1, 2, and 3 were statistically similar by multiple comparisons.

The end-systolic volume was significantly higher ($P<.01$) in condition 3 than in all other conditions. The end-systolic volume in conditions 1, 2, and 4 were statistically similar. When compared with baseline (condition 1), there was a decrease in CO and stroke volume only when PEEP and pneumoperitoneum were applied simultaneously (condition 4). There was a significant reduction in $V\text{CO}_2$ only when PEEP and IAP were applied together ($P = .04$).

COMMENT

Previous studies have shown that humans require IAPs of greater than 25 mm Hg during laparoscopy to suffer hemodynamic consequences.[6,7] The present study demonstrates that 15 mm Hg of IAP can cause hemodynamic consequences if 10 cm H_2O of PEEP is applied simultaneously. Previous studies of the hemodynamic effects of intra-abdominal hypertension have provided reasons why this may be the case. Toomasian et al[18] demonstrated that increased IAP causes a decrease in vena cava flow and an increase in intracavitary right and left atrial pressures. Positive end-expiratory pressure also decreases vena cava flow.[19,20] It is possible that PEEP and IAP are additive in their effects on preload.

Hypovolemia also decreases venous return. Only 20 to 40 mm Hg of IAP is required to reduce the CO in hypovolemic dogs.[2,18] We maintained normovolemia in our patients so that we could specifically look at the effects of PEEP and IAP in the normovolemic human. Because data were obtained after the patients had been given their initial crystalloid bolus and all data acquisition occurred during the first 15 minutes after induction, all patients were considered normovolemic in condition 1. The small increase in either PEEP (10 cm H_2O) or IAP (15 mm Hg) alone was well tolerated in these normovolemic patients. The end-diastolic volume decreased in condition 4 most likely because of decreased venous return resulting from the combination of elevated PEEP and IAP.

We used TEE instead of Swan-Ganz catheterization to estimate preload in this study for several reasons. When PEEP is elevated, wedge pressure may correlate poorly with CO.[21,22] The LVEDV is accurately measured by TEE[23] and may correlate better with CO than does right ventricular end-diastolic volume measured by volumetric Swan-Ganz catheters.[21] Estimating preload by means of wedge pressure in the experiment by Burchard et al[10] may have led to an incorrect conclusion. In their study, hemodynamics were monitored in dogs while the dogs received various PEEPs and IAPs. The wedge pressure increased with increasing IAP and PEEP, leading to the conclusion that the diminished CO in animals receiving PEEP and elevated IAP resulted from depressed cardiac function. In our study, the decrease in LVEDV in those with elevated PEEP and IAP suggests that CO decreased because of an additive effect of PEEP and IAP in decreasing venous return. The ejection fraction remained the same in all 4 conditions, and the Ees actually increased in condition 4, indicating that depressed myocardial contractility is not the reason for the low CO. The increase in Ees in condition 4 suggests that these patients increased their myocardial contractility to compensate for their low preload and CO.

The decrease in $V\text{CO}_2$ in condition 4 was most likely caused by reduction in CO. Without PEEP the $V\text{CO}_2$ is expected to increase by as much as 75% because of CO_2 absorption of the pneumoperitoneum when the abdomen is insufflated to 15 mm Hg of pressure. This increase in $V\text{CO}_2$ starts after 30 minutes of insufflating the abdomen.[3] However, the $V\text{CO}_2$ did not

Table 2. Abdominal and Thoracic Pressures of 9 Patients at 4 Conditions of PEEP and IAP Obtained by Pneumoperitoneum*

	Mean ± SD			
Pressures†	**Condition 1**	**Condition 2**	**Condition 3**	**Condition 4**
Set PEEP	0.0 ± 0.0	10.0 ± 0.0	0.0 ± 0.0	10.0 ± 0.0
AutoPEEP	2.8 ± 4.9	3.4 ± 6.0	0.9 ± 2.2	3.3 ± 5.1
Total PEEP	2.8 ± 4.9	13.4 ± 6.0	0.9 ± 2.2	13.3 ± 5.1
IAP	0.8 ± 1.7	. . .‡	15.0 ± 0.0	15.0 ± 0.0

*PEEP indicates positive end-expiratory pressure; IAP, intra-abdominal pressure. Condition 1 was PEEP of 0 cm H_2O and IAP of 0 mm Hg; condition 2, 10 cm H_2O and 0 mm Hg; condition 3, 0 cm H_2O and 15 mm Hg; and condition 4, 10 cm H_2O and 15 mm Hg.

†See "Patients and Methods" section for an explanation of set PEEP and autoPEEP.

‡Intra-abdominal pressure was not measured in condition 2.

Table 3. Cardiopulmonary Variables of 9 Patients at 4 Conditions of PEEP and IAP Obtained by Pneumoperitoneum*

	Mean ± SD			
Variables	**Condition 1**	**Condition 2**	**Condition 3**	**Condition 4**
End-diastolic volume, mL	89 ± 27	85 ± 30	92 ± 26	62 ± 20
End-systolic volume, mL	45 ± 10	46 ± 23	59 ± 18	37 ± 18
Ejection fraction, %	46 ± 12	41 ± 9	40 ± 10	46 ± 16
Stroke volume, mL	44 ± 20	38 ± 19	33 ± 13	27 ± 8
Cardiac output, L/min	3.6 ± 2.1	3.0 ± 1.7	2.3 ± 1.4	1.6 ± 1.0
Systolic blood pressure, mm Hg	113 ± 7	101 ± 7	102 ± 6	104 ± 8
Heart rate, beats/min	78 ± 6	77 ± 6	74 ± 6	70 ± 5
Ees, mm Hg/mL	2.77 ± 1.05	3.22 ± 2.13	2.00 ± 0.59	4.12 ± 2.27
Exhaled CO_2, mL/min	215.4 ± 17.8	201.6 ± 11.6	181.5 ± 56.2	156.2 ± 46.7
Dead space to tidal volume ratio	0.223 ± 0.028	0.213 ± 0.040	0.214 ± 0.018	0.230 ± 0.050
Pulmonary compliance, mL/cm	42.2 ± 10.3	43.8 ± 14.0	39.1 ± 8.4	30.0 ± 9.4
Peak airway pressure, cm H_2O	25.7 ± 4.2	28.1 ± 6.5	32.8 ± 6.3	32.9 ± 3.2
Mean airway pressure, cm H_2O	9.8 ± 1.0	3.5 ± 1.6	11.6 ± 4.6	15.3 ± 4.0

*PEEP indicates positive end-expiratory pressure; IAP, intra-abdominal pressure; Ees, ventricular end-systolic elastance (a measure of myocardial contractility); CO_2, carbon dioxide. See the first footnote to Table 2 for definitions of conditions.

change in any condition other than condition 4, which was the last manipulation. In this condition the V_{CO_2} decreased, most likely because of the fall in CO noted by echocardiography in condition 4. If CO remained constant, V_{CO_2} would probably have remained similar in all 4 conditions until 30 minutes after pneumoperitoneum, at which time V_{CO_2} would rise if there were no ventilator changes. Therefore, it is unlikely that acidemia and hypercapnea caused by CO_2 absorption were responsible for hemodynamic changes, because data were acquired early after insufflation, the respiratory rate and tidal volume were not changed, and the V_{CO_2} did not rise.

There is a potential problem with interpreting the data of these 4 conditions in which there were sequential manipulations. The most obvious problem is that we intended that there be 0 cm H_2O of PEEP in condition 3 within minutes of decreasing the PEEP from 10 cm H_2O in condition 2. Therefore, it is important to measure the total PEEP (set PEEP + autoPEEP). In condition 3 the average total PEEP was only 0.9 cm H_2O when the set PEEP was 0 cm H_2O. Because the autoPEEP was similar in all 4 conditions, sequential manipulations did not confound this aspect of the data. Sequential manipulations are not as much a problem with respect to IAP because no IAP was applied in the first 2 conditions and because, as IAP was applied, it was continuously measured to ensure an accurate estimate of IAP during each condition. Not all IAPs are 0 mm Hg before insufflation. Therefore, we measured the initial IAP before insufflation.

Table 4. Multiple Comparisons of the 4 Conditions of PEEP and IAP for the Variables in Table 3*

Variable	**Multiple Comparisons† of Conditions 1, 2, 3, and 4**
End-diastolic volume	4<1, 2, 3
End-systolic volume	1, 2, 4<3
Ejection fraction	No differences
Stroke volume	4<1
Cardiac output	4<1
Systolic blood pressure	No differences
Heart rate	No differences
Exhaled CO_2 per minute	4<1
Ratio of dead space to tidal volume	No differences
Pulmonary compliance	No differences
Peak airway pressure	1<3, 4
Mean airway pressure	1<4
AutoPEEP‡	No differences
Myocardial contractility (Ees)	4>3

*PEEP indicates positive end-expiratory pressure; IAP, intra-abdominal pressure; and CO_2, carbon dioxide. See the first footnote to Table 2 for definitions of conditions.

†According to the Tukey method.

‡See the "Patients and Methods" section for an explanation.

CONCLUSIONS

An IAP of 15 mm Hg in the normovolemic human can result in a significant reduction of preload and CO in the presence of 10 cm H_2O of PEEP. The cardiac and pulmonary effects of 15 mm Hg of IAP without PEEP are well tolerated. Consideration should be given to avoiding the combination of these 2 pressures in clinical practice. In situations where this combination cannot be avoided, care should be taken to closely monitor the heart and to optimize preload.

Reprints: Eric J. Kraut, MD, Department of Surgery, University of California, Davis, Health System, 4301 X St, Sacramento, CA 95817-2214 (e-mail: EKraut1@aol.com).

REFERENCES

1. Safran DB, Orlando R III. Physiologic effects of pneumoperitoneum. *Am J Surg.* 1994;167:281-286.
2. Kashtan J, Green J, Parsons E, Holcroft J. Hemodynamic effects of increased abdominal pressure. *J Surg Res.* 1981;30:249-255.
3. Ho H, Saunders C, Gunther R, Wolfe B. Effector of hemodynamics during laparoscopy: CO_2 absorption or intra-abdominal pressure? *J Surg Res.* 1995;59:497-503.
4. Burchard KW, Slotman GJ, Jed E, Singh AK, Gann DS. Positive pressure respirations and pneumatic antishock garment application: hemodynamic response. *J Trauma.* 1985;25:83-89.
5. Gaffney FA, Thal ER, Taylor WF, et al. Hemodynamic effects of medical antishock trousers (MAST garment). *J Trauma.* 1981;21:931-937.
6. Kelman GR, Swapp GH, Smith I, Denzie RJ, Gordon NL. Cardiac output and arterial blood-gas tension during laparoscopy. *Br J Anaesth.* 1972;44:1155-1162.
7. Motew M, Ivankovich AD, Bieniarz J, Albrecht RF, Zahad B, Scommegna A. Cardiovascular effects and acid-base blood gas changes during laparoscopy. *Am J Obstet Gynecol.* 1973;115:1001-1012.
8. Cullen DJ, Coyle JP, Teplick R, Long MC. Cardiovascular, pulmonary, and renal effects of massively increased intra-abdominal pressure in critically ill patients. *Crit Care Med.* 1989;17:118-121.
9. Meldrum DR, Moore FA, Moore EE, Franciose RJ, Sauaia A, Burch JM. Prospective characterization and selective management of the abdominal compartment syndrome. *Am J Surg.* 1997;174:667-673.
10. Burchard KW, Ciombor D, McLeod MK, Slothman GJ, Gann DS. Positive end expiratory pressure with increased intra-abdominal pressure. *Surg Gynecol Obstet.* 1985;161:313-318.
11. Ishizaki Y, Bandai Y, Shimomura K, Abe H, Ohtomo Y, Idezuki Y. Safe intraabdominal pressure of carbon dioxide pneumoperitoneum during laparoscopic surgery. *Surgery.* 1993;114:549-554.
12. Bednarz JE, Marcus RH, Lang RM. Technical guidelines for performing automated border detection studies. *J Am Soc Echocardiogr.* 1995;8:293-305.
13. Arnold JH, Thompson JE, Arnold LW. Single breath CO_2 analysis: description and validation of a method. *Crit Care Med.* 1996;24:96-102.
14. Fowler WS. Lung function studies, V: respiratory dead space in old age and in pulmonary emphysema. *J Clin Invest.* 1950;29:1439-1444.
15. Fletcher R, Jonson B, Cumming G, Brew J. The concept of deadspace with special reference to the single breath test for carbon dioxide. *Br J Anaesth.* 1981;53:77-88.
16. Chang MC, Mondy JS, Meredith JW, Miller PR, Owings JT, Holcroft JW. Clinical application of ventricular end-systolic elastance and the ventricular pressure-volume diagram. *Shock.* 1997;7:413-419.
17. Dawson-Saunders B, Trapp RG. Comparing three or more means. In: *Basic and Clinical Biostatistics.* Norwalk, Conn: Appleton & Lange; 1994:134-135.
18. Toomasian JM, Glavinovich G, Johnson MN, Gazzaniga AB. Hemodynamic changes following pneumoperitoneum and graded hemorrhage in the dog. *Surg Forum.* 1978;29:32-33.
19. Jardin F, Farcot JC, Boisante L, Curien N, Margairaz A, Bourdarias JP. Influence of positive end-expiratory pressure on left ventricular performance. *N Engl J Med.* 1981;304:387-392.
20. Powers SR Jr, Mannal R, Neclerio M, et al. Physiologic consequences of positive end-expiratory pressure (PEEP) ventilation. *Ann Surg.* 1973;173:265-272.
21. Kraut EJ, Owings JT, Anderson JT, et al. Right ventricular volumes overestimate left ventricular preload in critically ill patients. *J Trauma.* 1997;42:839-846.
22. Durham R, Neunabar K, Vogler G, et al. Right ventricular end diastolic volume as a measure of preload. *J Trauma.* 1995;39:218-224.
23. Marcus RH, Bednarz J, Coulden R, et al. Ultrasonic backscatter system for automated on-line endocardial boundary detection: evaluation by ultrafast computed tomography. *J Am Coll Cardiol.* 1993;22:839.

Relationship of Systemic Inflammatory Response Syndrome to Organ Dysfunction, Length of Stay, and Mortality in Critical Surgical Illness

Effect of Intensive Care Unit Resuscitation

Mia Talmor, MD; Lynn Hydo, BS; Philip S. Barie, MD, FCCM

Background: A systemic proinflammatory response has been implicated in the pathogenesis of organ dysfunction. The effects of surgery, surgical stress, anesthesia, and subsequent intensive care unit (ICU) resuscitation may affect the components of the systemic inflammatory response syndrome (SIRS) score (temperature, heart rate, respiratory rate, and white blood cell count). Any SIRS scores calculated within 24 hours after surgery or at the onset of nonoperative resuscitation may overestimate the proinflammatory response itself, making quantitation of SIRS at that time potentially too sensitive. We hypothesized that SIRS attributable to ICU resuscitation can be quantitated, and that SIRS after the first day of therapy in the ICU correlates with several outcomes.

Methods: Prospective analysis of 2300 surgical ICU admissions during a 49-month period. Acute Physiology and Chronic Health Evaluation III (APACHE III) scores were recorded after 24 hours. Daily and cumulative multiple organ dysfunction scores (0-4 points for each of 6 organs, 24 points total) and SIRS scores (1 point for each parameter, 4 points total) were recorded. Defined end points were hospital mortality, days in the ICU, and organ dysfunction.

Results: On day 1, 49.4% of patients had SIRS (score $\geq$2), whereas 34.5% of patients who remained in the ICU had SIRS (score $\geq$2) on day 2 ($P<.001$). The SIRS score decreased by a mean of 0.8 points from day 1 to day 2, regardless of the type of admission. A SIRS score that decreased on day 2, in comparison with the score on day 1, resulted in less mortality than a unchanged or higher score on day 2 (11% vs 18% vs 22%, $P<.001$). Systemic inflammatory response scores were higher for nonsurvivors than survivors on each of the first 7 days in the ICU. The day 2 SIRS score correlated well with the admission APACHE III score ($P<.001$) and all defined end points (all $P<.001$). The day 2 SIRS score also correlated with the day 2 multiple organ dysfunction score ($P<.001$). By multiple logistic regression, APACHE III ($P<.001$), day 2 SIRS score ($P<.01$) (but not day 1 SIRS score, $P=.99$), and day 2 multiple organ dysfunction score ($P<.001$) (but not day 1 multiple organ dysfunction score, $P=.81$) predicted mortality.

Conclusions: Systemic inflammatory response syndrome attributable to surgery or surgical stress can be quantitated. Twenty-four hours of ICU resuscitation results in a decline in the SIRS score. The magnitude of the proinflammatory response on the second ICU day may be a useful predictor of outcome in critical surgical illness.

Arch Surg. 1999;134:81-87

THE SYSTEMIC inflammatory response syndrome (SIRS) is a clinical response to an inflammatory or traumatic stimulus of unspecified etiology. As defined by the American College of Chest Physicians/Society of Critical Care Medicine consensus conference in 1992, SIRS is diagnosed if 2 or more of the following criteria are met: (1) temperature greater than 38°C or less than 36°C; (2) heart rate greater than 90 beats per minute; (3) respiratory rate greater than 20/min or a Pa_{CO_2} less than 32 mm Hg; or (4) white blood cell count greater than 12.0×10^9/L or less than 4.0×10^9/L or the presence of more than 10 immature bands.[1] The consensus stipulated that these changes should represent an acute alteration from baseline in the absence of other known causes for such abnormalities, such as chemotherapy-induced leukopenia. Although these diagnostic criteria were established via consensus rather than quantitative study, subsequent investigations have validated their usefulness in predicting groups of patients with an increased risk of mortality.[2-4]

The effect of SIRS on mortality in a mixed population of medical and surgical patients in the intensive care unit (ICU) has been studied[2] but the differential responses to surgical stress and anesthesia were not quantitated. The effects of sur-

From the Department of Surgery, Joan and Sanford I. Weill Medical College of Cornell University, and the Anne and Max A. Cohen Surgical ICU, New York Presbyterian Hospital–Cornell Medical Center, New York.

PATIENTS AND METHODS

This study was conducted during a 49-month period in the general surgical ICU of an urban university tertiary care medical center that provides surgical care to its local community and to tertiary care referrals, and functions also as a level I trauma center. Although the institution serves as a regional center for burn care and cardiothoracic surgery, those patients are cared for in separate, dedicated units and thus are excluded from this analysis.

All variables analyzed in this study were calculated prospectively, with the exception of SIRS scores, which were calculated retrospectively from raw data collected prospectively. Acute Physiology and Chronic Health Evaluation II and III (APACHE II and APACHE III) scores were calculated manually as described in the original reports[9,10] and reported for our patient population previously.[11] The worst physiologic values during the first 24 hours of critical care were used for calculation of the APACHE scores. All patients were analyzed until hospital discharge or death. In circumstances where a patient was readmitted to the surgical ICU during the same hospital stay, all admissions were included for the ICU length of stay analysis, but hospital mortality was calculated as a percentage of patients.

The MOD score of Marshall et al[12] was calculated daily and a maximal score was also determined. The MOD score grades increasing severity of dysfunction of 6 organ systems (cardiac, central nervous system, hematologic, hepatic, pulmonary, and renal) on a 4-point scale, so that a maximum of 24 points can be accrued. The maximal MOD score was calculated by summing the individual worst values at any time during the ICU stay for each of the 6 organ systems described. Therefore, the maximal MOD score could only increase for the duration of observation, whereas the daily MOD score would flucuate with clinical improvement or deterioration. Patients were considered to have some degree of organ dysfunction if the MOD score was 1 point or higher. This system was compared previously with that of Knaus and Wagner,[13] which considers organ failure to be an all-or-nothing phenomenon, and was found to correlate closely.[14]

The SIRS scores were calculated similarly. The SIRS score assigns 1 point for each parameter (temperature, white blood cell count, heart rate, and respiratory rate), so that a maximum of 4 points can be accrued. A maximal SIRS score was calculated by summing the individual worst value in each of the 4 parameters.[7] Thus, a patient might have a maximal SIRS score of 4, even if the patient had scored 1 point in each different parameter at different points in the ICU admission. A daily SIRS score, which fluctuates on a day-to-day basis similar to the daily MOD score, was also calculated each day of the ICU stay.

The ICU length of stay, hospital length of stay, and maximal MOD score were assessed for each daily SIRS score group (eg, day 1 vs day 2, 3, and so on), and compared using a 1-way analysis of variance (ANOVA) with repeated measures. Differences between groups were identified using the Tukey post hoc test. Mortality rates and the incidences of MOD were compared using a χ^2 contingency table analysis for multiple group comparisons. Comparison of group mean data for continuous variables between survivors and nonsurvivors was made using an unpaired nonparametric Wilcoxon analysis. Subset analyses were performed on survivors vs nonsurvivors, and of elective or emergent operative vs nonoperative admissions. Patients admitted electively were those who underwent a scheduled operation on the day of admission, according to the published operating room schedule. These patients were considered to be elective if the ICU admission followed a destabilizing event during surgery or in the postanesthesia care unit. Nonoperative patients were those admitted with illness or injury (eg, pancreatitis or multiple trauma) or those who sustained a superimposed insult (eg, myocardial infarction or pulmonary embolism) necessitating ICU care at least 24 hours after surgery. Multivariate assessments of the effect of independent variables on dependent outcome variables (magnitude of MOD, length of stay, and mortality) were made with a multivariate logistic regression analysis.

All statistical analyses were performed by microcomputer using commercial software (StatView 4.0.1 with SuperANOVA 1.1.1, Abacus Concepts Inc, Berkeley, Calif). Statistical significance was determined at an α level of .05. Group mean data are expressed as mean±SE.

gical stress, anesthesia, postoperative pain, and subsequent resuscitation may affect the components of the SIRS score. Critics have argued that SIRS scores, when calculated in the immediate postoperative period, may overestimate the proinflammatory response, making quantitation of SIRS at that time potentially too sensitive.[5,6] Pittet et al[4] investigated the epidemiology of SIRS in a population of 170 patients admitted to the surgical ICU and found that the score was too sensitive, precluding its usefulness for prediction of outcome. We subsequently performed a prospective analysis of 2218 surgical ICU patients[7] and found that the development of SIRS over the entire duration of the ICU stay correlated with an increase in the incidence of multiple organ dysfunction (MOD), longer hospital stays, and increased mortality.

The purpose of this study was to determine the effect of surgical stress and ICU resuscitation on SIRS. We hypothesized that SIRS attributable to surgery or resuscitation can be quantitated, and that failure of the SIRS score to decrease after day 1, reflective of the true proinflammatory state, would correlate with a higher MOD score and, hence, prolonged length of stay as well as increased mortality.[8]

RESULTS

Data from 2300 consecutive admissions for critical surgical illness, postoperative complications, or postoperative care were evaluated. The composition of the population within the ICU during the first week of care is depicted in **Figure 1**. The mean age for the group was 64.6 ± 0.3 years, the mean APACHE II score was 13.9 ± 0.2, and the mean APACHE III score was 44.2 ± 0.6. Mean ICU length of stay was 5.5 ± 0.2 days, and average hospital length of stay was 22.4 ± 0.6 days. Forty-nine per-

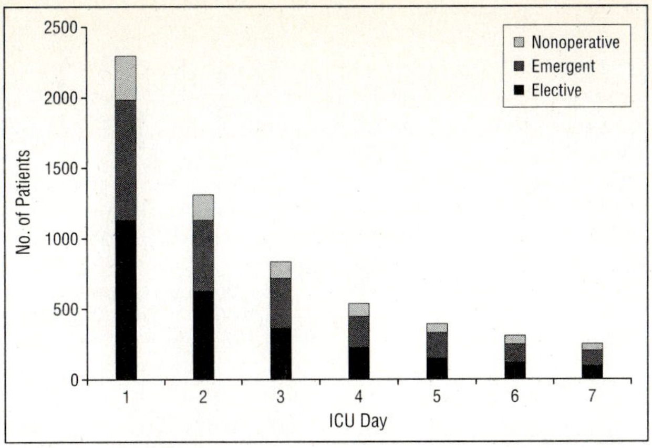

Figure 1. *Composition of patients in the intensive care unit (ICU) during the first week. Note that whereas the number of patients remaining in the ICU decreases progressively with each ICU day, the relative composition of the groups remains proportionate for the first 2 days (see legend to Figure 7).*

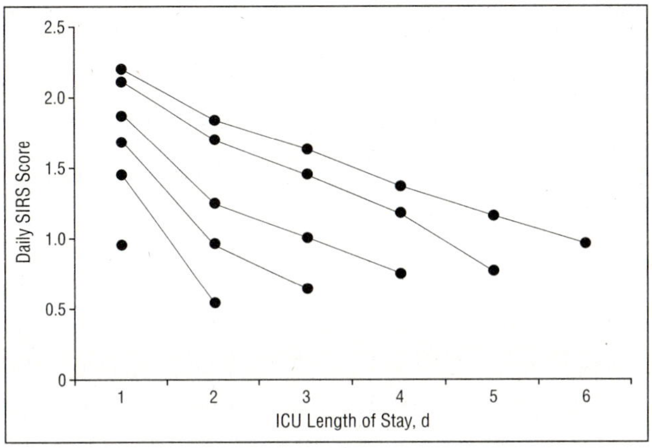

Figure 2. *Daily systemic inflammatory response syndrome (SIRS) scores are depicted as a function of the ultimate length of stay in the intensive care unit (ICU). The mean daily SIRS score is higher on day 1 for each successive length-of-stay group, but the resolution of SIRS (declination of the score in each group) is similar, so that the SIRS score has declined to less than 1 point on the day of discharge for each group. For example, the patients discharged on day 5 had a mean SIRS score of 0.8 on that day, whereas the patients discharged on day 6 had a mean SIRS score of 1.2 on day 5, which decreased to 0.95 on day 6. The relationship does not hold for ICU stays of 7 days or longer, partly because of small sample sizes. All points are statistically discrete (P<.01); error bars are obscured by the points themselves.*

cent of patients developed some degree of organ dysfunction, and hospital mortality for the entire group was 8.3%. The mean maximal SIRS score for the group was 1.9 ± 0.1. On day 1, 49.4% of patients had SIRS (≥2 criteria), whereas 34.5% of patients who remained in the ICU had SIRS on day 2 (*P*<.001). The SIRS scores on successive days, as a function of ultimate ICU length of stay, are depicted in **Figure 2**. The day 1 SIRS scores were successively higher (*P*<.01) for patients who were destined for longer ICU length of stay, but the rate of resolution of SIRS was similar. On average, the SIRS score on the day of discharge from the ICU was 0.5 to 0.95.

Mean daily SIRS scores are depicted (**Figure 3**) for survivors and nonsurvivors for the first 7 days of the ICU stay. This analysis is not based on the day of discharge, therefore patients with multiday stays were considered

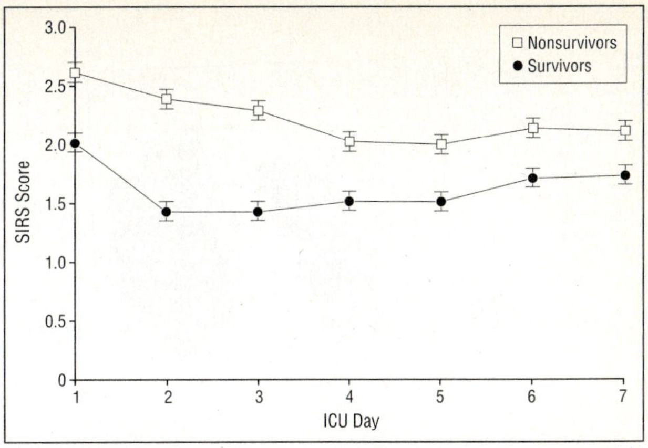

Figure 3. *Mean daily systemic inflammatory response syndrome (SIRS) scores are depicted for survivors and nonsurvivors for the first 7 days of the intensive care unit (ICU) stay. This analysis is not based on the day of discharge; therefore, patients with multiday stays were considered repetitively. The SIRS score was significantly higher (P<.01) for nonsurvivors on each day.*

Table 1. Characteristics Associated With Day 2 SIRS Scores*

SIRS Score	Admission APACHE III Score†	ICU Length of Stay†	MOD Score†	Mortality, %†
0	47.6 ± 1.8	4.0 ± 0.4	3.6 ± 0.2	3.8
1	51.8 ± 1.7	7.0 ± 0.7	4.5 ± 1.2	8.2
2	60.3 ± 1.9	11.3 ± 1.0	7.0 ± 0.3	18.4
3	58.0 ± 2.3	12.6 ± 1.4	7.5 ± 0.5	24.2
4	78.5 ± 4.9	9.8 ± 2.1	8.5 ± 0.6	40.0

**Data are presented as mean ± SE unless otherwise indicated. SIRS indicates systemic inflammatory response syndrome; APACHE III, Acute Physiology and Chronic Health Evaluation III; ICU, intensive care unit; and MOD, multiple organ dysfunction.*

†*P<.001.*

repetitively. The SIRS score was significantly higher (*P*<.01) for nonsurvivors on each day, as were age, APACHE II and III scores, ICU length of stay, and hospital length of stay (all *P*<.001) (data not shown). The APACHE III scores, ICU length of stay, MOD score, and mortality rate all increased with higher day 2 SIRS scores (*P*<.001) (**Table 1**). In actuality, a higher SIRS score related to higher mortality for each of the first 4 days in the ICU (*P*<.001) (**Figure 4**). Mortality was negligible for patients who never had any component of SIRS, but increased progressively (*P*<.01) for higher scores as the ICU stay became prolonged. Mortality was highest (38% and 45%, respectively) for patients with a SIRS score of 4 on day 2 or day 3.

Among patients who had an ICU length of stay of 2 days or more, a decreased day 2 SIRS score, compared with the same-patient SIRS score on day 1, resulted in less mortality than an unchanged or positive score (11% vs 18% vs 22%, *P*<.001). In contrast, the mean SIRS score of patients discharged in less than 24 hours was 1.0 ± 0.1 and mortality was 3.8%, due in part to 22 patients who died within the first 24 hours.

A subset analysis of elective or emergent operative vs nonoperative admissions was performed (**Figure 5** and **Figure 6**). Whereas the mean SIRS score on day 1

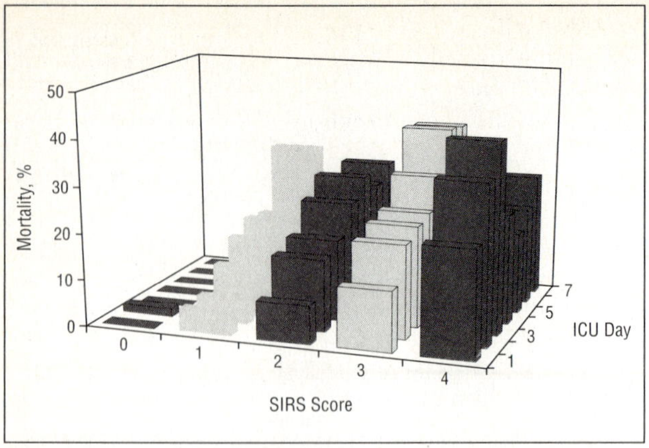

Figure 4. *The mortality rate is depicted as a function of the systemic inflammatory response syndrome (SIRS) score for each of the first 7 days of the intensive care unit (ICU) stay. Mortality was negligible for patients who never had any component of SIRS, but increased progressively (*P<.01*) for higher scores as the ICU stay became prolonged. This analysis considers repetitive scores in patients, so the increased SIRS score may reflect either persistence or worsening. The highest mortality rates (38% and 45%, respectively) were noted for patients with a SIRS score of 4 on day 2 or 3, suggesting the importance of failure of early resuscitation to ameliorate the proinflammatory response in critically ill patients.*

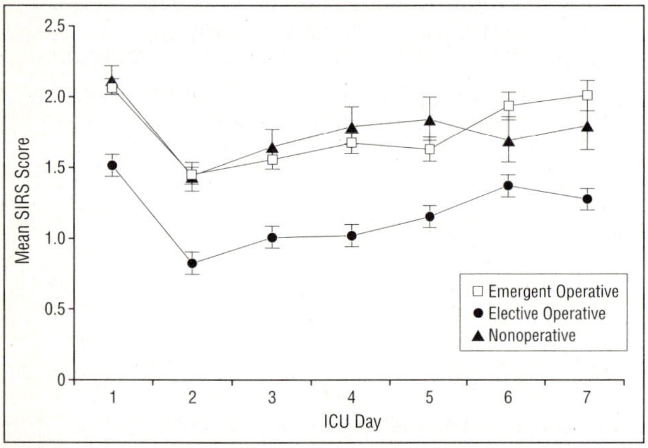

Figure 5. *Subset analysis of systemic inflammatory response syndrome (SIRS) scores in emergent vs nonemergent admissions and operative vs nonoperative admissions. This analysis excludes patients who stayed in the intensive care unit (ICU) for less than 24 hours. Although the SIRS score was always lower (*P<.001*) in the elective patients, note that the response to 24 hours of ICU care was identical (a mean decrease of 0.8 points).*

in the elective group (1.5 ± 0.1) was lower than in the emergent or nonoperative groups (both 2.1 ± 0.1) (*P*<.001), the decrease in SIRS by 0.8 points from day 1 to day 2 was identical (Figure 5). From a nadir on day 2, SIRS scores increased in aggregate on each subsequent day, reflective of the illness severity that prolongs ICU length of stay. Similarly, MOD scores were higher in relation to prolonged ICU length of stay (Figure 6). The increase in SIRS and MOD scores was related to ICU length of stay, in each subset of patients, and in inverse relation to the number of patients remaining in the ICU (**Figure 7**).

The multivariate analysis of the data is summarized in **Table 2**. The APACHE III score (*P*=.01), day 2 SIRS score (*P*<.001) (but not day 1 SIRS score, *P*=.88) and day 2 MOD score (*P*<.001) (but not day 1 MOD score, *P*=.62) were independent predictors of mortality.

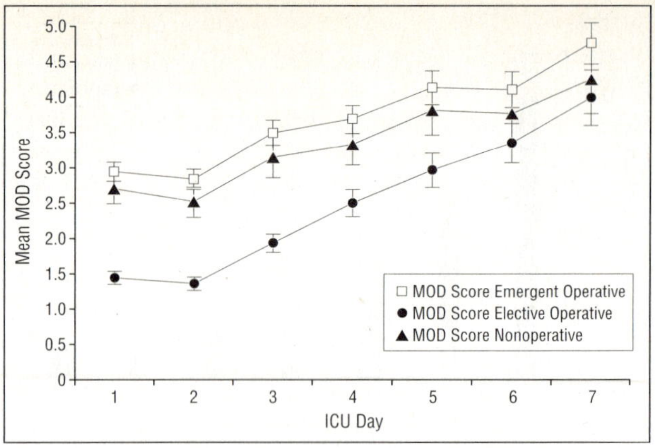

Figure 6. *Subset analysis of multiple organ dysfunction (MOD) scores for the same groups depicted in Figure 5. A longer intensive care unit (ICU) length of stay was associated with more MOD (*P<.001*), although elective surgical admissions had less MOD (*P<.001*) regardless of the length of the ICU stay.*

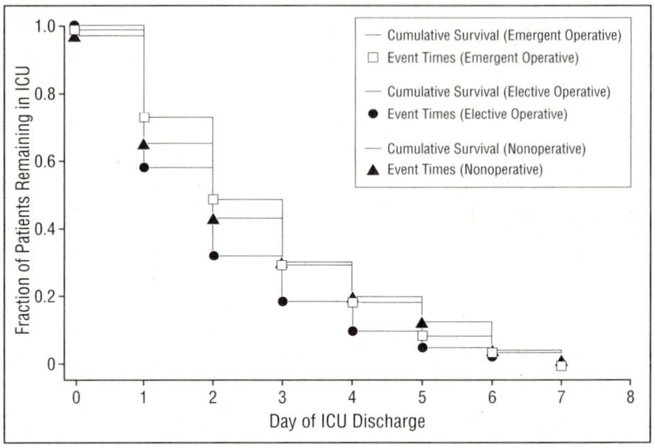

Figure 7. *Kaplan-Meier plot of the number of patients remaining in the intensive care unit (ICU) with respect to time. As length of stay increases to 7 days, elective surgery patients remain in the ICU at a rate equivalent to the other groups (approximately 3% each).*

Table 2. Multiple Logistic Regression Analysis of Early-Stay ICU Severity Scores and Effect on Mortality*

Score	*P*	β-Coefficient	SE	95% CI
APACHE II day 1	.84	.0075	0.0375	−0.0660 to 0.0809
APACHE III day 1	.01	.0244	0.0097	0.0053 to 0.0435
SIRS score day 1	.88	−.0210	0.1413	−0.3051 to 0.2638
SIRS score day 2	<.001	.4607	0.1350	0.1960 to 0.7253
MOD score day 1	.62	.0360	0.0714	−0.1040 to 0.1759
MOD score day 2	<.001	.2621	0.0674	0.1299 to 0.3942

**ICU indicates intensive care unit; CI, confidence interval; APACHE, Acute Physiology and Chronic Health Evaluation; SIRS, systemic inflammatory response syndrome; and MOD, multiple organ dysfunction.*

COMMENT

The data indicate that SIRS attributable to surgical stress and ICU resuscitation can be quantitated. Regardless of admission type, the mean SIRS score decreased by 0.8 points from day 1 to day 2 of the ICU stay, reflective of ICU resuscitation. Elevated day 1 SIRS scores are largely artifact in elective surgery patients because the mean score decreased by 50% to only 0.8 ± 0.1 points on day 2. Furthermore, the SIRS score decreased by an identical amount from day 1 to day 2 in emergent operative and nonoperative patients, making it plausible that the similarity of responses reflects either resuscitation to comparable end points or adherence to similar principles (eg, pain control, suppression of tachycardia),[15] despite the ostensible dissimilarity of the groups.

In 1995, Pittet et al[4] investigated the epidemiology of SIRS in a population of 170 surgical ICU patients. The SIRS criteria (≥2) were met by 93% of the patients, whereas only 8.2% died. The authors concluded that because of very high sensitivity and poor specificity, SIRS did not identify those patients who died ultimately. They did not investigate the relationship of SIRS to the incidence or magnitude of MOD. In a critique of Pittet et al, Sibbald et al[5] suggested that the high rate of SIRS reported by Pittet et al could be explained by differences in definitions for SIRS proposed by the American College of Chest Physicians/Society of Critical Care Medicine panelists and those used by the authors. Illustrating their point, Sibbald et al[5] suggested that in postoperative patients, the American College of Chest Physicians/Society of Critical Care Medicine criteria would not have defined SIRS on ICU admission because the acute alteration from baseline occurred due to another known cause (namely, the surgery). Sibbald et al suggested further that by 12 hours postoperatively, ongoing abnormalities are referable to a baseline (ICU admission) and a diagnosis of SIRS may be confirmed once the effects of anesthesia several hours before had subsided. Menger and Vollmar[6] concurred in principle, but argued that patients might be affected by major surgery for several days, and that major surgical tissue injury, as with entities such as trauma, might be an important factor in the development of SIRS and severe sepsis.

Indeed, the quantitation of SIRS is potentially overly sensitive in surgical populations. Major surgical stress, anesthesia, and postoperative pain can result in a systemic response (temperature >38°C, leukocytosis, tachypnea, and tachycardia) that can mimic acute inflammation, but the response should be short-lived if resuscitation is adequate. Therefore, a SIRS score obtained within 24 hours of ICU admission is a poor predictor of outcome, as Sibbald et al[5] suggested. However, contrary to the contention of Menger and Vollmar,[6] this proinflammatory response seems to be pathological if it persists beyond 24 hours. In this study, an elevated SIRS score obtained between 24 and 48 hours after admission, despite aggressive resuscitation, predicted an increased mortality. Moreover, it is not only the day 2 score in isolation, but failure of the score to decrease or indeed to increase during the second 24 hours (which indicates an ongoing or superimposed proinflammatory response) that is important.

Haga et al[16] retrospectively studied 292 ICU patients after gastrointestinal tract surgery. They found that not only the number of positive SIRS criteria but also the duration of SIRS correlated with an adverse outcome. These authors examined a surgical stress parameter (blood loss indexed to body mass), operative time, and serum C-reactive protein concentrations and documented that surgery itself can lead to a proinflammatory state, as had been hypothesized.[5,6] However, patients who recovered from early postoperative SIRS had a lower incidence of MOD than did those in whom SIRS persisted. Specifically, SIRS (≥2 criteria) continuing consecutively for 2 days after postoperative day 3 had a higher incidence of both infectious and noninfectious postoperative complications, as well as a higher incidence of MOD. We agree that persistent SIRS is deleterious, but our data indicate that the magnitude of SIRS on the second postoperative day (3 days before the study of Haga et al) correlates strongly with adverse outcomes.

Our findings support the current theories regarding the pathogenesis of SIRS and organ dysfunction syndrome popularized by Bone.[17,18] An elevated day 1 SIRS score may be secondary to a local proinflammatory coping reaction. However, by day 2, if a putative anti-inflammatory response has not balanced the proinflammatory response, SIRS persists, resulting in an increased incidence of MOD and death. Our findings also support those who point to the narrow time window for effective resuscitation after surgical or traumatic stress. Abramson et al[19] showed that trauma patients who were resuscitated adequately within 24 hours (measured by normalization of serum lactate levels) all survived. In contrast, only 75% of patients survived if their lactate levels normalized within 24 to 48 hours, and 14% of patients survived if their lactate levels did not normalize within 48 hours. Similarly, a decreased day 2 SIRS score (presumably reflective of adequate resuscitation and postoperative care) correlates with a significantly lower mortality than an increased or unchanged score.

The effect of 24 hours of ICU resuscitation for both operative as well as nonoperative patients is clear from our data. Whereas patients admitted emergently had higher SIRS scores than those admitted electively on day 1, the decrease in SIRS from day 1 to day 2 by 0.8 points was identical regardless of the cause for admission, reflecting the effect of consistent ICU resuscitation. For this reason, SIRS scores calculated prior to resuscitation may result in artificially elevated scores that correlate poorly with outcome.

Current hypotheses of the pathogenesis of MOD may need to be reexamined. In the classic paradigm that affects most patients, organ failure develops catastrophically as a late consequence of critical illness, as induced by a "2-hit" phenomenon.[20] The 2-hit phenomenon represents priming of the inflammatory response by a primary insult (eg multiple trauma), followed by activation of the response by a secondary insult (eg, pneumonia). This study and our previous data indicate that clinically meaningful derangements are present and detectable very early in the course of critical illness.[8] Sequential elements necessary for the development of SIRS or MOD may occur within hours rather than days.[21] The importance of early, aggressive resuscitation is underscored, but the time window for successful intervention may be narrow.

Presented at the 18th Annual Meeting of the Surgical Infection Society, New York, NY, May 2, 1998.

Statement of Clinical Relevance

The early identification of seriously ill patients at risk for an adverse outcome would yield several benefits. Patient triage and resource utilization will become more efficient, and accurate prognostic information would enhance the dialogue with patient or family regarding the plan of care and the expected result. A simple-to-calculate indicator that correlates closely with outcomes in groups of patients has the advantage of ease of use, but is not yet significantly robust for outcome assessments in individuals. Of equal importance is the recognition that physiologic responses so early (day 2) in the ICU stay reflect outcomes. In contrast to the long-standing observation that organ dysfunction occurs as a late, catastrophic event, meaningful derangements are detectable early, and the window for successful resuscitation appears to be narrow.

Reprints: Philip S. Barie, MD, FCCM, Department of Surgery, The New York Presbyterian Hospital–Cornell Medical Center, 525 East 68th St, New York, NY 10021.

REFERENCES

1. American College of Chest Physicians/Society of Critical Care Medicine Consensus Conference. Definitions for sepsis and organ failure, and guidelines for the use of innovative therapies in sepsis. *Crit Care Med.* 1992;20:864-874.
2. Rangel-Frausto MS, Pittet D, Costigan M, et al. The natural history of the systemic inflammatory response syndrome. *JAMA.* 1995;273:117-123.
3. Knaus WA, Harrell FE, Fisher CJ, et al. The clinical evaluation of new drugs for sepsis: a prospective study design based on survival analysis. *JAMA.* 1993;270:1233-1241.
4. Pittet D, Rangel-Frausto S, Li N, et al. Systemic inflammatory response syndrome, sepsis, severe sepsis, and septic shock: incidence, morbidities and outcomes in surgical ICU patients. *Intensive Care Med.* 1995;21:302-309.
5. Sibbald WJ, Doig G, Inman KJ. Sepsis, SIRS and infection. *Intensive Care Med.* 1995;21:299-301.
6. Menger MD, Vollmar B. Systemic inflammatory response syndrome (SIRS) and sepsis in surgical patients. *Intensive Care Med.* 1996;22:616-617.
7. Talmor M, Hydo L, Lu A, Barie PS. Interrelationships between systemic inflammatory response syndrome (SIRS) and multiple organ dysfunction syndrome (MODS) in critical surgical illness: impact on outcome [abstract]. *Crit Care Med.* 1998;26:A125.
8. Barie PS, Hydo LJ. Influence of multiple organ dysfunction syndrome on duration of critical illness and hospitalization. *Arch Surg.* 1996;131:1318-1325.
9. Knaus WA, Draper EA, Wagner DP, et al. APACHE II: a severity of disease classification system. *Crit Care Med.* 1985;13:818-824.
10. Knaus WA, Wagner DP, Draper EA, et al. The APACHE III prognostic system: risk prediction of hospital mortality for critically ill hospitalized patients. *Chest.* 1991;100:1619-1636.
11. Barie PS, Hydo L, Fischer E. Comparison of APACHE II and III scoring systems for mortality prediction in critical surgical illness. *Arch Surg.* 1995;130:77-82.
12. Marshall JC, Sibbald WJ, Cook DA, et al. The multiple organ dysfunction (MOD) score: a reliable indicator of a complex clinical outcome. *Crit Care Med.* 1995;23:1638-1652.
13. Knaus WA, Wagner DP. Multiple systems organ failure: epidemiology and prognosis. *Crit Care Clin.* 1989;2:221-232.
14. Barie PS, Hydo L, Fischer E. A prospective comparison of two different multiple organ failure/dysfunction scoring systems for prediction of mortality in critical surgical illness. *J Trauma.* 1994;37:660-666.
15. Mangano DT, Layug EL, Wallace A, Tateo I. Effect of atenolol on mortality and cardiovascular morbidity after noncardiac surgery: Multicenter Study of Perioperative Ischemia Research Group. *N Engl J Med.* 1996;335:1713-1720.
16. Haga Y, Beppu T, Doi K, et al. Systemic inflammatory response syndrome and organ dysfunction following gastrointestinal surgery. *Crit Care Med.* 1997;25:1994-2000.
17. Bone RC. Sir Isaac Newton, sepsis SIRS and CARS. *Crit Care Med.* 1996;24:1125-1128.
18. Bone RC. Toward a theory regarding the pathogenesis of the systemic inflammatory response syndrome: what we do and do not know about cytokine regulation. *Crit Care Med.* 1996;24:163-172.
19. Abramson D, Scalea TM, Hitchcock R, Trooskin SZ, Henry SM, Greenspan J. Lactate clearance and survival following injury. *J Trauma.* 1993;35:584-588.
20. Moore FA, Moore EE. Evolving conceots in the pathogenesis of post injury multiple organ failure. *Surg Clin North Am.* 1995;72:257-277.
21. Godin PJ, Buchman TG. Uncoupling of biological oscillators: a complementary hypothesis concerning the pathogenesis of multiple organ dysfunction syndrome. *Crit Care Med.* 1996;24:1107-1116.

DISCUSSION

David Spain, MD, Louisville, Ky: I would like to congratulate Dr Talmor on an excellent presentation. In this prospective study it was hypothesized that the SIRS score attributable to ICU resuscitation could be quantified and that failure to reduce your SIRS score in 24 hours in the ICU would correlate with MOD score, ICU length of stay, and mortality. All of these did prove to be true. I have 3 straightforward issues to address.

First, your data show that the SIRS score was as good as the MOD score and the APACHE III in predicting mortality. This suggests that the tried and true parameters of temperature, heart rate, respiratory rate, and white blood cell count, are still reliable indicators of the degree of critical illness and that it's best to look at them "once the dust has settled." This appeals to my somewhat simplistic tendencies and confirms my suspicion that sick people don't do well. Should we abandon the more complex APACHE III and other scoring systems, especially when stratifying patients for clinical studies, and start using the SIRS score? This would keep me from having to take my laptop computer to the ICU.

Second, the decrease in SIRS from ICU day 1 to day 2 was attributable to the ICU resuscitation. This implies that a patient had an inadequate intraoperative resuscitation. Was this assessed? Secondly, do you have a standard resuscitation protocol in your ICU, and how is the adequacy of your resuscitation assessed? Do you use routine vital signs and urine output or was base deficit or lactate clearance used? When were invasive monitors used and was oxygen delivery optimized? And did the patients who had a pulmonary artery catheter inserted have different outcomes; ie, were they more likely to lower their SIRS score postoperatively? Obviously there would be a selection bias toward the sicker patients getting pulmonary artery catheters, but with such a large database you may be able to answer this question.

As you alluded to, does failure to decrease your SIRS score from ICU day 1 to day 2 truly reflect the degree of a proinflammatory state or is this just another marker of inadequate resuscitation? I think that this may be a mixed population of 2 types of patients. If I did my math correctly, approximately 390 of your patients in the ICU on day 2 had a SIRS score greater than or equal to 2. Is there any way to differentiate these 2 patient populations and allow appropriate therapeutic intervention? That is, patients who are underresuscitated could be further resuscitated, while patients who are truly proinflammatory may need further operative care or then could be eligible for clinical drug investigations.

Attempts at curbing the proinflammatory response with pharmacologic agents have been largely disappointing, and this study begins to highlight the importance and impact of resuscitation on the systemic inflammatory response. I congratulate the authors and would like to thank the Surgical Infection Society for the privilege of discussing this paper.

Dr Talmor: With regard to your first question, I think that the SIRS score is a simplified severity of illness score much like the APACHE III and APACHE II scoring systems. It would be very convenient for all of us involved if the SIRS score did yield a meaningful prediction, and it might, but having not performed receiver operating characteristic curves or goodness-of-fit testing for SIRS versus APACHE, I would not recommend abandonment of a more sophisticated system that has been proven to work.

We did perform a multivariate analysis, and the results of this analysis suggest that if gone head-to-head the APACHE III score would prove a stronger system to use.

We have no fixed protocol for resuscitation in our ICU, in response to your second question, but having worked many months in that ICU I can tell you that Dr Barie does give us all special high-intensity training, and we are sort of all on the same page as far as that goes. We use heart rate monitoring, urine output, the standard monitoring as appropriate. We do have a high incidence of elderly patients and, because of this, a high incidence of coronary disease, and we do tend to use invasive monitoring, though we like many others have come away from using Swans, for obvious reasons, as often as we can. I think given the size of the database we might be able to determine a difference in our patients who were Swan vs those who weren't, but I am not sure that this would have any clinical significance or importance.

And finally, I think in answer to your question about separating patients who were inadequately resuscitated and those in whom a proinflammatory state exists, I think it is difficult to separate the 2. It probably is a mixed population and would be very difficult to extrapolate the 2 separate populations, but I do think that the adequacy of the resuscitation in these postoperative patients may be a determinant of the balance between the anti-inflammatory response and the proinflammatory response.

Mark A. Malangoni, MD, Cleveland, Ohio: This is a fascinating study and your work is very interesting. What it brought to mind was in a lot of other scoring systems that have multiple elements, there is one element or sometimes a few elements but not all that really make the difference. Earlier in this meeting, there was discussion about the lack of sensitivity of fever. Have you looked at that particular parameter or tried to look at each of these individual components of SIRS, and if you have, can you tell us which one is the most important and are there certain elements of SIRS that perhaps we could just quit looking at?

Dr Talmor: We actually are very interested in that point ourselves. There have been several papers, especially recently, looking at heart rate, for example, as a predictor of outcome, and studies have shown that patients who are treated postoperatively with β-blockade have done better than those who aren't. In fact we also stipulated that perhaps a combination of 2 of these criteria would portend a worst outcome, such as fever and white blood cell count, which seem to me most predictive of sepsis, and in just starting these subset analyses, which obviously involve very, very complicated statistical analyses in these 2300 patients that we have accumulated, it does seem to point to the fact that heart rate will be the most significant predictor of the 4, which is not what we would have necessarily predicted, but the analyses aren't complete at this point.

Per-Olof Nystrom, MD, PhD, Linkoping, Sweden: Well, since all the SIRS criteria are contained in the APACHE II and especially APACHE III scoring, I am very happy to learn that you think we should not substitute those more sophisticated scores in terms of using them for outcome prediction; however, that begs the question, why should we use the SIRS score? What purpose, what does it tell us about patients? And I wish you could speculate a little about why you use it.

Dr Talmor: I don't think that the SIRS score tells us more about the patient obviously than the APACHE II or the APACHE III scores, which are far more sophisticated, but as Dr Spain alluded, those of us who are calculating these APACHE scores, by hand in our situation because the software is prohibitively expensive to do this, the calculation of the scoring is extremely tedious. If we could go to a patient's bedside, look at the bedside monitor and immediately know what the SIRS score was, and if this did give us an accurate prediction that would allow us to have a dialogue with the patient and the family regarding outcome, I think it would be a very powerful tool for us, and that is what we are hoping to do.

CLINICAL OBSERVATION

Perforation of the Sigmoid Colon Due to Geophagia

Alexander Woywodt, MD; Akos Kiss, MD, FCSSA

G*eophagia*, the habit of eating earth, soil, or clay, is common among African women and frequently encountered during pregnancy. The condition is relatively benign; grave surgical complications are infrequently observed. We describe an adult, nonpregnant, African woman with sigmoid colon perforation and fatal peritonitis due to geophagia. Geophagia is a rare cause of colonic perforation and peritonitis and a high degree of suspicion must be employed to identify this disorder.

Arch Surg. 1999;134:88-89

Throughout the world, *geophagia* (the deliberate consumption of earth, soil, or clay), has been practiced from antiquity to the present. Apart from being a culturally sanctioned practice, this custom may also occur in the mentally handicapped, during pregnancy, or as a feature of iron-deficiency anemia. There is reason to believe that geophagia is not rare, but rarely reported, since many patients are reluctant to volunteer a history of eating earth, soil, or clay and many physicians are generally unaware of the disorder. Therefore, a high degree of suspicion is necessary to suspect geophagical habits and tact must be employed to obtain such information. We describe a 45-year-old African woman who presented with a surgically acute abdomen and a plain abdominal x-ray film that was, in retrospect, highly suggestive of geophagia. It was not until a laparotomy was performed that a diagnosis of geophagia was made, and the patient died of "soil" peritonitis caused by perforation of the sigmoid colon. There was no evidence of any other pathologic condition, particularly diverticular disease or malignancy, that could have accounted for perforation. We believe that knowledge of the disorder and a timely diagnosis might have prompted more aggressive surgical management, although it is unclear whether this would have improved the outcome. Surgeons need to be more familiar with geophagia, since grave complications such as perforation of the sigmoid colon, may occur. We discuss another fatal case of geophagia that emphasizes the complications, diagnosis, and management of this remarkable disorder.

From the Department of Surgery, Chris Hani Baragwanath Hospital, Soweto, University of the Witwatersrand, Johannesburg, Republic of South Africa.
Dr Woywodt is now with the Franz-Volhard-Clinic, Humboldt University, Charité Campus Berlin Buch, Berlin, Germany.

REPORT OF A CASE

A 45-year-old Sowetan woman consulted her physician complaining of constipation and severe abdominal pain that had gradually increased during the past 3 days. There were no precipitating or aggravating factors. She denied having any medical history and was not receiving any medication, but did have a history of anorexia and amenorrhea, and had felt increasingly ill for 6 months. The patient was a housewife and had 4 pregnancies with uneventful deliveries. Her physician noted a mass on the left iliac fossa and she was admitted to the hospital.

On physical examination, the patient was pale, emaciated, and appeared acutely ill. She was pyrexial, with a temperature of 37.9°C, and her abdomen was distended with guarding to palpation in the right iliac fossa. A pregnancy test was negative. An abdominal x-ray film (**Figure**) showed free intraperitoneal air, and the entire colon appeared to be filled with radiopaque material.

A laparotomy was performed and showed the entire large bowel to be fragile and densely impacted with solid material. Generalized peritonitis originated from a sigmoid colon perforation, resulting in a mesenteric abscess that had perforated into the abdominal cavity. There was no evidence of a malignant neoplasm or diverticular disease. Resection, Hartmann procedure of the sigmoid colon, and colotomy of the transverse colon were performed to evacuate the impacted colonic contents that eventually

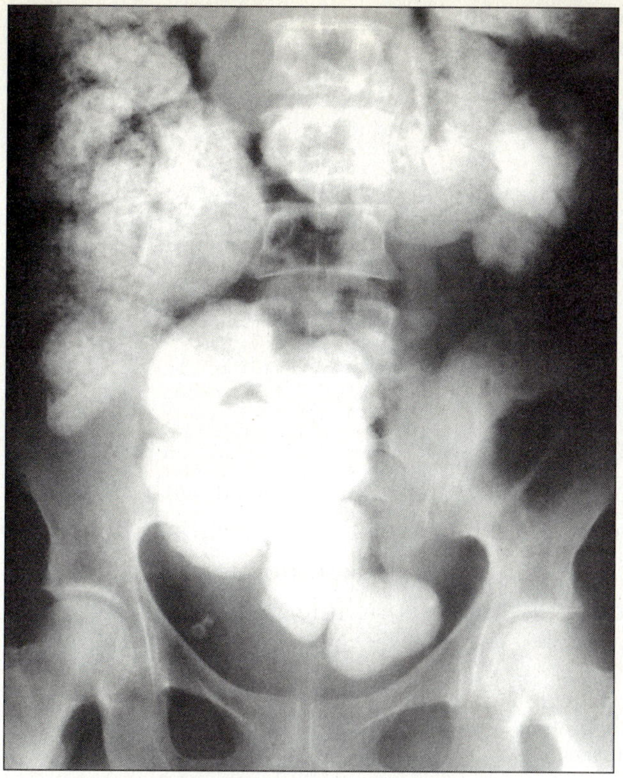

Plain abdominal x-ray film of the patient on admission to the hospital. Free intra-abdominal air is present and the entire colon appears to be densely impacted with radiopaque material that proved to be dry soil.

proved to be dry, feculent soil. Histological examination confirmed peritonitis, with no evidence of malignant neoplasm or colitis. Intensive care was unavailable and the patient eventually died of septic shock as a result of feculent peritonitis on the second postoperative day.

COMMENT

Pica (derived from the Latin word *Pica pica* for magpie, a bird known for its indiscriminate eating habits) is a persistent eating of nonnutritive substances beyond occasional childhood habits or culturally sanctioned practices. Geophagia is a subset of pica and is the habit of eating earth, soil, or clay.[1] The disorder is frequently encountered among natives of Africa and their descendants throughout the world.[2] Women are predominantly affected and the condition is particularly common during pregnancy. Less often, geophagia may occur due to iron deficiency. There is sufficient reason to believe that both pica and geophagia are underdiagnosed.

Complications of geophagia include parasitic infestation, electrolyte disturbance, and intestinal obstruction. Colonic perforation, however, has also been reported.[3] In a review of surgical complications in 44 patients with pica, geophagia accounted for 11 of 31 patients who required laparotomy.[4] Maternal death due to sigmoid perforation and peritonitis in a 31-year-old pregnant black woman has also been described.[5] Our patient's prognosis underscores geophagia as a rare cause of surgical acute abdomen due to colonic perforation and "soil" peritonitis, but seems unique in that her entire colon was densely packed with solid material.

Little is known about the pathogenesis of perforation in geophagia. Infection with anaerobic organisms may play a role[3] although many cases, like our patient, lack histological evidence for colitis. It may be reasonable to assume that chronic mechanical damage to colonic mucosa by progressive accumulation of dry, solid material in the lumen is a crucial factor.[4] A colon densely filled with solid material may represent the end stage of an insidious process, with increased luminal pressures causing mucosal ulceration, necrosis, and perforation.

The diagnosis of geophagia rests on a history of ingesting earth, soil, or clay. Patients may be reluctant to volunteer such information and many physicians fail to inquire into this habit. Therefore, a high degree of suspicion and tact are necessary to elicit a history of geophagia. Plain abdominal x-ray films are the diagnostic procedure of choice for patients who deny geophagical habits.[1] An x-ray film showing colonic filling with radiopaque material, is specific for geophagia, provided that recent application of contrast material can be ruled out.

Little information is available regarding the management of obstruction in geophagia; however, disimpaction of rectal contents by irrigation or mechanical removal is beneficial in rectosigmoid obstruction.[6] Successful resection and primary anastomosis have also been reported.[3] In our patient, sigmoid resection and Hartmann procedure were performed instead of primary anastomosis because of the vulnerable colon, including the resection margins. In retrospect, we believe that total colectomy may have been warranted and easy to perform in this emaciated patient, since the dense, full-length, colonic impaction was impossible to evacuate both manually and by colotomy.

CONCLUSION

We report a case of fatal soil peritonitis due to perforation of the sigmoid colon in a 45-year-old African woman suffering from geophagia. If sought, geophagia is still common throughout the world, particularly among natives of Africa and their descendants, especially those with iron deficiency or who are pregnant. Colonic perforation is a rare but potentially fatal complication of this peculiar habit and necessitates early diagnosis and aggressive surgical management.

Reprints: Alexander Woywodt, MD, Franz-Volhard-Clinic, Charité Campus Berlin-Buch, Humboldt-University, Wiltbergstrasse 50, 13125 Berlin, Germany (e-mail: woywodt@aol.com).

REFERENCES

1. Hawass NED, Alnozha MM, Kolawole T. Adult geophagia—report of three cases with review of the literature. *Trop Geogr Med.* 1987;39:191-195.
2. Vermeer DE, Frate DA. Geophagia in rural Mississippi: environmental and cultural contexts and nutritional implications. *Am J Clin Nutr.* 1979;32:2129-2135.
3. Delaitre B, Lemaigre G, Acar JF, Atsamena M, Bouhroum A. Entérite nécrosante et géophagie. *Nouv Presse Méd.* 1976;5:1743-1746.
4. Anderson JE, Akmal M, Kittur DS. Surgical complications of pica: report of a case of intestinal obstruction and a review of the literature. *Am Surg.* 1991;57:663-667.
5. Key TC, Horger EO, Miller JM. Geophagia as a cause of maternal death. *Obstet Gynecol.* 1982;60:525-526.
6. Ginaldi S. Geophagia: an uncommon cause of acute abdomen. *Ann Emerg Med.* 1988;17:979-981.

Transection of the Appendix

A Seat Belt Injury

Robert A. Edwards, DO; Douglas B. Paul, DO; Gary L. Anderson, DO; Mary C. McCarthy, MD

Blunt appendiceal injuries are uncommon. The recent care of a patient with an appendiceal transection following vehicular trauma led us to review the existing English literature. The presence of an abdominal wall contusion, in conjunction with a typical mesenteric tear and appendiceal transection, led us to conclude that the seat belt contributed to the injury.

Arch Surg. 1999;134:90-91

Blunt abdominal trauma has been hypothesized to contribute to the development of traumatic appendicitis and direct injury to the appendix; however, only 40 cases of injuries to the appendix due to blunt trauma have been reported.[1] The recent care of a patient who had experienced blunt abdominal trauma and a resulting appendiceal injury led us to review the existing English literature and to propose a possible mechanism for some cases of direct appendiceal trauma.

REPORT OF A CASE

A 41-year-old man was involved in a head-on, motor vehicle collision in which he was a restrained driver. He was taken to a local emergency department. On initial presentation, he complained only of a headache; his vital signs were stable; his Glasgow Coma Scale score was 15; and he was alert and afebrile. Seat belt abrasions and tenderness in the area of contusion were noted across the lower abdomen. No other injuries were identified.

He was transferred to a trauma center with computed tomographic scan capabilities, where he began to complain of increased lower abdominal pain. There were no peritoneal signs. A computed tomographic scan of the abdomen and pelvis showed a small amount of free fluid without solid organ injury. Following the scan, the patient's abdominal tenderness became more pronounced and an urgent laparotomy was performed.

Exploration of the abdomen revealed a 6-cm mesenteric injury at the ileocecal junction. Active bleeding was immediately controlled. The distal ileum and cecum were mobile and appeared ischemic, and a 2-cm appendiceal stump was attached to the base of the cecum. The distal appendix and its mesentery were avulsed and attached to the pelvic peritoneum (**Figure**). There was no fecal spill. An ileocecal resection with a primary anastomosis was performed and a serosal tear of the sigmoid colon was noted and repaired.

The patient had an uneventful postoperative course. He remained afebrile, tolerated advancement of his diet, and was discharged from the hospital on the fourth postoperative day. His incision was closed primarily and healed without signs of infection. Pathologic evaluation revealed a free portion of the appendix with hemorrhage, congestion, and fecal material in the lumen. Mild inflammation of the cecum and hemorrhage of the terminal ileum and mesentery was also reported.

COMMENT

Abdominal trauma has been implicated in the development of a syndrome of posttraumatic appendicitis. Mechanisms can include a sudden increase in intraluminal pressure with displacement of feces and gas into the appendix and mucosal injury, displacement of mobile viscera with

From the Departments of Surgery, Grandview Hospital (Drs Edwards, Paul, and Anderson), Wright State University School of Medicine (Drs Paul, Anderson, and McCarthy), and Miami Valley Hospital (Drs Paul, Anderson, and McCarthy), Dayton, Ohio.

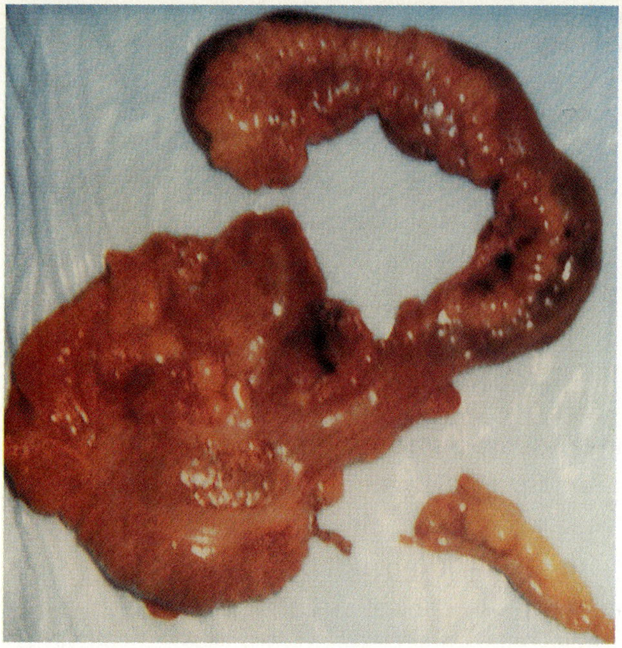

View of a pathologic specimen of the distal ileum, appendix, and cecum. The distal appendix and mesentery are avulsed, with a 2-cm appendiceal stump attached to the base of the cecum.

traction at fixed points, or direct traumatic injury.[2] In a review of reported cases, Serour et al[1] identified only 40 cases of posttraumatic appendicitis that presented symptoms between a few hours and 3 days after the traumatic event. Signs of local trauma were noted in 8 patients.

Blunt abdominal trauma may cause direct appendiceal injury. Two cases reported following motor vehicle collisions may help elucidate the mechanism of injury in the patient described herein. In 1956, Gatewood and Russum[3] reported a case of complete transection of the appendix following blunt abdominal trauma. The patient, a 39-year-old woman involved in a motor vehicle collision, complained of abdominal pain after 3 hours of observation. Seat belt use was not recorded; however, the right rectus muscle had been torn across, as may be seen in a seat belt injury. At laparotomy, a 30-cm laceration of the mesentery at the terminal ileum was noted. A free-floating appendix was recovered. The mechanism of transection was believed to be due to a fixed cecum with a tangential force compressing the appendix and ileal mesentery against the retroperitoneum or spine.

In 1975, Geer et al[4] described a 39-year-old man who presented with abdominal pain following an automobile collision. It was not recorded whether the patient was wearing a seat belt. He presented 24 hours after the accident with rebound tenderness in both lower quadrants. At laparotomy, the appendix was avulsed from the mesoappendix but in continuity with the cecum. The distal two thirds of the appendix was necrotic and appendectomy was performed. A 4-cm tear in the mesentery of the distal ileum was also repaired. The patient's postoperative course was uneventful.

In our patient, who was restrained, the presence of an abdominal seat belt contusion and free intra-abdominal fluid without solid organ injury were important indicators of potential visceral injury. Indeed, at the time of laparotomy, mesenteric injury and appendiceal transection were found. The presence of a sigmoid deserosalization also corroborates the seat belt mechanism of injury.

CONCLUSION

Direct appendiceal trauma is a rare event. In our patient, complete appendiceal transection due to a motor vehicle collision occurred. To our knowledge, there has only been one previous report of this mechanism of injury. Direct seat belt injury may be a factor in addition to deceleration forces applied to fixation points of mobile viscera. Posttraumatic appendicitis must also be considered in patients presenting with pain following blunt abdominal trauma.

Corresponding author: Mary C. McCarthy, MD, Wright State University School of Medicine Department of Surgery, 1 Wyoming St, Suite 7000 CHE, Dayton, OH 45409.

REFERENCES

1. Serour F, Efrati Y, Klin B, Shikar S, Weinberg M, Vinogard I. Acute appendicitis following abdominal trauma. *Arch Surg.* 1996;131:785-786.
2. Fowler RH. The rare incidence of acute appendicitis resulting from external trauma. *Ann Surg.* 1938;107:529-539.
3. Gatewood JW, Russum WJ. Injuries to the appendix secondary to blunt trauma. *Am J Surg.* 1956;91:558-560.
4. Geer DA, Armanini G, Guernsey JM. Trauma to the appendix: a report of two cases. *Arch Surg.* 1975;110:446-447.

Surgery in the Netherlands

H. Jaap Bonjer, MD, PhD; Hajo A. Bruining, MD, PhD

Surgery in the Netherlands is performed by 700 surgeons in 148 hospitals that serve a population of more than 15 million. Surgical standards are high and among the best in Western medicine. Training in surgery requires 6 years. In 1998, one third of the medical doctors applying to the surgical training program were women. The practice of surgery and surgical training are under pressure by the government to limit the working hours of residents, to reduce the number of hospitals, and to reduce medical budgets.

Arch Surg. 1999;134:92-98

Surgery in the Netherlands has a long history dating back to the 12th century. The French and German surgical schools have served an important role in the development of Dutch surgery through the centuries. During the second half of the 20th century, health care in the Netherlands has been subjected to strict organization and regulation by the government. Health care is available for all Dutch citizens on an equal basis. However, governmental involvement in health care also has resulted in the reduction of hospital beds, a severe reduction in the working hours of residents, and restricted medical budgets. This article reviews the evolution of surgery in the Netherlands, its current status, and perspectives.

HISTORY

The Netherlands is a small European country with a population of 15 million, surrounded by Germany, Belgium, and the water of the North Sea. The boundaries of the Netherlands have changed continuously during many centuries. Early in the 12th century, the Low Countries were divided into the Northern and Southern Netherlands, separated by the river Maas. Flanders (the northern province of contemporary Belgium), Brabant, and Zeeland composed the Southern Netherlands. Trade and industry flourished in the Southern Netherlands in the 12th and 13th centuries owing to transit trade with England and the manufacturing of English wool into cloth. Holland, the western part of the Northern Netherlands was economically unimportant in those days. Utrecht, Tiel, and the Hanseatic towns along the river Yssel (towns banded together for mutual protection and trade advantages) were the major trading centers of the Northern Netherlands.

The first report of surgery in the Low Countries dates back to the middle of the 12th century. Count Arnold I of Flanders suffered from a bladder stone. Several surgeons gathered at the court to relieve the count of his ailment. However, despite a public demonstration of their skills, the count declined surgical treatment. During the 13th and 14th centuries, the cities of the Low Countries appointed town-surgeons to provide care for the poor.[1] The town-surgeons also were required to treat persons who had undergone corporal punishment and to accompany the militia. The salary of the town-surgeons was in coins, fabric, and an exemption from the excise on spirits.

During the 15th century, an important role began for Holland and Zeeland in the shipping traffic with the Baltic countries and the industrial countries in western Europe. Amsterdam was among the flourishing cities in Holland, although it was merely a small fishing village during the 12th century. During the 15th century, Charles V inherited from his parents and his Hapsburg grandfather, Maximilian I of Austria, the southern Dutch Provinces and Austria. Charles V also acquired Spain from his mother, the Span-

From the Department of Surgery, University Hospital Rotterdam Dijkzigt, Rotterdam, the Netherlands.

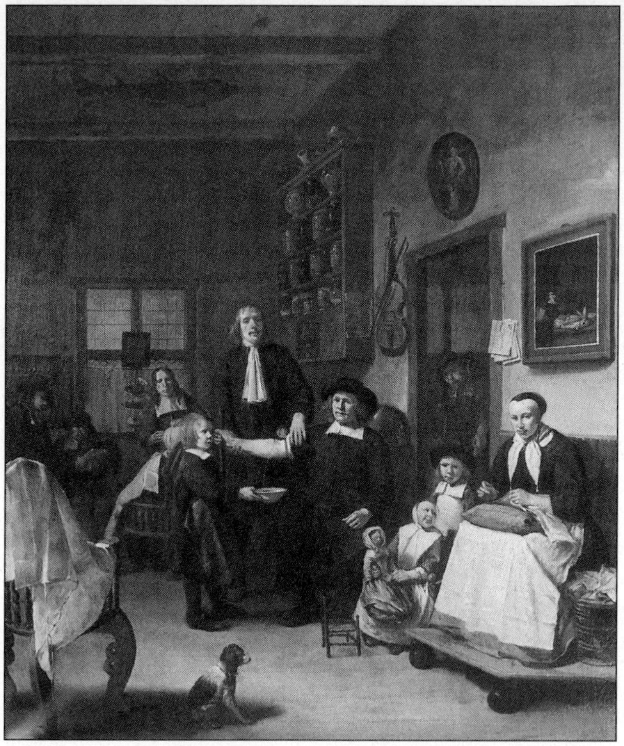

Figure 1. *Egbert van Heemskerck (1634-1704),* The Surgeon Jacob Fransz Hercules With His Family at Work in His Shop, *oil on canvas. 70 × 59 cm. Courtesy of the Amsterdam Historisch Museum, Amsterdam, the Netherlands. While the surgeon is performing a phlebotomy, the apprentice is barbering.*

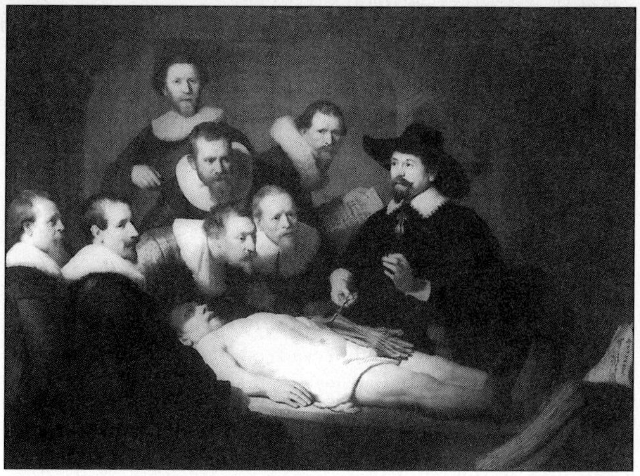

Figure 2. *Rembrandt van Rijn (1606-1669),* The Anatomy Lesson of Dr Nicolaes Tulp, *oil on canvas. 169.5 × 216.5 cm. Courtesy of the Mauritshuis, The Hague, the Netherlands.*

ish princess Joanna of Castile. The northern Dutch Provinces were forced to acknowledge Charles V.

During the 1460s, the surgeons were organized by the town councils into guilds whose membership also was open to women. Passing the master's examination, which assessed one's capability to perform phlebotomy and to manufacture and sharpen lancets, was mandatory to become a member of the guild. Joining a guild was obligatory when one intended to practice surgery, which included hairdressing and barbering. Initially, phlebotomy was the main surgical skill that the town-surgeons were required to master; however, the barber work prevailed in the practice of these medieval surgeons. During the 16th century, trephination of the skull and knowledge of fractures, dislocations, wounds, growths, and ulcers were added to the armamentarium of the surgeon-barbers.

During the 16th century, the son and heir of Charles V, Philip II, strove for an integration of the Low Countries and the Spanish-Hapsburg monarchy. Stadtholders were appointed for each province. William of Orange became the stadtholder of Holland, Zeeland, and Utrecht. The Protestants in this region were oppressed by the Catholic Spanish troops. Philip II responded to the iconoclastic fury in 1566 by sending a strong army to the Netherlands, commanded by the Duke of Alva, who installed a ruthless regime. The rebellious Dutchmen were led by William of Orange. In 1572, these Dutch Sea Beggars captured Brielle in Zeeland and some other cities. A long war between the Dutch and the Spanish troops followed. In 1574, Alkmaar and Leyden were besieged by the Spanish but withstood despite many deaths due to starvation. Because of this, Leyden was rewarded with the first university (including a medical school) in the Netherlands in 1575.[1] The Republic of Seven Provinces was then formed. In 1648, the war with the Spanish ended, and each Province was permitted to have one university. Amsterdam could not have a university because the province of Holland already had its university in Leyden. Therefore, the Athenaeum Illustre was founded in Amsterdam.

During the 17th century, women were no longer permitted to join the guilds. Religion was another cause of exclusion; only surgeons who belonged to the Reformed Church were eligible for guild membership. Catholics were not accepted. In the countryside, guilds did not exist. Often surgeons trained to work on ships, who had completed a training period of only 2 years, practiced in the rural areas. The guilds in the cities had their own surgeon's halls, which contained the surgical instruments and library. Apprenticeship in surgery lasted 4 to 5 years. The apprentice was required to pay the tuition during the first years of his training. During the surgeon's training, barbering and domestic duties consumed most of the time of the apprentice before phlebotomy and trephination of the skull became part of the surgeon's role (**Figure 1**).

During the 17th century, the importance of anatomy was acknowledged at the universities of medicine and in the practical surgical training. In Leyden in 1593, Professor Pieter Pauw built an anatomical theater with 6 galleries holding 400 spectators. The anatomical demonstrations were open to the public on payment of an admission fee. Rembrandt painted an anatomical demonstration by Dr Nicolaes Tulp which is known as the *Anatomy Lesson* (**Figure 2**).

Hospitals have existed in the Netherlands since the 12th century. These hospitals usually were referred to as "guesthouses," since they acted simultaneously as almshouses, nursing homes, and orphanages. The surgeons were subordinate to the physicians who supervised the hospitals. During 1554, the first operation was performed at a hospital in the Netherlands. With the permission of the town authorities, several toes were amputated by 3 master surgeons in the presence of 2 medical doctors at a hospital in Amsterdam.

The Seven Provinces of the Netherlands were weakened severely by their consecutive wars with the Spanish. Four Anglo-Dutch naval wars left the Provinces in dire straits, and the armies of the French Revolution took over the country in 1795. The Batavian Republic was declared as a unified state with a central government in The Hague.

EIGHTEENTH-CENTURY surgery in the Netherlands is considered the French period. A small number of Dutch surgeons observed the work of French surgeons and paid steep fees. After their study period in France, they adopted the title "French master." During the 18th century, the training of surgeons by the guilds changed little. Surgeons, however, attempted to acquire university doctorates to attain equal footing with physicians (ie, internists). The public discriminated a clear difference in status between physicians and surgeons; the physicians usually were categorized in the upper class, while the surgeons were categorized in the lower middle class.[1]

Major operations were rarely performed during the 1700s. In Amsterdam, which had a population of around 200 000 people at that time, not more than 4 lithotomies per year were performed, while a herniotomy to relieve a strangulated hernia or amputation of a leg was even more scarce.

The Netherlands were annexed by Napoleon to the French Empire in 1810. Although the trading opportunities for the Dutch became scarce, some French measures were to the advantage of the Netherlands. Registries of births, marriages, and deaths and cowpox vaccinations were introduced. The French degraded the universities of Utrecht, Franeker, and Harderwijk to *ecoles secondaires,* while Leyden and Groningen were designated as *Academies de l'Universite Imperiale.* The government effected its first medical constitution in the history of the Netherlands. Enrollees in university medical education were divided into 3 groups: doctors of medicine, doctors of surgery, and doctors of obstetrics. The government also divided surgeons into city surgeons, country surgeons, and obstetricians.

During the early 1800s, the surgical guilds started to crumble. In Amsterdam, the municipal government installed the Committee of Medical Supervision to replace the guild administration, which was known as the *Collegium Chirurgicum.* Barbering was separated from surgery in most cities.

During 1813, Napoleon was defeated in Leipzig by Austria, Russia, Prussia, and Sweden. Upon liberation from the French, a monarchial form of government was initiated in the Netherlands. In 1828, training schools for surgeons, known as "clinical schools," were established in several cities in the Netherlands. These clinical schools were linked to hospitals and funded by the municipalities. The candidates for the clinical schools were expected to be able to read and write and to have some knowledge of Latin. The training for city surgeons and country surgeons was of 4 years' duration.

During the 19th century, which was marked by the technological development of new power sources and epidemics of smallpox, scarlet fever, and cholera throughout Europe, major changes occurred in surgery. Until the 19th century, pain during operations could be limited only by operating at high speed with razor-sharp instruments. The American invention of anesthesia was of paramount importance for the development of surgery. Horace Wells, a dentist in Hartford, Conn, discovered the anesthetic value of laughing gas in 1844, and William Morton, Boston, Mass, succeeded in inducing general anesthesia with the inhalation of ether in 1846.[2] These developments rapidly spread to Europe. In 1847, the first operation under general anesthesia in the Netherlands was performed in The Hague.

In 1852, the Dutch military surgeon, Mathijsen, invented the modern plaster bandage to immobilize fractures. Antisepsis was, in addition to anesthesia, the other revolutionary change in surgery. Inspired by the fundamental research of the French chemist Louis Pasteur, who showed that unicellular microorganisms caused putrefaction, Joseph Lister (a professor of surgery in Glasgow, Scotland) used carbolic acid for the disinfection of wounds, surgical instruments, and surgeons' hands.[2] The use of antisepsis was first used in the Netherlands in 1874.

During the second half of the 19th century, Germany became an important power owing to its high degree of industrialization. Germany also expanded its scientific knowledge. Training in surgery and surgical practices in Germany were organized in a very disciplined manner. German medical textbooks were progressively used in the Netherlands. Dutch surgeons visited the meetings of the German surgical association, the *Deutsche Gesellschaft für Chirurgie.* Chairs at various Dutch universities were held at the turn of the 19th century by Germans, Austrians, and the Swiss. Among them were pupils of the famous Theodor Billroth from Vienna, Austria, and Theodor Kocher from Bern, Switzerland.

Performing major operations remained rare during the 19th century. In 1891, the first herniotomy for a nonstrangulated hernia was performed in Utrecht. Appendectomy and other abdominal operations were performed later. Otto Lanz, who was a pupil of Kocher from Bern, introduced thyroid surgery in the Netherlands in 1902. During that same year, the Dutch Surgical Society was founded.

During 1865, the Dutch government ended surgical training outside the universities. However, specialization in surgery was not structured. Candidates would serve as assistants at a hospital in the Netherlands or abroad for a self-determined term. Gynecology and surgery were frequently combined as a double specialty. Until 1931, all physicians had the right to perform surgical procedures.

During 1930, the Dutch Medical Association, which was formed in 1849, decided to start registering specialists. The duration required for the surgeon's training was established at 3 years. This remained the required period until 1948.

The occupation of the Netherlands by the Germans during World War II interfered greatly with the education at the universities, since only those who supported the German regime could attend the university. Medical research was performed in secrecy during the war. During 1942, however, Willem Johan Kolff designed an artificial kidney for extracorporeal dialysis. In Nijmegen, which was in the front line of battle in 1944 and 1945, the intramedullary Küntscher nail was used for the first time in the Netherlands to treat femoral fractures. In 1948, the Dutch Surgical Society established a council from among its members, the *Concilium Chirurgicum*. Today, the Concilium Chirurgicum, in Utrecht, still delineates the training requirements and supervises the training at the teaching hospitals. In 1948, this council extended the surgical specialty training from 3 to 6 years. During the 1950s, thoracic and vascular surgery were first performed. In 1961, the first kidney from a living donor was successfully transplanted. In 1979, the first liver transplantation was performed in Groningen, while the first heart was transplanted in 1984 in Rotterdam.

MEDICAL SCHOOLS

The 8 medical schools in the Netherlands are located in Amsterdam (2 schools), Groningen, Leyden, Maastricht, Nijmegen, Rotterdam, and Utrecht. Yearly, approximately 1600 candidates start medical school. The selection of candidates for medical school is determined by chance and by the mean grade of the final examinations at high school. More than 60% of all Dutch medical students are women. The annual tuition for medical school is only $1000 (US dollars) owing to vast governmental subsidies. The medical curriculum is a 6-year program divided into 2 phases: a first phase of 4 years and a second phase of 2 years. The education during the first phase is moving away from teaching large groups of students toward the interactive teaching of small groups of students. Medical problem solving and integration of courses have become the priorities instead of acquisition of medical knowledge.[3]

On completion of the first phase, the master's degree is acquired. The second phase is solely practical, involving rotations in almost all medical specialties. At the end of the second phase, the medical doctor degree is awarded.

SURGICAL TRAINING

In the Netherlands, training in general surgery requires 6 years. Candidates applying for the training in general surgery should have completed medical school. Foreign medical graduates from countries in the European community also are permitted to apply for surgical training in the Netherlands. However, command of the Dutch language is a prerequisite. The number of applicants has been relatively constant during the last few years, averaging around 220 per year. The proportion of female applicants is increasing. In 1998, one third of the candidates were women.

The surgical training in the Netherlands is organized into 8 regions. Each region consists of 1 university hospital and 4 or 5 affiliated community hospitals. The candidates may indicate 3 regions of preference, and the assignment is made based on these preferences. In each region, a regional training committee, with the directors of surgical training of the hospitals as members, selects and interviews residents. In some regions, a surgical resident is a member of the regional training committee. The number of residents permitted to start the training in general surgery is determined every year, based on the expected number of retiring surgeons and the expected greater demand for surgical care owing to the aging population, by the Central Admittance Committee, which is appointed by the Dutch Surgical Society to supervise the selection of surgical residents. Limiting the inflow of surgical residents was started in 1980 when the number of recently qualified surgeons without a permanent position increased steadily.[4] Yearly questionnaires among surgeons who have just completed the training assess the current employment market. At present, the market for surgeons seems to be in balance in the Netherlands.

The surgical training in the Netherlands usually takes place within 1 region. Surgical residents are trained at the university hospital and at the community hospitals. Most of them spend 3 years at a community hospital and 3 years at a university hospital, although other schedules are also possible. Half a year of the 6-year curriculum may be devoted to research in the Netherlands or abroad. The training schedule is determined by the individual regions. The Dutch Surgical Society has set 600 as the minimum number of operations that a surgical resident should have performed by the end of the training period. To ensure a good balance between simple and complex surgical procedures, the procedures have been divided into 7 categories. For instance, repair of an umbilical hernia is considered category I, while total thyroidectomy is considered category VI. Category I operations are appropriate for the first-year resident, category II for the second-year resident, and so on. Category VII, which includes procedures such as renal transplantation, is intended for surgeons in a fellowship who are "superspecializing." However, the categories are not used rigidly. The distribution of the 600 operations within the categories should be as follows: I through III, 375; IV, 125; V, 75; and VI and VII, 25.

During the training, the surgical resident rotates through all divisions of general surgery. In some regions, specific rotations at a pediatric hospital and a cancer institute exist. Specific rotations through the departments of thoracic surgery, plastic and reconstructive surgery, urology, and orthopedic surgery are no longer part of the training. The majority of pulmonary surgery in the Netherlands is performed by general surgeons at community hospitals, so surgical residents may participate in pulmonary surgery during their period at the community hospitals. An official fellowship in pulmonary surgery is available for general surgeons. The Netherlands is one of the few countries in which trauma care is provided by the general surgeon. During the training in general surgery in the Netherlands, the resident is trained to diagnose and treat almost the entire spectrum of fractures.

In the Netherlands, the departments of surgery display a high degree of unity despite various divisions. Most meetings are attended by all members of the department. The average day begins with a meeting of the entire department during which residents who have been on duty report clinical activities during the past night or weekend. At the end of the afternoon, another general meeting takes place during which the operations of that day are reported. Furthermore, medical students or surgical residents present the medical cases of patients who have been scheduled for an operation the next day. Morbidity and mortality meetings are held weekly.

The surgical resident must pass 2 examinations in preoperative and postoperative care, intensive care, and oncology during the first 2 years of training. During the following 4 years, mandatory specialized courses on various topics are taught twice a year. These courses are organized by the Dutch Surgical Society. During the surgical training program, all residents attend the basic osteosynthesis course, based on the "Allgemeiner Osteosynthesis" principles from the Swiss school of fracture treatment, and an advanced trauma life support course. Surgical residents are assessed yearly by the director of surgical training. This assessment is discussed with the resident. A resident deemed unqualified for continuation or completion of the residency can be transferred to another hospital for a second assessment. There is no final examination at the end of the surgical training.

An important recent change in surgical training in the Netherlands is the regulation of the working hours of residents. During the early 1990s, Dutch surgical residents worked between 80 and 100 hours per week. The government determined that the long working hours compromised the quality of health care and the well-being of residents, and it intervened. Within a few years, the working hours of residents were reduced to 48 hours per week. In addition, strict rules indicate the number of consecutive hours that a resident is permitted to work. Although the basic principles of limiting working hours are admirable, the extent of the reduction of hours has met great opposition in the medical field. However, a law has been passed obligating hospitals to follow the regulations, and violation results in steep fines. Surprisingly, the working hours of specialists have not been subjected to governmental intervention. The consequences of the reduced work week are far reaching. Continuity of patient care is deregulated, attendance at meetings of the department of surgery is fragmented, and, foremost, the available time for training has become less. Considering this fact and the increasing specialization in various fields of surgery, the format of the training in general surgery will be adjusted. In 1999, the sixth year of residency will be designated the "differentiation year." Four differentiations are possible: surgical oncology, gastrointestinal tract surgery, vascular surgery, and trauma care. The future will show whether the quality of the surgical training suffers owing to the reduced working hours.

During the 1950s, about 75% of the population had medical care that was subsidized by the government ("sickness funds").[5] Considering the major role of the government in health care, an organization for training in specialties was founded in 1961 that comprised specialists, government representatives, and hospital representatives. The Central Board, with medical representatives from university and nonuniversity hospitals, representatives from hospital associations, and representatives of the Ministry of Education and the Ministry of Public Health, determines the institution of new specialties and establishes the requirements for trainers, training institutions, and residents. The Committee for Specialist Registration, with members from all recognized specialties and hospital associations, implements the decisions of the Central Board. The Committee for Specialist Registration grants permits to teachers and training centers and oversees their inspection by committees of inspectors, who are recruited from the councils of the specialist associations. Training hospitals are inspected at least every 5 years. If the conditions established by the Central Board are not met, a reinspection is ordered by the Committee for Specialist Registration after 2 years. The permit for training can be withdrawn at reinspection.

SURGICAL SOCIETIES AND RESEARCH

The Dutch Surgical Society has more than 1100 members. Within the Dutch Surgical Society are societies for vascular surgery, gastrointestinal tract surgery, surgical oncology, trauma care, pediatric surgery, thoracic surgery, endoscopic surgery, endocrine surgery, and tropical diseases. The Dutch Surgical Society organizes 2 meetings per year with free attendance at presentations of papers and invited lectures. The societies organize courses and workshops in addition to these meetings.

The Dutch Surgical Society publishes 2 official journals. The *Nederlands Tijdschrift voor Heelkunde* is a national journal of the society in the Dutch language. The *Netherlands Journal of Surgery* joined the *Acta Chirurgica Scandinavica* to form the *European Journal of Surgery*.

Research in surgery, both clinical and experimental, is performed extensively in the Netherlands. Clinical research has focused in the past on randomized clinical trials. Such trials are feasible in the Netherlands since Dutch patients, by choice, do not have an outspoken opinion about the kind of treatment they desire when they visit the medical specialist. Cooperation with the Scandinavian countries in randomized trials is frequently sought because of their many similarities with the Netherlands in the outlook toward and the organization of health care. Follow-up in the Netherlands is feasible since traveling time is limited by the size of the country. Another advantage for follow-up studies is the registration of all citizens, which facilitates the tracking of patients. All hospitals have medical ethics committees that assess the clinical value, statistical methods, and ethical aspects of clinical trials.

Experimental research is concentrated at the university hospitals. Most university hospitals have facilities for experimental animal work. Research with experimental animals is bound by strict regulations. Researchers are required to complete a course on animal handling and ethics before they are permitted to work with experimental animals. Experimental research projects must be approved by animal ethics committees.

Funding for research is provided by governmental subsidies, charity funds, or funds from the medical industry. The funding by the government has decreased during past years.

DISEASE PATTERNS AND THEIR INFLUENCE ON SURGICAL PRACTICE

The Netherlands has the highest population density of all European countries. Every square kilometer has a mean population of 442. Owing to a high birth rate during the 1950s and 1960s, the proportion of inhabitants 65 years or older is only 13%. However, the population is aging, with an annual increase of 1.3% in the group older than 65 years.[6] Of the Dutch population, 4.8% are not of the Dutch nationality. The majority of these are Turkish or Moroccan. Another 4.7% was not born in the Netherlands but acquired the Dutch nationality. Most originate from former Dutch colonies, such as Indonesia, Suriname, and the Dutch Antilles.

Cardiovascular disease accounts for 38% of mortality in the Netherlands.[7] Ischemic heart disease and cerebrovascular disease are the most common cardiovascular events. Malignant tumors are the second major cause of death (30%).[6] In men, 25% of deaths are due to lung cancer, while prostate cancer (14%) and colorectal cancer (12%) are other common causes of death. In women, breast cancer is the most frequent cause of death (32%). Colorectal cancer (14%), lung cancer (5%), endometrial cancer (5%), and ovarian cancer (5%) are other frequent malignant tumors in Dutch women.

Mortality due to traffic accidents decreased greatly after the introduction of maximum speed limits, safety belts, crash barriers, and mandatory helmet use for motorcyclists and moped riders during the 1970s. The annual mortality due to traffic accidents decreased from 3181 in 1970 to 1334 in 1995.[8] Considering the growth of the population and the increase in the number of vehicles during this period, the value of safety measures in traffic is evident. Of the 1334 traffic casualties in 1995, 267 were cyclists, and 118 were moped riders. Bicycles and mopeds are commonly used for transportation in the Netherlands.

The acquired immunodeficiency syndrome was the cause of death of 418 people in 1990. In 1996, this number had decreased to 208.[9]

The total annual number of operations in the Netherlands has remained relatively constant during the last few years.[10] An average of 225 000 operations is performed per year. Repair of hernias (13%), venous and arterial procedures (12.3%), operative treatment of fractures (9%), breast surgery (8%), and gallbladder surgery (8%) are the most common in the Dutch surgical practice.

Endoscopic techniques were introduced into Dutch surgical practice in 1990.[11] In 1995, 70% of all cholecystectomies were performed laparoscopically, as were 50% of all antireflux operations (Nissen fundoplications) and 13% of all inguinal hernia repairs.[12]

HEALTH CARE PROVISION

Dutch citizens have equal access to health care in the Netherlands. Dutch legislation requires that every citizen have health insurance. Of the population, 63% is covered by sickness funds,[9] a type of health insurance that is subsidized by the government. The remaining 37% of the Dutch population is insured by private companies. The annual salary of a person determines the eligibility for sickness funds or private insurance. Almost 9% of the gross national product was spent on health care in the Netherlands in 1995.[9]

General practitioners have a vital role in Dutch health care. When ill, the patient must first consult the general practitioner. If the general practitioner determines that referral to a medical specialist is indicated, the patient is referred to a hospital. Direct consultation of a medical specialist by a citizen is impossible except for the treatment of traumatic lesions, for which patients are permitted to visit the emergency room of a hospital within 24 hours of the injury. The government designates general practitioners as the gatekeepers in health care to limit costs.

Before 1983, hospitals were financed based on their production output,[13] and the costs of health care had increased steadily during previous decades. In 1983, to control the costs of health care, the Dutch government introduced hospital budgeting. A global budget based on previous years was calculated for each hospital. If expenses exceeded the budget by 5% or more without an evident explanation, the budget was decreased the following year. This measure has stimulated growth of outpatient care. In 1985, only 204 000 outpatient admissions were registered; this number more than tripled, to 644 000, in 1995.[9] The mean length of hospital stay has decreased gradually from 18 days in 1970 to 10 days in 1995. Another important change in medical finances is the recent change in the rates for medical care. Until 1997, different rates existed for patients with sickness funds than for those with private insurance. In 1997, the rates were equalized. The rates for surgical procedures are determined by a national committee composed of representatives of the government, health care insurance companies, and hospitals. Medical specialists are not permitted to set their own rates.

In an attempt to limit the costs of health care and increase the effectiveness of hospitals, the Dutch government has closed more than 25% of the hospitals in the Netherlands since 1985.[9] At present, 148 hospitals remain. The number of hospital beds decreased from 68 461 in 1985 to 60 489 in 1995.[9]

The number of nursing staff has been reduced, and the working hours have been reduced to 36 hours per week. At present, particularly in the western part of the Netherlands, there is a shortage of operative nurses and anesthesiology nurses. Low salaries, limited career prospects, and inadequate opportunities for part-time jobs seem to be the causative factors.

The aforementioned developments have resulted in growing waiting lists for medical procedures. The waiting time for orthopedic procedures and eye surgery at many hospitals exceeds 1 year. General surgical procedures, such as inguinal hernia repair and laparoscopic cholecystectomy, also face these waiting times, particularly at the university hospitals. Local collaboration projects between hospitals and large companies to guarantee short waiting times for the employees of the companies have been initiated. However, the Ministry of Health is opposed to such arrangements because they could conflict with the principle of equal access to health care for all Dutch citizens.

THE FUTURE

The future of surgery in the Netherlands harbors several uncertainties. The first uncertainty is the extent to which surgery can remain a general profession. Initiatives to isolate vascular surgery, trauma surgery, and other subspecialties are commonplace. The increasing complexity of specific procedures and the growing quest of patients for quality care will make general surgeons a rare species. The second uncertainty is the quality of care. Considering the reduced income of surgeons, it is likely that surgeons will limit their work week according to the working hours that have been implemented for the majority of the Dutch working population. This will undoubtedly affect the care for the patient. Another uncertainty is whether the quality of surgical training will deteriorate owing to the decreased number of work hours. What will be the role of women in surgery? Will female surgeons outnumber male surgeons in several years? Will surgery become a part-time job? Will private hospitals have an important role in health care in the near future? Time will answer these questions.

Corresponding author: H. Jaap Bonjer, MD, PhD, Department of Surgery, University Hospital Rotterdam Dijkzigt, Dr Molewaterplein 40, 3015 GD Rotterdam, the Netherlands (e-mail: bonjer@hlkd.azr.nl).

REFERENCES

1. De Moulin D. *A History of Surgery.* Dordrecht, the Netherlands: Martinus Nijhoff Publishers; 1988.
2. Lindeboom GA. *Inleiding tot de geschiedenis der geneeskunde.* Rotterdam, the Netherlands: Erasmus Publishing; 1993.
3. Bouman LN, Metz JCM. Medisch onderwijs van morgen: een blik in de (naaste) toekomst. *Ned Tijdschr Geneeskd.* 1997;141:2575-2579.
4. Keeman JN, Lagaay MB. Selectie van assistent-geneeskundigen voor de opleiding heelkunde in Nederland. *Ned Tijdschr Geneeskd.* 1989;133:2239-2242.
5. den Otter G. The training of a surgeon in the Netherlands. *Arch Chir Neerl.* 1978;30:199-206.
6. Visser O, Coebergh JWW, Schouten LJ, eds. *Incidence of Cancer in the Netherlands 1991.* Utrecht, the Netherlands: SIG Health Care Information; 1991.
7. Dalstra JAA, Reitsma JB, eds. *Hart en vaatziekten in Nederland 1997.* Mouthaan, the Netherlands: Hendrik Ido Ambacht; 1997.
8. Centraal Bureau voor de Statistiek. *Statistiek van de verkeersongevallen op de openbare weg 1995.* Voorburg/Heerlen, the Netherlands: Centraal Bureau voor de Statistiek; 1996.
9. *Statistisch Jaarboek 1997.* Nijmegen, the Netherlands: GJ Thieme BV; 1998.
10. Hesselink EJ. *Trends in Surgery 1984-1993: SIG Health Care Information.* Utrecht, the Netherlands: SIG Health Care Information; 1995.
11. van Erp WFM, Bruyninckx CMA. De eerste ervaringen met de laparoscopische cholecystectomie. *Ned Tijdschr Geneeskd.* 1991;135:272-276.
12. Bonjer HJ, Cuesta MA, Bemelman WA, Janssen IMC, de Brauw LM, de Wit LT. Diffusion of endoscopic surgery in the Netherlands [abstract]. *Surg Endosc.* 1997;11:257.
13. Casparie AF, Hoogendoorn D. Effects of budgeting on health care services in Dutch hospitals. *Am J Public Health.* 1991;81:1442-1447.

IN OTHER AMA JOURNALS

ARCHIVES OF INTERNAL MEDICINE

Impact of Major Cardiovascular Disease Risk Factors, Particularly in Combination, on 22-Year Mortality in Women and Men

Lynn P. Lowe, PhD; Philip Greenland, MD; Karen J. Ruth, MS; Alan R. Dyer, PhD; Rose Stamler, MA; Jeremiah Stamler, MD

Background: The appropriateness of current cardiovascular disease (CVD) risk factor guidelines in women continues to be debated.
Objective: To present new data on the appropriateness of current CVD risk factor guidelines, for women and men, from long-term follow-up of a large population sample.
Methods: Cardiovascular disease risk factor status according to current clinical guidelines and long-term impact on mortality were determined in 8686 women and 10 503 men aged 40 to 64 years at baseline from the Chicago Heart Association Detection Project in Industry; average follow-up was 22 years.
Results: At baseline, only 6.6% of women and 4.8% of men had desirable levels for all 3 major risk factors (cholesterol level, <5.20 mmol/L [<200 mg/dL]; systolic and diastolic blood pressure, <120 and <80 mm Hg, respectively; and nonsmoking). With control for age, race, and other risk factors, each major risk factor considered separately was associated with increased risk of death for women and men. In analyses of combinations of major risk factors, risk increased with number of risk factors. Relative risks (RRs) associated with any 2 or all 3 risk factors were similar: for coronary heart disease mortality in women, RR = 5.72 (95% confidence interval [CI], 2.35-13.93), and in men, RR = 5.51 (95% CI, 3.10-9.77); for CVD mortality in women, RR = 4.54 (95% CI, 2.33-8.84), and in men, RR = 4.12 (95% CI, 2.56-6.37); and for all-cause mortality in women, RR = 2.34 (95% CI, 1.73-3.15), and in men, RR = 3.20 (95% CI, 2.47-4.14). Absolute excess risks were high in women and men with any 2 or all 3 major risk factors.
Conclusions: Combinations of major CVD risk factors place women and men at high relative, absolute, and absolute excess risk of coronary heart disease, CVD, and all-cause mortality. These findings support the value of (1) measurement of major CVD risk factors, especially in combination, for assessing long-term mortality risk and (2) current advice to match treatment intensity to the level of CVD risk in both women and men. *(1998;158:2007-2014)*

Reprints: Philip Greenland, MD, Department of Preventive Medicine, Northwestern University Medical School, 680 N Lake Shore Dr, Suite 1102, Chicago, IL 60611 (e-mail: p-greenland@nwu.edu).

Laparoscopic Splenectomy

Richard T. Schlinkert, MD; Sumeet S. Teotia, MD

Laparoscopic splenectomy is emerging as the procedure of choice for splenic removal in patients with hematologic disorders and normal to moderately enlarged spleens. We herein describe our technique for laparoscopic splenectomy. Alternative techniques are also discussed, with detailed modifications of techniques for patients with splenomegaly.

Arch Surg. 1999;134:99-103

Laparoscopic splenectomy (LS) has been shown to decrease postoperative discomfort and shorten hospital stays, compared with open splenectomy.[1-5] Laparoscopic splenectomy has been performed for immune thrombocytopenic purpura (ITP) in most cases. There have been few conversions, and results demonstrate more than 90% initial response of platelet counts, as well as long-term effects comparable with those of open splenectomy.[6,7] The spleen in ITP is of normal size with normal vasculature, and there is generally not an associated coagulopathy. Therefore, these are the spleens with which surgeons should begin their LS experience. Spleens have been removed for a variety of other disease states, including massive enlargement (up to 26 cm, with weights >2500 g in our series).

See Invited Critique at end of article

The following discussion describes our technique for LS. The major steps of the procedure are detailed, with particular attention to the techniques for the patient with ITP. Alternative techniques are discussed also in an effort to provide the surgeon with options, should the primary approach not work for a particular patient or surgeon. In addition, the modifications, which may be applied to patients with massive splenomegaly, are highlighted.

PREOPERATIVE PREPARATION

All patients undergoing splenectomy should be immunized against encapsulated bacteria, and coagulopathies should be corrected. Although the absolute value of platelet count required for safe splenectomy is not known, we have frequently performed LS for patients with platelet counts of 20×10^9/L or even lower without sequelae. As with laparoscopic cholecystectomy, we have noticed decreased oozing during LS, perhaps related to the increased intra-abdominal pressure related to the pneumoperitoneum. Platelets are, therefore, used selectively, and only if signs of bleeding are evident or if the counts are extremely low.

Patients who have received corticosteroids within the previous year should be treated with perioperative steroids to prevent acute adrenocortical insufficiency.

The use of preoperative angiographic ablation of the spleen[8] has been abandoned. Embolization led to severe pain in many patients and to splenic venous thrombosis in 1 of our patients. Blood loss without this is minimal and does not justify embolization, even for patients with splenomegaly. If, however, one chooses to perform embolization preoperatively, it should be done with anesthesia support and an operating room waiting so patients are spared the pain related to splenic infarction.

POSITIONING

The patient is placed in the right lateral semidecubitus position (rotated slightly back) from a full decubitus position, approximately 80° from supine (**Figure 1**). An axillary roll is placed, and the arms are secured on an arm board positioned as far superiorly as possible. The right knee is bent, and the left is straight. This increases working space at the surgical field. The patient is appropriately padded and secured. For splenomegaly, the patient is positioned in a 40° to 60° semidecubitus posi-

From the Department of Surgery, Mayo Clinic Scottsdale, Scottsdale, Ariz.

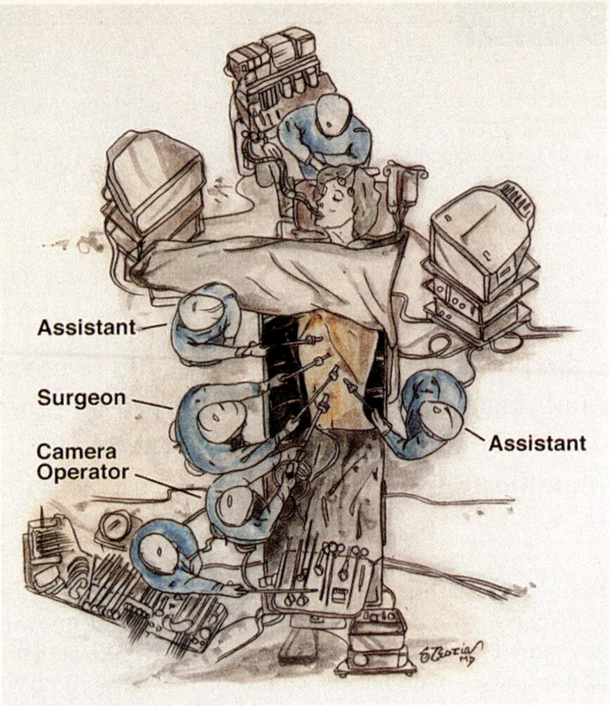

Figure 1. *Operating room setup.*

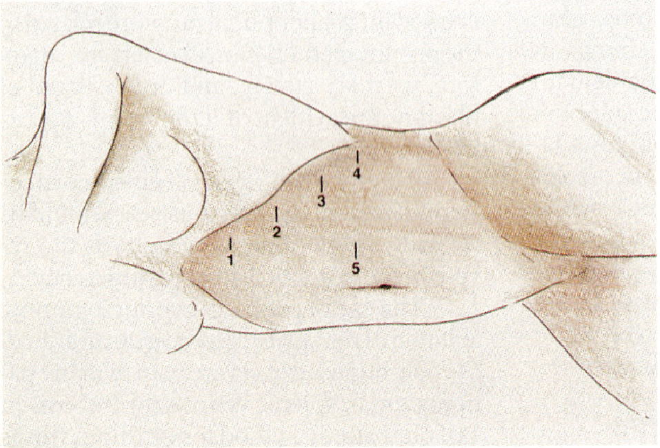

Figure 2. *Trocar placement. Ports 1 and 4 are 5 mm, ports 2 and 3 are 12 mm, and port 5 is 11 mm in diameter. Port 5 should be placed to visualize the spleen between ports 2 and 3.*

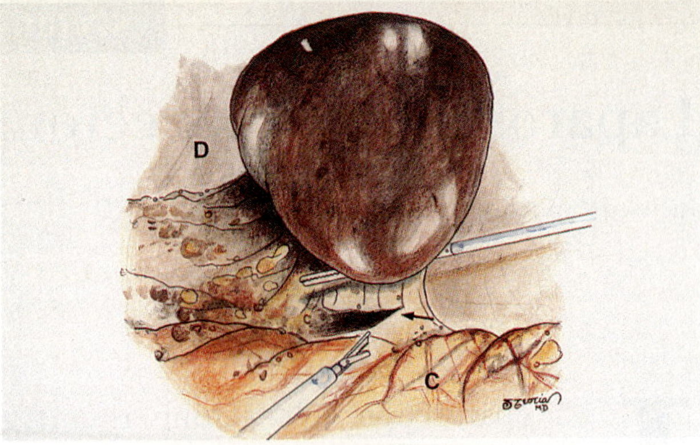

Figure 3. *After exploration, the dissection of the splenic attachments is begun with the splenocolic ligament (arrow). Traction is always placed toward the spleen with countertraction, if necessary. C indicates colon; D, diaphragm.*

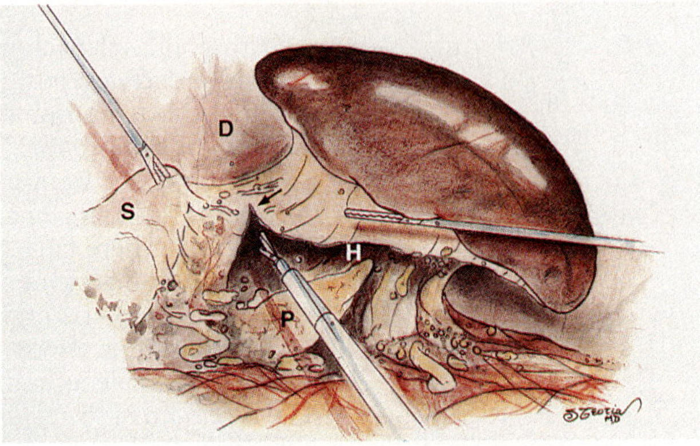

Figure 4. *The gastrosplenic ligament is divided (arrow). Dissection is begun at the inferior aspect and continued until all short gastric vessels are divided. The superior medial aspect of the splenophrenic ligament is also divided. S indicates stomach; P, pancreas; D, diaphragm; and H, hilum.*

tion. This facilitates retraction of the heavy spleen and exposure of the vasculature.

TROCAR PLACEMENT

Trocar port sites are numbered in **Figure 2**. This numbering will be used to identify sites in the remaining discussion. An incision is made over the costal cartilage at port site 2. Pneumoperitoneum is instituted using an open or a closed technique. As the abdomen expands, this initial incision will be drawn down over the abdominal cavity. After a 12-mm trocar is inserted at port site 2, the camera port is placed at site 5 under direct vision. This port should be placed to allow the spleen to be visualized between ports 2 and 3. A 5-mm trocar is placed at port site 1. Adhesions, which are usually present near the splenic flexure of the colon, are then lysed to allow insertion of a 12-mm trocar at port site 3 and a 5-mm trocar at port site 4. In splenomegaly, ports 4 and 5 will need to be placed more inferiorly, and the operative ports (2 and 3) may need to be moved anteriorly to allow dissection without hindrance from the spleen.

EXPLORATION

Identification of accessory splenic tissue is crucial to the success of LS. Abdominal exploration is somewhat limited in the semidecubitus position. However, excellent visualization of the left upper quadrant is possible. The transverse colon is elevated to examine the left side of the transverse mesocolon. The omentum is examined also. During the course of the remaining steps, careful attention is paid to the tissues in an effort to identify accessory splenic tissue.

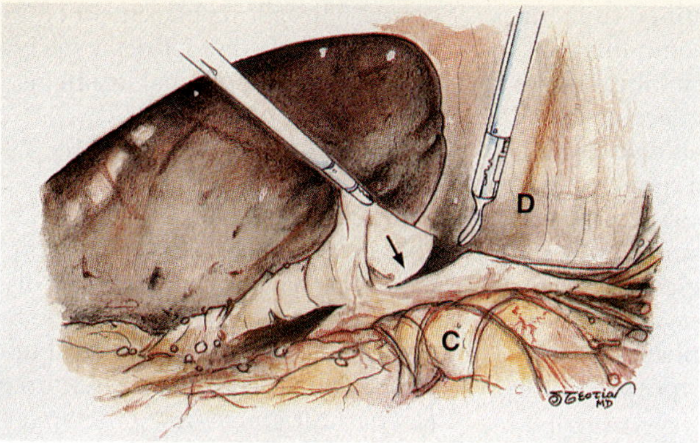

Figure 5. *The splenorenal ligament (arrow) is divided, retracting the spleen anteriorly. Areolar connective tissue between this ligament and the splenic hilum is gently divided. C indicates colon; D, diaphragm.*

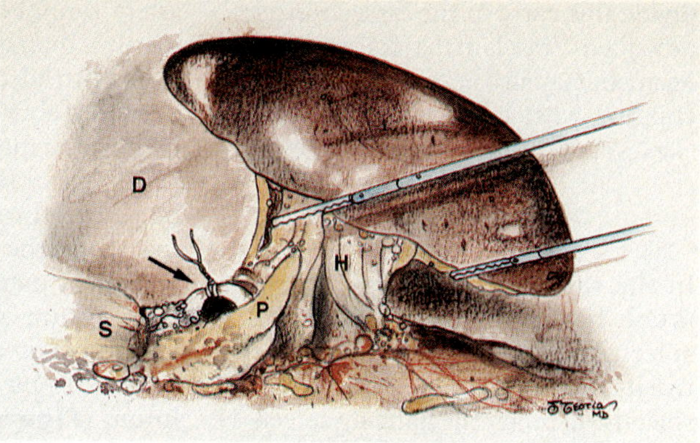

Figure 7. *If the splenic artery can be identified superior to the tail of the pancreas, it is ligated (arrow). S indicates stomach; D, diaphragm; P, pancreas; and H, hilum.*

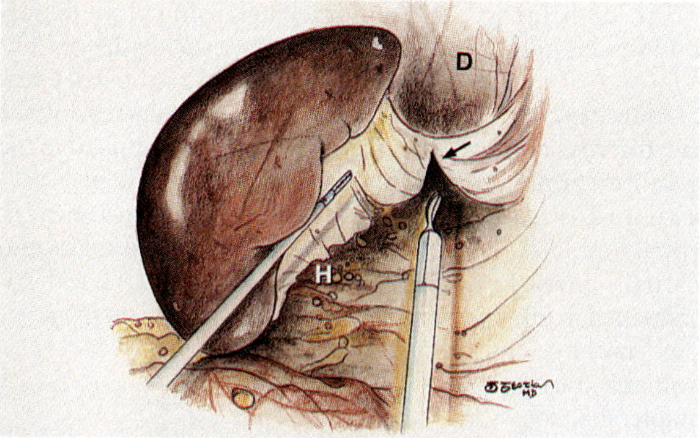

Figure 6. *The gastrophrenic ligament is divided (arrow), and areolar connective tissue again is dissected. At the completion of this step, the splenic hilum has been mobilized circumferentially. D indicates diaphragm; H, hilum.*

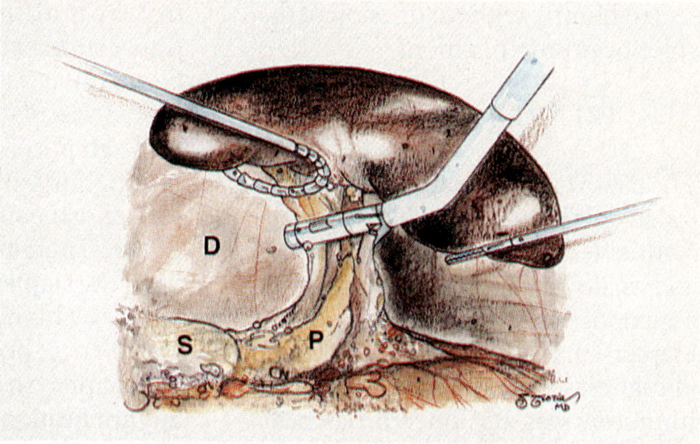

Figure 8. *The splenic hilum is now divided with the spleen retracted far into the left upper quadrant. After transection, the spleen is placed in a bag, morcellated, and removed. P indicates pancreas; D, diaphragm; and S, stomach.*

MOBILIZATION

Skandalakis et al[9] provided an excellent review of splenic anatomy. This may prove useful to the surgeon embarking on LS. The division of the splenic ligaments proceeds in an orderly fashion. The object of this mobilization is the circumferential isolation of the splenic hilum before hilar vascular transection. The inferior tip of the spleen is initially elevated with a grasper, which holds the tissues adjacent to the spleen. Traction is always placed toward the spleen to prevent a capsular tear. The splenocolic ligament is then divided (**Figure 3**) with a commercially available shears (Harmonic Shears; Ethicon, Cincinnati, Ohio). Electrocautery may also be used. A vessel to the inferior pole of the spleen may be encountered and may require clips if it is large enough. As few clips as possible are used, however, as these may interfere with the use of vascular staplers on the splenic hilum.

The gastrosplenic ligament is then divided beginning at the inferior border (**Figure 4**). The lesser sac is entered early during this maneuver, exposing the pancreas and splenic hilum at the posterior aspect of the sac. Dissection is performed between the stomach and the spleen, and all short gastric vessels are divided. The advantages of the shears used for this dissection have been published.[10] Dissection continues as far as possible superior to the spleen, dividing the upper portions of the splenophrenic ligament.

Attention is now turned to the splenorenal ligament. The spleen is reflected anteriorly, and the splenorenal ligament is grasped and pulled toward the spleen for exposure. The ligament is divided 1 to 2 cm away from the spleen (**Figure 5**). Scissors with electrocautery have worked well here. This dissection is continued onto the splenophrenic ligament (**Figure 6**) and eventually should communicate with the previous dissection superior to the spleen. The areolar connective tissue located between the posterior aspect of the splenic hilum and the posterior splenic ligaments is taken down with a gentle sweeping motion and judicious use of electrocautery or harmonic oscillation. The splenic hilum should now be exposed circumferentially.

Alternative

Some authors have preferred the "hanging spleen" technique[11] and have applied it with excellent results. With this variation, the splenophrenic ligament is not divided until the hilum is transected. We do not use this technique unless the patient has significant splenomegaly. We believe that we can expose the hilum better using traction to elevate the spleen rather than just allowing it to hang. In addition, should bleeding occur in the hilum, the splenophrenic ligament often has to be divided to control the hemorrhage. Instead, it would seem easier to us to divide this early in the dissection as described. Vessels in the gastrosplenic ligament may also be divided between clips or with endoscopic vascular staples at the discretion of the surgeon.

Splenomegaly

In the case of splenomegaly, it is much harder to manipulate the spleen and to elevate it or to control its rotation. Therefore, for these spleens we prefer the hanging spleen technique. The splenocolic and gastrosplenic ligaments are divided as described above. The tissues posterior to the splenic hilum are dissected bluntly without division of the splenophrenic ligament.

HILAR DISSECTION

The use of vascular staplers to transect the splenic hilum has resulted in a substantial reduction in operating times and yielded excellent hemostasis in our experience (unpublished data, 1996). Staplers may be placed across individual vessels or used to transect the hilum en masse. Concern has been raised about the potential for the development of arteriovenous fistulas with the en masse technique. To date, such a fistula has not been documented in a human, although arteriograms have not been performed routinely. As a precaution, we try to place a ligature about the main splenic artery before mass hilar transection.

The spleen is reflected posteriorly, and the splenic artery can be seen pulsating just superior to the tail of the pancreas. The artery often has a prominent knuckle and is mobilized at this point (**Figure 7**). The vessel is exposed, and an instrument is placed around the artery. A tie is brought in through a separate port and placed around the dissected vessel. The tie is then brought out through the initial port. (The use of a grasper as a fulcrum protects the artery from the sawing motion of the tie during this maneuver.) The tie is secured with an extracorporeal tie. (We have found this to be more secure than an intracorporeal tie on this major vessel.) A large clip may be used also; however, this may necessitate use of a clip applier, which would not otherwise have been opened. At times the camera may need to be moved to a different site to visualize the artery. If the artery cannot be identified (uncommonly), then we will omit this step.

With adequate mobilization, as described above, the spleen now may be elevated into the left upper quadrant. A flexible 5-mm retractor may be placed through port 3 and used to encircle the hilum and elevate the spleen in patients with a normal-sized hilum. Graspers and retractors to balance the spleen also may be used to provide exposure of the hilum (**Figure 8**).

Ideally, the tail of the pancreas should be identified. However, if the pancreas is not well seen, one must at least be certain there is nothing along the line of hilar transection except blood vessels and connective tissue.

A vascular stapler is now inserted through port 3 and placed across the hilum. It usually will require 2 applications of the stapler for a normal-sized hilum. There is a potential for bleeding if the stapler only partially crosses a vessel. This has not happened in our experience; however, we have a second stapler cartridge available during any application of the stapler that does not completely cross the hilum. Should bleeding occur, the site would be temporarily occluded with a grasper while the cartridge is rapidly changed and the stapler is reapplied. Any tissue left superior to the hilum is divided with cautery or harmonic oscillation.

Alternative

Vessels within the splenic hilum also may be controlled and divided individually. We used this technique early in our experience and found it to be quite tedious without depth perception. In addition, should bleeding ensue within the hilum, we frequently had to revert to the use of staplers to control it. Application of the staplers was hindered by the presence of previously placed clips. Therefore, we now prefer to use staplers initially. Excellent results, however, may be obtained with individual vessel ligation.

Splenomegaly

Hilar dissection is similar for splenomegaly in that we prefer to ligate the splenic artery initially. Tissues posterior to the hilum are then bluntly dissected. This allows placement of the staplers without division of the splenophrenic and splenorenal ligaments.

SPECIMEN REMOVAL

A number of plastic bags are available now to facilitate specimen removal, each with advantages and disadvantages. No incisions need to be enlarged for specimen removal unless an intact specimen is required for pathologic review (the specimen need not be intact for ITP).

Once the specimen is in the bag, the open end of the bag is brought out through trocar port 3. The spleen is then morcellated using blunt dissection with clamps, a sucker tip, or a finger, and the pieces are removed. Great care is exercised to prevent tearing the bag. Traction should be applied to the contents rather than the bag.

Following specimen removal, the abdomen is insufflated again, and hemostasis is checked. The abdomen is irrigated before closure.

Alternative

Port sites may be enlarged to aid removal; however, this generally results in increased postoperative pain, and there is little to be gained.

Splenomegaly

Techniques are not altered for mild to moderate degrees of splenomegaly. Patients with massive splenomegaly, however, pose unique challenges. A counterincision may be made low on the abdomen for specimen removal. However, this will often need to be substantial in its length, thus negating many of the benefits gained from the laparoscopic dissection. Placing the truly massive spleen into a bag for removal is frequently futile, even if one is using a hand-assisted technique. This has led some to divide the spleen within the abdomen and to place the pieces in separate bags. Although this may seem objectionable initially, it may be justified in select cases. First, spread of disease is unlikely. There is a great deal of experience with incisional biopsies of intra-abdominal lymphomas, and these are performed without fear of spread (lymphoma being a systemic disease). Second, although splenosis is a concern, this should be preventable. The abdomen is irrigated copiously after splenic removal and aspirated with a 10-mm suction tip. At the conclusion of this, there should be no visible splenic tissue within the abdomen. Finally, most of these patients undergo operation for symptoms of splenomegaly and not hyperfunction. Therefore, it is unlikely that splenic implants would cause significant morbidity, even if they were to occur. Long-term review of patients will be required to substantiate the use of this maneuver; however, it may be reasonable to use it now. Patients are informed of these options preoperatively. This maneuver should never be used for conditions such as ITP or hemolytic anemia, as splenic implants might cause recurrence of the disease.

CLOSURE

Trocars are removed under direct vision, and we close the fascia of all trocar ports 10 mm in diameter or larger. In the obese patient, we use a fascial closure device, and a number of these are available. Subcutaneous tissues are irrigated before skin closure. Sites may also be injected with a long-acting local anesthetic.

POSTOPERATIVE CARE

Patients are allowed to take liquids later the same day and progress to a regular diet the following day. Approximately 75% of our patients are discharged on the day after surgery. Most patients require little or no parenteral narcotics, and oral pain medications frequently suffice. The risk for bleeding from open procedures on the night of surgery is well known. Postoperative bleeding likely will occur, on rare occasions, following LS. Therefore, we have elected not to perform LS as an outpatient procedure at this time.

CONCLUSIONS

Current techniques for LS have been discussed. These techniques allow for a systematic and controlled dissection and have led to high success rates for the procedure. However, minimally invasive surgery is still a new discipline, and these techniques will likely be improved in the future.

Reprints: Richard T. Schlinkert, MD, Department of Surgery, Mayo Clinic Scottsdale, 13400 E Shea Blvd, Scottsdale, AZ 85259 (e-mail: schlinkert.richard@mayo.edu).

REFERENCES

1. Schlinkert RT, Mann D. Laparoscopic splenectomy offers advantages in selected patients with immune thrombocytopenic purpura. *Am J Surg.* 1995;170:624-627.
2. Poulin EC, Thibault C, Mamazza J. Laparoscopic splenectomy. *Surg Endosc.* 1995;9:172-177.
3. Watson DI, Coventry BJ, Chin T, Gill PG, Malycha P. Laparoscopic versus open splenectomy for immune thrombocytopenic purpura. *Surgery.* 1997;121:18-22.
4. Phillips EH, Carroll BJ, Fallas MJ. Laparoscopic splenectomy. *Surg Endosc.* 1994;8:931-933.
5. Kathouda N, Waldrep DJ, Feinstein D, et al. Unresolved issues in laparoscopic splenectomy. *Am J Surg.* 1996;72:1-5.
6. Tsiotos G, Schlinkert RT. Laparoscopic splenectomy for immune thrombocytopenic purpura. *Arch Surg.* 1997;132:642-646.
7. Harold KL, Schlinkert RT, Mann D, et al. Long-term results of laparoscopic splenectomy for immune thrombocytopenic purpura. *Mayo Clin Proc.* In press.
8. Poulin E, Thibault C, Mamazza J, Girotti M, Cote G, Renaud A. Laparoscopic splenectomy: clinical experience and the role of preoperative splenic artery embolization. *Surg Laparosc Endosc.* 1993;3:445-450.
9. Skandalakis PN, Colborn GL, Skandalakis LJ, Richardson DD, Mitchell WE, Skandalakis JE. The surgical anatomy of the spleen. *Surg Clin North Am.* 1993;73:747-768.
10. Laycock WS, Trus TL, Hunter JH. New technology for the division of short gastric vessels during laparoscopic Nissen fundoplication. *Surg Endosc.* 1996;10:671-673.
11. Delaitre B. Laparoscopic splenectomy: the "hanged spleen" technique. *Surg Endosc.* 1995;9:528-529.

Invited Critique

Different techniques of laparsocopic splenectomy have been described previously. Drs Schlinkert and Teotia provide us with a concise presentation of their version of it. Clearly one technique does not apply to spleens of all sizes and types of anatomy.

Lessons learned from other laparoscopic operations should be applied to splenectomy as well. Anytime an operation traditionally performed using the open technique is approached laparoscopically, one should make every effort not to alter the key components of the operation. In the current report, an en masse ligation of the splenic artery and vein using a stapling device is recommended. This approach is only acceptable if the surgeon routinely does not identify and ligate the splenic artery and vein separately during open splenectomy. Additionally, the authors suggest division of the "massive" spleen into pieces within the peritoneal cavity to facilitate its retrieval. This maneuver clearly violates the principles of oncologic surgery and should rarely be considered.

If the steps used in open splenectomy must be modified for laparoscopic splenectomy, I have my own biases. First, I too am a proponent of the "hanging spleen" technique, which advocates devascularization of the spleen prior to division of the lateral ligamentous attachments. I believe this technique minimizes the risk of inadvertent loss of control of the hilar vessels and therefore reduces operative blood loss.

Second, to reduce the size of the "massive spleen," controlled venous back-bleeding into the splenic fossa has been previously reported. This technique undoubtedly results in additional blood loss, and also violates good surgical principles. Alternatively, one may ligate (but not divide) the splenic artery early and complete the operation with late ligation of the splenic vein, followed by division of both structures.

Vafa Shayani, MD
Maywood, Ill

Necessity Is the Mother of Invention

DURING MY surgical residency at the University of Cincinnati, Cincinnati, Ohio, in the 1950s, in addition to the daily duties required by the training program, I was involved with the development of the first successful bubble oxygenator for total bypass of the heart and lungs.[1] The project was the brainchild of Leland Clark, Jr, PhD, a biochemist at the Fels Institute at Antioch College in Yellow Springs, Ohio, who led the research team with James Helmsworth, MD, a thoracic surgeon, and Samuel Kaplan, MD, a cardiologist. Thomas Larsen, MD, was a surgical resident on rotation with the laboratory service.

In the early phase of our experiments with the oxygenator, it was crucial to determine the degree of blood oxygenation in dogs undergoing bypass at any given time during the bypass period. The only method for measuring the oxygen content of blood available then was the Van Slyke apparatus, a time-consuming, complicated procedure. During the bypass procedure, we drew venous and arterial blood from the animal and recorded intervals to be analyzed later and correlated with the stage of the experiment when drawn.

After the experiment was complete, there was always a period of anxious waiting for our faithful laboratory assistant Zena Taylor to report the results of the Van Slyke analysis of our samples. Until these results were in, we had no knowledge of the efficiency with which our pump could oxygenate the blood during the procedure.

Late one night, after our daily experimental bypass had been completed, Dr Clark and I were sitting in the laboratory, patiently waiting for the results of the laborious Van Slyke analysis. Dr Clark slowly opened a package of cigarettes while we waited and said, "Did you know that oxygen tension in clear solutions can be determined polarographically, but not in blood because the red cells cluster around the cathode, preventing an accurate reading?" He turned the cellophane cigarette wrapping over in his hands and said, "I think that if the cathode is wrapped with cellophane, the red cells might be kept from fouling the cathode, yet oxygen could still diffuse through the cellophane permitting an accurate measurement of oxygen tension in blood."

A few days later, we incorporated the first prototype of Dr Clark's polarographic electrode into our oxygenator and were able to continuously and immediately monitor oxygen tension during the bypass period.[2]

I did not realize it then, of course, but I had been privileged to witness the discovery of the Clark oxygen electrode for the polarographic measurement of oxygen tension in blood, a device that has been so important for the management of patients and has contributed immeasurably to the development of modern-day critical care and many other invaluable adjuncts to patient care.

Roger T. Sherman, MD
Atlanta, Ga

REFERENCES

1. Helmsworth JA, Clark LC Jr, Kaplan S, Sherman RT, Largen T. Artificial oxgenation and circulation during complete by-pass of the heart. *J Thoracic Surg.* 1953;24:117.
2. Clark LC Jr, Helmsworth JA, Kaplan S, Sherman RT, Taylor Z. Polarographic measurement of oxygen tension in whole blood and tissues during total by-pass of the heart. *Surg Forum.* 1953;93.

Henry H. Smith's *A System of Operative Surgery*

The son of a lawyer, Henry Hollingsworth Smith was born in Philadelphia on December 10, 1815. He attended the University of Pennsylvania, Philadelphia, where he also completed his medical studies (1837), and at the same time served as a private student of William Horner (1793-1853), professor of anatomy and dean of the school. Following graduation, Smith took a position as resident physician of Pennsylvania Hospital for 2 years. Believing his medical background to be incomplete, he spent 1840 and 1841 in Europe. Intending to make surgery his specialty, Smith returned to Philadelphia in the fall of 1841, where he began to teach private classes in minor surgery.

The growth of Smith's practice was slow, such that he was able to devote much time to his work as a medical author. During that first year he translated from the French Jean Civiale's (1792-1867) *Treatise on the Medical and Prophylactic Treatment of Stone and Gravel*. In 1843, Smith prepared under the supervision of Homer an *Anatomical Atlas, Illustrative of the Structure of the Human Body*. Smith and Horner's relationship was strengthened no doubt by the former's marriage in October of that year to the latter's eldest daughter. Smith's first solo book length volume was also published in 1843, *A Treatise on Minor Surgery*. The following year Smith helped edit the fourth edition of his father-in-law's *The United States Dissector, or, Lessons in Practical Anatomy*.

It was not unexpected that with his large literary output, the presentation of numerous lectures, and a little bit of nepotism, Smith was elected a surgeon to St Joseph's Hospital, Philadelphia, in 1849. This was soon followed by the Episcopal and Blockley Hospitals in 1854. For several years he was also an assistant lecturer on clinical surgery in his alma mater and, in 1855, was named professor of surgery. During the 1850s, Smith authored 2 well-known textbooks, *A System of Operative Surgery* (1852) and *A Treatise on the Practice of Surgery* (1856). His *A System of Operative Surgery* was a massive compendium of various surgical operations and would prove particularly important to the photographic history of American medicine because it was the country's first surgical textbook to have illustrations based on daguerreotypes. In addition, Smith provided an extremely detailed introductory section describing the progress of American surgical history, a bibliographical index of American surgical writers with a list of their works by subject, and an extensive alphabetical list of American surgeons including the titles of their most important papers.

At the beginning of the Civil War, Smith was selected by the governor of Pennsylvania to reorganize the hospital department of the state and received the title of Surgeon-General of Pennsylvania. Returning to civilian life in late 1862, Smith found that the fifth edition of his *Minor Surgery*, the second edition of *A System of Operative Surgery*, and the first edition of his *A Treatise on the Practice of Surgery* had been completely sold out. Through an arrangement with J. B. Lippincott, it was decided to revise all 3 works and publish them together as a new 2-volume set, *The Principles and Practice of Surgery Embracing Minor and Operative Surgery* (1863). The work was an immediate success and is historically important because it represents the only systematic textbook of surgery to be authored by an American surgeon during the Civil War.

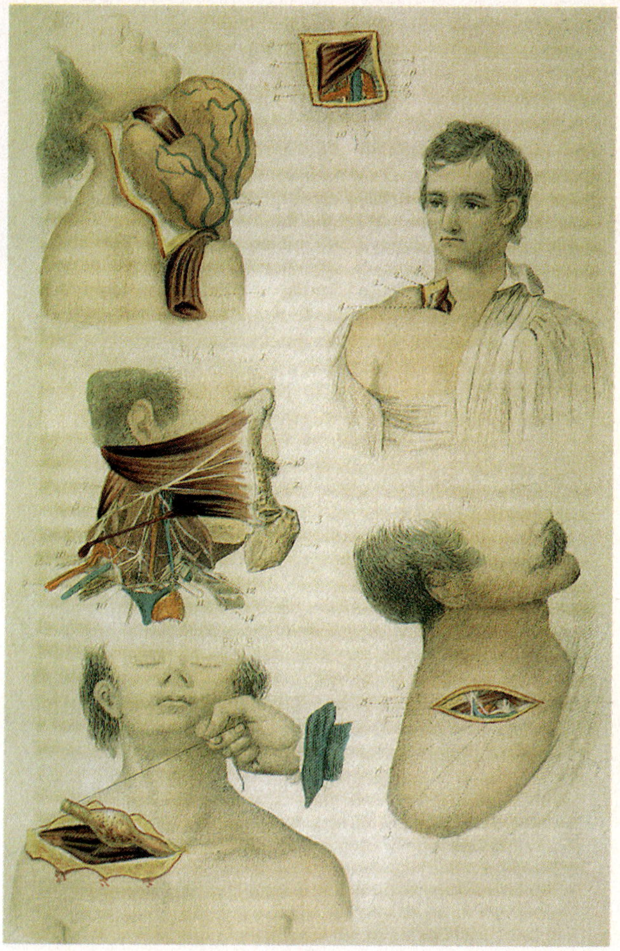

A limited number of Smith's A System of Operative Surgery *were produced with "colored to life" plates. The shading helped highlight certain aspects of surgical technique, in this particular case "operations practiced at the lower portion of the neck."*

Following his retirement from active academic life (1871), Smith continued a private surgical practice while participating in the politics of organized medicine. In 1878, he became president of the Philadelphia County Medical Society. Five years later, Smith was elected president of the Medical Society of the State of Pennsylvania. In 1887, he was named chairman of the Section of Military and Naval Surgery and Medicine of the Ninth International Medical Congress, conducted in Washington, DC. Smith died on April 11, 1890.

Ira M. Rutkow, MD, MPH, DrPH

PRODUCTS & SERVICES

The information given here is supplied by the companies cited. Publication of these notices does not imply endorsement or warranty by the American Medical Association, publishers of the *Archives of Surgery*.

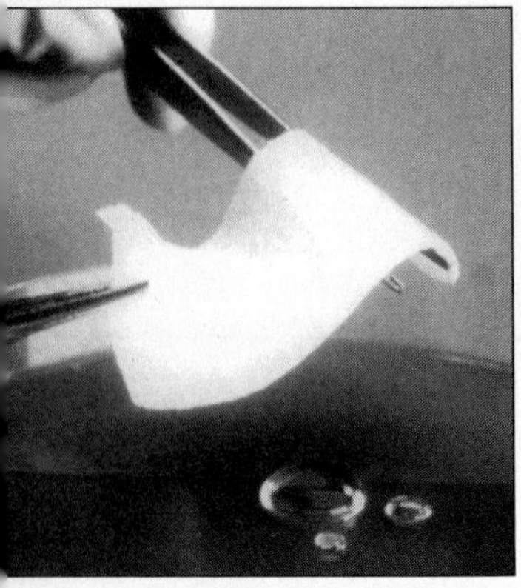

SURGICAL PRODUCT —

AlloDerm, an acellular dermal graft derived from human donor skin, is the first soft tissue implant to regenerate normal soft human tissue. A product of LifeCell Corporation, AlloDerm can be used for both surface grafting and repair and replacement of integumental tissue defects.

AlloDerm is created via a revolutionary process that removes from dermal tissue the cellular components that are prone to a rejection response and preserves the essential biochemistry of the dermal matrix. The benefits are numerous and offer many advan tages over traditional soft tissue alternatives including no need to harvest autologous tissue for soft tissue reconstructive procedures and a minimized need for harvesting autologous tissue for grafting procedures, reducing surgery time as well as donor site morbidity.

LifeCell employs stringent donor screening, including medical and social history as well as serological testing for many diseases. AlloDerm is one of the most commonly used acellular dermal grafts in the US and has been used in more than 40 000 surgical procedures with excellent cosmetic and functional results.

For information write
LIFECELL CORPORATION
3606 Research Forest Drive
The Woodlands, TX 77381

Call toll free
800-367-5737

Fax
281-363-3360

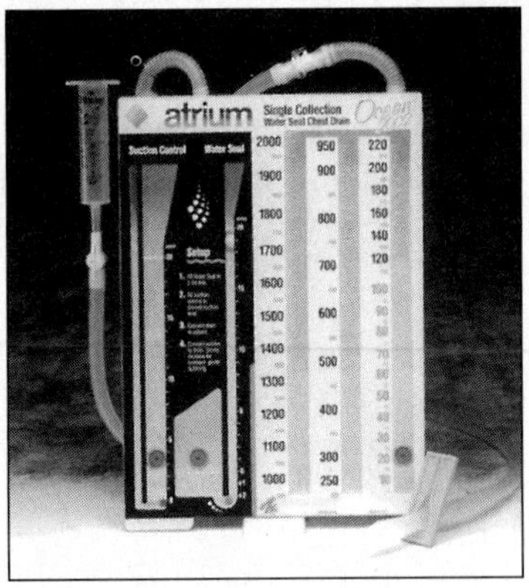

SURGICAL PRODUCT —

Atrium Medical Corporation is pleased to announce the transition to latex-free tubing for their entire line of wet and dry chest drainage products. This product enhancement has been made in response to an overwhelming demand for latex-free medical products from the global marketplace.

Atrium latex-free chest drains are currently being manufactured and will be made available at no additional cost as existing supply channel inventories are depleted.

Atrium Medical Corporation is a leading international supplier of medical products, including chest drains, thoracic catheters, vascular grafts, and surgical mesh.

For information write
ATRIUM MEDICAL CORPORATION
Attn: Craig Weimer
5 Wentworth Drive
Hudson, NH 03051

Call toll free
800-370-7899 x5210

Fax
603-880-4545

E-mail
cweimer@atiummed.com

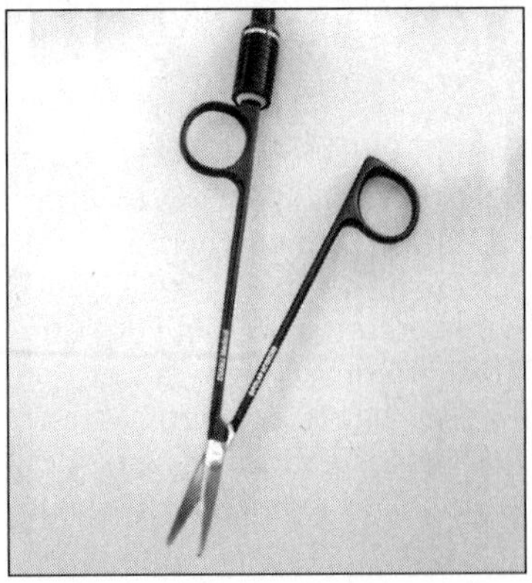

SURGICAL INSTRUMENT —

Enable Medical Corporation has just released a revolutionary new product, the Enable Bipolar Scissors (EBS) consisting of a computer machined reusable scissors and a disposable bipolar cartridge pair which snap onto the scissors' blades.

The surgeon activates bipolar energy using a foot pedal, and the energy flows along the edge of each scissors blade coagulating tissue before it is cut.

This unique product allows the surgeon to perform the multiple tasks of dissecting, cutting, and coagulating tissue with a single instrument and may significantly reduce the use of sutures and clips.

The EBS scissors have applications in virtually every open surgical procedure, including general, plastic, ENT, head and neck, gynecological, oncological, and cardiac surgery. The EBS scissors are being used for harvesting of the saphenous vein and other vessels for open-heart surgery.

For information write
ENABLE MEDICAL CORPORATION
Attn: Michael Hooven
6345 Centre Park Drive
West Chester, OH 45069-3863

Phone
513-755-7600 x711

Fax
513-755-7676

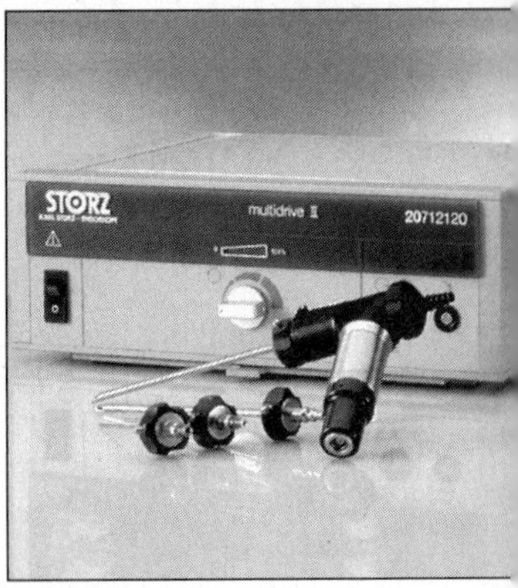

SURGICAL INSTRUMENT —

Karl Storz Endoscopy-America, Inc introduces the Paranasal Sinus Shaver System for endoscopic sinus procedures. Engineered for maximum surgical efficiency and effectiveness, the Paranasal Sinus Shaver System features a uniquely designed ergonomic handpiece angled at 90° to provide comfort for users. The cutting and suction aperture is infinitely rotatable by 360° without repositioning the instrument handle.

Unobstructed and optimum suction is produced by a centrally configured, straight, in-line vacuum channel. Continuously adjustable suction is controlled by a rotatable mechanism on the handpiece and provides maximum control.
By working with constant suction, the sinus shaver helps reduce instrument passes.

Markings on the outer sheath allow the physician to monitor depth of penetration during surgery.
A quick-release mechanism ensures safe, fast replacement of shaver blades. Reusable blades are available in serrated, concave, smooth and abrading designs. Disposable blades are available in an aggressive saber tooth bullet design with or without irrigation or in an abrader burr design.

For information write
KS ENDOSCOPY-AMERICA, INC
600 Corporate Pointe
Culver City, CA 90230-7600

Call toll free
800-421-0837

Web site
www.karlstorz.com

MANUSCRIPT CRITERIA AND INFORMATION

Manuscripts are to be sent by first-class or overnight express mail to Claude H. Organ, Jr, MD, Editor, *Archives of Surgery,* c/o Dept of Surgery, University of California–Davis, East Bay, 1411 E 31st St, Oakland, CA 94602. All materials requested must be enclosed to ensure prompt review and publication consideration in the *Archives of Surgery*. Use the checklist to ensure completeness.

Rejected manuscripts will no longer be returned to the authors owing to the increasing cost of postage and the widespread use of computers and photocopy machines. To ensure confidentiality, the manuscripts will be destroyed. Outside peer reviewers are directed to destroy these manuscripts after their review to protect the authors' confidentiality and ownership. Original figures and photographs, however, will be returned to the authors.

Manuscript Preparation

The original typescript plus 3 high-quality copies must be submitted, including legends, tables, and references. All copy, including references, legends, and tables, must be typed double-spaced on 8½×11-in, heavy-duty white bond paper. Margins must be at least 1 in. **Do *not* use justified right margins.** All illustrations must be originals, not copies.

Abstract. Include a *structured abstract* of no more than 250 words for reports of original articles and reviews. For detailed instructions, see pages 112-115.

Copyright. A copyright release form dated and signed by *all* authors of manuscripts, brief communications, and correspondence is required by the Copyright Revision Act of 1976. The following statement may be used: "**In consideration of the American Medical Association's taking action in reviewing and editing my submission, the undersigned author(s) hereby transfers, assigns, or otherwise conveys all copyright ownership to the AMA in the event that such work is published by the AMA.**

I certify that I (1) have participated sufficiently in this work to take public responsibility for the content of this manuscript; (2) believe the experimental design and method as well as the collection, analysis, and interpretation of the data are sound; and (3) have reviewed the final version of the manuscript and approve it for publication. This manuscript has not been published and is not being considered for publication elsewhere except as described in an attachment hereto."

US Federal Employees. If this manuscript was prepared as a federal employee, please so indicate by signing the following statement: "**I was an employee of the US federal government when this work was investigated and prepared for publication.**"

Financial Disclosure. All authors are required to sign the following statement: "**I certify that all affiliations with or involvement in any organization or entity with a direct financial interest in the subject matter or materials discussed in the manuscript (eg, employment, consultancies, stock ownership, honoraria) have been disclosed in an attachment. I understand that such affilation(s) will not affect consideration of the manuscript but may be published as a footnote if the manuscript is accepted.**"

References. *References* should be listed in *consecutive numerical order* as they are cited in the text, *not alphabetically*. Once a reference is cited, all subsequent citations should be to the original number. All references must be cited in the text or tables. Unpublished data and personal communication are not encouraged and may not be listed as references. References to journal articles should include, in this order, (1) authors (list all authors and/or editors up to 6; if more than 6, list the first 3 and "et al"), (2) title, (3) journal name as abbreviated in *Index Medicus*, (4) year, (5) volume number, and (6) inclusive

Checklist for Authors

Send:

- ☐ One original and 3 copies of manuscript, including abstract, legends, and tables, each **stapled** as a complete unit.
- ☐ Four sets of all illustrations, clearly labeled as described in the instructions, all submitted in original format and not copied.
- ☐ Number all pages.
- ☐ Double-space manuscript (text and references), and leave right margins **unjustified** (ragged)
- ☐ On the title page, designate a corresponding author and provide a complete address, telephone and fax numbers, and e-mail address.
- ☐ Statements, signed by each author, for authorship responsibility, financial disclosure, and copyright transfer or federal employment.
- ☐ Disk for all book reviews, editorials, commentaries, and letters to the editor. List make of computer (IBM or Macintosh) and software program and version.
- ☐ Disk for original articles and clinical observations only when revised manuscript is being submitted.
- ☐ Check references for accuracy, completeness, and proper format in numerical order.
- ☐ Include written permission from publisher to reproduce or adapt previously published illustrations and tables.
- ☐ Informed consent forms for identifiable patient descriptions, photographs, and pedigrees.
- ☐ Send to Claude H. Organ, Jr, MD
Editor
Archives of Surgery
1411 E 31st St
Oakland, CA 94602

page numbers. References to books should include (1) authors (list all authors and/or editors up to 6; if more than 6, list the first 3 and "et al"), (2) chapter title, if any, (3) editor, if any, (4) title of book, (5) year, (6) city, and (7) publisher. Volume and edition numbers, specific pages, and name of translator should be included when appropriate.The author is responsible for the accuracy and completeness of the references and for their correct text citation.

Author Responsibility. Please designate 1 author as the *corresponding author*, with his or her address, telephone and fax numbers, and e-mail address. All correspondence and copyediting will be forwarded to this author. The corresponding author will receive an edited typescript rather than galley proofs for approval. The authors are responsible for all statements in their work, including changes made by the copy editor. Reprint order forms are included with the edited typescript sent for approval to the corresponding author. Reprints are shipped 3 weeks after publication.

Group Authorship. If authorship is attributed to a group (either solely or in addition to 1 or more individual authors), all members of the group must meet the full criteria and requirements for authorship (copyright, authorship responsibility, and disclosure). One or more authors may take responsibility "for" a group, in which case the other group members are not authors, but may be listed in an acknowledgment.

Titles. *The title* must be *short*, specific, clear, and not exceed 42 characters per line, including punctuation and spaces (2-line limitation). The title page should include the **complete** names, academic affiliations, and highest academic degrees of all authors. Please limit the number of authors to a maximum of 8. If the manuscript was presented at a meeting, indicate the name of the organization, the location, and the date of presentation.

SI Units. Use Système International (SI) measurements.

Illustrations. Submit 4 **original** illustrations, unmounted and untrimmed. They should clarify and augment the text. Do not send original artwork. Send high-contrast glossy prints (not photocopies). Computer-generated graphics produced by high-quality laser printers are acceptable for black-and-white line art only. Type the figure number, name of senior author, and arrow indicating "top" on a gummed label and affix to the back of each illustration. All lettering in illustrations must be legible after reduction to column size. Illustrations should preferably be in a proportion of 5×7 in. *Color illustrations* are accepted for publication if the editors believe that color will add significantly to the manuscript. The ARCHIVES will pay only part of the expense of color reproduction and printing of color illustrations. The author's share of the expense is $400 for up to 6 square finished illustrations that can be arranged on a 1-page layout. Additional illustrations or special effects will be billed to the author at cost. Positive color transparencies (35 mm preferred) must be submitted for an evaluation. Color prints must be accompanied by original transparencies. Computer-generated graphics produced by high-quality laser printers are not acceptable.

Legends. Type all legends consecutively and double-spaced. Please limit each legend to a maximum of 40 words.

Tables. Each table must be typed double-spaced, including all headings, on a separate sheet of 8½×11-in paper. Do not use larger-sized paper. If a table must be continued, use a second sheet and repeat all heads and stubs. Each table must have a title.

Manuscript Acceptance. Accepted manuscripts become the permanent property of the ARCHIVES and may not be published elsewhere without permission from the publisher (AMA). Send all requests for copyright permissions to: Office of Copyrights and Permissions, American Medical Association, 515 N State St, Chicago, IL 60610.

Instructions for Preparing Reports of Randomized Controlled Trials

The checklist on page 107 should be used as a guideline and submitted with the manuscript. In addition, include a flow diagram illustrating the progress of patients throughout the trial (see Figure below for example).

The checklist and flow diagram will be reviewed along with the manuscript. If the manuscript is accepted, the flow diagram will be published.

Profile of a Randomized Controlled Trial

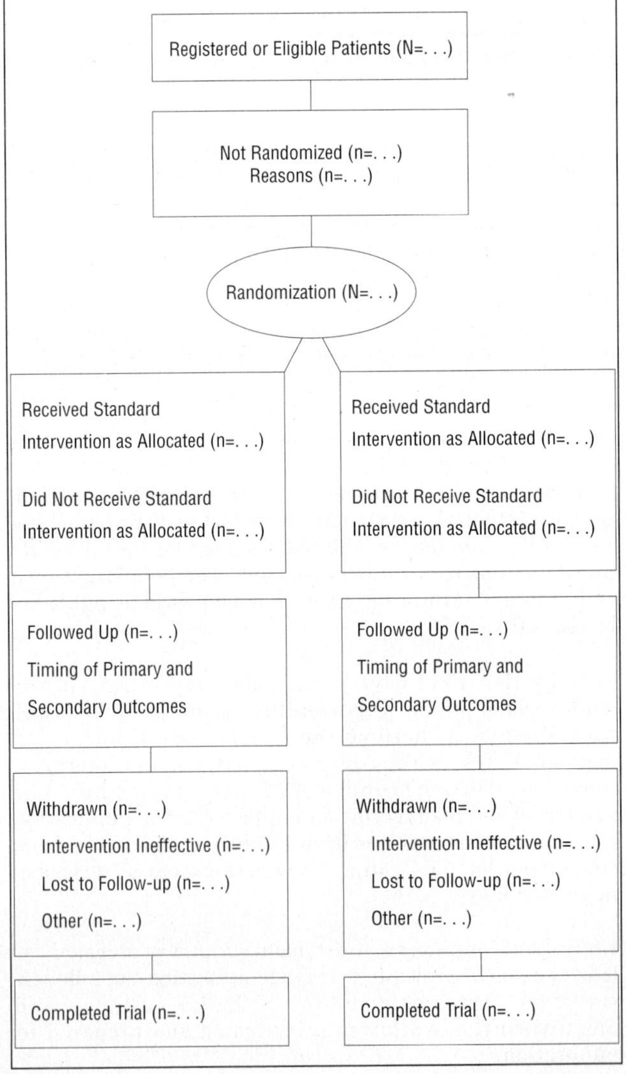

OTHER INFORMATION

Clinical Notes. The ARCHIVES will consider Clinical Notes for review. These reports should provide a new or unique contribution and consist of 800 words or less, 4 references, and 1 illustration. The synopsis-abstract may not exceed 80 words.

Correspondence or Brief Communications. The Editor is pleased to receive letters that pertain to material published in the ARCHIVES. Such contributions should be 250 words or less, typewritten, double-spaced without an abstract, and clearly marked "for publication," with no more than 2 references.

Operative Techniques. The *Archives of Surgery* is instituting a new section, Operative Techniques, wherein a variety of simple and complex procedures will be presented. Drawings of operative photographs should clearly illustrate sequential steps in the procedure. Each drawing should be accompanied by a legend and sufficient descriptive text so that the reader is taken through the procedure in an orderly fashion. Color drawings or photographs may be utilized if they would clearly enhance the reader's understanding of the procedure.

Acknowledgments. Illustrations from other publications must be acknowledged to include author(s), title of article, title of journal or book, volume number, pages, and month and year and submitted with the publisher's permission to the ARCHIVES when the manuscript has been formally accepted.

Statistical Review. Manuscripts containing statistical evaluation should include the name and affiliation of the statistical reviewer. The Editor may request that the author provide a statistical review prior to final acceptance.

Informed Consent. Manuscripts reporting the results of experimental investigations on human subjects must include a statement in the "Methods" section that the institutional review board has approved the project and/or that informed consent was obtained from all adult participating subjects and from parents or legal guardians for minors.

Reference to Patients. Patients may be referred to by number or, in anecdotal reports, by fictitious names. Real names or initials must not be used in the text, tables, or illustrations.

Animal Experiments. When reporting experiments on animals, please indicate that the institution's or the National Research Council's guide for or any national law on the care and use of laboratory animals was followed.

Photographic Consents. A letter of consent must accompany all photographs of patients in which a possibility of identification exists. It is *not* sufficient to simply cover the eyes to mask identity.

Checklist for Authors Submitting Reports of Randomized Controlled Trials to *Archives of Surgery**

First Author's Name and Manuscript Title ______________________________

Heading	Subheading	Descriptor	Was It Reported? Yes or No	If Yes, What Page No.?
Title		1. Identify the study as a randomized trial.	______	______
Abstract		2. Use a structured format.	______	______
Introduction		3. State prospectively defined hypothesis, clinical objectives, and planned subgroup or covariate analyses.	______	______
Methods	Protocol	Describe		
		4. Planned study population, together with inclusion/exclusion criteria.	______	______
		5. Planned interventions and their timing.	______	______
		6. Primary and secondary outcome measure(s) and the minimum important difference(s), and how the target sample size was projected.	______	______
		7. Rationale and methods for statistical analyses, detailing main comparative analyses and whether they were completed on an intention-to-treat basis.	______	______
		8. Prospectively defined stopping rules (if warranted).	______	______
	Assignment	Describe		
		9. Unit of randomization (eg, individual, cluster, geographic).	______	______
		10. Method used to generate the allocation schedule.	______	______
		11. Method of allocation concealment and timing of assignment.	______	______
		12. Method to separate the generator from the executor of assignment.	______	______
	Masking (Blinding)	13. Describe mechanism (eg, capsules, tablets); similarity of treatment characteristics (eg, appearance, taste); allocation schedule control (location of code during trial and when broken); and evidence for successful masking (blinding) among participants, person doing intervention, outcome assessors, and data analysts.	______	______
Results	Participant Flow and Follow-up	14. Provide a trial profile (see Figure of flow diagram on page 952) summarizing participant flow, numbers and timing of randomization assignment, interventions, and measurements for each randomized group.	______	______
	Analysis	15. State estimated effect of intervention on primary and secondary outcome measures, including a point estimate and measure of precision (confidence interval).	______	______
		16. State results in absolute numbers when feasible (eg, 10/20, not 50%).	______	______
		17. Present summary data and appropriate descriptive and inferential statistics in sufficient detail to permit alternative analyses and replication.	______	______
		18. Describe prognostic variables by treatment group and any attempt to adjust for them.	______	______
		19. Describe protocol deviations from the study as planned, together with the reasons.	______	______
Comment		20. State specific interpretation of study findings, including sources of bias and imprecision (internal validity) and discussion of external validity, including appropriate quantitative measures when possible.	______	______
		21. State general interpretation of the data in light of the totality of the available evidence.	______	______

**This checklist of 21 items is intended to assist authors, editors, and reviewers by ensuring that information pertinent to the trial is included in the study report. Adapted from Begg C, Cho M, Eastwood S, et al. Improving the quality of reporting of randomized controlled trials: the CONSORT statement.* JAMA. *1996;276:637-639.*

AUTHORSHIP RESPONSIBILITY, FINANCIAL DISCLOSURE, AND ASSIGNMENT OF COPYRIGHT

Each author must read and sign (1) the statement on authorship responsibility; (2) the statement on financial disclosure; and (3) either the statement on copyright transfer or the statement on federal employment. If necessary, photocopy this document to distribute to coauthors for their signatures. Please return all copies to *Archives of Surgery*, 1411 E 31st Street, Oakland, CA 94602.

Manuscript No. and/or Title: ____________________

1. Authorship Responsibility

I certify that I (1) have participated sufficiently in this work to take public responsibility for the content of this manuscript; (2) believe the experimental design and method as well as the collection, analysis, and interpretation of the data are sound; and (3) have reviewed the final version of the manuscript and approve it for publication. This manuscript has not been published and is not being considered for publication elsewhere except as described in an attachment hereto.

Author(s) Signature(s)	Date	Author(s) Signature(s)	Date

2. Financial Disclosure

All authors are required to sign the following statement: "I certify that all affiliations with or involvement in any organization or entity with a direct financial interest in the subject matter or materials discussed in the manuscript (eg, employment, consultancies, stock ownership, honoraria) have been disclosed in an attachment. I understand that such affiliation(s) will not affect consideration of the manuscript but may be published as a footnote if the manuscript is accepted."

Author(s) Signature(s)	Date	Author(s) Signature(s)	Date

3. Copyright

In consideration of the action of the AMA in reviewing and editing my submission, the author(s) undersigned hereby transfer(s), or otherwise convey(s) all copyright ownership to the AMA in the event that such work is published by the AMA.

Author(s) Signature(s)	Date	Author(s) Signature(s)	Date

US Federal Employees: I was an employee of the US federal government when this work was conducted and prepared for publication. Therefore, it is not protected by the Copyright Act and there is no copyright, thus ownership cannot be transferred.

Author(s) Signature(s)	Date	Author(s) Signature(s)	Date

All manuscripts that are (1) reports of original data or (2) reviews, including meta-analyses, should be submitted with structured abstracts as described below. For other types of articles, submit a narrative abstract of no more than 135 words.

Reports of Original Data

Authors submitting manuscripts reporting original data should prepare an abstract of no more than 250 words under the following headings: Hypothesis, Design, Setting, Patients (or Other Participants), Interventions (if any), Main Outcome Measure(s), Results, and Conclusions. The content following each heading should be as follows:

1. **Hypothesis.** The abstract should begin with a clear statement of the precise hypothesis addressed in the report. If more than one hypothesis is addressed, the main proposition should be indicated. If an a priori hypothesis was tested, it should be stated.

2. **Design.** The basic design of the study should be described. The duration of follow-up, if any, should be stated. As many of the following terms as apply should be used.

A. Intervention studies: randomized control trial (see Glossary for the definition of this and other technical terms); nonrandomized control trial; double-blind; placebo control; crossover trial; before-after trial.

B. For studies of screening and diagnostic tests: criterion standard (that is, a widely accepted standard with which a new or alternative test is being compared; this term is preferred to "gold standard"); blinded or masked comparison.

C. For studies of prognosis: inception cohort (subjects assembled at a similar and early time in the course of the disorder and followed thereafter); cohort (subjects followed forward in time, but not necessarily from a common starting point); validation cohort or validation sample if the study involves the modeling of clinical predictions.

D. For studies of causation: randomized control trial; cohort; case-control; survey (preferred to "cross-sectional study").

E. For descriptions of the clinical features of medical disorders: survey; case series.

F. For studies that include a formal economic evaluation: cost-effectiveness analysis; cost-utility analysis; cost-benefit analysis. For new analyses of existing data sets, the data set should be named and the basic study design disclosed.

3. **Setting.** To assist readers to determine the applicability of the report to their own clinical circumstances, the study setting(s) should be described. Of particular importance is whether the setting is the general community, a primary care or referral center, private or institutional practice, ambulatory or hospitalized care.

4. **Patients or Other Participants.** The clinical disorders, important eligibility criteria, and key sociodemographic features of patients should be stated. The numbers of participants and how they were selected should be provided (see below), including the number of otherwise eligible subjects who were approached but refused. If matching is used for comparison groups, characteristics that are matched should be specified. In follow-up studies, the proportion of participants who completed the study must be indicated. In intervention studies, the number of patients withdrawn for adverse effects should be given.

For selection procedures, these terms should be used, if appropriate: random sample (where "random" refers to a formal, randomized selection in which all eligible subjects have a fixed and usually equal chance of selection); population-based sample; referred sample; consecutive sample; volunteer sample; convenience sample. These terms assist the reader to determine an important element of the generalizability of the study. They also supplement (rather than duplicate) the terms used by professional indexers when articles are entered into computerized databases.

5. **Intervention(s).** The essential features of any interventions should be described, including their method and duration of administration. The intervention should be named by its most common clinical name (for example, the generic term "chlorthalidone"). Common synonyms should be given as well to facilitate electronic text-word searching. This would include the brand name of a drug if a specific product was studied.

6. **Main Outcome Measure(s).** The primary study outcome measurement(s) should be indicated as planned before data collection began. If the paper does not emphasize the main planned outcomes of a study, this fact should be stated and the reason indicated. If the hypothesis being reported was formulated during or after data collection, this information should be clearly stated.

7. **Results.** The main results of the study should be given. Measurements that require explanation for the expected audience of the manuscript should be defined. Important measurements not included in the presentation of results should be declared. As relevant, it should be indicated whether observers were blinded to patient groupings, particularly for subjective measurements. Due to the current limitations of retrieval from electronic da-

Adapted from Haynes RB, Mulrow CD, Huth EJ, Altman DG, Gardner MJ. More informative abstracts revisited. Ann Intern Med. *1990;113:69-76.*

tabases, results must be given in narrative or point form rather than tabular form if the abstract is to appear in computerized literature services such as MEDLINE. If possible, the results should be accompanied by confidence intervals (for example, 95%) and the exact level of statistical significance. For comparative studies, confidence intervals should relate to the differences between groups. For nonsignificant differences for the major study outcome measure(s), the clinically important difference sought should be stated and the confidence interval for the difference between the groups should be given. When risk changes or effect sizes are given, absolute values should be indicated so that the reader can determine the absolute as well as relative impact of the finding. Approaches such as "number needed to treat" to achieve a unit of benefit are encouraged when appropriate; reporting of relative differences alone is usually inappropriate. If appropriate, studies of screening and diagnostic tests should use the terms "sensitivity," "specificity," and "likelihood ratio." If predictive values or accuracy is given, prevalence or pretest likelihood should be given as well. No data should be reported in the abstract that do not appear in the rest of the manuscript.

8. **Conclusions.** Only those conclusions of the study that are directly supported by the evidence reported should be given, along with their clinical application (avoiding speculation and overgeneralization), and indicating whether additional study is required before the information should be used in usual clinical settings. Equal emphasis must be given to positive and negative findings of equal scientific merit.

To permit quick and selective scanning, the headings outlined above should be included in the abstract. For brevity, parts of the abstract can be written in phrases rather than complete sentences. (For example: "2. *Design*. Double-blind randomized trial," rather than "2. *Design*. The study was conducted as a double-blind, randomized trial.") This technique may make reading less smooth but facilitates selection scanning and allows more information to be conveyed per unit of space.

Review Manuscripts (Including Meta-analyses)

Authors submitting review manuscripts and reports of the results of meta-analyses should prepare an abstract of no more than 250 words under the following headings: Objective, Data Sources, Study Selection, Data Extraction, Data Synthesis, and Conclusions. The content following each heading should be as follows:

1. *Objective*. The abstract should begin with a precise statement of the primary objective of the review. The focus of this statement should be guided by whether the review emphasizes factors such as cause, diagnosis, prognosis, therapy, or prevention. It should include information about the specific population, intervention, exposure, and test or outcome that is being reviewed.

2. *Data Sources*. A succinct summary of data sources should be given, including any time restrictions. Potential sources include experts or research institutions active in the field, computerized databases and published indexes, registries, abstract booklets, conference proceedings, references identified from bibliographies of pertinent articles and books, and companies or manufacturers of tests or agents being reviewed. If a bibliographic database is used, the exact indexing terms used for article retrieval should be stated, including any constraints (for example, English language or human subjects).

3. *Study Selection*. The abstract should describe the criteria used to select studies for detailed review from among studies identified as relevant to the topic. Details of selection should include particular populations, interventions, outcomes, or methodologic designs. The method used to apply these criteria should be specified (for example, blind review, consensus, multiple reviewers). The proportion of initially identified studies that met selection criteria should be stated.

4. *Data Extraction*. Guidelines used for abstracting data and assessing data quality and validity (such as criteria for causal inference) should be described. The method by which the guidelines were applied should be stated (for example, independent extraction by multiple observers).

5. *Data Synthesis*. The main results of the review, whether qualitative or quantitative, should be stated. Methods used to obtain these results should be outlined. Meta-analyses should state the major outcomes that were pooled and include odds ratios or effect sizes and, if possible, sensitivity analyses. Numerical results should be accompanied by confidence intervals, if applicable, and exact levels of statistical significance. Evaluations of screening and diagnostic tests should address issues of sensitivity, specificity, likelihood ratios, receiver operating characteristic curves, and predictive values. Assessments of prognosis could include summarizations of survival characteristics and related variables. Major identified sources of variation between studies should be stated, including differences in treatment protocols, co-interventions, confounders, outcome measures, length of follow-up, and dropout rates.

6. *Conclusions*. The conclusions and their applications should be clearly stated, limiting generalization to the domain of the review. The need for new studies may be suggested.

Glossary of Methodologic Terms

BEFORE-AFTER TRIAL. Investigation of therapeutic alternatives in which individuals of one period and under one treatment are compared with individuals at a subsequent time, treated in a different fashion. If the disorder is not fatal and the "before" treatment is not curative, the same individuals may be studied in the before and after periods, strengthening the design through increased group comparability for the two periods. See also CROSSOVER TRIAL.

BLIND or BLINDED. Masked. Unaware. The term may be modified according to the purpose of the blinding. For example, clinicians or patients can be blind to the treatments that patients are receiving and observers can be blind to each other's assessments, making their observations uninfluenced by one another (see also

DOUBLE-BLIND). To avoid confusion, the term MASKED is preferred in studies in which vision loss of patients is an outcome of interest.

CASE-CONTROL STUDY (CASE-REFERENT OR CASE-COMPARISON STUDY). Study generally used to test possible causes of a disease or disorder, in which individuals who have a designated disorder are compared with individuals who do not have the disorder with respect to previous current exposure to a putative causal factor. For example, persons with hepatic cancer (cases) are compared with persons without hepatic cancer (controls) and history of hepatitis B is determined for the two groups. A CASE-CONTROL STUDY is often referred to as a RETROSPECTIVE STUDY (even if patients are recruited prospectively) because the logic of the design leads from effect to cause.

CASE SERIES. A series of patients with a defined disorder. The term is usually used to describe a study reporting on a consecutive collection of patients treated in a similar manner, without a concurrent control group. For example, a surgeon might describe the characteristics of and outcomes for 100 consecutive patients with cerebral ischemia who received a revascularization procedure. See also CONSECUTIVE SAMPLE.

COHORT. A group of persons with a common characteristic or set of characteristics. Typically, the group is followed for a specified period to determine the incidence of a disorder or complications of an established disorder (that is, prognosis), as in COHORT ANALYTIC STUDY (prospective study) (see also INCEPTION COHORT).

COHORT ANALYTIC STUDY. Prospective investigation of the factors that might cause a disorder in which a cohort of individuals who do not have evidence of an outcome of interest but who are exposed to the putative cause are compared with a concurrent cohort who are also free of the outcome but not exposed to the putative cause. Both cohorts are then followed to compare the incidence of the outcome of interest.

CONFOUNDER, CONFOUNDING VARIABLE. A factor that distorts the true relationship of the study variables of central interest by virtue of being related to the outcome of interest but extraneous to the study question and unequally distributed among the groups being compared. For example, age might confound a study of the effect of a toxin on longevity if individuals exposed to the toxin were older than those not exposed.

CONSECUTIVE SAMPLE. Sample in which the units are chosen on a strict "first come, first chosen" basis. All individuals who are eligible should be included as they are seen.

CONVENIENCE SAMPLE. Individuals or groups selected at the convenience of the investigator or primarily because they were available at a convenient time or place.

COST-BENEFIT ANALYSIS. A form of economic assessment, usually from society's perspective, in which the costs of medical care are compared with the economic benefits of the care, with both costs and benefits expressed in units of currency. The benefits typically include reductions in future health care costs and increased earnings due to the improved health of those receiving the care.

COST-EFFECTIVENESS ANALYSIS. An economic evaluation in which alternative programs, services, or interventions are compared in terms of the cost per unit of clinical effect (for example, cost per life saved, cost per millimeter of mercury of blood pressure lowered, or cost per quality-adjusted life-year gained). The last form of measuring outcomes (and equivalents such as "healthy days of life gained") gives rise to what is also referred to as COST-UTILITY ANALYSIS.

COST-UTILITY ANALYSIS. See COST-EFFECTIVENESS ANALYSIS.

CRITERION STANDARD. Preferred term to "gold standard." A method having established or widely accepted accuracy for determining a diagnosis, providing a standard to which a new screening or diagnostic test can be compared. The method need not be a single or simple procedure but could include follow-up of patients to observe the evolution of their conditions or the consensus of an expert panel of clinicians, as is frequently used in the study of psychiatric conditions. CRITERION STANDARD can also be used in studies of the quality of care to indicate a level of performance, agreed to by experts or peers, to which the performance of individual practitioners or institutions can be compared.

CROSSOVER TRIAL. A method of comparing two or more treatments or interventions in which subjects or patients, on completion of the course of one treatment, are switched to another. Typically, allocation to the first treatment is by random process. Participants' performance in one period is used to judge their performance in others, usually reducing variability. See also BEFORE-AFTER TRIAL.

DATA-SET. Raw data gathered by investigators.

DOUBLE-BLIND or DOUBLE MASK. (1)Neither the subject nor the study staff (those responsible for patient treatment and data collection) are aware of the group or intervention to which the subject has been assigned. (2) Any condition in which two different groups of persons are purposely denied access to information in order to keep that information from influencing some measurement, observation, or process.

ECONOMIC EVALUATION. Comparative analysis of alternative courses of action in terms of both their costs and consequences.

END POINT. See OUTCOMES.

GOLD STANDARD. See CRITERION STANDARD.

INCEPTION COHORT. A designated group of persons, assembled at a common time early in the development of a specific clinical disorder (for example, at the time of first exposure to the putative cause or at the time of initial diagnosis), who are followed thereafter (see also COHORT).

LIKELIHOOD RATIO. For a screening or diagnostic test (including clinical signs or symptoms), expresses the relative odds that a given test result would be expected in a patient with (as opposed to one without) a disorder of interest.

MASKED. See BLIND.

MATCHING. The deliberate process of making a study group and a comparison group comparable with respect to factors that are extraneous to the purpose of the investigation but that might interfere with the interpretation of the study's findings (for example, in case-control studies, individual cases might be matched or paired with a specific control on the basis of comparable age, gender, clinical features, or a combination).

NONRANDOMIZED CONTROL TRIAL. Experiment in which assignment of patients to the intervention groups is at the convenience of the investigator or according to a preset plan that does not conform to the definition of RANDOM. See also RANDOMIZED CONTROL TRIAL.

OUTCOMES. All possible changes in health status that may occur in following subjects or that may stem from exposure to a causal factor or from preventive or therapeutic interventions. The narrower term END POINTS refers to health events that lead to completion or termination of follow-up of an individual in a trial or cohort study, for example, death or major morbidity, particularly related to the study question.

PRIMARY CARE. Medical care provided by the clinician of first contact for the patient. Typically, the primary care physician is a general practitioner, family practitioner, primary care internist, or primary care pediatrician. Primary care may also be administered by health professionals other than physicans, notably, specially trained nurses (nurse practitioners) and paramedics. Usually, a general practitioner, family practitioner, nurse practitioner, or paramedic provides only primary care services but a person with specialty qualifications may provide primary care, alone or in combination with referral services (see also REFERRED CARE). Thus, it is the nature of the contact (first compared with referred) that determines the care designation rather than the qualifications of the practitioner.

PRIMARY CARE CENTER, PRIMARY CARE SETTING. Medical care facility that offers first-contact health care only. Patients requiring specialized medical care are referred elsewhere. Some primary care centers provide a mixture of primary and referred care. Thus it is the nature of the service provided (first contact) rather than the setting per se that distinguishes primary from more advanced levels of care. See also PRIMARY CARE, REFERRED CARE, TERTIARY CARE CENTER.

PROSPECTIVE STUDY. See COHORT and COHORT ANALYTIC STUDY.

RANDOM. Governed by a formal chance process in which the occurrence of previous events is of no value in predicting future events. The probability of assignment of, for example, a given subject to a specified treatment group is fixed and constant (typically 0.50) but the subject's actual assignment cannot be known until it occurs.

RANDOM SAMPLE. A sample derived by selecting sampling units (for example, individual patients) such that each unit has an independent and fixed (generally equal) chance of selection. Whether a given unit is selected is determined by chance (for example, by a table of randomly ordered numbers).

RANDOMIZATION, RANDOM ALLOCATION. Allocation of individuals to groups by chance, usually done with the aid of a table of random numbers. Not to be confused with systematic allocation (for example, on even and odd days of the month) or allocation at the convenience or discretion of the investigator.

RANDOMIZED TRIAL (RANDOMIZED CONTROL[LED] TRIAL, RANDOMIZED CLINICAL TRIAL, RCT). Experiment in which individuals are randomly allocated to receive or not receive an experimental preventive, therapeutic, or diagnostic procedure and then followed to determine the effect of the intervention.

REFERRED CARE. Medical care provided to a patient when referred by one health professional to another with more specialized qualifications or interests. There are two levels of referred care: secondary and tertiary. Secondary care is usually provided by a broadly skilled specialist such as a general surgeon, general internist, or obstetrician. Tertiary care is provided on referral of a patient to a subspecialist, such as an orthopedic surgeon, neurologist, or neonatologist. See also TERTIARY CARE CENTER.

RETROSPECTIVE STUDY. See CASE-CONTROL STUDY.

SECONDARY CARE. See REFERRED CARE.

SENSITIVITY. The sensitivity of a diagnostic or screening test is the proportion of people who truly have a designated disorder who are so identified by the test. The test may consist of or include clinical observations.

SEQUENTIAL SAMPLE. See CONSECUTIVE SAMPLE.

SPECIFICITY. The specificity of a diagnostic or screening test is the proportion of people who are truly free of a designated disorder who are so identified by the test. The test may consist of or include clinical observations.

SURVEY. Observational or descriptive, nonexperimental study in which individuals are systematically examined for the absence or presence (or degree of presence) of characteristics of interest.

TERTIARY CARE. See REFERRED CARE.

TERTIARY CARE CENTER. A tertiary care center is a medical facility that receives referrals from both primary and secondary care levels and usually offers tests, treatments, and procedures that are not available elsewhere. Most tertiary care centers offer a mixture of primary, secondary, and tertiary care services so that it is the specific level of service rendered rather than the facility that determines the designation of care in a given study. See also REFERRED CARE.

Classified Advertising

Academic/Faculty
Cardiovascular/Thoracic Surgery
CME Corner
Chiefs/Department Heads/ Directors
Courses/Symposia/Seminars
Facial Plastic Surgery
Graduate Training/ Residencies/Fellowships
Locum Tenens Wanted
Multiple Specialties/Group Practice
Neurosurgery
Notices
Othopedic Surgery
Pediatric Surgery
Plastic Surgery
Practices For Sale
Surgical Specialities
Thoracic Surgery
Vascular Surgery

Sales Information

1999 CLASSIFIED ADVERTISING RATES

Regular	1x 1.65/wd	*3x 1.55/wd
Bold	1x 1.85/wd	*3x 1.75/wd

*In order to receive the 3-time frequency price, the request must be made upon initial placement. The minimum charge is 20 words. A word consists of one or more letters surrounded by space on each side. For information on display advertising and our network buys contact an account representative.

POLICY

Orders for classified advertising must be submitted in writing. Although the American Medical Association believes the classified advertisements in these pages to be from reputable sources, the Association does not investigate the offers made and assumes no liability concerning them. Acceptance of advertising is restricted to professional opportunities, practices for sale, and medical office space available. The Association reserves the right to decline, withdraw, or edit advertisements at its discretion. Every care is taken to avoid mistakes but responsibility cannot be accepted by the Association for clerical or printer's errors.

REPLY BOX SERVICE

Confidential box numbers are available for an additional $25 per issue, plus the words: Box ________, c/o SUR. When responding to a box number, please send to Archives of Surgery, Box ________, c/o SUR, 515 N State St, Chicago, IL 60610.

CANCELLATIONS/CHANGES

Cancellations/changes must be received in writing at least 25 days prior to the date of the issue. In order to expedite, please fax to 312-464-5909 to the attention of your account representative.

GENERAL INFORMATION

To contact a Classified Advertising account representative, call 312-464-2475/2490/2491/4485 or 800-AMA-2260. Or fax your insertion order to 312-464-5909. Mail your materials to AMA Classified Advertising, 12th Floor, 515 N State St, Chicago, IL 60610.

ACADEMIC/FACULTY

FULLY ACCREDITED UNIVERSITY affiliated surgical residency program seeks Assistant/Associate in Surgical education. Parent hospital a 601-bed tertiary medical center, part of the Carilion Health System. Interest in resident and medical student education, participation in clinical activities including resident cases, trauma services, vascular non-invasive lab interpretation required. Competitive salary and benefits for experienced board certified surgeon. Direct curriculum vitae/inquiries to Ross S. Davies, MD, Director of Surgical Education, Carilion Roanoke Memorial Hospitals, PO Box 13367, Roanoke, VA 24033.

GRADUATE TRAINING/ RESIDENCIES/FELLOWSHIPS

STANFORD UNIVERSITY BREAST SURGERY FELLOWSHIP: One year clinical training in breast surgery and multidisciplinary breast cancer treatment. Start July 1999. Must be license eligible and have completed a general surgery residency. Will obtain experience in sentinel node biopsy, endoscopic axillary dissection, breast ultrasound, mammographically-directed large core biopsy, interventional breast MR techniques, and clinical trials research. Send CV to Stefanie S. Jeffrey, MD, Attn: Elizabeth Spence, Division of Surgical Oncology, Medical School Office Bldg X-300, Stanford Medical Center, Stanford, CA 94305-5414. Fax: 650-725-3918. E-mail: espence@leland.stanford.edu

LEGAL SERVICES

MALPRACTICE CASE EVALUATION
Board-certified medical experts needed. All specialties. All locations. Defense and plaintiff cases. Excellent remuneration. Send CVs to:
Barry Gustin, MD, MPH, FACEP
AMERICAN MEDICAL FORENSIC SPECIALISTS, Inc
2991 Shattuck Ave, Ste 302
Berkeley, CA 94705

LOCUM TENENS WANTED

HKA LOCUM TENENS is looking for quality surgical specialty physicians to do Locum Tenens. We have opportunities coast-to-coast. We furnish Occurrence Malpractice Insurance (no tail necessary). Please call HKA LOCUM TENENS at (800) 226-6347, Extension AM7.1.

MULTIPLE SPECIALTIES/ GROUP PRACTICE

WEST VIRGINIA, KANSAS, ILLINOIS, NEBRASKA: IMs, FPs, OB/GYN, Urologist, GENSUR. Call Mariana with Medfinder's: 888-666-5110, Fax: CV 561-997-9672. E-mail: Medfinders@aol.com or visit our web site at www.medfinders.com

PEDIATRICS

PEDIATRIC SURGERY OPPORTUNITY An excellent pediatric surgery opportunity is now available in a beautiful, affordable area of California with the nation's largest freestanding children's hospital west of the Mississippi River. Enjoy unparalleled support and services and a new 216-bed, $176 million facility. Highly competitive compensation and benefits package. Contact Clint Scott, Medical Doctor Associates, 800-932-1023.

POSITIONS WANTED

BE GENERAL SURGEON: Excellent training in Laparo-endoscopy, General Vascular, Trauma/ Critical care seeks employment in health manpower shortage area for J-1 waiver. Reply to Box 1030, c/o SUR, 515 N State St, 12th Fl, Chicago, IL 60610.

PROFESSIONAL/TECHNICAL

EARN AN ADDITIONAL $100,000.00: Seeking doctors to serve on medical advisory board of company going public. Compensation up to $100,000.00. No business experience necessary. Call 800-321-2778 Monday thru Friday 9-5 EST.

SURGERY: GENERAL

BOSTON SUBURB: Excellent opportunity for BC/ BE General and Vascular Surgeon to join 3 well-trained surgeons in established practice. Practice includes all aspects of general surgery in addition to general vascular surgery and advanced laparoscopy. The group is affiliated with a progressive healthcare system. Opportunity exists to establish a center for breast disease. Please forward CV to Recruiter, 43 Riverside Ave #81, Medford, MA 02155-4605. Fax: 781-396-2545.

FLORIDA CENTRAL EAST COAST: Expanding general surgery practice seeking to add recently trained BC/ BE surgeon. Must have vascular experience. Excellent location in family oriented coastal community. Competitive financial package and direct path to partnership. Send CV to Box 410670, Melbourne, FL 32941.

GENERAL SURGERY, PORTLAND, OREGON: Northwest Permanente, PC, a physician-managed, multispecialty group serving the members of Kaiser Permanente in the Northwest Division, has an excellent opportunity for a BC/BE general surgeon. Our new associate will practice with the 21 general surgeons at Kaiser Permanente's affiliated hospitals in Portland. The Northwest Division has a total of 24 general surgeons providing quality care to over 430,000 plan members in Oregon and Washington. Ours is a collegial and professionally stimulating practice in one of the most successful managed care programs in the country. In addition to a lifestyle inherent to the beautiful Pacific Northwest, we offer a predictable work schedule and a competitive salary and benefit package which includes professional liability coverage, a comprehensive pension program, sabbatical leave and more. For additional information, please forward CV to A. S. Weiland, MD, Regional Medical Director, NORTHWEST PERMANENTE, PC, 500 NE Multnomah, Suite 100, Portland, OR 97231-2099. EOE.

OPPORTUNITY IN NORTHEASTERN OKLAHOMA LAKE COUNTRY: Strong 70 bed JCAHO accredited not-for-profit hospital has an opportunity for 1 general surgeon. General surgery service area of 60,000+. 12 BC physicians on staff including an anesthesiologist. 40 minutes from Tulsa. Negotiable financial arrangements. Call Stan Schuermann at INTEGRIS Baptist Medical Center at 800-332-8663.

OPPORTUNITY FOR SEASONED, progressive, board certified general surgeon to immediately join busy, well established, private surgical practice. Located in Northern Michigan on the Great Lakes. Spectacular four season recreation, safe, caring, family oriented community. Supportive and friendly hospital and professional staff with over forty referring physicians and excellent ER, ICU, and diagnostic imaging support. Efficient, state-of-the-art office suite in new medical office building connected to hospital. Competitive salary with full benefits. Send cover letter and curriculum vitae to T. M. Burandt, DO & Associates, PC, 810 South Main Street, Suite#1, Cheboygan, MI 49721, Facsimile: 616-627-7758, E-mail: tburandt@cdimed.com

---

OUTSTANDING GENERAL SURGERY OPPORTUNITIES. Two excellent opportunities to join a premier GS group in the beautiful Southeast or join a highly respected general surgeon in a premier private multi-specialty group in the piney woods of the South. These communities will offer you excellent schools and great housing choices. All opportunities are accompanied by a highly competitive financial package that includes bonuses, full benefits and partnership potential. Contact Brian White, Medical Doctor Associates, 800-932-1023.

WELL ESTABLISHED BUSY SURGICAL PRACTICE: Seeking Board Eligible/Board Certified General Surgeon with Vascular Surgery experience to join a four surgeon General/Vascular/Trauma practice. Opportunity for partnership. Practice located approximately one and one-half hours drive from Baltimore/Washington area in Western Maryland. Appalachian Trail, Potomac River and ski resorts in local area. Position available July 1999. For more information, contact or send Curriculum Vitae to Hagerstown Surgical Clinic, 11110 Medical Campus Road, Suite 100, Hagerstown, MD 21742. Telephone: 301-714-4325, Fax: 301-714-4326.

WISCONSIN: General/vascular surgeon sought for two-surgeon group. Must be willing to do general and vascular, but fellowship training not required. Community of 100,000 only 1 1/2 hours from Minneapolis/St Paul. Prefer a '99 resident. $150,000 salary, bonus, benefits and partnership. Contact Todd Dillon, 800-883-7345, ID#6338AR, Fax: 810-603-2942, e-mail: tdillon@cejka.com Visit our website: www.cejka.com

---

WILLAMETTE VALLEY, OREGON: Opportunity available for BC/BE General Surgeon. Join 3-member department within large physician-owned multi-specialty group. Corvallis is home to Oregon State University, town of 45,000, located in heart of beautiful Willamette Valley wine country; one hour from coast, two hours from Cascade Mountains ski and recreation areas. Guaranteed salary, incentive bonus, and excellent benefits. Position is available April 1999. Send CV and cover letter to, Medical Director, The Corvallis Clinic, PC, 444 NW Elks Dr, Corvallis, OR 97330, Fax: 541-757-1847.

EVANSVILLE, IN: A prestigious clinic needs an additional General Surgeon. Call 1:5. Competitive income guarantee package. Live in a safe, family oriented community. Two universities. Cultural activities: music, theatre and dance. Numerous parks & recreational centers offer everything from ice hockey to golf courses. Call Anne Sheahan 800-765-3055 x3478. Fax CV to 314-726-3009 or e-mail: asheahan@cejka.com ID#6345AR; Visit our website at www.cejka.com

SURGERY: ORTHOPEDIC

OPPORTUNITY IN NORTHEASTERN OKLAHOMA LAKE COUNTRY: Strong not-for-profit hospital has an opportunity for 1 orthopedic surgeon. Orthopedic surgery service area of 60,000+. 70 bed JCAHO accredited hospital with 12 BC physicians on staff including an anesthesiologist. 40 minutes from Tulsa. Negotiable financial arrangements. Call Stan Schuermann at INTEGRIS Baptist Medical Center at 800-332-8663.

SURGERY: SURGICAL SPECIALTIES

BC/BE SURGEON: every fourth night for Indian Health Service facility with state of the art laparoscopic and endoscopic equipment. College town 1 hour from metro area. Ideally located at base of Ozark Mountains with abundant four season recreational opportunities. Salary negotiable, excellent benefits, loan repayment. We are an equal opportunity employer. Contact Lisa Spry at 918-458-3360.

SURGERY: THORACIC

SOUTH FLORIDA: BC/BE Non Cardiac-Thoracic Surgeon to join multispecialty surgical group. Interest/ability in vascular or general surgery a strong plus. Salary guarantee plus incentive with benefit package. CV to Dexter Sereda, MD, Surgery Associates, 1150 N 35th Ave, Suite 490, Hollywood, FL 33021.

TRAUMA/CRITICAL CARE

TRAUMA SURGEON: The Department of Surgery, Wright State University School of Medicine in Dayton, Ohio seeks a trauma attending surgeon at Miami Valley Hospital, a Level I Trauma Center. The appointee will assist in patient care, educational activities, research, injury prevention and development of a regional trauma system. Applicants must have completed an accredited surgical residency program and a fellowship in trauma/critical care. Board eligibility/certification in general surgery and critical care is required. Must be licensable to practice medicine in Ohio. Faculty appointment at the instructor/assistant/associate professor rank commensurate with experience. All applications received by February 15, 1999 will be considered. If the position is not filled from these, applications will be considered until the position is filled. Applicants should submit a curriculum vitae and three references to Mary C. McCarthy, MD, Professor, WSU Department of Surgery, Director of Trauma, Miami Valley Hospital, One Wyoming St, Ste 7000CHE, Dayton, OH 45409. Wright State University is an Affirmative Action/Equal Opportunity employer.

THE UNIVERSITY OF MICHIGAN SURGICAL BREAST ONCOLOGY FELLOWSHIP

The University of Michigan Medical School, Section of General Surgery, seeks MD candidate for a Breast Oncology Fellowship in the Division of Surgical Oncology. Applicants should be board certified or board eligible by the American Board of Surgery and have a demonstrated interest in the multidisciplinary approach to the treatment of breast cancer and breast related diseases. Responsibilities include breast surgery, teaching and research.

Please send curriculum vitae and cover letter to:

Helen A. Pass, MD
Director, Breast Care Center
University of Michigan Health Service
1500 E Medical Center Drive
CGC-3302, Box 0932
Ann Arbor, MI 48109-0932

The University of Michigan is a non-discriminatory/ Affirmative Action employer and strongly encourages females and minorities to apply.

THE DEPARTMENT OF SURGERY AT THE UNIVERSITY OF CALIFORNIA, DAVIS

wishes to recruit, at the Assistant, Associate or Professor level, a general surgeon with a special interest in gastrointestinal disease. A special interest in colon and rectal surgery is preferred but not required. Appointment will be at the Assistant, Associate or Professor level in either the in-residence or clinical series according to the training, clinical experience and academic achievement of the applicant. This individual must have a commitment to teaching in the clinical arena. Licensure in the State of California is required. A letter outlining research and teaching background, a complete Curriculum Vitae and the names and addresses of five references should be forwarded to:

James E. Goodnight, Jr, MD, PhD
Chairman, Department of Surgery
UC Davis Medical Center
4301 X Street
Room 2310
Sacramento, CA 95817

This position will remain open until filled but no later than September 1, 1999. All applications must be received no later than September 1, 1999.

The University of California is an Affirmative Action/ Equal Opportunity Employer.

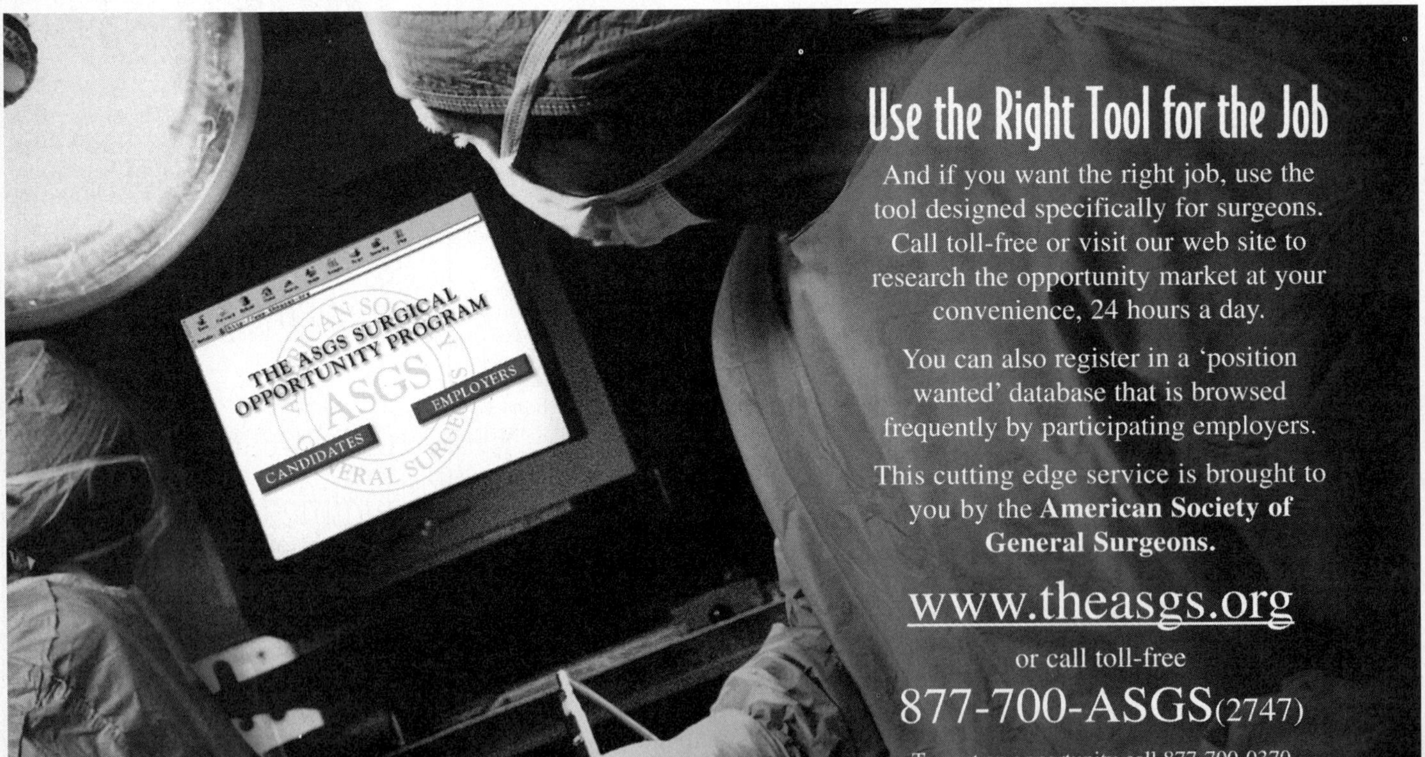

CHAIR

Department of Surgery

The New York University School of Medicine has begun a search for an individual to assume the Chairmanship of our Department of Surgery. The new Chair will succeed Dr. Frank Spencer, the George David Stewart Professor of Surgery, who has chaired the department with distinction for the past 32 years and has stepped down.

The Department is poised to undergo a major growth phase designed to further strengthen its clinical and research programs. It is expected that the individual who is selected for this position will be Board Certified in Surgery and have a distinguished record of clinical and research excellence with the leadership skills necessary to develop and manage a complex, multifaceted academic department.

Please consider this opportunity and recommended potential candidates by replying to:

Joseph D. Zuckerman, M.D.
Chair, Department of Orthopedic Surgery
Chair, Department of Surgery Search Committee
New York University School of Medicine
550 First Avenue, New York, N.Y. 10016

SCHOOL OF MEDICINE
NEW YORK UNIVERSITY

New York University is an Equal Opportunity Employer.

Index of Advertisers

BRAINTREE LABORATORIES
Nulytely Cover4

CLASSIFIED ADVERTISING 116-119
http://www.ama-assn.org

PFIZER, US PHARMACEUTICAL GROUP
http://www.pfizer.com
Diflucan .... Cover 2-1

While every precaution is taken to ensure accuracy, we cannot guarantee against the possibility of an occasional change or omission in the preparation of this index.

ARCHIVES OF SURGERY

FEBRUARY 1999

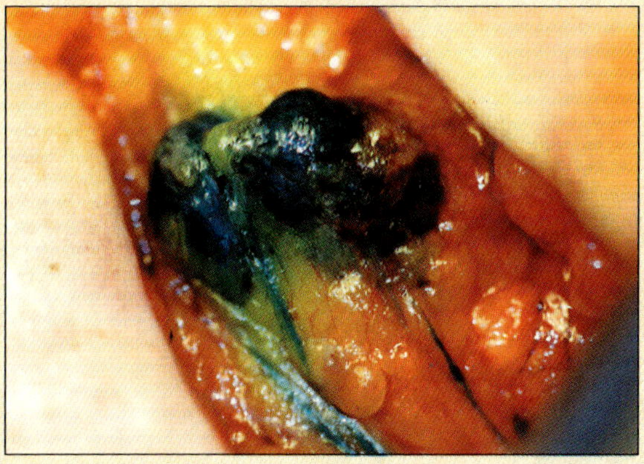

Sentinel node biopsy. See page 195.

SHOULD GENERAL SURGEONS PROVIDE CRITICAL CARE?

LAPAROSCOPIC GASTROSTOMY AND JEJUNOSTOMY

SUBTOTAL PANCREATODUODENECTOMY

SURGICAL TREATMENT OF HYDATID DISEASE OF THE LIVER

ANATOMIC SITE OF PRIMARY MELANOMA IS ASSOCIATED WITH DEPTH OF INVASION

MAPPING A PATHWAY FOR AXILLARY STAGING

COMPLETE TABLE OF CONTENTS INSIDE

American Medical Association
Physicians dedicated to the health of America

www.ama-assn.org/surgery

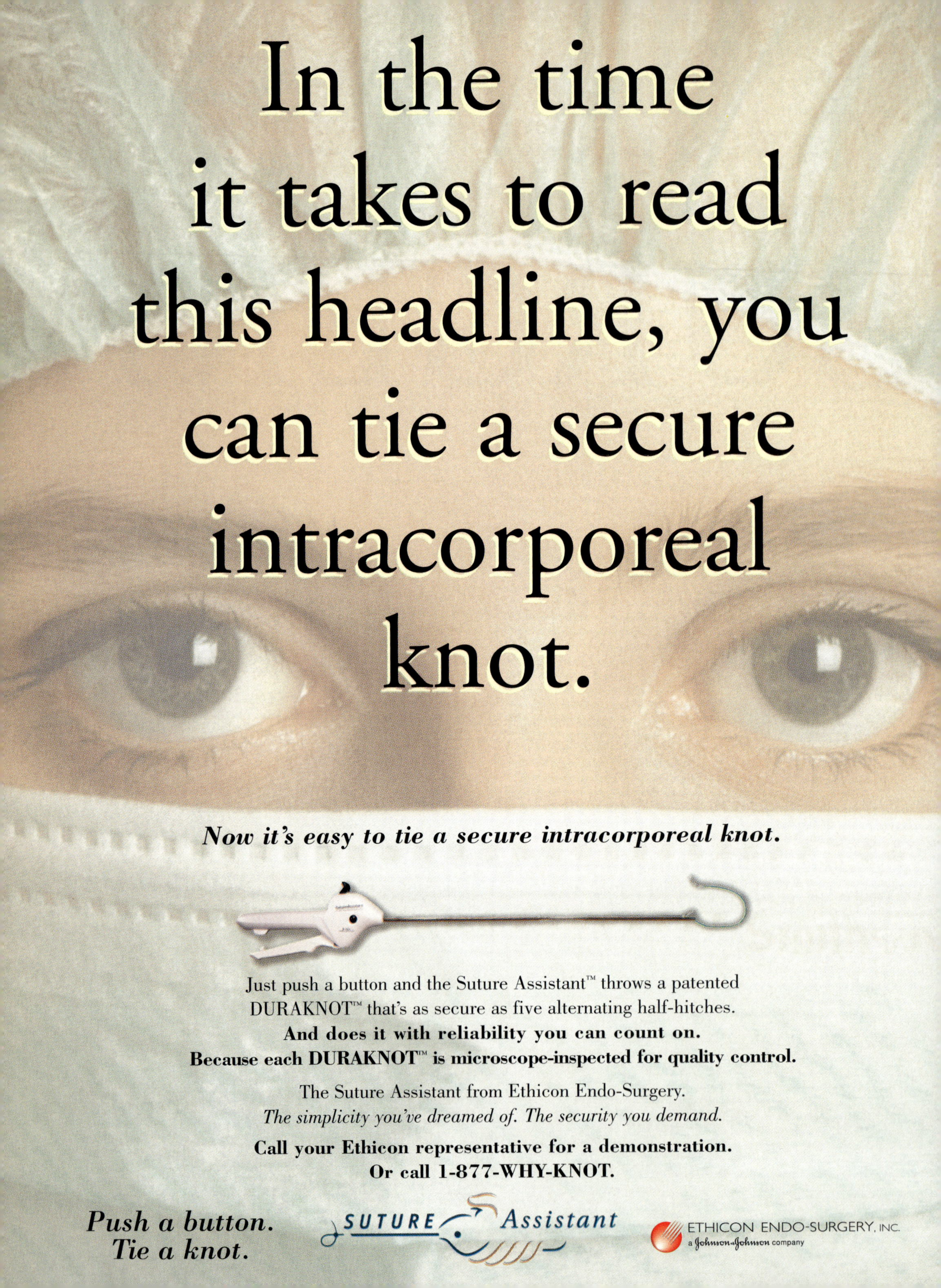
In the time it takes to read this headline, you can tie a secure intracorporeal knot.
Now it's easy to tie a secure intracorporeal knot.
Just push a button and the Suture Assistant™ throws a patented DURAKNOT™ that's as secure as five alternating half-hitches.
And does it with reliability you can count on.
Because each DURAKNOT™ is microscope-inspected for quality control.
The Suture Assistant from Ethicon Endo-Surgery.
The simplicity you've dreamed of. The security you demand.
Call your Ethicon representative for a demonstration.
Or call 1-877-WHY-KNOT.
Push a button. Tie a knot.
SUTURE Assistant
ETHICON ENDO-SURGERY, INC.
a Johnson & Johnson company

ARCHIVES OF SURGERY

The ARCHIVES OF SURGERY is a member of the consortium of AMA journals listed below. The complete text of all AMA journals is available online from Dialog Information Services and Information Access Company.

The Journal of the American Medical Association (JAMA)
Archives of Dermatology
Archives of Facial Plastic Surgery
Archives of Family Medicine
Archives of General Psychiatry
Archives of Internal Medicine
Archives of Neurology
Archives of Ophthalmology
Archives of Otolaryngology–Head & Neck Surgery
Archives of Pathology & Laboratory Medicine
Archives of Pediatrics & Adolescent Medicine
Archives of Surgery

The ARCHIVES OF SURGERY (ISSN 0004-0010) is published monthly by the American Medical Association, 515 N State St, Chicago, IL 60610, and is an official publication of the Association. The ARCHIVES OF SURGERY reaches more than 19 000 readers in over 69 countries each month. Periodicals postage paid at Chicago, IL, and at additional mailing offices. GST registration number 12622 5556 RT. Canada Post International Publications Mail (Canadian Distribution) Sales Agreement No. 319309.

Printed in the USA.

Official Publication of the New England Surgical Society, Pacific Coast Surgical Association, Surgical Infection Society, Western Surgical Association.

SUBSCRIPTION RATES—The personal subscription rates for the ARCHIVES OF SURGERY are $145 for 1 year (12 issues) in the United States and US possessions; $195 in the Americas; £125 outside the Americas. The institution rates for 1 year are $245 in the US; $345 in the Americas; £195 outside the Americas. Special rates for residents and medical students are available. Address all subscription communications to: Subscriber Services Center, American Medical Association, PO Box 10946, Chicago, IL 60610-0946. Phone: (800) 262-2350. Fax: (312) 464-5831. E-mail: ama-subs@ama-assn.org. For mailing addresses outside the United States and US possessions, see International Subscription Information.

CHANGE OF ADDRESS—POSTMASTER, send all address changes to ARCHIVES OF SURGERY, c/o Subscriber Services, American Medical Association, 515 N State St, Chicago, IL 60610. Please notify us of address change at least 6 weeks in advance to ensure uninterrupted service. Include both old and new addresses, a recent mailing label, and new ZIP code. For mailing addresses outside the United States and US possessions, see International Subscription Information.

SUBSCRIBER SERVICES—For information about subscribing to any of the AMA publications, change of address, missing issues, or purchasing back issues, please contact Subscriber Services Center, American Medical Association, PO Box 10946, Chicago, IL 60610-0946, or call (800) 262-2350 or (312) 670-SUBS (670-7827) between 8:30 AM and 4:30 PM CST. Fax: (312) 464-5831. E-mail: ama-subs@ama-assn.org. For mailing addresses outside the United States and US possessions, see International Subscription Information.

INTERNATIONAL SUBSCRIPTION INFORMATION—Subscriptions outside the United States and US possessions are served according to geographic region. Please address correspondence to the following 2 offices based on delivery address: (1) For delivery in North America, Central America, and South America, contact Subscriber Services, AMA, PO Box 10946, Chicago, IL 60610-0946. Phone: (312) 670-7827. Fax: (312) 464-5831. E-mail: ama-subs@ama-assn.org. (2) For delivery outside the Americas contact JAMA & Archives Journals, Reader Services Centre, PO Box 299, London WC1H 9TD, England. Phone: +44 (0)171-383-6270. Fax: +44 (0)171-383-6402. E-mail: jama-archives@dial.pipex.com.

REPRINTS—Authors place their reprint order at the time the edited typescript is reviewed and should allow 4 to 6 weeks for delivery following publication. Requests for individual reprints should be sent directly to the author at the address shown in the article.

For bulk reprint orders for distribution by commercial organizations, please contact Wanda Bartolotta, 500 Fifth Ave, #2210, New York, NY 10110. Phone: (212) 354-0050. Fax: (212) 354-1169. E-mail: wanda_bartolotta@ama-assn.org. For reprint orders in limited quantities for distribution by educational organizations and for author reprints, please contact Joseph R. Rekash, 515 N State St, Chicago, IL 60610. Phone: (312) 464-4594. Fax: (312) 464-4849.

WORLD WIDE WEB ADDRESS—http://www.ama-assn.org.

SURGERY HOME PAGE—http://www.ama-assn.org/surgery.

PERMISSIONS—Contact Ada Jimenez-Walker, Permissions Assistant, 515 N State St, Chicago, IL 60610. Phone: (312) 464-2513.

ADVERTISING PRINCIPLES—Each advertisement in this issue has been reviewed and complies with the principles governing advertising in AMA scientific publications. A copy of these principles is available on request. The appearance of advertising in AMA publications is not an AMA guarantee or endorsement of the product or the claims made for the product by the manufacturer.

ARCHIVES OF SURGERY

www.ama-assn.org/surgery

VOL 134 NO. 2, FEBRUARY 1999

MISSION STATEMENT

To promote the art and science of surgery by publishing relevant peer-reviewed clinical and basic science information to assist the surgeon in optimizing patient care. The *Archives of Surgery* will also serve as a forum for the discussion of issues that involve ethics, teaching, surgical history, and socioeconomic concerns.

*Approved by the Editorial Board, *Archives of Surgery*, July 19, 1996.

COMMENTARY

Should General Surgeons Provide Critical Care? 125
Frederick A. Moore, MD

ORIGINAL ARTICLES

Thyroid Cancer With Concurrent Hyperthyroidism 130
Tzu-Chieh Chao, MD, PhD; Jen-Der Lin, MD; Long-Bin Jeng, MD; Miin-Fu Chen, MD

Subtotal Pancreatoduodenectomy: Use of a Defunctionalized Loop for Pancreatic Stump Drainage 135
John D. Papadimitriou, MD; Alex C. Fotopoulos, MD; Basil Smyrniotis, MD; Andreas A. Prahalias, MD; Georgia Kostopanagiotou, MD; Lila J. Papadimitriou, MD

Bronchoscopic Staging of Squamous Cell Carcinoma of the Upper Thoracic Esophagus 140
Alessandro Baisi, MD; Luigi Bonavina, MD; Alberto Peracchia, MD

The Blood Supply of the Sternocleidomastoid Muscle and Its Clinical Implications 144
Antonius C. Kierner, MD; Martin Aigner, MD; Irmgard Zelenka, MD; Gunther Riedl; Martin Burian, MD

Anatomic Site of Primary Melanoma Is Associated With Depth of Invasion 148
Yoram Hemo, MD; Mordechai Gutman, MD; Joseph M. Klausner, MD

American Medical Association

Physicians dedicated to the health of America

All articles published, including editorials, letters, and book reviews, represent the opinions of the authors and do not reflect the policy of the American Medical Association, the Editorial Board, or the institution with which the author is affiliated, unless this is clearly specified.

E. Ratcliffe Anderson, Jr, MD
Executive Vice President, Chief Executive Officer

Lynn Jensen, PhD
Chief Operating Officer

Robert L. Kennett
Interim Senior Vice President, Publishing & Business Services

Peter L. Payerli
Publisher

Peter G. Messina
National Sales Manager

Geoffrey A. Flick
Manager, Marketing Services

Cheryl Iverson
Director, Editorial Processing Division

Vanessa Hayden
Director, Production & Distribution Division

James A. Skowrenski
Director, Circulation & Content Marketing Division

Advertising Office: J. P. Cahill & Associates, 341 S Waiola Ave, La Grange, IL 60525 (708) 352-0322.

AMA Classified Advertising Department: Thalia Moss, 800-262-2260.

Laparoscopic Gastrostomy and Jejunostomy: Safety and Cost With Local vs General Anesthesia 151
Quan-Yang Duh, MD; Andrea L. Senokozlieff-Englehart, RN, MS; Yong S. Choe, MAS; Allan E. Siperstein, MD; Kathleen Rowland, BSN, RN; Lawrence W. Way, MD

Lymphangiosis as a Predictor of Outcome in Patients With Primary Diffusely Infiltrative Adenocarcinoma of the Colon and Rectum 157
Reiping Tang, MD; Jeng-Yi Wang, MD; Kuo-Chien Tsao, BS; Yat-Sen Ho, MD

INTERNATIONAL MEETING SUMMARY

Summary of the 115th Annual Meeting of the German Society of Surgery: Berlin, April 28 to May 2, 1998 161
Ernst Klar, MD

ORIGINAL ARTICLES

Surgical Treatment of Hydatid Disease of the Liver: Review of 304 Cases 166
Ahmet A. Balik, MD; Mahmut Başoğlu, MD; Fehmi Çelebi, MD; Durkaya Ören, MD; K. Yalçin Polat, MD; S. Selçuk Atamanalp, MD; Müfide N. Akçay, MD

Invited Critique 169
Kazutomo Inoue, MD

Selective Decontamination of the Digestive Tract in Surgical Patients: A Systematic Review of the Evidence 170
Avery B. Nathens, MD, PhD, FRCSC; John C. Marshall, MD, FRCSC

Isolated Limb Perfusion With High-Dose Tumor Necrosis Factor α and Melphalan for Kaposi Sarcoma 177
Dina Lev-Chelouche, MD; Subhi Abu-Abeid, MD; Ofer Merimsky, MD; Josephine Isakov, MD; Yoram Kollander, MD; Isaac Meller, MD; Joseph M. Klausner, MD; Mordechai Gutman, MD

Pathologic Features of Prognostic Significance for Adrenocortical Carcinoma After Curative Resection 181
Lawrence E. Harrison, MD; Paul B. Gaudin, MD; Murray F. Brennan, MD

Invited Critique 185
Andrew Saxe, MD

Lung-Sparing Surgery After Penetrating Trauma Using Tractotomy, Partial Lobectomy, and Pneumonorrhaphy 186
George C. Velmahos, MD, PhD; Craig Baker, MD; Demetrios Demetriades, MD, PhD; Jeremy Goodman; James A. Murray, MD; Juan A. Asensio, MD

ARCHIVES OF SURGERY

Multifactorial Analysis of Long-term Follow-up (More Than 5 Years) of Primary Extremity Sarcoma 190
Jonathan J. Lewis, MD, PhD; Denis Leung, PhD; Ephraim S. Casper, MD; James Woodruff, MD; Steven I. Hajdu, MD; Murray F. Brennan, MD

COMMENTARY

Mapping a Pathway for Axillary Staging: A Personal Perspective on the Current Status of Sentinel Lymph Node Dissection for Breast Cancer 195
Armando E. Giuliano, MD

BASIC SCIENCE FOR SURGEONS

Vascular Endothelial Growth Factor Is More Important Than Basic Fibroblastic Growth Factor During Ischemic Wound Healing 200
Claudio J. Corral, MD; Aamir Siddiqui, MD; Liancun Wu, MD; Catherine L. Farrell, PhD; David Lyons, PhD; Thomas A. Mustoe, MD

SPECIAL ARTICLE

Surgery in Nigeria 206
Olajide Olaolu Ajayi, FRCS, FWACS, FMCS(Nig); Clement Adebayo Adebamowo, FWACS

SURGICAL TECHNIQUE

Laparoscopic Adrenalectomy 212
Roberto V. Barresi, MD; Richard A. Prinz, MD

BOOK REVIEWS

Fundamentals of Plastic Surgery 218
Claude H. Organ, Jr, MD

Colon and Rectal Surgery 218
John M. MacKeigan, MD, FRCSC

CORRESPONDENCE AND BRIEF COMMUNICATIONS

Methods of Surgical Training 220
Sylvanus Oyogoa, MD, MSc; Ian Komenaka, MD

SURGICAL REMINISCENCES

O. H. Wangensteen, MD, PhD 221
J. Bradley Aust, MD, PhD

MOMENTS IN SURGICAL HISTORY

The Surgeon's Glove 223
Ira M. Rutkow, MD, MPH, DrPH

DEPARTMENTS

Surgical Anatomy 194

Products & Services 224

Classified Advertising 225

Index to Advertisers 228

Instructions for Authors— See January 1999 issue, page 107, or visit the Web site at http://www.ama-assn.org/surgery.

About the Cover

Please refer to the Commentary on page 195 by Dr Armando E. Giuliano titled "Mapping a Pathway for Axillary Staging: A Personal Perspective on the Current Status of Sentinel Lymph Node Dissection for Breast Cancer."

Should General Surgeons Provide Critical Care?

A BASIC tenet of general surgery training is that the best perioperative care is provided by a well-trained general surgeon. Consequently, providing optimal care to patients in the intensive care unit (ICU) has been an integral component of surgical education and practice.[1-5] Dedication to providing optimal ICU care has allowed general surgeons to contribute heavily to the evolving field of critical care medicine. Much of our current understanding of shock resuscitation, inflammatory response, wound healing, immunosuppression, nutritional support, treatment of infections, and many other topics were derived from research done by general surgeons. General surgeons rightfully deserve continued leadership in critical care and the professional recognition that they are more than operating room technicians. Unfortunately, many nonsurgeons view the aforementioned as unfounded surgical rhetoric. In fact, most practicing surgeons (with the exception of those involved in trauma and burn care) have abdicated their ICU responsibilities to nonsurgeons.[6,7] For a variety of reasons, the traditional involvement of general surgeons in critical care has eroded. An explosion of knowledge and technology has promoted organ-specific medical specialization (eg, pulmonary, cardiology, renal, and infectious diseases), and general surgery has been partitioned into areas of special regional interests (colorectal, vascular, thoracic, endocrine, breast, and hepatopancreatobiliary). Due to a lack of ongoing exposure, some surgeons are intimidated by the ever-changing ICU environment. Additionally, the "global surgery" fee forbids extra payment for high-acuity ICU care. Since there is no financial penalty, many surgeons consult organ-specific medical specialists to provide routine critical care, allowing for increased operating room participation and more billing opportunities. Unfortunately, this also resulted in the loss of surgical autonomy and increases ICU expenses with unnecessary tests and professional fees. Intensive care units are expensive cost centers that must be controlled, and surgeons are not providing the leadership. Board-certified intensivists are becoming increasingly vocal that they are better qualified to provide ICU care for surgical patients and that they can do it more cheaply. This commentary will address these issues and suggest potential solutions.

EDUCATION AND RESEARCH

Critical care is a broad and complex body of knowledge that crosses specialty interests. No one specialty can claim it as their sovereign domain.[8-12] The future ICU practitioners will come from the specialties that provide essential training. Traditionally, the ICU has been an invaluable resource for surgical training programs, providing continued exposure to a variety of patients with complex medical problems. This forces trainees to be physiologically orientated and to be able to integrate multiple problems into a unified treatment plan. Many general surgery training programs have formal critical care rotations. This is generally 2 to 3 months in duration and done at the postgraduate year 2 level. This is a good start, but continued exposure is needed to produce competent critical care physicians. Unfortunately, as general surgery residents advance to more senior levels, they rotate on specialized surgical services (eg, vascular, oncology, colorectal, thoracic, endoscopy, and minimally invasive surgery). This provides good technical training and a high volume of index cases, but the specialty attending surgeons are not actively involved in critical care. Subliminally, general surgery residents are being taught to provide specialized technical services and let someone else take care of the patients. Once they are done with general surgery training, their professional interests match financial reality. Interest in critical care evaporates along with critical care skills.

The solution for general surgery residents is straightforward. If our goal is to train competent critical care physicians, then they need to be actively involved in ICU care throughout their training. When rotating on specialty surgical services, they cannot be relegated to a "visiting observer" status in regards to their ICU patients. The attending surgeons need to recognize that they are training general surgeons (not regional surgeons).

Maintaining the competence of practicing surgeons is more problematic. The first obstacle is to create a financial incentive. The current global surgery fee does not do this. The second obstacle is to maintain the skills of practicing surgeons who have limited their practice so they rarely have patients in the ICU. The third obstacle is to provide ongoing education for evolving management strategies that cross over into other specialty interests. Critical care should be an integral component of a postgraduate surgeon's continuing medical educa-

This article is also available on our Web site: www.ama-assn.org/surgery.

tion, but surgeons need to participate in multidisciplinary educational forums.

General surgeons also need to maintain scientific legitimacy by performing high-quality research in surgical ICUs. A cadre of experts are needed. Traditionally, these individuals have come from the specialists who care for a high-volume of ICU patients (eg, trauma and burn surgeons). The more recent alternative is formal critical care training that qualifies the participants to earn an added qualification certificate. Additionally, surgeons need to communicate their unique surgical insights. In the past, this has permitted noteworthy observations that have had huge effects on patient care. These observations should not only be presented at surgical meetings, but also need to be presented at multidisciplinary education and research forums.

GLOBAL SURGERY FEES

Traditionally, surgeons have offered a package deal to their patients: if they perform a procedure, routine perioperative services are included in the fee. Unfortunately, many surgeons collect global surgery fees, but provide less than global care. Economic pressures are unlikely to allow this behavior to persist. Specifically, on January 1, 1992, a new Medicare fee schedule was implemented.[13] This is the most comprehensive reform in the Medicare program since its inception in 1965. The major goal is to make physician payments more rational and equitable by a budget-neutral redistribution of payments. Specialties that provide cognitive-based services will gain at the expense of those who provide procedure-based services. The integral component of the new Medicare fee schedule is the resource-based relative value scale that classifies each service in the physician's *Current Procedure Terminology* according to the amount of work (relative value units) required by the physician; however, the Medicare fee schedule has maintained the global surgery fee as a strategy to limit payments. How this applies to ICU care has been an ongoing source of confusion. First, it is important to recognize that while the Health Care Financing Administration has attempted to clarify their rules of what is included in this package, the *Current Procedure Terminology* rules are different and less defined. Unfortunately, when billing an insurance company, it is unclear which set of rules apply and it is in their best interest if this issue remains obtuse. Second, even when we know that the Health Care Financing Administration rules apply, irrationalities and inequalities exist. For example, if a patient has a complicated postoperative course that requires high-cognitive ICU care, the general surgeon cannot bill for it. But, if the same patient requires a second operation, the general surgeon can bill for it. Is time spent in the operating room different than the time spent in the ICU? After considerable pressure, the Health Care Financing Administration now permits trauma and burns surgeons (but not general surgeons who have the same training) to use the critical care codes 99291 and 99292 for the advanced postoperative ICU care they provide. To use these critical care codes, however, the trauma and burn surgeon must provide at least 30 minutes of documented constant attention unrelated to the specific injuries that required a surgical procedure and use coding modifier 24 that will increase the likelihood of a manual review by the local insurance carrier. The alternative for trauma and burn surgeons is to consult a nonsurgeon who can use a variety of codes for the services provided and is more likely to get paid without any questions. Why are the trauma and burn surgeons and their patients being penalized? Clearly, the continuity and quality of care is better if the trauma or burn surgeon who provides initial emergency department and/or operating room management also provides the early ICU care. Another contentious example is the surgical subspecialist who performs high-risk, regional surgical procedures that routinely place patients in the ICU. They are paid impressive professional fees, but have no intention of providing routine, postoperative ICU care. Do they deserve to be paid the full global fee? These are questions that need to be answered if there is to be financial incentive for general surgeons to maintain a role in ICU care. An alternative is to unbundle ICU care, but this would not be attractive to the Health Care Financing Administration or the insurance companies because more professional fees would need to be paid.

MULTIPLE CONSULTANT SYNDROME

As the field of critical care medicine has become more complex, organ-specific specialists have prospered; it is not unusual for patients in the ICU to have multiple consultants. There is no financial penalty to the surgeon. It is an effective strategy for surgeons to generate reciprocal consultations from the medical specialists. It also increases operating room time availability and diffuses medicolegal responsibility. While most patients receive reasonable care with this model, complex patients do not. The term "consultarrhea" amply describes a critically ill patient in evolving organ failure who can have a half-dozen, organ-specific specialists ordering many tests and conflicting therapies, with no one really in control. This is poor patient care. The bedside nurses know it, the residents know it, and the patient's families know it. This practice also promotes unnecessary expenses for tests and professional fees. Hospital administrators and insurance carriers are beginning to understand this issue.

One alternative is to have a qualified general surgeon as the ICU director. This surgeon's responsibility would be to create an optimal patient care environment where surgeons can care for their patients by developing management guidelines that can be driven by existing nonphysician ICU personnel (eg, nurses, respiratory therapists, and pharmacists). Standardized care can be assessed and modified to maximize quality and cost-effectiveness. It also reduces the need for multiple physician consultants. Larger institutions need to embrace the concept of a critical care team of multidisciplinary practitioners (nurses, respiratory therapists, and pharmacists led by an intensivist (perhaps a surgeon).[14] It is important that this team functions as an extension of the attending surgeon by implementing standard care and serving as surrogate when the attending surgeon is not available, but deferring critical decisions to the attending surgeon. Data are emerging in the literature that document this approach and are finding (not surprisingly), that it is more efficient than the use of multiple consultants.[15-17] If we do not adopt this collaborative approach, it will be imposed on us and we will not control it. The ICUs will be "closed." Surgical patients will no longer be admitted under the operating surgeon, but rather the intensivist will assume primary responsibility. This is the model used in many medical ICUs and would be the natural evolution if nonsurgeons assume primary responsibility for surgical ICUs.

ICUs ARE EXPENSIVE COST CENTERS

Hospitals recognize that ICUs are expensive cost centers that must be controlled if further cost reductions are to occur. Recent cost data for trauma reporting line at Hermann Hospital illustrates this nicely. Over the past 3 years, the trauma service has been restructured to be more cost-effective, with a core group of trauma surgeons working with clinical specialists and case managers to develop and implement management guidelines and transfer agreements. The primary goal is to facilitate daily plans and appropriate early discharge from the hospital. A designated administrator designs ongoing performance improvement projects and provides monthly status reports as feedback. Our financial report card is depicted in the **Figure**. Case mix index is obtained using diagnosis related groups cost weights, cost per case is obtained by Transition Systems Inc, and the University Hospital Consortium expected cost (ie, the benchmark) is obtained using the University Hospital Consortium clinical database. Over 30 months, we have observed that: (1) the length of stay has steadily decreased; (2) less severely injured patients are being discharged from the hospital earlier and the case mix index has steadily increased; and (3) the bottom line (cost per case adjusted by case mix index) has steadily decreased. In the first quarter of fiscal year 1996 (October-December 1995), our mean ± SEM cost per case was \$7981 ± \$579. This was significantly above University Hospital Consortium expected (\$5810 ± \$420). By the fourth quarter of fiscal year 1997 (July-September 1997), our cost per case dropped significantly to \$5908 ± \$338. In fiscal year 1998, however, our costs did not decrease. As expected, we have "hit the wall." Facilitating care plans of the less severely injured patients so that

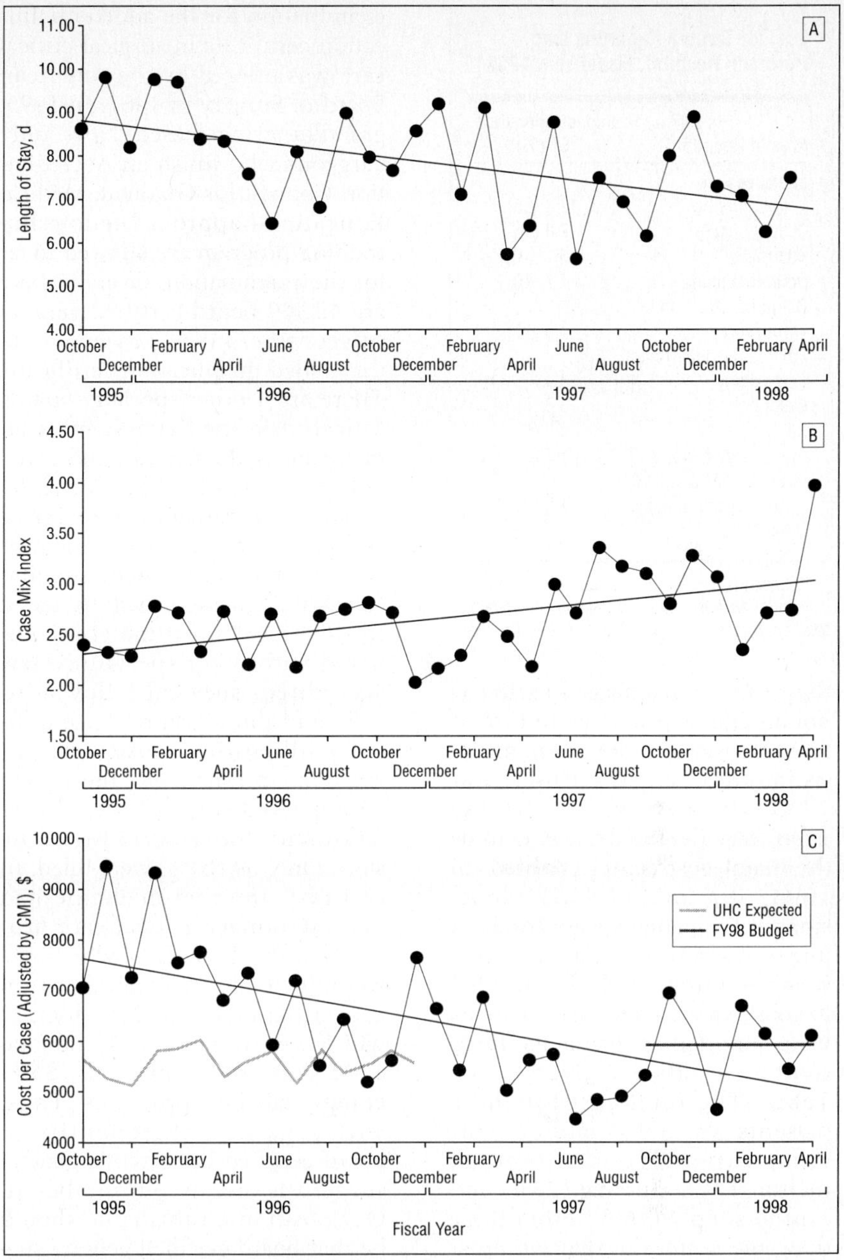

Our financial report card for 30 months detailing the case mix index obtained using diagnosis related groups cost weights for fiscal years (FY) 1996-1998. The cost per case was obtained by Transition Systems Inc, and University Hospital Consortium (UHC) expected cost was obtained using the University Hospital Consortium clinical database. Length of stay and the cost per case adjusted by the case mix index (CMI) has steadily decreased and the case mix index has increased due to earlier discharge from the hospital for less severely injured patients.

Cost for Trauma Reporting Line, Hermann Hospital, Fiscal Year 1998*

Area of Hospital	Budget Allocation, $† (%)
Intensive care unit nursing	12.4 (25)
Central supply	7.8 (16)
Pharmacy	5.1 (10)
Routine nursing	4.7 (10)
Operating room and recovery	4.6 (10)
Emergency department/ life flight	4.4 (9)
Laboratory	3.8 (8)
Radiology	3.0 (6)
Respiratory therapy	1.7 (3)
Physical, occupational, and speech therapy	1.0 (2)
Other costs	0.7 (1)

**Hermann Hospital is located in Houston, Tex.*
†Dollar amount indicates millions of dollars; total cost for fiscal year 1998 was $49.5 million.

they can be discharged earlier is not an effective strategy to further reduce costs. A more recent analysis for our cost data for fiscal year 1998 (October 1997-September 1998) has identified the ICU to be the major cost center (**Table**). In 1998, of a total of 4083 admissions, 1272 patients were admitted under observation status (23 hours was the anticipated time needed for observation) and 2811 patients were admitted as inpatients. Inpatient cost data are given in the Table. The total cost for these patients was $49.5 million. Our most expensive components included ICU nursing (25%) and central supply (16%). From these data, we conclude that we must shift our focus of cost reduction efforts to the ICU. The 2 options are to either decrease the daily cost or decrease the number of days spent in the ICU. We believe the latter strategy will be most effective and will focus on methods to reduce ICU stay over the next fiscal year.

BOARD-CERTIFIED INTENSIVISTS

After failure in the early 1980s to create a multidisciplinary board certification for critical care, individual specialty boards developed their own training programs and certification processes. The first examination for the added qualification certificate in surgical critical care was offered by the American Board of Surgery in 1987. In 1995, grandfathering ceased. Now, only surgeons who finish an Accreditation Council for Graduate Medical Education– approved fellowship training program are allowed to sit for the examination. Overall, there are 42 389 board-certified general surgeons 1573 (4%) of whom hold this added qualification certificate. There are 4 other specialty boards (anesthesia, pediatrics, internal medicine, and obstetrics and gynecology) that offer pathways by which their trainees can be board certified in critical care. In the near future, emergency medicine and osteopathic medicine will be added to this list. Unfortunately, compared with other specialties, few accredited, surgical fellowships exist and those that do have difficulty filling their positions. For example, in June 1996, there were 62 approved surgical critical care fellowships offering 114 training slots. Only 69 (61%) were filled. In contrast, internal medicine had 108 pulmonary critical care programs with 813 slots, of which 777 were filled and 65 medical critical care programs with 269 slots, of which 236 were filled. Of the total 1082 slots, 909 individuals (84%) completed their programs. Thus, with regard to the quantity of board-certified intensivists, general surgery is clearly outnumbered. Our position on this issue should be that board-certified general surgeons are capable of providing critical care. The purpose for the added qualification certificate is to maintain a cadre of surgical experts who can serve as ICU directors, perform high-quality ICU research, and be responsible for surgical education. We also need to acknowledge that the intensivist (surgeon or nonsurgeon) can play an important role in postoperative ICU care, but it is the operating surgeon's responsibility to be involved in important decisions. We must recognize that the quality of critical care is not determined by board certification, but rather by a commitment to provide high-quality care. If the operating surgeon is not qualified or available, an intensivist is the best alternative for the patient.

CONCLUSIONS

General surgery first needs to answer the question "Should general surgeons provide critical care?" If the answer is no, then our course is already set. General surgeons will become progressively less involved in the ICU. Nonsurgeons will provide more postoperative ICU care and global surgery fees will decrease. Only high-volume surgical physicians in regional trauma and burn centers will continue to provide surgical critical care. The added qualification certificate will be needed to verify their critical care skills because general surgery programs will no longer provide the essential training. On the other hand, if the answer to the question is yes, then important initiatives include (1) ensuring that general surgeons remain competent in critical care through ongoing education; (2) providing financial incentive for continued involvement by clarifying the global surgery fee so that care provided above and beyond routine postoperative care can be billed by the operating surgeon (ie, unbundle ICU care); (3) maintaining scientific legitimacy by performing high-quality research in surgical ICUs; (4) abandoning multiple consultants and embrace the critical care team that functions as an extension of the surgeon; and (5) providing leadership in ICU cost reduction.

Frederick A. Moore, MD
Department of Surgery
University of Texas-Houston Medical School
Hermann Hospital
Houston, Tex

Dr Moore is the James H. "Red" Duke Professor and Vice Chair of the Department of Surgery, University of Texas-Houston Medical School.

Corresponding author: Frederick A. Moore, MD, Department of Surgery, University of Texas-Houston Medical School, 6431 Fannin, Suite 4.264, Houston, TX 77030.

REFERENCES

1. Sugerman HJ. Surgeons and the surgical intensive care unit. *Arch Surg.* 1982;117:391-392.
2. Walt AJ. The training and role of the surgeon in the intensive care unit. *Surg Clin North Am.* 1985; 65:753-762.
3. Meyer AA, Fakhry SM, Sheldon GF. Critical care education in general surgery residencies. *Surgery.* 1989;106:392-399.
4. Higgins GA. Evolution of the healing room. *Arch Surg.* 1990;125:1101-1102.
5. Holcroft JW. Who should be responsible for care of the critically ill surgical patient? *Arch Surg.* 1990; 125:1103-1104.
6. Trask AL, Faber DR. The intensive care unit—who's in charge? *Arch Surg.* 1990;125:1105-1108.
7. Fakhry SM, Buehrer JL, Sheldon GF, Meyer AA. A comparison of intensive care unit care of surgical patients in teaching and nonteaching hospitals. *Ann Surg.* 1991;214:19-23.
8. Weil MH, Shubin H. The practice of critical care medicine: is it viable? *Crit Care Med.* 1975;3:173-174.
9. Weil MH, Shoemaker WC, Rackow EC. Training and certification of critical care medicine in the United States. *Chest.* 1988;93:1122-1123.
10. King EG, Sibbald WJ. The territorial imperative. *Chest.* 1988;93:1121-1122.
11. Holcroft JW. Who should be responsible for care of the critically ill surgical patient? *Arch Surg.* 1990; 125:1103-1104.
12. Haupt MT, Grenvik A, Rogers PL. Physician education and training in critical care medicine. *New Horiz.* 1998;6:235-311.
13. Moore FA, Moore EE, Read RA, Ogunkeye JO. Medicare's resource-based relative value scale fee schedule portends a gloomy future for trauma surgery. *J Trauma.* 1993;34:900-907.
14. Ivy ME, Bonnell BW, Angood PB. Characterizing the practice of surgical critical care fellowship graduates: what's a fellow to do? *Current Surgery.* In Press.
15. Pollack MM, Katz RW, Ruttimann UE, Getson PR. Improving the outcome and efficiency of intensive care: the impact of an intensivist. *Crit Care Med.* 1988;16:11-17.
16. Brown JJ, Sullivan G. Effect of ICU mortality of a full-time critical care specialist. *Chest.* 1989;96: 127-129.
17. Roberts DE, Ball DD, Ostryzniuk T, et al. Eliminating needless testing in intensive care: an information-based team management approach. *Crit Care Med.* 1993;21:1452-1458.

IN OTHER AMA JOURNALS

JAMA

Postoperative Radiotherapy in the Treatment of Single Metastases to the Brain: A Randomized Trial

Roy A. Patchell, MD; Phillip A. Tibbs, MD; William F. Regine, MD; Robert J. Dempsey, MD; Mohammed Mohiuddin, MD; Richard J. Kryscio, PhD; William R. Markesbery, MD; Kenneth A. Foon, MD; Byron Young, MD

Context: For the treatment of a single metastasis to the brain, surgical resection combined with postoperative radiotherapy is more effective than treatment with radiotherapy alone. However, the efficacy of postoperative radiotherapy after complete surgical resection has not been established.
Objective: To determine if postoperative radiotherapy resulted in improved neurologic control of disease and increased survival.
Design: Multicenter, randomized, parallel group trial.
Setting: University-affiliated cancer treatment facilities.
Patients: Ninety-five patients who had single metastases to the brain that were treated with complete surgical resections (as verified by postoperative magnetic resonance imaging) between September 1989 and November 1997 were entered into the study.
Interventions: Patients were randomly assigned to treatment with postoperative whole-brain radiotherapy (radiotherapy group, 49 patients) or no further treatment (observation group, 46 patients) for the brain metastasis, with median follow-up of 48 weeks and 43 weeks, respectively.
Main Outcome Measures: The primary end point was recurrence of tumor in the brain; secondary end points were length of survival, cause of death, and preservation of ability to function independently.
Results: Recurrence of tumor anywhere in the brain was less frequent in the radiotherapy group than in the observation group (9 [18%] of 49 vs 32 [70%] of 46; $P<.001$). Postoperative radiotherapy prevented brain recurrence at the site of the original metastasis (5 [10%] of 49 vs 21 [46%] of 46; $P<.001$) and at other sites in the brain (7 [14%] of 49 vs 17 [37%] of 46; $P<.01$). Patients in the radiotherapy group were less likely to die of neurologic causes than patients in the observation group (6 [14%] of 43 who died vs 17 [44%] of 39; $P=.003$). There was no significant difference between the 2 groups in overall length of survival or the length of time that patients remained functionally independent.
Conclusions.—Patients with cancer and single metastases to the brain who receive treatment with surgical resection and postoperative radiotherapy have fewer recurrences of cancer in the brain and are less likely to die of neurologic causes than similar patients treated with surgical resection alone. *(1998;280:1485-1489)*

Reprints: Roy A. Patchell, MD, Neurosurgery Division, University of Kentucky Medical Center, 800 Rose St, Lexington, KY 40536-0084 (e-mail: RPatchell@aol.com).

Thyroid Cancer With Concurrent Hyperthyroidism

Tzu-Chieh Chao, MD, PhD; Jen-Der Lin, MD; Long-Bin Jeng, MD; Miin-Fu Chen, MD

Objective: To study the clinical manifestation, outcome, and factors predicting metastases in patients with thyroid cancer and concurrent hyperthyroidism.

Design: Retrospective study of 37 thyrotoxic patients with differentiated carcinomas of the thyroid who were operated on between 1979 and 1995. The follow-up period ranged from 562 days to 14 years 9 months (mean ± SE, 2093 ± 201 days).

Setting: University hospital with an annual performance rate of about 700 thyroid operations.

Patients: Thyroidectomy was performed in 37 patients (31 women and 6 men), including 33 papillary carcinomas and 4 follicular carcinomas. The mean ± SE age of the patients was 38.6 ± 2.2 years.

Results: The mean ± SE diameter of tumors was 13.2 ± 0.9 mm (range, 2-67 mm). The tumor size in 25 patients (68%) was 10 mm or smaller. Subtotal thyroidectomy (21 patients), total thyroidectomy (8 patients), near-total thyroidectomy (4 patients), and completion thyroidectomy (4 patients) were performed. Twenty-eight patients underwent postoperative sodium iodide I 131 (^{131}I) ablation for thyroid remnant. There was 1 local recurrence, 3 metastases to regional neck lymph nodes, and 3 distant metastases. A patient with follicular carcinoma died of metastases at 3 years 4 months after thyroidectomy. Age, sex, duration of thyrotoxic symptoms, tumor size, histopathological findings, type of goiter, extent of surgery, ^{131}I ablation, and 6-week postoperative serum concentrations of thyroglobulin or thyrotropin were not significant factors in predicting metastases. Serum levels of triiodothyronine and thyroxine before antithyroid treatment in the patients with metastases were significantly higher than in those without metastases.

Conclusion: The majority of patients with thyroid cancer and concurrent hyperthyroidism have small carcinomas.

Arch Surg. 1999;134:130-134

From the Division of General Surgery, Department of Surgery (Drs Chao, Jeng, and Chen), and the Division of Endocrinology and Metabolism, Department of Medicine (Dr Lin), Chang Gung University College of Medicine and Chang Gung Memorial Hospital, Taipei, Taiwan.

IT HAS been reported that thyroid cancer occurs in 0.76% to 8.7% of the glands removed for treatment of thyrotoxicosis.[1-5] Although recent reports have found higher rates of thyroid cancer associated with hyperthyroidism, earlier reports emphasize the rarity of these 2 conditions occurring simultaneously. Controversy surrounds the disease course of thyroid cancer with concurrent hyperthyroidism. Belfiore et al[6] and Ozaki et al[2] have reported that thyroid cancer associated with Graves disease had an aggressive course. In contrast, other investigators did not highlight the aggressive characteristics.[5,7,8] The discrepancies of the results are probably due to geographic, racial, or other unknown factors. To better understand the association of thyroid cancer with hyperthyroidism, we retrospectively reviewed the data of patients who had thyroid cancer with concurrent hyperthyroidism. In the present study, clinical manifestations, treatment, outcome, and factors predicting metastases are presented.

RESULTS

Goiter types of 37 patients with hyperthyroidism with thyroid cancer were toxic diffuse goiter (30 patients, 81%), toxic multinodular goiter (6 patients, 16%), and toxic adenoma (1 patient, 3%). Two of 30 patients with toxic diffuse goiter and 1 of 6 patients with toxic multinodular goiter were found to have papillary carcinoma by preoperative fine-needle aspiration cytology. The mean diameter of malignant tumors was 13.2 ± 0.9 mm (range, 2-67 mm). Twenty-five patients (68%) had a small tumor (≤10 mm) and 12 (32%) had a large tumor (>10 mm). The mean diameter of small tumors and large tumors was 6.4 ± 0.9 mm (range, 2-10 mm) and 30.0 ± 4.9 mm (range, 12-62 mm), respectively.

Thirty-one patients were women and 6 patients were men (ratio, 5.2:1). The age ranged from 20 to 82 years, with a mean ± SE age of 38.6 ± 2.2 years. The mean age of female patients was 37.5 ± 2.4 years (range, 20-82 years) and male

PATIENTS AND METHODS

During a 17-year period from 1979 to 1995, 1013 patients with thyroid cancer were treated at the Division of General Surgery, Chang Gung Memorial Hospital, Taipei, Taiwan. There were 741 papillary carcinomas (73.1%), 168 follicular carcinomas (16.6%), 21 medullary carcinomas (2.1%), 48 anaplastic carcinomas (4.7%), and 35 carcinomas of other histological types (3.5%). During the same period, 3502 patients underwent thyroidectomy for thyrotoxicosis at our hospital. Hyperthyroidism was diagnosed on the basis of elevated triiodothyronine (T_3), elevated thyroxine (T_4), and low thyrotropin (TSH) levels in combination with hyperthyroid clinical symptoms. Of 3502 patients with hyperthyroidism, there were 2934 toxic diffuse goiters (Graves disease) (83.8%), 303 toxic multinodular goiters (8.7%), and 265 toxic adenoma (toxic autonomously functioning thyroid nodule) (7.6%). Patients were treated with carbimazole, methimazole, or propylthiouracil preoperatively. They also received Lugol iodine solution for 7 to 10 days before surgery. The indications for surgery were (1) recurrent thyrotoxicosis, (2) adverse effects of antithyroid medications, (3) patient unlikelihood or inability to take medications, (4) presence of cold nodules within toxic glands on thyroid scanning, (5) unusually large diffuse or multinodular goiters, (6) malignancy or fine-needle aspiration biopsy findings suggestive of thyroid cancer, and (7) autonomously functioning nodules.

Of 3502 patients with hyperthyroidism, 41 (1.2%) were identified to have thyroid cancer. Thirty (1.0%) of 2934 patients with toxic diffuse goiter, 6 (2.0%) of 303 patients with toxic multinodular goiter, and 1 (0.4%) of 265 patients with toxic adenoma had malignant neoplasms of the thyroid. The histopathological type of the thyroid cancer associated with hyperthyroidism included 34 papillary thyroid carcinomas (83%), 4 follicular carcinomas (10%), 2 medullary carcinomas (5%), and 1 Hürthle cell carcinoma (2%). Tumor diameter was the maximum diameter measured on pathological examination or by ultrasonography. In carcinomas with multiple foci, the maximum diameter of tumor foci was used as the diameter of tumor. Small tumor was defined as a tumor measuring 10 mm or less and a large tumor, greater than 10 mm. The patients with medullary carcinoma and Hürthle cell carcinoma and a patient who died 30 days after surgery (papillary carcinoma) were excluded from the present study. Data from the remaining 37 patients were retrospectively reviewed. Results are presented as mean ± SE.

patients was 44.5 ± 6.2 years (range, 24-69 years). Although women, on average, were 7 years younger than men, the difference was not statistically significant.

The duration of hyperthyroid clinical symptoms ranged from 30 days to 6 years (693 ± 122 days). Mean serum levels of T_3 and T_4 before administration of antithyroid medications were 5.78 ± 0.53 nmol/L (range, 2.73-12.01 nmol/L) and 232 ± 9 nmol/L (range, 172-320 nmol/L), respectively. Serum level of TSH was less than 200 µIU/L in each patient. Comparison of data between patients with small tumors and large tumors is shown in **Table 1**. There were no differences in age, sex, duration of thyrotoxic symptoms, serum levels of T_3 and T_4 before taking antithyroid medications, and 6-week postoperative serum thyroglobulin level between the 2 groups. However, 6-week postoperative serum TSH level in the group with small tumor was significantly ($P<.05$) lower than that in the group with large tumor. This difference could be attributed to the fact that most small tumors were treated with subtotal thyroidectomy (**Table 2**).

Twenty-five patients underwent technetium Tc 99m pertechnetate thyroid scanning, including those with toxic diffuse goiter (19 patients), toxic multinodular goiter (5 patients), and toxic adenoma (1 patient). Four of 19 patients with toxic diffuse goiter and 2 of 5 with toxic multinodular goiters had coexistent cold nodules on thyroid scanning. Thyroid ultrasonography with fine-needle aspiration cytology was performed in 5 patients with cold nodule on thyroid scanning and 8 patients with clinically palpable nodule. Only 3 of these patients had evidence of papillary carcinoma. Fourteen patients underwent intraoperative frozen section biopsy, including 5 with toxic diffuse goiter, 3 with toxic diffuse goiter with cold nodules on thyroid scan, 2 with toxic diffuse goiter with a solid nodule on ultrasonogram, 2 with multinodular goiter, and 2 with multinodular goiter with a cold nodule on scan. Frozen sections disclosed malignant neoplasms in 12 patients (86%). Two false-negative case results included 1 toxic diffuse goiter and 1 multinodular goiter.

Operative methods are shown in Table 2. Subtotal thyroidectomy was performed in 21 patients (57%), including 19 patients with toxic diffuse goiter and 2 with toxic multinodular goiter. Total thyroidectomy (6 patients) and near-total thyroidectomy (6 patients) were performed after confirmation of thyroid cancer by frozen section biopsy. One patient with a huge multinodular goiter was primarily treated with total thyroidectomy and postoperative pathological evaluation revealed a small papillary carcinoma. Most patients (n = 18; 49%) with small tumor underwent subtotal thyroidectomy. Three patients underwent completion total thyroidectomy after postoperative pathological confirmation of malignancy. Of these 3 patients, initial subtotal thyroidectomy was performed for toxic diffuse goiter (1 patient) and toxic multinodular goiter (2 patients). The overall postoperative complications were transient hypoparathyroidism (1 patient, 3%), permanent hypoparathyroidism (2 patients, 5%), and transient recurrent laryngeal nerve palsy (2 patients, 5%).

Whole-body scanning with 18 mBq sodium iodide I 131 (^{131}I) was performed on 29 patients 6 weeks after thyroidectomy. Of these 29 patients, 28 underwent subsequent ^{131}I ablation of thyroid remnant (13 subtotal thyroidectomies, 7 total thyroidectomies, 4 completion thyroidectomies, 4 near-total thyroidectomies) since thyroid tissue capable of ^{131}I uptake over a 24-hour period was greater than 1%. The overall mean dosage of ^{131}I radiation for ablation was 3182 ± 407 mBq (range, 1100-7400 mBq). The average ablation dosage of ^{131}I for the patients undergoing subtotal thyroidectomy was 3330 ±

Table 1. Data of the Patients With Small and Large Thyroid Cancers*

	Small Tumors	Large Tumors	*P*
Age, y	39.4 ± 3.0 (20-82)	36.7 ± 2.7 (24-49)	.97†
Sex, F/M	22:4	9:2	1.00‡
Duration of symptoms, d	757.7 ± 141.7 (120-2196)	498.6 ± 242.6 (30-1825)	.16†
Serum T_3,§ nmol/L	5.96 ± 0.71 (2.73-12.01)	5.17 ± 0.68(3.02-7.25)	.87†
Serum T_4,§ nmol/L	238 ± 12 (178-320)	210 ± 14 (172-250)	.20†
Postoperative thyroglobulin, µg/L	20.5 ± 9.4 (1-139)	56.8 ± 48.7 (1.4-300)	.49†
Postoperative serum TSH,‖ µIU/L	6150 ± 2340 (40-35 600)	27 340 ± 13 000 (390-94 700)	.05†

*Data are expressed as mean ± SE (range) except for sex. T_3 indicates triiodothyronine; T_4, thyroxine; and TSH, thyrotropin.
†Mann-Whitney *U* test.
‡Fisher exact test.
§Measured before antithyroid treatment.
‖Six-week postoperative serum TSH level was measured in 24 patients.

Table 2. Operative Methods

	No. of Patients		
Surgery	Small Tumors	Large Tumors	Total
Subtotal thyroidectomy	18	3	**21**
Near-total thyroidectomy	3	3	**6**
Total thyroidectomy	3*	4	**7**
Completion thyroidectomy	1	2	**3**

*One patient underwent total thyroidectomy for a huge toxic multinodular goiter and postoperative pathological evaluation showed a small papillary carcinoma.

407 mBq (range, 1110-3700 mBq). On the other hand, ablation dosage of ^{131}I for those with near-total or total thyroidectomy was 3219 ± 666 mBq (range, 1110-7400 mBq). These 28 patients also had thyroxine suppression treatment. Postoperative ^{131}I whole-body scanning and thyroid ablation were not performed on 8 patients with small tumors who underwent subtotal thyroidectomy. The mean tumor diameter of these 9 patients was 4.9 ± 0.7 mm (range, 2-8 mm).

The follow-up period ranged from 562 days to 14 years 9 months (2093 ± 201 days). Initial 6-week postoperative ^{131}I whole-body scan or chest x-ray films did not reveal tumor metastases. A recurrence of cancer at the thyroid bed occurred 2 years 6 months after a near-total thyroidectomy for a 3.5-cm follicular carcinoma. Distant metastases (2 papillary carcinomas and 1 follicular carcinoma) or metastases to regional neck lymph nodes (3 papillary carcinomas) occurred 20.5 ± 4.7 months (median, 17.5 months) after initial thyroidectomy (**Table 3**). The patient with follicular carcinoma died of metastases to the lungs, bone, and leptomeninges 3 years 4 months after thyroidectomy.

The patient age, tumor size, and 6-week postoperative serum levels of thyroglobulin and TSH in the patients with metastases were not different from those without metastases. However, mean serum levels of T_3 and T_4 in the patients with metastases were significantly greater than those in the patients without metastases (**Table 4**). To examine the factors capable of predicting metastases, various parameters were compared. Age, sex, duration of thyrotoxic symptoms, tumor size, histopathological tumor type, type of goiter, extent of surgery, ^{131}I ablation, 6-week postoperative serum levels of thyroglobulin or TSH were not significant factors in predicting metastases (**Table 5**). However, when patients were divided into 2 groups according to the median serum levels of T_3 (6.93 nmol/L) and T_4 (277 nmol/L) before initiation of antithyroid medications, T_3 and T_4 were significant factors in predicting metastases. Four (50%) of 8 patients with a T_4 level higher than 277 nmol/L had metastases and 4 (44.4%) of 9 patients with a T_3 level higher than 6.93 nmol/L had metastases.

COMMENT

In the present study, serum concentrations of T_3 and T_4 before antithyroid treatment were found to be significant prognostic factors in predicting metastases in patients with differentiated thyroid carcinoma with concurrent hyperthyroidism. To our knowledge, similar findings have never been reported. Serum concentrations of TSH are suppressed in patients with hyperthyroidism with elevated serum concentrations of T_3 and T_4. On the other hand, serum TSH concentrations become normal or elevated after surgery. It is not clear whether T_3 or T_4 influences the growth of normal thyroid or thyroid tumors. However, experimental data and clinical reports suggest that TSH not only stimulates normal thyroid cell growth and function[9] but also the growth of thyroid tumors.[10] Normal thyroid and benign and malignant thyroid tumors express TSH receptors on the plasma membrane.[11] Thyrotropin interacts with TSH receptors and is primarily transducted via the TSH-receptor-adenylate cyclase pathway.[9] Suppression of TSH by thyroid hormones has been used clinically to prevent the recurrence of thyroid cancer after surgery.[12-15] Therefore, elevated serum TSH concentrations in the postoperative period might stimulate the growth of residual thyroid cancer cells, eventually leading to local recurrence or metastases. However, as shown in the present study, postoperative TSH level is higher in patients with a tumor larger than 10 mm, but it is not a significant predictor of metastases in differentiated thyroid carcinoma with concurrent hyperthyroidism. This suggests that other factors may influence the prognosis of patients with thyroid cancer and concurrent hyperthyroidism. The presence of TSH receptor antibodies in the blood has been noted to be one of the causes of Graves disease.[16,17] Like TSH, TSH receptor antibodies (thyroid-stimulating immunoglobulins) interact with TSH receptors and stimulate thyroid growth and func-

Table 3. Patient and Clinical Characteristics of Metastatic Thyroid Carcinoma

Histopathology	Patient Age, y/Sex	Tumor Size, mm	Goiter Type	Surgery*	Metastasis	Time After Surgery
Papillary carcinoma	33/F	8	Diffuse	NT	Lung	2 y
Papillary carcinoma	35/F	4	Diffuse	ST	Neck lymph nodes	11 mo
Papillary carcinoma	20/F	2, multicentric	Diffuse	ST	Neck lymph nodes	2 y 3 mo
Papillary carcinoma	49/M	20	Diffuse	NT	Neck lymph nodes	11 mo
Papillary carcinoma	26/F	67	Diffuse	CT	Lung	11 mo
Follicular carcinoma	82/F	. . .	Multinodular	ST	Lung, bone, leptomeninges	3 y 3 mo†

*NT indicates near-total thyroidectomy; ST, subtotal thyroidectomy; CT, completion thyroidectomy; and ellipses, not described in the medical chart.
†This patient died of metastases at 3 years 4 months after the initial surgery.

Table 4. Parameters in Patients With Thyroid Cancer With Metastases or Without Metastases*

	Metastases	No Metastases	*P*†
Age, y	40.8 ± 9.2 (20-82)	38.2 ± 2.1 (21-69)	.83
Tumor size, mm	20.2 ± 12.1 (2-67)	11.8 ± 2.4 (2-51)	.82
Serum T_3,‡ nmol/L	8.07 ± 0.75 (6.38-10.39)	5.18 ± 0.60 (2.73-12.01)	.02
Serum T_4,‡ nmol/L	272 ± 15 (226-317)	221 ± 10 (172-320)	.04
Postoperative thyroglobulin, µg/L	77.2 ± 49.6 (1-300)	11.8 ± 3.4 (1.2-57.5)	.87
Postoperative serum TSH,§ µIU/L	6300 ± 4100 (200-14 100)	13 200 ± 5000 (40-94 700)	1.00

*Data are expressed as mean ± SE (range). T_3 indicates triiodothyronine; T_4, thyroxine; and TSH, thyrotropin.
†Mann-Whitney U test.
‡Measured before antithyroid treatment.
§Six-week postoperative serum TSH level was measured in 24 patients.

tion.[18,19] Thyrotropin receptor–stimulating immunoglobulins have been found in the serum of patients with metastatic thyroid carcinomas and hyperthyroidism[18] and of patients with thyroid carcinoma and concurrent hyperthyroidism.[2,6] However, it has not yet been directly proven that TSH receptor–stimulating antibodies can stimulate the growth of thyroid carcinoma cells.

Although some authors have reported that some occult (≤1 cm) thyroid papillary carcinomas had an aggressive propensity,[20,21] the concept that small thyroid carcinomas are associated with an excellent prognosis is widely accepted.[22-25] Hay et al[25] have reported a 6% recurrence rate after 20 years in 535 patients with papillary carcinoma of 1.0 cm or less in diameter. Only 2 patients died of small papillary carcinoma in their series. As shown in the present study and the literature,[2,7] most carcinomas associated with hyperthyroidism are small and found incidentally, during pathological examination of the thyroid and during surgery. One major question is what must be done when a small carcinoma is found postoperatively on pathological examination after subtotal thyroidectomy for hyperthyroidism. Although total or near-total thyroidectomy is generally recommended for differentiated thyroid carcinoma,[26-29] many investigators believe that patients with occult papillary carcinoma or follicular carcinoma with minimal capsular invasion can be treated with limited surgery, such as lobectomy and isthmectomy.[22-24,30,31] This is based on the findings that extent of surgery did not influence the outcome of patients with small differentiated thyroid carcinomas. In the present study, extent of thyroidectomy did not influence the incidence of metastases (Table 5). Grant et al[30] have reported that there were no differences in local recurrence and survival rates of patients with thyroid cancer when subtotal thyroidectomy was compared with total thyroidectomy. Vickery et al[31] have demonstrated that no patient with a small carcinoma experienced recurrence in the resected thyroid bed or contralateral lobe after subtotal thyroidectomy or lobectomy. In a retrospective study of 867 patients with thyroid carcinomas smaller than 10 mm by Schroeder et al,[23] 416 patients (48.0%) were operated on with a preoperative diagnosis of Graves disease. The majority of patients underwent subtotal thyroidectomy, lobectomy, or partial lobectomy. The type of thyroidectomy did not affect patient survival. Therefore, thyrotoxic patients with occult differentiated thyroid cancer may be treated with limited surgery without influencing the prognosis.

In the present study, ^{131}I ablation did not influence the incidence of metastases. Ablation of thyroid remnant with ^{131}I is generally performed after total or near-total thyroidectomy for well-differentiated thyroid carcinoma.[32,33] Recent reports have shown a significant reduction in recurrence and cancer-related deaths for patients treated with ^{131}I ablative therapy.[34,35] However, most investigators would not recommend the routine administration of ^{131}I to patients with small tumor confined to the thyroid bed.[36] In the study by Schroder et al,[23] postoperative ^{131}I ablation was not administered to the patients in the absence of metastases and the recurrence-free 20-year survival rate was high. Similar findings were reported by Hay et al[25] Therefore, routine ^{131}I ablation is not indicated in the patients with small differentiated thyroid carcinoma.

Table 5. Factors Predicting Metastases of Thyroid Cancer Associated With Hyperthyroidism*

Factor	No. (%) of Patients		
	Metastasis	No Metastasis	P†
Age, y			
≤25	1 (3)	2 (5)	.42
>25	5 (14)	29 (78)	
Sex			
Female	5 (14)	26 (70)	1.00
Male	1 (3)	5 (14)	
Duration of symptoms, y			
≥2	3 (8)	11 (30)	.65
<2	3 (8)	20 (54)	
Serum T_4 level,‡ nmol/L			
≥277	4 (11)	4 (11)	.01
<277	2 (5)	27 (73)	
Serum T_3 level,‡ nmol/L			
≥6.93	4 (11)	5 (14)	.02
<6.93	2 (5)	26 (70)	
Tumor size, mm			
≤10	4 (11)	22 (60)	1.00
>10	2 (5)	9 (24)	
Histopathology			
Papillary carcinoma	5 (14)	28 (76)	.52
Follicular carcinoma	1 (3)	3 (8)	
Hyperthyroidism§			
Diffuse goiter	5 (14)	25 (69)	1.00
Multinodular goiter	1 (3)	5 (14)	
Surgery			
Subtotal thyroidectomy	3 (8)	18 (49)	1.00
Total or near-total thyroidectomy	3 (8)	13 (35)	
Iodine 131 ablation			
Ablation	6 (16)	22 (60)	.30
No ablation	0	9 (24)	
Postoperative thyroglobulin, µg/L			
>52	2 (5)	2 (5)	.12
≤52	4 (11)	29 (78)	
Postoperative TSH,‖ µIU/L			
≥3250	2 (8)	10 (42)	1.00
<3250	1 (4)	11 (46)	

*T_4 indicates thyroxine; T_3, triiodothyronine; and TSH, thryrotropin.
†Fisher exact test.
‡Measured before antithyroid treatment.
§A toxic adenoma was not included.
‖Postoperative serum TSH level was measured in 24 patients.

In conclusion, the tumor size of the majority of patients with thyroid cancer and concurrent hyperthyroidism is 1 cm or smaller. Cold nodules on thyroid scanning might suggest the presence of thyroid carcinoma in thyrotoxic patients. Age, sex, tumor size, extent of surgery, or ^{131}I ablation do not influence the prognosis. Patients with thyroid cancer with higher serum concentrations of T_3 or T_4 before antithyroid treatment have an aggressive tumor course as compared with those with lower concentrations.

Reprints: Tzu-Chieh Chao, MD, PhD, Department of Surgery, Chang Gung Memorial Hospital, 199 Tung Hwa North Rd, Taipei, Taiwan (e-mail: ischen01@ms15.hinet.net).

REFERENCES

1. Shapiro ST, Friedmann NB, Perzik SL, Catz B. Incidence of thyroid carcinoma in Graves' disease. *Cancer.* 1970;26:1261-1270.
2. Ozaki O, Ito K, Kobayashi K, Toshima K, Iwasaki H, Yashiro T. Thyroid carcinoma in Graves' disease. *World J Surg.* 1990;14:437-441.
3. Wahl RA, Goretzki P, Meybier H, Nitschke J, Linder M, Roher H-D. Coexistence of hyperthyroidism and thyroid cancer. *World J Surg.* 1982;6:385-390.
4. Rieger R, Pimpl W, Money S, Rettenbacher L, Galvan G. Hyperthyroidism and concurrent thyroid cancer. *Surgery.* 1989;106:6-10.
5. Behar R, Arganini M, Wu T-C, et al. Graves' disease and thyroid cancer. *Surgery.* 1986;100:1121-1127.
6. Belfiore A, Garofalo MR, Giuffrida D, et al. Increased aggressiveness of thyroid cancer in patients with Graves' disease. *J Clin Endocrinol Metab.* 1990;70:830-835.
7. Hales IB, McElduff A, Crummer P, et al. Does Graves' disease or thyrotoxicosis affect the prognosis of thyroid cancer. *J Clin Endocrinol Metab.* 1992;75:886-889.
8. Edmonds CJ, Tellez M. Hyperthyroidism and thyroid cancer. *Clin Endocrinol.* 1988;28:253-259.
9. Dumont JE, Lamy F, Roger P, Maenhaut C. Physiological and pathological regulation of thyroid cell proliferation and differentiation by thyrotropin and other factors. *Physiol Rev.* 1992;72:667-697.
10. Doniach I. The effect of radioactive iodine alone and in combination with methylthiouracil upon tumor production in the rat's thyroid gland. *Br J Cancer.* 1953;7:181-202.
11. Ichikawa Y, Saito E, Abe Y, Homma M, Muraki T, Ito K. Presence of TSH receptor in thyroid neoplasms. *J Clin Endocrinol Metab.* 1976;42:395-398.
12. Pujol P, Daures J-P, Nsakala N, Baldet L, Bringer J, Jaffiol C. Degree of thyrotropin suppression as a prognostic determination in differentiated thyroid cancer. *J Clin Endocrinol Metab.* 1996;81:4318-4323.
13. Rossi RL, Cady B, Silverman ML, et al. Surgically incurable well-differentiated thyroid carcinoma: prognostic factors and results of therapy. *Arch Surg.* 1988;123:569-574.
14. Simpson WJ, Panzarella T, Carruthers JS, Gospodarowicz MK, Sutcliffe SB. Papillary and follicular thyroid cancer: impact of treatment of 1578 patients. *Int J Radiat Oncol Biol Phys.* 1988;14:1063-1075.
15. Cunningham MP, Duda RB, Recant W, Chmiel JS, Sylvester J, Fremgen A. Survival discriminants for differentiated cancer. *Am J Surg.* 1990;160:344-347.
16. Rees Smith B, McLachlan SM, Furmaniak J. Autoantibodies to the thyrotropin receptor. *Endocr Rev.* 1988;9:106-121.
17. Sugino K, Mimura T, Ozaki O, et al. Early recurrence of hyperthyroidism in patients with Graves' disease treated by subtotal thyroidectomy. *World J Surg.* 1995;19:648-652.
18. Filetti S, Belfiore A, Amir SM, et al. The role of thyroid-stimulating antibodies of Graves' disease in differentiated thyroid cancer. *N Engl J Med.* 1988;318:753-759.
19. Di Paola R, Menzaghi C, De Filippis V, Corda D, Di Cerbo A. Cyclooxygenase-dependent thyroid cell proliferation induced by immunoglobulins from patients with Graves' disease. *J Clin Endocrinol Metab.* 1997;82:670-673.
20. Miki H, Oshimo K, Inoue H, et al. Diagnosis and surgical treatment of small papillary carcinomas of the thyroid gland. *J Surg Oncol.* 1993;54:78-81.
21. Allo MD, Christianson W, Koivunen D. Not all "occult" papillary carcinomas are "minimal." *Surgery.* 1988;104:971-976.
22. Wanebo HJ, Andrews W, Kaiser DL. Thyroid cancer: some basic considerations. *Am J Surg.* 1981;142:474-479.
23. Schroder DM, Chambors A, France CJ. Operative strategy for thyroid cancer: is total thyroidectomy worth the price? *Cancer.* 1986;58:2320-2328.
24. Farrar WB, Cooperman M, James AG. Surgical management of papillary and follicular carcinoma of the thyroid. *Ann Surg.* 1980;192:701-704.
25. Hay ID, Grant CS, van Heerden JA, et al. Papillary thyroid microcarcinoma: a study of 535 cases observed in a 50-year period. *Surgery.* 1992;112:1139-1147.
26. Clark OH, Levin K, Zeng Q-H, Greenspan FS, Siperstein A. Thyroid cancer: the case for total thyroidectomy. *Eur J Cancer Clin Oncol.* 1988;24:305-313.
27. Levin KE, Clark AH, Duh Q-Y, Demeure M, Siperstein AE, Clark OH. Reoperative thyroid surgery. *Surgery.* 1992;111:604-609.
28. Ley PB, Roberts JW, Symmonds RE Jr, et al. Safety and efficacy of total thyroidectomy for differentiated thyroid carcinoma: a 20-year review. *Am Surg.* 1993;59:110-114.
29. Hamming JF, Van de Velde CJ, Goslings BM, et al. Prognosis and morbidity after total thyroidectomy for papillary, follicular and medullary thyroid cancer. *Eur J Cancer Clin Oncol.* 1989;25:1317-1323.
30. Grant CS, Hay ID, Gough IR, Bergstralh EJ, Goellner JR, McConahey WM. Local recurrence in papillary thyroid carcinoma: is extent of surgical resection important? *Surgery.* 1988;104:954-962.
31. Vickery ALJ, Wang C-A, Walker AM. Treatment of intrathyroid papillary carcinoma of the thyroid. *Cancer.* 1987;60:2587-2595.
32. Van De Velde CJH, Hamming JF, Goslings BM, et al. Report of the consensus development conference on the management of differentiated thyroid cancer in the Netherlands. *Eur J Cancer Clin Oncol.* 1988;24:287-292.
33. Baldet L, Manderscheid JC, Glinoer D, et al. The management of differentiated thyroid cancer in Europe in 1988: results of an international survey. *Acta Endocrinol.* 1989;120:547-558.
34. Mazzaferri EL, Jhiang SM. Long-term impact of initial surgical and medical therapy on papillary and follicular thyroid cancer. *Am J Med.* 1994;97:418-428.
35. Attie JN, Bock G, Moskowitz GW, Margouleff D, Dubner S. Postoperative radioactive iodine evaluation of total thyroidectomy for thyroid carcinoma: reappraisal and therapeutic implications. *Head Neck.* 1992;14:297-302.
36. Schlumberger M, Parmentier C, de Vathaire F, Tubiana M. Iodine-131 and external radiation in the treatment of local and metastatic thyroid cancer. In: Falk SA, ed. *Thyroid Disease: Endocrinology, Surgery, Nuclear Medicine, and Radiotherapy.* 2nd ed. Philadelphia, Pa: Lippincott-Raven; 1997:601-617.

ORIGINAL ARTICLE

Subtotal Pancreatoduodenectomy

Use of a Defunctionalized Loop for Pancreatic Stump Drainage

John D. Papadimitriou, MD; Alex C. Fotopoulos, MD; Basil Smyrniotis, MD; Andreas A. Prahalias, MD; Georgia Kostopanagiotou, MD; Lila J. Papadimitriou, MD

Background: Since its introduction, pancreaticoduodenal resection for periampullary cancer has undergone numerous modifications. As a result, there has been a dramatic decline in the mortality rate. However, a high morbidity rate, mainly due to pancreatic fistula formation, is still reported.

Objective: To evaluate the results of the use of a defunctionalized jejunal loop in patients undergoing pancreatoduodenectomy to minimize both the frequency and severity of anastomotic leak.

Setting: Second Surgical Department, Athens University, Aretaieon Hospital, Athens, Greece.

Design: A series of retrospective cases from February 1990 to December 1997.

Patients: One hundred five patients who underwent pancreatoduodenectomy and had the pancreatic stump drained in a defunctionalized jejunal loop.

Methods: To avoid problems related to fistula formation due to erosion of the anastomoses from activated pancreatic enzymes, a defunctionalized jejunal loop was constructed and the pancreatic stump was invaginated into the end of this loop.

Results: Using the defunctionalized jejunal loop, the mean (± SD) hospitalization was 7.57 ± 1.42 days, the morbidity rate was 11.2%, and the mortality rate was 0.95%.

Conclusions: A modification of pancreatoduodenectomy for the treatment of pancreatic cancer resulted in an improvement in the immediate results of subtotal pancreatoduodenectomy. Careful detachment of the posterior surface of the pancreas from the anterior surface of the portal vein and performance of pancreaticojejunal anastomosis to a defunctionalized jejunal loop results in lower mortality and morbidity rates, thus making pancreatoduodenectomy a safe procedure.

Arch Surg. 1999;134:135-139

From the Second Surgical Department (Drs J.D. Papadimitriou, Fotopoulos, Smyrniotis, and Prahalias) and the Anesthesiology Unit (Drs Kostopanagiotou and L.J. Papadimitriou), University of Athens, Aretaieon Hospital, Athens, Greece.

INCREASING AT an annual rate of 6% for men and 3% for women, pancreatic carcinoma is the seventh leading cause of cancer death in Greece.[1] Pancreatoduodenectomy became the operation of choice after Whipple and colleagues[2] described this procedure.

A surgeon performing pancreatoduodenectomies for cancer of the head of the pancreas faces the following main problems: (1) how to perform a safe dissection between the neck of the pancreas and the portal and superior mesenteric veins, and (2) how to seal the pancreaticojejunal anastomosis.

After the 1960s, many authors[3,4] suggested that this procedure should be abandoned owing to a high operative mortality rate ranging from 20% to 40% and postoperative morbidity rates ranging from 40% to 60%. Leakage at the pancreaticojejunostomy is responsible for approximately 30% of operative mortality.[3,5,6] A decline in both mortality and morbidity rates has recently been reported.[7]

In the present study, we report the results of a technique that secures and simplifies subtotal pancreatoduodenectomy.

RESULTS

The mortality rate in this series was 0.95%. Since submission of this article, 10 more cases have been added with no deaths, reducing the mortality rate to 0.86%. The patient who died was 72 years old and had developed acute respiratory distress syndrome and multiple organ failure.

Twelve patients had various complications (morbidity rate, 11.42%). Bile leakage was noticed in 2 patients (1.9%). Six patients had septic complications: 3 (2.85%) had an abscess formation, which was treated by computed tomography–guided drainage and the other 3 (2.85%)

PATIENTS AND METHODS

CLINICAL FEATURES

The hospital records of 105 consecutive patients (61 men and 44 women with a mean age of 54.1 years [range, 28-76 years]) who underwent subtotal pancreatoduodenectomy for pancreatic cancer between February 1990 and December 1997 at the Second Surgical Department of the University of Athens, Aretaieon Hospital, Athens, Greece, were reviewed.

The most common symptom was weight loss (mean [± SD], 8.4 ± 1.1 kg), which occurred in 79 patients (75.2%), followed by jaundice, which occurred in 74 patients (70.5%). Fifty-four patients (51.4%) experienced pain. The mean (± SD) duration of symptoms was 6.9 ± 0.8 weeks.

DIAGNOSIS

Various diagnostic modalities were used to preoperatively evaluate the patients. During the early period, computed tomography, endoscopic retrograde cholangiopancreatography, or percutaneous transhepatic cholangiography were the most common imaging procedures used. From 1992 onward, numerous patients underwent magnetic resonance imaging, magnetic resonance cholangiopancreatography, and transoperative ultrasonography.

OPERATIVE PROCEDURES

Resection

After the duodenum was mobilized and the head of the pancreas thoroughly palpated, a firm decision with regard to operability was made; to this end, transoperative ultrasonography gave additional information (**Figure 1**). Then, the common bile duct or the common hepatic duct as well as the gastroduodenal artery were dissected and divided. Next, the lower stump of the bile duct and the gastroduodenal artery were retracted downward (**Figure 2**), and, under direct vision, the anterior surface of the portal vein was dissected from the duodenum and the posterior surface neck of the pancreas. Any small veins were carefully ligated.

As the operation continues, dissection of the lower part of the surface of the neck of the pancreas and the superior mesenteric vein was completed by inserting the index finger downward (**Figure 3**). Following this maneuver, division of the pancreas was an easy task.

Reconstruction

After the cut surface of the distal pancreatic stump was prepared, an isolated jejunal loop was created and a Roux-en-Y anastomosis was performed (**Figure 4**). The pancreaticojejunal anastomosis was attached to a defunctionalized jejunal loop to provide a total diversion of the pancreatic juice from the hepaticojejunal and gastrojejunal anastomoses. The pancreaticojejunal anastomosis was done in an end-to-end fashion in 2 layers so that the pancreatic stump could be intussuscepted into the free end of the jejunal loop (**Figure 5**). The cut end of the pancreatic duct must be anastomosed using 4 to 6 interrupted polyglactin 910 (Vicryl; Ethicon Inc, Somerville, NJ) suture stitches to the intestinal mucosa using loops when necessary.

Anesthetic Management

Careful anesthetic management was of paramount importance. In addition to thorough clinical and laboratory investigation, preoperative care included correction of coagulopathy, nutritional and electrolyte abnormalities, as well as measures for autotransfusion.

In most cases epidural analgesia was planned and insertion of the catheter prior to induction of anesthesia was necessary. Since pancreatic surgery may be associated with major fluid shift, monitoring was required, especially in patients with cardiopulmonary compromise and renal dysfunction.

developed wound infection. One patient (0.95%) had upper gastrointestinal tract bleeding and another (0.95%) had intra-abdominal bleeding; on reoperation, however, no visible bleeding was found. One patient developed renal insufficiency (0.95%), and another patient developed respiratory insuffiency (0.95%).

In 12 patients, various other complications, such as fever of unknown origin, cystitis, pleural effusion, superficial thrombophlebitis, transient renal insufficiency, and paralytic ileus, were recorded.

Some patients had more than 1 complication. No leaking from the pancreaticojejunal anastomosis was observed. The mean (± SD) length of hospitalization of the patients was 7.57 ± 1.42 days.

COMMENT

Since 1935, when Whipple et al[2] documented a 2-stage pancreatoduodenectomy for ampullary cancer, this procedure[8] became the treatment of choice for pancreatic cancer. However, enthusiasm waned during the 1960s, when numerous centers reported operative mortality rates as high as 40%[7] and morbidity rates ranging from 40% to 60%.[4,9,10]

In the last few years, there has been a dramatic drop in perioperative mortality, which has been reported to be in the range of 1% to 2%, creating renewed interest in subtotal pancreatoduodenectomy.[11,12] Better perioperative care, accumulative experience on the part of surgeons, refinement of surgical materials, improved anesthesiologic management, and a better understanding of patients' nutritional needs have all contributed to the decline of perioperative mortality rates.[7]

Although mortality rates are within an acceptable range, high complication rates still remain a problem and range from 25% to 39%.[7,12,13] Pancreatic fistula presents the most frequent postoperative complication, with an incidence of 5% to 20%.[7] Leakage of the pancreaticojejunal anastomosis has been reported to account for the majority of deaths.[3,6] Hicks and

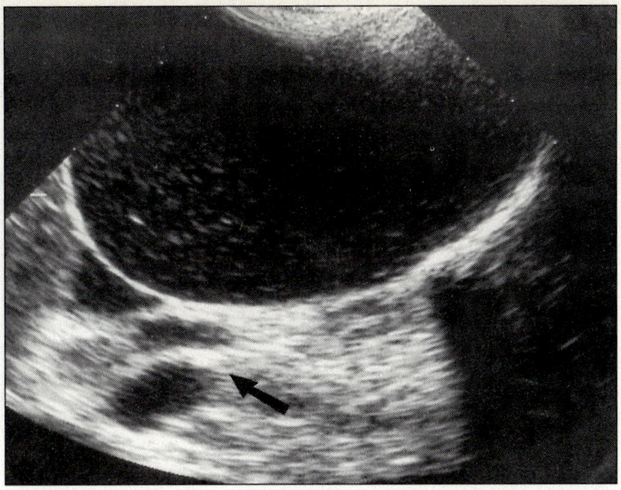

Figure 1. *Transoperative ultrasonography may be helpful in determining operability. Arrow shows relation between the portal vein and pancreas.*

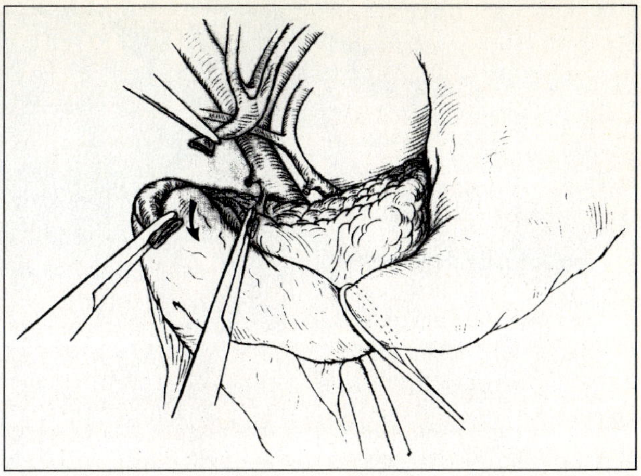

Figure 2. *After the common hepatic duct and the gastroduodenal artery have been divided, the duodenum and pancreas are retracted downward (arrow) so that, under direct vision, the portal vein is dissected from the neck of the pancreas.*

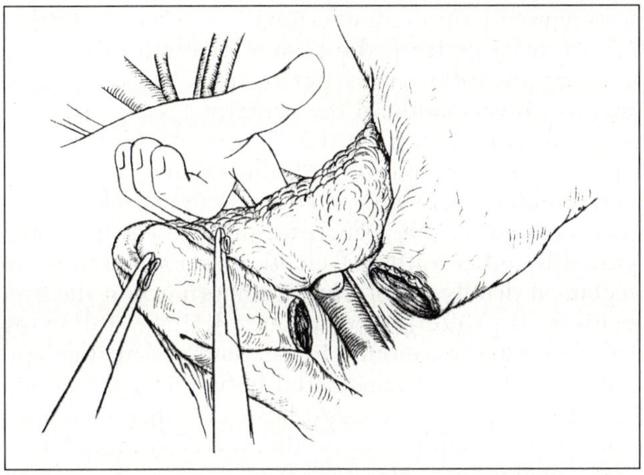

Figure 3. *Dissection of the posterior face of the pancreas from the portal vein is completed using the index finger.*

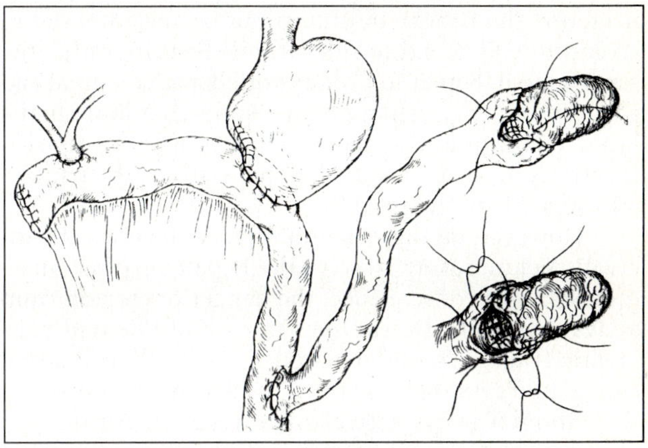

Figure 4. *Reconstruction is performed using a Roux-en-Y loop. The pancreaticojejunal anastomosis is accomplished by intussuscepting the pancreatic stump into the defunctionalized jejunal loop end.*

Brooks[6] reported that in patients undergoing pancreatoduodenectomy, the operative mortality rate was 18%, and this was mainly due to leakage from the anastomosis of the pancreatic remnant. In addition, Monge et al[5] reported an overall operative mortality of 12%, and 50% of the deaths were due to bleeding; they concluded that the greatest postoperative danger was from autodigestion of the tissues near the pancreaticojejunal stoma with resultant hemorrhage. Lerut et al[14] reported that pancreatic fistula was the most common and most important complication in pancreatoduodenectomy, accounting for 75% of early complications. Moreover, pancreatic fistula accounted for 55% of postoperative deaths. Apart from bleeding, pancreatic fistula was also implicated in infective complications.[12] Intra-abdominal sepsis, which was probably related to biliary or pancreatic leaks, was responsible for most of the fatalities after pancreatoduodenectomy.[15]

The aim of the many modifications of the procedure introduced by Whipple et al[2] is the control of the anastomotic leak. Placement of drains to control the anastomotic leak in the area of pancreatic anastomosis may minimize morbidity.[7] However, intensive supportive measures, namely, parenteral nutrition and daily care of the skin around the tube to avoid skin excoriation, are necessary.[7] The use of somatostatin[16] and octreotide[17] is an additional measure in the armamentarium of the physician managing pancreatic fistula.[16] Even reoperation and complete resection of the pancreatic remnant have been suggested[18] in cases of prolonged pancreatic drainage. However, the golden rule in surgery is to anticipate rather than treat a complication. Operative management of the pancreatic duct remains the most important factor in preventing complications after pancreatoduodenectomy. A number of techniques to secure the pancreaticojejunostomy have been described in the literature: an oversewn pancreatic duct resulted in a 50% to 79% rate of fistula occurrence,[19-21] and stenting of the pancreatic duct is still a useful technique,[19] resulting in a lower mortality rate. Because of the high mortality associated with treatment of complicated pancreatic leakage,[14,19] the morbidity rate remains high.[11]

Much attention has been paid to the management of pancreaticojejunal anastomosis, aiming at the prevention of this complication. In subtotal pancreatoduode-

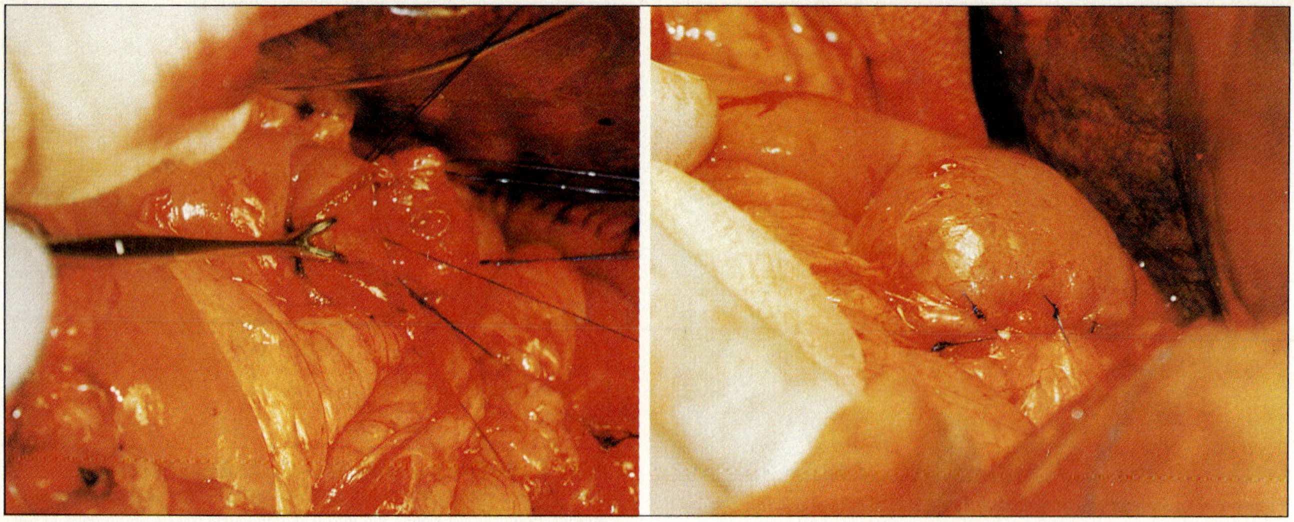

Figure 5. *Pancreaticojejunal anastomosis in the surgical field. Left, The first posterior layer. Right, After intussusception is completed.*

nectomy, the pancreatic stump can be anastomosed in an end-to-end or end-to-side fashion, by using either the same jejunal loop in continuity with hepaticojejunal and gastrointestinal anastomoses or a Roux-en-Y loop. In the latter technique, the hepatic duct is usually anastomosed to an isolated jejunal loop distally to the pancreaticojejunal anastomosis.[22]

However, all these methods place the critical pancreaticojejunostomy close to the hepaticojejunal anastomosis. As a consequence, the danger of erosion from activated pancreatic enzymes in case of bile and pancreatic leakage is not obviated. Some authors[23] advocate pancreaticogastrostomy to avoid activation of trypsinogen to its active form, trypsin. Additional advantages of this technique include the thickness of the gastric wall and the anatomic proximity of the 2 organs. However, according to Yeo et al,[24] the incidence of leakage in pancreaticogastrostomy is not lower compared with pancreaticojejunostomy. The incidence of pancreatic fistula for the former was 11.7%, compared with 12.3% for the latter. Mason[25] concluded that pancreaticogastrostomy is a satisfactory alternative technique that is similar to pancreaticojejunostomy for deconstruction after pancreatoduodenectomy.

Some investigators[26,27] have advocated total pancreatectomy for carcinoma of the head of the pancreas to eliminate the morbidity associated with pancreaticojejunostomy. Nonetheless, in a later study[12] it was proved that this procedure was associated with a 14% mortality rate and a morbidity rate as high as 59%. Herter et al[15] stated that in comparison to pancreatoduodenectomy, total pancreatectomy had a significantly worse prognosis, with a complication rate of 42% and a postoperative mortality rate of 23%.

Total pancreatectomy may be reserved only for patients whose tumors are spread across the line of resection or whose pancreatic remnant is friable and thus predisposed to complications.[28]

Our present data indicate that a significant improvement in the morbidity rate may be achieved by anastomosing the pancreatic stump to a defunctionalized jejunal loop in an end-to-end fashion. To further secure leakage from the pancreaticojejunostomy, a 2-layer anastomosis is performed; the technique involves invagination of the pancreatic stump into the isolated jejunal loop. In the 2-layer anastomosis, the outer layer is completed with interrupted silk sutures and the inner layer with interrupted absorbable sutures incorporated into the pancreatic duct, as has been suggested by other authors.[7] Gentleness and attention to technical details are of utmost importance in the prevention of prolonged pancreatic drainage following pancreatoduodenectomy. End-to-end pancreaticojejunal invagination is considered to be the safest option even in patients at high risk; however, when combined with hepaticojejunostomy, the rate of complications and reoperations is about 6%.[21]

The low morbidity and mortality rates in this series are attributed to the safeguards taken while dissecting the posterior surface of the pancreas from the anterior surface of the portal vein and the superior mesenteric vein, the integrity of the pancreaticojejunal anastomosis, which was confirmed by magnetic resonance cholangiopancreatography, and to the diversion of the pancreatic secretions to the intestinal tract away from other anastomoses.

Reprints: John D. Papadimitriou, MD, 8 Iassiou St, GR-115 21 Athens, Greece (e-mail: johnpap@aretaieio.uoa.gr).

REFERENCES

1. Katsougianni K, Kogevinas M, Dontas N, Maissonneuve P, Boyle P, Trichopoulos D. *Mortality From Malignant Neoplasms in Greece.* Athens, Greece: Hellenic Anticancer Society; 1990:20.
2. Whipple AO, Parsons WB, Mullins CR. Treatment of carcinoma of the ampulla of Vater. *Ann Surg.* 1935;102:763-779.
3. Gudjonsson B, Livstone EM, Spiro HM. Cancer of the pancreas: diagnostic accuracy and survival statistics. *Cancer.* 1978;42:2494-2506.
4. Lansing PB, Blalock JB, Oschner JL. Pancreaticoduodenectomy: a retrospective review, 1949-1967. *Ann Surg.* 1972;28:79-86.
5. Monge JJ, Judd ES, Gage RP. Radical pancreaticoduodenectomy: a 22-year experience with complications, mortality rate and survival rate. *Ann Surg.* 1964; 160:711-719.

6. Hicks RE, Brooks JR. Total pancreatectomy for ductal carcinoma. *Surg Gynecol Obstet.* 1971;133:16-20.
7. Lillemoe KD. Current management of pancreatic carcinoma. *Ann Surg.* 1995; 221:133-148.
8. Peters JH, Carfey LC. Historical review of pancreaticoduodenectomy. *Am J Surg.* 1991;161:219-225.
9. Gilsdorf RB, Spanos P. Factors influencing morbidity and mortality in pancreaticoduodenectomy. *Ann Surg.* 1973;177:332-337.
10. Shapiro TM. Adenocarcinoma of the pancreas: a statistical analysis of biliary bypass vs Whipple resection in good risk patients. *Ann Surg.* 1975;182:715-721.
11. Cameron JL, Crist DW, Sitzmann JV, et al. Factors influencing survival following pancreaticoduodenectomy for pancreatic cancer. *Am J Surg.* 1991;161:120-125.
12. Grace PA, Pitt HA, Tompkins RK, DenBesten L, Longmire WP Jr. Decreased morbidity and mortality after pancreatoduodenectomy. *Am J Surg.* 1986;151:141-148.
13. Crist DW, Sitzmann JV, Cameron JL. Improved hospital morbidity, mortality and survival after the Whipple procedure. *Ann Surg.* 1987;206:358-365.
14. Lerut JP, Gianello PR, Othe JB, Kestens PJ. Pancreaticoduodenal resection: surgical experience and evaluation of risk factors in 103 patients. *Ann Surg.* 1984; 199:432-437.
15. Herter FP, Cooperman AM, Ahlborn TN, Antinori C. Surgical experience with pancreatic and periampullary cancer. *Ann Surg.* 1982;195:274-281.
16. Kwan D, Aufses AH. Short-term administration of SMS-201-995 in the management of an external pancreatic fistula. *Am J Gastroenterol.* 1989;84:326-328.
17. Büchler M, Friess H, Klempa I, et al. Role of octreotide in the prevention of postoperative complications following pancreatic resection. *Am J Surg.* 1992;163: 125-131.
18. van Berger Henegouwen MI, De Wit LT, Van Gulik TM, Obertop H, Gouma DJ. Incidence, risk factors and treatment of pancreatic leakage after pancreaticoduodenectomy: drainage versus resection of the pancreatic remnant. *J Am Coll Surg.* 1997;185:18-24.
19. Aston SJ, Longmire WP Jr. Pancreaticoduodenal resection: twenty years' experience. *Arch Surg.* 1973;106:813-817.
20. Papachristou DN, D'Agostino H, Fortner JG. Ligation of the pancreatic duct in pancreatectomy. *Br J Surg.* 1980;67:260-262.
21. Marcus SG, Cohen H, Ranson JHC. Optimal management of the pancreatic remnant after pancreaticoduodenectomy. *Ann Surg.* 1995;221:635-648.
22. Ligidakis NJ, Brummelkap WH. A new approach for the reconstruction of continuity of the alimentary tract after pancreaticoduodenectomy. *Surg Gynecol Obstet.* 1988;160:453-458.
23. Pikarsky AJ, Muggia-Sullam M, Eid A, et al. Pancreaticogastrostomy after pancreatoduodenectomy. *Arch Surg.* 1997;132:296-299.
24. Yeo CJ, Cameron JL, Maher MM, et al. A prospective randomized trial of pancreaticogastrostomy versus pancreaticojejunostomy or pancreaticoduodenectomy. *Ann Surg.* 1995;222:580-588.
25. Mason GR. Invited Commentary. *Arch Surg.* 1997;132:299.
26. Romine WH, Priestley JT, Judd ES, King JN. Total pancreatectomy. *Ann Surg.* 1970;172-595-604.
27. Brooks JR, Calebras JM. Cancer of the pancreas: palliative operation: Whipple procedure or total pancreatectomy? *Am J Surg.* 1976;131:516-520.
28. Trede M. Treatment of pancreatic carcinoma: the surgeon's dilemma. *Br J Surg.* 1987;74:79-80.

IN OTHER AMA JOURNALS

JAMA

Mortality Differences Between Men and Women Following First Myocardial Infarction

Jaume Marrugat, MD, PhD; Joan Sala, MD, PhD; Rafel Masiá, MD; Marco Pavesi, PhD; Ginés Sanz, MD, PhD; Vicente Valle, MD; Lluis Molina, MD, PhD; Lluis Serés, MD; Roberto Elosua, MD, PhD; for the RESCATE Investigators

Context: Mortality after acute myocardial infarction is worse in women than in men, even after adjustment for comorbidity and age dissimilarities between sexes.
Objective: To assess the influence of sex on survival after acute myocardial infarction.
Design: Inception cohort obtained in a prospective registry of patients with acute myocardial infarction from 1992 through 1994.
Setting: Four teaching hospitals in northeastern Spain.
Patients: All consecutive patients aged 80 years or younger with first acute myocardial infarction. A total of 331 women and 1129 men were included.
Main Outcome Measure: Survival at 28 days and mortality or readmission at 6 months.
Results: Women were older (mean, 68.6 vs 60.1 years), presented more often with diabetes (52.9% vs 23.3%), hypertension (63.9% vs 42.3%), or previous angina (44.6% vs 37.4%), and developed more severe myocardial infarctions than men (acute pulmonary edema or cardiogenic shock occurred in 24.8% of women and 10.5% of men) (all $P<.02$). Men were more likely than women to receive thrombolytic therapy (41.3% vs 23.9%; $P<.001$), but rates of percutaneous transluminal angioplasty and coronary artery bypass graft surgery at 28 days were similar among men and women. The 28-day mortality rate was significantly higher among women (18.5% for women, 8.3% for men; $P<.001$). Revascularization procedures at 6 months were performed in a similar proportion of women and men. However, women had higher 6-month mortality rates (25.8% in women, 10.8% in men; $P<.001$) and readmission rates (23.3% for women, 12.2% for men; $P<.001$). After adjustment, women had greater risk of death than men at 28 days (odds ratio [OR], 1.72; 95% confidence interval [CI], 1.12-2.65) and at 6 months (OR, 1.73; 95% CI, 1.18-2.52).
Conclusions: In this study population, women experienced more lethal and severe first acute myocardial infarction than men, regardless of comorbidity, age, or previous angina.(*1998;280:1405-1409*)

Reprints: Jaume Marrugat, MD, PhD, Unitat de Lipids i Epidemiologia Cardiovascular, Institut Municipal d'Investigació Mèdica, Dr Aiguader 80, E-08003 Barcelona, Spain (e-mail: jaume@imim.es).

ORIGINAL ARTICLE

Bronchoscopic Staging of Squamous Cell Carcinoma of the Upper Thoracic Esophagus

Alessandro Baisi, MD; Luigi Bonavina, MD; Alberto Peracchia, MD

Objective: To identify bronchoscopic findings that predict resectability of squamous cell carcinoma of the upper thoracic esophagus.

Design: Tracheobronchoscopy was performed in patients with squamous cell carcinoma of the thoracic esophagus to assess the infiltration of the tracheobronchial tree by the tumor and predict the resectability. Bronchoscopic records were matched with clinical outcome and intraoperative findings.

Setting: University hospital, tertiary care referral center.

Patients: A total of 113 patients with supracarinal esophageal carcinoma underwent bronchoscopy as part of the preoperative staging. In 47 patients the bronchoscopy was repeated after a regimen of neoadjuvant chemotherapy.

Intervention: A total of 160 bronchoscopies performed by the same operator.

Main Outcome Measures: Bronchoscopic records matched with clinical outcome and intraoperative findings.

Results: Including patients before and after neoadjuvant chemotherapy, 27 of the 46 with no bronchoscopic abnormalities were operated on: in 24 (89%) of them radical surgical resection was possible. Among the 22 patients with a slight compression on the tracheobronchial tree admitted to surgery, a radical surgical resection was possible in 20 cases (91%). In none of the 5 patients with compression/deviation associated with fixation of the tracheobronchial tree but no mucosal infiltration who underwent surgery was a radical surgical resection possible because of tracheobronchial infiltration.

Conclusions: Compression of the tracheobronchial tree does not necessarily mean infiltration by esophageal carcinoma. If the compression is slight and the mobility of the tracheobronchial tree is normal, a radical esophagectomy is possible in 91% of patients.

Arch Surg. 1999;134:140-143

From the Institute of General Surgery and Oncological Surgery, Università degli Studi di Milano-Ospedale Maggiore Policlinico, Milan, Italy.

BETWEEN 40% and 60% of esophageal carcinomas are unresectable at presentation.[1,2] A number of diagnostic tools such as barium swallow, upper gastrointestinal tract endoscopy, bronchoscopy, computed tomographic scan, magnetic resonance imaging, and endoscopic ultrasonography are available to stage the tumor and to establish the involvement of any of the surrounding mediastinal structures with the disease.[3,4] If involvement exists, a radical surgical resection is unlikely.

Bronchoscopy plays an important role in staging esophageal carcinoma by assessing whether the tumor involves the tracheobronchial tree. The Consensus Conference of the International Society for Diseases of the Esophagus held in Milan, Italy, in August 1995 suggested that all patients with squamous cell carcinoma of the supracarinal esophagus undergo bronchoscopy as part of the disease's staging.[5]

However, to our knowledge, very little has been written about the incidence and degree of bronchoscopic abnormalities in patients with esophageal carcinoma and how these findings relate to surgical resectability of the tumor and the patient's clinical outcome.[1,3,6-8] Our purpose was to present a classification of bronchoscopic findings that we found able to predict tumor resectability and patient outcome in patients with supracarinal esophageal carcinoma.

RESULTS

In 2 patients (1.8%) a synchronous bronchogenic carcinoma was found. The category of bronchoscopic abnormalities

PATIENTS, MATERIALS, AND METHODS

Between November 1, 1992, and May 31, 1997, 113 patients (97 men, 16 women; mean age, 59.8 years [age range, 19-80 years]) with supracarinal esophageal carcinoma underwent bronchoscopy as part of the preoperative staging that also included barium esophagogram, upper gastrointestinal tract endoscopy, and chest computed tomographic scan. In 47 patients, the bronchoscopy was repeated after a regimen of neoadjuvant chemotherapy (CHT). A total of 160 bronchoscopies were performed.

A flexible videobronchoscope (Olympus CV-200, Olympus Optical Co, Ltd, Tokyo, Japan) was used. The examination was performed under topical anesthesia by spraying 10 to 20 mL of 2% lidocaine. No systemic premedication was used. Pulse oximetry was performed in all patients. Supplemental oxygen was seldom necessary. All bronchoscopies were performed by the same operator (A.B.). The examination was always extended to the peripheral bronchial tree to exclude the presence of a synchronous bronchogenic carcinoma. No complications occurred.

Bronchoscopic findings were graded according to the following classification. Category I: no abnormalities. Category IIa: slight compression on the posterior wall of the trachea or left bronchus; normal mobility of the tracheobronchial wall; and parallel and regular longitudinal folds of the pars membranacea. Category IIb: impingement or deviation of the trachea or left bronchus or widening of the carina, with or without narrowing, associated with a reduction in mobility during breathing and coughing (ie, fixation of the involved tracheobronchial segment). The mucosa is still normal, but the longitudinal folds of the pars membranacea may be widened. Category III: mucosal irregularities or tracheoesophageal fistula. Mucosal brushing or biopsies were performed whenever mucosal abnormalities were suspected; a positive finding for cancer cells on specimens graded the patient as having a category III classification.

Bronchoscopic records were matched with clinical outcome and intraoperative findings.

was related to the length of the tumor measured on the barium swallow; results of this test are reported in **Table 1**. The sites of tracheobronchial abnormalities are as follows:

Site of Lesion	No. (%) of Patients
Trachea carina	41 (25.6)
Left bronchus	41 (25.6)
Left bronchus + trachea	31 (19.3)
Right bronchus	1 (0.6)
Right bronchus + trachea	2 (1.2)
None	44 (27.5)

Bronchoscopic findings of the 113 patients with squamous cell carcinoma of the supracarinal thoracic esophagus who underwent bronchoscopy at first observation were graded according to the category classification given in the "Patients, Materials, and Methods" section: 33 cases (30%) were in category I; 17 (15%), in category IIa; 57 (50%), in category IIb; and 6 (5%), in category III.

Table 1. Length of the Esophageal Tumor and Category of Bronchoscopic Abnormalities

Length, mm	Total No.	Category, No. (%)			
		I	IIa	IIb	III
≤50	**75**	30 (65)	23 (66)	20 (38)	2 (25)
>50	**85**	16 (35)	12 (34)	51 (72)	6 (75)

Bronchoscopic staging was related to clinical outcome (**Table 2**). Fifteen patients with the category I grade were operated on, and in 14 a radical resection was performed. Six patients with the category IIa grade underwent surgery, and in all a radical resection was possible. One patient with the category IIb grade underwent surgery; a nonradical resection was done because of tracheobronchial infiltration.

Forty-seven of the 113 patients underwent neoadjuvant CHT. After the treatment, patients again underwent bronchoscopy (**Table 3**). Thirteen of them were classified as having category I; 18, category IIa; 14, category IIb; and 2, category III grades (**Figure**). Twelve patients with a category I and 16 with a category IIa classification were operated on and in 10 and 14, respectively, a radical resection was possible. Four patients with a category IIb classification were operated on and in none was a radical resection possible.

On the whole, including patients before and after neoadjuvant CHT, 27 of the 46 staged as category I were operated on: in 24 (89%) of them, radical surgical resection was possible; in 3 (11%), a nonradical resection as a result of aortic infiltration was done. Among the 22 patients staged as having a category IIa grade who were admitted to surgery, a radical surgical resection was possible in 20 cases (91%), while a nonradical surgical resection was done in 2 (9%) because of aortic[1] or tracheobronchial[1] infiltration. In none of the 5 patients with a category IIb classification who underwent surgery was a radical surgical resection possible because of tracheobronchial infiltration.

COMMENT

Bronchoscopy allows direct inside visualization of the tracheobronchial tree and plays a key role in evaluating its involvement by carcinoma of the thoracic esophagus.[1,5,6] In this report, we did not consider patients with infracarinal squamous cell carcinoma or adenocarcinoma because in these patients bronchoscopy is seldom performed.[5]

In 1984, Choi et al[1] proposed a classification of bronchoscopic findings in patients with esophageal carcinoma. This classification includes patients with no abnormalities in the category I, those with impingement and no mucosal changes in the category II, and those with mucosal invasion in the category III classifications.[1,3] There is no doubt as to the surgical

Table 2. Bronchoscopic Staging Related to Clinical Outcome and Intraoperative Findings of Patients Who Underwent Bronchoscopy at First Observation for Squamous Cell Carcinoma of the Supracarinal Thoracic Esophagus

Bronchoscopic Staging Category	Total No.	Not Operated on (Age or Poor General Condition)	Not Operated on (Local Advanced or Distant Metastases)	Not Operated on (Bronchial Carcinoma)	Neoadjuvant Chemotherapy	Radical Resection	Nonradical Resection (Aorta)	Nonradical Resection (Tracheobronchial)
I	**33**	12	3	1	2	14	1	0
IIa	**17**	4	3	0	4	6	0	0
IIb	**57**	5	10	1	40	0	0	1
III	**6**	0	5	0	1	0	0	0

Table 3. Bronchoscopic Staging Related to Clinical Outcome and Intraoperative Findings of Patients With Supracarinal Esophageal Carcinoma Who Underwent Bronchoscopy After a Neoadjuvant Chemotherapy Regimen

Bronchoscopic Staging After Neoadjuvant Chemotherapy, Category	Total No.	Not Operated on (Age or Poor General Condition)	Not Operated on (Local Advanced or Distant Metastases)	Not Operated on (Bronchial Carcinoma)	Radical Resection	Nonradical Resection (Aorta)	Nonradical Resection (Tracheobronchial)
I	**13**	0	1	0	10	2	0
IIa	**18**	1	1	0	14	1	1
IIb	**14**	0	10	0	0	0	4*
III	**2**	0	2	0	0	0	0

** Two explorative thoracotomies.*

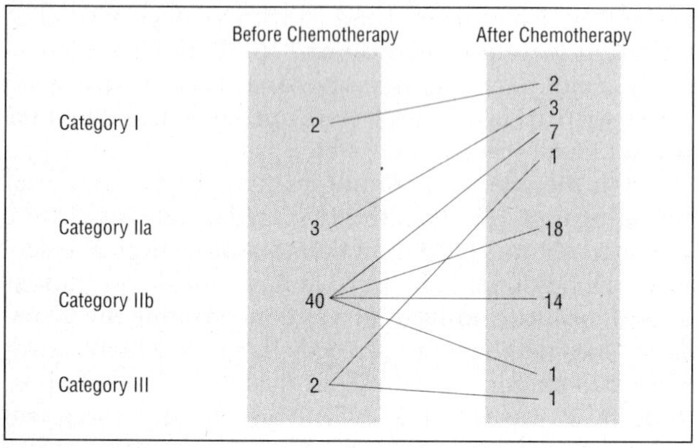

Bronchoscopic findings in patients with squamous cell carcinoma before and after neoadjuvant chemotherapy.

indications in patients with category I and in those with category III classifications. Conversely, category II includes a large group of patients with evidence of impingement and no mucosal invasion. As stated by Choi et al[1] in their original article, the likelihood of performing a surgical radical resection in these patients is open to question because the impingement can be because of either a simple compression with no infiltration of the neoplastic mass that is adjacent to the tracheobronchial tree or early infiltration.[1,3] In the former instance, a surgical radical resection can be performed; in the latter, this is unlikely. Since 1992 we divided category II into 2 subcategories: IIa and IIb. In category IIa we included patients with simple compression and no tumorous infiltration of the tracheobronchial tree. This group of patients can be identified because the compression on the involved tracheobronchial tree is usually slight and its mobility is normal. In category IIb we included those patients with compression in which the fixation of the tracheobronchial tree suggests tumorous invasion. Other abnormalities that classify patients as having the category IIb grade are widening of the carina and deviation of the trachea or bronchi, with or without narrowing.

To assess the value of this modified classification, we related bronchoscopic results to clinical outcome and to intraoperative findings of patients who underwent surgery. As expected, a radical resection was possible in most of the patients with a category I classification who underwent surgery. In those patients in whom a surgical radical resection was not feasible, it was because of infiltration of mediastinal structures other than the tracheobronchial tree. Also in patients with category IIa grade, the infiltration of the tracheobronchial tree at surgical exploration was very rare, thus demonstrating that in these patients esophageal carcinoma had compressed but not infiltrated the tracheobronchial tree, as suggested by its normal mobility. Conversely, only 5 patients with category IIb staging underwent surgery, and a surgical radical resection was never possible because of tracheobronchial infiltration. The indicators for surgery were findings seen on the computed tomographic scan or the young age of the patient.

According to our experience, category IIa identifies a subgroup of patients with fairly advanced tumor in which the tracheobronchial tree is not yet involved and a radical resection is possible. Their clinical outcome and intraoperative findings are similar to those of patients with no abnormalities at bronchoscopic examination (category I). It must be emphasized that only 17 of the 113 patients who underwent bronchoscopy at first observation were included in category IIa. Patients with a category IIa classification have been seen more frequently as a result of downstaging after neoadjuvant CHT. In this latter group of patients, the chances of a surgical radical resection have been the same as in patients classified as having category IIa staging at first observation.

The length of the esophageal tumor seems poorly related to the category of bronchoscopic findings.[6] Some carcinomas have a tendency to infiltrate surrounding structures in the early stage of development, regardless of their overall length. As expected, the sites esophageal carcinoma most frequently involved have been the trachea and the left main bronchus.

The results of this study show that bronchoscopy is very useful in the tumor staging of patients with esophageal carcinoma. Compression of the tracheobronchial tree at bronchoscopic examination does not necessarily mean infiltration by esophageal carcinoma. There is a group of patients (those with a category IIa classification) in whom the tracheobronchial tree is only compressed and not infiltrated by the tumor, thus making a radical resection possible. Conversely, in patients with a category IIb classification, there is a frank infiltration of the tracheobronchial tree and a radical resection is unlikely. These patients can be downstaged by appropriate neoadjuvant CHT that would then make radical resection feasible. Accurate bronchoscopic examination with special attention to the mobility of the tracheobronchial tree allows the distinction to be made between patients with category IIa and those with category IIb classifications with a high degree of accuracy, even after neoadjuvant CHT.

Reprints: Alessandro Baisi, MD, Istituto di Chirurgia Generale ed Oncologia Chirurgica, Università degli Studi di Milano-Ospedale Maggiore Policlinico, Via F. Sforza, 35 20122 Milan, Italy (e-mail: PeracchiaAlberto @unimi.it).

REFERENCES

1. Choi TK, Siu FS, Lam K, Wong J. Bronchoscopy and carcinoma of the esophagus, I: findings of bronchoscopy in carcinoma of the esophagus. *Am J Surg.* 1984; 147:757-759.
2. Mandard AM, Chalse J, Villedieu B, et al. Autopsy findings in 111 cases of esophageal cancer. *Cancer.* 1981;48:329-335.
3. Choi TK, Siu FS, Lam K, Wong J. Bronchoscopy and carcinoma of the esophagus, II: carcinoma of the esophagus with tracheobronchial involvement. *Am J Surg.* 1984;147:760-762.
4. Mori SM, Kasai M, Watanabe T, Shibuya I. Preoperative assessment of resectability for carcinoma of the thoracic esophagus. *Ann Surg.* 1979;190: 100-105.
5. Bumm R. Staging and risk analysis in esophageal carcinoma. *Dis Esophagus.* 1996;9(suppl 1):20-29.
6. Benchimol D, Mouroux J, Limouse B, Bernard JL, Lemoigne F, Richelme H. Que faut-il attendre de la fibroscopie tracheo-bronchique dans le bilan d'un cancer de l'oesofage? *Ann Chir.* 1990;44:471-474.
7. Watanabe A, Saka H, Sakai S, Hirao T, Hattori T, Shimokata K. Bronchoscopic and cytopathological findings of tracheobronchial involvement in esophageal carcinoma. *Endoscopy.* 1990;22:273-275.
8. Argyros GJ, Torrington KG. Fiberoptic bronchoscopy in the evaluation of newly diagnosed esophageal carcinoma. *Chest.* 1995;107:1447-14449.

Announcement

The *Archives of Surgery* will give priority review and early publication to seminal works. This policy will include basic science advancements in surgery and critically performed clinical research.

The Blood Supply of the Sternocleidomastoid Muscle and Its Clinical Implications

Antonius C. Kierner, MD; Martin Aigner, MD; Irmgard Zelenka, MD; Gunther Riedl; Martin Burian, MD

Background: The knowledge of the exact anatomy of the sternocleidomastoid (SCM) muscle and its nerve and blood supply must be considered a basic prerequisite for its use as a pedicle muscle flap.

Objective: To give an exact description of the courses and variability of all vessels supplying the SCM muscle.

Design: Anatomic analysis of all arteries supplying the SCM muscle.

Setting: The blood supply of the SCM muscle was studied by dissecting bilaterally the anterior regions of the neck of 31 perfusion-fixed human cadavers of both sexes aged 50 to 94 years (mean, 78 years).

Results: The blood supply to the SCM muscle can be divided into 3 parts: upper, middle, and lower. The upper third of the SCM muscle was found to be constantly supplied by branches of the occipital artery. According to their courses, these branches are categorized into types 1, 2a, 2b, and 3. The middle third of the SCM muscle receives its blood supply from a branch of the superior thyroid artery (42%), the external carotid artery (23%), or branches of both (27%). In most cases, the lower third of the muscle was supplied by a branch arising from the suprascapular artery (>80%), which has not been described until now.

Conclusions: In contrast to available data, the arterial blood supply of the lower third of the SCM muscle is constantly provided by a branch of the suprascapular artery. Since the SCM muscle flap is used in reconstructive surgery of the neck, the exact knowledge of its blood supply may help to minimize the risk of flap necrosis after surgical procedures.

Arch Surg. 1999;134:144-147

From the Institute of Anatomy 2 (Drs Kierner, Aigner, and Zelenka and Mr Riedl) and University Clinic of Otolaryngology (Dr Burian), University of Vienna, Vienna, Austria.

AT THE beginning of this century, Jianu[1] first described the applicability of the sternocleidomastoid (SCM) muscle for locoregional tissue transfer. Later, the SCM muscle had been used to reconstruct defects after resection of the mandible, the floor of the mouth, and the tongue, or to close pharyngoesophageal and tracheal fistulae.[2-8] The SCM muscle has offered vascular neck protection after radical lymph node dissection of the neck and also may help to prevent Frey syndrome in cases of facial paralysis.[9,10] There are several reasons for the application of the SCM muscle for tissue repair: (1) the muscle is richly vascularized, (2) it can be used as a myocutaneous flap, (3) each of its 2 heads can be shifted separately, and (4) the cosmetic results are satisfactory. However, the success rate of the SCM muscle flap lags behind other frequently used flaps in head and neck surgery.[10] It has been shown that necrosis of the SCM muscle flap due to insufficient perfusion limits its use in reconstructive surgery.[11-13] Therefore, it is of importance to have a thorough understanding of the anatomy and vascular supply of the SCM muscle. Although many authors have mentioned the arterial blood supply of the SCM muscle, we found no detailed anatomically based work on this subject. Most notably, available data about the vessels supplying the lower third of the muscle are incomplete, confusing, and sometimes contradictory.[14-17] Therefore, the aim of this study was to further improve the success rate of this flap by determining the exact courses and variability of vessels supplying the SCM muscle.

RESULTS

The blood supply to the SCM muscle can be divided into 3 parts: an upper, a middle, and a lower part, each being supplied by at least 1 main artery (**Figure 1**).

The upper third of the muscle was supplied by branches of the occipital artery. These branches can be further divided into 3 categories[18]: smaller upper branches (**Figure 2**, A, 1), which were present in 26 right and 27 left preparations, represent-

MATERIALS AND METHODS

Thirty-one necks (61 preparations) taken from 31 human bodies of both sexes (20 male and 11 female), aging from 50 to 94 years (mean, 78 years), donated to our institute were dissected. The cadavers were fixed by perfusion through the femoral artery with a mixture of 4% phenolic acid and 0.5% formaldehyde as standard for dissection methods. Individuals with any signs of severe disease or previous operation on the neck were excluded from this study. The anterior and posterior triangles of the neck were completely dissected by one of us (A.C.K. or M.A.), who documented his findings immediately. Results were reviewed by the other authors independently. In addition, sketches were drawn of all preparations and photographs were taken of all representative cases as well as exceptional cases.

ing 87% for each side. In addition to these tiny branches, a single well-developed branch was found in 10 cases (33%) on the right side and in 12 cases (39%) on the left side (Figure 2, A, 2). In 8 specimens on the right side and 6 specimens on the left side, this artery takes a course parallel to the spinal accessory nerve. In 1 right and 1 left preparation there existed a lower branch (Figure 2, A, 3).

The middle third of the SCM muscle mostly receives its blood supply from 1 branch of the superior thyroid artery and the external carotid artery. In nearly one third of the specimens (8 [27%] on the right side and 8 [26%] on the left), these 2 arteries almost equally shared the blood supply. In the remaining 45 cases, a single branch of either the superior thyroid artery (12 [40%] on the right side and 14 [45%] on the left) or the external carotid artery (23% each side [7 cases each]) was the only nutritive vessel for this part of the muscle (Figure 2, B). In 12 preparations, the branch arising from the external carotid artery had a very characteristic course. Ascending for a short distance in a cranial direction, it wound around the hypoglossal nerve loop and descended subsequently along the anterior margin of the SCM muscle for approximately 2 cm. In most of the cases (n = 10), it entered the muscle between its upper and its middle third parts (Figure 2, B).

In 1 case, the blood supply of the midportion of the SCM muscle was provided by a branch of the lingual artery and the external carotid artery. Both arteries take the characteristic course around the loop of the hypoglossal nerve. In this particular case no branch of the superior thyroid artery was observed.

In 34 preparations we took special attention to branches arising from the ascending cervical artery. Since some of these branches are very thin, this step of preparation was done by means of a microscope. However, in 26 preparations (77%), a few very tiny branches heading toward the SCM muscle could be found.

The lower third of the SCM muscle showed a unique blood supply. We found a branch of the suprascapular artery that showed a well-defined topographical course in 24 right (80%) and 25 left (81%) preparations (Figure 2, C).

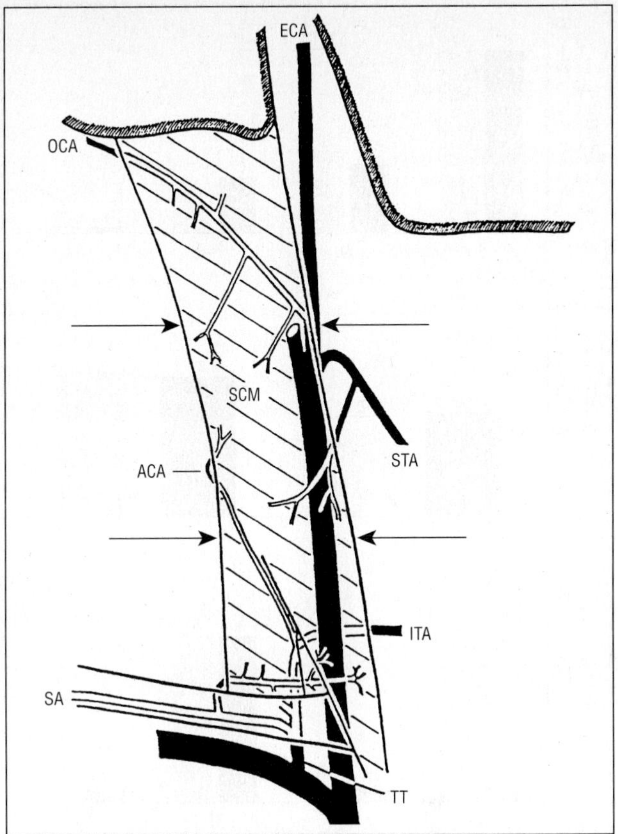

Figure 1. *Schematic illustration of all arteries supplying the sternocleidomastoid (SCM) muscle. Arrows indicate the estimated borders between the upper, middle, and lower thirds of the SCM muscle. OCA indicates occipital artery; ECA, external carotid artery; STA, superior thyroid artery; ACA, ascending cervical artery; ITA, inferior thyroid artery; SA, suprascapular artery; and TT, thyrocervical trunk.*

The caliber of this artery is comparable with those of the other main arteries that supply the SCM muscle. Under cover of the clavicle, it originates from the suprascapular artery behind the clavicular head of the SCM muscle. After ascending for about 1 cm, it bends around the lateral border of the pretracheal lamina of the cervical fascia that is attached between the omohyoid muscles. Running right between the fascia and the SCM muscle in a medial direction it supplies both heads of the muscle with several branches (**Figure 3**). One of these small muscular branches is constantly found between 2 muscular layers of the clavicular head of the SCM muscle. Furthermore, there are very tiny branches to the clavicle and to the sternum. In 2 cases, this suprascapular branch was found to take its lateromedial course superficial to the SCM muscle, being covered only by the superficial cervical fascia and the platysma.

In cases in which the branch of the suprascapular artery is remarkably thin or does not exist, either a longer branch from the superior thyroid artery descended caudally (4 cases) or a branch from the transverse or superficial cervical artery (5 cases each) supplied the lower third of the muscle.

The most important difference between the 2 types of blood supply (one arising from the suprascapular artery and the other arising from the transverse cervical artery) to the lower third of the SCM muscle seems to be their topography. The branches of the transverse or the

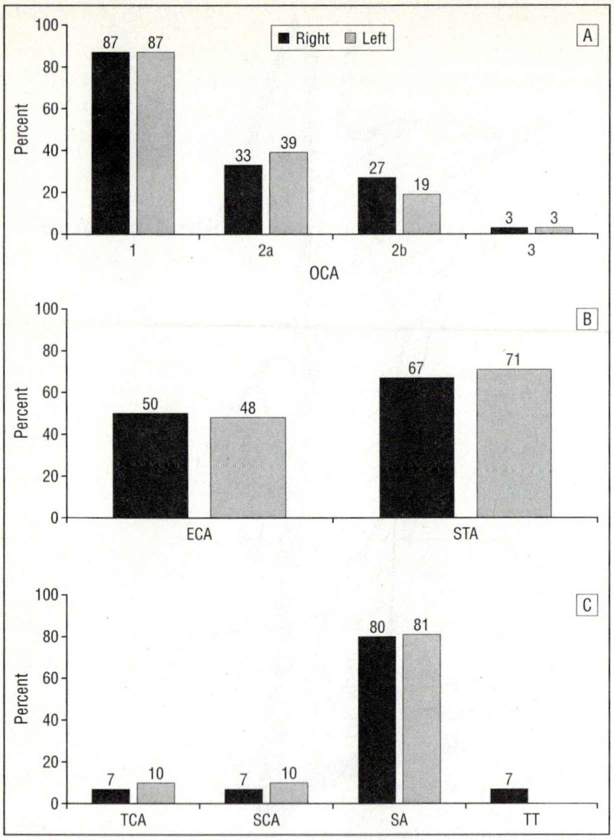

Figure 2. *Arteries supplying the sternocleidomastoid (SCM) muscle in percentage incidence of supplying vessels (n = 61). A, The upper third of the SCM muscle. 1, 2a, 2b, and 3 refer to the categorization of the branches arising from the occipital artery (OCA) given in the text. B, The middle third of the SCM muscle. ECA indicates branches arising directly from the external carotid artery; STA, branches arising from the superior thyroid artery. C, The lower third of the SCM muscle. TCA indicates branches arising from the transverse cervical artery; SCA, branches arising from the superficial cervical artery; SA, branches arising from the suprascapular artery; and TT, branches arising directly from the thyrocervical trunk. Right indicates right side of the neck; left, left side of the neck.*

superficial cervical artery have to be expected approximately 1.5 cm more cranial than that of the suprascapular artery (**Figure 4**).

In 2 cases (7%), the artery supplying the lower third of the SCM muscle arose directly from the thyrocervical trunk.

COMMENT

In general, our findings are in agreement with the traditional view that the blood supply of the SCM muscle originates from 3 main arteries.[3,15,18] However, a main artery supplying the lower third of the SCM muscle has not been described up to now. Data on the variability and the frequency of the vessels under consideration could not be found in the literature. The main task of many investigations on the SCM muscle is to clarify the usefulness of the muscle as a pedicle flap.[3,10,14,16,19] Since these investigations are aimed at clinical questions, the detailed description of the SCM muscle's blood supply seems to be of secondary importance. Only a few authors have done studies using cadaver dissection to address this question.[15,16] Yet, the data presented are sometimes incomplete, possibly due to the small numbers of bodies dissected. The majority of investigators, however, cite old textbooks of anatomy.[20,21] Because the field of plastic and reconstructive surgery has advanced greatly over the past few decades, descriptions given therein may no longer be sufficient.

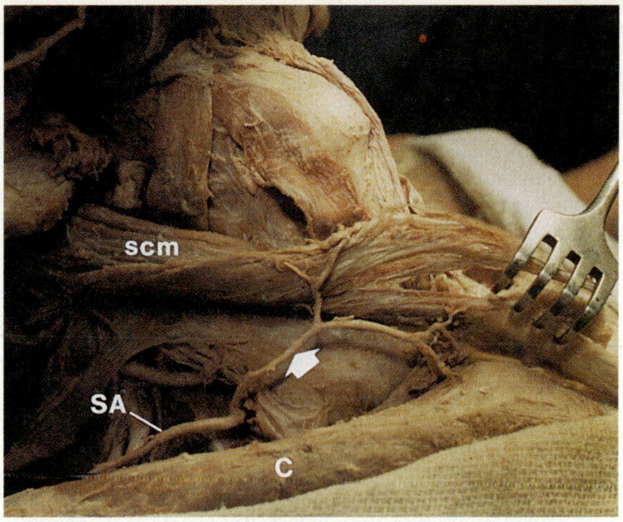

Figure 3. *Preparation of the right side of a neck. The clavicular head of the sternocleidomastoid muscle (scm) is cut and held upward. The arrow indicates the branch of the suprascapular artery (SA); C, clavicle.*

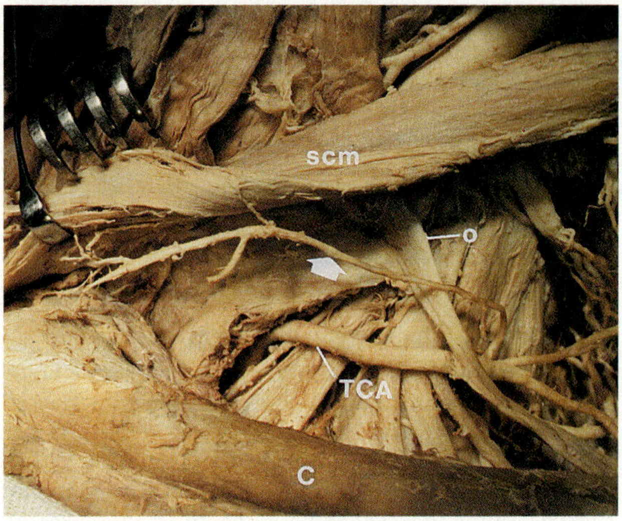

Figure 4. *Preparation of the left side of a neck. The clavicular head of the sternocleidomastoid muscle (scm) is cut and held upward. The arrow indicates the branch arising from the transverse cervical artery (TCA) bending around the omohyoid muscle (o); C, clavicle.*

Agossou-Voyenne et al[17] tried to avoid these problems by investigating the blood supply of 40 SCM muscles by means of angiography. This method has at least 2 problems: first, vessels of this size may refuse filling during angiography unless a selective catheter is used, and, second, in our opinion only vessels that are already known can be reliably described from an angiogram. Therefore, this method does not seem appropriate for discovering arteries that have never been described before.

In addition, the variety of applications for the SCM muscle flap makes it nearly impossible to compare results with each other. This might be one of the reasons why there are still doubts about the reliability of the use of the SCM muscle for reconstructive procedures. Marx and McDonald,[22] for example, who used the SCM muscle as a muscular or myocutaneous flap for oral and facial reconstruction in 16 patients, described 4 cases of necrosis, representing a failure rate of 25%. Tivari[12] reported 3 failures of 9 cases, therefore raising the question whether the vascularity of the muscle is adequate for reconstruction. Furthermore, he considers the occipital artery to be the major blood supply of the SCM muscle and disagrees that splitting of the muscle could be an attractive alternative. According to our findings, we do not believe that the occipital artery is the main source of blood supply to the whole SCM muscle. Larson and Goepfert[11] also considered the occipital artery to be the major blood supply and stated that although the SCM muscle might be used to close pharyngocutaneous fistulae, it is of more limited usefulness than reported in earlier studies. Furthermore, they report on 4 failures, 3 of which had to be revised, of a total of 12 cases. Yet, in transferring the whole SCM muscle, they complained about the "bulky flap," which requires later revision. As our findings indicate and other authors already have shown, this problem can be solved by using only 1 head of the muscle (preferably the clavicular one) for transposition. Friedman et al,[7,8] who used the SCM muscle for repair of subglottic and tracheal defects, have shown that the muscle can meet requirements in selected cases. Siemssen et al,[23] who were the first to transfer only the clavicular head of the SCM muscle, reported 1 case of necrosis of 18 cases, which seems to be a very good result. Tovi,[5] following Siemssen et al's concept for the repair of laryngeal and tracheal defects, succeeded in all 3 of his cases. Alvarez et al,[24] who used a split SCM myocutaneous flap, reported 2 complete failures of 11 cases. They considered this technique (leaving the sternal head in situ) a viable alternative to other procedures. One of the most comprehensive descriptions of muscles used in plastic and reconstructive surgery of the head and neck is by Conley.[14] Although he stated that the SCM muscle has a limited and specific applicability, he does not doubt its usefulness overall.[3] A good overview about the concept and the outcome of SCM muscle transfer in various studies has been given by Yugueros and Woods.[10] They emphasize the advantages of this technique, but in contrast to our findings, state that the lower third of the muscle lacks a constant vascular anatomy.

Additionally, the sometimes inconsistent taxonomy of the vessels under consideration in the literature makes a comparison between the various surgical procedures even more difficult. For that reason we categorized the SCM branches of the occipital artery. To estimate the frequency of different types of blood supply to the SCM muscle we determined the percentage incidence of all supplying vessels. Our results indicate that only the middle third of the SCM muscle shows some variability in its blood supply. The external carotid artery and the superior thyroid artery are able to supply this part of the muscle either together or on their own. The blood supply of the lower third of the SCM muscle, however, is quite constant.

CONCLUSIONS

The demand for plastic and reconstructive surgery has been increasing quickly within the last years. The SCM muscle flap represents a considerable opportunity for reconstructions after resections within the upper aerodigestive tract. The exact knowledge of the blood supply of the SCM muscle helps to avoid muscle necrosis after transposition and will further increase the success rate of this surgical procedure. Moreover, the unique possibility of rotating either of the 2 heads of the muscle allows an aesthetic as well as functionally satisfactory result.

We thank Robert Mayr, MD, for his support and critical comment, and Roland Blumer, MD, and Christl Krivanek for their technical help and assistance.

Reprints: Antonius C. Kierner, MD, Anatomisches Institut, 2 Unterrichtseinheit, Waehringerstrasse 13/3, A-1090 Vienna, Austria (e-mail: antonius.kierner@univie.ac.at).

REFERENCES

1. Jianu J. Die chirurgische Behandlung der Facialislähmung. *Deutsche Z Chir.* 1909; 102:377-386.
2. Owens N. Compound neck pedicle designed for the repair of massive facial defects. *Plast Reconstr Surg.* 1955;15:369-389.
3. Conley J, Gullane PJ. The sternocleidomastoid muscle flap. *Head Neck Surg.* 1980; 2:308-311.
4. Eliachar I, Moscona AR. Reconstruction of the laryngotracheal complex in children using the sternocleidomastoid myocutaneous flap. *Head Neck Surg.* 1981;4:16-21.
5. Tovi F. Sternocleidomastoid myoperiosteal flap for the repair of laryngeal and tracheal defects. *Head Neck Surg.* 1983;5:447-451.
6. Rubin JS. Sternocleidomastoid myoplasty for the repair of chronic cervical esophageal fistulae. *Laryngoscope.* 1986;96:834-836.
7. Friedman M, Toriumi DM, Strorigl T, Chilis T, Skolnik E. The sternocleidomastoid myoperiosteal flap for esophagopharyngeal reconstruction and fistula repair: clinical and experimental study. *Laryngoscope.* 1988;98:1084-1091.
8. Friedman M, Toriumi DM, Owens R, Grybauskas V. Experience with the sterno-cleido-mastoid myoperiosteal flap for reconstruction of subglottic and tracheal defects: modification of technique and long-term results. *Laryngoscope.* 1988; 98:1003-1011.
9. Casler JD, Conley J. Sternocleidomastoid muscle transfer and superficial musculoaponeurotic system plication in the prevention of Frey's syndrome. *Laryngoscope.* 1991;101:95-100.
10. Yugueros P, Woods JE. The sternocleidomastoid flap: a reappraisal. *Br J Plast Surg.* 1996;49:93-96.
11. Larson DL, Goepfert H. Limitations of the sternocleidomastoid musculocutaneous flap in head and neck cancer reconstruction. *Plast Reconstr Surg.* 1982;70:328-335.
12. Tivari R. Experiences with the sternocleidomastoid muscle and myocutaneous flaps. *J Laryngol Otol.* 1990;104:315-321.
13. Friedman M, Mayer AD. Laryngotracheal reconstruction in adults with the sterno-cleido-mastoid myoperiosteal flap. *Ann Otol Rhinol Laryngol.* 1992;101:897-908.
14. Conley JJ. *Concepts in Head and Neck Surgery.* Stuttgart, Germany: Georg Thieme Verlag; 1970.
15. Ariyan S. One-stage reconstruction of defects of the oral cavity with the sterno-cleidomastoid pedicle musculocutaneous flap. *Plast Reconstr Surg.* 1979;63: 618-625.
16. Jabaley ME, Heckler FR, Wallace WH, Knott LH. Sternocleidomastoid regional flaps: a new look on an old concept. *Br J Plast Surg.* 1979;32:106-113.
17. Agossou-Voyenne AK, Hureau J, Germain MA. Vascularisation et innervation du muscle sterno-cleido-mastoidien et de son revetement cutane: bases anatomiques de son utilisation en chirurgie plastique. *Ann Chir Plast Esthet.* 1991;36: 108-115.
18. Williams PL, Warwick R, Dyson M, Bannister LH. *Gray's Anatomy.* 37th ed. London, England: Churchill Livingstone; 1989:583f.
19. Glenwood AC, Hamaker RC, Singer MI. Sternocleidomastoid myocutaneous flap. *Laryngoscope.* 1987;97:970-974.
20. Spalteholz W. *Hand Atlas of Human Anatomy.* Philadelphia, Pa: JB Lippincott Co; 1921.
21. Lanz TV, Wachsmuth W. *Praktische Anatomie.* Berlin, Germany: Springer Verlag; 1955.
22. Marx RE, McDonald DK. The sternocleidomastoid muscle as a muscular or myocutaneous flap for oral and facial reconstruction. *J Oral Maxillofac Surg.* 1985; 43:155-162.
23. Siemssen SO, Kirkby B, O'Connor TPF. Immediate reconstruction of a resected segment of the lower jaw using a compound flap of clavicle and sternomastoid muscle. *Plast Reconstr Surg.* 1978;61:724-735.
24. Alvarez GE, Escamilla JT, Carranza A. The split sternocleidomastoid myocutaneous flap. *Br J Plast Surg.* 1983;36:183-186.

Anatomic Site of Primary Melanoma Is Associated With Depth of Invasion

Yoram Hemo, MD; Mordechai Gutman, MD; Joseph M. Klausner, MD

Background: The prognosis of melanoma is correlated to the stage of the primary lesion. Tumor site has also been implicated, with locations such as the trunk carrying a worse prognosis than others (such as limbs).

Hypothesis: To determine if tumor thickness correlates with location in a nonvisible body area.

Design and Setting: Retrospective medical record review of all patients with stage I melanoma treated in our medical center between 1986 and 1994. Demographic data as well as primary tumor characteristics were recorded.

Methods: The skin's surface was divided into occult and exposed areas. Exposed indicated visible to the patient during routine activities; occult areas included posterior aspect of the neck, back, posterior aspect of the thigh, calf, and plantar region. Data were analyzed for significance using the χ^2 test.

Results: Of the 178 patients with stage I melanoma analyzed, 51.1% had limb, 35.9% trunk, and 12.9% head and neck lesions. Depth of invasion was less than 0.76 mm in 32.6%, 0.76 to 1.5 mm in 25.2%, and more than 4 mm in 7.9%. In 87 patients the tumor occurred in occult areas and in 91 patients in exposed areas. Comparing the depth of invasion in these 2 groups disclosed that thin (<0.76 mm) melanomas occurred in 20.7% of occult areas compared with 44% of exposed areas ($P<.05$). Deeper melanomas (>2.50 mm) occurred in 28.7% of occult areas compared with 12.1% of exposed areas ($P<.05$).

Conclusions: Tumors in less-visible body areas are significantly thicker at the time of diagnosis than those occurring in more highly visible areas. Delayed detection may be responsible for this finding.

Arch Surg. 1999;134:148-150

MALIGNANT melanoma was once named "the fatal black tumor" owing to its totally unpredictable biological behavior. However, since the introduction of microstaging methods by Clark et al[1] and Breslow,[2] more accurate predictions can be made regarding prognosis.[3-6] Numerous studies have shown that while thin (<1.25 mm) melanomas are considered curable by simple excision alone, deeply invasive lesions have probably metastasized by the time of diagnosis.[7]

The high curability rate of early melanoma has increased public awareness to the issue of their early detection, and although the incidence of melanoma is rising faster than that of any other cancer,[8,9] an increasing number of patients are being diagnosed at an early stage.[10]

Other than depth of invasion of the primary lesion, one tumor characteristic that has been suggested as an independent prognostic factor is body location.[11-17] It has long been known that for some locations, such as the trunk, the prognosis is worse than for limb lesions.[18,19] However, whether these differences are due to the tumor's biological behavior or simply to the time of diagnosis, meaning that lesions located in less-visible body regions are diagnosed late and therefore carry a worse prognosis, has not been investigated. Our study was designed to answer this question.

From the Department of Surgery, Tel Aviv Sourasky Medical Center, Sackler Faculty of Medicine, Tel Aviv University, Tel Aviv, Israel.

RESULTS

One hundred seventy-eight patients with stage I melanoma were analyzed. There were 95 men (53.4%) and 83 women (46.6%). The average age was 57 years (range, 14-81 years). In 91 patients (51.1%) the melanoma occurred in the limb, in 64 (35.9%) in the trunk, and in 23 (12.9%) in the neck and head region (**Figure 1**). The depth of invasion was less than 0.76 mm in 32.6% of patients, 0.76 to 1.49 mm in 25.2%, 1.5 to 2.4 mm in 21.9%, 2.5 to 3.99 mm in 12.3%, and more than 4 mm in 7.9% (**Table** and **Figure 2**).

PATIENTS AND METHODS

The medical records of all patients with stage I cutaneous melanoma treated at the Tel Aviv Sourasky Medical Center, Tel Aviv, Israel, between 1986 and 1994 were retrospectively analyzed. Patients with multiple primary tumors or those with incomplete records of their primary tumor were excluded. The data included age, sex, tumor site, and microstaging according to Breslow.[2]

The skin's surface was divided into occult and exposed areas. *Occult areas* referred to those body regions not visible to patients during normal activities and included the scalp and posterior aspect of the neck, back, posterior aspect of the thigh, posterior aspect of the calf, foot (plantar aspect), and posterior aspect of the arm. *Exposed areas* included the face and anterior aspect of the neck, chest and abdomen, anterior aspect of the thigh (including medial and lateral aspects), anterior aspect of the calf and foot (ventral), arm (ventral), forearm, and hand.

These data were analyzed for significance using the χ^2 test.

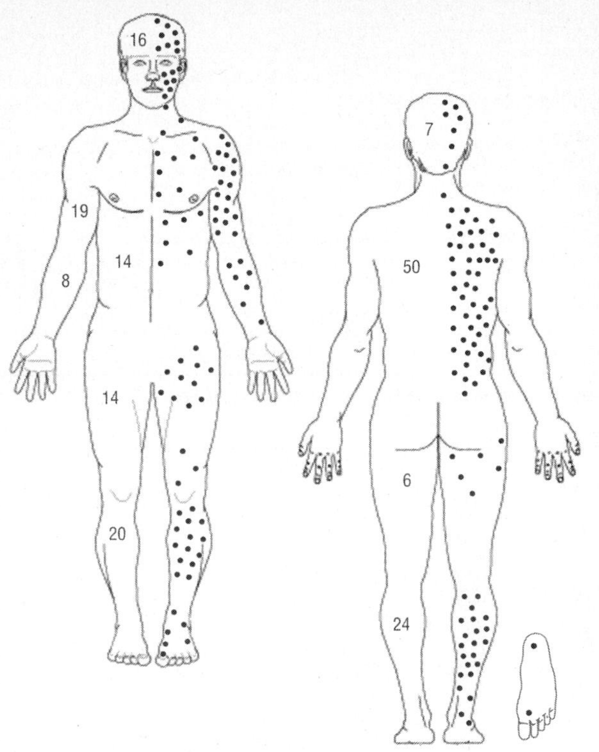

Figure 1. *Location of primary tumor in 178 melanoma patients.*

Thickness of Primary Tumor

Location	Depth of Invasion, No. (%)					Total, No. (%)
	<0.75 mm	0.76-1.49 mm	1.50-2.49 mm	2.50-3.99 mm	>4.00 mm	
Occult area						
Back	12 (24)	17 (34)	10 (20)	6 (12)	5 (10)	**50 (100)**
Scalp and posterior aspect of the neck	1 (14)	1 (14)	3 (43)	1 (14)	1 (14)	**7 (100)**
Posterior aspect of the thigh	0 (0)	1 (17)	3 (50)	1 (17)	1 (17)	**6 (100)**
Exposed area						
Posterior aspect of the leg and plantar region	5 (21)	3 (12)	6 (25)	6 (25)	4 (17)	**24 (100)**
Abdomen and chest	7 (50)	4 (29)	3 (21)	0 (0)	0 (0)	**14 (100)**
Anterior aspect of the thigh	3 (21)	5 (36)	2 (14)	3 (21)	1 (7)	**14 (100)**
Anterior aspect of the leg and foot	9 (45)	7 (35)	4 (20)	0 (0)	0 (0)	**20 (100)**
Upper limb and shoulder, face, and anterior aspect of the neck	21 (49)	7 (17)	8 (19)	5 (12)	2 (5)	**43 (100)**
Total	**58** (33)	**45** (25)	**39** (22)	**22** (12)	**14** (8)	**178 (100)**

An analysis of tumor site according to a patient's ability to see it disclosed that in 87 patients the lesion was located in occult areas, while in 91 it was diagnosed on exposed body regions (Figure 1). Comparing the depth of invasion in these 2 groups of patients disclosed that 20.7% of melanomas occurring in occult areas were less than 0.75 mm, as compared with 44% in exposed areas ($P<.05$). In the deeply invasive groups, (2.50-3.99 and >4.0 mm), 28.7% occurred in occult and only 12.1% in exposed areas of the body ($P<.05$) (**Figure 3**). In melanomas measuring 0.76 to 2.49 mm, there was no significant difference between exposed and occult body regions (Figure 3). These differences were more pronounced in women; 15.6% of tumors measuring less than 0.75 mm were found in occult areas as compared with 46.2% in exposed body regions. In the deep (>4 mm) group, 18.8% were in occult areas and only 1.9% in exposed body regions ($P<.05$).

An analysis of the data according to the various body regions disclosed that in half of the exposed regions, there was no single lesion measuring more than 2.5 mm in depth, while there were such lesions in each of the occult regions (Table).

COMMENT

Early detection plays a pivotal role in the management of malignant melanoma. Patients diagnosed with thin lesions are usually cured by surgery alone, while those with deep lesions frequently develop metastases.[7] Melanoma usually arises on a cutaneous surface. It is an unusual ex-

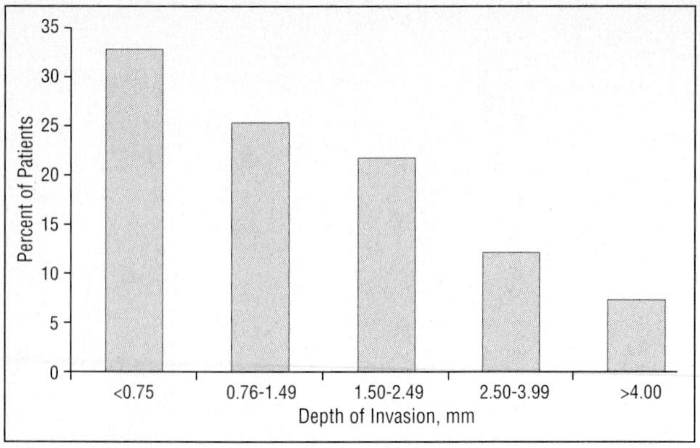

Figure 2. *Depth of invasion in 178 melanoma patients.*

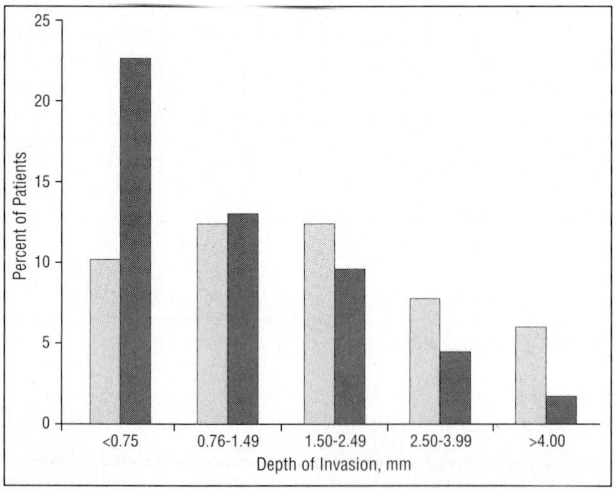

Figure 3. *Stage I melanomas in occult (light-shaded bars) and exposed (dark-shaded bars) body regions.*

ample of a potentially fatal neoplasm that is often visible to the naked eye. However, not all body regions are equally visible during routine daily activities. In this study, we have demonstrated that tumors presenting in occult body regions have a greater average Breslow thickness. This finding helps explain the worse prognosis associated with certain anatomic locations.

The body location of the primary tumor in melanoma has long been recognized as an important prognostic factor.[11-19] Although some studies have shown in a mathematical model that once tumor thickness and ulceration are determined other tumor characteristics such as location lose their significance,[20,21] others, using multivariant analysis, have shown that tumor location is an independent prognostic factor[22] with trunk lesions considered to have a poorer prognosis than limb lesions. Many studies have addressed this issue but, except for tumors occurring in the plantar or palmar skin, which have an especially poor prognosis,[18] the differences in prognosis could not be explained.

Our study offers a partial explanation for the different site-related prognoses of melanoma. The fact that melanoma occurring in occult body regions were thicker implies that delay in diagnosis may be responsible for the worse prognosis of tumors in these locations. A prospective study involving a large group of patients who receive skin cancer screening at regular intervals would help to answer this question.

Skin cancer screening programs, which include examination of nonvisible body regions, have the potential to decrease the morbidity and mortality associated with late detection. Because approximately 1% of the population will develop melanoma,[23] public education regarding self-examination of the skin and screening conducted by trained professionals should be emphasized.

Corresponding author: Mordechai Gutman, MD, Surgical Unit for Regional Chemotherapy, Department of Surgery, Tel Aviv Sourasky Medical Center, 6 Weizmann St, Tel Aviv 64239, Israel.

REFERENCES

1. Clark WH Jr, From L, Bernardino EA, Mihm MC. The histogenesis and biologic behavior of primary human malignant melanoma of the skin. *Cancer Res.* 1969; 29:705-727.
2. Breslow A. Thickness, cross-sectional areas, and depth of invasion in the prognosis of cutaneous melanoma. *Ann Surg.* 1970;172:902-908.
3. Mihm MC Jr, Fitzpatrick TB, Brown MM, Raker JW, Malt RA, Kaiser JS. Early detection of primary cutaneous malignant melanoma. *N Engl J Med.* 1973;289:989-996.
4. Sober AJ, Fitzpatrick TB, Mihm MC Jr, et al. Early recognition of cutaneous melanoma. *JAMA.* 1979;242:2795-2799.
5. Breslow A. Prognostic factors in the treatment of cutaneous melanoma. *J Cutan Pathol.* 1979;6:208-212.
6. Balch CM, Soong S-J, Milton GW. A comparison of prognostic factors and surgical results in 1786 patients with localized melanoma treated in Alabama USA and New South Wales, Australia. *Ann Surg.* 1982;196:677-684.
7. Rhodes AR, Weinstock MA, Fitzpatrick TB, Mihm MC Jr, Sober AJ. Risk factors for cutaneous melanoma: a practical method of recognizing predisposed individuals. *JAMA.* 1987;258:3146-3154.
8. Silverberg E, Lubera J. Cancer statistics, 1987. *CA Cancer J Clin.* 1987;37:2-19.
9. Glass AG, Hoover RN. The emerging epidemic of melanoma and squamous cell skin cancer. *JAMA.* 1989;262:2097-2100.
10. Balch CM, Soong SJ, Milton GW, et al. Changing trends in cutaneous melanoma over a quarter century in Alabama, USA, and New South Wales, Australia. *Cancer.* 1983;52:1748-1753.
11. Rogers GS, Kopf AW, Rigel DS, et al. Effect of anatomical location on prognosis in patients with clinical stage I melanoma. *Arch Dermatol.* 1983;119:644-649.
12. Blois MS, Sagebiel RW, Abarbanel RM, Caldwell TM, Tuttle MS. Malignant melanoma of the skin, 1: the association of tumor depth and type, and patient age, sex and site with survival. *Cancer.* 1983;52:1330-1341.
13. Shaw H, McGovern V, Milton GW, Farago GA, McCarthy WH. Malignant melanoma: influence of site of lesion and age of patient in the female superiority in survival. *Cancer.* 1980;46:2731-2735.
14. Garbe C, Butyner P, Bertz J, et al. Primary cutaneous melanoma: identification of prognostic groups and estimation of individual prognosis for 5093 patients. *Cancer.* 1995;75:2484-2491.
15. Thorn M, Adami HO, Ringborg U, Bergstrom R, Krusemo U. The association between anatomic site and survival in malignant melanoma: an analysis of 12,353 cases from the Swedish Cancer Registry. *Eur J Cancer Clin Oncol.* 1989;25:483-491.
16. Day CL, Mihm MC, Sober AJ, et al. Prognostic factors for melanoma patients with lesions 0.76 to 1.69 mm in thickness. *Ann Surg.* 1982;195:30-34.
17. Weinstock MA, Morris BT, Lederman JS, et al. Effect of BANS location on the prognosis of clinical stage I melanoma. *Br J Dermatol.* 1987;116:303-310.
18. Gutman M, Klausner JM, Inbar M, Skornick M, Baratz M, Rozin RR. Acral (volar subungual) melanoma. *Br J Surg.* 1985;72:610-613.
19. Day CA, Sober AJ, Kopf AW, et al. A prognostic model for clinical stage I melanoma of the lower extremity: location on foot as independent risk factor for recurrent disease. *Surgery.* 1981;89:599-603.
20. Clark WH, Elder DE, Guerry D, et al. Model predicting survival in stage I melanoma based on tumor progression. *J Natl Cancer Inst.* 1989;81:1893-1904.
21. Schuchter L, Schultz DJ, Synnestvedt M, et al. A prognostic model for predicting 10-year survival in patients with primary melanoma. *Ann Intern Med.* 1996; 125:369-375.
22. Soong S-J. A computerized mathematical model and scoring system for predicting outcome in patients with localized melanoma. In: Balch CM, Houghton AN, Milton GW, Sober A, Soong S-J, eds. *Cutaneous Melanoma.* Philadelphia, Pa: JB Lippincott Co; 1992:200.
23. Roush GC, Schymura MJ, Holford TR. Risk for cutaneous melanoma in recent Connecticut birth cohorts. *Am J Public Health.* 1985;75:679-682.

ORIGINAL ARTICLE

Laparoscopic Gastrostomy and Jejunostomy

Safety and Cost With Local vs General Anesthesia

Quan-Yang Duh, MD; Andrea L. Senokozlieff-Englehart, RN, MS; Yong S. Choe, MAS; Allan E. Siperstein, MD; Kathleen Rowland, BSN, RN; Lawrence W. Way, MD

Background and Hypothesis: General anesthesia is used for laparoscopic enteral access because pneumoperitoneum requires relaxation of the abdominal muscles. We wanted to determine whether these procedures could be performed with similar results and cost under local anesthesia.

Design: Randomized controlled study with 30-day follow-up including a cost-benefit analysis.

Setting: University-affiliated hospitals.

Patients: Forty-eight patients (32 men, 16 women; mean age, 67 years) undergoing laparoscopic gastrostomies (n = 32) and jejunostomies (n = 16).

Intervention: Twenty-four patients underwent laparoscopic gastrostomy (n = 15) and jejunostomy (n = 9) under local anesthesia with intravenous conscious sedation and monitored anesthesia care. Twenty-four patients had general anesthesia.

Main Outcome Measures: Conversion to general anesthesia, complications, and cost.

Results: Ten patients under local anesthesia had periods of deep sedation and 1 required conversion to general anesthesia. One patient under general anesthesia required conversion to open gastrostomy. No patients had intraoperative aspiration; however, 4 aspirated after the procedure. One patient died of myocardial infarction during the 30-day follow-up. We found no significant difference in the total mean cost and actual procedure time. The surgeon's fee accounted for 31% of the total cost.

Conclusions: Some patients undergoing laparoscopic enteral access may require deep sedation and a rare patient may require general anesthesia. Clinical conditions and surgeon preference, therefore, should determine whether local anesthesia is suitable for laparoscopic gastrostomies and jejunostomies, and in what setting, since there is no difference in success rate or complications when compared with general anesthesia. Potential savings are possible from the operating room (26% of total cost) or anesthesiologist (12% of total cost) if these procedures are performed in an endoscopy suite without monitored anesthesia care.

Arch Surg. 1999;134:151-156

WE AND others have previously shown that gastrostomies and jejunostomies can be performed safely with laparoscopic techniques using the T fasteners to retract and anchor the bowel.[1-9] Relaxation of the abdominal muscles is required for adequate pneumoperitoneum. Therefore, general anesthesia is used for most patients who undergo laparoscopic feeding tube placement.

Other techniques, such as open surgical gastrostomy or jejunostomy, percutaneous endoscopic gastrostomy[10-12] or jejunostomy,[13] and percutaneous feeding tube placement by interventional radiologists, can be performed in most patients under local anesthesia with conscious sedation. For laparoscopic techniques to be a true alternative for placing feeding tubes, local anesthesia with conscious sedation needs to be an option, especially for patients who are at very high risk for general anesthesia.

We therefore undertook a multi-institutional prospective randomized study to determine whether laparoscopic gastrostomy or jejunostomy can be performed safely in most patients under local anesthesia with conscious sedation as compared with under general anesthesia. We studied how often local anesthesia is successful without the need to convert to general anesthesia, how often the laparoscopic cases required conversion to open procedures, and whether the rates of complications or costs differ between cases performed under local vs general anesthesia.

From the Surgical Service, Veterans Affairs Medical Center, San Francisco, and the Department of Surgery, University of California, San Francisco (Drs Duh and Way); Mount Zion Medical Center, University of California, San Francisco (Dr Siperstein); and Medical Nutrition Research and Development, Ross Products Division, Abbott Laboratories, Columbus, Ohio (Mss Senokozlieff-Englehart and Rowland and Mr Choe).

PATIENTS AND METHODS

PATIENTS AND RANDOMIZATION

The protocols were reviewed and approved by the institutional review boards of the 6 participating institutions (Veterans Affairs Medical Center, San Francisco, Calif; Duke Medical Center, Durham, NC; Creighton University, Omaha, Neb; University of California, San Francisco; University of Nebraska Medical Center, Omaha; and University of California, Davis). A signed informed consent was obtained from each patient.

All the participating surgeons were experienced laparoscopic surgeons who had participated in prior studies of laparoscopic feeding tube placement. Each surgeon was required to have performed at least 2 cases of laparoscopic gastrostomy or jejunostomy under local anesthesia and sedation before starting the study.

To achieve true randomization, the surgeon, anesthesiologist, and patient all had to agree to either general or local anesthesia before the patient was enrolled in the study. Thus, patients were excluded if they had other specific indications for general anesthesia (because of other concomitant operations or inability to cooperate) or local anesthesia (because the cardiopulmonary risk was too high for general anesthesia).

Patients were randomized to receive local or general anesthesia by a predetermined randomization schedule in sealed envelopes. The assignment to gastrostomy or jejunostomy, however, depended on the clinical indications. Jejunostomies were performed only when gastrostomies were contraindicated (gastroparesis, gastrectomy, or gastroesophageal reflux). Because of this, twice as many patients underwent gastrostomy as jejunostomy.

Forty-eight patients requiring 32 feeding gastrostomies and 16 jejunostomies were randomized to undergo the procedure laparoscopically under local anesthesia with intravenous conscious sedation (16 men, 8 women; mean age, 65 ± 4 years; range, 17-86 years) or under general anesthesia (16 men, 8 women; mean age, 69 ± 2 years; range, 47-89 years).

The indications for feeding tube placement were malnutrition and potential malnutrition, most commonly caused by cancer and neurologic disease. Twenty-three patients had neurologic dysfunction, such as stroke or Parkinson disease. Twenty-four patients had cancers of the head and neck or esophagus (including 3 patients who also had neurologic deficit). Four patients had other causes of malnutrition.

The mean serum albumin level was 30 g/L (reference range, 35-50 g/L) for both groups of patients (local anesthesia and general anesthesia). The mean serum prealbumin level was 119 g/L (reference range, 160-400 g/L) for patients randomized to local anesthesia and 161 g/L for those randomized to general anesthesia.

There were no differences between those randomized to local anesthesia vs those randomized to general anesthesia in age, sex, primary diagnosis, or American Society of Anesthesiologists (ASA) classification. Of the 24 patients who were randomized to local anesthesia, 17 were ASA class 3 and 7 were ASA class 4. Of the 24 patients who were randomized to general anesthesia, 18 were ASA class 3 and 6 were ASA class 4.

SURGICAL TECHNIQUES

Laparoscopic gastrostomy and jejunostomy were performed using the T-fastener techniques as previously described.[1,2] These procedures were performed by experienced laparoscopic surgeons who had already performed at least 2 laparoscopic gastrostomies and 2 laparoscopic jejunostomies under local anesthesia.

Because the abdominal muscles need to be relaxed for adequate laparoscopy, the patient needs to be kept relatively pain-free and without anxiety. Shoulder pain from

RESULTS

RESPONSE TO ANESTHESIA

Although 10 of the 24 patients randomized to local anesthesia and intravenous sedation had periods of deep sedation (level 2), none became unconscious (level 3) (**Table 1**). One patient, however, was converted to general anesthesia. This was an 86-year-old man who received 1 mg of midazolam and 80 mg of propofol over 91 minutes for jejunostomy. He developed cardiac arrhythmia associated with oxygen desaturation (cutaneous Po_2 <90 mm Hg), and was intubated to protect the airway. One other patient developed intraoperative oxygen desaturation because of an unexpected need for extensive lysis of adhesions, but the jejunostomy was completed without conversion to general anesthesia.

CONVERSIONS AND INTRAOPERATIVE COMPLICATIONS

One patient undergoing laparoscopic gastrostomy under general anesthesia had perforation of the posterior stomach wall, which was recognized intraoperatively. The procedure was converted to open gastrostomy and the perforation repaired.

Although 10 patients had a history of aspiration pneumonia before the procedure, none had intraoperative aspiration. There were no intraoperative complications.

PROCEDURE TIME

Table 2 summarizes the total procedure time (time in the operating room) and actual procedure time (skin incision to wound closure). The total procedure time included 8 concurrent procedures: 3 tracheostomies, 2 central line placements, and 1 each of lysis of adhesions, skin graft, and epigastric hernia repair. None of these procedures, by themselves, would have dictated general anesthesia.

POSTOPERATIVE COMPLICATIONS

Major postoperative complications occurred in 5 patients (11%). Four patients had aspiration pneumonia and 1 patient had bleeding.

diaphragmatic irritation by carbon dioxide is the most common discomfort that is felt by patients undergoing laparoscopic procedures under local anesthesia. This can be partially alleviated by decreasing the pneumoperitoneum pressure. Too low a pressure, however, makes laparoscopic visualization difficult. The optimal pneumoperitoneum pressure is usually 6 to 8 mm Hg, but needs to be adjusted according to the clinical situation.

ANESTHESIA

The protocols for anesthesia were prospectively reviewed by and agreed to by the anesthesiologists. All procedures were performed in the operating room with an anesthesiologist who administered either the general anesthesia or the intravenous sedation and monitored the patient throughout the procedure. Local anesthesia was administered by the surgeon. Patients who were randomized to local anesthesia received injection of lidocaine or bupivacaine without epinephrine, optional intravenous conscious sedation as per the individual institution's protocol, and/or monitored anesthesia care. Patients who were randomized to general anesthesia received general anesthesia that is routine at each institution and endotracheal intubation. They also received injection of lidocaine or bupivacaine without epinephrine for the trocar sites and stoma sites. Patients were routinely monitored by continuous pulse oximetry.

For patients undergoing local anesthesia, the depth of sedation was controlled by the anesthesiologist using intravenous sedation and titrated to a level that was considered safe for the patient but sedated enough for the procedure. Sedation levels were classified according to the standard developed by the American Dental Association in 1984: level 1 (conscious sedation), level 2 (deep sedation), or level 3 (unconscious). Patients who could not tolerate the procedure under local anesthesia and intravenous sedation, or who could not protect their airway, were intubated and converted to general anesthesia.

Total procedure time (from the time patient arrived in the operating room to the time the patient left, including the time required for concurrent procedures) and actual procedure time (from skin incision to wound closure) were recorded. Patients were reevaluated at 24 hours, 2 weeks, and 30 days after the procedure for postoperative complications and outcomes. Length of hospitalization after the procedure was also recorded.

STATISTICAL ANALYSIS

Analysis of variance (ANOVA) was used to compare patient groups. Differences are considered significant if $P<.05$. The comparison between the local anesthesia group and the general anesthesia group was made on the basis of initial randomization (intent). Thus, the patient who was converted from local to general anesthesia was included in the local anesthesia group for data analysis. Unless otherwise indicated, data are presented as mean ± SEM.

COST ANALYSIS

We prospectively collected hospital and professional charges and other billing information. These charges were converted to cost and then analyzed by Vector Research Inc, Ann Arbor, Mich. The hospital charges were converted to cost, using institution-specific cost-to-charge ratios calculated by Hospital Cost Investment Analysis Inc, Baltimore, Md. Professional charges for the surgeon, anesthesiologist, and nurse anesthetist, were converted to cost, using national-level data from the American Medical Association, Chicago, Ill, and Medical Group Management Association, Englewood, Colo. We only calculated the cost for the procedure and not that for total hospitalization. The cost was analyzed from the perspective of the hospital.

Because the Veterans Affairs Medical Center does not charge patients or provide cost information, the cases from that institution were excluded from cost analysis.

Although 7 of 24 local anesthesia patients and 3 of 24 general anesthesia patients had a history of aspiration pneumonia, only 1 patient in the local anesthesia group and 3 patients in the general anesthesia group had aspiration pneumonia after the procedure. Three of the 4 patients with postoperative aspiration pneumonia did not have a history of aspiration before the procedure. These patients developed aspiration pneumonia 14 to 30 days after the procedure. One patient, who had a rectus abdominus flap to cover a surgical neck wound, required suture ligation for bleeding of his muscle flap near the gastrostomy site 30 days after laparoscopic gastrostomy.

Minor postoperative complications occurred in 10 patients (6 from the local anesthesia group and 4 from the general anesthesia group). Seven patients had T-fastener or stoma site irritation that resolved with local care. Three tubes required replacement.

Eleven patients (23%) died within 30 days of the procedure. One was an 86-year-old man with congestive heart failure and an inoperable abdominal aortic aneurysm who died of a myocardial infarction 1 day after undergoing laparoscopic jejunostomy under local anesthesia. Postmortem investigation showed the jejunostomy tube to be in a good position without leakage. The other 10 patients died of underlying diseases.

There were no differences in the rate of major postoperative complications and 30-day mortality between the group randomized to local anesthesia and those randomized to general anesthesia.

LENGTH OF HOSPITAL STAY

Length of postoperative hospital stay, from the day of feeding tube placement to the day of discharge, did not differ for those randomized to local anesthesia (6 ± 1 days) and those randomized to general anesthesia (8 ± 2 days). As expected, the length of hospitalization was mainly due to the underlying diseases and not due to the procedure or anesthesia.

COST OF PROCEDURES

Analysis of the cost for the procedure showed that major components were the surgeon (31%), operating room (26%), and anesthesiologist (12%) (**Figure 1**). There

Table 1. Levels of Sedation for 48 Patients Who Underwent Laparoscopic Gastrostomies and Jejunostomies Under Local or General Anesthesia

Level of Sedation (ADA)*	Gastrostomy		Jejunostomy		Total	
	Local	General	Local	General	Local	General
Conscious (level 1)	7	0	7	0	**14**	0
Deep (level 2)	8	0	2†	0	**10**	0
Unconscious (level 3)	0	17	0	7	0	**24**

*ADA indicates American Dental Association.
†Both patients had oxygen desaturation and 1 was converted to general anesthesia (see "Results" section).

Table 2. Actual (Skin Incision to Wound Closure) and Total (Time in Operating Room) Procedure Times for 48 Patients Undergoing Laparoscopic Gastrostomies and Jejunostomies Under Local or General Anesthesia*

	Total Procedure Time, min	Actual Procedure Time, min
Gastrostomy		
Local (n = 15)	88 ± 7	54 ± 5
General (n = 17)	95 ± 9	52 ± 3
Jejunostomy		
Local (n = 9)	119 ± 23	81 ± 16
General (n = 7)	98 ± 7	55 ± 8
Gastrostomy (n = 32)	92 ± 5	53 ± 3
Jejunostomy (n = 16)	110 ± 13	70 ± 10
Local anesthesia (n = 24)	100 ± 10	64 ± 7
General anesthesia (n = 24)	96 ± 6	53 ± 3

*Data are presented as mean ± SEM.

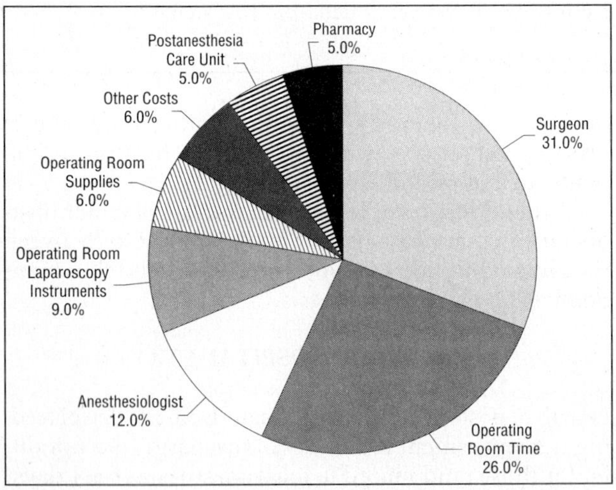

Figure 1. *Distribution of total cost of laparoscopic gastrostomy and jejunostomy.*

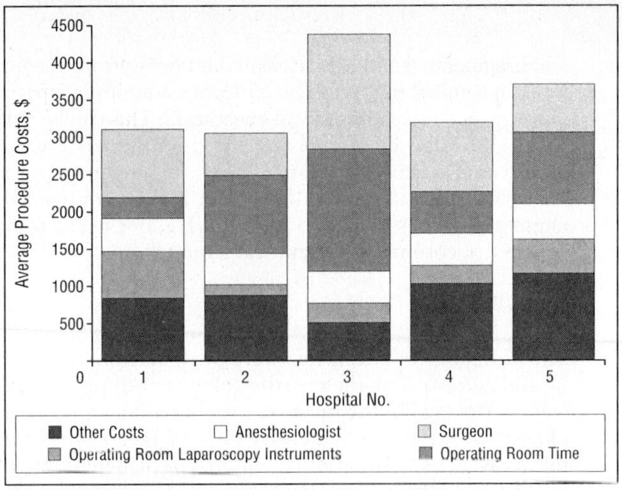

Figure 2. *Variations among 5 hospitals in total and component costs for laparoscopic gastrostomy and jejunostomy. Hospital 1 indicates Duke Medical Center, Durham, NC; hospital 2, Creighton University, Omaha, Neb; hospital 3, University of California, San Francisco; hospital 4, University of Nebraska Medical Center, Omaha; and hospital 5, University of California, Davis.*

Table 3. Cost of Procedures for 42 Patients Undergoing Laparoscopic Gastrostomies and Jejunostomies Under Local or General Anesthesia*

	Cost, $		
	Total	Professional	Institutional
Gastrostomy			
Local (n = 15)	3567 ± 585	1591 ± 286	1976 ± 442
General (n = 13)	3584 ± 649	1553 ± 298	2031 ± 545
Jejunostomy			
Local (n = 8)	3813 ± 1264	1924 ± 486	1889 ± 937
General (n = 6)	4304 ± 809	1883 ± 488	2422 ± 470
Gastrostomy (n = 28)	3575 ± 604	1573 ± 287	2001 ± 484
Jejunostomy (n = 14)	4023 ± 1084	1907 ± 468	2117 ± 795
Local anesthesia (n = 23)	3652 ± 861	1707 ± 392	1945 ± 637
General anesthesia (n = 19)	3812 ± 763	1657 ± 387	2155 ± 542

*Veterans Affairs Medical Center (San Francisco, Calif) patients are excluded from analysis. Data are presented as mean ± SD.

were marked variations in total cost and its components among the 5 hospitals studied (**Figure 2**).

The cost of procedures as calculated using the charge-to-cost ratios is summarized in **Table 3**. The cost for laparoscopic jejunostomy was higher than for laparoscopic gastrostomy. This was primarily due to the higher professional cost for jejunostomy. There was no difference between the cost of cases performed under local anesthesia and those performed under general anesthesia (power >0.80 [type II error <0.20, type I error = 0.05]) to detect a 20% difference.

COMMENT

Laparoscopic gastrostomies and jejunostomies have been shown by multiple studies to be safe and effective.[3,4] In this prospective randomized study, we found that these procedures can be performed as safely under local anesthesia as under general anesthesia, and for similar cost.

We did not choose regional anesthesia as an option in this randomized study. Regional anesthesia is very rarely used in laparoscopic procedures because it has the disadvantage of not completely relaxing the abdominal wall without the advantage of minimal anesthesia of local anesthesia with sedation. Also, one of the purposes of the study was to prepare for a comparative study between laparoscopic gastrostomy and jejunostomy vs percutaneous endoscopic gastrostomy, which is performed under local anesthesia and sedation.

The finding that no clinically or statistically significant difference was found between the local anesthesia and general anesthesia groups for laparoscopic feeding tube placement is not surprising, since these procedures are relatively simple in the spectrum of laparoscopic operations[13] and we and others have successfully used local anesthesia previously in selected cases.[14,15] In addition, many laparoscopic gynecological procedures are routinely performed under local anesthesia[16-19] and laparoscopic hernia repair has been performed successfully under local anesthesia.[20]

Technical advances simplify laparoscopic feeding tube placement. T fasteners, for example, obviated the need for laparoscopic suturing and shortened the procedure time. Other advances, such as small-bore needletrocars used with microendoscopes and micrograspers,[15] could also decrease patient discomfort. The main source of patient discomfort while under local anesthesia, however, seemed to be the diaphragmatic irritation due to carbon dioxide pneumoperitoneum. Using nitrous oxide pneumoperitoneum[20] or the gasless technique[21] may decrease the amount of intravenous sedation required and may have avoided the deeper (level 2) sedation that occurred in 10 of our patients.

In this study, the cost of procedures under local anesthesia was not different from the cost of procedures under general anesthesia. Other randomized studies of simple laparoscopic procedures have found local anesthesia to be less expensive. For example, a randomized study of laparoscopic sterilization found the local anesthesia group to have a shorter operating time, less discomfort, and lower cost than the general anesthesia group.[19] Our study has a greater than 80% chance of detecting a 20% difference in cost.

One reason for finding no difference in cost between the local and general anesthesia groups is the requirement of our protocol to perform the procedures in the operating room (accounting for 26% of total cost) and to have an anesthesiologist for monitoring (accounting for 12% of total cost). These are areas of potential savings if laparoscopic feeding tubes can be safely placed in an endoscopy suite with monitoring by a nurse (as is usually done for percutaneous endoscopic gastrostomy). These potential savings will not be realized, however, if the rate of conversion from local to general anesthesia or from laparoscopic to open is too high and therefore unsafe for outside the operating room. Our study did not address whether it is safe to place laparoscopic feeding tubes in patients outside the operating room without the help of an anesthesiologist.

We also confirmed prior findings that laparoscopic feeding tube placement is relatively safe and associated with acceptable morbidity and mortality rates.[1-9] The 30-day postoperative mortality rate is high (23%) in this study, but it is not unexpected for similar patients who require feeding tube placement.[22] All our patients were relatively high risk, at least ASA class 3, and many were ASA class 4. All the deaths can be attributed to underlying diseases.

Although we found no difference in procedure time between local anesthesia and general anesthesia groups, the procedures were technically more challenging when performed under local anesthesia. It is more difficult to perform a thorough diagnostic laparoscopy because of a more limited exposure under local anesthesia. Some patients were unable to relax the abdominal muscles because of discomfort from carbon dioxide pneumoperitoneum, and some would only tolerate a lower pneumoperitoneum pressure (4-6 mm Hg). The requirement for deeper sedation in 10 of our patients reflects the inadequacy of conscious sedation in this group of patients.

We conclude that laparoscopic gastrostomy or jejunostomy can be performed with the patient under local anesthesia and intravenous conscious sedation with similar success as under general anesthesia and for similar cost. There may be potential savings by eliminating the cost of the operating room or the anesthesiologist. Some patients, however, may require deep sedation and rare cases may need to be converted to general anesthesia or to an open procedure. Clinical conditions and surgeon preference, therefore, should determine whether local anesthesia is used and in what setting, since there is no observed difference in success rate or complications when compared with general anesthesia.

This study was supported in part by the Medical Research Service of the Veterans Affairs Medical Center, San Francisco, Calif, and the Ross Product Division, Abbott Laboratories, Columbus, Ohio.

Drs Duh and Way developed the procedure for creating laparoscopic enterostomies using the T-fastener technique. The Regents of the University of California, San Francisco, hold the patent to this technique (US patent No. 5 151 086). The Regents of the University of California have licensed Abbott Laboratories to use this patent for laparoscopic enterostomy kits. Drs Duh and Way may be entitled to a share of the royalties. Ms Senokozlieff-Englehart, Mr Choe, and Ms Rowland are employees of Abbott Laboratories.

Special thanks to the following investigators for their participation in this project: John P. Grant, MD, Duke Medical Center, Durham, NC; Robert J. Fitzgibbons Jr, MD, Creighton University, Omaha, Neb; Kenric M. Murayama, MD, University of Nebraska Medical Center, Omaha; and Bruce M. Wolfe, MD, University of California, Davis.

Reprints: Quan-Yang Duh, MD, Surgical Service 112, Veterans Affairs Medical Center, San Francisco, CA 94121 (e-mail: Quan-Yang-Duh@med.va.gov).

REFERENCES

1. Duh QY, Way LW. Laparoscopic gastrostomy using T-fasteners as retractors and anchors. *Surg Endosc.* 1993;7:60-63.
2. Duh QY, Way LW. Laparoscopic jejunostomy using T-fasteners as retractors and anchors. *Arch Surg.* 1993;128:105-108.
3. Duh QY, Senokozlieff-Englehart AL, Siperstein AE, et al. Prospective evaluation of the safety and efficacy of laparoscopic jejunostomy. *West J Med.* 1995;162: 117-122.
4. Murayama KM, Schneider PD, Thompson JS. Laparoscopic gastrostomy: a safe method for obtaining enteral access. *J Surg Res.* 1995;58:1-5.
5. Sangster W, Swanstrom L. Laparoscopic-guided feeding jejunostomy. *Surg Endosc.* 1993;7:308-310.

6. Modesto VL, Harkins B, Calton WC Jr, Martindale RG. Laparoscopic gastrostomy using four-point fixation. *Am J Surg.* 1994;167:273-276.
7. Edelman DS, Unger SW. Laparoscopic gastrostomy. *Surg Gynecol Obstet.* 1991; 173:401.
8. Reiner DS, Leitman IM, Ward RJ. Laparoscopic Stamm gastrostomy with gastropexy. *Surg Laparosc Endosc.* 1991;1:189-192.
9. Wu TK, Pietrocola D, Welch HF. New method of percutaneous gastrostomy using anchoring devices. *Am J Surg.* 1987;153:230-232.
10. Gauderer MWL, Ponsky JL, Izant RJ Jr. Gastrostomy without laparotomy: a percutaneous endoscopic technique. *J Pediatr Surg.* 1980;15:872-875.
11. Ponsky JL, Gauderer MD. Percutaneous endoscopic gastrostomy: indications, limitations, techniques and results. *World J Surg.* 1989;13:165-170.
12. Jarnagin WR, Duh Q-Y, Mulvihill SJ, Ridge JA, Schrock TR, Way LW. The efficacy and limitations of percutaneous endoscopic gastrostomy. *Arch Surg.* 1992; 127:261-264.
13. DiSario JA, Foutch PG, Sanowski RA. Poor results with percutaneous endoscopic jejunostomy. *Gastrointest Endosc.* 1990;36:257-260.
14. Ng PC. Laparoscopic gastrostomy: a simple way to feed. *Surg Laparosc Endosc.* 1994;4:463-464.
15. Sylvester KG, Paskin DL, Schuricht AL. Combined laparoscopic-endoscopic gastrostomy. *Surg Endosc.* 1994;8:1072-1075.
16. Schlinkert RT, Sarr MG, Donohue JH, Thompson GB. General surgical laparoscopic procedures for the "nonlaparologist." *Mayo Clin Proc.* 1995;70:1142-1147.
17. Munk T, Kjer JJ. Laparoscopic sterilization under local anesthesia. *Acta Obstet Gynecol Scand.* 1994;73:347-348.
18. Gupta SP. Experience in 4500 cases of laparoscopic sterilization. *Int Surg.* 1993; 78:76-78.
19. Bordahl PE, Raeder JC, Nordentoft J, Kirste U, Refsdal A. Laparoscopic sterilization under local or general anesthesia? a randomized study. *Obstet Gynecol.* 1993;81:137-141.
20. Pendurthi TK, DeMaria EJ, Kellum JM. Laparoscopic bilateral inguinal hernia repair under local anesthesia. *Surg Endosc.* 1995;9:197-199.
21. Viani MP, Poggi RV, Pinto A, Fusai G, Andreani SM, Marvotti RA. Gasless laparoscopic gastrostomy. *J Laparoendosc Surg.* 1995;5:245-249.
22. Wolfsen HC, Kozarek RA, Ball TJ, Patterson DJ, Botoman VA, Ryan JA. Long-term survival in patients undergoing percutaneous endoscopic gastrostomy and jejunostomy. *Am J Gastroenterol.* 1990;85:1120-1122.

IN OTHER AMA JOURNALS

ARCHIVES OF GENERAL PSYCHIATRY

Familial Transmission of Substance Dependence: Alcohol, Marijuana, Cocaine, and Habitual Smoking: A Report From the Collaborative Study on the Genetics of Alcoholism

Laura Jean Bierut, MD; Stephen H. Dinwiddie, MD; Henri Begleiter, MD; Raymond R. Crowe, MD; Victor Hesselbrock, PhD; John I. Nurnberger, Jr, MD, PhD; Bernice Porjesz, PhD; Marc A. Schuckit, MD; Theodore Reich, MD

Background: Alcoholism and substance dependence frequently co-occur. Accordingly, we evaluated the familial transmission of alcohol, marijuana, and cocaine dependence and habitual smoking in the Collaborative Study on the Genetics of Alcoholism.
Methods: Subjects (n = 1212) who met criteria for both *DSM-III-R* alcohol dependence and Feighner definite alcoholism and their siblings (n = 2755) were recruited for study. A comparison sample was also recruited (probands, n = 217; siblings, n = 254). Subjects were interviewed with the Semi-Structured Assessment for the Genetics of Alcoholism. The familial aggregation of drug dependence and habitual smoking in siblings of alcohol-dependent and non–alcohol-dependent probands was measured by means of the Cox proportional hazards model.
Results: Rates of alcohol, marijuana, and cocaine dependence and habitual smoking were increased in siblings of alcohol-dependent probands compared with siblings of controls. For siblings of alcohol-dependent probands, 49.3% to 50.1% of brothers and 22.4% to 25.0% of sisters were alcohol dependent (lifetime diagnosis), but this elevated risk was not further increased by comorbid substance dependence in probands. Siblings of marijuana-dependent probands had an elevated risk of developing marijuana dependence (relative risk [RR], 1.78) and siblings of cocaine-dependent probands had an elevated risk of developing cocaine dependence (RR, 1.71). There was a similar finding for habitual smoking (RR, 1.77 in siblings of habitual-smoking probands).
Conclusions: Alcohol, marijuana, and cocaine dependence and habitual smoking are all familial, and there is evidence of both common and specific addictive factors transmitted in families. This specificity suggests independent causative factors in the development of each type of substance dependence. *(1998;55:982-988)*

Reprints: Laura Jean Bierut, MD, Department of Psychiatry, Washington University School of Medicine, 4940 Children's Pl, St Louis, MO 63110 (e-mail: laura@newhar.wustl.edu).

Lymphangiosis as a Predictor of Outcome in Patients With Primary Diffusely Infiltrative Adenocarcinoma of the Colon and Rectum

Reiping Tang, MD; Jeng-Yi Wang, MD; Kuo-Chien Tsao, BS; Yat-Sen Ho, MD

Objective: To investigate the relationships between outcome and clinicopathological factors, DNA flow cytometrical characteristics, and postoperative adjuvant therapy in patients with primary diffusely infiltrative colorectal adenocarcinoma.

Design: Inception cohort study.

Setting: A medical center that offers a mixture of primary, secondary, and tertiary care services.

Patients: Among 7035 patients undergoing resection of primary colorectal adenocarcinoma from 1980 to 1996, 37 patients with a pathological diagnosis of primary diffusely infiltrative tumor were selected. All patients had received regular follow-up until February 28, 1998, or until death.

Main Outcome Measures: Cancer-specific survival compared by log-rank test and Cox regression model.

Results: Univariate analyses revealed tumor stage (stages II-III vs stage IV, $P=.01$) and severity of lymphangiosis (absent/mild vs moderate/severe, $P=.04$) were significant in predicting outcome. A proliferative index of greater than 20% was insignificant ($P=.08$) in predicting outcome. In a Cox regression model, TNM stage and lymphangiosis were independently correlated with a worse outcome. When compared with tumors having less severe lymphangiosis, the odds ratio of death due to cancer in cases of tumors with moderate to severe lymphangiosis was 2.4 (95% confidence interval, 1.0-5.6; $P=.05$).

Conclusion: Lymphangiosis and TNM stage were independently predictive of outcome in patients with primary diffusely infiltrative colorectal cancer.

Arch Surg. 1999;134:157-160

DIFFUSELY INFILTRATIVE carcinoma mainly spreads beneath the mucosal layer, produces minimal mucosal alterations, and transforms the affected organ into a rigid, contracted tubular structure.[1] The terms *linitis plastica*[2-9] and *scirrhous carcinoma*[10-12] are used interchangeably to describe the same type of disease. Laufman and Saphir[2] first described this type of disease in the colon in 1951. Although diffusely infiltrative carcinoma was originally believed to mainly consist of poorly differentiated or signet ring cell carcinoma,[2,3,5] moderately differentiated tumor has been reported.[9,13] Because of the relative mucosal sparing and varied histologic pattern, diagnosis is based on exclusion of metastasis from cancer of other organs and on its characteristic morphologic appearance. The prognosis of patients with diffusely infiltrative carcinoma is generally reported to be poor.[3,5,13] Nevertheless, the association between the prognosis of patients and variable factors, including clinicopathological factors, DNA flow cytometrical variables, and postoperative adjuvant therapy, is unknown. This study sought to assess whether any clinicopathological factors, DNA flow cytometrical variables, or postoperative adjuvant therapy correlate with outcome in patients with diffusely infiltrative carcinoma.

From the Departments of Colorectal Surgery (Drs Tang and Wang) and Pathology (Drs Tsao and Ho), Chang Gung Memorial Hospital, Taipei, Taiwan.

RESULTS

CLINICAL FINDINGS

Among 7035 cases of primary colorectal carcinoma, 37 (0.53%) were of the primary diffusely infiltrative type. Twenty patients (54.1%) were female. The average age at diagnosis was 48.1 years (SD, 18.4 years). Eighteen tumors (48.6%) were located in the rectum. All 37 patients had at least 1 of the following complaints: diarrhea, changes in bowel habits, abdominal pain, or rectal bleeding. None of the 37 patients had a history of chronic ulcerative colitis.

PATIENTS AND METHODS

PATIENTS

A total of 7035 patients underwent resection of primary colorectal adenocarcinoma at Chang Gung Memorial Hospital, Taipei, Taiwan, a privately run medical center, from 1980 to 1996. Thirty-seven of these patients (those with a histologic diagnosis of primary diffusely infiltrative tumor) were selected for study. Signet ring cell rectal adenocarcinoma that was initially suspected to be metastatic was diagnosed in 3 of these patients after vigorous surveillance failed to find another primary origin. Paraffin-embedded tissue blocks of resected specimens from each of the 37 cases were used for DNA analysis and were reexamined by a pathologist (without knowledge of clinical data) to determine pathological features, including histologic grade,[14] presence of intracellular or extracellular mucin, resection margin, involvement of lymph nodes, lymphangiosis, and TNM stage.[15] Lymphangiosis was scored as negative, mild, moderate, or severe.[13] An average of 10 slides were examined per tumor. Clinical and demographic data including tumor location, sex, age, symptoms, and status of follow-up were obtained from medical records and/or the Registry of Colorectal Cancer, Chang Gung Memorial Hospital. Hematogenous spread at diagnosis included metastasis to liver, lung, bone, or peritoneum. Tumors with a lower edge within 15 cm of the anal verge were designated as rectal.

Radiotherapy and/or fluorouracil-based chemotherapy had been performed within 4 to 6 weeks of resection. All patients had received regular follow-up with serum carcinoembryonic antigen testing, physical examinations every 3 to 6 months, annual chest x-ray, abdominal computed tomography (or sonography of liver), and colonoscopic examinations until February 28, 1998, or until death. Cancer-related death was defined as death due to metastatic disease or treatment of the disease.

DNA FLOW CYTOMETRY

DNA flow cytometrical analysis was performed as previously described.[16] The prepared tissue samples were analyzed with a FACS Analyzer (Becton Dickinson, San Jose, Calif). A DNA histogram was generated using a computer with CellFIT Cell-Cycle Analysis software (Version 2.02; Becton Dickinson). The nondiploid histogram included aneuploid and tetraploid histograms. A high proliferative index was defined as 20% or more nuclei in the S and G2M phases. An unfavorable cell kinetic profile included nondiploid histograms and histograms with a high proliferative index.[17]

STATISTICAL ANALYSIS

Differences in the clinicopathological variables were compared in 2 groups using the Student t, χ^2, or Fisher exact test. Survival curves were constructed by the Kaplan-Meier method[18] and were compared by the log-rank test.[19] A 95% confidence interval (CI) was obtained using the Greenwood formula.[20] Survival time was measured in months. The Cox multiple regression analysis was used to adjust simultaneously for all covariates.[21] The end point was cancer-related death (cancer-specific survival). The survival time was 0 months for postoperative death. The type I error was set at 0.05. All analyses were performed using the statistical package SPSS for Windows, release 6.0 (SPSS Inc, Chicago, Ill).

PATHOLOGICAL FEATURES

Macroscopically, all the 37 lesions showed a pipelike appearance with a stenotic lumen and a rigid, thickened wall in the long segment. The average tumor size was 8.3 cm (SD, 2.3 cm; range, 5-15 cm) in axial length and 4.1 cm (SD, 1.1 cm; range, 2-7 cm) in transverse length. The ratio of axial to transverse length was 2.2 (SD, 0.8; range, 1-5). Nineteen tumors had a flattened and finely granular mucosal surface with tiny diffuse ulcerations or a cobblestone, edematous mucosa without obvious ulceration. The mucosa was spared from tumor involvement. Eighteen tumors had a single ulcer that varied in size (ranging from 1-4 cm in the axial length), usually located in the center of the lesion. The margins of these ulcers were not elevated. Their remaining peripheral portions were covered by intact, atrophic, or edematous mucosa. Diffuse infiltration through all layers of the wall with sparing of the mucosal layer and into the surrounding tissues was observed in all cases. Microscopically, cancer cells were composed of moderately to poorly differentiated cells. Twenty-one patients (57%) had intracellular (signet ring cell) or extracellular mucin-producing tumors. Eighteen (49%) tumors had moderate to severe lymphangiosis (**Figure 1**). Frequently, overlying mucosa of the lesion was not involved by tumor cells (**Figure 2**).

SURVIVAL ANALYSIS

Three patients (8.1%) had stage II tumors (2 with transmural invasion and 1 with contiguous organ involvement), 7 (18.9%) had stage III tumors, and 27 (73.0%) had stage IV tumors. One patient died of sepsis 2 weeks after surgery. The overall median cancer-specific survival time was 12 months (SE, 1 month; 95% CI, 11-13 months). Univariate analyses (**Table**) revealed tumor stage (stages II-III vs stage IV, P=.01) and severity of lymphangiosis (absent/mild vs moderate/severe, P=.04; **Figure 3**) were significant in predicting outcome. Proliferative index (low vs high, P=.08) was not correlated with prediction of outcome. All 3 of these variables were entered into the Cox regression model. Stage IV tumor and moderate to severe lymphangiosis were associated with a worse outcome. When compared with tumor stages II to III, the odds ratio of death from cancer for stage IV was 3.9 (95% CI, 1.4-10.6; P=.007). When compared with tumors of less severe lymphangiosis, the odds ratio of death from cancer in cases of tumors with moderate to severe lymphangiosis was 2.4 (95% CI, 1.0-5.6; P=.05).

Of 19 patients with colon tumor, 18 had data regarding the status of chemotherapy. Eleven had received chemotherapy while 7 had not. The outcome was not related to the adjuvant therapy. The respective me-

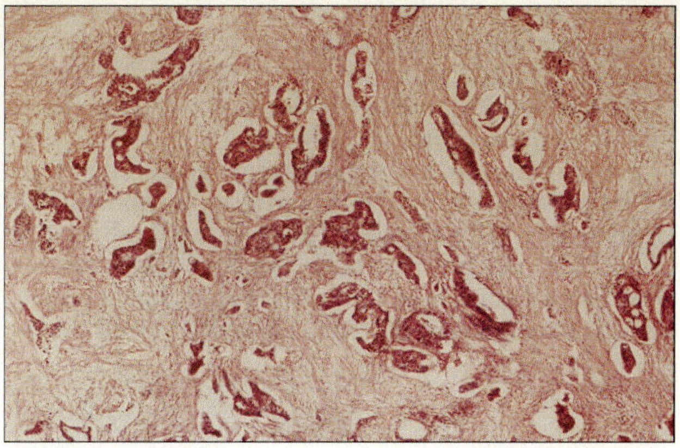

Figure 1. *Microscopic view of lesion showing marked lymphatic permeation (severe lymphangiosis) of moderately differentiated cells in submucosal layer. Severe desmoplastic reaction is also observed (hematoxylin-eosin, original magnification ×100).*

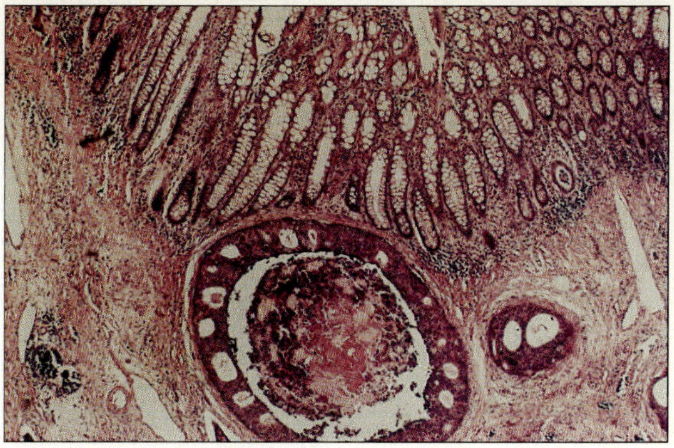

Figure 2. *Microscopic view of lesion showing comedolike lymphatic permeation of moderately differentiated cancer cells in the submucosal layer. The overlying mucosa is not involved by the tumor cells (hematoxylin-eosin, original magnification ×100).*

dian survival was 13 months (95% CI, 8-18 months) for patients who received chemotherapy and 14 months (95% CI, 8-20 months) for those who did not (*P*=.86). Of 18 patients with rectal cancer, 7 (including 1 postoperative death) had no adjuvant therapy, 6 had single-modality chemotherapy, 2 had single-modality radiotherapy, and 3 had combined chemotherapy and radiotherapy. Chemotherapy (with or without radiotherapy) was associated with a longer survival time (*P*=.007). The median survival was 14 months (95% CI, 5-23 months) for patients who received chemotherapy and 6 months (95% CI, 4-8 months) for those who did not. Radiotherapy was not associated with a better outcome. The respective median survival for patients with radiotherapy and those without was 14 and 10 months (*P*=.83). The survival times for the 3 patients who received combined chemotherapy and radiotherapy was 14, 30, and 72 months, respectively. Six of 9 patients with rectal cancer who received chemotherapy had stage IV tumors, compared with 6 of 8 patients who did not receive chemotherapy (*P*=.71). Adjusted by stage in a Cox regression model, chemotherapy was still important in predicting outcome. The likelihood of death due to cancer in patients who did not receive chemotherapy was 5 times greater than for those who received chemotherapy (95% CI, 1.5-15.3; *P*=.009).

COMMENT

Among the clinicopathological and DNA flow cytometrical variables studied, only tumor stage and lymphangiosis were important in predicting outcome of patients with primary diffusely infiltrative colorectal cancer. The odds of death for patients with a stage IV tumor was 4-fold compared with those with a less advanced tumor. The risk of death for patients with a tumor of moderate to severe lymphangiosis was 2.4 times that of patients with a tumor of milder lymphangiosis. The median survival was 11 months (95% CI, 9-13 months) for patients with moderate to severe lymphangiosis compared with 14 months (95% CI, 10-18 months) for patients with milder lymphangiosis (*P*=.04). In the study of Nakahara et al,[13] the median survival time was 7 months for 11 patients with moderate to severe lymphangiosis, compared with 24.5

Clinicopathological Factors and DNA Content Analysis vs Cancer-Specific Survival in Patients With Primary Diffusely Infiltrative Colorectal Cancer

		Median Survival		
Factor	No. of Patients	Months (SE)	95% Confidence Interval	*P*
Sex				
F	20	11 (3)	5-17	.87
M	17	12 (1)	9-15	
Age, y				
≤50	19	12 (2)	8-16	.32
>50	18	12 (1)	10-14	
Duration of symptoms, mo				
≤3	25	10 (2)	6-14	.10
>3	11	17 (4)	9-25	
Tumor location				
Colon	19	13 (2)	10-16	.21
Rectum	18	11 (1)	8-14	
Axial-transverse ratio				
≤2	22	12 (2)	9-15	.40
>2	15	12 (3)	7-17	
Mucin secretion				
Absent	16	7 (1)	4-10	.12
Intracellular	11	14 (2)	10-18	
Extracellular	10	12 (1)	10-14	
Lymphangiosis				
Absent/mild	19	14 (2)	10-18	.04
Moderate/severe	18	11 (1)	9-13	
Histologic grade				
Moderate	12	11 (8)	0-26	.87
Poor	25	12 (1)	11-13	
TNM stage				
II-III	10	23 (4)	15-31	.01
IV	27	10 (1)	8-12	
DNA content analysis				
Ploid status				
Diploid	20	12 (1)	10-14	.41
Nondiploid	13	14 (2)	11-17	
Proliferative index, %				
≤20	13	19 (4)	11-27	.08
>20	20	11 (1)	8-14	
Cellular kinetics				
Favorable	11	14 (2)	11-17	.29
Unfavorable	22	12 (1)	10-14	

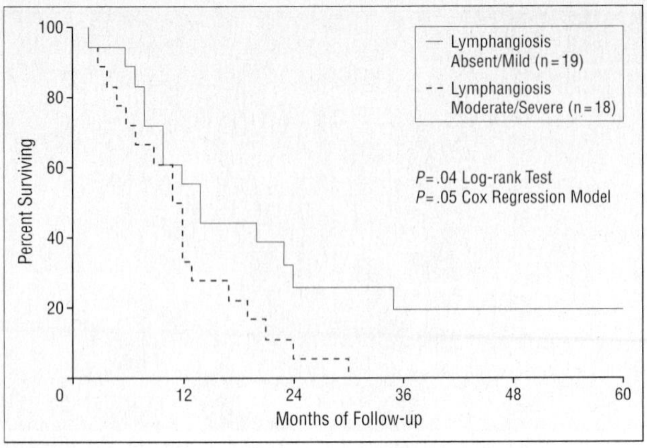

Figure 3. *Overall cancer-specific survival of patients with primary diffusely infiltrative carcinoma of the colon and rectum (n=37) by lymphangiosis. Patients with a tumor of moderate to severe lymphangiosis had a significantly decreased overall survival compared with those with a tumor of milder lymphangiosis.*

months for 4 patients with mild lymphangiosis. The degree of lymphatic permeation is also reported to be an important prognostic factor in patients with other morphologic types of stage III rectal tumor.[22]

In the present study, 37 (0.53%) of 7035 cases with primary colorectal carcinoma were the primary diffusely infiltrative type. This incidence is similar to that of the series of Nakahara (0.64%).[13] Twelve (32.4%) moderately differentiated tumors were found in 37 cases. The reported incidence of moderately differentiated tumor varied from 25% to 52%.[9,13] The wide variation may be due to a small sample size of each study. The average age of the 37 patients was 47.4 years in the current study—10 years younger than those with other morphologic types of colorectal cancer.[16] The earlier age at diagnosis of cancer may be due to more rapid tumor progression and/or different pathogenesis. Although Anderson and Hansen[6] found chronic ulcerative colitis in 25% of reviewed cases, both our study and the study of Nakahara et al[13] found no chronic ulcerative colitis in cases of primary diffusely infiltrative tumor. This may be explained by the higher prevalence of chronic ulcerative colitis in the Western countries than in Asia.[23] Some patients with long-standing chronic ulcerative colitis may develop colorectal carcinoma,[24] which tends to be infiltrative and scirrhous.[25]

The grave prognosis of patients with primary diffusely infiltrative colorectal cancer is well documented.[3,4,13,26] Radical resection was not possible in 73% of our patients because of disseminated disease or extensive locoregional invasion. This finding of late diagnosis is in accordance with other studies.[4,5] In an earlier study of 538 stage III tumors, we also found that the odds of death for patients with such tumors was 11-fold that of patients with other morphologic types of tumors.[27] The average duration of symptoms of 3.1 months prior to diagnosis and the higher prevalence of cases with stage IV disease at the time of diagnosis in the current study suggest that the grave prognosis of primary diffusely infiltrative colorectal cancer is caused by both the higher aggressiveness of these tumors and the insidious nature of their growth, which causes minimal symptoms until an advanced stage is reached.

It is interesting that postoperative chemotherapy prolonged the median survival time in patients with rectal tumors, but not in those with colon tumors. The causes of differential response to chemotherapy between colon and rectal cancers are not known.

In conclusion, both lymphangiosis and tumor stage were the independent factors in determining outcome in patients with diffusely infiltrative colorectal cancer. Our results also suggest that fluorouracil-based postoperative chemotherapy might provide a better chance for survival in patients with diffusely infiltrative rectal cancer.

Reprints: Reiping Tang, MD, Department of Colorectal Surgery, Chang Gung Memorial Hospital, 199 Tung Hwa North Rd, Taipei, Taiwan (e-mail: rptang@ms11.hinet.net).

REFERENCES

1. Fahl JC, Dockerty MB, Judd ES. Scirrhous carcinoma of the colon and rectum. *Surg Gynecol Obstet.* 1960;3:759-766.
2. Laufman H, Saphir O. Primary linitis plastica type of carcinoma of the colon. *Arch Surg.* 1951;62:79-91.
3. Stevens WR, Ruiz P. Primary linitis plastica carcinoma of the colon and rectum. *Mod Pathol.* 1989;2:265-269.
4. Amorn Y, Knight WA Jr. Primary linitis plastica of the colon: report of two cases and review of the literature. *Cancer.* 1978;4:2420-2425.
5. Nadel L, Mori K, Shinya H. Primary linitis plastica of the colon and rectum: report of two cases. *Dis Colon Rectum.* 1983;26:736-740.
6. Andersen JA, Hansen BF. Linitis plastica of the colon and rectum: report of two cases. *Dis Colon Rectum.* 1972;15:217-221.
7. Rao TR, Hambrick E, Abcarian H, Salgia K, Recant WM. Colorectal linitis plastica. *Dis Colon Rectum.* 1982;25:239-244.
8. Papp JP Jr, Levine EJ, Thomas FB. Primary linitis plastica carcinoma of the colon and rectum. *Am J Gastroenterol.* 1995;90:141-145.
9. Shirouzu K, Isomoto H, Morodomi T, Ogata Y, Akagi Y, Kakegawa T. Primary linitis plastica carcinoma of the colon and rectum. *Cancer.* 1994;74:1863-1868.
10. McQueeney AJ, Olson RW, Medwid A. Primary scirrhous carcinoma of colon: roentgenologic diagnosis. *AJR Am J Roentgenol.* 1967;101:306-310.
11. Carlson DH, Feen D, Simon H. Primary scirrhous adenocarcinoma of the colon (signet-ring cell type). *South Med J.* 1981;74:1525-1529.
12. Balthazar EJ, Siegel SE, Megibow AJ, Scholes J, Gordon R. CT in patients with scirrhous carcinoma of the GI tract: imaging findings and value for tumor detection and staging. *AJR Am J Roentgenol.* 1995;165:839-845.
13. Nakahara H, Ishikawa T, Itabashi M, Hirota T. Diffusely infiltrating primary colorectal carcinoma of linitis plastica and lymphangiosis types. *Cancer.* 1992;69:901-906.
14. Morson BC, Sobin LH. *Histological Typing of Intestinal Tumours.* Geneva, Switzerland: World Health Organization; 1976. Technical report No. 15.
15. Hermanek P, Sobin LH, eds. *TNM Classification of Malignant Tumors.* 4th ed. Berlin, Germany: Springer-Verlag; 1987:47-49.
16. Tang R, Ho YS, You YT, et al. Prognostic evaluation of DNA flow cytometric and histopathologic parameters of colorectal cancer. *Cancer.* 1995;76:1724-1730.
17. Witzig TE, Loprinzi CL, Gonchoroff NJ, et al. DNA ploidy and cell kinetic measurements as predictors of recurrence and survival in stages B2 and C colorectal adenocarcinoma. *Cancer.* 1991;68:879-888.
18. Kaplan EL, Meier P. Nonparametric estimation from incomplete observations. *J Am Stat Assoc.* 1958;53:457-481.
19. Peto R, Peto J. Asymptoticaly efficient rank invariant test procedures. *J R Stat Soc.* 1972;135:185-198.
20. Lee ET. *Statistical Methods for Survival Data Analysis.* Belmont, Calif: Lifetime Learning Publications; 1980:96.
21. Cox DR. Regression models and life tables. *J R Stat Soc.* 1972;34:1987-2002.
22. Shirouzu K, Isomoto H, Morodomi T, Kakegawa T. Carcinomatous lymphatic permeation, prognostic significance in patients with rectal carcinoma: a long term prospective study. *Cancer.* 1995;75:4-10.
23. Kirsner JB, Shorter RG. Recent developments in nonspecific inflammatory bowel disease: part II. *N Engl J Med.* 1982;306:837-848.
24. Ohman U. Colorectal carcinoma in patients with ulcerative colitis. *Am J Surg.* 1982;144:344-349.
25. Corman ML. *Colon and Rectal Surgery.* 2nd ed. Philadephia, Pa: JB Lippincott Co; 1989:794-795.
26. Henrion J, de Neve A, Sergent H, Schmitz A, Heller F. Primary linitis plastica of the rectum and colon. *Gastroenterol Clin Biol.* 1984;8:814-818.
27. Tang R, Wang JY, Chen JS, et al. Survival impact of lymph node metastasis in TNM stage III carcinoma of the colon and rectum. *J Am Coll Surg.* 1995;180: 705-712.

Your best medical information source...

ARCHIVES OF SURGERY

from the
American Medical Association

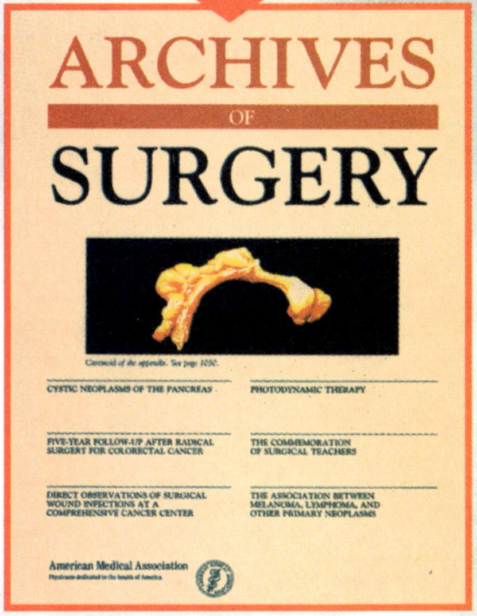

Archives of Surgery is the best read journal representing a full range of specialty interests. Original submissions, the best papers from surgical societies, stringent statistical reviews, invited commentaries and a greater use of illustration set the standard in its field.

Enter a personal subscription — send in a reply card today!

ARCHIVES OF SURGERY — SUBSCRIPTION ORDER FORM

☑ **YES!** Enter my personal subscription to ***Archives of Surgery*** at the special money saving rate checked below:

- ❑ AMA Member rate: One year (12 issues) — $95*.
- ❑ Individual non-member rate: One year (12 issues) — $145*.
- ❑ Corporate/Institutional rate: One year (12 issues) — $245.
- ❑ *My personal check in U.S. $ is enclosed. (Make check payable to *American Medical Association*).
- ❑ Charge my personal credit card: ❑ VISA ❑ MASTERCARD ❑ AMEX ❑ OPTIMA

Card No.______ Exp. Date______ Signature______

Name (Please print) ______

Address ______

City______ State/Province______ Zip/Postal Code ______

Phone______ Fax______ e-mail ______

IMPORTANT: The individual non-member rate is available in the U.S. and Canada only. Payment must accompany order. Corporate/Institutional checks are not accepted for personal subscriptions. Canada residents add 7% GST. GST # (12622 5556 RT). **I9X2DZ**

ARCHIVES OF SURGERY — SUBSCRIPTION ORDER FORM

☑ **YES!** Enter my personal subscription to ***Archives of Surgery*** at the special money saving rate checked below:

- ❑ AMA Member rate: One year (12 issues) — $95*.
- ❑ Individual non-member rate: One year (12 issues) — $145*.
- ❑ Corporate/Institutional rate: One year (12 issues) — $245.
- ❑ *My personal check in U.S. $ is enclosed. (Make check payable to *American Medical Association*).
- ❑ Charge my personal credit card: ❑ VISA ❑ MASTERCARD ❑ AMEX ❑ OPTIMA

Card No.______ Exp. Date______ Signature______

Name (Please print) ______

Address ______

City______ State/Province______ Zip/Postal Code ______

Phone______ Fax______ e-mail ______

IMPORTANT: The individual non-member rate is available in the U.S. and Canada only. Payment must accompany order. Corporate/Institutional checks are not accepted for personal subscriptions. Canada residents add 7% GST. GST # (12622 5556 RT). **I9X2DZ**

ARCHIVES OF SURGERY — SUBSCRIPTION ORDER FORM

☑ **YES!** Enter my personal subscription to ***Archives of Surgery*** at the special money saving rate checked below:

- ❑ AMA Member rate: One year (12 issues) — $95*.
- ❑ Individual non-member rate: One year (12 issues) — $145*.
- ❑ Corporate/Institutional rate: One year (12 issues) — $245.
- ❑ *My personal check in U.S. $ is enclosed. (Make check payable to *American Medical Association*).
- ❑ Charge my personal credit card: ❑ VISA ❑ MASTERCARD ❑ AMEX ❑ OPTIMA

Card No.______ Exp. Date______ Signature______

Name (Please print) ______

Address ______

City______ State/Province______ Zip/Postal Code ______

Phone______ Fax______ e-mail ______

IMPORTANT: The individual non-member rate is available in the U.S. and Canada only. Payment must accompany order. Corporate/Institutional checks are not accepted for personal subscriptions. Canada residents add 7% GST. GST # (12622 5556 RT). **I9X2DZ**

NO POSTAGE
NECESSARY
IF MAILED
IN THE
UNITED STATES

BUSINESS REPLY MAIL
FIRST-CLASS MAIL PERMIT NO. 1376 CHICAGO IL

POSTAGE WILL BE PAID BY ADDRESSEE

SUBSCRIBER SERVICES CENTER
AMERICAN MEDICAL ASSOCIATION
PO BOX 10945
CHICAGO IL 60610-9902

NO POSTAGE
NECESSARY
IF MAILED
IN THE
UNITED STATES

BUSINESS REPLY MAIL
FIRST-CLASS MAIL PERMIT NO. 1376 CHICAGO IL

POSTAGE WILL BE PAID BY ADDRESSEE

SUBSCRIBER SERVICES CENTER
AMERICAN MEDICAL ASSOCIATION
PO BOX 10945
CHICAGO IL 60610-9902

ARCHIVES OF SURGERY

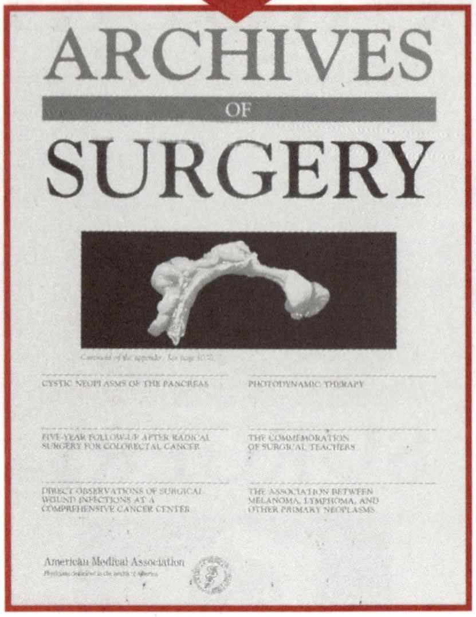

Essential reading to stay on the cutting-edge of clinical developments...

SUBSCRIBE NOW!

NO RISK GUARANTEE:

If you are not completely satisfied with your first issue, you may cancel and receive a full refund of your subscription payment. Or, if at any time, *Archives of Surgery* stops meeting your needs, you may cancel and receive a full refund of all unmailed issues.

Summary of the 115th Annual Meeting of the German Society of Surgery

Berlin, April 28 to May 2, 1998

Ernst Klar, MD

The annual meeting of the German Society of Surgery is equivalent to the meeting of the American College of Surgeons. More than 4800 surgeons, internists, and basic scientists gathered in Berlin. All major issues of modern surgery were adressed in 785 oral presentations and more than 270 posters with special emphasis on progress in surgical technique, transatlantic cooperation, improvement in quality management between surgery and anesthesia, and the mainstay of surgical research—microcirculation and molecular biology. The following summary conveys an impression of the current fields of reassesssment and progress in German surgery.

"HUMANITY AND SCIENCE" PRESIDENTIAL ADDRESS BY CHRISTIAN HERFARTH, MD, HEIDELBERG, GERMANY

Humanity is independent from science, but without humanity, science turns senseless. *Evidence-based surgery* is a typical modern term that was initially used with great enthusiasm to imply perfect patient care. There is no doubt that surgical decision making has to be primarily based on study results. However, it soon had to be realized that the surgeon's experience and intuition are similarly called for. The dualism is especially exemplified by oncological surgery: evidence-based prognostic factors and the patients' characteristics in the wider sense determine the choice of therapy: age, tumor type, and grade of disease are objective parameters. Biological age, mental vigor, psychosocial background, family infrastructure, different effect of alternative therapy will be considered equally on the subjective base of the experienced surgeon to reach the best decision regarding quality, profit, consumption, or waste of the remaining life span. A purely scientific approach can undermine intuition and experience to the point of collapse. The paradox between science and humanity creates the incentive for the progress of surgery.

Nowadays the progress of science in surgery is influenced and characterized by mutual interdisciplinary exchange. The interventional treatment of portal hypertension by transjugular intrahepatic portosystemic stent shunt has challenged surgeons to reassess indications for and technique of shunt surgery, to clearly define disadvantages of the less invasive technique, and to prevent transgression of the optimal timing for liver transplantation. Endovascular therapy of aortic aneurysms represents another example that surgery must encourage cooperation in the new field of combined disease approach rather than try and hinder other specialties to deal with disease entities formerly reserved for operative therapy. In this sense surgeons also have a gatekeeper function in participating in the evolvement of techniques that are often looked at with uncritical acceptance due to minimal invasiveness.

One main concern is the adequate representation of scientific data in Germany, the solution of which is probably a double strategy. It is self-evident that original data should be published in high-ranking international journals, even more so, if representing basic sciences. However, a German publishing culture has to be maintained at the same time aiming at the national dis-

From the Department of General Sugery, University of Heidelberg, Heidelberg, Germany.

tribution of research results especially for clinical education. University and medical center hospitals have to account for continuous progress especially in the respective main area to increase transparency for appropriate referrals. Therefore, the classical impact factor is not the main yardstick of scientific prowess for most German medical faculties and an internal journal ranking has become the basis for academic promotion in many institutions. (German faculties define an "internal" impact factor since the national importance of several German journals is not reflected by the official impact factor.)

THE AMERICAN EXPERIENCE—MOTIVATION AND IMPETUS TO REFLECT

Samuel A. Wells, MD, St Louis, Mo, outlined the education of the surgical scientist emphasizing that a surgical career in clinical research must be thoroughly prepared in the method and process of laboratory research at a young age starting during medical school training. The most productive research experience should be gained as a house officer during the second or third clinical year. Wells advocated that this period of research be of sufficient length (2 or 3 years) and that the laboratory project be of relevance to the young surgeon's area of clinical interest. The house officer should join the research team of an experienced senior scientist who will provide adequate mentorship. After completing the residency, the future staff position must provide a protected time for laboratory research and an environment of collaborative interaction with distinguished scientists. An obstacle to this logical concept is the diminishing volume of grant support for surgical projects compared with internal medicine and basic sciences that applies to the United States as well as Germany. Continuity of research activity seems to be a prerequiste for success. The same principle was underlined in the analysis of transatlantic cooperation between Andrew L. Warshaw, MD, Harvard Medical School, Massachusetts General Hospital, Boston, and our institution, which has been fruitful over a decade due to a continuous and overlapping integration of research fellows from Heidelberg in Boston. The efficiency of laboratory work was guaranteed by an experienced mentor, compelling laboratory work within a functioning infrastructure, the mutual transfer of ideas, and the additive application of different techniques specific for the respective laboratory to build up a coherent line of investigation. However, it was stated that, in general, transatlantic cooperation is lacking a true exchange of fellows. The reluctance for Americans to come to Germany is only partly explained by language problems. The main reason may lie in high university fees in the United States leaving many young physicians with the committment to pay back a considerable bank loan and the desire to finish residency within the shortest possible time. John Cameron, MD, Baltimore, Md, analyzed the question: General surgery, visceral surgery, or further specialization? Eighty-two percent of the operative spectrum in general surgery consist of gastrointestinal (GI)-surgery supporting the statement that general surgery in the United States is in fact alimentary tract surgery. After analyzing the training profile of 1000 young surgeons in 1994, it became apparent that at qualification after a 5-year training period only few candidates had ever performed major operations like esophagectomy, total gastrectomy, hemihepatectomy, or Kausch-Whipple procedure. Moreover the spectrum of operations performed at recertification 10 years later did not differ significantly in the vast majority of surgeons. Thus, the general surgeon seems to be sufficiently prepared for the standard requirements regarding GI-surgery and there is no need for general generic GI-fellowships. In addition a GI-fellowship would destroy the general surgery program due to the large overlap. However, Cameron emphasized that special fellowships must be provided for the complex and more advanced surgical procedures. There are hard data that show that the volume of cases and surgical experience can change the outcome. Therefore, to guarantee a sufficient number of operations, there are individual fellowships offered, eg, hepatobiliary-pancreatic, at institutions outstanding in this field but by no means covering the whole field of GI-sugery in a countrywide standardized fashion.

SPECIALIZATION IN SURGERY AND THE REORGANIZATION OF THE GERMAN SOCIETY OF SURGERY

The current surgical training program in Germany was reconstituted 5 years ago and is based on the standards of the European community. It consists of a 5-year basic training period, to which a 3-year special education program can be added in the following specialties: visceral, vascular, thoracic, and trauma surgery.

At this year's annual meeting, the German Society of Visceral Surgery was founded, a step that represents the final recognition that visceral surgery is a highly specific specialty and not just a constituent of general surgery a designation that used to be applied for virtually all areas of surgery without a properly defined advanced training program. Subspecialization to the present degree is widely agreed on by the German surgeons. However, it seems important to guarantee that the position of the German Society of Surgery is not compromised. The influence of politics for quality assessment, cost-benefit analysis, and training can only be controlled by an influencial roof organization that acts on behalf of all surgical disciplines. The attraction of the annual meeting of the German Society of Surgery is at stake due to additional high-level congresses of the different disciplines. Planning for the near future comprises a day-by-day representation of each surgical field that will reduce the historical preponderance of GI surgery. In addition to the main fields of surgery mentioned the 3 separate disciplines—pediatric, plastic, and cardiac surgery—will also be integrated in the annual meeting resulting in a similar structure to the "Surgical Week." Another example of organ-specific specialization is the diminishing influence of pediatric surgery in Germany. In 1967 the first chair was established at the University of Heidelberg followed by a total of 18 throughout the country. The growing tendency toward a treatment of highly specific pediatric diseases by the most experienced surgeons in the respective field like pediatric coloanal, endocrinologic, urological, or cardiac surgery may lead to a remnant of inguinal and minor GI pathologic features to deal with for the pediatric surgeon proper, resulting in a downgrading of the academic position in many cases.

SURGICAL RESEARCH

Microcirculation and molecular biology can be considered as 2 main components of surgical research. The understanding of organ microcirculation was only made possible by the development of different models of intravital microscopy that was initialized by K. Meßmer, Institute for Surgical Research, Munich, Ben W. Zweifach, PhD, and Marcos Intaglietta, PhD, AMES Bioengineering Institute, La Jolla, San Diego, Calif, exactly 20 years ago. The standard of today comprises a description of the angioarchitecture of most parenchymal organs and the quantification of microvessel perfusion and the analysis of blood cell-endothelium interaction with special reference to leukocytes and thrombocytes. The microcirculatory effect of systemic inflammatory response opened new insight into the sepsis syndrome. In addition the analysis of microvascular perfusion failure in surgical disease states lead to new therapeutic concepts. During the last 15 years it has been shown that the mortality rate of acute pancreatitis could be considerably reduced by the recognition that the early phase of the disease is the main field of intensive care unit therapy directed at a reversal of microcirculatory breakdown especially in the pancreas. The establishment of necroses can be counteracted and better demarcation of already existing necroses facilitates surgical debridement. Thus a decreasing number of operations at a later stage of the disease was the logical consequence of perceiving microcirculatoty events and has been confirmed as a major therapeutical progress. In the field of liver surgery better knowledge of ischemia-reperfusion injury has a great potential effect on surgical decision making. Hepatic resection for primary tumors or metastatic disease has been extended during the last years regarding the indication for resection and the volume of removed tissue resulting in a prolonged warm ischemia time and a marginal liver remnant. Therefore, it may be significant to reduce warm ischemia/reperfusion injury. A promising line of investigation is preconditioning of the liver before resection, ie, to induce adaptive mechanisms by short-time ischemia before induction of the main ischemic period. To define the time frame with regard to duration of preconditioning, length, and frequency of reperfusion intravital microscopy is used as the optimal tool. Surprisingly, a variety of attempts to reduce ischemia/reperfusion injury in transplantation surgery have been shown to be effective experimentally, the clinical transposition, nevertheless, has been insufficient. Either only observation studies have been reported or randomization of only few patients without stratification concerning graft function was performed. Recently, thermodiffusion (as used in our institution) offers the possibility to quantify hepatic microcirculation as the main determinant of graft quality in patients thus providing a quantifiable parameter of graft quality with a pathophysiological key role.

The analysis of microcirculation would be confined to pure phenomenology if molecular biology did not provide the respective techniques to describe the underlying mechanisms. The interaction of blood cells and vascular endothelium plays a central role in the chain of pathophysiological events. Although the location of adhesion molecules has been previously detected by other conventional methods like immunohistochemistry, the modern techniques of molecular biology allow for a more accurate quantification of ligand/receptor expression by Northern or Western blot, a more specific description of the role of defined mediators by gene knock-out animals and a pinpointed blockade of receptor/ligand interactions by anti–sense messenger RNA inactivation. Conversely, tumor immunotolerance may be a topic to exemplify how molecular biology can benefit from advances in microcirculation. The knowledge of tumor microvessel organization as well as structure and function of the endothelial barrier helps to understand and to modify transmigration of immunocompetent cells from the bloodstream as first event of tumoricidal action.

SURGICAL FORUM

The surgical forum was integrated into the annual meeting in 1972 under the presidency of Fritz Linder, MD, Heidelberg, to emphasize the surgeon's key position in research. Compared with other disciplines, the therapeutic approach to disease in surgery is most direct and invasive. For the patients' benefit a free flow of scientific questions and solutions from the bedside to the laboratory and vice versa is mandatory and can only be guaranteed by an institutionalized surgical research. Throughout Germany there are 5 chairs for surgical research and 10 positions associated with the chair of surgery, providing the opportunity for young residents to spend a research fellowship at the same insitution. This structure has the advantage that there is continuity and close cooperation even after the fellows return to clinical work.

Statistics concerning the Surgical Forum show increasing research activity in Germany. The number of submitted abstracts fluctuated around 200 from 1972 to 1982 gradually increasing to more than 470 this year; the rate of acceptance ranged between 30% to 36%. Concerning the proportion of submitted abstracts according to the different surgical specialties there was a distinct shift toward the representation of general/visceral surgery. Heart, lung, and vascular surgery decreased from 19% in 1972 to actually 5% and traumatology from 13% to 5%, whereas visceral surgery increased from 34% to 72%. This may only partly reflect overall research activities and could be an indicator for the tendency that the different surgical specialties divert some of their scientific presentations away from the German Society of Surgery to their own annual meetings. Concerning the presentation of scientific papers, interest and participation of the broad surgical community became an overt problem to an extent that requires reorganization. At our annual meeting and during the meeting of the Society for Surgery of the Alimentary Tract in New Orleans, La, the auditorium in several scientific sessions was limited to not more than 20 people. The prevention of simultaneous clinical sessions and the addition of invited commentaries by opinion leaders in the respective field might help to restore adequate appreciation.

This year's award session consisted of the 12 highest ranking abstracts, 2 of which were selected for the Forum Prize. Celik et al from the Institute of Theoretical Surgery, Marburg, Germany, presented a complex animal model featuring clinical variability and the principles of a randomized, controlled, clinical trial to evaluate the effect of different drug combinations (ie, clinical modeling randomized trial). To demonstrate the practicability of the model different combinations of histamine$_2$-receptor blockers were evaluated for prophylaxis during the induction phase of anesthesia. In 4 groups of 15 animals each it could be demonstrated that the combination of dimethindene maleate/cimetidine and dimethindene/famotidine showed an effectiveness similar to the randomized clinical trial. With dimethindene/ranitidine no significant prophylactic effect was documented. It was concluded that clinical modeling randomized trials in animals are able to answer clinical questions that could only be solved by complex clinical studies otherwise. Clinical modeling randomized trials can be performed faster than comparable studies under clinical conditions. The second award study investigated the resuscitation of livers procured from non–heart beating donors after 1 hour of cardiac arrest in a pig transplantation model. By venous systemic oxygen gas persufflation via the suprahepatic vena cava during hypothermic storage graft ischemia/reperfusion injury could be minimized to a comparable degree to the experimental group that had not been subjected to warm ischemia prior to liver explantation (S. Saad, MD, Köln, Germany).

THE EFFECT OF MOLECULAR BIOLOGY ON SURGICAL DECISION MAKING

Molecular biology was newly introduced as a separate session into the surgical forum in 1995. This year 25% of all accepted forum presentations dealt with molecular mechanisms or were based on molecular biological techniques. Beyond the surgical forum the main emphasis throughout the meeting was put on the question: to what extent clinical concepts and surgical decisions are influenced by the latest advances of molecular biology.

The effect of molecular biological evaluation on hereditary nonpolyposis colon cancer (HNPCC) for preventive surgery was outlined by H. T. Lynch, MD, Houston, Tex. Focusing on clinical and histomorphological characteristics, HNPCC tumors were identified as inducing a profound lymphoid reaction and resulting in a better prognosis than demonstrated for sporadic colon cancer. Undoubtedly, frequent colonoscopic surveillance is indicated in patients who tested positive for any HNPCC-associated mismatch repair gene mutation. It is yet too early to give a general recommendation concerning prophylactic colectomy. Growing knowledge of the clinical and pathological characteristics of HNPCC tumors will ultimately help to define patients who will benefit from prophylactic colectomy.

The value of immunochemistry to prescreen for mismatch repair gene defects in patients with potential HNPCC syndrome was underlined by an analysis of 30 patients suspected to have HNPCC on clinical grounds (S. Vossen, MD, Düsseldorf, Germany). By 3 independent investigators immunochemistry was shown to be an excellent screening method to identify patients with HNPCC who then could be further analyzed by DNA sequencing.

In a cooperative contribution from Düsseldorf and the Mayo Clinic (Rochester, Minn) families with HNPCC syndrome were analyzed for the occurrence of rectal carcinoma since general recommendations suggest ileorectal anastomosis as the therapy of choice for HNPCC-positive patients. The incidence of rectal carcinoma was 29% in 42 patients with HNPCC fulfilling Amsterdam criteria. Therefore, the authors (G. Möslein, MD, and S. Thibodeau, MD) conclude that restaurative proctocolectomy with ileoanal pouch anastomosis seems to be the therapy of choice for patients with HNPCC at least when rectal cancer can be excluded at the time of therapeutical intervention.

In 1996, Vasen et al [*Lancet*. 1996;348:433] suggested ileorectal anastomosis instead of restorative proctocolectomy with ileoanal pouch anastomosis in patients with familial adenomatous polyposis if the mutation in the *APC* gene was located 5′ of codon 1250. In contrast to the reported findings, analysis from our familial adenomatous polyposis register (Martina Kadmon, MD, Heidelberg) did not demonstrate a favorable prognosis for patients with mutations at this location. Therefore we suggested that restorative proctocolectomy with ileoanal pouch anastomosis remains the therapy of choice for all patients with familial adenomatous polyposis.

Detection and eradication of disseminated neoplastic cells that are the reason for tumor recurrence after curative resection was another main topic in the molecular biology session. In comparison to immunohistochemistry reversed transcriptase-polymerase chain reaction (RT-PCR) assays have profoundly improved sensitivity and specificity of tumor cell detection in blood and bone marrow samples and are also applied to achieve a more accurate staging of lymphatic tumor spread. Jürgen Weitz, MD, Heidelberg, used cytokeratin 20–RT-PCR for the detection of isolated disseminated tumor cells of colorectal cancer in lymph nodes. Tumor progression after R0-resection in patients with colorectal cancer stage UICC I and II could be caused by isolated disseminated tumor cells in lymph nodes, which are not detected by current staging methods. With the established cytokeratin 20–RT-PCR tumor cells were detected in 32 of 107 histopathologically negative lymph nodes from patients with colorectal cancer. Thus, lymphogenic tumor cell dissemination seems more common in early colorectal cancer than previously acknowledged. These results underline the therapeutic importance of meticulous lymph node dissection in colorectal tumor surgery.

Since disseminated tumor cells are predominantly nondividing cells (dormant tumor cells), conventional chemotherapy is probably ineffective. Relevant strategies for therapeutical interventions were the application of antibodies (17-1A, 425), peptide vaccination (17-1A, MUC-1, *ras*, p53) for the induction of a T-cell reaction, in vivo or in vitro prodrug gene therapy, and the reconstitution of wild type tumor suppressor genes (H. Kalthoff, MD, Kiel, Germany).

One of the basis of surgery, the treatment of wounds and the correction of disturbances in wound healing, has previously been a less prominent topic in academic surgery. However, the options of a basic understanding of cell function and interaction provided by molecular biology techniques revitalized the effort to improve patient care in this field. R. Hanselmann, MD (Homburg, Germany), pointed out, that influencing late wound healing and especially prolonged healing of fractures would have a major effect for the individual patient and the socioeconomic consequences of extended healing processes. In various animal models and phase 1 clinical trials, a stable expression of transgenes in wound tissue and areas of fracture defects has been demonstrated. Since the expression of transgenes was restricted to the defect location the gene therapy vectors applied can be regarded as reasonably safe for the transfection of therapeutc genes. The genes presently tested include growth hormones and factors influencing angiogenesis. Further development of tissue specific promoters should facilitate an isolated transduction of therapeutic genes in target cells thereby increasing the efficacy and safety of gene therapy protocols.

Another topic with dramatic socioeconomic impact is the prevention of aortic aneurysms affecting as many as 5% of men older than 60 years. J. Powell, PhD (London, England), stressed the influence of the matrix metalloproteinases and plasmin together with inflammation and neovascularization as the precursors of medial thinning and consecutive aortic aneurysm formation. Her provocative message to the molecular biologist was, that analyzing the inflammatory and proteolytic processes may lead to earlier therapeutic options than evaluating the genetic basis of aneurysm formation in the elderly. Whether the presence of *Chlamydia pneumoniae* DNA in as many as 50% of the aneurysms represents an epiphenomenon or plays a causative role remains to be evaluated.

MULTIMEDIA TRAINING

The significance of new media for basic and advanced training was analyzed on a broad scale by representatives of the German Society of Surgery and of the Board of German Surgeons as well as by leading scientific publishers, authors, information scientists, software and hardware engineers, and experts on didactics. Virtual reality is still in the early stage of development and will be used in the future not only to increase manual skills but also to convey theoretical knowledge as a textbook equivalent. Currently CD-ROM technology is generally agreed on as a most effective, feasible multimedia training tool. A high level of interactivity represents a main advantage compared with the classical video presentation. Problem-based training is facilitated due the fast selection of specific topics within the main subject of the respective CD-ROM. According to a survey among the participants of the multimedia session CD-ROM technology is used for the following applications: the collection of slides by 93% of institutions, animated pictures (80%), the presentation of congress or symposium material (80%), the collection of video clips (67%), demonstration of case reports (43%), and simple text storage (40%). As overlapping technical alternative the Internet was referred to in 33%, the digital video disc technology in 20%, online services and conventional data banks, respectively, in 15%. The major concern centered around loosing personal contact and exchange in medical training by the use of computers.

THE GREAT FINISH: ROWING

After the scientific meeting had come to an end the congress moved to the historical rowing track in Berlin-Grünau. Forty-two teams from surgical institutions all over Germany took part in the first German Surgical Rowing Competition. In an enchanting and relaxed atmosphere competitiveness was left to the rowing crews. After 2 hours of qualifications, the finals for fours and eights cox revealed the Universities of Ulm, Heidelberg, and Kiel as most persistent, women and men alike.

Corresponding author: Ernst Klar, MD, Chirurgische Universitätsklinik, Im Neuenheimer Feld 110, 69120 Heidelberg, Germany.

Surgical Treatment of Hydatid Disease of the Liver

Review of 304 Cases

Ahmet A. Balik, MD; Mahmut Başoğlu, MD; Fehmi Çelebi, MD; Durkaya Ören, MD; K. Yalçin Polat, MD; S. Selçuk Atamanalp, MD; Müfide N. Akçay, MD

Hypothesis: To review the results of different modalities of treatment of hydatid disease of the liver.

Design: Retrospective study of 304 patients.

Setting: A university hospital in Turkey.

Patients: Three hundred four patients with hepatic hydatid disease who underwent operation between 1981 and 1996.

Main Outcome Measures: Mortality and morbidity.

Results: Two hundred thirty-eight patients had a cyst on the right lobe, 41 patients had a cyst on the left lobe, and 25 patients had a cyst on both lobes. Forty-five patients had multiple hepatic cysts and 18 patients had coexisting cysts in other intra-abdominal organs. Surgical procedures were tube drainage, capitonnage, omentoplasty, cystectomy, segmentectomy, and cystoenterostomy. Of the patients with tube drainage, 36 developed an infection of the remaining cavity, 10 developed long-lasting biliary fistula, 8 developed cholangitis, and 6 developed septicemia. Four patients died of unreleated complications. Of the patients with capitonnage, 7 developed cholangitis and 3 developed an infection of the remaining cavity. Of the patients with omentoplasty, 1 developed an infection of the remaining cavity and 1 developed cholangitis. One patient who underwent segmentectomy developed pulmonary complications. Of the patients with cystoenterostomy, 1 developed cholangitis, 1 developed septicemia, and 1 developed pulmonary complications.

Conclusion: For management of hydatid disease of the liver, capitonnage, omentoplasty, cyst excision, segmentectomy, or cystoenterostomy are all superior to tube drainage.

Arch Surg. 1999;134:166-169

HUMAN HYDATID disease or echinococcosis, caused by the larval form of *Echinococcus granulosus*, has a worldwide distribution and is endemic in many countries in the Mediterranean region, the Middle and Far East, and South America.[1]

See Invited Critique at end of article

The adult *E granulosus* is a worm that resides in the jejenum of dogs and other canines and produces eggs that are passed in the stool. Eggs ingested by intermediate hosts (cows, sheep, mice, caribou, and humans) liberate an embryo in the duodenum, which passes through the intestinal mucosa to enter portal circulation. Most of these embryos are trapped in the liver; the rest pass through the liver and are scattered to other organs and develop into hydatid cysts. The hydatid cyst of the liver has 2 layers; the ectocyst, a dense fibrous host reaction to the parasite, and the parasite-derived endocyst, which has an outer laminated and an inner germinal layer. The single-celled germinal membrane gives rise to brood capsules, which contain the scoleces, and daughter cysts, which float freely in the clear cyst fluid.[2-7]

Uncomplicated hydatid cysts are usually asymptomatic. Symptoms are produced by 2 mechanisms: a generalized toxic reaction due to the presence of the parasite itself and local or mechanical symptoms depending on the location of the cyst.[4] The mechanical symptoms also depend on the size and number of the cysts. In more than 40% of cases, the complications precede the diagnosis of the disease. Rupture, secondary infection, and suppuration are the most common complications.[3]

Plain abdominal x-ray films may show a calcification in the right upper quadrant

From the Department of General Surgery, Atatürk University School of Medicine, Erzurum, Turkey.

PATIENTS AND METHODS

Three hundred four patients with hepatic hydatidosis were treated surgically between 1981 and 1996. One hundred ninety-nine were women and 105 were men. The mean age was 40.4 years (range, 4-82 years). The most common complaints were pain in the right upper quadrant and epigastrium and abdominal mass, which were present in 74% and 55% of the cases, respectively. Symptoms at clinical presentation are summarized in **Table 1**. Fifteen patients had previous surgery for hydatid disease before being referred to our center.

The Casoni test was positive in 187 of 204 patients and the Weinberg test was positive in 149 of 197 patients.

Plain abdominal x-ray films, ultrasonography, and computed tomography were used as imaging techniques (**Table 2**). Plain x-ray films of the abdomen showed calcification in 48 (19.4%) of 247 patients, which is a suggestive finding of hydatid disease of the liver. Ultrasonography and computed tomography demonstrated cystic lesions in both intrahepatic and extrahepatic locations in many cases.

Cysts were found in the right lobe in 238 patients (78.3%), in the left lobe in 41 patients (13.5%), and bilaterally in 25 patients (8.2%). Forty-five patients (14.8%) had multiple cysts in the liver, and 18 patients (5.9%) had coexisting cysts in the spleen (3 patients), pancreas (2 patients), adrenal gland (2 patients), mesocolon (4 patients), ovaries (1 patient), retroperitoneum (4 patients), and abdominal wall (2 patients). The diameter of the cysts was smaller than 5 cm in 13 patients (4.3%), 5 to 10 cm in 106 patients (34.9%), and larger than 10 cm in 185 patients (60.8%). Thirty-five patients (11.5%) had infected cysts.

Forty-six patients recieved mabendazole (50 mg/kg of body weight) and 56 patients recieved albendazole (10 mg/kg of body weight) perioperatively for 1 month in cases of abdominal hydatidosis or suspicion of intraoperative spillage.

For the tube drainage procedure, after the abdominal cavity had been isolated with compresses soaked in 20% hypertonic saline solution, the cyst was punctured and hydatid fluid aspirated to reduce the tension within the cyst. Cysts were then widely deroofed by excising the projecting part of the pericyst and evacuating its contents. The remaining cavity was irrigated with a scolocidal agent. Sterile hypertonic saline, 95% ethanol, or povidone-iodine were used as scolocidal agents. External drainage of the residual cavity was done using a wide-gauge rubber tube brought out through a stab wound and connected with a bag for gravity drainage; suprahepatic and subhepatic spaces are also drained in some cases. Tubes were removed within a few days in the absence of bile leakage or any discharge. To obliterate the remaining cavity, a portion of omentum with a good blood supply was sutured into the cavity (omentoplasty), or remaining walls of the cavity were brought together with a series of purse-string or mattress sutures starting from the bottom and working outward (*capitonnage*). If obliteration of the remaining cavity was not possible, Roux-en-Y cystojejunostomy was performed by a wide anastomosis between pericystic opening and jejenum. In the instance of cystobiliary communication, treatment included closure of the communications with fine absorbable sutures. In our series, tube drainage was performed in 122 patients (40.1%), capitonnage in 100 patients (32.9%), omentoplasty in 40 patients (13.2%), cystectomy in 22 patients (7.2%), segmentectomy in 10 patients (3.3%), and cystoenterostomy in 10 patients (3.3%). Because of intrabiliary rupture, in 18 patients migrated hydatid material was cleared from the common bile duct through a choledochotomy and choledochostcopy was performed in those patients. After the common bile duct had been cleared, T tube drainage was performed in 13 patients and choledochoduodenostomy was performed in 5 patients. Coexistent cysts were treated by splenectomy, oophorectomy, and cyst excision.

Statistical analyses were performed using the Student *t* test for postoperative hospital stay and χ^2 test for morbidity. $P \leq .05$ was considered significant.

that is a suggestive finding of hydatid disease of the liver. Ultrasonography and computed tomography are highly sensitive in the diagnosis of hepatic hydatid cysts. The positivity of Casoni and Weinberg tests in hydatid disease is 87% and 69%, respectively.[3,8] Of the serological tests, the indirect hemaglutination test is more sensitive than the complement fixation test.[9]

Although medical treatment with mabendazole[10] or albendazole[11] has been reported to be effective in some cases, little objective evidence is available to support these claims. Treatment of hydatid disease consists either of surgery or percutaneous drainage. A variety of surgical procedures have been described,[4,8] but there are basically 2 surgical alternatives—resection or conservative procedures.[2] Resection of small or pedunculated cysts may be simple and safe, but in most cases cystectomy involves a major resection, with its attendant increase in operative risk. Conservative procedures are easier to perform, but the rate of postoperative complications and the duration of hospital stay are not always satisfactory.[1-3] In this article, we have retrospectively reviewed results of different surgical procedures in 304 patients with hepatic hydatid disease in a 15-year period.

RESULTS

The most common complication was postoperative infection in the remaining cavity. Of the patients with tube drainage, 36 (29.5%) developed infection of the remaining cavity, 8 (6.6%) developed cholangitis, 6 (4.9%) developed septicemia, and 10 (8.2%) developed long-lasting biliary fistula (2-4 months). All those fistulas were closed spontaneously. Four patients received octreotide because of high-volume fistula (1000 mL/d). Of the patients with capitonnage, 7 (7%) developed cholangitis, 3 (3%) developed infection of the remaining cavity, and 2 (2%) developed septicemia. Of the patients with omentoplasty, 1 (4.5%) developed infection of the remaining cavity and 1 (4.5%) developed cholangitis. One patient (10%) in the segmentectomy group developed pulmonary complications. In the cystoenterostomy group, 1 patient developed cholangitis, 1 patient developed septicemia, and 1 patient developed pulmonary complications. Infection of the remaining cavity and biliary fistula were significantly more frequent ($P<.05$) in the tube drainage group as compared with the other groups, and there

Table 1. Clinical Presentation

Presenting Sign or Symptom	No. (%) of Patients
Abdominal pain	225 (74)
Abdominal mass	167 (55)
History of fever	69 (22.7)
History of jaundice	18 (5.9)
Acute abdomen	3 (1)
Asymptomatic	29 (9.5)

Table 2. Imaging Techniques

	No. of Patients	No. Positive	Sensitivity, %
Plain abdominal x-ray film	243	28	11.5
Ultrasonography	304	297	97.7
Computed tomography	154	154	100.0

were no significant differences between groups other than tube drainage ($P>.05$).

Postoperative hospital stay is summarized in **Table 3**. The average hospital stay was longer in the tube drainage group as compared with the other groups ($P<.01$), and there were no significant differences between groups other than tube drainage ($P>.05$).

Four patients (1.3%) died of cardiopulmonary complications. No recurrence was seen in follow-up lasting from 3 months to 6 years.

COMMENT

Hydatid disease is still a problem in developing countries. Although the disease is often asymptomatic for many years owing to slow growth of the cyst, complications including infection, obstructive jaundice, and rupture could cause serious problems. In our series there were 35 patients (11.5%) with infected cysts, 18 patients (5.9%) with obstructive jaundice, and 3 patients (0.98%) with cyst rupture.

The diagnosis of hydatid disease of the liver had previously been based on history and clinical findings that are compatible with the disease. The clinical findings are too nonspecific to be diagnostic. Skin tests and serological tests are helpful in diagnosis. In our series, the Casoni test was positive in 187 (91.7%) of 204 patients and the Weinberg test was positive in 149 (75.6%) of 197 patients. Altough it has been reported that the Casoni test can cause anaphylaxis, in our series this was not seen. In all patients Casoni and Weinberg tests were performed after the cyst had been diagnosed by imaging techniques, so we are not able to discuss the false-positivity of those tests.

Ultrasonography and computed tomography are highly sensitive in the diagnosis of hepatic hydatid disease. In our series, sensitivities were 97.7% and 100% for ultrasonography and computed tomography, respectively.

Percutaneous drainage is helpful in diagnosis and is a good alternative to surgery in treatment of hepatic hydatidosis.[12,13]

The first step in hydatid surgery is evacuation and irrigation of the cyst cavity. To prevent peritoneal contamination, the peritoneal cavity must be carefully protected during cyst evacuation. After evacuation, the remaining cavity must be irrigated with scolocidal agents. There are many scolocidal agents available. Years ago, formalin was used for inactivation, but it has beeen abandoned because of sclerosing cholangitis[14,15] and systemic reactions.[16] Many agents, such as chlorheximide, 80% ethanol, hypertonic saline, and 0.5% cetrimide are effective scolocidals.[8] We used 20% saline, 95% ethanol, and povidone-iodine as scolocidal agents. Although it was reported that hypertonic saline solution could cause sclerosing cholangitis,[14] in our series this complication was not present.

Table 3. Postoperative Hospital Stay

Type of Treatment	Mean ± SD Hospital Stay, d
Tube drainage (infected)	27.9 ± 7.9
Tube drainage (uncomplicated)	16.1 ± 3.0
Capitonnage	11.2 ± 2.8
Omentoplasty	11.2 ± 2.6
Cystectomy	9.5 ± 1.9
Lobectomy	11.1 ± 2.6
Cystoenterostomy	12.8 ± 1.7

The second step is management of the cyst cavity. If possible the cyst cavity should be obliterated by capitonnage[4] or omentoplasty,[17] but if it is not, drainage procedures such as tube drainage or marsupialization could be performed. If the cyst is peripheral or pedunculated, cystectomy or lobectomy could be performed. We do not recommend hepatic resection if the cyst location is central. In our series segmentectomy was performed for cysts located on the left lobe.

In cases of suppuration, marsupialization or tube drainage is unavoidable.[3] In these cases the duration of hospitalization is long because of complications, especially infection and biliary drainage. In our series, tube drainage was performed in 87 patients with uncomplicated cysts. The average hospital stay was shorter in patients with uncomplicated cysts as compared with patients with complicated cysts ($P<.05$).

In our series, surgical strategy varied over the 15 years. Tube drainage had previously been preferred, especially in patients who had concomitant medical illness. However, since 1986, radical procedures have been performed in most cases. Since 1991, percutaneous drainage has been performed in 101 selected cases. Percutaneous drainage was performed in patients who had type 1 or type 2 hydatid cysts according to the description of Gharbi et al.[18] In this procedure, after percutaneous aspiration of the cyst fluid, the cyst cavity is irrigated with a scolocidal agent and the catheter is removed. Thus, complications such as infection of the remaining cavity or biliary fistula are not seen in patients treated with percutaneous drainage.

We concluded that omentoplasty, cystectomy, capitonnage, lobectomy, and cystoenterostomy are superior to external drainage. In uncomplicated cysts these procedures had a shorter duration of hospitalization as compared with tube drainage. In this respect, marsupialization or tube drainage should be avoided as much as possible.

Corresponding author: Ahmet A. Balik, MD; Atatürk University School of Medicine, Erzurum, Turkey (e-mail: abalik@hotmail.com).

REFERENCES

1. Eckert J, Gemmel MA, Matyas Z, Saulsby EJ. *Guidelines for Surveillance, Prevention and Control of Echinococcosis/hydatidosis.* Geneva, Switzerland: World Health Organization; 1984:1-5.
2. Langer CJ, Rose DB, Keystone JS, et al. Diagnosis and management of hydatid disease of the liver. *Ann Surg.* 1984;199:412-417.
3. Sayek I, Yalýn R, Sanaç Y. Surgical treatment of hydatid disease of the liver. *Arch Surg.* 1980;115:847-850.
4. Romero-Torres R, Campbell JR. An interpretive review of the surgical treatment of hydatid disease. *Surg Gynecol Obstet.* 1965;121:851-864.
5. Lewis JW, Koss N, Kersein MD. A review of echinococcal disease. *Ann Surg.* 1975; 181:390-396.
6. Pissiotis CA, Wander JV, Condon RE. Surgical treatment of hydatid disease. *Ann Surg.* 1972;104:454-459.
7. Walt JA. Cysts and benign tumors of the liver. *Surg Clin North Am.* 1977;57:449-464.
8. Barnes SA, Lillemoe KD. Liver abscess and hydatid cyst disease. In: Zinner JZ, ed. *Maiongot's Abdominal Operations.* 10th ed. Hartford, Conn: Appleton & Lange; 1997:1513-1545.
9. Chematai AK, Bowry TR, Ahmad Z. Eveluation of five immunodiagnostic tecniques in echinococcosis patients. *Bull World Health Organ.* 1981;59:767-772.
10. Bekhti A, Schaaps JP, Capron M, et al. Treatment of hepatic hydatid disease with mabendasole: preliminary results in four cases. *BMJ.* 1977;2:1047-1051.
11. Saimot AT, Meulemans A, Cremieux AC, et al. Albendasole as a potential treatment for human hydatozis. *Lancet.* 1983;17:652-656.
12. Khuroo MS, Zargar SA, Mahajan R. *Echinococcus granulosus* cyst in the liver: management with percutaneous drainage. *Radiology.* 1991;180:141-145.
13. Filice C, Pirola F, Brunetti E, et al. A new therapeutic approach for hydatid liver cysts: aspiration and alcohol injection under sonographic guidance. *Gastroenterology.* 1990;98:1366-1368.
14. Belghiti J, Benhamou JP, Houry S, et al. Causting sclerosing cholangitis. *Arch Surg.* 1986;121:1162-1165.
15. Houry S, Languille O, Hugier M, et al. Sclerosing cholangitis induced by formaldehyde solution injected into the biliary tree of rats. *Arch Surg.* 1990;125: 1059-1061.
16. Hankins JR. Management of complicated hepatic hydatid cysts. *Ann Surg.* 1963; 158:1020-1024.
17. Papadimetriou J, Mandrekas A. The surgical tratment of hydatid disease of the liver. *Br J Surg.* 1970;57:431-433.
18. Gharbi HA, Hassine W, Brauner MW, Dupuch K. Ultrasound examination of the hydatid liver. *Radiology.* 1981;139:459-463.

Invited Critique

This article represents a retrospective study on the results of different modalities of treatment of hydatid disease of the liver, concluding that capitonnage, omentoplasty, cystectomy, lobectomy, and cystoenterostomy are superior to tube drainage and that marsupialization or tube drainage should be avoided as much as possible. Human hydatid disease, an endemic disease in many countries, is caused by a parasite that is identified as *Echinococcus granulosus* or *Echinococcus multilocularis*. Most of the embryos are trapped in the liver and the rest pass through the liver and are scattered to other organs such as the lung, brain, or spleen, where they develop into hydatid cysts. Although the proliferation and differentiation of germinal cells of *E multilocularis* are presumed to be deeply involved in the incidence of this disease, the clinocopathologic features of the disease are not well established. Chemotherapy is reportedly not effective in most cases.

This article emphasizes that the first step in hydatid surgery of the liver is evacuation and irrigation of the cystic cavity, followed by management of the cyst cavity. Rupture of the cyst, secondary infection, and suppuration are the most common complications. The rate of postoperative complications and the duration of hospital stay are not always satisfactory when conservative procedures are chosen; nevertheless, the mortality rate is low.

On the other hand, hydatid disease of the liver in Hokkaido (northern Japan) behaves like a malignant neoplasm and is often fatal. Hydatid disease in this area in Japan can be controlled only by complete resection of the lesions. Conservative therapies are not effective in patients with nonresectable lesions. Causes of death are liver failure, disseminated intravascular coagulation, and multiple organ failure due to biliary sepsis. The clinicopathologic features of this disease in the northern hemisphere seem to be somewhat different from what is observed in southern or southeastern areas.

Establishment of an in vitro primary culture of germinal cells of *E multilocularis* is considered to be indispensable for elucidation of the clinicopathologic feautres and improvement of the prognosis of this disease.

Kazutomo Inoue, MD
Kyoto, Japan

Selective Decontamination of the Digestive Tract in Surgical Patients

A Systematic Review of the Evidence

Avery B. Nathens, MD, PhD, FRCSC; John C. Marshall, MD, FRCSC

Objective: To determine the comparative efficacy of selective decontamination of the digestive tract in critically ill surgical and medical patients, and in selected subgroups of surgical patients with pancreatitis, major burn injury, and those undergoing major elective surgery and transplantation.

Data Sources: The MEDLINE database was searched from January 1966 to December 1996 using the terms "decontamination or prophylaxis," "intensive care units," and "antibiotics." The search was limited to English-language studies evaluating the efficacy of selective decontamination of the digestive tract in human subjects.

Study Selection: The primary review was restricted to prospective randomized trials.

Data Extraction: End points of interest included rates of nosocomial pneumonia, bacteremia, urinary tract infection, wound infection, mortality, and length of intensive care unit stay. Methodologic quality of individual studies was assessed using a previously described model.

Data Synthesis: Odds ratios (ORs) together with their (95% confidence interval [CIs]) were reported and determined using the Mantel-Haenszel method. Mortality was significantly reduced with the use of selective decontamination of the digestive tract in critically ill surgical patients (OR, 0.7; 95% CI, 0.52-0.93), while no such effect was demonstrated in critically ill medical patients (OR, 0.91; 95% CI, 0.71-1.18). The greatest effect was demonstrated in studies where both the topical and systemic components of the regimen were used. Rates of pneumonia were reduced in both subsets of patients, while those of bacteremia were significantly reduced only in surgical patients.

Conclusions: Selective decontamination of the digestive tract notably reduces mortality in critically ill surgical patients, while critically ill medical patients derive no such benefit. These data suggest that the use of selective decontamination of the digestive tract should be limited to those populations in whom rates of nosocomial infection are high and in whom infection contributes notably to adverse outcome.

Arch Surg. 1999;134:170-176

SELECTIVE decontamination of the digestive tract (SDD) is an infection prophylaxis regimen that employs topical and oral nonabsorbable antibiotics to eradicate pathogenic organisms from the gastrointestinal (GI) tract. The regimen was first used in patients with neutropenic leukemia undergoing induction therapy with promising results.[1] In 1983, Stoutenbeek et al[2] adapted the technique of SDD to patients in an intensive care unit (ICU) setting; the first clinical trial in a homogeneous group of multiple trauma patients was described the following year.[3] Since then, at least 25 controlled clinical trials and 4 meta-analyses[4-7] evaluating the technique have been reported; however, although SDD is widely used in European ICUs, it has not found favor in North America.

The microbiologic rationale for SDD derives from clinical and experimental studies on the normal GI tract flora and its changes in critical illness. The indigenous flora of the oropharynx and GI tract is remarkably constant over time. Mechanisms preventing overgrowth with potentially pathogenic organisms include salivary flow,[8] gastric acidity,[9] bile acids,[10] secretory IgA,[11] and peristalsis. In addition, obligate anaerobic bacteria contribute to the prevention of colonization of the digestive tract by facultative anaerobic and potentially pathogenic bacteria and yeasts, a phenomenon referred to as colonization resistance.

In the critically ill patient, the mechanisms limiting overgrowth of potentially pathogenic organisms are compromised by the underlying disease processes, instrumentation, and medication that result in

From the Division of General Surgery, The Toronto Hospital (Dr Marshall), and the Department of Surgery, University of Toronto (Dr Nathens), Toronto, Ontario.

MATERIALS AND METHODS

The MEDLINE database from January 1966 to December 1996 was searched using the search terms "decontamination or prophylaxis," "intensive care units," and "antibiotics." Titles and abstracts were also searched during this period for the term "decontamination." Additional citations were obtained from several recent meta-analyses[4-6] and through personal communications from other investigators involved in primary studies. The primary review was restricted to prospective, randomized, or consecutive trials. Studies using historic controls were reviewed only in patient populations where limited data exist. Studies were considered to have enrolled surgical patients if at least 75% of the subjects evaluated had been admitted following trauma or major surgery. Studies were considered to have enrolled medical patients when fewer than 25% of patients met this criterion.

Methodologic quality of the studies selected for this systematic review was evaluated using a model previously described by Heyland et al[29] (**Table 1**). Odds ratios (ORs) and pooled ORs together with their 95% confidence intervals (CIs) were reported and determined using the Mantel-Haenszel method. An OR of less than 1.0 suggests that SDD results in a reduction in the relative odds of dying or developing a nosocomial infection.

impairment of salivary flow, gastric alkalization, cholestasis, and intestinal ileus. In addition, the use of broad-spectrum antibiotics eradicates the anaerobic flora, leading to a loss of colonization resistance. The net result is that within days of admission to an ICU, the relatively avirulent indigenous flora is replaced by a variety of potentially pathogenic species. Abnormal gastric colonization develops within days in more than two thirds of patients admitted to an ICU; the most common isolates include *Candida albicans*, *Escherichia coli*, *Klebsiella pneumoniae*, *Pseudomonas aeruginosa*, *Enterococcus*, and coagulase-negative *Staphylococcus*,[12,13] the predominant infecting species of nosocomial ICU-acquired infection.

Many descriptive studies have shown an association between pathologic, oropharyngeal, and gastric colonization and the development of nosocomial infection.[14-17] Interventional studies in which normal gastric acidity is maintained by the use of cytoprotective agents support, but do not confirm, a role for altered gastric flora in the pathogenesis of ventilator-associated pneumonia.[18,19] Aspiration of contaminated upper GI tract fluid is the most plausible and readily demonstrable mechanism of infection with proximal gut organisms.[20,21] Alternatively, proximal GI tract colonization may lead to translocation of viable organisms through an intact gut wall. Although a well-established phenomenon in animal models,[22,23] translocation has not been conclusively demonstrated in humans.[24]

The standard SDD regimen consists of 2 components. Topical, nonabsorbed polymyxin E, tobramycin, and amphotericin B, a combination active against essentially all aerobic gram-negative bacteria and fungi.[25] These antibiotics have limited activity against the normal anaerobic flora and maintain normal colonization resistance.[26] In addition, intravenous cefotaxime sodium is administered until surveillance cultures demonstrate adequate decontamination of the GI tract, generally 4 days following the initiation of SDD. Cefotaxime treats early established infection by community-acquired pathogens, particularly *Streptococcus pneumoniae* or *Haemophilus influenzae*, that may be aspirated during intubation, and temporizes until the enterally administered antibiotics have adequately decontaminated the GI tract. Selective decontamination of the digestive tract is initiated as soon as possible following admission and is continued until cessation of mechanical ventilation or discharge from the ICU.

The disparate results of clinical trials in different patient populations suggest that the practice may benefit select groups of patients. Its role in surgical patients has not been explicitly evaluated, although surgical patients might be anticipated to show particular benefit. Rates of nosocomial pneumonia seem to be higher in critically ill surgical patients than in patients admitted to a medical ICU, and the mortality attributable to nosocomial pneumonia is notably greater in the surgical subpopulation.[27] On the other hand, concerns have been voiced that a reduction in rates of pneumonia in SDD studies does not seem to result in improved outcome and that widespread adoption of the technique may contribute to the emergence of antibiotic resistance.

To evaluate the utility of SDD in surgical patients, we conducted a formal, systematic, English-literature review using an evidence-based methodology[28] that generates recommendations based on the strength of positive evidence provided by clinical studies. Grade A recommendations are supported by level I evidence that reflects statistically significant conclusions from randomized, controlled trials and provides a strong argument for adopting the therapy evaluated. Grade B recommendations are supported by level II evidence; and grade C recommendations, by level III, IV, or V evidence. Grade B and C recommendations provide less convincing evidence of therapeutic efficacy and justify either adoption or withholding of the therapy in question. Notable differences in the response to SDD in surgical, as compared with medical, ICU patients are evident, justifying a grade A recommendation in support of the use of routine SDD prophylaxis in critically ill surgical patients. Selective decontamination of the digestive tract shows evidence of clinical benefit in subpopulations of surgical patients as well, although the limited sample sizes of published studies preclude definitive conclusions regarding its use in specific subgroups.

RESULTS

SDD IN CRITICALLY ILL SURGICAL PATIENTS

Eleven randomized prospective studies have been published on the use of SDD in surgical ICU patients.[30-40] All of the available studies are limited in their sample size, and thus have insufficient power to detect even

Table 1. Criteria Used to Assess Methodologic Quality*

	Score 0	Score 1	Score 2
Methods			
Randomization	Not randomized	...	Truly randomized
Blinding	Not blinded	Double blinded	...
Analysis	Other	...	Intention to treat
Population			
Patient selection	Selected patients or cannot tell	Consecutive eligible patients	...
Comparability of groups of baseline	No or not sure	Yes	...
Extent of follow-up, %	<100	100	...
Intervention			
Treatment protocol	Poorly described	Reproducibly described	...
Cointerventions†	Not described	Described but not equal or not sure	Well described and equal
Crossovers, %	Not described	>10	<10

*Variables were dichotomous variables scored on a 3-point scale with no middle value. Ellipses indicate no middle value.
†From Heyland et al.[29]

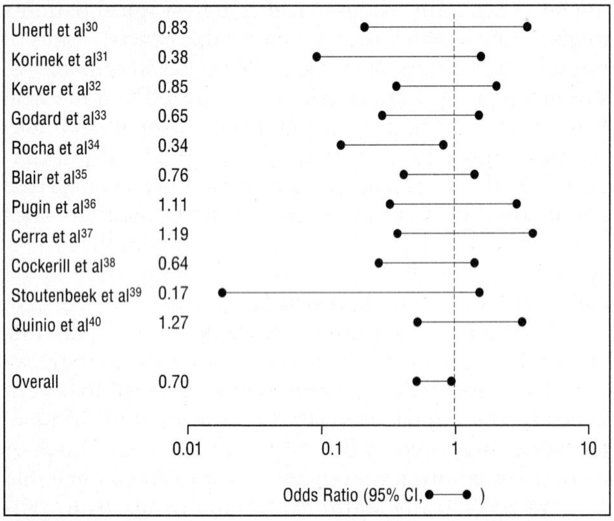

Figure 1. *The effect of selective decontamination of the digestive tract on mortality in critically ill surgical patients. Odds ratios and the 95% confidence intervals (CI) in 11 studies with more than 75% postoperative or trauma patients are demonstrated.*

modest reductions in mortality. The OR for mortality in patients treated with SDD was less than 1 in 8 of the 11 trials, with 1 demonstrating a significant reduction in mortality[34] (**Figure 1**). The pooled OR for these 11 trials is 0.70, with CIs indicating at worst a 7% and at best a 48% reduction in the odds of death in surgical ICU patients treated with SDD (**Table 2**). Separate analysis of studies in which systemic antimicrobial therapy was administered[32,34,35,38,40] compared with those with only the topical components of the regimen[30,31,33,36,37,39] demonstrated the greatest survival benefit in the former group. The effect of SDD on rates of nosocomial infection in surgical patients is similarly evident. Nine of 10 assessable trials demonstrated a statistically significant reduction in the rate of nosocomial pneumonia, with a pooled OR of 0.19. There is a significant reduction in bacteremic episodes and urinary tract infections in patients treated with SDD while wound infection rates are unaffected (Table 2). Only 1 of 8 assessable studies demonstrated a clear reduction in length of ICU stay,[37]

Table 2. Efficacy on Mortality and Nosocomial Infection Rates of Selective Decontamination of the Digestive Tract, Surgical vs Medical Intensive Care Units

Characteristics	Odds Ratio (95% CI*) Surgical	Medical
Mortality		
Overall	0.70 (0.52-0.93)	0.91 (0.71-1.18)
Topical and systemic	0.60 (0.41-0.88)	0.75 (0.53-1.06)
Topical only	0.86 (0.51-1.45)	1.14 (0.77-1.68)
Nosocomial Infection		
Pneumonia	0.19 (0.15-0.26)	0.45 (0.33-0.62)
Bacteremia	0.51 (0.34-0.75)	0.77 (0.43-1.36)
Urinary tract infection	0.51 (0.34-0.76)	0.51 (0.32-0.82)
Wound infection	0.56 (0.23-1.37)	...

*CI indicates confidence interval; ellipses, no analysis performed.

although there is a significant reduction in the pooled length of stay in these 8 studies (for control patients, 16.9 ± 13 days vs 15.2 ± 12.5 days for SDD patients; $P<.05$, t test). All values are expressed as mean ± SD.

SDD IN CRITICALLY ILL MEDICAL PATIENTS

Ten prospective, randomized, controlled clinical trials of SDD have been carried out in critically ill medical patients.[41-50] Similar to the trials in critically ill surgical patients, almost all of the studies lack sufficient power to detect a clinically significant reduction in mortality. Only 1 study (445 evaluable patients) had adequate power to detect a 25% reduction in mortality. This trial failed to demonstrate any notable survival benefit in patients receiving SDD.[43] In contrast to most of the other studies, systemic antimicrobial therapy was not administered. The pooled OR for a reduction in mortality using SDD prophylaxis in medical patients is 0.91 with the upper limit of the CI being more than 1.0 (**Figure 2**). Even if the analysis is limited to studies in which systemic antimicrobials are administered,[41,42,44,46,47,49] the effect on survival fails to reach statistical significance (Table 2). Selective decontamination of the digestive tract had a significant effect in reducing episodes of nosocomial pneumonia and urinary tract infections in medical patients (Table 2); however, there was no reduction in the risk of bacteremia (OR, 0.77) or length of ICU stay (for controls patients, 16.7 ± 16 days vs 16.8 ± 13 days for SDD patients).

To rule out the possibility that differences in the methodologic quality of the clinical trials evaluating medical and surgical patients accounted for the differential benefit seen in surgical patients, a formalized assessment of the quality of the individual trials was performed as described in the "Materials and Methods" section. Methodologic quality scores were similar in medical (7.6 ± 1.9) and surgical trials (7.9 ± 2.3), suggesting that the conduct of the study did not account for the differential results observed.

Data from meta-analyses and from subset analysis of critically ill medical and surgical patients provide sufficient level I and II evidence for a grade A recommendation for the use of SDD in critically ill surgical patients as a prophylactic measure to reduce mortality. Topical antimicrobial therapy should be used in conjunction with a short course of systemic antibiotics.

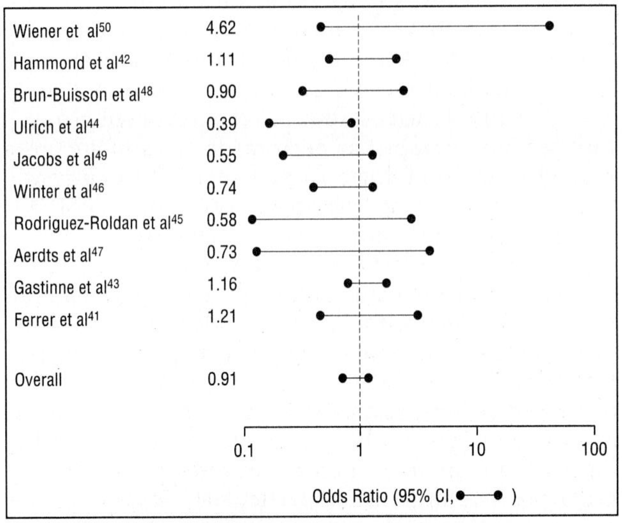

Figure 2. *The effect of selective decontamination of the digestive tract on mortality in critically ill medical patients. Odds ratios and the 95% confidence intervals (CIs) in 10 studies with 25% or fewer postoperative or trauma patients are demonstrated.*

SDD IN TRANSPLANTATION

Infection contributes to mortality in patients undergoing solid-organ transplantation.[51] Selective decontamination of the digestive tract has only been formally evaluated in patients undergoing orthotopic liver transplantation. Case series and retrospective studies suggest a reduction in rates of infection when compared with historic controls.[52-55] There are 3 randomized prospective studies of SDD in liver transplantation[56-58] (**Table 3**) that show a reduction in rates of nosocomial infection and a modest improvement in survival. Support for the use of SDD in liver transplantation is based on level II evidence and is given a grade B recommendation. Further studies are required in both liver transplant and other solid-organ recipients to provide adequate power to determine whether a true survival benefit exists.

SDD IN MAJOR ELECTIVE SURGERY

Selective decontamination of the digestive tract has been most extensively studied in cardiac surgical patients, a homogeneous group of patients undergoing major elective surgery.[59-62] Randomized trials show a reduction in rates of infection, but not mortality, in a group of patients with a low baseline mortality rate[59-61] (Table 3), and reduced levels of endotoxin and interleukin 6 in the postoperative period.[61]

The role of SDD vs standard perioperative antibiotic prophylaxis in patients undergoing elective esophageal resection for carcinoma has been examined in a prospective, randomized study.[63] Selective decontamination of the digestive tract resulted in a significant reduction in rates of pneumonia (14% vs 2%) and wound infections (35% vs 11%) without a reduction in the length of hospital stay or mortality (2% vs 3%). The effectiveness of SDD in patients undergoing total gastrectomy and esophagojejunal anastomosis has been evaluated in a designed prospective multicenter study.[64] Selective decontamination of the digestive tract initiated the evening prior to the procedure resulted in a significant reduction in the rate of anastomotic leaks (10.9% vs 2.9%), pneumonia (22.3% vs 8.8%), and mortality (10.6% vs 4.9%).

Although SDD can reduce the incidence of postoperative infection in patients undergoing cardiac surgery, its routine use is probably unnecessary. Risk factors for

Table 3. Randomized Trials of Selective Decontamination of the Digestive Tract (SDD) in Liver Transplantation and Cardiac Surgery*

	Mortality, %			Infection, %		
Source, y	**Placebo**	**SDD**	**Pooled Odds Ratio (95% CI)**	**Placebo**	**SDD**	**Pooled Odds Ratio (95% CI)**
			Liver Transplantation			
Smith et al,[57] 1993	17	11		61	17	
Bion et al,[56] 1994	16	0	0.29 (0.06-1.47)	39	14	0.44 (0.23-0.87)
Arnow et al,[58] 1996	...	...		42	39	
			Cardiac Surgery			
Zobel et al,[59] 1991	8	12		36	8	
Flaherty et al,[60] 1990	2	0	0.68 (0.19-2.50)	27	12	0.28 (0.12-0.67)
Martinez-Pellus et al,[61] 1993	8	3		...	...	

**CI indicates confidence interval; ellipses, no analysis performed.*

infection and mortality in cardiac surgery have been clearly elucidated, and include Acute Physiology and Chronic Health Evaluation II scores greater than 19 in the first 24 hours,[65] prolonged use of an intra-aortic balloon pump,[66] and prolonged mechanical ventilation (>72 hours).[67] It is recommended that SDD be considered for high-risk cardiac surgical patients. This is a grade B recommendation based on 4 level II clinical trials. The use of SDD as a method of infection prophylaxis in patients undergoing esophageal and gastric resection seems promising. Although these data cannot necessarily be extrapolated to all patients undergoing operations on the GI tract, it would seem that patients undergoing upper GI tract surgery derive benefit through a reduction in the risk of aspiration pneumonia. It is recommended that SDD be considered for patients undergoing upper GI tract surgery as a form of infection prophylaxis. This is a grade B recommendation based on level II data.

SDD IN THERMAL INJURY

The development of gram-negative bacteremia or nosocomial pneumonia following thermal injury is associated with an increased risk of death.[68,69] To our knowledge, there are no prospective randomized studies evaluating the efficacy of SDD in burn patients. Mackie et al[70] described a series of 31 consecutive patients with burns of greater than 30% of total body surface area who were treated with SDD, comparing them with a group of 33 historic controls. The incidence of respiratory tract infections (27.3% vs 6.5%) and bacteremias (24.2% vs 3.2%) was reduced, with a concomitant reduction in mortality (21.2% vs 3.2%); however, there was no reduction in length of hospital stay. Although promising, data on the role of SDD prophylaxis following thermal injury are retrospective and must be interpreted with due consideration. On the basis of level IV evidence, the use of SDD in patients with significant thermal injury is awarded a grade C recommendation. There is a need for well-designed prospective studies in this patient population.

SDD IN ACUTE PANCREATITIS

In a prospective randomized trial of SDD in acute pancreatitis, Luiten et al[71] demonstrated a 50% reduction in the incidence of infected pancreatic necrosis (38% vs 18%). Patients receiving SDD required fewer laparotomies and had a significant reduction in mortality when stratified by Imrie score, with Imrie scores of 3 or higher obtaining the greatest survival benefit. A small, retrospective study[72] of critically ill patients receiving mechanical ventilation examined the effects of SDD on patients with pancreatitis compared with historic controls. This study demonstrated a reduction in the incidence of bacteremia and nosocomial pneumonia in patients poorly matched for both Acute Physiology and Chronic Health Evaluation score and Ranson criteria. It is recommended that SDD be considered in patients with severe acute pancreatitis. This grade B recommendation is based on a single level I study.

COMMENT

The results of this meta-analysis show that the technique of SDD can benefit surgical patients. Selective decontamination of the digestive tract reduces rates of nosocomial pneumonia and bacteremia and nosocomial infections at remote sites. More importantly, it has a statistically significant effect on mortality. The best estimate for this effect is a 30% reduction in ICU mortality with CIs narrow enough to all but exclude the possibility of a type I error. This mortality effect is larger than that seen with other prophylactic modalities that have become standard care in surgical practice, including those that prevent deep venous thrombosis and pulmonary embolism[73] or surgical wound infections.[74]

Nonetheless, SDD has not been widely adopted as a prophylactic measure. There are several possible explanations for this. Pharmaceutical-grade preparations of polymyxin E and amphotericin B for topical use are not readily available. As a result, centers that have adopted the SDD technique have had to use intravenous preparations at substantially greater cost and local hospital pharmacies must prepare the SDD paste and suspension. The cost of SDD in the ICU setting has received only passing attention. In the 21 studies evaluating the efficacy of SDD in the ICU, 6 make no reference to overall antibiotic use.[33,36,41,45,48,49] In 4 studies, overall antibiotic costs were higher in patients receiving SDD.[34,42,43,50] In only 1 study was total antibiotic cost lower in the treatment group.[39] Further, no attempt has been made to estimate costs related to microbiologic surveillance. With currently available data, it is not possible to conclude that SDD is a cost-effective, infection prevention strategy.

Although available data show no increase in the prevalence of resistant gram-negative organisms in patients managed with SDD (and indeed SDD has been promoted as a potential method of decontaminating patients with resistant gram-negative organisms[48]), its safety in centers where resistant gram-positive organisms are common has not been established. Several studies have documented an increase in rates of isolation of gram-positive organisms, particularly *Staphylococcus aureus*,[37,42,43] coagulase-negative *Staphylococcus*, and *Enterococcus*[34,37,38] when SDD is implemented. The spectrum of resistance is poorly reported. Gentamicin sulfate–resistant enterococci were prevalent in one study; however, surveillance cultures were not performed on the control group.[38] In another study, a notable increase in methicillin-resistant *S aureus* colonization in patients receiving SDD compared with controls was documented.[42] Resistant gram-negative organisms seem to be less of a concern; however, tobramycin-resistant, aerobic, gram-negative bacilli have been reported in 2 studies.[34,35] Although notably overt infection with resistant organisms has not been reported with the use of SDD, this potential exists, and routine surveillance cultures may be necessary to allow for the early detection of antimicrobial resistance.

Meta-analyses show that SDD has a favorable effect on both nosocomial infection and ICU mortality when it is used as standard prophylactic therapy for critically ill surgical patients. Yet the technique is not widely employed in North America but rather viewed with suspicion and skepticism by many. The appropriate resolution of such a state of clinical equipoise is a randomized, double-blind, placebo-controlled, clinical trial,[75] and we believe it is important that such a trial be undertaken. This trial should evaluate a homogeneous group of patients at high risk for infection-related morbidity and mortality; for example, victims of multiple trauma or patients undergoing solid-organ transplantation. It must have an objective primary end point, namely, ICU mortality, and be adequately powered to include or exclude a clinically important mortality effect. It must also incorporate the microbiologic surveillance that will permit definitive conclusions regarding the effect of SDD on the microbial ecology and resistance patterns in patients undergoing cardiac surgery. Finally, the study should incorporate a control group of patients receiving systemic but not topical prophylaxis. A prospective, randomized trial of SDD in trauma patients showed comparable outcomes in a control group receiving systemic antimicrobial prophylaxis alone.[76]

Corresponding author: John C. Marshall, MD, FRCSC, The Toronto Hospital, EN 9-234, 200 Elizabeth St, Toronto, Ontario, Canada M5G 2C4 (e-mail: jmarshall@torhosp.toronto .on.ca).

REFERENCES

1. Sleifer DT, Mulder NH, de Vries-Hospers HG, et al. Infection prevention in granulocytopenic patients by selective decontamination of the digestive tract. *Eur J Cancer.* 1980;16:859-868.
2. Stoutenbeek CP, Van Saene HK, Miranda DR, Zandstra DF. A new technique of infection prevention in the intensive care unit by selective decontamination of the digestive tract. *Acta Anaesthesiol Belg.* 1983;34:209-221.
3. Stoutenbeek CP, Van Saene HKF, Miranda DR, Zandstra DF. The effect of selective decontamination of the digestive tract on colonisation and infection rate in multiple trauma patients. *Intensive Care Med.* 1984;10:185-192.
4. Selective Decontamination of the Digestive Tract Trialists' Collaborative Group. Meta-analysis of randomised controlled trials of selective decontamination of the digestive tract. *BMJ.* 1993;307:525-532.
5. Heyland DK, Cook DJ, Jaeschke R, Griffith L, Lee HN, Guyatt GH. Selective decontamination of the digestive tract: an overview. *Chest.* 1994;105:1221-1229.
6. Kollef MH. The role of selective digestive tract decontamination on mortality and respiratory tract infections: a meta-analysis. *Chest.* 1994;105:1101-1108.
7. D'Amico R, Pifferi S, Leonetti C, Torri V, Tinazzi A, Liberati A, for the study investigators. Effectiveness of antibiotic prophylaxis in critically ill adult patients: systematic review of randomized controlled trials. *BMJ.* 1998; 316:1275-1285.
8. Gibson G, Barrett E. The role of salivary function on oropharyngeal colonization. *Spec Care Dentist.* 1992;12:153-156.
9. Driks MR, Craven DE, Celli BR, et al. Nosocomial pneumonia in intubated patients given sucralfate as compared with antacids or histamine type 2 blockers: the role of gastric colonization. *N Engl J Med.* 1987;317:1376-1382.
10. Floch MH, Gershengoren W, Elliott S, Spiro HM. Bile acid inhibition of the intestinal microflora: a function for simple bile acids. *Gastroenterology.* 1971;61:228-233.
11. Mcloughlin GA, Hede JE, Temple JG, Bradley J, Chapman DM, McFarland J. The role of IgA in the prevention of bacterial colonization of the jejunum in the vagotomized subject. *Br J Surg.* 1978;65:435-437.
12. Cade JF, McOwat E, Siganporia R, Keighley C, Presneill J, Sinickas V. Uncertain relevance of gastric colonization in the seriously ill. *Intensive Care Med.* 1992; 18:210-217.
13. Marshall JC, Christou NV, Horn R, Meakins JL. The microbiology of multiple organ failure: the proximal gastrointestinal tract as an occult reservoir of pathogens. *Arch Surg.* 1988;123:309-315.
14. Johanson WG, Pierce AK, Sanford JP, Thomas GD. Nosocomial respiratory infections with gram-negative bacilli. *Ann Intern Med.* 1972;77:701-706.
15. du Moulin GC, Hedley-White J, Paterson DG, Lisbon A. Aspiration of gastric bacteria in antacid-treated patients: a frequent cause of postoperative colonization of the airway. *Lancet.* 1982;1:242-244.
16. Simms HH, DeMaria E, McDonald L, Peterson D, Robinson A, Burchard KW. Role of gastric colonization in the development of pneumonia in critically ill trauma patients: results of a prospective randomized trial. *J Trauma.* 1991;31:531-537.
17. Marshall JC, Christou NV, Meakins JL. The gastrointestinal tract: the "undrained abscess" of multiple organ failure. *Ann Surg.* 1993;218:111-119.
18. Cook DJ, Laine LA, Guyatt GH, Raffin TA. Nosocomial pneumonia and the role of gastric pH: a meta-analysis. *Chest.* 1991;100:7-13.
19. Cook DJ, Guyatt GH, Marshall JC, et al, for the Canadian Critical Care Trials Group. A randomized trial of sucralfate versus ranitidine for stress ulcer prophylaxis in critically ill patients. *N Engl J Med.* 1998;338:791-797.
20. Kingston GW, Phang PT, Leathley MJ. Increased incidence of nosocomial pneumonia in mechanically ventilated patients with subclinical aspiration. *Am J Surg.* 1991;161:589-592.
21. Torres A, Serra-Batlles J, Ros E, et al. Pulmonary aspiration of gastric contents in patient receiving mechanical ventilation: the effect of body position. *Ann Intern Med.* 1992;116:540-543.
22. Deitch EA, Winterton J, Berg R. The gut as a portal of entry for bacteremia. *Ann Surg.* 1987;205:681-692.
23. Jones WG, Minei JP, Barber AE, Rayburn JL, Fahey TJ, Shires GT. Bacterial translocation and intestinal atrophy after thermal injury and burn wound sepsis. *Ann Surg.* 1990;211:399-405.
24. Moore FA, Moore EE, Poggetti R, et al. Gut bacterial translocation via the portal vein: a clinical perspective with major torso trauma. *J Trauma.* 1991;31: 629-638.
25. Van Saene HK, Stoutenbeek CP, Hart CA. Selective decontamination of the digestive tract (SDD) in intensive care patients: a critical evaluation of the clinical, bacteriological and epidemiological benefits. *J Hosp Infect.* 1991;18:261-277.
26. van der Waaij D, Aberson J, Thijm HA, Welling GW. The screening of four aminoglycosides in the selective decontamination of the digestive tract in mice. *Infection.* 1982;10:35-40.
27. Cunnion KM, Weber DJ, Broadhead WE, Hanson LC, Pieper CF, Rutala WA. Risk factors for nosocomial pneumonia: comparing adult critical-care populations. *Am J Respir Crit Care Med.* 1996;153:158-162.
28. Cook DJ, Guyatt GH, Laupacis A, Sackett DL. Rules of evidence and clinical recommendations on the use of antithrombotic agents. *Chest.* 1992;102:305S-311S.
29. Heyland DK, Cook DJ, King D, Kernerman P, Brun-Buisson C. Maximizing oxygen delivery in critically ill patients: a methodologic appraisal of the evidence. *Crit Care Med.* 1996;24:517-524.
30. Unertl K, Ruckdeschel G, Selbmann HK, et al. Prevention of colonization and respiratory infections in long-term ventilated patients by local antimicrobial prophylaxis. *Intensive Care Med.* 1987; 13:106-113.
31. Korinek AM, Laisne MJ, Nicolas MH, Raskine L, Deroin V, Sanson-Lepors MJ. Selective decontamination of the digestive tract in neurosurgical intensive care unit patients: a double-blind, randomized, placebo-controlled study. *Crit Care Med.* 1993;21:1466-1473.
32. Kerver AJ, Rommes JH, Mevissen-Verhage EA, et al. Prevention of colonization and infection in critically ill patients: a prospective randomized study. *Crit Care Med.* 1988;16:1087-1093.
33. Godard J, Guillaume ME, Bachmann B, et al. Intestinal decontamination in a polyvalent ICU: a double-blind study. *Intensive Care Med.* 1990;16:307-311.
34. Rocha LA, Martin MJ, Pita S, et al. Prevention of nosocomial infection in critically ill patients by selective decontamination of the digestive tract: a randomized, double blind, placebo-controlled study. *Intensive Care Med.* 1992;18: 398-404.
35. Blair P, Rowlands BJ, Lowry K, Webb H, Armstrong P, Smilie J. Selective decontamination of the digestive tract: a stratified, randomized, prospective study in a mixed intensive care unit. *Surgery.* 1991;110:303-310.
36. Pugin J, Auckenthaler R, Lew DP, Suter PM. Oropharyngeal decontamination decreases incidence of ventilator-associated pneumonia: a randomized, placebo-controlled, double-blind clinical trial. *JAMA.* 1991;265:2704-2710.
37. Cerra FB, Maddaus MA, Dunn DL, et al. Selective gut decontamination reduces nosocomial infections and length of stay but not mortality or organ failure in surgical intensive care unit patients. *Arch Surg.* 1992;127:163-169.
38. Cockerill FR, Muller SR, Anhalt JP, et al. Prevention of infection in critically ill patients by selective decontamination of the digestive tract. *Ann Intern Med.* 1992; 117:545-553.
39. Quinio B, Albanese J, Bues-Charbit M, Viviand X, Martin C. Selective decontamination of the digestive tract in multiple trauma patients. *Chest.* 1996;109: 765-772.
40. Stoutenbeek CP, Van Saene HKF, Zandstra DF. Prevention of multiple organ system failure by selective decontamination of the digestive tract in multiple trauma patients. In: Faist E, Baue AE, Schildberg FW, eds. *The Immune Consequences of Trauma, Shock and Sepsis—Mechanisms and Therapeutic Approaches.* Berlin, Germany: Pabst Science Publishers; 1996:1055-1066.

41. Ferrer M, Torres A, Gonzalez J, et al. Utility of selective digestive decontamination in mechanically ventilated patients. *Ann Intern Med.* 1994;120:389-395.
42. Hammond JM, Potgieter PD, Saunders GL, Forder AA. Double-blind study of selective decontamination of the digestive tract in intensive care. *Lancet.* 1992; 340:5-9.
43. Gastinne H, Wolff M, Delatour F, Faurisson F, Chevret S. A controlled trial in intensive care units of selective decontamination of the digestive tract with nonabsorbable antibiotics. *N Engl J Med.* 1992;326:594-599.
44. Ulrich C, Harinck-de Weerd JE, Bakker NC, Jacz K, Doornbos L, de Ridder VA. Selective decontamination of the digestive tract with norfloxacin in the prevention of ICU-acquired infections: a prospective randomized study. *Intensive Care Med.* 1989;15:424-431.
45. Rodriguez-Roldan JM, Altuna-Cuesta A, Lopez A, et al. Prevention of nosocomial lung infection in ventilated patients: use of an antimicrobial pharyngeal nonabsorbable paste. *Crit Care Med.* 1990;18:1239-1242.
46. Winter R, Humphreys H, Pick A, MacGowan AP, Willatts SM, Speller DC. A controlled trial of selective decontamination of the digestive tract in intensive care and its effect on nosocomial infection. *J Antimicrob Chemother.* 1992;30:73-87.
47. Aerdts SJA, van Dalen R, Clasener HAL, Festen J, van Lier HJJ, Vollaard EJ. Antibiotic prophylaxis of respiratory tract infection in mechanically ventilated patients. *Chest.* 1991;100:783-791.
48. Brun-Buisson C, Legrand P, Rauss A, et al. Intestinal decontamination for control of nosocomial multiresistant Gram-negative bacilli. *Ann Intern Med.* 1989; 110:873-881.
49. Jacobs S, Foweraker JE, Roberts SE. Effectiveness of selective decontamination of the digestive tract in an ICU with a policy encouraging a low gastric pH. *Clin Intensive Care.* 1992;3:52-58.
50. Wiener J, Itokazu G, Nathan C, Kabins SA, Weinstein RA. A randomized, double-blind, placebo-controlled trial of selective decontamination in a medical-surgical intensive care unit. *Clin Infect Dis.* 1995;20:861-867.
51. Cuervas-Mons V, Matinez AJ, Dekker A, Starzl TE, Van Thiel DH. Adult liver transplantation: an analysis of the early causes of death in 40 consecutive cases. *Hepatology.* 1986;6:495-501.
52. Cuervas-Mons V, Barrios C, Garrido A, et al. Bacterial infections in liver transplant patients under selective decontamination with norfloxacin. *Transplant Proc.* 1989;21:3558
53. Raakow R, Steffen R, Lefebre B, Bechstein WO, Blumhardt G, Neuhaus P. Selective bowel decontamination effectively prevents gram-negative bacterial infections after liver transplantation. *Transplant Proc.* 1990;22:1556-1557.
54. Rosman C, Klompmaker IJ, Bonsel GJ, Bleichrodt RP, Arends JP, Sloof MJH. The efficacy of selective bowel decontamination as infection prevention after liver transplantation. *Transplant Proc.* 1990;22:1554-1555.
55. Weisner RH, Hermans PE, Rakela J, et al. Selective bowel decontamination to decrease Gram-negative aerobic bacterial and candidal colonization and prevent infection after orthotopic liver transplantation. *Transplantation.* 1988;45:570-574.
56. Bion JF, Badger I, Crosby HA, Hutchings P, et al. Selective decontamination of the digestive tract reduces Gram-negative pulmonary colonization but not systemic endotoxemia in patients undergoing elective liver transplantation. *Crit Care Med.* 1994;22:40-49.
57. Smith SD, Jackson RJ, Hannakan CJ, Wadowsky RM, Tzakis AG, Rowe MI. Selective decontamination in pediatric liver transplants. *Transplantation.* 1993;55: 1306-1309.
58. Arnow PM, Carandang GC, Zabner R, Irwin ME. Randomized controlled trial of selective bowel decontamination for prevention of infections following liver transplantation. *Clin Infect Dis.* 1996;22:997-1003.
59. Zobel G, Kuttnig M, Grubbauer HM, Semmelrock HJ, Thiel W. Reduction of colonization and infection rate during pediatric intensive care by selective decontamination of the digestive tract. *Crit Care Med.* 1991;19:1242-1246.
60. Flaherty J, Nathan C, Kabins SA, Weinstein RA. Pilot trial of selective decontamination for prevention of bacterial infection in an intensive care unit. *J Infect Dis.* 1990;162:1393-1397.
61. Martinez-Pellus AE, Merino P, Bru M, et al. Can selective digestive decontamination avoid the endotoxemia and cytokine activation promoted by cardiopulmonary bypass. *Crit Care Med.* 1993;21:1684-1691.
62. Fox MA, Peterson S, Fabri BM, Van Saene HK. Selective decontamination of the digestive tract in cardiac surgical patients. *Crit Care Med.* 1991;19:1486-1490.
63. Tetteroo GW, Wagenvoort JH, Castelein A, Tilanus HW, Ince C, Bruining HA. Selective decontamination to reduce gram-negative colonisation and infections after oesophageal resection. *Lancet.* 1990;335:704-707.
64. Schardey HM, Joosten U, Finke U, et al. The prevention of anastomotic leakage after total gastrectomy with local decontamination: a prospective, randomized, double-blind, placebo-controlled multicenter trial. *Ann Surg.* 1997;225:172-180.
65. Kreuzer E, Kaab S, Pilz G, Werdan K. Early prediction of septic complications after cardiac surgery by APACHE II score. *Eur J Cardiothorac Surg.* 1992;6:524-528.
66. Asnes J, Abdelnoor M, Berge V, Fjeld NB. Risk factors of septicemia and perioperative myocardial infarction in a cohort of patients supported with intra-aortic balloon pump (IABP) in the course of open heart surgery. *Eur J Cardiothorac Surg.* 1993;7:153-157.
67. Kollef MH, Wragge T, Pasque C. Determinants of mortality and multiorgan dysfunction in cardiac surgery patients requiring prolonged mechanical ventilation. *Chest.* 1995;107:1395-1401.
68. Shirani KZ, Pruitt BA, Mason AD. The influence of inhalation injury and pneumonia on burn mortality. *Ann Surg.* 1987;205:82-87.
69. Sittig K, Deitch EA. Effect of bacteremia on mortality after thermal injury. *Arch Surg.* 1988;123:1367-1370.
70. Mackie DP, van Hertum WA, Schumburg T, Kuijper EC, Knape P. Prevention of infection in burns: preliminary experience with selective decontamination of the digestive tract in patients with extensive injuries. *J Trauma.* 1992;32:570-575.
71. Luiten EJT, Hop WCJ, Lange JF, Bruining HA. Controlled clinical trial of selective decontamination for the treatment of severe acute pancreatitis. *Ann Surg.* 1995; 222:57-65.
72. Mclelland P, Murray A, Yaqoob M, Van Saene HKF, Bone JM, Mostafa SM. Prevention of bacterial infection and sepsis in acute severe pancreatitis. *Ann R Coll Surg Engl.* 1992;74:329-334.
73. Collins R, Schrimgeour A, Yusuf S, Peto R. Reduction in fatal pulmonary embolism and venous thrombosis by perioperative administration of subcutaneous heparin. *N Engl J Med.* 1988;318:1162-1173.
74. Kaiser AB. Antimicrobial prophylaxis in surgery. *N Engl J Med.* 1986;315:1129-1138.
75. Freedman B. Equipoise and the ethics of clinical research. *N Engl J Med.* 1987; 317:141-145.
76. Lingnau W, Berger J, Javorsky F, Lejeune P, Mutz N, Benzer H. Selective intestinal decontamination in multiple trauma patients: prospective, controlled trial. *J Trauma.* 1997;42:687-694.

ORIGINAL ARTICLE

Isolated Limb Perfusion With High-Dose Tumor Necrosis Factor α and Melphalan for Kaposi Sarcoma

Dina Lev-Chelouche, MD; Subhi Abu-Abeid, MD; Ofer Merimsky, MD; Josephine Isakov, MD; Yoram Kollander, MD; Isaac Meller, MD; Joseph M. Klausner, MD; Mordechai Gutman, MD

Background: Although the classic form of Kaposi sarcoma is considered indolent and benign, at times its evolution is more severe, with an acute onset and debilitating complications necessitating aggressive treatment and even amputation.

Objective: To evaluate the efficacy of hyperthermic isolated limb perfusion (ILP) with tumor necrosis factor α and melphalan as a limb-sparing modality for extensive regional Kaposi sarcoma.

Setting: University hospital and national referral center.

Patients: Five patients, aged 60 to 82 years, with extensive, symptomatic, classic Kaposi sarcoma of the lower limb were operated on. All were candidates for amputation owing to debilitating symptoms.

Interventions: Patients underwent ILP through the iliac (n = 2), femoral (n = 2), and popliteal (n = 1) vessels. Tumor necrosis factor α, 4 mg, and melphalan, 1.5 mg/kg body weight, were perfused for an overall time of 90 minutes. The limb was heated to 40°C. Clinical and pathological responses were recorded for all patients after 6 to 8 weeks.

Results: The overall response rate was 100%: 1 of 5 patients had complete response and 4 of 5 had partial response. Two patients had progression of disease 2 months after ILP but one of them was asymptomatic and did not require any further treatment. The second patient underwent amputation. Thus, limb preservation was achieved in 80% (4 of 5 patients). Median follow-up was 24 months. There were no deaths associated with treatment or major system complications. Local complications were all reversible.

Conclusion: These findings suggest that hyperthermic ILP with tumor necrosis factor α and melphalan can be considered an effective palliative and limb-sparing treatment modality for extensive Kaposi sarcoma.

Arch Surg. 1999;134:177-180

From the Departments of Surgery (Drs Lev-Chelouche, Abu-Abeid, Klausner, and Gutman), Oncology (Dr Merimsky), and Orthopedic Oncology (Drs Isakov, Kollander, and Meller), Tel Aviv Sourasky Medical Centre, Tel Aviv University, Tel Aviv, Israel.

THE INTEREST in Kaposi sarcoma has escalated during the last decade because it has become the most frequent malignancy associated with the acquired immunodeficiency syndrome. However, the classic form of this disease was first described more than 100 years ago by Kaposi as a rare multifocal neoplasm. This form is an infrequent cutaneous angiolymphoproliferative disease that usually involves the lower limbs, and mainly affects people of Mediterranean, Eastern European, or Jewish heritage.[1] It occurs most frequently in men after the sixth decade of life. Unlike other forms, classic Kaposi sarcoma usually has a chronic course following an indolent and benign clinical course. It is not generally life-threatening, and thus may not require specific therapy early in its course. However, at times it can result in local aggressive lesions, causing pain, edema, ulceration, and bleeding, which seriously impair the quality of life.[2,3]

Currently, treatment options are confined to old modalities, mainly radiotherapy and various chemotherapeutic agents, and some new experimental therapies based on biomodulators such as interferons.[4-7] In numerous studies, some of these treatment options achieved palliation but this was mostly temporary at the expense of major toxic effects. Because the population most commonly afflicted with this form of Kaposi sarcoma is elderly and often affected with concomitant disease (mainly of the cardiovascular and respiratory systems), and because toxicity must be kept to a minimum, it seems an ideal setting for using local treatments.[8] To date, different local therapies have been used for the treatment of Kaposi sarcoma, including simple excision, cryotherapy, laser treatment, and intralesional therapy, and, although these therapies are easy to perform, relatively safe, and often sufficient for a very localized small tumor burden,

PATIENTS AND METHODS

PATIENTS

Between June 1994 and November 1997, 5 patients with advanced Kaposi sarcoma were treated with TNF-α and melphalan via ILP (**Table 1**). All were men, with an age range of 60 to 82 years (mean age, 73 years). All had very extensive recurrent disease confirmed histologically (**Figure 1**). Except for 1 patient with 1 very large lesion located on the ankle that was not amenable for resection, the remaining 4 patients all had more than 20 lesions. All patients had symptoms due to their Kaposi sarcoma: pain (5 patients), bleeding (2 patients), and infected necrotic lesions (2 patients). Previous therapy had failed in all patients, with either a short-lived response or no response at all: radiotherapy (4 patients), systemic chemotherapy (2 patients), and photodynamic therapy (1 patients) At the stage when they were referred to us, they were all considered absolute candidates for some form of amputation.

The study was conducted within the framework of an "investigator's own responsibility study," which was approved by the National Helsinki (Finland) committee. Informed consent was obtained from all patients.

ILP WITH RECOMBINANT TNF-α AND MELPHALAN

The technique of hyperthermic ILP with high-dose recombinant TNF-α and melphalan is described elsewhere.[13] Briefly, to isolate the limb, the main artery and vein are dissected and all collaterals ligated. The vessels are cannulated and connected to a pump oxygenator similar to that used in cardiopulmonary bypass. A tourniquet (200-400 mm Hg) or Esmarch band is applied to the root of the limb to ascertain complete vascular isolation and to ensure that all tumors lie within the perfused area and receive adequate drug dosing. The temperature of the perfused limb is maintained at 39° to 40°C during the entire procedure by using both external heating and warming of the perfusate.

Systemic leakage from the perfused limb is monitored continuously by using technetium Tc 99–radiolabeled human serum albumin injected into the perfusate. Radioactivity above the precordial area is recorded using a Geiger counter.

DRUG ADMINISTRATION

Recombinant TNF-α was administered at a dose of 4 mg as a bolus into the arterial line of the perfusate. Melphalan (Alkeran, Glaxco Wellcome, Research Triangle Park, NC) was administered at 1 mg/kg body weight 30 minutes after recombinant TNF-α administration and perfusion was continued for a further 60 minutes.

RESPONSE EVALUATION

Evaluation of response according to Union Internationale Contre le Cancer criteria was performed 6 to 8 weeks after ILP and included clinical response assessed by counting and measuring the lesions and a pathological estimation assessed by multiple incisional biopsy specimens from the remaining tumors or tumor bed (**Figure 2**).

they are not a feasible treatment for an extensive disease with dozens of lesions. Kaposi sarcoma is a highly radiosensitive neoplasm and thus local radiation has been widely used for control of individual problem-causing lesions with complete regression rates of up to 80% to 90%.[9,10] However, recurrences are frequent, and this modality is limited and cannot be used repeatedly. At times, failure of all other treatment options makes amputation inevitable.

Isolated limb perfusion (ILP) is a form of regional therapy that enables the administration of chemotherapeutic agents at a dose of up to 20 times the maximally tolerated systemic dose while avoiding exposing the entire body to major side effects of these agents. High-dose recombinant tumor necrosis factor α (TNF-α) administered in combination with the cytotoxic drug melphalan via ILP resulted in remarkable response rates for melanoma and nonresectable soft tissue sarcoma confined to the limb, with a limb-sparing rate of more than 90%.[11-13]

Because Kaposi sarcoma can evolve into a major local problem in the inflicted limb, this study evaluated the role of ILP with TNF-α and melphalan in the palliation and limb preservation for such patients.

RESULTS

Patients underwent ILP via the iliac (n = 2), femoral (n = 2), and popliteal (n = 1) vessels (**Table 2**).

COMPLICATIONS

There were no deaths associated with the treatment. None of the patients experienced any form of systemic complication. Local limb complications assessed according to Wieberdink et al[14] manifested as redness in 3 patients (grade 2) and blisters in 4 (grade 3). No patient experienced neuropathy and none necessitated amputation.

RESPONSE

The overall response rate was 100% (5/5). One patient (20%) achieved complete response and 4 patients (80%) achieved partial response. Within the limitations of a short follow-up (3-42 months; median, 24 months), local recurrence occurred in 2 patients within 2 months. One patient required amputation due to recurrent lesions that became necrotic and infected. In the second patient, the lesions reappeared but because they were asymptomatic, to date, he has not required any further treatment. Thus, limb preservation was achieved in 4 of 5 patients who were previously all candidates for amputation.

One patient died during the follow-up (36 months) of a myocardial infarction.

COMMENT

Tumor necrosis factor α has long been recognized for its antineoplastic properties, which have been demonstrated re-

Table 1. Patient and Clinical Data

Patient No./ Sex/Age, y	Duration of Disease, y	Location of Disease	No. of Lesions	Prior Therapy
1/M/82	7	Calf and ankle	20	Radiation and chemotherapy
2/M/76	1	Leg	>100	Radiation
3/M/60	11	Ankle	1	Radiation
4/M/64	3	Leg	>100	Radiation and chemotherapy
5/M/82	4	Foot and ankle	30	Photodynamic therapy

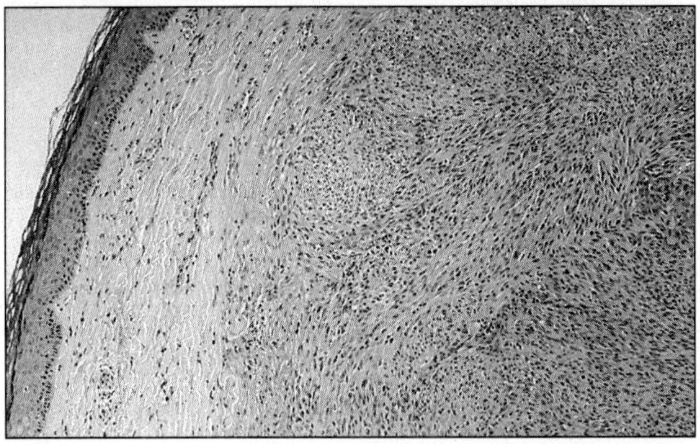

Figure 1. *Biopsy specimen of skin with Kaposi sarcoma showing numerous tumor cells occupying the entire subcutaneous layer (hematoxylin-eosin, ×200).*

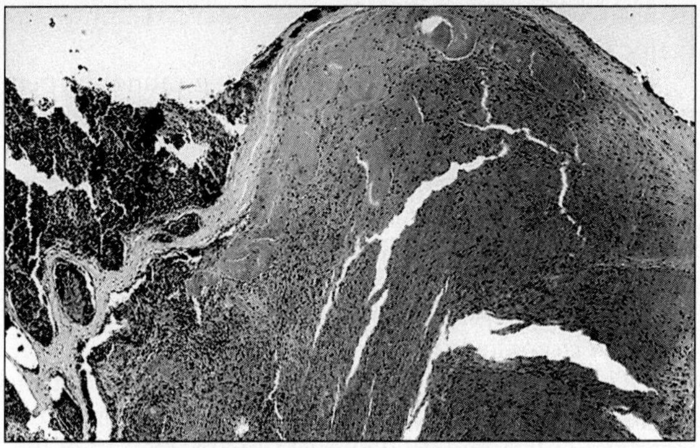

Figure 2. *Cross section of a Kaposi sarcoma lesion 6 weeks after isolated limb perfusion with tumor necrosis factor and melphalan showing necrosis and dense inflammatory infiltration with no evidence of tumor cells (hematoxylin-eosin, ×200).*

Table 2. Results and Follow-up of Treatment

Patient No.	Vascular Approach	Response	Limb Salvage	Local Recurrence	Follow-up
1	Femoral	Partial	No*	2 mo	Died, 36 mo†
2	Iliac	Partial	Yes	2 mo	Alive, 42 mo
3	Femoral	Complete	Yes	None	Alive, 24 mo
4	Iliac	Partial	Yes	None	Alive, 14 mo
5	Popliteal	Partial	Yes	None	Alive, 3 mo

*Amputation performed 3 months after treatment.
†Died of myocardial infarction.

peatedly in various in vitro and in vivo studies.[15,16] The effect of TNF-α on tumor vasculature, and its role as an important mediator in the immune system generating many different kinds of cytokines and mediators, makes Kaposi sarcoma an ideal target for its antitumoral effect. Kaposi sarcoma is assumed to be a neoplasm of vascular origin and thus contains numerous amounts of endothelial cells and blood vessels. Using its procoagulant properties,[17-19] TNF-α activates specific adhesion molecules on the surface of endothelial cells within the tumor and membranal receptors on macrophages and leukocytes. Rapid migration of leukocytes to the tumor capillary bed leading to adhesion to the endothelium, release of oxygen free radicals and other cytokines, and extensive local inflammatory reaction may result in obstruction of the tumor's capillary bed. This TNF-α–induced endothelial damage is exclusive to tumor vasculature, whereas normal vasculature is spared.

A link between the development of Kaposi sarcoma and a suppressed immune system was suspected for a long time since it occurs more commonly in conditions of iatrogenic immunosuppression,[20] in transplant recipients,[21] in patients with hematological malignant neoplasms,[22] and in the elderly who have a more deficient immune system. This speculation has received major support with the emergence of human immunodeficiency virus (HIV)–associated Kaposi sarcoma. Tumor necrosis factor α has the ability to modulate the immune functions and induce the generation of many cytokines,[23,24] such as interleukin 1, interleukin 6, interleukin 8, interferon, oxygen free radicals, and arachidonic acid products, some of which have a definite anticancer effect.

However, systemic administration of TNF-α cannot be clinically implemented for patients with Kaposi sarcoma in the same way as for patients with other malignant disease since the dose required to achieve its anticancer effect is 10 times higher than the maximal tolerated systemic dose in humans. Immediately on its systemic administration, TNF-α leads to marked hypotension and septic shocklike syndrome and eventually to multiorgan failure.[25] This effect provided the rationale for a trial evaluating direct intratumoral injection of TNF-α, [26] and, although regression of lesions was observed in 94% of cases, systemic toxicity was common and limited the clinical usefulness of TNF-α.

Our growing experience of ILP with TNF-α and melphalan for treatment of patients with melanoma and soft tissue sarcoma,[13] and the understanding that TNF-α in high doses might achieve a major response and thus limb preservation in patients with Kaposi sarcoma who were candidates for amputation, led us to implement this method.

All 5 patients responded to the treatment, with more than 50% regression of the tumor mass. Although this is only a small group of patients, it is essential to remember that all had very extensive and mutilating disease, and that these results were obtained despite the fact that previous treatment modalities had failed, such as chemotherapy and irradiation. Four of the 5 patients, including 1 in whom the tumor recurred a few months after treatment, achieved limb salvage and are asymptomatic. There was no evidence of leakage of TNF-α to the systemic circulation due to meticulous isolation of the limb and thus no systemic side effects of TNF-α administration. These results are encouraging and suggest that hyperthermic ILP with TNF-α and melphalan can be considered as an effective treatment for limb salvage in patients with extensive Kaposi sarcoma not limited by major side effects.

Considering the entire procedure, it cannot be postulated that the TNF-α is the only effective factor since it is given in combination with the alkylating agent melphalan. However, from past experience with other malignant tumors such as soft tissue sarcoma, ILP with chemotherapeutic agents alone resulted in a low response rate, and the addition of TNF-α showed marked improvement. Moreover, there is a clear synergism between TNF-α and various cytotoxic drugs, among them melphalan.[27]

The other factor is hyperthermia. Throughout the procedure, the limb is heated to about 40°C. Several studies in patients with HIV demonstrated regression of disseminated lesions of Kaposi sarcoma when treated with low-flow extracorporeal perfusion hyperthermia.[28,29] Hyperthermia by itself is also known to potentiate the activity of melphalan and TNF-α and may be partly responsible for the observed efficiency of the treatment.[27,30]

The fact that 2 of our patients had relapse of disease early after the procedure might indicate that at least in some patients control of disease is only temporary, and an additional treatment modality should be considered to achieve a sustained response.

One possibility is to exchange the chemotherapeutic drug melphalan with one of the vinka alkaloids or antibiotics, which have a known effect on Kaposi sarcoma.[31]

Recently, biomodulators such as interferons are being studied for their effect on Kaposi sarcoma.[7,32,33] The interferons are a group of naturally occurring proteins that inhibit the growth of tumors in vivo and of many transformed cells in vitro. Limited information is available to assess the efficacy of interferons of different types, mainly interferon alfa, at different doses, in the treatment of Kaposi sarcoma. However, these studies do demonstrate therapeutic benefits of such treatment.

Combining TNF-α with interferon appears logical, since TNF-α itself potentiates the action of different interferons. These and other biological agents in combination with TNF-α via ILP should be studied in the near future.

Liposomal daunorubicin hydrochloride, a newly described agent, shows promising primary results in the treatment of classic and HIV-associated Kaposi sarcoma.[34,35] Further studies are needed to compare its efficacy with that of ILP and TNF-α or even to combine both treatment modalities for a long-standing response.

The long-term effect of ILP and TNF-α in patients with Kaposi sarcoma is as yet unknown; however, it seems to be a safe and effective treatment for classic Kaposi sarcoma, and might even be considered a palliative method for HIV-related Kaposi sarcoma.

Reprints: Mordechai Gutman, MD, Department of Surgery, Tel Aviv Sourasky Medical Centre, 6 Weizmann St, Tel Aviv 64239 Israel.

REFERENCES

1. Cox FH, Helwig EB. Kaposi's sarcoma. *Cancer.* 1959;12:289-298.
2. Zafari B, Anhalt TS. Kaposi's saroma. *Semin Dermatol.* 1984;3:69-77.
3. Tappero JW, Conant MA, Wolfe SF, Berger TG. Kaposi's sarcoma: epidemiology, pathogenesis, histology, clinical spectrum, staging criteria and therapy. *J Am Acad Dermatol.* 1993;28:371-395.
4. Krown SE, Myskowski PL, Paredes J. Kaposi's sarcoma. *Med Clin North Am.* 1992;76:235-252.
5. Martin RW, Hood AF, Farmer ER. Kaposi's sarcoma. *Medicine.* 1993;72:245-261.
6. Northfeld DW. Treatment of Kaposi's sarcoma: current guidelines and future prospectives. *Drugs.* 1994;48:569-582.
7. Rybojod M, Borradai L, Verola O, Zeller J, Puissant A, Morel P. Non-AIDS associated Kaposi's sarcoma (classical and endemic African types): treatment with low doses of recombinant interferon-alpha. *J Invest Dermatol.* 1990;95:1765-1795.
8. Tur E, Brenner S. Treatment of Kaposi's sarcoma. *Arch Dermatol.* 1996;132:327-331.
9. El Akkad S, Bull CA, El-Senaissi MA, Griffin JT, Anner M. Kaposi's sarcoma and its management by radiotherapy. *Arch Dermatol.* 1986;122:1396-1399.
10. Cooper JS, Sacco J, Newall Y. The duration of local control of classic (non-AIDS–associated) Kaposi's sarcoma by radiotherapy. *J Am Acad Dermatol.* 1988;19:59-66.
11. Lienard D, Ewelenko P, Delmotte JJ, Renard N, Lejeune FJ. High-dose recombinant tumor necrosis factor alpha in combination with interferon gamma and melphalan in isolation perfusion of the limbs for melanoma and sarcoma. *J Clin Oncol.* 1992;10:52-60.
12. Eggermont AMM, Schraffordt-Koops H, Klausner JM, et al. Isolated limb perfusion with tumor necrosis factor and melphalan for limb salvage in 186 patients with locally advanced soft tissue extremity sarcomas: the cumulative multicenter European experience. *Ann Surg.* 1996;6:756-765.
13. Gutman M, Inbar M, Lev-Shlush D, et al. High-dose tumor necrosis factor-α and melphalan administered via isolated limb perfusion for advanced limb soft tissue sarcoma results in >90% response rate and limb preservation. *Cancer.* 1997;79:1129-1137.
14. Wieberdink J, Benckhuysen C, Braat RP, et al. Dosimetry in isolation perfusion of the limbs by assessment of perfused tissue volume and grading of toxic tissue reactions. *Eur J Cancer Clin Oncol.* 1982;18:905-910.
15. Haranak K, Satomi N, Sukari A. Antitumor activity of murine tumor necrosis factor against transplanted murine tumors and heterotransplanted human tumors in nude mice. *Int J Cancer.* 1984;34:263-267.
16. Asher AL, Mule JY, Reichert CM, Shiloni E, Rosenberg SA. Studies of the antitumor efficacy of systemically administered recombinant tumor necrosis factor against several murine tumors in vivo. *J Immunol.* 1987;138:963-974.
17. Wantanabe N, Niitsu Y, Umeno H, et al. Toxic effect of TNF on tumor vasculature in mice. *Cancer Res.* 1988;49:2179-2183.
18. Nawroth PP, Stern DM. Modulation of endothelial cell hemostatic properties by tumor necrosis factor. *J Exp Med.* 1986;163:740-745.
19. Bevilacqua MP, Pober JS, Majeau GR, Fiers W, Cotran RS, Gimbrone MA Jr. Recombinant tumor necrosis factor induces procoagulant activity in cultured human vascular endothelium: characterization and comparison with actions of interleukin-1. *Proc Natl Acad Sci U S A.* 1986;83:4533-4537.
20. Klein MB, Pereira FA, Kantor I. Kaposi's sarcoma complicating systemic lupus erythematosus treated with immunosuppression. *Arch Dermatol.* 1974;110:602-604.
21. Penn I. Kaposi's sarcoma in organ transplant recipients: report of 20 cases. *Transplantation.* 1979;27:8-11.
22. Kapadia SB, Krause JR. Kaposi's sarcoma after long-term alkylating agent therapy for multiple myeloma. *South Med J.* 1977;70:1011-1013.
23. Beutler B, Cerami A. Tumor necrosis, cachexia, shock and inflammation: a common mediator. *Ann Rev Biochem.* 1988;57:505-518.
24. Quinn TD, Polk HC Jr, Edwards MJ. Hyperthermic isolated limb perfusion increases circulating levels of inflammatory cytokines. *Cancer Immunol Immunother.* 1995;40:272-275.
25. Tracey KY, Beutler B, Lowry SF, et al. Shock and tissue injury induced by recombinant human cachectin. *Science.* 1986;234:470-473.
26. Kahn JO, Kaplan LD, Volberding PA, et al. Intralesional recombinant tumor necrosis factor-α for AIDS-associated Kaposi's sarcoma: a randomized, double-blind trial. *J AIDS.* 1989;2:217-223.
27. Krosnick JA, Mule JJ, McIntosh JK, Rosenberg SA. Augmentation of antitumor efficacy by the combination of recombinant tumor necrosis factor and chemotherapeutic agents in vivo. *Cancer Res.* 1989;49:3729-3733.
28. Alonso K, Potiggia P, Nardi C, Sabato A, Cuppone CF. Systemic hyperthermia in the treatment of HIV-related Kaposi's sarcoma: a phase I study. *Biomed Pharmacother.* 1992;46:21-24.
29. Alosno K, Ponfiggia P, Sabato A, et al. Systemic hyperthermia in the treatment of HIV-related disseminated Kaposi's sarcoma: long-term follow-up of patient with low-flow extracorporeal perfusion hyperthermia. *Am J Clin Oncol.* 1994;17:353-359.
30. Robbins HJ, d'Oleire F, Kutz M, et al. Cytotoxic interactions of tumor necrosis factor, melphalan and 41.8°C hyperthermia. *Cancer Lett.* 1995;89:55-62.
31. Brambilla L, Boneschi IV, Beretta G, Finzi AF. Chemotherapeutic approach to Kaposi's sarcoma. In: Cerimele D, ed. *Kaposi's Sarcoma.* New York, NY: Spectrum; 1985:137-148.
32. Real FX, Herbert HF, Krown SE. Kaposi's sarcoma and the acquired immune deficiency syndrome: treatment with high and low doses of recombinant leukocyte A interferon. *J Clin Oncol.* 1986;4:544-551.
33. Krown SE, Real FX, Vadhan-Ray S, et al. Kaposi's sarcoma and the acquired immune deficiency syndrome: treatment with recombinant interferon alpha and analysis of prognostic factors. *Cancer.* 1986;57:1662-1665.
34. Gottlieb JJ, Washenik K, Chachoua A, et al. Treatment of classic Kaposi's sarcoma with liposomal encapsulated doxorubicin. *Lancet.* 1977;350:1363-1364.
35. Fournier S, Dupont B, Gialoux G, et al. Efficacy and tolerance of liposomal daunorubicin in Kaposi sarcoma associated with human immunodeficiency virus infection. *Arch Dermatol.* 1997;133:918-919.

Pathologic Features of Prognostic Significance for Adrenocortical Carcinoma After Curative Resection

Lawrence E. Harrison, MD; Paul B. Gaudin, MD; Murray F. Brennan, MD

Objective: To identify the pathologic features of prognostic significance in patients with resectable adrenocortical carcinomas.

Design: Retrospective review.

Setting: Tertiary referral center.

Patients: Review of the Memorial Sloan-Kettering Cancer Center prospective adrenocortical carcinoma database from 1986 through 1996 identified 46 patients who underwent curative adrenalectomy for primary disease. All cases were reviewed by a single pathologist and each primary tumor was characterized by 16 separate pathologic parameters.

Main Outcome Measure: Overall survival rates in the patient population.

Results: The 5-year overall survival rate for the entire cohort was 36% (median survival rate, 28 months). Of the pathologic factors analyzed, tumor size, number of mitotic figures, and the presence of intratumoral hemorrhage were independent prognostic factors. Patients presenting with primary tumors larger than 12 cm (n=30) had a worse outcome compared with those with smaller tumors (n=16) (5-year survival rate: 53% vs 22%, $P<.05$). Mitotic count (≥6 per 10 high-power fields) was a negative prognostic feature (n=15) with a 5-year survival rate of 13% vs 51% for 0 to 6 mitotic figures per 10 high-power fields (n=31, $P<.05$). Intratumoral hemorrhage (n=23) was also a negative prognostic factor compared with no evidence of intratumoral hemorrhage (n=23) (5-year survival rate, 53% vs 22%, $P<.05$). Overall survival rates were also calculated based on the number of pathologic risk factors. Patients with no risk factors had an 83% 5-year survival rate, which decreased to 42% with 1 factor, 33% with 2 factors, and 0% with all 3 risk factors.

Conclusions: Tumor size, hemorrhage, and mitotic count correlate with survival rates for patients undergoing curative resection. Based on these pathologic factors, adrenocortical carcinomas may be divided into low- and high-risk groups.

Arch Surg. 1999;134:181-185

The outcome for patients with adrenocortical carcinoma is dismal, with the reported 5-year survival rate ranging from 16% to 23%.[1] One reason for this poor outcome is the inclusion of a large number of patients with advanced disease. These patients significantly skew survival rates since resectability and stage at presentation are powerful independent prognostic factors.[2-4] Importantly, studies evaluating pathologic features of prognostic significance often include patients with resectable and unresectable disease.

See Invited Critique at end of article

The subset of patients with resectable adrenocortical carcinomas represents a select group with a better prognosis; however, even in this group, some patients will subsequently die of recurrent disease. For these patients, age, functional status of the tumor, and completeness of resection have been reported to be independent clinical prognostic factors.[3] While these clinical factors have been reported, pathologic predictors for patients undergoing curative resection are not well documented. Our purpose is to identify the pathologic features of prognostic significance in patients with resectable adrenocortical carcinomas. These factors may be important in predicting who is at high risk for recurrence and cancer-related death after curative resection.

From the Division of Surgical Oncology, Department of Surgery, University of Medicine and Dentistry of New Jersey, New Jersey Medical School, Newark (Dr Harrison); and the Departments of Pathology (Dr Gaudin) and Surgery (Dr Brennan), Memorial Sloan-Kettering Cancer Center, New York, NY.

RESULTS

Of the 46 patients, 30 were women and 16 were men. There was no difference in the

PATIENTS AND METHODS

A review of the Memorial Sloan-Kettering Cancer Center's prospective adrenocortical carcinoma database identified 103 patients from 1986 through 1996. Of these patients, 46 underwent curative adrenalectomy for primary disease and constitute the group analyzed for pathologic prognostic factors. All cases were reviewed by a single pathologist (P.B.G.) and each primary tumor was characterized by 16 separate pathologic parameters, including size, invasion, growth pattern, hemorrhage, venous invasion, nuclear grade, mitotic figures, and necrosis (**Table**). Survival was calculated by the Kaplan-Meier method and compared by log-rank test with statistical significance defined as $P<.05$.

laterality of tumor, with 22 presenting on the right and 24 presenting on the left. The median age at diagnosis was 49 years (age range, 22-77 years). The median tumor size was 15 cm (range, 2.5-27 cm).

The median follow-up time for the entire cohort was 20 months (range, 1-101 months). The 5-year overall survival rate for the entire cohort was 36% (median survival rate, 28 months) (**Figure 1**). Of the 16 pathologic factors analyzed, tumor size, number of mitotic figures, and the presence of intratumoral hemorrhage were independent prognostic factors (Table). Patients with primary tumors larger than 12 cm (n=30) had a worse outcome compared with those with smaller tumors (n=16) (5-year survival rate, 53% vs 22%, $P<.05$) (**Figure 2**). Mitotic count (≥6 per 10 high-power fields) was a negative prognostic feature (n=15) with a 5-year survival rate of 13% vs 51% for 0 to 6 mitotic figures per 10 high-power fields (n=31, $P<.05$) (**Figure 3**). Hemorrhage into the tumor (n=23) was also a negative prognostic factor compared with no evidence of intratumoral hemorrhage (n=23) (5-year survival rate, 53% vs 22%, $P<.05$) (**Figure 4**). Overall survival rate was also calculated based on the number of pathologic risk factors. Patients with no risk factors had an 83% 5-year survival rate that decreased to 42% with 1 risk factor, 33% with 2, and 0% with all 3 ($P<.02$) (**Figure 5**).

Pathologic Parameters of Primary Tumors in Patients With Adrenocortical Carcinoma After Curative Resection, 1986 to 1996*

Characteristics	No. of Patients	Median Survival, mo	5-y Survival Rate, %	P
Size, cm				
≤12	16	101	66	.03
>12	30	26	23	
Local invasion				
No	31	28	38	>.05
Yes	13	18	32	
Diffuse growth pattern				
No	2	...	100	>.05
Yes	44	28	34	
Necrosis				
No	4	100	...	.06
Yes	42	26	30	
Fibrous bands				
No	4	56	33	>.05
Yes	42	28	39	
Capsular invasion				
No	3	28	0	>.05
Yes	43	28	37	
Hemorrhage				
No	23	101	53	.05
Yes	23	20	22	
Myxoid				
No	33	28	41	>.05
Yes	13	32	45	
Venous invasion				
No	9	32	43	>.05
Yes	37	21	42	
Sinusoidal invasion				
No	2	28	0	>.05
Yes	44	28	38	
Nuclear pleomorphism				
No	4	...	67	>.05
Yes	42	28	34	
Nuclear grade				
<4	16	32	47	>.05
4	29	30	26	
Abnormal mitotic figures				
No	2	...	...	>.05
Yes	44	28	34	
Mitotic index				
0-6	31	59	51	.003
>6	15	15	13	
Nuclear hyperchromasia				
No	1	...	...	>.05
Yes	45	34	28	
Nucleoli				
No	1	...	...	>.05
Yes	45	35	28	

**Ellipses indicate that there were too few patients to evaluate statistically.*

COMMENT

Adrenocortical carcinoma is a rare tumor (annual incidence, 0.5-2 cases per million[1]) but a highly lethal disease, with a mortality rate of more than 50%. Patients able to undergo complete resection have a better prognosis, with 5-year survival rates up to 50% after removal of localized disease[2-5]; however, even after curative resection, many die of recurrent disease. Routine adjuvant chemotherapy is not indicated, as its value for adrenocortical carcinoma has not been proven and its most active agent, mitotane, has significant side effects. Identifying patients with a poor prognosis after curative resection may be useful to select those who may benefit from adjuvant chemotherapy.

A variety of histologic indices of adrenal malignancy has been proposed based on the presence of a diffuse growth pattern, nuclear pleomorphism, tumor necrosis, intratumoral fibrous bands, mitotic figures, vascular, capsular, or sinusoidal invasion, and less than 25% of clear cells.[6,7] The distinction of adrenocortical carcinoma from adenoma can usually be made based on these pathologic features; however, these same factors may be useful in selecting a high-risk group of patients after curative resection. Our study evaluated the pathologic features of 46 patients who underwent curative

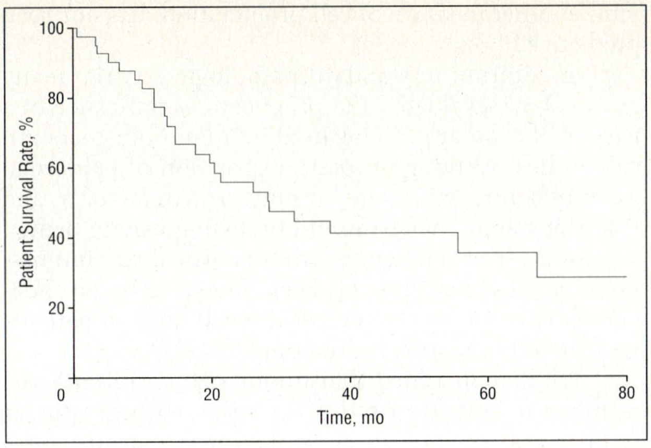

Figure 1. *The overall 5-year survival rates for the entire cohort of 46 patients was 36% (median survival, 28 months).*

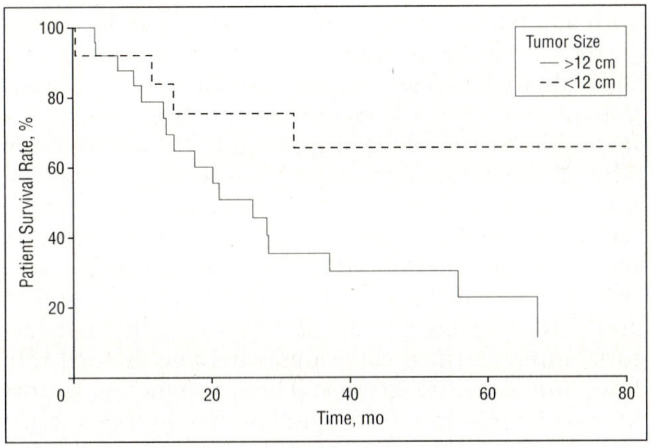

Figure 2. *Patients with primary tumors larger than 12 cm (n=30) had a worse outcome compared with those with smaller tumors (n=16) (5-year survival rates, 53% vs 22%,* P<.05*).*

resection for primary adrenocortical carcinoma and correlated these pathologic factors with survival rates. We demonstrated that tumor size, the presence of mitotic figures, and tumor hemorrhage were independent prognostic factors for this select group.

In our study our patients with tumors larger than 12 cm had a worse outcome compared with patients with smaller tumors. While tumor size has been shown to be a predictor of adrenal malignancy, it has not been reported as a predictor of survival rates after resection. This may be explained by the fact that most studies use a 5-cm cut-off for comparison based on the staging of adrenocortical carcinomas. Most studies do not report survival rate differences between stage I (<5 cm, node negative) and stage II (>5 cm, node negative) disease[2,3] and, in fact, most large studies group stages I and II together as 1 stage.[2,4,8] Stage is based not only on size, but on nodal status, local invasion (stage III), and the presence of metastatic disease (stage IV). In our series, complete pathologic staging was not possible since lymph node specimens were sampled in only 18 patients (39%). This lack of nodal information in our data set may represent either the absence of clinically involved lymph nodes at resection or that no nodes were resected. Others have reported this lack of pathologic nodal information. Lee et al[5] reported the results of 23 patients who underwent primary surgical resection for an adrenocortical carcinoma, and lymph nodes were identified in only 5 specimens (22%). Other groups reported a higher incidence of evaluable nodes.[3,4] This may represent institutional bias to perform regional lymphadenectomy with resection, although this has not been shown to improve survival or recurrence rates. There was no correlation in tumor size with lymph node status cases where lymph nodes were identified ($P<.05$, Mann-Whitney *U* test). Since lymph node evaluation is not reliably available, tumor size represents a dependable and important prognostic component for resected adrenocortical carcinoma.

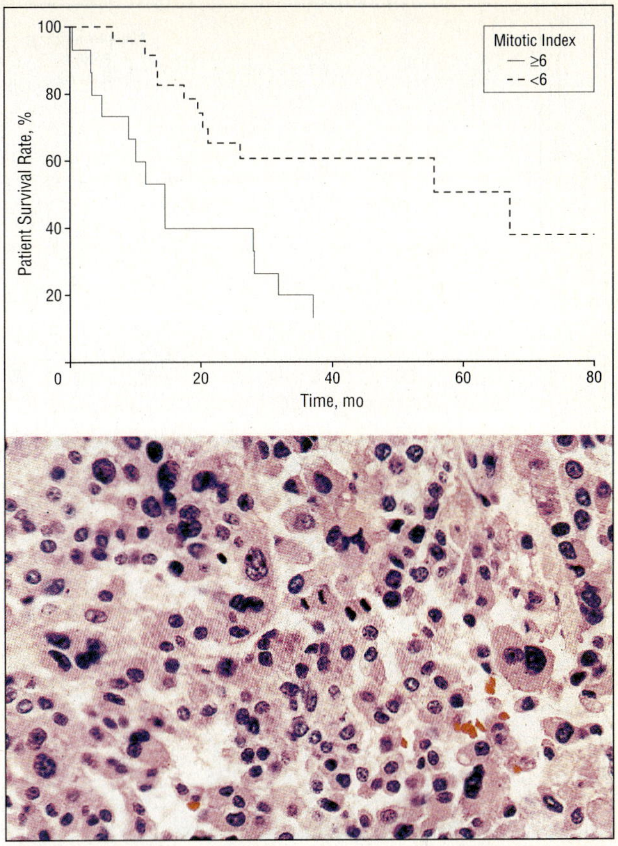

Figure 3. *Mitotic count (≥6 per 10 high-power fields) was a negative prognostic factor (n=15) with 5-year survival rates of 13% vs 51% for mitotic figures of less than 6 per 10 high-power fields (n=31,* P<.05*). Top, Survival curve. Bottom, Histologic example of abnormal mitotic figures.*

Our data suggest that mitotic rate is a predictor of the survival rate in the subset of patients undergoing curative resection (Figure 3). The presence of mitotic figures has been used as a major criterion to separate benign from malignant cortical tumors.[7,9,10] In addition, mitotic rate has been reported as a predictor of survival rate in patients with adrenocortical carcinoma. Analyzing patients who underwent resection and those who did not, Weiss et al[6] reported that mitotic rate had a strong statistical association with outcome. Patients whose tumors had greater than 20 mitoses per 50 high-power fields had a median survival rate of 14 months, while those with less than 20 mitoses had a median survival rate of 58 months. Similar results have been

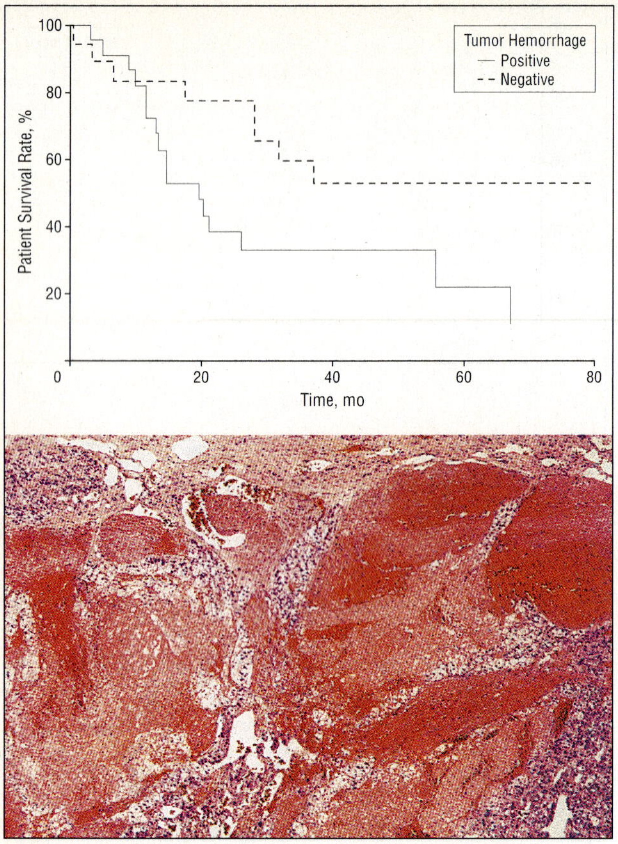

Figure 4. *Intratumoral hemorrhage (n=23) was a negative prognostic factor compared with no evidence of intratumoral hemorrhage (n=23) (5-year survival rates, 53% vs 22%,* P<.05*). Top, Survival curve. Bottom, Histologic example of intratumoral hemorrhage.*

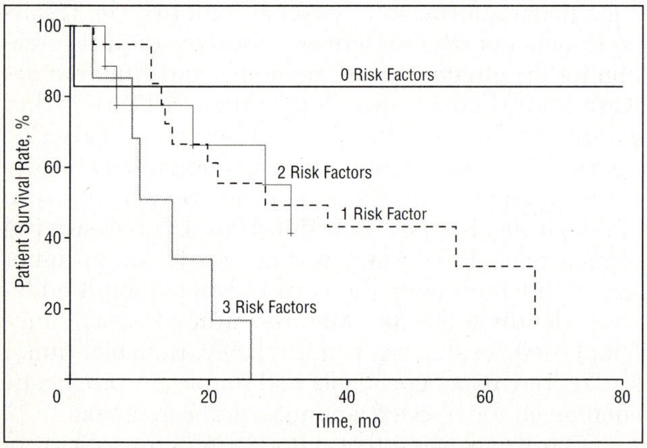

Figure 5. *Patients with no risk factors (>12 cm, no hemorrhage, mitotic figures ≥6/high-power fields) (n=6) had an 83% 5-year survival rate that decreased to 42% with 1 risk factor (n=10), 33% with 2 (n=23), and 0% with all 3 (n=7,* P<.02*).*

reported by Van Slooten et al.[7] Evans and Vassilopoulou-Sellin[11] also report that mitotic rate was a significant predictor of outcome. Like the above studies, they included all stages in their analysis. When patients with metastatic disease were excluded, there was a trend toward shorter survival rates with higher (n=14) compared with lower mitotic rates (n=25), although this was not statistically significant. Interestingly, DNA content, another measure of cell proliferation, has not been predictive of outcome.[5,12]

In addition to standard pathologic criteria, many groups have evaluated the prognostic significance of a variety of cellular proteins used in immunohistochemical studies. Although protein expression of epidermal growth factors, p53, transforming growth factor α, and P-glycoprotein, may be useful in distinguishing benign adenomas from malignant adrenocortical carcinomas, none of these markers has been shown to be an independent prognostic factor for survival rates in patients with an adrenocortical carcinoma.[13-16]

We demonstrated that tumor size (>12 cm), the number of mitotic figures (≥6 per 10 high-power fields), and intratumoral hemorrhage can predict a lower survival rate in patients undergoing curative resection for adrenocortical carcinoma. The presence of tumor necrosis nearly reached significance (*P*=.06), and with additional numbers, may also be an independent predictor. As the number of pathologic risk factors for individuals increase, overall survival rates decrease. Patients with no risk factors demonstrated relatively favorable 5-year survival rates (83%). Benefits from adjuvant chemotherapy may be difficult to establish; however, none of the patients whose tumors had all 3 pathologic risk factors was alive at 5 years despite undergoing a "curative" resection. Patients with 1 or 2 risk factors shared a similar 5-year survival rate of 42% and 33%, respectively. Based on these pathologic factors, adrenocortical carcinomas may be divided into low- and high-risk groups. These prognostic factors may be helpful in dictating follow-up strategies, especially since resection for recurrent adrenocortical carcinoma may lead to higher long-term survival rates. High-risk patients may be considered for adjuvant treatment in an attempt to improve their survival rates.

Corresponding author: Murray F. Brennan, MD, chair, Department of Surgery, Memorial Sloan-Kettering Cancer Center, 1275 York Ave, New York, NY 10021 (e-mail: mbrennan@mskcc.org).

REFERENCES

1. Pommier R, Brennan M. Management of adrenal neoplasms. *Curr Probl Surg.* 1991;28:659-739.
2. Pommier R, Brennan M. An eleven-year experience with adrenocortical carcinoma. *Surgery.* 1992;112:963-971.
3. Icard P, Chapuis Y, Andreassian B, Bernard A, Proye C. Adrenocortical carcinoma in surgically treated patients: a retrospective study on 156 cases by the French Association of Endocrine Surgery. *Surgery.* 1992;112:972-980.
4. Crucitti F, Bellatone R, Ferrante A, Boscherini M, Crucitti P, for the Italian Registry Group. The Italian registry for adrenal cortical carcinoma: analysis of a multiinstitutional series of 129 patients. *Surgery.* 1996;119:161-170.
5. Lee J, Berger D, el-Naggar A, et al. Surgical management, DNA content and patient survival in adrenal cortical carcinoma. *Surgery.* 1995;118:1090-1098.
6. Weiss L, Medeiros L, Vickery A. Pathologic features of prognostic significance in adrenocortical carcinoma. *Am J Surg Pathol.* 1989;13:202-206.
7. Van Slooten H, Schaberg A, Smeenk D, Moolenaar A. Morphologic characteristics of benign and malignant adrenocortical tumors. *Cancer.* 1985;55:766-773.
8. Luton JP, Cerdas S, Billaud L, et al. Clinical features of adrenocortical carcinoma, prognostic factors, and the effects of mitotane therapy. *N Engl J Med.* 1990;322:1195-1201.
9. Weiss L. Comparative histologic study of 43 metastasizing and nonmetastasizing adrenocortical tumors. *Am J Surg Pathol.* 1984;8:163-169.

10. Hough A, Hollifield J, Page D, Hartmann W. Prognostic factors in adrenal cortical tumors: a mathematical analysis of clinical and morphologic data. *Am J Clin Pathol.* 1979;72:390-399.
11. Evans H, Vassilopoulou-Selin R. Adrenal cortical neoplasms: a study of 56 cases. *Am J Clin Pathol.* 1996;105:76-86.
12. Cibas E, Medeiros L, Weinberg D, Gelb A, Weiss L. Cellular DNA profiles of benign and malignant adrenocortical tumors. *Am J Surg Pathol.* 1990;14:948-955.
13. Flyn S, Murren J, Kirby W, Honig J, Kan L, Kinder BK. P-glycoprotein expression and multidrug resistance in adrenocortical carcinoma. *Surgery.* 1992;112:981-986.
14. Reincke M, Karl M, Travis W, et al. p53 Mutation in human adrenocortical neoplasms: immunohistochemical and molecular studies. *J Clin Endocrinol Metab.* 1994;78:790-794.
15. Sasano H, Suzuki T, Shizawa S, Kato K, Nagura H. Transforming growth factor alpha, epidermal growth factor, and epidermal growth factor receptor expression in normal and diseased human adrenal cortex by immunohistochemistry and in situ hybridization. *Mod Pathol.* 1994;7:741-746.
16. Schroder S, Padberg B, Achilles E, Holl K, Dralle H, Kloppel G. Immunocytochemistry in adrenocortical tumours: a clinicomorphological study of 72 neoplasms. *Virchows Arch A Pathol Anat Histopathol.* 1992;420:65-70.

Invited Critique

Harrison et al have built on Brennan's long-standing interest in adrenocortical carcinoma, using the Memorial Sloan-Kettering Cancer Center's extensive experience and detailed database to compile a unique report. This series correlates histologic features of resected tumors with clinical outcome, but only in patients undergoing curative surgery. As they properly point out, other investigators have made the same correlation, but not in reports restricted to patients treated with curative surgery. Series "contaminated" by patients undergoing palliative surgery who received adjuvant therapy may obscure more subtle findings that should more properly influence the use of adjuvant therapy. Some may argue that the issue is moot without effective adjuvant agents. Although mitotane has been almost uniformly disappointing, there is hope that taxanes may be effective.

In addition to recording their statistically significant predictors of prognosis, the authors provide other information of interest to me but not emphasized in the article. Although the MacFarlane staging system (introduced in 1958) is the most frequently employed for adrenocortical carcinoma, it is widely criticized because it creates stages I and II based on a cutpoint in size (≤5 cm vs >5 cm, both node negative) that is not useful. Harrison et al provide 2 types of data that indict this staging system. They confirm that the cutoff of 5 cm is of little use and they document how frequently nodal status is unknown. Limited utility of a staging system is a powerful incentive to investigate tumor-related factors that predict prognosis.

We are indebted to Harrison et al for advancing our understanding of the highly lethal adrenocortical carcinoma. If only we could make similar progress in recognizing those patients with adrenocortical carcinoma among the multitude of patients with incidentalomas.

Andrew Saxe, MD
Detroit, Mich

ORIGINAL ARTICLE

Lung-Sparing Surgery After Penetrating Trauma Using Tractotomy, Partial Lobectomy, and Pneumonorrhaphy

George C. Velmahos, MD, PhD; Craig Baker, MD; Demetrios Demetriades, MD, PhD; Jeremy Goodman; James A. Murray, MD; Juan A. Asensio, MD

Objective: To evaluate the role of lung-sparing surgical techniques in the surgical management of penetrating pulmonary injuries.

Design: Retrospective case series.

Setting: Academic level I trauma center.

Patients and Methods: Forty patients underwent thoracic surgery for penetrating lung injuries during a 63-month period from January 1993 to March 1997. Five (12.5%) underwent anatomical lobectomy, 3 (7.5%) pneumonorrhaphy, 9 (22.5%) stapled wedge resection, and 23 (57.5%) stapled tractotomy. In total, 34 patients (85%) were treated with stapling techniques (1 anatomical lobectomy, 1 pneumonorrhaphy, 9 stapled wedge resections, and 23 stapled tractotomies) and 35 (87.5%) underwent had lung-sparing surgery for trauma.

Results: Morbidity and mortality rates were 40% and 5%, respectively. Patients who underwent anatomical lobectomy required longer mechanical ventilatory support, intensive care unit stay, and hospital stay and had a higher morbidity rate compared with patients who underwent lung-sparing surgery for trauma but had central and extensive pulmonary injuries. Stapled tractotomy was efficient in controlling bleeding and bronchial leaks, but, in 3 patients, parts of the divided lung parenchyma were devascularized and had to be resected.

Conclusions: Lung-sparing surgery for trauma with the use of staplers can be used in the majority of patients with penetrating pulmonary injuries requiring operation. Stapled tractotomy is a rapid and effective method for controlling hemorrhage and air leaks.

Arch Surg. 1999;134:186-189

THE MAJORITY of injuries to the lung are managed by tubal thoracostomy.[1] The combination of lung expansion, low intravascular pressures, and high concentration of tissue thromboplastin provides adequate hemostasis in most instances.[2] Thoracotomy to control bleeding is reserved for approximately 10% to 15% of penetrating thoracic injuries.[1,2] In contrast with the abdominal cavity, where surgical exploration is frequently mandated by abdominal tenderness even in the presence of hemodynamic stability, operations in the chest are almost exclusively done for severe intrathoracic blood loss affecting the vital signs. Therefore, rapid bleeding control with the least possible physiologic insult is highly desirable.

Anatomical or nonanatomical lung resections and suturing superficial lacerations are the main techniques used to achieve hemostasis.[2-7] An alternative method has been suggested to achieve the same goals without destroying lung parenchyma. Wall et al[8] described tractotomy, the opening of the pulmonary injury tract over vascular clamps and the selective ligation of bleeding vessels, as a safe and straightforward procedure. Our group has practiced this technique by using linear staplers instead of vascular clamps to expedite and simplify the procedure.[9] Lung-sparing surgery can be performed by using techniques such as tractotomy, wedge resection, and pneumonorrhaphy as alternatives to anatomical resection. The purposes of this study were to analyze our experience with pulmonary tractotomy and evaluate the role of lung-sparing techniques in pulmonary surgery for trauma.

RESULTS

Of 40 patients, 5 (12.5%) underwent AL (1 underwent a pneumonectomy) and 35 underwent lung-sparing surgery: PR in 3 (7.5%), SWR in 9 (22.5%), and ST in 23 (57.5%). Linear stapling devices were used in 1 AL, 1 PR, and all SWRs and STs. The mean age and score on the Injury Severity Scale for the group was 27 years and 17, respectively. Additional injuries to the chest included lacerations to the heart (4 patients) and subclavian artery (1 patient). Twenty-two patients (55%) un-

From the Department of Surgery, University of Southern California and the Los Angeles County and University of Southern California Medical Center, Los Angeles.

PATIENTS AND METHODS

Forty patients (38 male and 2 female) who underwent surgery between January 1993 to March 1997 for a penetrating injury to the lung (32 gunshot wounds and 8 stab wounds) were included in this study. Patients who underwent thoracic procedures for isolated vascular or cardiac injuries and those who underwent thoracotomies in the emergency department but did not survive the procedure were excluded.

All patients admitted to the Los Angeles County and University of Southern California Medical Center, Los Angeles, are treated by a dedicated trauma team. Attending physicians provide in-house, around-the-clock coverage and participate in all resuscitations and surgical interventions. Patients with hemodynamic instability due to blood loss were taken immediately to the operating room. An immediate chest tube output of more than 1000 to 1500 mL was an additional indication for surgical exploration. However, rigid adherence to numbers was avoided; the decision for operative or expectant management was usually made by combining information on the hemodynamic status of the patient, thoracostomy tube outputs, and clinical and radiographic findings.

Emergent surgical access to the injured lung was usually achieved by anterolateral thoracotomy (27 patients), unless suspected heart injury prompted a median sternotomy (3 patients). One of these 3 patients received both incisions, since manipulation of the lung through the sternotomy, which is done for an associated cardiac injury, was followed by desaturation and hemodynamic instability. Two patients underwent bilateral anterolateral thoracotomies. Posterolateral thoracotomy was reserved for 11 patients who were hemodynamically stable and had bullet or knife trajectories that clearly excluded the probability of associated injuries in other body cavities. Single-lumen endotracheal intubation was used in most patients (37) due to the need for rapid airway access. Once the thoracic cavity was entered, the injury to the lung was evaluated. In the presence of profuse bleeding or significant air leakage from central cavities, the corresponding hilar pedicle was cross-clamped (9 patients). Stapled tractotomy (ST) was the preferred method of operative management by a technique previously described (**Figure 1** and **Figure 2**).[9] In short, a stapler (GIA [gastrointestinal anastomosis] stapler 55 or 75, US Surgical Corp, Norwalk, Conn) was used to open the tract, and individual ligation of exposed vessels and bronchi was used to control bleeding or air leaks. Peripheral injuries were frequently controlled by stapled wedge resections (SWRs). Central injuries were managed by anatomical lobectomy (AL) only if they were extensive and therefore not amenable to tractotomy or if they involved hilar vessels. Oversewing (pneumonorrhaphy [PR]) was reserved only for superficial lacerations. The entry and exit sites of a trajectory were never oversewn, since oversewing leaves the central cavity as a source of uncontrolled bleeding or air embolism.

Data on injury characteristics, management, and outcome were collected from the patients' medical records and the trauma registry. Statistical analysis was performed using the Student *t* test, Fisher exact test, and analysis of variance. *P* values of less than .05 were considered significant.

derwent an additional laparotomy for abdominal tenderness, bleeding, or inability to evaluate the abdomen. In 16 of these patients, injuries to intra-abdominal structures such as the liver (3), spleen (3), stomach (3), small bowel (2), colon (2), pancreas (1), or retrohepatic inferior vena cava (1) were identified and repaired. All but one patient required admission to the intensive care unit (ICU), with an average ICU length of stay of 7 days. Complications developed in 16 patients (40%) and were related to the lung surgery in 11 (27.5%). Two patients (5%) died. One of these patients underwent a thoracotomy in the emergency department, where a gunshot wound through the hilar region with profuse bleeding was discovered. After achieving temporary control of the bleeding, he was taken to the operating room, where a pneumonectomy was performed with a stapler (TA90, US Surgical Corporation). During the operation he experienced cardiac arrest twice and was resuscitated. The bleeding was controlled, but he experienced cardiogenic shock in the ICU later that day. The other patient had multiple truncal and extremity gunshot wounds. A laparotomy revealed injuries to the liver and retrohepatic inferior vena cava that were controlled by total liver isolation, primary vascular repair, and packing. Bilobular lacerations to the right lung were managed by SWR. The patient died in the ICU on the third postoperative day owing to fulminant multiple organ failure. The mean hospital stay among survivors was 15 days.

Table 1 shows injury characteristics and physiologic parameters in patients who underwent ST, SWR, PR, or AL. Although statistical comparisons are limited by the low number of patients in the various groups, it appears that these parameters were not different. All injuries that required lobectomy were close to the pulmonary hilum. Of the 35 patients who underwent lung-sparing surgery, 14 (39%) had extrathoracic injuries requiring exploration compared with 2 (40%) of 5 patients who underwent lobectomies. The latter group required a higher median volume of intraoperative fluid (8600 vs 5000 mL) and blood resuscitation (7 vs 12 U) compared with the former group. The number of days on which mechanical ventilation was used, the duration of tubal thoracostomy, the number of days spent in the ICU and hospital, and the morbidity rates were different between the 2 groups (**Table 2**).

There were 10 complications that were directly related to the type of lung surgery (**Table 3**). Seven (20%) occurred in the lung-sparing group and 3 (67%) in the lobectomy group. Two patients developed empyema, which was drained percutaneously using computed tomographic guidance in both cases. All 4 persistent air leaks were sealed using expectant management within 11 to 15 days. Three patients required reoperation. Two of these patients underwent ST as the primary procedure. One patient underwent reoperation the same day for recurrent bleeding. No bleeding source was identified, and he subsequently recovered. The second patient underwent reoperation for sepsis on the 13th day after a middle- and upper-lobe ST of the right side. A large segment of the divided upper lobe was necrotic and, for this reason, was resected by linear staplers. The patient was discharged from the hospital after 50 days. The third patient initially underwent a middle lobectomy of the right side but developed sepsis on the basis of unexplained occlusion of the right upper bronchus with interruption of blood flow to the corresponding lobe. Reexploration on the third postoperative day revealed an upper lobe torsion in the right side. The lobe was resected, but the patient had a difficult postoperative course complicated by pneumonia and respiratory failure. He was eventually discharged from the hospital 52 days after admission. In 2 more patients (not included in the postoperative morbidity list), portions of devascularized lung after ST were resected at the primary operation.

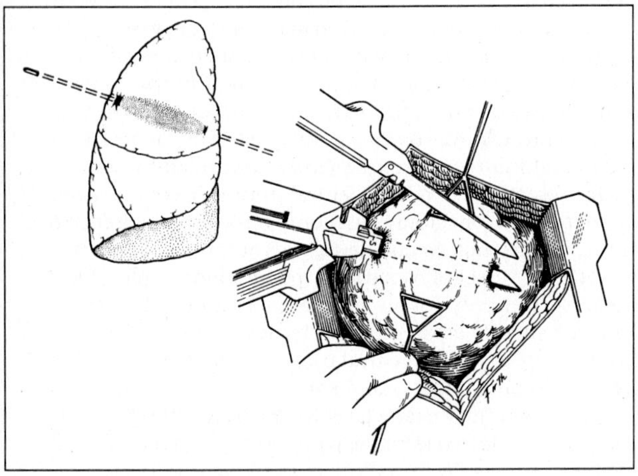

Figure 1. *Placement of stapler through bullet trajectory.*

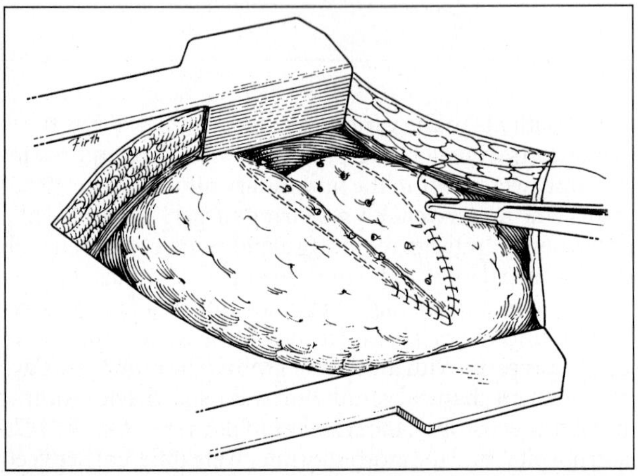

Figure 2. *Opening the tract, individually ligating vessels, and, if necessary, oversewing the staple line.*

COMMENT

There has been a remarkable change in the types of operations for lung trauma in the last decade.[10-14] Although older reports[10,11] recommend lobectomy as the typical operative management of pulmonary injuries, more recent experience[13,14] suggests that the use of lung-sparing techniques is equally effective. Stapling devices play a central role in such management as they facilitate and expedite the execution of these techniques.[12,13] In our series, 34 (85%) of 40 patients were treated using staplers: tractotomy in 23, partial resection in 9, PR in 1, and pneumonectomy in 1.

Tractotomy has been identified as an easy and rapid method of controlling bleeding without subjecting the patient to unnecessary lung resection.[8,9] The technique was first described by Wall et al,[8] who reported excellent results in 16 patients with penetrating lung injuries. Our modification includes the application of a stapler (GIA) through the injurious weapon's trajectory to visualize the bleeding areas and allow direct ligation.[9] The use of staplers makes the procedure easier and faster. Oversewing the staple line is not necessary unless it is thought that the tissue incorporated in the staples is too thick, which may occur with central trajectories. During tractotomy, a portion of the divided tissue may become ischemic due to interruption of its vascular supply. Careful inspection at the end of the procedure to detect and resect such areas is essential. In our series, 1 patient required reoperation for removal of a necrotic part of the tractotomized upper lobe. For the same reason, 2 more patients underwent small wedge resections during the initial operation following tractotomy.

Although with increasing experience the appropriate procedure is selected as soon as the site and severity of injury is recognized, bleeding control by expeditious stapled tractotomy can be attempted initially for most injuries. However, in cases where bleeding cannot be satisfactorily controlled by this technique—usually due to a central location of the injury with larger vessels or bronchi involved—conversion to some form of resection should be done early. Partial lobectomies are easily done with the use of staplers. We used a linear stapling device in all 9 patients in our study who required a partial lobectomy. Even ALs or pneumonectomies have been described with the use of staplers.[15,16] The rapidity in completion of the procedure is the main advantage for patients who are bleeding severely. However, there are concerns on the appropriateness of en masse sta-

Table 1. Injury Characteristics and Physiologic Data in Patients Who Underwent Different Types of Lung Surgery for Penetrating Pulmonary Injuries*

	Stapled Tractotomy (n = 23)	Stapled Wedge Resection (n = 3)	Pneumonorrhaphy (n = 5)	Anatomical Lobectomy (n = 5)
Injury Severity Score	16 ± 8	19 ± 7.5	10 ± 0.5	20 ± 12
Abbreviated Injury Score (chest)	3.4 ± 0.7	3.3 ± 0.7	3.0 ± 0.0	3.8 ± 0.8
Gunshot wound, %	78	90	66	80
Systolic blood pressure on admission, mm Hg	104 ± 33	115 ± 30	116 ± 16	98 ± 60
Hematocrit level on admission	0.34 ± 0.05	0.34 ± 0.07	0.31 ± 0.07	0.35 ± 0.04
Lowest pH level	7.2 ± 0.1	7.2 ± 0.1	7.2 ± 0.1	7.0 ± 0.1
Lowest mean arterial oxygen saturation, %	96	98	97	97

Data are presented as mean ± SD unless indicated otherwise. The P values were not significant; P values less than .05 were considered significant.

Table 2. Comparison of Outcome Parameters Between the Patients Who Underwent Either Lung-Sparing Surgery or Anatomical Lobectomy*

	Lung-Sparing Group (n = 35)	Lobectomy Group (n = 5)	P
Duration of mechanical ventilation, d	4 ± 6	19.5 ± 17	<.0001
Intensive care unit stay, d	5 ± 7	21.5 ± 20	<.0001
Hospital stay, d	14 ± 13	36 ± 24	<.0001
Duration of tubal thoracostomy, d	9 ± 9	24 ± 13	.002
Mortality, No. (%)	1 (3)	1 (20)	.24
Total morbidity, No. (%)	12 (35)†	4 (100)‡	.03
Lung-related morbidity, No. (%)§	7 (21)	3 (75)	.09

Data are presented as mean ± SD unless indicated otherwise. P *values less than .05 were considered significant.*

†*Calculated on 34 survivors.*

‡*Calculated on 4 survivors.*

§*Excluding pneumonia.*

Table 3. Complications Related to Lung Surgery*

	No. (%) of Patients		
	Stapled Tractotomy (n = 23)	Stapled Wedge Resection (n = 9)	Anatomical Lobectomy (n = 5)
Empyema	1 (4)	1 (11)	. . .
Air leak ≥10 d after surgery	2 (9)	1 (11)	1 (20)
Reoperation	2 (9)†	. . .	1 (20)‡
Other	. . .	. . .	1 (20)§
Total	**5** (22)	**2** (22)	**3** (67)

Ellipses indicate not applicable.

†*One operation for bleeding and 1 for partial lobar necrosis.*

‡*One operation for right upper lung torsion.*

§*Persistent lower lobe collapse that required reintubation and prolonged positive pressure ventilation.*

pling together of the pulmonary hilum, including vessels and bronchi. Our experience is limited. We performed a stapled pneumonectomy on an exsanguinating patient who had a gunshot wound in the right side of the chest and had a cardiac arrest after arriving at the hospital. Although the bleeding was controlled, the combined cardiorespiratory burden of the injury and the traumatic pneumonectomy did not allow him to survive beyond 24 hours. After the end of the study, we performed 1 more stapled pneumonectomy. In this anecdotal case, the stapler was fired close to the mediastinum, the stapled stump was retracted backward, and the patient began to bleed uncontrollably. If a stapling device is used for traumatic lobectomy or pneumonectomy, we recommend firing the stapler twice before transecting the lung and leaving a long stump.

Only 3 patients in our study underwent PR. One of these injuries was controlled by stapling. We believe that this technique has a role only in superficial lacerations that can be sutured or stapled closed without leaving a cavity behind. As such wounds are unlikely to require surgical management, PR is not commonly used. Leaving a cavity predisposes the patient to recurrent bleeding and, more importantly, to air embolism, a potentially lethal complication.[17,18] For this reason, transpulmonary wounds should never be managed by oversewing the entry and exit sites without controlling bleeding and air leaks from the tract.

Finally, hemostasis should not be the sole end point in pulmonary surgery for trauma. Identification and repair of significant bronchial leaks are important to avoid persistent postoperative bronchopleural fistulae. At the end of the procedure, the lung should be fully reinflated by manual ventilation and thoroughly inspected for the presence of recurrent bleeding, residual air leaks, or failures of staple lines. Careful repositioning in the thoracic cavity without twisting the hilar region is essential to avoid pulmonary torsion.[19] Anchoring the remaining lobes together or against the interior thoracic wall by a suture is advisable for the same purpose.[19]

Although the majority of lung injuries can be managed nonoperatively, severe bleeding may still require expeditious thoracic surgery. Lung-sparing surgery can be frequently done by using stapling devices with good results. In particular, stapled pulmonary tractotomy is becoming the preferred technique for the management of a notable number of penetrating lung injuries.

Corresponding author: George C. Velmahos, MD, Los Angeles County and the University of Southern California Medical Center, 1200 N State St, Room 9900, Los Angeles, CA 90033 (e-mail: velmahos@hsc.usc.edu).

REFERENCES

1. Richardson JD. Secondary assessment: thorax. In: RR Ivatury, CG Cayten, eds. *The Textbook of Penetrating Trauma.* Baltimore, Md: Williams & Wilkins; 1996:273-280.
2. Rodriquez A, Thomas MD, Shillinglaw WRC. Organ system injuries: lung and tracheobronchus. In: RR Ivatury, GC Cayten, eds. *The Textbook of Penetrating Trauma.* Baltimore, Md: Williams & Wilkins; 1996:531-554.
3. Carillo EH, Block EF, Zeppa R, Sosa JL. Urgent lobectomy and pneumonectomy. *Eur J Emerg Med.* 1994;1:126-130.
4. Boyd AD, Glassman LR. Trauma to the lung. *Chest Surg Clin N Am.* 1997;7:263-284.
5. Vasquez JC, Castaneda E, Bazan N. Management of 240 cases of penetrating thoracic injuries. *Injury.* 1997;28:45-49.
6. Tominaga GT, Waxman K, Scannell G, Annas G, Ott RA, Gazzaniga AB. Emergency thoracotomy with lung resection following trauma. *Am Surg.* 1993;59:834-837.
7. McSwain NE Jr. Blunt and penetrating chest injuries. *World J Surg.* 1992;16:924-929.
8. Wall MJ Jr, Hirshberg A, Mattox KL. Pulmonary tractotomy with selective vascular ligation for penetrating injuries to the lung. *Am J Surg.* 1994;168:665-669.
9. Asensio JA, Demetriades D, Berne JD, et al. Stapled pulmonary tractotomy: a rapid way to control hemorrhage in penetrating pulmonary injuries. *J Am Coll Surg.* 1997;185:486-487.
10. Thompson DA, Rowlands BJ, Walker WE, et al. Urgent thoracotomy for pulmonary or tracheobronchial injury. *J Trauma.* 1988;28:276-279.
11. Robinson PD, Harman PK, Trinkle JK, Grover FL. Management of penetrating lung injuries in civilian practice. *J Thorac Cardiovasc Surg.* 1988;95:184-188.
12. Wall MJ Jr, Soltero E. Damage control for thoracic injuries. *Surg Clin North Am.* 1997;77:863-878.
13. Mattox KL, Wall MJ Jr. Newer diagnostic measures and emergency management. *Chest Surg Clin N Am.* 1997;7:213-226.
14. Richardson JD, Miller FB, Carrillo EH, Spain DA. Complex thoracic injuries. *Surg Clin North Am.* 1996;76:725-748.
15. Goins WA. Morbidity and mortality after traumatic pneumonectomy: the effect of compromised oxygenation and cardiac function. *J Intensive Care Med.* 1995;10:193-199.
16. Baumgartner F, Omari B, Lee J, et al. Survival after trauma pneumonectomy: the pathophysiologic balance of shock resuscitation with right heart failure. *Am Surg.* 1996;62:967-972.
17. Chiu CJ, Golding MR, Linder JB, Fries CC. Pulmonary venous air embolism: a hemodynamic reappraisal. *Surgery.* 1967;61:816-819.
18. Estrera AS, Pass LJ, Platt MR. Systemic arterial air embolism in penetrating lung injury. *Ann Thorac Surg.* 1990;50:257-959.
19. Velmahos GC, Frankhouse HJ, Ciccolo M. Pulmonary torsion of the right upper lobe following right middle lobectomy for a stab wound to the chest. *J Trauma.* 1998;44:920-922.

ORIGINAL ARTICLE

Multifactorial Analysis of Long-term Follow-up (More Than 5 Years) of Primary Extremity Sarcoma

Jonathan J. Lewis, MD, PhD; Denis Leung, PhD; Ephraim S. Casper, MD; James Woodruff, MD; Steven I. Hajdu, MD; Murray F. Brennan, MD

Background: The majority of survival studies in patients with extremity soft tissue sarcoma have focused on early recurrence and mortality. There are few data addressing long-term follow-up and survival.

Objective: To analyze survival and recurrence in patients with extremity soft tissue sarcoma who survive for more than 5 years.

Methods: Patients who underwent treatment for primary tumors (July 1982 to July 1994) and were followed up for more than 5 years were the subject of study. Disease-specific and disease-free survival were determined actuarially. Significance was evaluated using log-rank testing for univariate analysis and Cox model stepwise regression for multivariate analysis.

Results: A total of 495 patients with primary extremity tumors were treated before July 1989 and eligible for 5-year follow-up. Of these, 282 have been followed up for more than 5 years (median follow-up, 84.4 months). Actuarial disease-specific survival of patients who survive for longer than 5 years was 79% ± 7% (±SEM) at 10 years, and of those who were metastasis free at 5 years was 91% ± 4% at 10 years. On univariate analysis, post–5-year disease-specific survival was influenced by positive microscopic margin and initial tumor size of 5 cm or greater. On multivariate analysis, post–5-year disease-specific survival was influenced only by positive margins.

Conclusions: Based on these analyses, 21% of patients with primary extremity sarcoma who survive for 5 years will die of disease within 5 years. Even of those who are metastasis free at 5 years, 9% will die of disease within 5 years. In contrast to early mortality, tumor grade has no influence on post–5-year prognosis. Patients with positive microscopic margins are at risk for post–5-year disease-specific mortality and therefore require long-term follow-up and consideration for investigational therapy.

Arch Surg. 1999;134:190-194

SOFT TISSUE sarcomas are rare and unusual neoplasms, with an annual incidence in the United States of approximately 5000 to 6000 persons. Although these tumors may develop in any anatomic site, approximately 50% will occur in the extremities. Current staging systems for extremity sarcomas, based on short-term outcome, focus on histological grade of the tumor, the size of the primary tumor, and the presence or absence of metastasis.[1,2] Histological grade is a major prognostic determinant and is based on differentiation, cellularity, mitotic activity, presence of necrosis, stromal content, and vascularity. Low-grade lesions are assumed to have a low (<15%) risk of subsequent metastasis and the high-grade lesions a high (>50%) risk of subsequent metastasis. Although size has historically been considered a less important determinant of biologic behavior, this bias is predicated on measurement of early recurrence and mortality events. It would appear that grade is a factor in early metastasis and size is a feature of more delayed metastasis.[2]

The majority of survival and biology studies in patients with extremity soft tissue sarcoma focus on early recurrence and mortality, and there are few data addressing long-term follow-up and survival.[3] Furthermore, the relatively small number of cases and their diversity in anatomic location, histological appearance, and biologic behavior make the comparative analysis of survival difficult. The objective of this study was to analyze disease-specific and disease-free survival in patients, treated and followed up at a single institution, who survive for more than 5 years. In addition, we compared these long-term survivors with patients who died of their disease within 5 years.

From the Departments of Surgery (Drs Lewis and Brennan), Biostatistics (Dr Leung), Medicine (Dr Casper), and Pathology (Drs Woodruff and Hajdu), Memorial Sloan-Kettering Cancer Center, New York, NY. Dr Hajdu is now with the Department of Pathology, North Shore University Hospital, Manhasset, NY.

PATIENTS AND METHODS

PATIENTS

A prospective database of all adult patients (>16 years) with soft tissue sarcoma, treated at Memorial Sloan-Kettering Cancer Center, New York, NY, was established in July 1982. This database is defined by the accrual and entry of clinical, pathologic, and treatment data of all consecutive patients at the time of initial presentation, with patients then prospectively followed up for recurrence and survival. Patients who underwent treatment for primary extremity soft tissue sarcoma before July 1989 and were therefore eligible for longer than 5-year follow-up (through July 1994) or those who died of disease within 5 years were the subject of this study. Clinical and pathologic variables were correlated with survival end points. Patient variables analyzed included age at diagnosis (<60 or ≥60 years), sex, and race. Tumor variables included size (<5 or ≥5 cm), histological grade (low or high), depth (superficial or deep), microscopic margins (negative or positive), and histological subtype. The histopathologic subclassification has been monitored by 2 pathologists (J.W. and S.I.H.) during this time. Histological grade was divided into low or high, distinct from other aspects of intermediate transition.[2,4] Depth was defined by the relationship of the tumor to the deep fascia. Because treatment was not prospectively randomized, but included both patients prospectively randomized in trials[5,6] and those given standard of care based on prognosis,[3] the inclusion of treatment variables in any of the analyses would confound the effects of other factors. Therefore, while we report the treatment data, we have chosen not to include them in any of the analyses.

STATISTICS

Pre– and post–5-year disease-specific and disease-free survivals were modeled with the Kaplan-Meier method.[7] Deaths that were confirmed to be caused by the disease were treated as an end point for disease-specific survival; other deaths were treated as censored observations. Disease-free survival was segregated into local recurrence-free and metastasis-free survival. Survival curves were compared using log-rank testing for univariate analysis and Cox model stepwise regression for multivariate influence. To arrive at a parsimonious multivariate model, covariates were selected only if they contributed significantly to the fit of the model. The influence of time of metastasis on survival was analyzed using the approach of dynamic cohorts. Comparison between patient and tumor categorical variables in different groups was performed using the Fisher exact test for univariate analysis and logistic regression for multivariate analysis.

RESULTS

PATIENTS

During the period under study we treated 818 patients with extremity soft tissue sarcoma. This included 495 patients who presented with primary tumor and 323 patients who presented with recurrent tumor (initially treated either at a referring institution or at Memorial Sloan-Kettering Cancer Center before July 1982). The 495 patients with primary tumor constituted the study group. At 5 years' follow-up, 111 patients died of disease (early mortality), and 14 died with no evidence of disease. Eighty-eight patients were alive at last follow-up but did not complete 5-year follow-up. This included patients from out of state or from foreign countries who were lost to long-term follow-up. The median follow-up of this group was 3.4 years and they were excluded from analysis. There were 282 patients with greater than 5-year follow-up and this group constituted the long-term survivors. There were no significant differences in age or sex between the long-term survivor group and the early mortality group (**Table 1**). Distribution of primary surgical and adjuvant radiation treatment in long-term survivors is shown in **Table 2**, top.

TUMOR CHARACTERISTICS

Comparison of tumor characteristics between patients with early mortality (died of disease at <5 years) and long-term survivors (alive at >5 years) is summarized in Table 1. Not surprisingly, histological high grade, large size (≥5 cm), deep lesion, and positive microscopic margins, and not the histological subtype, were significant predictors on univariate analysis of early mortality. Logistic regression analysis of risk of death within 5 years, vs survival or death after 5 years, revealed histological high grade as the dominant risk factor ($P<.001$; odds ratio, 7.7).

DISEASE-SPECIFIC SURVIVAL

Of patients alive at 5 years, within a median follow-up time of 84.4 months, 23 patients died of disease. Actuarial survival for the group of 282 patients alive at 5 years was 79% ± 7% (±SEM) at 10 years. There was no difference in survival when patients with histological high-grade tumors were compared with those with low-grade tumors ($P=.80$). In contrast, both large size and positive microscopic margins adversely influenced survival. Patients with large (≥5 cm) tumors did worse compared with those with small (<5 cm) tumors ($P=.03$). Similarly, those with positive microscopic margins did worse compared with those with negative margins ($P=.01$; **Figure 1**). Results of a Cox model multivariate analysis, for disease-specific survival, are summarized in **Table 3**. Positive microscopic margin ($P=.02$; risk ratio, 2.7) was the dominant factor influencing long-term survival. Distribution of primary surgical and adjuvant radiation treatment in patients with positive microscopic margins is shown in Table 2, bottom.

DISEASE-FREE SURVIVAL

Disease-free survival was segregated into local recurrence-free and metastasis-free survival. Among the 282 long-term survivor patients, 23 had local recurrence without distant metastases, 20 developed distant metastases with-

Table 1. Clinical and Pathologic Characteristics From Patients Alive at 5 Years vs Those Dead of Disease Within 5 Years

	No. (%)		
	Alive >5 y	Dead <5 y	P*
Age, y			
<60	200 (71)	78 (70)	.20
≥60	82 (29)	33 (30)	
Sex			
Male	150 (53)	61 (55)	.30
Female	132 (47)	50 (45)	
Grade			
High	182 (66)	101 (92)	<.001
Low	95 (34)	9 (8)	
Size, cm			
≥5	153 (56)	84 (76)	.001
<5	118 (44)	27 (24)	
Margins			
Positive	56 (20)	33 (31)	.001
Negative	222 (80)	74 (69)	
Depth			
Deep	191 (68)	101 (94)	<.001
Superficial	88 (32)	6 (6)	
Histological subtype			
Liposarcoma	93 (33)	31 (28)	.20
Malignant fibrous histiocytoma	53 (19)	22 (20)	
Synovial	37 (13)	18 (16)	
Leiomyosarcoma	20 (7)	8 (7)	
Fibrosarcoma	19 (7)	5 (4)	
Malignant peripheral nerve sheath tumor	12 (4)	4 (4)	
Other	48 (17)	23 (21)	
Local recurrence†	23 (8)	10 (9)	.20

*Fisher exact test.
†Patients who had local recurrence without distant metastases.

out local recurrence, and 13 developed both local and distant disease. Local recurrence was predicted in patients with positive microscopic margins ($P = .01$ on both univariate and multivariate analyses; risk ratio, 2.1) and patients older than 60 years at time of diagnosis ($P = .03$ on multivariate analysis; risk ratio, 2.1). When other factors had been corrected for, development of local recurrence did not influence metastasis-free or disease-specific survival.

Of the 282 long-term survivors, 20 developed metastases within 5 years and 13 developed metastases after 5 years; actuarial 10-year metastasis-free survival was 75% ± 5%. Of the 262 patients alive and metastasis free at 5 years, 9 went on to die of sarcoma metastases after 5 years. The 10-year actuarial disease-specific survival of patients who were disease free at 5 years was 91% ± 4%. When measured as a function of time of metastasis, there was no difference in disease-specific mortality ($P = .13$) between those who had metastases before 5 years or those who had metastases after 5 years. There was no difference between small (<5 cm) and large (≥5 cm) tumors on metastasis-free survival ($P = .07$). This was in contrast to the significant influence of microscopic margins (**Figure 2**) on metastasis-free survival ($P = .009$). In a multivariate Cox model (Table 3), both

Table 2. Distribution of Primary Surgical and Adjuvant Radiation Treatment

Primary and Adjuvant Treatment	No. of Patients	>5-y Disease-Specific Death, No. (%)
In All >5-y Survivors (n = 282)		
Surgery		
Limb-sparing resection	249	20 (8)
Amputation	33	3 (9)
Brachytherapy*†		
Yes	81	6 (7)
No	201	17 (9)
External beam radiation*†		
Yes	26	3 (12)
No	256	20 (8)
In >5-y Survivors With Positive Microscopic Margins (n = 56)		
Surgery		
Limb-sparing resection	55	8 (15)
Amputation	1	0
Brachytherapy*†‡		
Yes	24	4 (17)
No	32	5 (16)
External beam radiation*†‡		
Yes	14	2 (14)
No	42	7 (17)

*Median dose of radiation for patients receiving brachytherapy was 45 Gy in patients with positive and negative margins.
†Median dose of radiation for patients receiving external beam radiation was 65 Gy in patients with positive and negative margins.
‡Not all patients with positive margins received adjuvant radiation treatment (as part of a prospective randomized trial).[5,6]

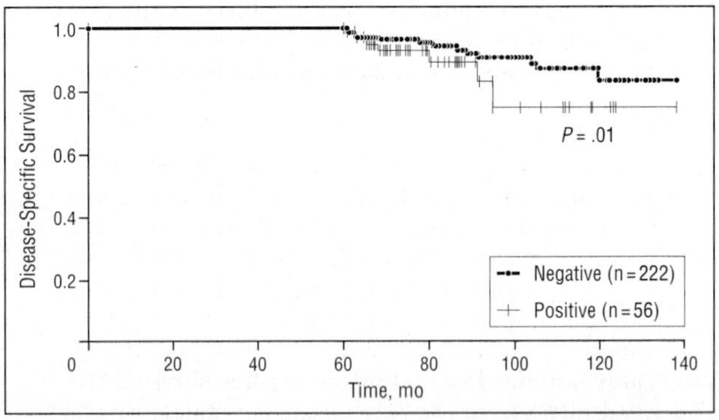

Figure 1. *Disease-specific survival for patients with extremity soft tissue sarcoma alive at 5 years, segregated by microscopic margins at primary resection. Post–5-year disease-specific survival was adversely impacted by positive microscopic margins.*

deep tumor ($P = .03$; risk ratio, 2.6) and positive microscopic margin ($P = .02$; risk ratio, 4.6) influenced metastasis-free survival.

COMMENT

The majority of survival and biology studies in patients with soft tissue sarcoma has focused on early recurrence and mortality, and there are few data addressing long-term follow-up and survival. This study analyzes disease-specific and disease-free survival in patients with primary extremity soft tissue sarcoma, treated at a single institution, who survived for more than 5 years. In addition, we have compared these long-term survivors with those

Table 3. Cox Model Analysis of Disease-Specific Survival and Disease-Free Survival in the >5-Year Survivors (n = 282)

	P	Risk Ratio (Confidence Interval)*
Disease-specific mortality		
Age (≥60 y)	.30	. . .
Grade (high)	.20	. . .
Depth (deep)	.20	. . .
Size (≥5 cm)	.07	. . .
Margin (positive)	.02	2.7 (1.1-6.5)
Local recurrence		
Age (≥60 y)	.03	2.1 (1.2-4.3)
Margin (positive)	.01	2.1 (1.0-3.9)
Metastatic recurrence		
Depth (deep)	.03	2.6 (1.2-5.3)
Margin (positive)	.02	4.6 (1.2-7.1)

*Ellipses indicate not predictive of risk.

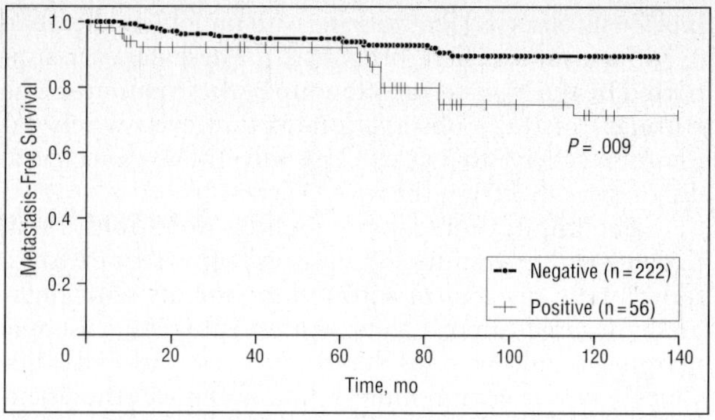

Figure 2. *Metastasis-free survival for patients with extremity soft tissue sarcoma alive at 5 years, segregated by microscopic margins at primary resection. Positive microscopic margin was a significant predictor for development of metastasis.*

who died of disease prior to 5 years. There are 3 novel and significant findings in this study. First, 21% of patients who are alive at 5 years will die of disease during the next 5 years; of those metastasis free at 5 years, 9% will die of disease during the next 5 years. Second, tumor histological grade, which is the pivotal variable influencing early outcome, has no influence on the subsequent survival of patients who are alive at 5 years. Third, positive microscopic margins, at the time of initial surgical resection, adversely impact the disease-specific survival of patients who are alive at 5 years.

From July 1982 to July 1989, we treated 818 patients with extremity soft tissue sarcoma. All patients were then prospectively followed up. Within this group, 495 patients were treated for primary tumor and of these 282 were alive at 5 years. The median follow-up time of the 282 patients was 84.4 months. After 5 years, 23 patients died of documented disease and the actuarial survival at 10 years was 79%. All disease-related deaths occurred in patients who had metastatic disease. Univariate analysis identified 2 prognostic variables for disease-specific mortality: tumor size of 5 cm or greater and microscopic margin of the resected specimen positive for tumor. Notable was the finding that histological high grade was not identified as a prognostic factor for disease-specific mortality after 5 years. Multivariate analysis revealed positive microscopic margin to be the dominant variable influencing post–5-year disease-specific survival. Positive microscopic margin and age older than 60 years at time of initial diagnosis predicted development of local recurrence. Development of local recurrence did not influence metastasis-free or overall survival. Positive microscopic margin did, however, predict the development of subsequent metastasis, both prior to and after 5 years.

The correlation between positive microscopic margin and local recurrence in extremity soft tissue sarcoma is well documented.[8-10] While some studies have reported a correlation between positive microscopic margins and metastasis and disease-specific mortality, the specific role of margins remains controversial.[9,11] Although it is apparent that positive margins are reflective of more aggressive tumor biologic behavior,[12-14] it is possible that residual microscopic disease may also represent a nidus for tumor dissemination.[15] The findings in our study suggest that microscopic margins are important predictors of metastasis, and disease-specific death, when patients are followed up long-term. Whether this is due to a biologic correlative epiphenomenon or residual nidus for subsequent tumor dissemination is speculative. The influence of local control on the margins, on disease biology, and on disease-specific survival for patients with extremity soft tissue sarcoma is unclear and controversial.[16,17]

Two prospective randomized trials have evaluated local control and survival in the context of defining treatment. In a randomized trial from the National Cancer Institute[8] comparing amputation vs conservative surgery plus radiation, local recurrence rates were 19% in the limb-sparing arm vs 6% in the amputation arm. Despite this observation, overall survival rates were equal at 70% (limb-sparing) vs 71% (amputation). In a randomized prospective trial from Memorial Sloan-Kettering Cancer Center[5,6] evaluating the role of brachytherapy in 126 patients with extremity sarcoma, adjuvant brachytherapy was found to substantially improve local control in patients with high-grade sarcomas. This improvement in local control, however, did not translate into any improvement in overall survival. Our present findings support those of these studies. Despite our observation that positive microscopic margin predicted the development of subsequent metastasis and mortality, development of local recurrence did not influence metastasis-free or overall survival. We did not include treatment variables in any of the analyses because treatment was not randomized in all long-term survivors.

The influence of histological tumor grade on early outcome is well established. Indeed, an earlier retrospective review from 13 institutions found the histological grade of the tumor to be the critical determinant of outcome.[1] We recently affirmed the remarkable discriminatory effect of grade, and it was our impression that grade is a factor in early metastasis.[2] Our present findings confirm these data. Multivariate analysis of risk of death within 5 years, vs survival or death after 5 years, revealed histological high grade as the dominant risk factor for early death. It is therefore not surprising that histological high grade has no influence on late survival. While large tumor size may be important in long-term survival, our sample was too small to get a clear answer. We have also previously observed that patients with tumors smaller than 5 cm have an excellent prognosis.[18] These data are supported by the long-term follow-up of these patients. The corollary of these observations is that even when patients do survive to 5 years, 21% will still be expected to die of disease during the next 5 years.

The implications of our findings are 3-fold. First, patients with extremity soft tissue sarcoma require long-term follow-up, and in addition to patients with high-grade or large tumors, those with positive microscopic margins should be considered for investigational adjuvant therapy. Second, interpretation of novel therapeutic interventions for extremity soft tissue sarcoma, while focusing on early outcome, must include long-term follow-up. Finally, prospective clinicopathologic databases, such as the one used in this study, expand our biologic understanding of the natural history of diseases and may benefit patient management considerably.

This work was supported by grant CA-47179 from the National Institutes of Health, Bethesda, Md.

Presented in part at the 48th Annual Cancer Symposium of The Society of Surgical Oncology, Boston, Mass, March 25, 1995.

Reprints: Jonathan J. Lewis, MD, PhD, Department of Surgery, Box 126, Memorial Sloan-Kettering Cancer Center, 1275 York Ave, New York, NY 10021 (e-mail: lewisj@mskcc.org).

REFERENCES

1. Russel WO, Cohen J, Enzinger F, et al. A clinical and pathological staging system for soft tissue sarcomas. *Cancer.* 1977;4:1562-1570.
2. Gaynor JJ, Tan CC, Casper ES, et al. Refinement of clinicopathologic staging for localized soft tissue sarcoma of the extremity: a study of 423 adults. *J Clin Oncol.* 1992;10:1317-1329.
3. Lewis JJ, Brennan MF. Soft tissue sarcomas. In: Sabiston D, ed. *The Biological Basis of Modern Surgical Practice.* 15th ed. New York, NY: WB Saunders Co; 1995:528-533.
4. Hajdu SI, Shiu MH, Brennan MF. The role of the pathologist in the management of soft tissue sarcomas. *World J Surg.* 1988;12:326-331.
5. Brennan MF, Casper ES, Harrison LB, Shiu MH, Gaynor J, Hajdu SI. The role of multimodality therapy in soft-tissue sarcoma. *Ann Surg.* 1991;214:328-336.
6. Pisters PWT, Harrison LB, Woodruff JM, Gaynor JJ, Brennan MF. A prospective randomized trial of adjuvant brachytherapy in the management of low grade soft tissue sarcomas of the extremity and superficial trunk. *J Clin Oncol.* 1994;12:1150-1158.
7. Kaplan EL, Meier P. Nonparametric estimation from incomplete observations. *J Am Stat Assoc.* 1958;53:457-462.
8. Rosenberg SA, Tepper J, Glatstein E, et al. The treatment of soft-tissue sarcomas of the extremities: prospective randomized evaluations of limb-sparing surgery plus radiation therapy compared with amputation and the role of adjuvant chemotherapy. *Ann Surg.* 1982;196:305-315.
9. Collin CF, Friedrich C, Godbold J, Hajdu S, Brennan MF. Prognostic factors for local recurrence and survival in patients with localized extremity soft tissue sarcoma. *Semin Surg Oncol.* 1988;4:30-37.
10. Singer S, Corson JM, Gonin R, Labow B, Eberlein TJ. Prognostic factors predictive of survival and local recurrence for extremity soft tissue sarcoma. *Ann Surg.* 1994;219:165-173.
11. Herbert SH, Corn BW, Solin LJ, et al. Limb-preserving treatment for soft tissue sarcomas of the extremities: the significance of surgical margins. *Cancer.* 1993;72:1230-1238.
12. Gustafson P, Rooser B, Rydholm A. Is local recurrence of minor importance for metastases in soft tissue sarcoma? *Cancer.* 1991;67:2083-2086.
13. Gustafson P, Dreinhofer KE, Rydholm A. Metastasis-free survival after local recurrence of soft-tissue sarcoma. *J Bone Joint Surg Br.* 1993;75:658-660.
14. Molls M, Feldmann HJ, Fuller J. Oxygenation of locally advanced recurrent rectal cancer, soft tissue sarcoma and breast cancer. *Adv Exp Med Biol.* 1994;345:459-463.
15. Suit HD. Local control and patient survival. *Int J Radiat Oncol Biol Phys.* 1992;23:653-660.
16. Emrich LJ, Ruka W, Driscoll DL, Karakousis CP. The effect of local recurrence on survival time in adult high-grade soft tissue sarcoma. *J Clin Epidemiol.* 1989;42:105-110.
17. Stotter AT, Ahern RP, Fisher C, Mott AF, Fallowfield ME, Westbury G. The influence of local recurrence of extremity soft tissue sarcoma on metastasis and survival. *Cancer.* 1990;65:1119-1129.
18. Geer RJ, Woodruff J, Casper ES, Brennan MF. Management of small soft-tissue sarcoma of the extremity in adults. *Arch Surg.* 1992;127:1285-1289.

Surgical Anatomy

The tubercle of Zuckerkandl is the most posterior extension of the lateral thyroid lobes.

1. Blackbourne LH, Fleischer KJ (eds). *Advance Surgical Recall.* Baltimore, Md: Williams & Wilkins: 1997:31.

Mapping a Pathway for Axillary Staging

A Personal Perspective on the Current Status of Sentinel Lymph Node Dissection for Breast Cancer

IN 1972, Haagensen[1] illustrated the axillary nodal uptake of a vital blue dye during mastectomy. In 1977 Cabanas[2] described the identification of nodal drainage pathways and a sentinel node (SN) from penile cancer. Fifteen years later, at the John Wayne Cancer Institute in Santa Monica, Calif, Morton et al[3] introduced intraoperative lymphatic mapping as a minimally invasive, practical means of identifying regional nodal metastases to eliminate routine lymph node dissection in patients with no evidence of metastases from cutaneous melanoma. Our group at the John Wayne Cancer Institute popularized the concept of an SN as the first regional lymph node to receive tumor cells that metastasize along the lymphatic drainage pathway from a primary tumor. The tumor status of this SN should therefore reflect the tumor status of the entire regional lymphatic drainage basin.

In October 1991, we began to test the feasibility of intraoperative lymphatic mapping and sentinel lymph node dissection (SLND) for patients with breast cancer. Our goal was to eliminate routine axillary lymph node dissection (ALND) without losing the staging advantage of axillary surgery. Three years later, we reported our cumulative experience in 174 patients with primary breast tumors (176 cases).[4] Intraoperative lymphatic mapping was performed with 1% isosulfan blue dye, and SLND was routinely followed by completion ALND (levels 1 and 2) to verify the procedure's accuracy. An SN was identified in 114 procedures (66%) and accurately predicted axillary status in 109 (96%) of 114 cases. Three of the 5 false-negative results were dye-stained axillary fat misidentified as an SN early in the series; this prompted the routine use of frozen sections to confirm lymph node recovery and prepare our pathologists for the review of frozen sections that, if tumor-free, would eventually obviate completion ALND. A fourth false negative was identified as a true positive when a tumor-free SN was reexamined using immunohistochemistry (IHC), a highly sensitive technique that has since become our routine for nodal specimens that do not contain metastases detectable with hematoxylin-eosin (HE).

To determine if the SN could predict axillary status by chance alone, we examined the ALND specimens of patients with SN that were found to harbor metastases on histologic examination. Of the 751 lymph nodes removed from 34 patients, 63 (8%) were SNs and 688 (92%) were non-SNs.[4] Tumors were found in 39 SNs (62%), compared with 93 non-SNs (14%) ($P<.001$). This suggests that a primary breast tumor spreads to the axilla along a specific pathway of lymph nodes that cannot be identified by random axillary sampling.

In 1995, we evaluated the first 162 patients who underwent successful SLND followed by completion ALND (SLND group) and compared them with 134 patients who underwent routine ALND alone (ALND group).[5] Each SN was evaluated by HE and anticytokeratin IHC staining; non-SNs were evaluated by HE alone. We detected a significantly higher incidence of axillary metastasis in the SLND group than in the ALND group (42% vs 28%; $P<.05$), which was primarily due to detection of more micrometastases ($\leq$2 mm) in SNs than in non-SNs (16% vs 3%; $P<.05$), particularly with IHC staining. We used these results to define our standard of focused histopathologic examination with IHC staining. This time-consuming and expensive technique is not practical for routine examination of the much larger ALND specimen; however, a focused examination of the lymph node most likely to contain cancer cells (the SN) may be more accurate than routine examination of all axillary lymph nodes and may enhance the staging accuracy of axillary surgery by detecting metastases that would be missed by routine tissue processing. Our painstaking IHC study of 1087 non-SNs confirmed that the SN is the first node to harbor tumor cells metastasizing from a primary breast lesion[6]; this study showed that when the SN is tumor free by both routine HE and IHC staining, the probability of the presence of a tumor in a non-SN is 1 in 1087, or .09%.

In the last few years, investigators at several other institutions have verified the existence of the SN in breast cancer. Krag et al[7] were the first to report radioguided SN identification in breast cancer using a gamma probe to follow the path of a radiolabeled isotope. In their 1993 pilot study[7] of probe-directed mapping, 22 patients received an injection of unfiltered technetium Tc 99m sulfur colloid 1 to 4 hours before surgery. No dye was used. The SN was identified in 18 patients (82%), and predicted the histopathologic status of the axilla in each case. A study by Albertini et al[8] combined isosulfan blue dye and filtered technetium Tc 99m sulfur colloid for lymphatic mapping. An SN was identified in 57 (92%) of 62 patients. Forty-five SNs were identified by both blue dye and

Studies Examining the Success Rate and Accuracy of SLND in Breast Cancer*

Study	No. of Cases Studied	Mapping Technique	Histopathologic Technique	Rate of SN Identification, No. (%)	Accuracy of SN as Indicator of Axillary Status, No. (%)	Average No. of SNs Examined	Rate of Metastasis to SNs Only, %
Krag et al[7]	22	Colloid	HE	18/22 (82)	18/18 (100)	NA	43
Giuliano et al[4]	174	Blue dye	HE	114/174 (66)	109/114 (96)	1.8	38
Albertini et al[8]	62	Blue dye and colloid	HE	57/62 (92)	57/57 (100)	2.2	67
Pijpers et al[10]	37	Colloid	HE	34/37 (92)	32/32 (100)†	2.2	64
Veronesi et al[9]	163	Colloid	HE	160/163 (98)	156/160 (98)	1.4	38
Giuliano et al[11]	107	Blue dye	HE and IHC	100/107 (94)	100/100 (100)	1.8	67
Guenther et al[12]	145	Blue dye	HE	103/145 (71)	100/103 (97)	NA	43
Dale and Williams[13]	21	Blue dye	HE	14/21 (67)	14/14 (100)	1.2	60
Borgstein et al[14]	130	Colloid	HE and IHC	122/130 (94)	103/104 (99)‡	1.2	59
Barnwell et al[15]	42	Blue dye and colloid	HE	38/42 (90)	38/38 (100)	1.0	33
O'Hea et al[16]	59	Blue dye and colloid	HE	55/59 (93)	52/55 (95)	2.2	41
Miner et al[17]	42	Colloid	HE	41/42 (98)	40/41 (98)	2.9	57
Offodile et al[18]	41	Colloid	HE and IHC	40/41 (98)	40/40 (100)	3.0	NA
Cox et al[19]	466	Blue dye and colloid	HE and IHC	440/466 (94)§	NA	1.9	NA
Koller et al[20]	98	Blue dye	NA	96/98 (98)	93/96 (97)'	2.7	27
Crossin et al[21]	50	Colloid	NA	42/50 (84)	41/42 (98)	2.0	NA

*SLND indicates sentinal lymph node dissection; SN, sentinal node; HE, hematoxylin-eosin; IHC, immunohistochemistry; and NA, not applicable.
†Two patients refused completion axillary lymph node dissection (ALND) and were removed from this analysis.
‡Eighteen patients refused completion ALND and were removed from this analysis.
§Most patients with tumor-negative SNs did not undergo completion ALND.

radiocolloid, and 12 were identified by colloid alone. Metastases were found in 18 SNs, all of which were identified by both dye and colloid. No patient had tumor-positive non-SNs if the SN was free of tumor. Albertini et al[8] concluded that the combination of dye and colloid increases identification of the SN, and in their hands this method is superior to colloid or dye alone. Veronesi et al[9] reported the results of probe-directed lymphatic mapping with technetium-labeled human serum albumin injected subdermally and superficial to the tumor. The SN was identified in 160 (98%) of 163 patients and was predictive of axillary status in 156 (97%) of 160 patients.

The **Table** summarizes results of numerous studies on the SN as a predictor of axillary status in patients with primary breast cancer.[4-22] Taken as a group, these studies confirm that lymphatic drainage of a breast cancer can be identified and traced to the SN intraoperatively, and that the histologic status of the SN accurately predicts the tumor status of the entire axilla. When these studies are considered individually, however, they illustrate the tremendous degree of variation in the SLND technique. The SN can be identified by radiocolloid alone, radiocolloid plus isosulfan blue dye, or blue dye alone. As of yet there is no standardization; the best technique depends on the experience and training of the surgeon and his or her team. Blue dye alone has been said to be too difficult for the beginner to use, and many neophytes prefer a combination of dye and colloid. However, adding a radiocolloid does not necessarily increase mapping accuracy and may introduce additional technical problems such as "shine-through" when the tumor is near the axillary nodal basin. In this case, an SN cannot be detected by the probe without special techniques such as removing the primary site or shielding the tumor from even the most collimated probe. Surgical fellows training at the John Wayne Cancer Institute generally learn dye-directed SLND after about 10 to 15 cases, and visiting surgeons who observe our technique usually find it easy to master when they return to their practice. Most surgeons just starting SLND will probably use both blue dye and radiocolloid, feeling more secure with a backup mapping agent that allows a second chance to identify the SN. This seems reasonable, but learning the procedure and assembling a committed team will not come easily regardless of the technique.

Our experience is primarily with blue dye; however, we now use both radiocolloid and blue dye for all medial hemisphere lesions. A preoperative lymphoscintigram is obtained to document axillary drainage from these tumors, and the intraoperative gamma counter is used to measure radioactivity over blue-stained and nonstained axillary lymph nodes. Although we have had excellent success with the probe, the technical details of our procedure are unlikely to be the same as those reported by other experienced investigators. Numerous variables must be considered. Some groups use peritumoral injection, while others use intratumoral or even subcutaneous or cutaneous injection. Some used filtered technetium Tc 99m sulfur colloid, some use unfiltered colloid, and others use radiolabeled albumin. In addition, the time from injection to operation varies widely among investigators using radiocolloid. A beginner is often unaware of these subtle technical variations and may be tempted to mix different techniques, not realizing that each technical variation (type of gamma counter, type of colloid, injection site, timing) gives rise to a whole new set of problems and may alter results. My initial experience with probe-directed lymphatic mapping was extremely unsatisfactory and I was unable to reproduce the results of others until I realized that I had mixed the technique described by Albertini et al[8] with that of Krag et al[7] and then added a few of my own modifications. The combination was not very successful, but was corrected and we are now content with radiocolloid and blue dye.

Axillary lymphatic mapping of the SN will not be successful unless it is initially performed exactly as reported. Results must be consistent and reproducible before any modifications can be considered. Our initial feasibility trial is often quoted as evidence for the difficulty of dye-directed lymphatic mapping. During that study we were constantly identifying and refining different aspects of our technique (volume of injectant, timing and site of injection, technique of dissection) until we developed a reliable, accurate protocol. Prior to this, there was no successful technique for breast cancer and we had to develop one from the very different melanoma protocol. We reported all cases leading up to our initial publication, even those cases that we now know were inappropriate, which is why the reported success rate was less than our current rate of success.

During the developmental phase of SLND and then for approximately 100 cases in which the mature technique was used, we did not consider abandoning routine completion ALND because we were still proving the accuracy of SLND. In 1997, we reported a series of 107 consecutive patients who underwent SLND routinely followed by completion ALND.[11] The rate of SN identification was 94% using dye alone, and there were no false-negative results—a sensitivity and specificity of 100%. Based on these results and the results of IHC on non-SNs,[6] in 1995 we abandoned ALND for node-negative patients and began a trial to study outcome and clinical recurrence rates in patients who underwent SLND followed by completion ALND *only* if the SN had tumor cells. Candidates for this trial were patients with clinically negative axillary lymph nodes and primary breast tumors no greater than 4 cm (T1 and T2). Currently, patients with primary tumors in the inner hemisphere must undergo preoperative lymphoscintigraphy to document axillary drainage. Sentinel lymph node dissection is performed using dye-directed mapping, except when inner hemisphere tumors are present, in which case both dye-directed and probe-directed mapping is used. The excised SN is intraoperatively examined by frozen section with HE or DiffQuik (Dade International, Miami, Fla); if it contains tumor, completion ALND is performed before the patient leaves the operating room. Immunohistochemistry staining, which is a 2-day process at our institution, is performed postoperatively on multiple levels of all SN that are tumor free by HE.

Because SLND is not a standard treatement, we did not begin our trial of SLND without routine completion ALND until we had discussed this new modality with the John Wayne Cancer Institute's bioethicist and had developed an informed consent process that would safeguard both the patient and the provider. All patients scheduled for SLND instead of routine ALND are given extensive written literature and counseled separately by the senior surgeon (A.E.G.) and by a research nurse about SLND, standard surgical practice, and the rationale for abandoning routine ALND. This lengthy informed consent is very important in establishing realistic expectations and ensuring that a patient is not agreeing to a new procedure without fully understanding its purpose and results. A patient who signs our informed consent document for SLND without routine completion ALND understands that in some cases the operation may leave metastases in the lymph nodes (a false-negative SN).

Our trial has now accrued more than 400 cases. In those patients who were followed up for at least 2 years, about 40% had SN metastases and underwent completion ALND; the remaining 60% had no evidence of SN metastases and therefore did not undergo ALND. No patient in either group has developed an axillary recurrence, and no patient in the SLND group has experienced lymphedema or numbness.

When we began this trial, we performed completion ALND as a second procedure whenever IHC staining revealed metastases. However, the data presented at the 1998 meeting of the Society of Surgical Oncology show that patients with HE-negative, IHC-positive SNs are unlikely to have HE-positive non-SNs when they undergo completion ALND.[23] Immunohistochemistry is not the standard of care and does not necessarily need to be performed outside a research setting. The clinical significance of metastases detected only by IHC is unclear, and studies on adjuvant therapy and staging have all been based on routine staining with HE.[24-28] From our own data, we suspect that completion ALND may not be necessary when tumor in the SN is micrometastatic and is detected only by IHC. A large prospective study is being undertaken by the American College of Surgeons to determine the importance of SN metastases detected only by IHC.

Clearly, there are patient incentives to undergo SLND without routine completion ALND. Removing only a few SNs is minimally invasive and has few complications. We have yet to see lymphedema in a patient undergoing SLND without ALND, although I suspect it will occur. As SLND becomes more widely publicized, more surgeons are confronted by patient requests for SLND instead of ALND. However, surgeons who are not yet proficient at SLND must not abandon routine completion ALND to satisfy consumer demand. Any surgeon interested in providing SLND as an alternative to ALND in node-negative women must establish an institutional protocol to accurately perform SLND; organize a committed team of pathologists, nuclear medicine physicians, nurses, and surgeons; and apply rigorous controls to assure proficiency at every stage of the technique. Once the team is trained, the surgeon should perform SLND followed immediately by completion ALND to test the accuracy of the procedure at that institution. Comparing the tumor status of SNs and non-SNs removed during SLND and ALND, respectively, will allow the surgeon and other members of the team to determine when they will be able to reproduce the excellent results reported in the literature.

This approach is illustrated by the results of an extremely important trial by Krag et al.[22] They report a well-done and relevant trial that is the first to examine the technique of SLND at multiple institutions with surgeons of different experience. This trial clearly identifies the promise and problems of the procedure. They reported SN dissections in 443 patients. An SN was identified in 405 patients who underwent completion ALND. Among these 405 patients, there were 114 node-positive women with 13 false-negative SNs, for a false-negative rate of 11%. Even with this high false-negative rate, which is similar to feasibility trials at single institutions, the overall staging accuracy of the procedure was 97%. However, among the 11 surgeons in the group, the SN identification rate varied from 79% to 98%, and the false-negative rate varied from 0% to 29%. These high failure rates among experienced surgeons are surprising, but may reflect the short learning curve (5 cases) necessary prior to entry into the trial. Clearly, even when a radioisotope is used, the technique requires substantial training, and results will vary according to an individual's surgical skill and experience. Surgeons must realize that, regardless of the technique used, a serious commitment toward learning the procedure must be undertaken. Routine completion ALND should not be abandoned until the entire team is able to achieve highly accurate results.

How many times must the surgeon perform SLND with completion ALND before switching to SLND alone? Morton[29] recently recommended performance of 60 to 80 procedures to develop an "acceptable level of technical skill (90% accuracy in identifying sentinel nodes)." He noted that the experience required to attain this level of proficiency exceeds the number of patients with breast cancer in most community practice situations or the number of breast operations performed by surgeons not working in major cancer centers. However, my estimate of the number of procedures that need to be performed to become proficient in identifying an SN is closer to 20 or 30. Both estimates are, of course, completely arbitrary. Surgeons who learn quickly and who have performed many axillary operations will master SLND after fewer cases, whereas others may never develop the skills necessary to accurately identify an SN. The multi-institutional study by Krag et al[22] confirms the marked variation in surgeons' ability to perform the procedure.

In an upcoming trial sponsored by the American College of Surgeons, patients with tumor-negative SNs are followed up without completion ALND, and patients with tumor-positive SNs are randomized to either completion ALND or no further axillary therapy. We have proposed that to participate in this trial, each institution's principal investigator must document a 90% accuracy rate in identifying the SN, and a 90% staging accuracy in at least 30 consecutive cases of SLND followed by completion ALND. Many surgeons feel that 30 cases is too many, but it is at least a reasonable starting point. The surgeon's skill in detecting an SN will increase with practice, regardless of what technique is used.

There is no doubt that SLND can accurately stage patients with breast cancer. The question is whether its potential can be fully translated into general practice. Each surgeon must learn how to do the procedure and assure that team members are cooperative in assuring accuracy, are committed to the procedure, and are skilled in their roles. Those teams who have performed a sufficient number of mapping procedures will be convinced of their own accuracy in identifying the SN and can comfortably abandon routine completion ALND. The literature shows that when the SN can be identified with accuracy, it can predict axillary status. Those surgeons who have not yet crested the SLND learning curve or whose institution has not yet formed a cohesive unit that can perform SLND should not abandon routine completion ALND. They should, however, work to develop the competence and confidence necessary to bring the advantage of this new technology to women with breast cancer.

Armando E. Giuliano, MD
Santa Monica, Calif

Supported by funding from the Ben B. and Joyce E. Eisenberg Foundation, Los Angeles, Calif, the Fashion Footwear Association of New York, New York City, and the Associates for Breast Cancer Research, Santa Monica, Calif.

Corresponding author: Armando E. Giuliano, MD, John Wayne Cancer Institute, 2200 Santa Monica Blvd, Santa Monica, CA 90404.

REFERENCES

1. Haagensen CD. Lymphatics of the breast. In: Haagensen CD, Feind CR, Herter FP, Slanetz CA, Weinberg JA. *The Lymphatics in Cancer.* Philadelphia, Pa: WB Saunders Co; 1972:300-398.
2. Cabanas RM. An approach for the treatment of penile carcinoma. *Cancer.* 1977;39:456-466.
3. Morton DL, Wen DR, Wong JH, et al. Technical details of intraoperative lymphatic mapping for early stage melanoma. *Arch Surg.* 1992;127:392-399.
4. Giuliano AE, Kirgan DM, Guenther JM, Morton DL. Lymphatic mapping and sentinel lymphadenectomy for breast cancer. *Ann Surg.* 1994;220:391-401.
5. Giuliano AE, Dale PS, Turner RR, Morton DL, Evans SW, Krasne DL. Improved axillary staging of breast cancer with sentinel lymphadenectomy. *Ann Surg.* 1995;222:394-401.
6. Turner RR, Ollila DW, Krasne DL, Giuliano AE. Histopathologic validation of the sentinel lymph node hypothesis for breast carcinoma. *Ann Surg.* 1997;226:271-278.
7. Krag DN, Weaver DL, Alex JC, Fairbank JT. Surgical resection and radiolocalization of the sentinel node in breast cancer using gamma probe. *Surg Oncol.* 1993;2:335-340.
8. Albertini JJ, Lyman GH, Cox C, et al. Lymphatic mapping and sentinel node biopsy in the patient with breast cancer. *JAMA.* 1996;276:1818-1822.
9. Veronesi U, Paganelli G, Galimberti V, et al. Sentinel-node biopsy to avoid axillary dissection in breast cancer with clinically negative lymph nodes. *Lancet.* 1997;349:1864-1867.
10. Pijpers R, Meijer S, Hoekstra OS, et al. Impact of lymphoscintigraphy on sentinel node identification with technetium-99m-colloidal albumin in breast cancer. *J Nucl Med.* 1997;38:366-368.
11. Giuliano AE, Jones RC, Brennan M, Statman R. Sentinel lymphadenectomy in breast cancer. *J Clin Oncol.* 1997;15:2345-2350.
12. Guenther JM, Krishnamoorthy M, Tan LR. Sentinel lymphadenectomy for breast cancer in a community managed care setting. *Cancer J Sci Am.* 1997;3:336-340.
13. Dale PS, Williams JT. Axillary staging utilizing selective sentinel lymphadenectomy for patients with invasive breast carcinoma. *Am Surg.* 1998;64:28-32.

14. Borgstein PJ, Pijpers R, Comans EF, et al. Sentinel lymph node biopsy in breast cancer: guidelines and pitfalls of lymphoscintigraphy and gamma probe detection. *J Am Coll Surg.* 1998;186:275-283.
15. Barnwell JM, Arredondo MA, Kollmorgen D, et al. Sentinel node biopsy in breast cancer. *Ann Surg Oncol.* 1998;5:126-130.
16. O'Hea BJ, Hill ADK, El-Shirbiny AM, et al. Sentinel lymph node biopsy in breast cancer: initial experience at Memorial Sloan-Kettering Cancer Center. *J Am Coll Surg.* 1998;186:423-427.
17. Miner TJ, Shriver CD, Jaques DP, et al. Ultrasonographically guided injection improves localization of the radiolabeled sentinel lymph node in breast cancer. *Ann Surg Oncol.* 1998;5:315-321.
18. Offodile R, Hoh C, Barsky SH, et al. Minimally invasive breast carcinoma staging using lymphatic mapping with radiolabeled dextran. *Cancer.* 1998;82:1704-1708.
19. Cox CE, Pendas S, Cox JM, et al. Guidelines for sentinel node biopsy and lymphatic mapping of patients with breast cancer. *Ann Surg.* 1998;227:645-653.
20. Koller M, Barsuk D, Zippel D, et al. Sentinel lymph node involvement—a predictor for axillary node status with breast cancer—has the time come? *Eur J Surg Oncol.* 1998;24:166-168.
21. Crossin JA, Johnson AC, Stewart PB, et al. Gamma-probe-guided resection of the sentinel lymph node in breast cancer. *Am Surg.* 1998;64:666-669.
22. Krag D, Weaver D, Ashikaga T, et al. The sentinel node in breast cancer: a multicenter validation study. *N Engl J Med.* 1998;339:941-995.
23. Chu KU, Bilchik A, Brennan M, Giuliano AE. Do all patients with sentinel node metastasis from breast carcinoma need complete axillary node dissection? Paper presented at: Society of Surgical Oncology; March 25-29, 1998; San Diego, Calif.
24. Nasser IA, Lee AKC, Bosari S, et al. Occult axillary lymph node metastases in "node-negative" breast carcinoma. *Hum Pathol.* 1993;24:950-957.
25. Chen ZL, Wen DR, Coulsen WF, et al. Occult metastases in the axillary lymph nodes of patients with breast cancer node negative by clinical and histologic examination and conventional histology. *Dis Markers.* 1991;9:239-248.
26. Hainsworth PJ, Tjandra JJ, Stillwell RG, et al. Detection and significance of occult metastases in node-negative breast cancer. *Br J Surg.* 1993;80:459-463.
27. Bettelheim R, Price KN, Gelber RD, et al. Prognostic importance of occult axillary lymph node micrometastases from breast cancer. *Lancet.* 1990;335:1565-1568.
28. De Mascarel I, Bonichon F, Coincre JM, Trojani M. Prognostic significance of breast cancer axillary lymph node micrometastases assessed by two special techniques: reevaluation with longer follow-up. *Br J Cancer.* 1992;66:523-527.
29. Morton DL. Intraoperative lymphatic mapping and sentinel lymphadenectomy: community standard care or clinical investigation? *Cancer J Sci Am.* 1997;3:328-330.

Vascular Endothelial Growth Factor Is More Important Than Basic Fibroblastic Growth Factor During Ischemic Wound Healing

Claudio J. Corral, MD; Aamir Siddiqui, MD; Liancun Wu, MD; Catherine L. Farrell, PhD; David Lyons, PhD; Thomas A. Mustoe, MD

Objectives: To test the influence of vascular endothelial growth factor (VEGF) on normal and ischemic wounds in a noncontractive dermal ulcer standardized model in the rabbit ear and to assay the levels of both VEGF and basic fibroblastic growth factor messenger RNA levels in normal and ischemic wounds at different intervals during the healing process.

Design and Interventions: Dermal ulcers were created in the normal and ischemic ears of 20 anesthetized young female New Zealand white rabbits. Either VEGF 121, VEGF 165 (30 µg per wound), or buffered saline solution alone was applied to each wound and covered. Wounds were harvested at day 7 or 10 and evaluated histologically. Twenty-four similar rabbits were wounded in the same manner and their untreated wounds were harvested at 1, 3, 7, and 10 days after wounding. The wounds were analyzed with reverse transcriptase polymerase chain reaction.

Main Outcome Measures: Histologic specimens were measured for amount of new epithelium and granulation tissue. Reverse transcriptase polymerase chain reaction was used to determine basic fibroblastic growth factor and VEGF messenger RNA expression.

Results: Both isoforms of VEGF improved granulation tissue formation in both normal and ischemic wounds with a magnitude similar to other vulnerary agents tested in the past. Vascular endothelial growth factor application had no effect on new epithelium formation. In contrast to basic fibroblastic growth factor, VEGF messenger RNA levels were induced 4 fold by ischemia alone and 6 fold by wounding in both ischemic and normal wounds.

Conclusion: Vascular endothelial growth factor seems to be more important than basic fibroblastic growth factor during ischemic wound healing. Treatment of ischemic wounds with VEGF improves the deficit in wound healing produced by ischemia.

Arch Surg. 1999;134:200-205

WOUND HEALING is characterized by an ordered sequence of events in response to injuries that ultimately result in tissue formation, reepithelialization, and scar formation. Angiogenesis is an integral part of this sequence of events and occurs during the proliferative phase of wound healing. It is characterized by new vessel formation and vascular hyperpermeability that improve tissue oxygenation and nutrient delivery and promote cellular and matrix deposition in the wound.[1]

Several growth factors have been implicated as possible mediators of angiogenesis during wound repair, including transforming growth factor beta-1, tumor necrosis factor α, epidermal growth factor, keratinocyte growth factor, interleukins 1, 6, and 8, basic fibroblastic growth factor (bFGF), platelet-derived growth factor (PDGF),[2,3] and most recently, vascular endothelial growth factor (VEGF).[4-6] These growth factors have angiogenic properties in vitro and in vivo. Their angiogenic properties have been traditionally categorized as either direct or indirect based on endothelial cell activation and mitogenesis.[7,8] Of these, only bFGF, PDGF, and VEGF have been shown to be directly mitogenic to endothelial cells[7,9,10]; however, it remains unclear which of these growth factors is the most important mediator of the angiogenic phase of healing. This question is of primary clinical importance, since improving the angiogenic response during wound healing using a single growth factor or in combination, may partially reverse the healing deficit observed in ischemic wounds.

Several authors have described possible mechanisms by which these growth factors are angiogenic.[7-9] There is evi-

From the Division of Plastic Surgery and Reconstructive Surgery, Northwestern University Medical School, Chicago, Ill (Drs Corral, Siddiqui, Wu, and Mustoe); and Amgen Inc, Thousand Oaks, Calif (Drs Farrell and Lyons).

MATERIALS AND METHODS

ANIMAL WOUNDING AND VEGF TREATMENT

Young adult female New Zealand white rabbits (New Franken Inc, New Franken, Wis) weighing 2.7 to 3.4 kg, were acclimated and housed under standard conditions and used in all experiments. All surgical procedures were performed under sterile conditions as previously described.[24] All animal protocols were approved by Northwestern University Animal Care and Use Committee.

Twenty rabbits were divided into ischemic and nonischemic groups. Rabbits were anesthetized with ketamine hydrochloride (60 mg/kg) and xylazine hydrochloride (5 mg/kg) prior to surgery. In the ischemic group, the ears were made ischemic by dividing the rostral and central arteries and the entire dermal circulation of the ear. Three full-thickness, 6-mm, dermal punches were made down to bare cartilage with the aid of a binocular microscope. In the nonischemic group, 4 wounds were similarly made in each ear. The wounds were treated at the time of wounding with either recombinant VEGF 121, VEGF 165 (30 μg per wound) (AMGEN Corp, Thousand Oaks, Calif), or phosphate-buffered saline solution vehicle. All wounds were covered with an occlusive dressing (Tagaderm; 3M, Minneapolis, Minn) for the duration of the experiment.

Ischemic wounds were harvested at day 10 and nonischemic wounds at day 7 as previously described.[25] All wounds were excised, bisected, and fixed in neutral buffered 10% formaldehyde solution (Sigma Chemical Co, St Louis, Mo). The specimens were then dehydrated in graded alcohol and xylene, embedded in paraffin, and sectioned (3 μm), taking care to obtain a cross section as near as possible to the center of the wound.

HISTOLOGICAL STAINING

All slides were stained with hematoxylin-eosin using standard protocols. The stained sections were analyzed under ×40 magnification. All slides were examined by 2 independent observers (C.J.C. and A.S.) with standard light microscopy under ×40 magnification. New granulation tissue formation and new epithelium were measured using a 100-μm lens redicle on the light microscope at ×40 magnification. The redicle was sectioned into 10-μm^2 squares, and the area occupied by the tissue was measured.

RNA EXTRACTION AND COMPETITIVE REVERSE TRANSCRIPTASE POLYMERASE CHAIN REACTION

After wounding, 24 rabbits were divided into 4 groups as to number of days after wounding: day 1, day 3, day 7 and day 10. All rabbits were wounded as above; however, only 1 ear was made ischemic. All wounds were left untreated and were covered with the occlusive dressing for the duration of the experiment. At the appropriate time, the rabbits were anesthetized and a 7-mm punch biopsy specimen of skin was obtained from each ear to serve as an ischemic and a normal skin control. Granulation tissue was harvested with a 7-mm punch biopsy specimen and immediately immersed in liquid nitrogen for later guanidine thiocyanate/phenol–based reagent to isolate RNA from the sample (TRI Reagent, Cincinnati, Ohio) as previously described.[26] Total RNA was pooled from each ear and quantified with a spectrophotometer (Genequant model 80-2103-98; Biochrom, Cambridge, England) prior to complementary DNA (cDNA) conversion. Five micrograms of total RNA was converted to cDNA using Maloney-Murine Leukemia Virus Reverse Transcriptase (M-MLV RT) and random primers (Gibco Biological Research Laboratories, Grand Island, NY) as previously described.[27]

Rabbit VEGF primers were designed from conserved Genbank sequences (AMGEN Corp). Amplimers obtained with these primers were sequenced to assure the correct target gene was being amplified. The FGF rabbit primers were obtained from a Genbank rabbit sequence (AMGEN Corp). Glutaraldehyde phosphate dehydrogenase rabbit primers were kindly donated by US Surgical Corporation, New Haven, Conn. Reverse transcriptase polymerase chain reaction was performed as previously described.[27,28] MIMICS for each primer set were designed as described by Siebert and Larrick.[27,28] Serial dilutions of MIMIC and constant concentration of cDNA were coamplified using a polymerase chain reaction. These products were run in a 2% agarose gel, photographed under UV light, and analyzed by densitometry (Imaging Densitometer GS-670; Bio Rad, Richmond, Calif). The ratio of target product to MIMIC was then obtained as previously described.[29] Glutaraldehyde phosphate dehydrogenase amplification was used as an external control of the reverse transcriptase reaction, and this was run in all cDNA samples tested. Each reaction was run in duplicate starting from the RNA to the cDNA step.

dence that suggests that not only the indirect angiogenic factors, but also bFGF and PDGF, may be acting in vivo through VEGF transcriptional regulation.[3,7,11-14] We have previously described the effects of transforming growth factor beta-1, PDGF, and bFGF in both ischemic and nonischemic wound healing.[15-17] These 3 growth factors improve wound healing and promote angiogenesis in the rabbit ear dermal ulcer model. The notable exception is bFGF, which failed to improve granulation tissue formation and epithelialization in ischemic wounds despite eliciting a marked local angiogenic response.[17]

Vascular endothelial growth factor is a heparin-binding dimeric glycoprotein and a member of the PDGF family of growth factors. It has 4 known homodimers of varying size and solubility (121, 165, 184 , and 209 kd). The isomers are generated by posttranscriptional splicing of a single *VEGF* gene.[18] Vascular endothelial growth factor receptors have been found primarily in vascular endothelium; however, they are also found in human melanoma cells, HeLa cells, and monocytes.[19] In contrast to bFGF, VEGF contains a typical signal sequence, can be secreted by intact cells, and is expressed in a variety of highly vascularized tissues, including the ovary, kidneys, brain, and solid tumors.[3,9] Vascular endothelial growth factor has been shown to directly induce mitogenesis and interstitial collagenase transcription in endothelial cells.[20] It has also been shown to upregulate in keratinocytes at the wound edges during wound healing

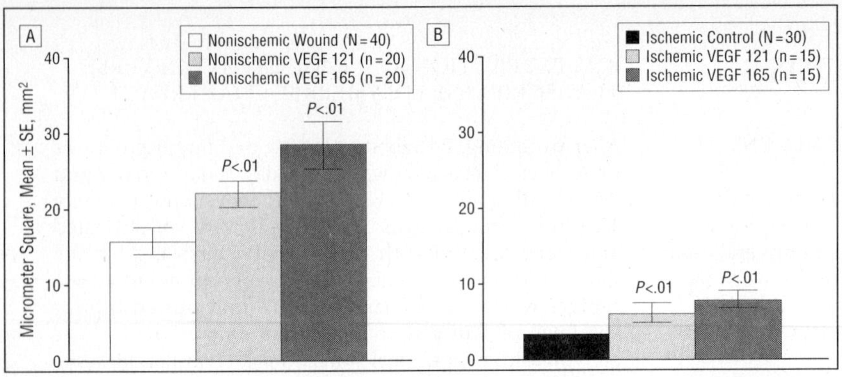

Figure 1. *New granulation tissue formation in response to 30 μg per wound of vascular endothelial growth factor (VEGF) in nonischemic (A) and ischemic (B) wounds. Note the difference in scale between the 2 graphs.*

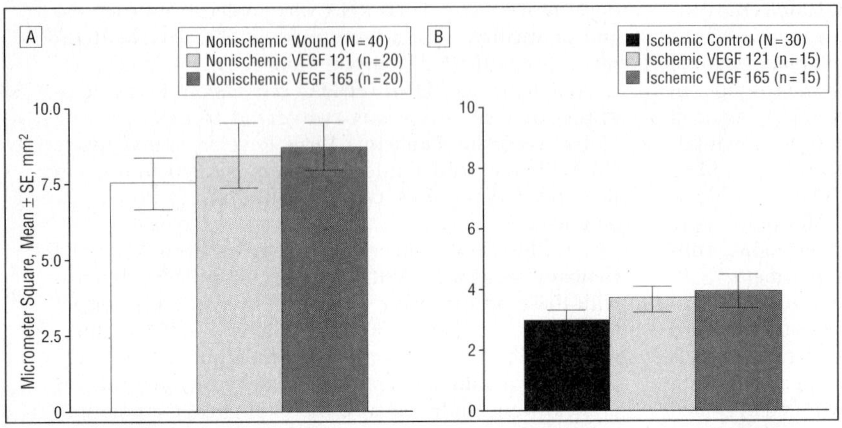

Figure 2. *New epithelium tissue formation in response to 30 μg per wound of vascular endothelial growth factor (VEGF) in nonischemic (A) and ischemic (B) wounds. Note the difference in scale between the 2 graphs. No significant differences were found.*

in rat and guinea pig skin.[4] In contrast to bFGF, VEGF has potent vascular hyperpermeability effects during wound healing that may enhance the delivery of nutrients to the site of repair.[4] More importantly, VEGF transcription has been shown to not only be up-regulated by ischemia both in vitro and in vivo, but also in response to a variety of growth factors and cytokines.[3,9] In addition, VEGF messenger RNA (mRNA) is stabilized in response to hypoxia, increasing the availability of VEGF transcripts during ischemic conditions.[21-23]

The precise role VEGF plays in the wound healing process is unknown; however, given its known biological activity, VEGF could potentially be playing a prominent role in the repair process. In the following set of experiments, we tested the effect of exogenous VEGF 121 or VEGF 165 treatment in both ischemic and nonischemic wounds in the rabbit ear dermal ulcer model. These 2 isomers were chosen since they are readily available and seem to be the most biologically active in vivo. We assayed VEGF and bFGF mRNA levels in normal and ischemic skin and in wounds to highlight any possible differences between these growth factors in their response to an ischemic event.

RESULTS

EFFECT OF EXOGENOUS VEGF ON WOUND HEALING

Treatment of rabbit ear wounds with 0.1, 1.0, and 10 μg per wound of either isomer of VEGF had no statistically significant effect (data not shown), although there was a trend with higher doses for 10% to 15% improvement in new granulation tissue formation. Single-dose treatment of rabbit ear wounds with VEGF 121 or VEGF 165 at 30 μg per wound improved granulation tissue formation in both ischemic and nonischemic wounds. Ischemic wounds had 100% and 150% more granulation tissue at day 10 when treated with VEGF 121 and VEGF 165, respectively. Nonischemic wounds had 50% and 70% more granulation tissue at day 10 when treated with VEGF 121 and VEGF 165, respectively. The effect was greater in ischemic wounds using either isomer, and the magnitude of the effect was always greater with VEGF 165 (**Figure 1**). Neither VEGF isomer had an effect on new epithelium formation (**Figure 2**). **Figure 3** shows a representative histological specimen.

EFFECT OF ISCHEMIA AND WOUNDING ON bFGF AND VEGF mRNA LEVELS

To control for the reverse transcriptase step in our polymerase chain reaction protocol, every cDNA sample was assayed for glutaraldehyde phosphate dehydrogenase expression.[27,29] We found no significant difference in glutaraldehyde phosphate dehydrogenase expression in any of the cDNA samples used (**Figure 4**). Ischemia up-regulated VEGF mRNA expression 3- to 5-fold over nonischemic skin. The effect was seen as early as 1 day following the onset of ischemia and lasted through the duration of the experiment with a trend toward normalization (Figure 4, B). Wounding the skin up-regulated VEGF mRNA expression 6- to 7-fold, irrespective of whether the wound was ischemic. This effect was also seen at day 1 after wounding and persisted for 10 days after wounding (**Figure 5**). Basic fibroblastic growth factor expression was not significantly induced by ischemia, in fact there was a 2-fold reduction of bFGF mRNA levels in ischemic skin with a trend toward normalization by day 10 after wounding. Wounding alone increased bFGF mRNA levels less than 2-fold over normal skin in both ischemic and nonischemic wounds (**Figure 6**).

COMMENT

During wound healing an ordered sequence of events takes place that promotes the repair of injured tissues. This cascade of events is triggered by injury and ultimately leads to tissue regeneration, matrix deposition, and scar formation. Angiogenesis is a critical component of the wound healing response, with several growth factors potentially mediating the angiogenic response.

We have previously shown that bFGF, PDGF-BB, and transforming growth factor beta-1 have angiogenic properties in healing wounds and also promote granulation tissue formation, matrix deposition, and reepithelialization through different mechanisms.[15-17] Of these, bFGF and PDGF have a direct mitogenic effect on the endothelial cell and are considered to have direct angiogenic properties.[7] We have also shown with exhaustive experiments that bFGF improves wound healing in nonischemic wounds, but fails to do so in ischemic wounds.[16,17] Thus, the role of bFGF in impaired wound healing remains controversial. Basic FGF seems to improve wound healing in nonischemic models of impaired healing such as diabetic mice and steroid-treated animals[30,31]; however, a large clinical trial of bFGF in leg ulcers was stopped because no therapeutic effect was detected.[32] In 1995, Richard et al[33] in 1995 concluded that topical application of bFGF had no advantage over placebo for healing chronic neuropathic diabetic ulcers of the foot. It seems that bFGF may not be effective in impaired models of healing where ischemia is the culprit of the impairment. In light of these data, VEGF may be a more important regulator of angiogenesis and may help to promote wound healing in ischemic wounds. As shown by others, we were also able to detect a 2-fold decrease in bFGF mRNA levels in response to ischemia, an observation that may provide clues as to why bFGF fails to enhance wound healing in ischemic wounds despite improved angiogenesis, and it suggests that bFGF is not the prime mediator of angiogenesis in ischemic conditions.[7,34] We have also previously observed that bFGF regained biological activity within ischemic wounds when the rabbits were treated with hyperbaric oxygen.[17] These findings imply that oxygen-dependent signaling mechanisms may be required for bFGF activity in hypoxic wounds, and they highlight the potential importance of VEGF as a hypoxia-inducible factor during wound healing.

Vascular endothelial growth factor has biological properties that make it a more attractive modulator during ischemic wound healing than either bFGF or PDGF. Vascular endothelial growth factor mRNA transcription is induced by a variety of growth factors and cytokines. We have shown that VEGF mRNA transcription is not only induced by ischemia in rabbit skin but is also induced to a greater extent by tissue injury. The levels of VEGF mRNA were higher in wounded tissue (6- to 8-fold), irrespective of the

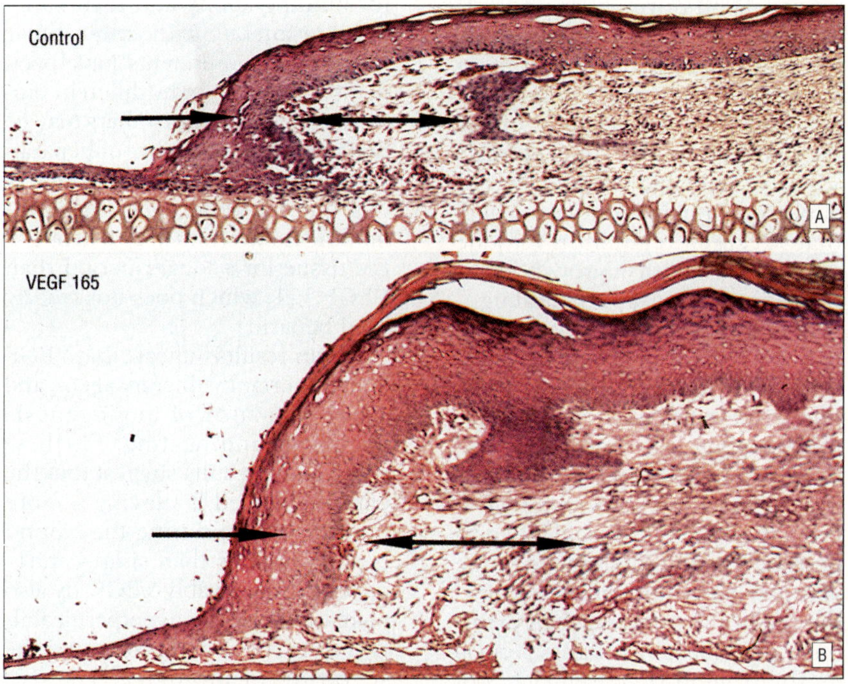

Figure 3. *Representative histological samples of each group. Top, Ischemic control group. Bottom, Ischemic wound treated with vascular endothelial growth factor 165. The single arrow points to new epithelium and the double arrow, granulation tissue.*

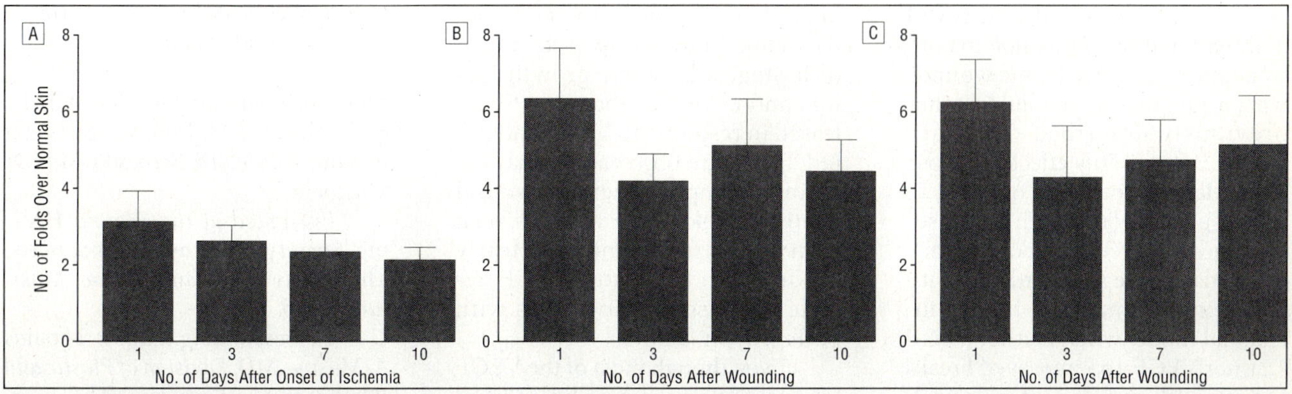

Figure 4. *A, Induction of vascular endothelial growth factor messenger RNA levels in response to ischemia. The y-axis is folded over nonischemic skin (n= 8 for each day,* P<.001 *for all days). B and C, Induction of vascular endothelial growth factor messenger RNA levels in response to wounding. B, Panel shows a nonischemic wound. C, Panel shows an ischemic wound. The y-axis is folded over nonischemic skin (n= 8 for each day,* P<.001 *for all days).*

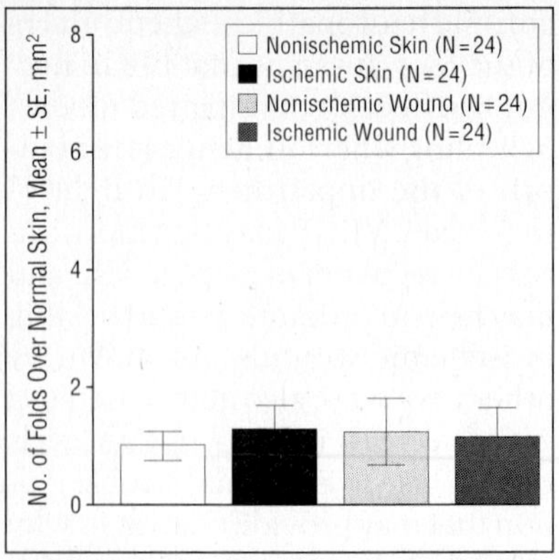

Figure 5. *Induction of glutaraldehyde phosphate dehydrogenase messenger RNA levels in response to ischemia and wounding. The y-axis is folded over nonischemic skin (n=8 for each day,* P<.001 *for all days).*

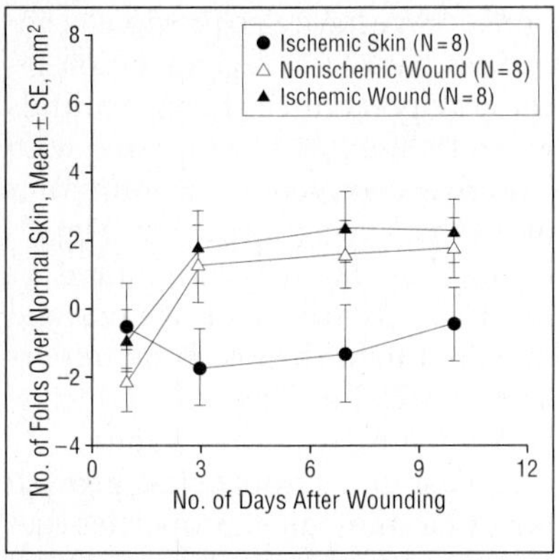

Figure 6. *Induction of basic fibroblastic growth factor messenger RNA levels in response to ischemia and wounding. The y-axis fold over nonischemic skin is increased (n=4 for each day). The only significant difference in this data is the fold increase in wounded tissue vs ischemic unwounded skin at days 3 and 7 (*P<.05*).*

tissue oxygen levels. Vascular endothelial growth factor is considered an important regulator of physiologic and pathologic angiogenesis and our data suggest that VEGF may also be an important modulator of ischemic wound healing.[21,34]

Exogenous VEGF improved granulation tissue formation in both ischemic and nonischemic wounds with a magnitude similar to other previously described vulnerary agents.[15-17,25,35] This effect was dose dependent, since doses of 0.1, 1.0, and 10 µg per wound with either isomer had no effect (data not shown). These data were in accordance with prior experiments done in a rat incisional model when neither VEGF 121 nor VEGF 165 improved breaking strength at day 7 after wounding with doses of 10 and 20 µg per wound (data not shown).[36]

All rabbit wounds treated with doses of either VEGF 121 or VEGF 165, of 30 µg per wound showed a notable increase over controls in the amount of granulation tissue formation. As expected, the magnitude of the effect was doubled in ischemic wounds. The fact that exogenous VEGF still had an effect on rabbit ear wounds despite maximal transcriptional up-regulation implies that either endogenous VEGF levels are not enough to saturate all VEGF receptors or exogenous VEGF has a local autoinductive effect on its own receptors at the wound site. Vascular endothelial growth factor receptors have been found to be up-regulated during wound healing[37] and have been shown to be up-regulated in the rat lung in response to ischemia.[38,39] Receptor up-regulation may account for the increased effect of exogenous VEGF in ischemic wounds. Recent data from our laboratory suggest that receptor regulation may be more important than growth factor regulation during wound healing.[29]

Increases in angiogenesis alone cannot entirely explain the observed improvement in granulation tissue, since bFGF fails to promote healing in ischemic wounds despite marked angiogenesis.[40] Among the other known biological properties of VEGF, vascular hyperpermeability in the wounded tissue may play a more prominent role during the healing process than previously described. Vascular hyperpermeability improves the efficiency of plasma protein delivery and cellular migration into the area of injury and is not a biological property of bFGF.[4,8,14] Moreover, the endothelial cell is known to secrete a host of biologically active growth factors and cytokines that may be released in response to VEGF and not bFGF. These 2 observations may explain the improvement in wound healing in ischemic wounds seen with VEGF treatment and clearly lacking with exogenous bFGF despite increased angiogenesis with both growth factors.

Even though most of the VEGF in wounds appears to be derived from dermal keratinocytes at the wound edge, VEGF did not notably affect epithelium formation in either ischemic or nonischemic wounds.[4,5] Unlike bFGF, which has a direct effect on dermal fibroblasts (the primary source of keratinocyte growth factor in the wound), VEGF affects only the endothelial cell that is not a keratinocyte growth factor–producing cell. This may explain in part the lack of effect seen with exogenous VEGF treatment in new epithelium formation.

We found that VEGF 165 was more potent than VEGF 121 in all parameters measured regardless of tissue ischemia. Although no biological differences between the 4 VEGF isoforms have been described, differences in their receptor-binding ability and their capability to interact with extracellular membrane components have been demonstrated.[19,41] The different bioactivity between the isomers may be due in part to the ability of heparan sulfates in the extracellular matrix to sequester VEGF 165, a heparin-binding isomer, and keep it active in the tissue for a longer period than VEGF 121, which does not readily bind heparin.

Our results indicate that VEGF is an important vulnerary agent, and a key regulator of angiogenesis during wound healing. Furthermore, these results suggest that the endothelial cell is playing a more prominent role during the wound healing process than simply mitogenesis. Conceivably VEGF, by also mediating vascular hyperpermeability in the tissue and promoting the secretion of biologically active growth factors and cytokines from the endothelial cell, has an important influence on the cascade of events necessary for normal and effective wound repair.

This work was supported in part by grant GM-41303, from the National Institutes of Health, Bethesda, Md (Dr Mustoe).

Presented at the Wound Healing Society Meeting, Minneapolis, Minn, May 1995, and Boston, Mass, June 1996.

Corresponding author: Thomas A. Mustoe, MD, Division of Plastic and Reconstructive Surgery, 707 E Fairbanks Ct, Suite 811, Chicago, IL 60611.

REFERENCES

1. Clark RF, Henson PM. *The Molecular and Cellular Biology of Wound Repair.* New York, NY: Plenum Publishing Corp; 1988.
2. Pierce GF, Mustoe TA. Pharmacologic enhancement of wound healing. *Ann Rev Med.* 1995;46:467-481.
3. Thomas KA. Vascular endothelial growth factor: a potent and selective angiogenic agent. *J Biol Chem.* 1996;271:603-606.
4. Brown LF, Yeo KT, Berse B, Morgentaler A, Dvorak HF, Rosen S. Expression of vascular permeability factor (vascular endothelial growth factor) by epidermal keratinocytes during wound healing. *J Exp Med* 1992;176:1375-1379.
5. Frank S, Hübner G, Breier G, Longaker MT, Greenhalh DG, Werner S. Regulation of vascular endothelial growth factor expression in cultured keratinocytes. *J Biol Chem.* 1995;270:12607-12613.
6. Detmar M, Yeo KT, Nagy JA, et al. Keratinocyte-derived vascular permeability factor (vascular endothelial growth factor) is a potent mitogen for dermal microvascular endothelial cells *J Invest Dermatol.* 1995;105:44-50.
7. Brogi E, Wu T, Namiki A, Isner JM. Indirect angiogenic cytokines upregulate VEGF and bFGF gene expression in vascular smooth muscle cells, whereas hypoxia upregulates VEGF expression only. *Circulation.* 1994;90:649-652.
8. Folkman J, Shing Y. Angiogenesis. *J Biol Chem.* 1992;267:10931-10934.
9. Leung DW, Cachianes G, Kuang WJ, Goeddel DV, Ferrara N. Vascular endothelial growth factor is a secreted angiogenic mitogen. *Science.* 1989;246:1306-1309.
10. Clauss M, Gerlach M, Gerlach H, et al. Vascular permeability factor: a tumor derived polypeptide that induces endothelial cell and monocyte procoagulant activity, and promotes monocyte migration. *J Exp Med.* 1990;172:1535-1545.
11. Pepper MS, Ferrara N, Orci L, Montesino R. Potent synergism between vascular endothelial growth factor and basic fibroblast growth factor in the induction of angiogenesis in vitro. *Biochem Biophys Res Commun.* 1992;189:824-831.
12. Goto F, Goto K, Weindel K, Folkman J. Synergistic effects of vascular endothelial growth factor and basic fibroblast growth factor on the proliferation of bovine capillary endothelial cells. *Lab Invest.* 1993;69:508-517.
13. Stavri GT, Zachary IC, Baskerville PA, Martin JF, Erusalimsky JD. Basic fibroblast growth factor upregulates the expression of vascular endothelial growth factor in vascular smooth muscle cells: synergistic interaction with hypoxia. *Circulation.* 1995;92:11-14.
14. Dvorak HF, Brown LF, Detmar M, Dvorak AM. Vascular permeability factor/vascular endothelial growth factor microvascular hyperpermeability, and angiogenesis. *Am J Pathol.* 1995:146:1029-1039.
15. Mustoe TA, Sang TA, Tarpley JE, Ahn ST, Pierce GF. Role of hypoxia in growth factor responses: differential effects of basic fibroblast growth factor and platelet-derived growth factor in an ischemic wound model. *Wound Repair Regeneration.* 1994;2:277-283.
16. Pierce GF, Tarpley JE, Yanagihara D, Mustoe TA, Fox GM, Thomason A. Platelet derived growth factor (BB homodimer), transforming growth factor beta-1 and basic fibroblast growth factor in dermal wound healing: neovessel and matrix formation and cessation of repair. *Am J Pathol.* 1992; 140:1375-1388.
17. Wu L, Pierce GF, Ladin DA, Zhao LL, Rogers D, Mustoe TA. Effects of oxygen in wound responses to growth factors: Kaposi's FGF, but not basic FGF stimulates repair in ischemic wounds. *Growth Factors.* 1995;12:29-35.
18. Ferrara N, Houck K, Jakeman L, Leung DW. Molecular and biological properties of the vascular endothelial growth factor family of proteins. *Endocr Rev.* 1992;13:18-32.
19. Cohen T, Gitay-Goren H, Sharon R, et al. VEGF 121, a vascular endothelial growth factor (VEGF) isoform lacking heparin binding ability, requires cell-surface heparan sulfates for efficient binding to the VEGF receptors of human melanoma cells. *J Biol Chem.* 1995;270:11322-11326.
20. Unemori EN, Ferrara N, Bauer EA, Amento EP. Vascular endothelial growth factor induces interstitial collagenase expression in human endothelial cells. *J Cell Physiol.* 1992;153:557-562.
21. Shweiki D, Itin A, Soffer D. Vascular endothelial growth factor induced by hypoxia may mediate hypoxia initiated angiogenesis. *Nature.* 1992;359:843-845.
22. Ikeda E, Achen MC, Breier G, Risau W. Hypoxia-induced transcriptional activation and increased mRNA stability of vascular endothelial growth factor in C6 glioma cells. *J Biol Chem.* 1995;270:19761-19766.
23. Levy AP, Levy NS, Goldberg MA. Post transcriptional regulation of vascular endothelial growth factor by hypoxia. *J Biol Chem.* 1996;271:2746-2753.
24. Ahn ST, Mustoe TA. Effects of ischemia on ulcer wound healing: a new model in the rabbit ear. *Ann Plast Surg.* 1990;24:17-23.
25. Mustoe TA, Pierce GF, Morishima C, Deuel TF. Growth factor-induced acceleration of tissue repair through direct and inductive activities in a rabbit dermal ulcer model. *J Clin Invest.* 1991;87:694-703.
26. Chomczynski P. A reagent for the single-step simultaneous isolation of RNA, DNA and proteins from cell and tissue samples. *Biotechniques.* 1993; 15:532-537.
27. Siebert PD, Larrick JW. Competitive PCR. *Nature.* 1992;359:557-558.
28. Siebert PD, Larrick JW. PCR MIMICS: competitive DNA fragments for use as internal standards in quantitative PCR. *Biotechniques.* 1993;14:244-249.
29. Brucker MJ, Gruskin E, Farrell CL, Siddiqui A, Mustoe TA. Differential expression of PDGF receptor-β in an aging model of wound repair. *Wound Repair Regeneration.* 1995;13:84.
30. Okumura M, Oruda T, Nakamura T, Yajima M. Effect of basic fibroblast growth factor on wound healing-impaired animal models. *Arzneimittelforschung.* 1996;45:547-551.
31. Tsuboi R, Rifkin DB. Recombinant basic fibroblast growth factor stimulates wound healing in healing-impaired db/db mice. *J Exp Med.* 1990; 172:245-251.
32. *Synergen Annual Report.* Boulder, Colo: Synergen Inc; 1992.
33. Richard JL, Parer-Richard C, Daures JP. Effect of topical basic fibroblast growth factor on the healing of chronic diabetic neuropathic ulcer of the foot: a pilot, randomized, double-blind, placebo-controlled study. *Diabetes Care.* 1995; 18:64-69.
34. Plate KH, Breier G, Millauer B, Ullrich A, Risau W. Up-regulation of vascular endothelial growth factor and its cognate receptors in a rat glioma model of tumor angiogenesis. *Cancer Res.* 1993;53: 5822-5827.
35. Pierce GF, Vande Berg J, Rudolph R, Trapley J, Mustoe TA. Platelet derived growth factor and transforming growth factor beta and selectively modulate glycosaminoglycans, collagens, and myofibroblasts in excisional wounds. *Am J Pathol.* 1991;138:629-646.
36. Mustoe TA, Pierce GF, Thomanson A, Gramates P, Sporn MB, Devel TF. Accelerated healing of incisional wounds in rats induced by transforming growth factor-beta. *Science.* 1987;237:1333-1336.
37. Peters KG, De Vries C, Williams LT. Vascular endothelial growth factor receptor expression during embryogenesis and tissue repair suggests a role in endothelial differentiation and blood vessel growth. *Proc Natl Acad Sci U S A.* 1993;90: 8915-8919.
38. Tuder RM. Flook BE, Voelkel NF. Increased gene expression for VEGF and the VEGF receptors KDR/Flk and Flt in lungs exposed to acute or to chronic hypoxia: modulation of gene expression by nitric oxide. *J Clin Invest.* 1995;95:1798-1807.
39. Plate KH, Breir G, Weich HA, Risau W. Vascular endothelial growth factor is a potential tumour angiogenesis factor in gliomas in vivo. *Nature.* 1992; 359:845-848.
40. Wu L, Zhao LL, Davidson DD, Wee SC, Roth SI, Mustoe TA. Effect of hyperbaric oxygen and growth factors on rabbit ear ischemic ulcers. *Arch Surg.* 1994;129:1043-1049.
41. Park JE, Keller GA, Ferrara N. The vascular endothelial growth factor (VEGF) isoforms: differential deposition into the subepithelial extracellular matrix and bioactivity of extracellular matrix-bound VEGF. *Mol Biol Cell.* 1993;4: 1317-1326.

Surgery in Nigeria

Olajide Olaolu Ajayi, FRCS, FWACS, FMCS(Nig); Clement Adebayo Adebamowo, FWACS

Nigeria, like most other developing countries, is today experiencing an increasing incidence of noncommunicable diseases and the unsolved problem of infectious diseases. The role of surgery in the management of these diseases has continued to increase. Surgical training has traditionally been of a high standard, and this has made it possible for surgeons trained in Nigeria to cope with this change in the spectrum of diseases. A low success rate at the diploma examinations and an increasing loss of local talent to foreign countries has increased calls for a modification of the training programs. There is a need to improve the working conditions and environment of surgeons to stem the attrition. Surgery in a poor resource environment demands more, rather than less, skill from the surgeon, and the training programs must ensure that the specialist is adequately equipped to deal with conditions that may not be considered general surgery. While the unavailability of modern technology has limited the scope of research, it is still possible to conduct appropriate, "low-tech," and relevant research that is subject to excellent study design, proper controls, and scientifically valid interpretations.

PREAMBLE

Nigeria is located in the Gulf of Guinea on the west coast of Africa. It has a land mass of 923 768 km^2 (about 356 669 sq mi), which makes it twice as large as California and 4 times the size of the United Kingdom. With a population estimated at 110 million, Nigeria is the most populous country in Africa. Selected health indicators from 1995 include an infant mortality rate of 87 per 1000 live births, a childhood mortality rate of 150 per 1000, a life expectancy at birth of 47.6 years, and a population growth rate of about 3%. The share of public health expenditure on health care in 1990 was 4.9%, which translates into 1.2% of the gross domestic product or gross national product. The physician-population ratio has fallen from 1:4300 in 1990 to 1:3707 in 1995. The population per hospital bed has risen from 1140 to 1477 during the same period.[1] The major causes of morbidity and mortality are malaria, dysentery, and pneumonia. With progressive industrialization and urbanization, Nigeria, like other developing countries, is experiencing an emerging pandemic of heart disease, cancer, hypertension, diabetes mellitus, sickle cell disease, and injuries.[2] Domestic, vehicular, and industrial injuries top the surgical problems in hospital practice. While there are about 14 000 health establishments in Nigeria, the centers where surgery is practicable are about 1100, excluding private clinics. These facilities include 15 accredited teaching hospitals associated with federal and state governments with an annually enrolled medical or health student population of more than 17 000. The teaching and specialist hospitals, of which there are currently 25, in addition to service and research, form the bastion of postgraduate medical education, which prepares candidates for the diploma of fellowship in surgery of the West African College of Surgeons and the Faculty of Surgery of the Nigerian National Postgraduate Medical College.

THE BEGINNING

The earliest recorded history of surgery in Africa dates back to Herophilus (circa 335-280 BC), who established the first medical school in the Alexandria of ancient Egypt. The early African practitioners of the art of

From the Department of Surgery, University College Hospital, Ibadan, Nigeria.

surgery founded the sciences of anatomy and physiology. They practiced such maneuvers as compression of the carotid arteries to induce loss of consciousness and of peripheral nerves to achieve regional analgesia. They described several surgical procedures for the management of injuries and ulcers, which were prevalent at that time.[3] Practices that were induced by social taboos and cultural demands also proliferated continentally. Many of these practices, like circumcisions, scarifications, and tattooing, cannot be considered surgery because they are not healing procedures by manipulation. Other procedures that were practiced include cataract extraction, cervical lymphadenectomy, and immobilization of limb fractures. Some other procedures were performed for dubious reasons, such as uvulectomy to treat a sore throat and clitoridectomy to ensure fidelity. It was the art without the science.

The first Portuguese expedition to West Africa in 1482 brought European medicine into contact with Africans for the first time. However, the European medicine of those days was largely empirical and not too different from the traditional practices prevalent in West Africa. The establishment of what could be identified as modern medicine did not take place until almost 400 years later when all European settlements in Nigeria passed to the British in 1850.[4] The initial health care service was devoted to the care of British soldiers, a process that accelerated when an epidemic destroyed the entire British garrison in 1756. With the formal colonization of Lagos, Nigeria, in 1850, health care services extended beyond military garrisons to colonial civil servants, excluding the local population. Missionary activities, however, resulted in increased health care services to ensure the good health of a select group of the local population, such as those working for the colonial government,[5] and also to ensure the propagation of religious faith.

UNDERGRADUATE TRAINING

The first recorded training of West African natives in Western medicine and surgery was in 1794 when a returned slave in Sierra Leone studied in the United Kingdom. He was Dr John Macauley Wilson. Two Nigerians were to follow more than 6 decades later: Dr William Broughton (of the Yoruba tribe), and Dr James Africannus Beale-Horton (of the Igbo tribe) who studied at the University of St Andrews and the University of Edinburgh in Scotland in 1858 and 1859, respectively.[4] The first attempt at local training followed in Nigeria with the formation of the first colonial hospital in 1861.[6] Of the initial intake of 4 trainees, 1 trainee became a medical practitioner in 1876. This program was probably not a formal training program and might have been the initiative of a colonial physician in search of assistants in the more mundane duties of a paramedical nature.

In 1932, the Higher College was established in Yaba, Lagos, with a medical program leading to a licentiate in medicine. The best students were enrolled there when the college took off in 1934. It was a peculiar institution in that the "pass list" was determined by the number of vacancies for assistant medical officers in the then colonial civil service.[7] Many of the successful students subsequently proceeded to the United Kingdom to sit for the licentiate of the Royal College of Physicians of London and the membership of the Royal College of Surgeons of England.

The Higher College was succeeded by the establishment of the University College in Ibadan, Nigeria, in 1948 as an affiliate of the University of London to award the degrees of bachelor of medicine and bachelor of surgery and other degrees. Local training was limited to the basic sciences, while the clinical part of the program was completed in various teaching hospitals in the United Kingdom pending the completion, equipment, and staffing of a teaching hospital (University College Hospital). By 1961, all parts of the training program were completed in Ibadan, and the students admitted from 1962 onward were awarded the MBBS degree of the University of Ibadan.

THE PROGRAM

With the advent of political independence in 1960, it became obvious that the workforce of the faculty of medicine in the University of Ibadan was never conceived to meet the health care needs of Nigeria. However, the proliferation of medical schools had to be tempered by the size of available funds. Equally important was the need to create a training program that was affordable and relevant to the health problems of the community and that would provide "sufficient acquaintance with fundamental principles of scientific methodology, some grounding in the art of clinical examination, a broad outline of human biology and the phenomenon of disease, an attitude of mind to learn on his own and an adequate sense of human values."[8] These broad objectives were pursued within the existing limitations and the realities of the policy so that by 1997, there were 15 medical schools in the country.

The curriculum of each medical school is the sole responsibility of the senate of the respective university. The law, however, empowers the Medical and Dental Council of Nigeria to provide guidelines on the minimum standards of medical education and accredit training institutions at prescribed intervals, ensuring the maintenance of such standards.[9] The council recognizes a clear distinction between basic medical sciences and the clinical sciences, although there are variations in some institutions that have integrated programs with a planned overlap between the 2 areas. The length of training is between 5 to 7 years depending on the student's educational level at entry into the course. The clinical part of the program lasts about 6 semesters, with at least a 2-month period spent working in a rural area. The surgery content of the course consists of 2 postings, each lasting at least 2 months, in general surgery: 1 posting in the surgical specialties, such as pediatric, cardiothoracic, urologic, neurologic, orthopedic, and plastic surgery and burns. Two postings are also undertaken in anesthesia, ophthalmology, and otorhinolaryngology. During the postings, the students are encouraged to have hands-on experience in every aspect of patient management. The period spent in rural settings provides the opportunity for more active involvement, decision making, and performing simple surgical procedures. The degree examination consists of 4 parts: Part I, anatomy, physiology, and biochemistry; Part II, pharmacology and pathology; Part III, pediatrics, obstetrics, and gynecology; and Part IV, surgery, medicine, and preventive and social medicine. To satisfy the examiners in each of the subjects, continuous assessment scores, which are based on attendance and participation in several clinical activities, and the marks earned at the end-of-postings tests are taken into consideration in determining the final results. Failure in the clinical part of the examination leads to failure of the whole examination.

POSTGRADUATE SURGICAL TRAINING

In the preindependence era and for about the following 2 decades, postgraduate certification in surgery could only be obtained in overseas institutions, particularly in the United Kingdom and the United States. Indeed, the first specialist surgeon in West Africa was a Nigerian who was admitted into the fellowship of the Royal College of Surgeons of Edinburgh in 1938.[4] The expanding health care services, the proliferation of medical schools, and the increasing reluctance of foreign institutions to accept a large number of trainees from the developing world forced a reappraisal of the strategies for postgraduate medical education in Nigeria. The need for self-reliance notwithstanding, the establishment of postgraduate medical education in Nigeria was also an opportunity to address the issues of training relevant to the environment, the development of skills appropriate to the socioeconomic status of the country, the availability of young trainees for service during the period of training, the opportunity to upgrade local facilities for service and research, and the containment of trained surgeons who remain in the overseas country of training.

The West African College of Surgeons grew from the Association of Surgeons of West Africa, which was founded in 1960. The decision to transform into a college was made in Accra, Ghana, in 1969. The association ceased to exist in 1973, when it transferred its assets and liabilities to the college in Benin City, Nigeria. The college prepared candidates and conducted examinations for the award of the fellowship diplomas of the college in anesthesia, dental surgery, obstetrics and gynecology, ophthalmology, otorhinolaryngology, radiology, and surgery. The programs in various faculties last 4 to 6 years depending on the areas of specialization and the availability of teachers in such specialties as neurosurgery and otorhinolaryngology. The program in surgery commences with the successful completion of the primary examinations, which consist of theory, practical, and oral examinations in anatomy, physiology, and pathology. The Part I examinations are taken at least 2 years later, after completing rotational posting in all the disciplines of surgery in accredited medical institutions anywhere in West Africa. The Part II examinations can be attempted after at least 2 more years of training, during which the candidate may opt for a particular specialty, such as urology, neurosurgery, orthopedic, pediatric, plastic, thoracic, and general surgery. The examinations in Parts I and II consist of written papers, multiple-choice questions, and clinical and oral sessions. No dissertation is required.

The Nigerian National Postgraduate Medical College was established by law in 1979 to be responsible for the postgraduate program of the Nigeria Medical Council, which had been in existence since 1970. The objective of the surgery component of the fellowship was "not to reproduce the University Postgraduate program in Surgery but to ensure a proficient training toward a specialist status in Surgery in Nigeria."[10] The diploma was acquired through a 5-year residency program that commenced after the compulsory preregistration year. The first 3 years were devoted to preliminary clinical training in the general principles of surgery apart from a 6-month course in basic sciences. The remaining 30 months were apportioned as follows: general and pediatric surgery (18 months); accident and emergency surgery (3 months); trauma and orthopedic surgery (3 months); ear, nose, and throat surgery (3 months); and neurosurgery and thoracic surgery (3 months). At the end of the postings, the candidate attempted the Part I examinations of the diploma of fellowship by writing 4 papers, with 3 hours for each paper, on the general principles of surgery, applied anatomy, applied physiology and biochemistry, and general principles of pathology. In addition, there was a clinical examination in surgery and an oral and practical examination in anatomy and physiology. The second phase of training leading to the Part II examinations was to specialize in a particular branch of surgery. The training period was for at least 2 years. At the end of this period, the candidate took an examination in general surgery, consisting of 2 written papers, with 3 hours for each paper, and clinical and oral examinations. Each candidate was required to present a dissertation or a casebook in the area of specialty, with comments on existing literature. The program has since been approximated to the West African college format except that a dissertation is still required. To supplement local training, a 1-year position at a surgical center abroad was undertaken, but this was difficult to organize and, in any case, has now become unaffordable in view of the present economic situation.

THE CONTENT

It is tempting to accept a surgical training program geared to the local circumstances and the local geographical pathologic conditions. The surgical training program in Nigeria strictly forbids this concept. One of us (O.O.A.) had the following to say on the matter more than a decade ago:

> To train a surgeon locally because he is expected to practice locally irrespective of the facilities available and without regard to a defined minimum standard is to destroy the image and value of surgical care. To base training only on local disease patterns is a failure to appreciate the "non-static" nature of geographical pathology. To equate training with practice is not to recognize that the latter is only partially the product of the former. The acquisition of basic knowledge and skills which allow for professional self-development and adaptation is the core of good training and it is independent of geographical pathology or the venue of training.[11]

The apparently comprehensive curriculum and the stiff examination processes result from the recognition that the poorer the available facilities, the greater the skills required in the practice of surgery. The surgeon working in isolation in a rural hospital with limited ancillary service triumphs only by a higher degree of technical competence, judgment, and experience. In addition to theoretical knowledge, the quality of clinical skills and evidence of adequate hands-on experience are keenly sought in prospective candidates for certification. To fail the clinical part of the examinations is tantamount to failure of the whole. The comprehensive education also explains the relative ease with which Nigerian-trained surgeons fit into a more sophisticated practice after becoming familiar with new technology.

THE CRITIQUE

It is the view of many that the demands of the surgical program cannot "appreciably increase the number of Fellows in the key disciplines in the future."[12] They further contend that the program "will ultimately be judged by its impact on the quality of healthcare in the country; not on how much expertise each of its products has." Even if the objective is to produce "mini-academicians," they think the current rate of production is outstripped by demand. Therefore, they advocate a "membership diploma" (as opposed to the current fellowship diploma) for successful candidates in the Part I examinations so that not becoming a fellow does not hinder "further career opportunities."[12]

The opposite view is that to lower the hurdle that has been set to meet the minimum standard of a Nigerian surgical specialist makes no sense since there is a need to set the minimum standard of surgical competence in the first place. Lowering the minimum standard might bring the art and science of surgery into public odium since the patients have no way of preselecting "well-baked" and "half-baked" surgeons. They averred that it would lead to a continual downward revision of standards and create a cycle of poor-quality surgeons to train even poorer-quality successors. To compromise the minimum desirable standard of postgraduate training, they argued, is to undermine the quality of surgical services, teaching, and research.[13] They contend that it would be socially divisive and would shift the focus from what we should be doing to correct the situation in the long term.

Both groups agree that what is required is a rational, pragmatic, sustainable, and balanced health care system that is adequately funded and efficiently administered. The answer would seem to be a higher investment in surgical training by upgrading the facilities and the provision of adequate remuneration and reward for the trainees and trainers. New knowledge in the health sciences, explosive advances in technology (with the consequential fragmentation and superspecialization in surgery), and a greater awareness of human rights in all communities of the world adds up to the need for higher, not lower, standards in training.

RESULTS

The high standards expected of successful candidates sitting for these examinations reflect the surgical needs of Nigeria and the circumstance of practice. A successful candidate has attained a consultant status in the practice of surgery, is potentially capable of further self-development, and is equipped to lead a health care team. In quantitative terms, the critics have a point, as evidenced by the examination results since inception. **Table 1** is particularly informative with respect to the West African College of Surgeons since the commencement of its examinations in 1979. The number of attempts does not correlate with the number of candidates because repeated efforts were plentiful. The situation is similar in the Faculty of Surgery of the Nigerian National Postgraduate Medical College. From the records available from 1972 to September 1997, a total of 2473 attempts were made at the primary examinations, while 1296 and 367 attempts were made in Part I and Part II of the examinations, respectively. The number of candidates who actually completed the program is 140. The total number of surgeons produced during the periods by the 2 examining bodies is not additive because some candidates successfully attempted both examinations. Many of the eligible candidates for the Part II examination did not sit for the examination since they may have recommenced training in Canada, the United States, and Europe in search of better remuneration and a much more "enabling environment" for training.[14] It is estimated that the Nigerian surgeons in practice in Canada, the United States, Europe, the Gulf states, and South Africa exceed the number of those in Nigeria.

THE SPECTRUM

The spectrum of surgical practice is a reflection of the disease pattern. The 3-tier stratification of the health care delivery system in Nigeria (primary, secondary, and tertiary care) corresponds to the level of surgical sophistication available at different levels. Gastroenterologic, urologic, orthopedic, cardiothoracic, oncologic, plastic and reconstructive, otorhinolaryngologic, endocrine, and vascular surgery are almost exclusively performed at tertiary health care centers, while primary health care surgery is limited to emergency first-aid care of minor trauma, suturing lacerations, splinting fractures, and incising and draining abscesses. The surgery often done is the surgery of trauma, infections, and neglect.[15] The largest group of surgical cases is found at the secondary level of health care. In a 14-year review of a secondary level surgical practice, external hernia repair constituted 56.1% of the procedures undertaken, excision of superficial lumps about 11.5%, and abdominal emergencies, such as intestinal obstruction, peritonitis, and ruptured spleen, about 7.7% (**Table 2**).[16] The broad-based training necessary for service in rural areas and those areas understaffed by physicians includes skills in cesarean sections, vesicovaginal fistula, and other gynecologic procedures. Surgery for tropical conditions, such as elephantiasis, chronic granulomatous diseases, ameboma, and African histoplasmosis, typically accounts for only 12% of operations.[17] Some of these conditions, though common in the tropics, are also seen in other parts of the world. What is characteristic of Nigeria is that patients with advanced disease tend to seek care in an environment where there are limited resources to cope with them.

Table 1. Number of Students Who Participated and Passed the Fellowship Examinations of the Faculty of Surgery, West African College of Surgeons, 1979-1997*

	No. of Students					
	Primary		Part I		Part II	
Year	Participated	Passed (%)	Participated	Passed (%)	Participated	Passed (%)
1979	27	2 (7.4)	. . .	. . .	. . .	. . .
1980	33	7 (21.2)	. . .	. . .	. . .	. . .
1981	56	13 (23.2)	4	2 (50.0)	. . .	. . .
1982	90	14 (15.5)	10	1 (10.0)	. . .	. . .
1983	109	11 (10.1)	15	5 (33.3)	. . .	. . .
1984	127	19 (15.0)	21	5 (23.8)	. . .	. . .
1985	118	19 (16.1)	21	5 (23.8)	3	1 (33.3)
1986	130	26 (20.0)	24	3 (12.5)	9	5 (55.6)
1987	197	36 (18.3)	32	10 (31.3)	10	6 (60.0)
1988	220	44 (20.0)	71	14 (19.7)	5	3 (60.0)
1989	204	22 (10.8)	114	38 (33.3)	11	2 (18.2)
1990	177	28 (15.5)	106	38 (35.8)	11	5 (45.5)
1991	184	51 (27.7)	93	18 (19.4)	26	9 (34.6)
1992	205	39 (19.0)	116	29 (25.0)	39	11 (28.2)
1993	209	38 (18.2)	122	35 (28.7)	56	19 (33.9)
1994	251	44 (17.5)	138	37 (26.8)	58	25 (43.1)
1995	196	47 (24.0)	122	35 (28.7)	49	16 (32.7)
1996	177	42 (23.7)	115	32 (27.8)	69	31 (44.9)
1997	218	64 (29.4)	134	33 (24.6)	71	22 (31.0)

**Source: Executive Secretary, West African Postgraduate Medical College, Lagos, Nigeria. Ellipses indicate that there were no candidates.*

Rural surgery is not primitive surgery or inferior surgery and may require more surgical capability beyond the conventional definition of the limits of general surgery. The absence of anesthetists adds to the professional competence required since all the procedures in the review were performed under spinal, intravenous, or local infiltration with lidocaine (Xylocaine; Astra USA Inc, Westboro, Mass).

RESEARCH

Without research, most of the diseases that are now well known and characterized in this environment would still be considered rare or nonexistent. Identifying local risk factors within the complex web of etiological factors in cross-cultural analytic studies is a worthwhile research activity even in a depressed economic situation. The unavailability of modern technology need not make impossible appropriate and relevant research that is subject to excellent study design, proper controls, and scientifically valid interpretations.[18] It did not require much, if any, technology to demonstrate the cost-effectiveness of the ambulatory management of spinal tuberculosis or the relative safety of outpatient surgery that was initially dictated by the necessity to control the cost of health care. The other areas of significant contributions are in neurosurgery (head injuries due to missiles and subgaleal dermoid cyst in children), oncologic surgery (Burkitt lymphoma and breast and malignant trophoblastic disease), endocrinologic surgery (thyroidectomy), plastic and reconstructive surgery (immunologic characteristics of keloid and craniofacial anomalies), and orthopedic surgery (sickle cell disease).

Although there is a national institute for medical research in Nigeria, research support for surgery has been minimal. Most research efforts are at the institutional level,

Table 2. Surgical Practice in Eruwa, 1983-1997*

Type of Operation	No. (%) of Procedures
External hernia repair	4190 (56.1)
Excision of lumps	860 (11.5)
Hydrocelectomy	450 (6.0)
Orchiopexy	70 (1.0)
Prostatectomy	227 (3.0)
Vagotomy and pyloroplasty or gastrojejunostomy	86 (1.2)
Thyroidectomy	71 (1.0)
Sequestrectomy	60 (0.8)
Nephrectomy	10 (0.1)
Cesarean section	490 (6.6)
Intestinal obstruction	130 (1.7)
Peritoneal abscesses and infections	440 (5.9)
Gynecologic procedures	175 (2.3)
Chest tube insertion	65 (1.0)
Management of major open fractures	35 (0.5)
Splenectomy	13 (0.1)
Others	100 (1.3)
Total	**7472 (100)**

**Adapted from Awojobi.[16]*

usually privately funded or funded in collaboration with nongovernmental international organizations. Yet the need for research is greater than ever before if only for the promotion of health, the prevention of disease, the identification of the changing pattern of disease, operational research for decision making, and the critical scientific appraisal of the value of some aspects of alternative medicine in surgical care. The forums for the exchange of information include organized scientific lectures under the aegis of professional associations, scientific meetings of the Nigerian Surgical Research Society, conferences of the West African College of Surgeons, the Nigerian National Postgraduate Medical College, and the Nigerian chapter of the International College of Surgeons, to mention a few. Dissemination of research findings is further promoted through publication in local journals, especially the *African Journal of Medicine and Medical Sciences*, the *Nigerian Journal of Surgery*, and the *West African Journal of Medicine*.

FINANCE

Since surgery is a hospital-based discipline, it is, unlike other interventionist options in health care, very expensive. Increasingly sophisticated surgery and biotechnology has been adding to the cost of health care, which developing countries cannot afford or contain.[19] The structural adjustment programs of international creditors, which are being imposed on poor countries with no structures to adjust, have further widened the gap between hope and reality.[20] Devaluation of national currencies and the collapse of apparently emerging markets have reduced social service expenditures in those countries to a trickle. The danger is that there may be no growth in surgical capabilities but, instead, a reduction to the level of an inglorious past. The large movement of people and material all over the world, the rapid changes in rural lifestyles, and increasing urbanization in developing countries are making new demands on sophisticated health care through changing geographical pathologic conditions. Cost-containment strategies will have to dictate the pattern of surgical services or further promote the rationing of surgical care. New indications for surgery are beginning to emerge from cost-effectiveness studies, cost-benefit analyses, and cost-containment activities.

Diminishing access to surgical care through prohibitive user fees have already altered the bed occupancy of teaching hospitals and changed the frequency ratios of diseases for the balanced instruction and experience of medical students and surgical trainees, respectively. In the socioeconomic circumstance of Nigeria, a meaningful health care standard, particularly in surgery, will depend on public funding for some time to come, notwithstanding the other options available for health care financing. In this situation, the state stands as the coordinator and guarantor of égalité and social justice in health care. Community involvement in the management of health care institutions will enhance efficiency and encourage patients to make financial contributions to their welfare while curtailing waste and abuse of the system. For the very poor and certain categories of patients (for example, children, pregnant women, and patients with communicable diseases), a system for exemptions will still be necessary.

CONCLUSION

This discourse on the current state of surgery in Nigeria is not meant to glorify the past, vilify the present, and destroy hope for the future. A forthright appraisal is the first step in determining the size of the problem and the prospect for a satisfactory amendment. No poor country has an excellent workforce development program or health care services. Economic prosperity must be sought before all other things can be added to it. Nigeria needs to accelerate relevant and appropriate development of the workforce, as it has done in the past, and create a scheme to safeguard its investment, as it has not done in the past, by measures suggested herein. Our training programs must be relevant, flexible, and adaptable to reflect our needs at all the 3 tiers of the health care system, and we cannot lose touch with new developments and technologies that can be used to manage the changing patterns of disease or the emergence of a new pandemic of diseases common in industrialized countries. The acquisition of management skills to ensure maximum returns from limited resources is an inevitable course for a brighter future. Specialization and new sophistication must be available to add to the skills of the Nigerian surgeon at the apex of the health care delivery system. Superspecialization and increasing fragmentation of surgical disciplines are not the pressing issues of surgical development in Nigeria at the moment. The reality of health care financing points to more effort at epidemiological and health care system research than laboratory animal research. The ability to make virtue out of necessity is the greatest and immediate challenge of all.

Reprints: Olajide Olaolu Ajayi, FRCS, FWACS, FMCS (Nig), Department of Surgery, University College Hospital, PMB 5116, Ibadan, Oyo State, Nigeria (e-mail: jide.ajayi@skannet.com.ng).

REFERENCES

1. United Nations Development Program. *Nigerian Human Development Report.* Lagos, Nigeria: United Nations Development Program; 1996.
2. Akinkungbe OO. *Non-communicable Diseases in Nigeria.* Lagos: Federal Ministry of Health and Human Services of Nigeria; 1992.
3. Solanke TF. Our surgical heritage. Ninth Sir Samuel Manuwa Memorial Lecture presented at: West African College of Surgeons; January 24, 1996; Lagos, Nigeria.
4. Easmon CO. The beginning. Second Sir Samuel Manuwa Memorial Lecture presented at: West African College of Surgeons; January 27, 1982; Lagos, Nigeria.
5. Ajayi OO. The irrelevancies of our endeavors. Lecture presented at: West African Society of Gastroenterology; May 10, 1990; Lagos, Nigeria.
6. Adeloye A. *African Pioneers of Modern Medicine.* Ibadan, Nigeria: University Press; 1985.
7. Majekodunmi MA. Health Services Administration in Nigeria. First Sir Samuel Memorial Lecture presented at: West African College of Surgeons; January 29, 1980; Enugu, Nigeria.
8. Esan GJF. *Priorities in National Health Planning: Proceedings of an International Symposium.* Akinkugbe OO, Olatunbosun D, Esan GJF, eds. Ibadan, Nigeria: 1973: 213-218.
9. *Guidelines on Minimum Standards of Medical Education.* Lagos: The Medical and Dental Council of Nigeria; 1984.
10. *Nigerian Medical Council (Postgraduate Examinations) Regulations, 1970.* Lagos: Nigerian Medical Council; 1970.
11. Ajayi OO. The effects of local pathology and disease patterns on the training and practice of surgery. *Trans Coll Med South Afr.* 1987;31:161-164.
12. Ikeme AC. The triumph of hope over experience. Fourteenth convocation lecture presented at: National Postgraduate Medical College; September 12, 1996; Lagos, Nigeria.
13. Ajayi OO. The life and times of Professor Abayomi Bandele Bandipo. First Bandele Bandipo Memorial Lecture presented at: Medical and Dental Consultants Association of Nigeria; November 6, 1996; Lagos, Nigeria.
14. Ajayi OO. Surgical training in 21st-century Africa. Keynote address presented at: Pan-African Association of Surgeons (PAAS); January 22, 1998; Abuja, Nigeria.
15. Barker EA. Surgical techniques and priorities. *Trop Doct.* 1995;25(suppl 1):27-29.
16. Awojobi OA. Principles of rural surgical practice. *Dokita.* 1998;25:161-162.
17. Holcombe C. Is experience overseas useful for the trainee surgeon? *Trop Doct.* 1995;25(suppl 1):73-76.
18. Lucas AO. *Health Research for Humankind.* Geneva, Switzerland: World Health Organization; 1996.
19. Gunn SWA. How can the World Health Organisation help? In: Cook J, ed. *The International Federation of Surgical Colleges Papers, 1958-1979.* Edinburgh, Scotland: The International Federation of Surgical Colleges; 1982:117-120.
20. Ajayi OO. The responsibility of established colleges to the developing world. *Aust N Z J Surg.* 1994;64:4-6.

Laparoscopic Adrenalectomy

Roberto V. Barresi, MD; Richard A. Prinz, MD

Advances in minimally invasive surgery have made it possible to remove solid organs such as the adrenal gland laparoscopically. Several studies have shown that when applied to appropriate operative candidates, laparoscopic adrenalectomy is a safe alternative to conventional open surgery with real advantages in terms of decreasing postoperative pain and length of hospital stay and allowing earlier return to normal activity. The indications for laparoscopic adrenalectomy are essentially the same as those described for open adrenalectomy. We do not recommend laparoscopic adrenalectomy for known primary or metastatic malignant tumors of the adrenal glands, because of the risk of tumor implantation that might compromise the patient's chance for cure, nor do we recommend it for lesions larger than 6 to 8 cm where the chance of malignancy is high. The preoperative preparation, laparoscopic instruments, operative techniques, and potential complications and their treatments are described in this review. Laparoscopic adrenalectomy is becoming the preferred method of surgically treating many adrenal problems. Although conventional surgical approaches will undoubtedly be required to treat certain adrenal lesions, surgeons with an interest in treating patients with adrenal disorders must become proficient in the technique of laparoscopic adrenalectomy. This will allow them to select the most appropriate operative approach for their patients' individual problems.

Arch Surg. 1999;134:212-217

Surgical removal of the adrenal glands has traditionally been undertaken with a reasonable degree of trepidation. These paired glands are small, friable, highly vascular, and positioned deep within the retroperitoneum.[1,2] They are situated between the level of the 11th thoracic and first lumbar vertebrae, and lie within the periadrenal adipose tissue. The right adrenal gland occupies a position superomedial to the right kidney, close to the bare area of the liver, and slightly lateral and posterior to the inferior vena cava. The left adrenal gland lies in a similar superomedial position to its corresponding kidney, in close proximity to the tail of the pancreas and splenic artery. As such, safe removal of the adrenal glands involves anatomical knowledge of, and careful attention to, the infradiaphragmatic great vessels and viscera.[3] Because of the difficulty in obtaining adequate exposure of these glands, several different surgical approaches have been used. Conventional means of gaining access to the adrenal glands have included the anterior (transabdominal), posterior (through the bed of the 12th rib), and lateral (thoracoabdominal) approaches.[4,5] While each of these operative methods has its respective merits and pitfalls, alternative approaches for safe adrenal surgery have long been sought.

In 1992, laparoscopic adrenalectomy was first described by Gagner et al[6] in 3 patients. A larger series soon validated the application of minimally invasive surgical techniques for the removal of the adrenal glands.[7] Numerous investigators have subsequently shown that this approach, when applied to appropriate operative candidates, is a safe alternative to conventional open surgery.[8]

In general, we have limited laparoscopic adrenalectomy to lesions that are smaller than 6 to 8 cm. With few excep-

From the Department of General Surgery, Rush-Presbyterian-St Luke's Medical Center, Chicago, Ill.

tions, indications for laparoscopic removal of the adrenal gland are essentially the same as those described for open adrenalectomy.[9] The indications for laparoscopic adrenalectomy are (1) Cushing syndrome due to a benign cortisol-producing adenoma; (2) Cushing disease that has not improved with other forms of therapy; (3) Conn syndrome, due to a unilateral adenoma; (4) benign-appearing pheochromocytomas that are located in the adrenal glands (although some surgeons have reported laparoscopic removal of extra-adrenal pheochromocytomas and malignant pheochromocytomas, we would caution against this because of variations in vascular anatomy in the former, and the possibility of inadequate curative resection in the latter); (5) nonfunctioning adenomas or incidentalomas that meet accepted criteria for open adrenalectomy, such as size between 4 and 6 cm or increase in size during observation; and (6) benign lesions, such as angiomyolipomas, that are symptomatic. We have not recommended laparoscopic adrenalectomy for primary or metastatic malignant tumors of the adrenal gland because of the risk of tumor implantation, which would compromise the patient's chance for cure.[10]

Preoperative imaging is critically important not only to demonstrate the size and location of the abnormality, but also the relationship to surrounding structures. For example, a large right lobe of the liver that extends down toward the pelvis may make access to the right adrenal gland difficult, if not impossible. Likewise, the variable location of the left adrenal gland can be better anticipated by preoperative imaging. Our preferred method of obtaining this information is spiral computed tomographic scanning. Although others may favor magnetic resonance imaging, we have not usually found that it adds any appreciable information. With hormone-producing lesions, the diagnosis should be secure, fluid and electrolyte deficits corrected, and the state of the hormone excess be reversed or blocked, if possible, prior to undertaking adrenalectomy.

SURGICAL TECHNIQUE

The necessary equipment for laparoscopic adrenalectomy includes standard television monitors (located on both sides of the operating table, toward the head of the patient), a high-volume insufflator, 10/11-mm trocars, a video camera, and a reliable irrigation/suction device. **Figure 1** demonstrates the standard operating room setup for the procedure. Additional equipment and instrumentation that may be needed include a 30° angled scope, 5-mm blunt "peanut"-type probes, a "fan"-type retractor, angled dissectors, blunt dissectors (large and small), and automatic clip appliers. An endovascular stapler is rarely needed, but should be available. Some surgeons find the "harmonic scalpel" to be useful, but we do not use it routinely. As with all laparoscopic surgical procedures, a complete laparotomy tray should be present in the operating room and available for immediate use, should there be a need to convert to an open procedure.

Laparoscopic adrenalectomy is performed under general anesthesia. The patient is intubated and anesthetized while supine, and then repositioned for the procedure. A Foley catheter, compression stockings for venous thrombosis prophylaxis, and any necessary invasive monitoring devices (arterial line, central venous pressure monitor, or pulmonary artery catheter) should be placed before positioning the patient for the operation. Prophylactic antibiotics are not indicated for this clean procedure. It is, however, prudent to perform mechanical bowel preparation since the colon will be mobilized and retracted in the course of the procedure. Just as for open adrenalectomy, there are a variety of minimally invasive approaches for laparoscopic adrenalectomy.[4] We favor the lateral transperitoneal approach as described by Gagner et al,[6,8] as it yields the most direct access to the ipsilateral gland and its attendant blood supply. The transperitoneal approach provides a large working space with anatomy that is familiar to most general surgeons. This approach reduces the need for extensive retraction of the inferior vena cava and precludes the need for broad mobilization of nearby organs.

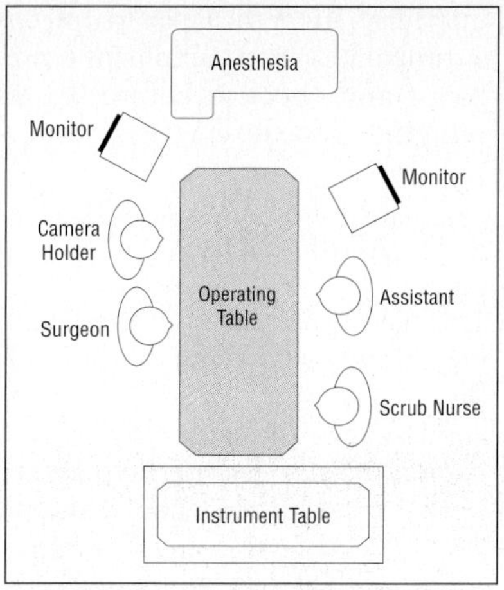

Figure 1. *The operating room setup for laparoscopic left adrenalectomy is depicted.*

Patient positioning is very important with the lateral transperitoneal approach. The patient is placed in the lateral decubitus position. This allows the viscera to fall away by gravity from the area of dissection. To maximize the region between the lower ribs and the iliac crest, the operating table should be flexed to stretch this area by lowering the head and legs. The table should have a kidney rest, and the patient's contralateral flank area between the 12th rib and the iliac crest should be positioned on it. The kidney rest should be elevated to magnify the flexion and push the adrenal gland and kidney on the side of the operation up and away from the other retroperitoneal structures. An axillary roll is placed, and careful padding of all pressure points is done to prevent any nerve or skin injury. Once the patient and the table are properly positioned, a safety belt or strap and wide adhesive tape are used to secure the patient on the operating table. This is important because the table will be rotated from side to side, and from Trendelenburg position to reverse Trendelenburg position, to use gravity and position for optimal retraction and exposure. The surgical drapes leave exposed the entire area between the spine laterally, the costal margin superiorly, just beyond the midline medially (including the periumbilical area in case an open trocar insertion at the navel is required), and the iliac crest inferiorly. All of the laparoscopic instrumentation and equipment is prepared and checked before beginning the procedure.

LEFT LAPAROSCOPIC ADRENALECTOMY

The patient is placed in the lateral decubitus position with the right side down. The surgeon stands on the right side of the table, as does the camera holder, facing the patient's anterior abdomen. The assistant stands on the left side. The table is then rotated slightly away from the surgeon. This places the left midclavicular line in a superior position. A Veress needle is placed into the peritoneal cavity approximately 1 to 2 cm below the costal margin. Three layers of fascia have to be penetrated. Standard methods of confirming the intraperitoneal position of the needle are performed before beginning insufflation. If there is difficulty placing the Veress needle, uncertainty about its position, or if the patient has undergone prior abdominal surgery, an open approach should be used, usually in the periumbilical region. Carbon dioxide pneumoperitoneum to a pressure of 15 mm Hg is then established. A 10/11-mm trocar is placed 1 finger breadth below the costal margin, in the midclavicular line. The laparoscope is passed through this trocar into the peritoneal cavity. A straight or angled scope can be used, depending on the operator's preference. The abdomen is surgically explored through this initial port. Under direct vision, 3 additional 10/11-mm trocars are placed in the anterior, mid, and posterior left axillary lines, just below the costal margin. **Figure 2** demonstrates the preferred positions of each of the trocars. The incisions for the trocars should be aligned, if possible, so they can be connected as a single incision should conversion to an open operation become necessary. While 4 trocars generally provide an adequate number of camera and operating ports, one should not hesitate to place an additional cannula if needed.

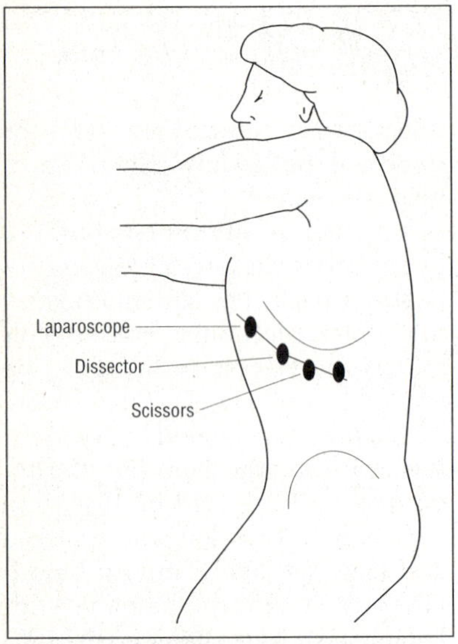

Figure 2. *The patient is placed in a lateral decubitus position for laparoscopic left adrenalectomy. Trocars (10/11 mm) are placed in the subcostal region in the midclavicular line and in the anterior, mid, and posterior axillary lines. Trocar incisions are placed along a line, allowing them to be connected by a single incision in the event that conversion to an open procedure becomes necessary.*

Using endoscopic scissors, blunt dissectors, and judicious use of electrocautery, the splenic flexure and descending colon are mobilized, as is the spleen (**Figure 3**). The splenocolic ligament is divided, displacing the spleen superiorly and medially, and the transverse colon and splenic flexure inferiorly and medially. This maneuver gains access to the retroperitoneum. The tail of the pancreas is usually visualized at this point (**Figure 4**). It can, however, be mistaken for the left adrenal gland. Obviously, it should be treated with respect and retracted gently. As the dissection proceeds, the left kidney and adrenal gland should come into view. In some instances, the left adrenal gland is not readily apparent within the substance of the periadrenal fat. We have found in such situations that the use of laparoscopic ultrasound is helpful in delineating the gland. Dissection of the adrenal gland begins at the superior pole, and moves in a superior to inferior direction. Moderate blunt dissection may be used in the areolar tissue surrounding the gland, but excessive manipulation is to be avoided. The inferior phrenic arterial branches supplying the adrenal gland are usually small enough to allow them to be safely transected with cautery. If they are larger, they can be clipped and divided. Some surgeons use the harmonic scalpel for

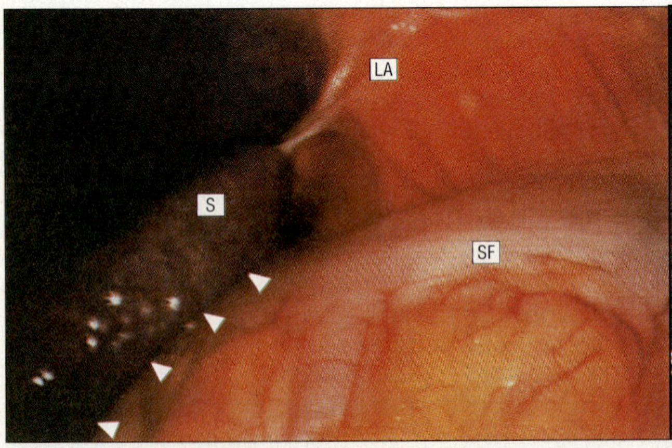

Figure 3. *Laparoscopic left adrenalectomy requires mobilization of several structures. Seen here are the spleen (S), its lateral attachments (LA), and the splenic flexure of the colon (SF). Entrance into the left retroperitoneum is achieved by dividing the splenocolic ligament (indicated by arrowheads). Division of the lateral attachments allows adequate splenic displacement.*

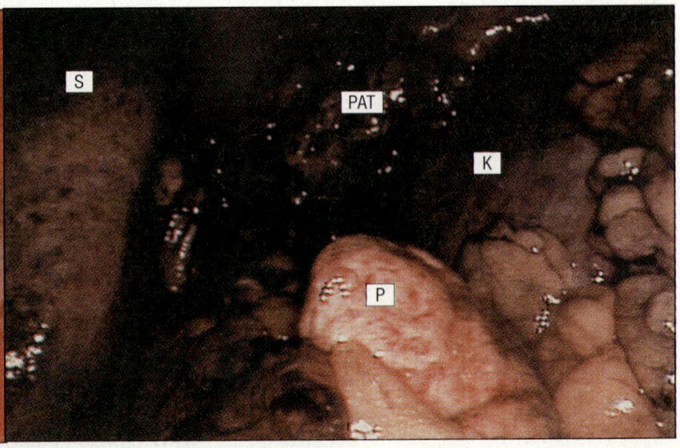

Figure 4. *Once the retroperitoneum is entered, the tip of the pancreas (P), kidney (K), and periadrenal adipose tissue (PAT) are seen. Note the superomedial displacement of the spleen (S).*

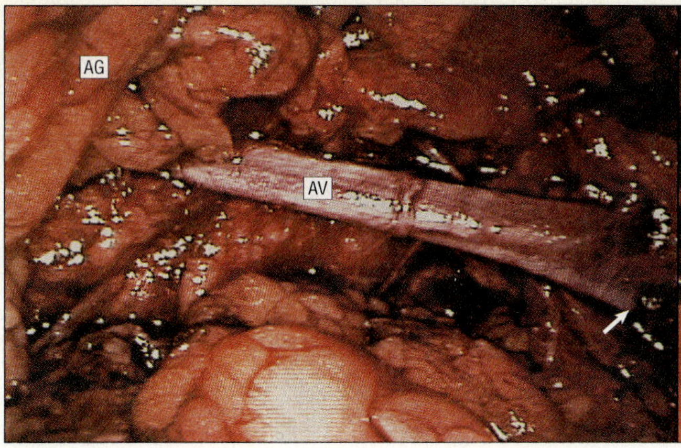

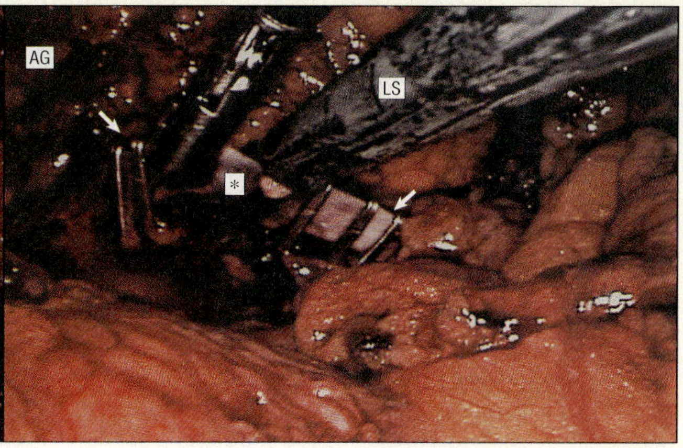

Figure 5. *The adrenal gland (AG) is identified within its periadrenal adipose tissue. The adrenal vein (AV) is well visualized as it enters the left renal vein (arrow). Caution must be exercised to avoid injury to the renal vessels at this point in the operation.*

Figure 6. *The adrenal gland (AG) and adrenal vein (asterisk) have been mobilized. Note the placement of the titanium clips (arrows)—3 on the side that enters the renal vein, 2 on the side of the specimen. The vein is then divided between clips with laparoscopic scissors (LS).*

this portion of the dissection, but we have not found it necessary. Dissection is continued to expose the arterial branches arising from the aorta, which are similarly divided with cautery. The central vein, often seen in its entirety as it joins the left renal vein, is likewise identified, clipped (or ligated), and divided (**Figure 5** and **Figure 6**). The surgeon must be careful not to mistake the renal vein for the adrenal vein and to avoid injury to the renal artery. The adrenal gland should not be grabbed or retracted directly. It is best to dissect in the periadrenal fat to be sure that the entire gland is removed and that the capsule is not entered. Once the gland has been completely mobilized and dissected from surrounding structures, it is removed by placing it into a sterile bag that has been placed into the abdomen through one of the port sites.

The importance of handling the gland gently throughout the entire operation cannot be overstated, as rupture of the gland may result in recurrence of disease (as with Cushing syndrome) or precipitation of a life-threatening alteration in blood pressure (as with pheochromocytomas). Similarly, this principle must be adhered to when removing the gland from the abdominal cavity through a port site. Rupture of the bag (especially if the gland is disrupted) can have detrimental consequences. If the gland is too large to remove directly through the cannula or trocar site itself without risk of rupturing the bag and spilling its contents, the incision should be enlarged to facilitate this process. For large glands that are likely difficult to remove, we use a heavy plastic bag that is much more resistant to rupture.

The operative field must be thoroughly inspected for hemostasis, and irrigation used to remove clots and any tissue debris before completing the operation. A drain is not necessary unless there is some concern about injury to the pancreas. All trocar sites should be closed at the level of the fascia with absorbable suture. Skin closure is done according to surgeon preference. Ours is to use a subcuticular closure with 5-0 polyglactin sutures. A long-acting local anesthetic (bupivicaine) is infiltrated around each trocar site, and sterile dressings are applied.

RIGHT LAPAROSCOPIC ADRENALECTOMY

The patient is placed in the lateral decubitus position with left side down. The surgeon and camera holder stand on the left side of the table facing the patient's anterior abdomen, and the assistant stands on the right side, facing the patient's back. The table is rotated slightly away from the surgeon to bring the right midclavicular line into a superior position. A Veress needle is advanced into the peritoneal cavity 1 to 2 cm below the costal margin, passing through 3 layers of fascia. Care must be taken to avoid injury to the liver. Once the position of the Veress needle is confirmed to be intraperitoneal, carbon dioxide pneumoperitoneum is established to a pressure of 15 mm Hg. As with the left side, if there are difficulties encountered with placement of the Veress needle, an uncertain position of the needle, or a patient with prior upper abdominal surgery, the recommended means of establishing pneumoperitoneum is via an open approach in the periumbilical region.

Once the abdomen is insufflated, a 10/11-mm trocar is then placed in each of the following locations: the midclavicular line (1 finger breadth below the costal margin), and the anterior, mid, and posterior axillary lines, just below the costal margin. The scope is then passed into the peritoneal cavity, and the abdomen is surgically explored (**Figure 7**). The dissection is begun by sharply incising the right triangular ligament. This allows the right lobe of the liver to be reflected medially and superiorly with a fan retractor. In displacing the right lobe of the liver, the superior pole of the right adrenal gland and the retrohepatic portion of the inferior vena cava (IVC) will be brought into view. Extreme caution is advised when approaching this portion of the IVC, as bleeding in this area is difficult to control. The IVC should be identified early in the course of the dissection, and its location should always be known to the surgeon throughout the procedure. In the event that exposure of the IVC and adrenal gland is suboptimal, a Kocher maneuver may be war-

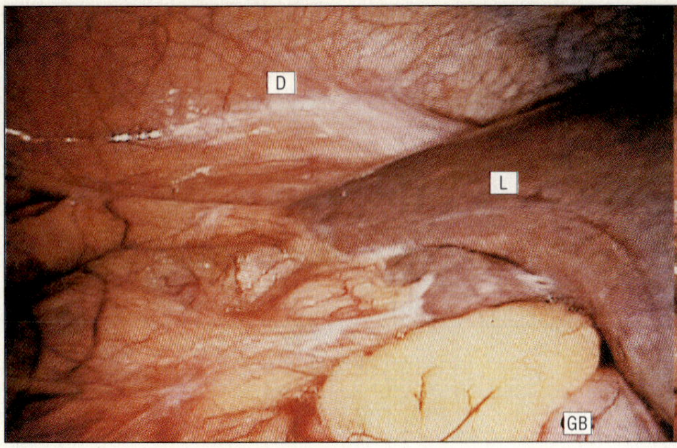

Figure 7. *The diaphragm (D), liver (L), and gallbladder (GB) are readily identified prior to dissection of the right adrenal gland.*

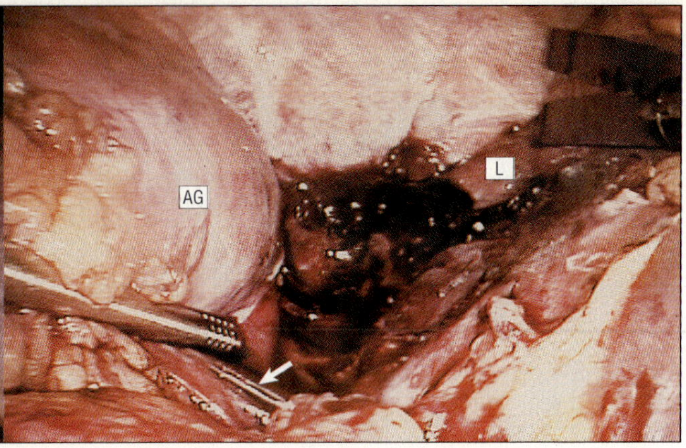

Figure 8. *The liver (L) is retracted medially, and the adrenal gland (AG) is well visualized. Note that the adrenal vein is seen here (arrow) as it courses toward the inferior vena cava.*

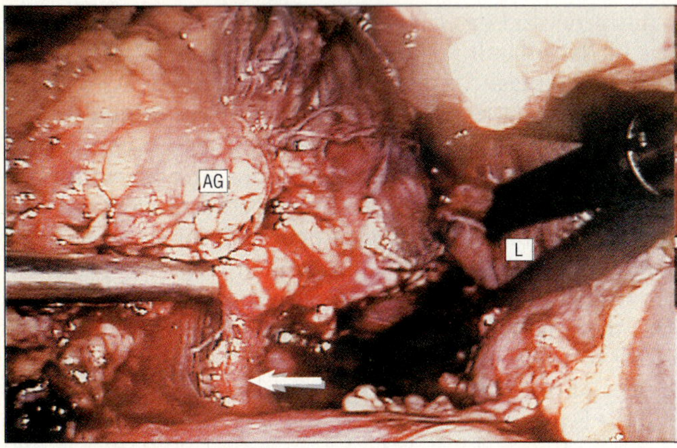

Figure 9. *The right adrenal gland (AG), containing a neoplasm in this case, is carefully dissected while maintaining medial retraction on the liver (L). The gray arrow identifies the right central adrenal vein as it courses toward the inferior vena cava.*

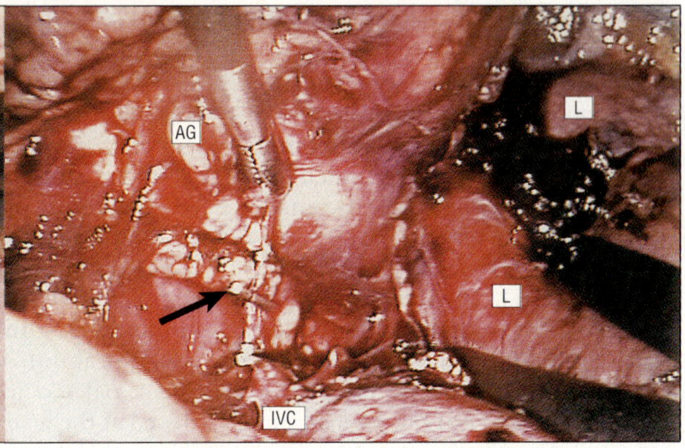

Figure 10. *The right adrenal vein has been safely mobilized between the adrenal gland (AG) and the inferior vena cava (IVC). The liver (L) is retracted medially. Note the titanium clips (arrow) that have been placed on the right adrenal vein prior to its division.*

ranted to better visualize these structures. The peritoneum overlying the adrenal gland and the IVC is then dissected along the medial border of each of these structures, and the retroperitoneal tissue is entered. The adrenal gland is displaced laterally and the IVC is gently retracted medially with a blunt probe, while maintaining gentle medial retraction on the liver (**Figure 8**). Dissection and mobilization of the adrenal gland is then undertaken in a superior to inferior direction. Gentle blunt dissection is begun in the perinephric fat, exposing the superior aspect of the gland. Arterial branches arising from the inferior phrenic artery and the aorta are usually quite small, and can often be transected with cautery. Larger vessels may need to be dissected, clipped, and divided carefully. Finally, the most critical step of the operation is performed. Cautious dissection is done to expose the central adrenal vein–vena cava junction. A caval injury at this point is difficult to control, and carries potentially disastrous consequences. The right adrenal vein should be dissected sufficiently to allow its safe transection (**Figure 9**). A laparoscopic right angle dissector is useful in mobilizing this vein completely. Titanium clips are then placed on the central vein, 3 on the caval side and 2 on the side of the gland (**Figure 10**). Although the right adrenal vein is relatively short, it is usually long enough to safely apply a sufficient number of clips. The vein can then be safely divided between the clips. If the adrenal vein is too large, or the operating space severely limited, an endovascular stapler may be used to divide the vein from the cava. Again, the gland is carefully removed from the retroperitoneum with the aid of a sterile laparoscopic bag as described for the left side. Similar attention is then paid to hemostasis, irrigation, and wound closure.

COMMENT

The most dangerous complication is uncontrolled hemorrhage. The location of the adrenal glands, deeply seated in the superior abdomen and in close proximity to the great vessels, makes vascular control difficult. Careful hemostasis must be maintained throughout the entire procedure, as an apparently minor amount of bleeding may impair the view of the operative field, creating a potentially hazardous situation. When bleeding becomes more pronounced, control may be temporarily achieved using direct pressure from forceps. If this lessens or halts the bleeding, the field can be irrigated, and inspected for possible definitive repair using intracoporeal suturing techniques or vascular clips. With massive and uncontrolled hemorrhage, the operation should be immediately converted to an open procedure to obtain vascular control and avoid further injury.

Other potential complications include injury to the adjacent viscera. On the right side, the organs at increased risk of injury include the liver, duodenum, hepatic flexure of the colon, and the right kidney. On the left side, the structures at risk include the spleen, splenic flexure of the colon, tail of the pancreas, stomach, and left kidney. Injury to solid organs, typically a small puncture or laceration incurred during retraction and dissection, can often be managed with local pressure, electrocautery, or suture. With injury to the pancreas, drains should be placed and not removed until the patient is eating and there is no evidence of pancreatic fluid leakage. If the injury is extensive, and hemorrhage becomes a problem, conversion to an open procedure is warranted and should be done without delay.

Injury to the diaphragm can occur with dissection of the adrenal glands high in the abdomen. The intra-abdominal pressure of the pneumoperitoneum can be transmitted into the chest. Tension pneumothorax may result from such an injury. Early recognition of diaphragmatic injury and release of the pneumoperitoneum will manage the acute problem until definitive repair can be performed.

Adrenalectomy, when indicated and appropriate, can be ideally suited for the laparoscopic approach. The location of the glands, their inherent friability, and their proximity to great vessels pose substantial challenges to the operating surgeon. With use of increased magnification, the greater capability of angled viewing scopes, and the capacity to work in a limited space with narrow instruments, this technique is becoming more widely used. While technically more demanding than the open operation, laparoscopic adrenalectomy offers patients decreased length of hospital stay, decreased pulmonary complications, reduced need for postoperative narcotic analgesics, earlier return to normal activity, and better cosmesis.

Conventional surgical approaches, particularly the transabdominal and thoracoabdominal approaches, will undoubtedly be required to treat certain lesions of the adrenal gland. This is especially true when dealing with larger tumors, and those suspicious for malignancy. Surgeons with an interest in treating patients with adrenal disorders must become proficient in the technique of laparoscopic adrenalectomy. This will allow them to offer their patients the most appropriate means of operative therapy suitable for their individual problems.

Corresponding author: Richard A. Prinz, MD, Department of General Surgery, Rush-Presbyterian-St Luke's Medical Center, 1653 W Congress Parkway, Chicago, IL 60612-3833 (e-mail: rprinz@rpslmc.edu).

REFERENCES

1. Prinz RA, Rao R. Minimally invasive endocrine surgery. In: Frantzides CT, ed. *Laparoscopic and Thoracoscopic Surgery.* St Louis, Mo: Mosby-Year Book; 1995.
2. Hansen P, Bax T, Swanstrom L. Laparoscopic adrenalectomy: history, indications, and current techniques for a minimally invasive approach to adrenal pathology. *Endoscopy.* 1997;29:309-314.
3. Fernandez-Cruz L, Saenz A, Benarroch G, Torres E, Astudillo E. Technical aspects of adrenalectomy via operative laparoscopy. *Surg Endosc.* 1994;8:1348-1351.
4. Prinz RA. A comparison of laparoscopic and open adrenalectomies. Arch Surg. 1995;130:489-494.
5. Staren ED, Prinz RA. Adrenalectomy in the era of laparoscopy. *Surgery.* 1996;120:706-711.
6. Gagner M, Lacroix A, Bolte E. Laparoscopic adrenalectomy in Cushing's syndrome and pheochromocytoma [letter]. *N Engl J Med.* 1992;327:1033.
7. Gagner M, Lacroix A, Prinz R, et al. Early experience with laparoscopic approach for adrenalectomy. *Surgery.* 1993;114:1120-1125.
8. Gagner M, Pompe A, Heniford BT, Pharand D, Lacroix A. Laparoscopic adrenalectomy: lessons learned from 100 consecutive procedures. *Ann Surg.* 1997;226:238-247.
9. MacFadyen BV Jr, Ponsky JL. Adrenalectomy. In: Petelin JB, ed. *Operative Laparoscopy and Thoracoscopy.* Philadelphia, Pa: Lippincott-Raven Publishers; 1996:497-520.
10. Jacobs JK, Goldstein RE, Geer RJ. Laparoscopic adrenalectomy: a new standard of care. *Ann Surg.* 1997;225:495-502.

Fundamentals of Plastic Surgery

by Malcolm W. Marks MD, and Charles Marks, MD, PhD, 412 pp, with 366 illus, $75, ISBN 0-7216-6449-0, Philadelphia, Pa, WB Saunders Co, 1997.

Fundamentals of Plastic Surgery, written by Marks and Marks, contains significant core information regarding plastic and reconstructive surgery. These 2 authors represent contrasting backgrounds, one a board-certified plastic surgeon and the other a thoracic and vascular surgeon with a PhD in anatomy. Although this book contains minimal new information, it is an excellent resource for medical students and residents. The chapters are written with clarity, and the black-and-white illustrations, graphs, and tables deserve commendation.

The chapters on skin grafting, flaps, tissue expansion, microvascular techniques and cleft lip/palate repairs are particularly well written and designed. The chapter on burns contains fundamental information that would be of less interest to practicing, experienced surgeons. The fundamentals of laser therapy (including biophysics) and its utilization, are both timely and needed. The chapter on head and neck surgery is designed to be of less depth in comparison with the remainder of the book; it does not carry the basic multidisciplinary approaches to diagnosis and management. Overall, the authors adhere to their theme of dealing with fundamentals.

Claude H. Organ, Jr, MD
Oakland, Calif

Colon and Rectal Surgery

4th ed, by Marvin L. Corman, MD, 1440 pp, with illus, $225, Philadelphia, Pa, Lippincott-Raven Publishers, 1998.

Marvin Corman's latest and fourth edition of *Colon and Rectal Surgery* should be on every surgeon's shelf and accessible to all general, colorectal, and gastroenterology residents.

The new text has added 13 new chapters and more than 200 new pages. This book's foundation is the work of Dr Corman, his fine writing style, and his interjection of personal opinion on controversial issues. This book has been improved and modified through 3 prior editions beginning in 1984. Until now it has been primarily the work of one well-respected colorectal surgeon. Dr Corman has now added 15 coauthors. These include new chapters on anatomy, physiology, analgesia, trauma, polypoid diseases and pathology, colorectal manifestations of human immunodeficiency virus infection, laparoscopic colectomy, and enterostomal therapy. Pediatric surgical problems are again well covered, as in the last edition, by Dr Alberto Pena.

The number and breadth of color plates has been expanded. All the chapters have been rewritten and references expanded. Despite the additional authors, the illustrations remain uniform and are of the same high quality. The addition of the anatomy and physiology chapters expands the book's usage to anyone in the medical field.

Specific chapters on setting up a colorectal physiology laboratory and colorectal manifestations of acquired immunodeficiency syndrome are well done and timely in light of recent interest in these subjects. As the use of laparoscopic surgery has grown since the last edition, a new chapter has been added for this subject alone.

The chapter on diet and drugs in colorectal surgery could be enhanced with a wider treatment of other disorders, and a section on the role of diet in preventive medicine may have been appropriate.

With 1400 pages and an enlarged page size, the book is not easily handled. Future printings may benefit from a 2-volume edition. However, its size speaks to its completeness and coverage of the subject material. The comprehensive coverage of the subject material has been the strength and reputation of prior Corman editions. This has been maintained and expanded with the added chapters and authors. I can not emphasize enough the high quality of the illustrations. Lois Barnes' work is well known to those in colorectal surgery and is often imitated.

The strength of single authorship in prior editions has not been lost in the current edition despite added authors. The uniformity of style, headlines, and illustrations is maintained.

I highly recommend this book on colon and rectal surgery. Its title belittles its comprehensive treatment of gastrointestinal disorders and anorectal problems including anatomy, function, and specific operative technique.

John M. MacKeigan, MD, FRCSC
Grand Rapids, Mich

Methods of Surgical Training

We read with interest the article by Ko et al[1] published in the August issue of the ARCHIVES. It is about time we take a hard look at US general surgery training, especially surgical resident training, and consider the effects of various subspecialties and newer technologies. Claude H. Organ, Jr, stated that, "Surgeons are completing their surgical training at an age later than the Jesuits are ordaining their priests! . . . Residents in training today must be competent in open and closed operative skills, which has added a new dimension to our educational process."

I currently hold the position of surgical chief resident. There are 3 chief residents within the surgical residency program at this hospital. One has already been accepted to a cardiothoracic surgery fellowship. The other is interested in a colorectal surgery fellowship. My interests lie in general surgery.

Residency review committee rules dictate that each chief resident must have an equal number of similar cases. I am interested primarily in general surgery. However, I still have to participate in the same number of pancreatic, gastric, colonic, head and neck, and vascular cases as my fellow chief residents interested in specializing in cardiothoracic and colorectal surgery.

I agree with those who propose that general surgery training should be extended to 6 years for better-qualified general surgeons. I also agree that the short-track method is best for those interested in other subspecialties such as cardiothoracic, vascular, or plastic surgery.

The results of the study by Ko et al demonstrate that most respondents developed interest in a surgical subspecialty during their junior residency years. This way, residents interested in other subspecialties would not have to share or detract cases from residents who are solely interested in general surgery.

With the finite number of teaching cases, some believe that general surgery is presently squandering precious training opportunities on residents who will practice in other fields, while graduating incompletely trained general surgeons.[2,3] The short-tracking system will be the best method for those interested in other specialties. A 6-year residency is needed for those completing general surgery training, with possibly 1 of those years spent in a surgical intensive care unit.

Sylvanus Oyogoa, MD, MSc
Ian Komenaka, MD
Brooklyn, NY

1. Ko CY, Whang EE, Karamanoukian R, Longmire WP, McFadden DW. What is the best method of surgical training? a report of America's leading senior surgeons. *Arch Surg*. 1998;133:900-905.
2. Way L. General surgery in evolution: technology and competency. *Am J Surg*. 1996;171:2-9.
3. Cameron J. Is fellowship training in alimentary tract surgery necessary? *Am J Surg*. 1993;165:2-8.

O. H. Wangensteen, MD, PhD

DURING MY long association with Dr Wangensteen, one of his attributes that I most admired was his ability to negotiate on behalf of his trainees. His success was legendary. There were only 3 paid general surgery faculty slots in the Department of Surgery at the University of Minnesota, Minneapolis, his and 2 others, yet the faculty always numbered 8 to 10. The additional faculty were supported by soft money, through scholarships, grants, advanced fellowships, or medical school endowments. For example, he secured 13 Markle Scholars, 4 American Heart Association fellows, and 2 scholars of the American Cancer Society, all with 5-year faculty stipends. His support and negotiation through the years helped 38 of his faculty and former residents attain departmental chair status and 31 become division heads.

Dr Wangensteen did not go to many committee meetings (he thought that "a committee is the unwilling appointing the inept to do the unnecessary"), but he did not miss the important ones and was very politically astute when he was involved in committee work. This political savvy affected me when Barney Zimmermann, MD, PhD, a faculty member who had been appointed cancer coordinator for the medical school of the University of Minnesota left to become chair of the Department of Surgery at West Virginia University Medical School, Morgantown. The position of cancer coordinator had been held in the Department of Surgery successively by Arnold Kremen, MD, PhD; George Moore, MD, PhD; and Dr Zimmermann. The presence of internal medicine in the field of oncology was coming to the fore and B. J. Kennedy, MD, was one of the leaders in that movement. Simultaneously, surgeons in Minnesota had become involved in cardiac surgery and were very prominent in activities relating to heart disease. The American Legion Heart Professorship had always been in the Department of Medicine. At this committee meeting, during which the successor to Dr Zimmermann as cancer coordinator was to be appointed, Cecil Watson, MD, PhD, made an impassioned plea to the effect that the position of cancer coordinator had always been in the Department of Surgery and he thought that it was time they considered an internist for the position—furthermore, he felt that Dr Kennedy was a very worthy successor to Dr Zimmermann. At this point, Dr Wangensteen rose graciously and said that he agreed that Dr Kennedy was a strong candidate for the position and that he also thought it was time for a surgeon to be considered for the American Legion Heart Professorship. Immediately following, Dr Watson nominated me as the next cancer coordinator. To a difficult faculty member Dr Wangensteen once said, "The Department of Surgery is like a boat at sea; I'm the captain and my responsibility is to steer. You are the oarsman; your responsibility is to furnish the power without rocking the boat too much." He was quite effective in steering his young men into academic careers.

J. Bradley Aust, MD, PhD
San Antonio, Tex

The Surgeon's Glove

ONCE ANTISEPTIC and aseptic techniques had been finally accepted as part of routine surgical practice (mid 1890s), it was inevitable that other elaborate operating room rituals would similarly take hold. The use of gloves, face masks, operating gowns, and caps naturally evolved. In 1843, along with other developments in rubber processing, the procedure of vulcanization (treating crude rubber with sulfur or its compounds and subjecting it to heat to make it nonplastic and increase its strength and elasticity) was patented and the use of rubber gloves became a possibility. However, surgeons were generally reluctant to use such devices, primarily because until the 1870s no truly flexible, functional glove had been designed. This situation changed in 1878, when Thomas Forster, an employee of the India-Rubber Works in Surrey, England, was granted both British and United States patents for the "manufacture of gloves for surgical operations."

As physicians and surgeons began to understand the bacteriologic research of Louis Pasteur (1822-1895), Robert Koch (1843-1910), and Joseph Lister (1827-1912), it was inevitable that hand coverings would be introduced. Not unexpectedly, the identity of the first surgeon who required that flexible rubber gloves be routinely worn for every surgical operation remains uncertain. However, it is known that as early as 1878, T. Gaillard Thomas (1831-1903), a New York City-based gynecologist was allowing select members of his surgical team to wear rubber gloves to protect their hands from the caustic effects of the various solutions used to clean the surgical instruments.

Eleven years later, it was such a dermatitis, produced by mercuric chloride solution on the arms and hands of William Halsted's (1852-1922) operating room nurse, that first brought rubber gloves into The Johns Hopkins Hospital, Baltimore, Md. Commonly regarded as the individual who popularized their use in the operating room, Halsted's interest in gloves was nothing more than accidental. For him, the operating in gloves was an evolution rather than an inspiration and like most surgeons in the 19th century represented a method to prevent a chemical-induced dematitis as opposed to the prevention of surgical infection. An element of romance interweaves itself throughout the story of Halsted and rubber surgical gloves: the operating room nurse for whom he had ordered the gloves made later became his wife.

By the mid 1890s, surgeons were becoming satisfied with their antiseptic methods and the attendant results. Wound infection was becoming less of a concern, although difficulties still existed. Rubber gloves remained a curiosity, however, and were not yet considered an integral part of surgical operative routine. Many surgeons insisted that they reduced the delicacy of touch and had their assistants wear them while they themselves remained barehanded. In the more extreme cases, surgeons countered the use of gloves by engaging in an elaborate ritual of hand washing that often required more time than the operation itself. This attitude would slowly begin to change, prompted by researchers as Bernard Krönig (1863-1917) of Germany, who scientifically examined the time-honored methods of hand washing by systematically spreading gas gangrene spores on the arms of cadavers of children (1894). He then applied various disinfecting agents. Scrapings from the skin were cultured and mice injected. As he expected, most of the animals died of gas gangrene. It is not difficult to imagine the stunned silence of the surgical community as Krönig told them that mechnical cleansing alone, even if carried out for half an hour, was insufficient to make their skin surfaces bacteria free. Despite his research, the international acceptance of rubber gloves as a necessary adjunct to any surgical operation would not occur until after World War I.

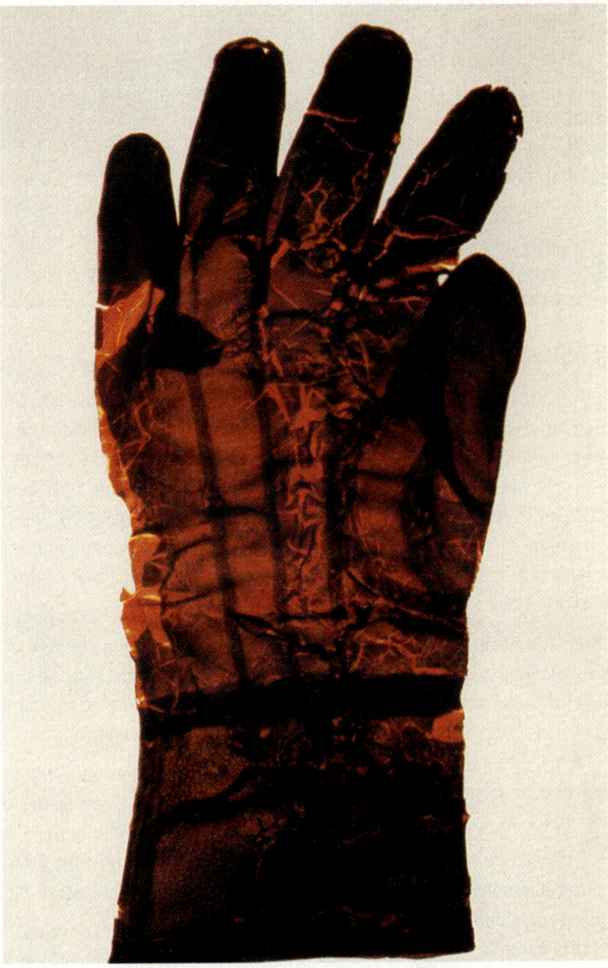

One of the original rubber surgical gloves (preserved in lucite) designed by William Halsted and fabricated by the Goodyear Rubber Company of New York City. (Courtesy of The Alan Mason Chesney Medical Archives of The Johns Hopkins Medical Institutions, Baltimore, Md.)

Ira M. Rutkow, MD, MPH, DrPH

The information given here is supplied by the companies cited. Publication of these notices does not imply endorsement or warranty by the American Medical Association, publishers of the *Archives of Surgery*.

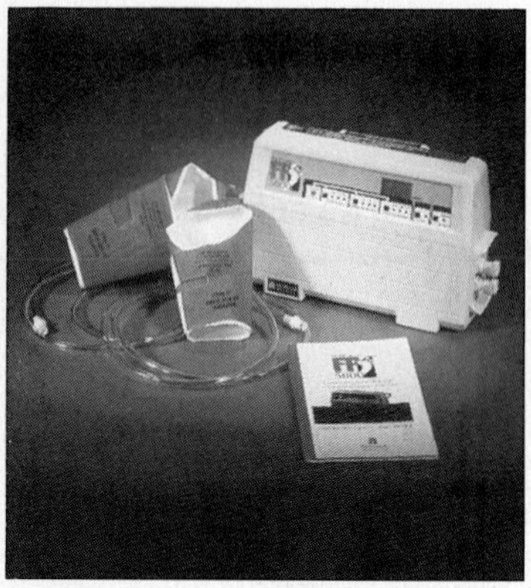

COMPRESSION PRODUCT —

Huntleigh Healthcare announces the launch of the FP5000™ System for external intermittent pneumatic compression of the foot. The FP5000™ Pump System is a non-invasive, mechanical prophylaxis system for reducing the incidence of deep vein thrombosis (DVT).

Other clinical applications include: prevention of venous stasis, enhancement of venous and arterial circulation, reduction of acute and chronic edema, reduction of lower limb pain due to trauma and surgery and reduction of compartmental pressures.

It is the ideal prophylactic modality when use of standard calf or thigh length garment are inappropriate. It allows the user to operate the pump in single leg mode and adjust the pressure settings with the press of a button. This system utilizes a new foot garment with cushioned foam dorsum and heel sections to protect skin integrity.

For information write
HUNTLEIGH HEALTHCARE INC.
227 Route 33 East
Manalapan, NJ 07726

Call toll free
800-223-1218

Fax
732-446-1938

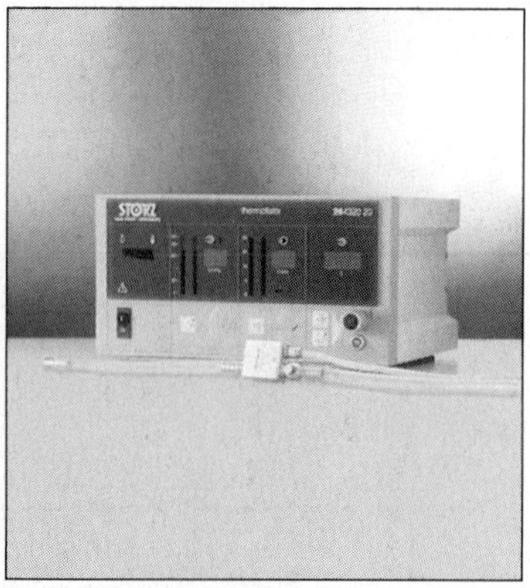

SURGICAL PRODUCT —

Karl Storz Endoscopy-America, Inc. introduces the Thermoflator, the only insufflaton device on the market today. It utilizes a unique OptiTherm heating system to warm CO_2 gas (37°C/99°F) immediately before it enters a patient's abdominal cavity.

Heated CO_2 helps maintain body temperature, lowering the risk of hypothermia and tissue damage during laparoscopic procedures, in addition to reducing endoscope fogging.

Thermoflator features user-adjustable gas flow rates. Three modes of insufflation are available: Semi-continous, normal intermittent flow and insufflation initialization mode.

The Thermoflator also contains many safety features, including the overpressure alarm that automatically relieves excess pressure through the SECUVENT safety valve.

For information write
KARL STORZ ENDOSCOPY-AMERICA, INC.
Attn: Cindy Monticue
600 Corporate Pointe
Culver City, California 90230-7600

Call toll free
800-421-0837

Fax
310-410-5527

Web site
www.karlstorz.com

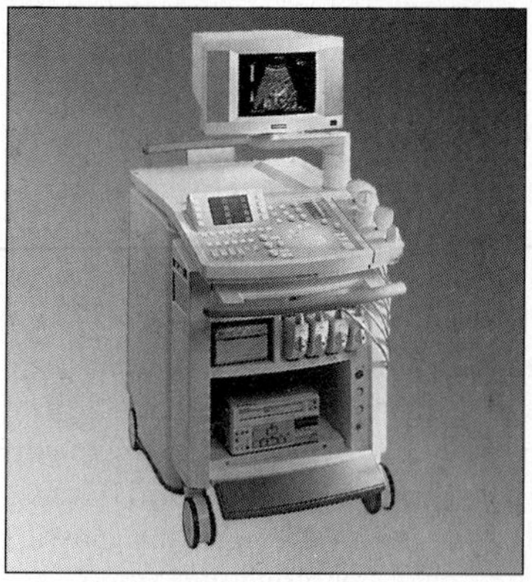

IMAGING SYSTEM —

Siemens Medical Systems, Inc., Ultrasound Group, introduces a new line of intraoperative, cardiac and specialty transducers for its premium performance platform, the SONOLINE® Versa Plus ultrasound imaging system.

The Version 3.0 software upgrade supports three new intraoperative transducers. These include LAP8-4 Laparoscope, 7.5L50-I and 7.5L50 -Q transducers.

The new intraoperative transducers allow doctors to gather accurate images during surgery. Intraoperative imaging allows surgeons to view images that are impossible to obtain with a conventional transducer outside the body.

The TEE transducer gives clinicians clear images of the heart without significant lung artifacts. The VF13-5 and the LB5-2 transducers enhance small parts and biopsy imaging capabilities. The VF13-5 transducer provides contrast-rich images from the skin-line. The LB5-2 transducer is designed to aid in safe, ultrasonically guided biopsy and/or aspiration procedures.

For information write
SIEMENS MEDICAL SYSTEMS, INC.
Attn: Sara Britton
22010 S.E. 51st St.
Issaquah, WA 98029-7002

Phone
206-448-1200

E-mail
britton@sqi.com

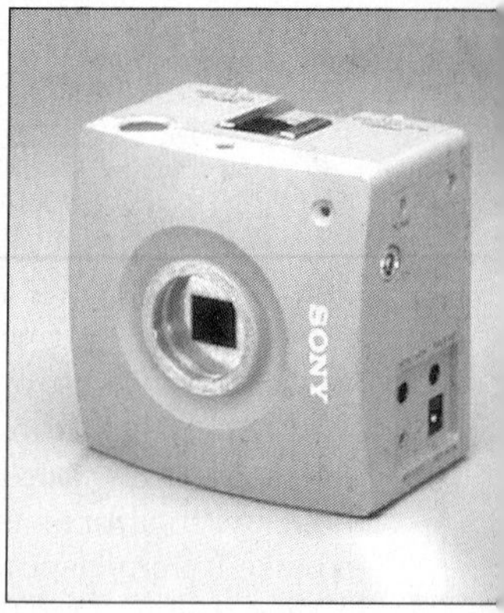

ELECTRONIC PRODUCT —

Sony Electronics introduces a new digital still camera (DKC-CM30) incorporating progressive scan technology, for use in applications including scientific research and analysis, documentation, and archiving medical student and patient education, medical publishing and web page design.

Compact and lightweight, the camera's overall design, and C-mount lens type for flexibility in lens selection make it a powerful and unique solution for the scientific imaging market.

The camera incorporates a 1/3" 350,000-pixel progressive scan CCD. Four MB of internal flash memory, electronic shutter and a two-inch, 100,000-pixel TFT color LCD monitor. Camera control is available by remote control unit or through a computer via an RS-232 interface.

Images stored in the DKC-CM30 can be transferred to a PC running Windows® 95 software with the supplied MGI® "PhotoSuite SE" software.

The DKC-CM30 is currently available at a suggested list price of $1,395

For information write
SONY ELECTRONICS INC.
1 Sony Drive
Park Ridge, New Jersey 07656-80

Call toll free
800-686-SONY

Web site
www.sony.com/news

Classified Advertising

Academic/Faculty
Cardiovascular/Thoracic Surgery
CME Corner
Chiefs/Department Heads/Directors
Courses/Symposia/Seminars
Facial Plastic Surgery
Graduate Training/Residencies/Fellowships
Locum Tenens Wanted
Multiple Specialties/Group Practice
Neurosurgery
Notices
Othopedic Surgery
Pediatric Surgery
Plastic Surgery
Practices For Sale
Surgical Specialities
Thoracic Surgery
Vascular Surgery

Sales Information

1999 CLASSIFIED ADVERTISING RATES

Regular	1x 1.65/wd	*3x 1.55/wd
Bold	1x 1.85/wd	*3x 1.75/wd

*In order to receive the 3-time frequency price, the request must be made upon initial placement. The minimum charge is 20 words. A word consists of one or more letters surrounded by space on each side. For information on display advertising and our network buys contact an account representative.

POLICY

Orders for classified advertising must be submitted in writing. Although the American Medical Association believes the classified advertisements in these pages to be from reputable sources, the Association does not investigate the offers made and assumes no liability concerning them. Acceptance of advertising is restricted to professional opportunities, practices for sale, and medical office space available. The Association reserves the right to decline, withdraw, or edit advertisements at its discretion. Every care is taken to avoid mistakes but responsibility cannot be accepted by the Association for clerical or printer's errors.

REPLY BOX SERVICE

Confidential box numbers are available for an additional $25 per issue, plus the words: Box ________, c/o SUR. When responding to a box number, please send to Archives of Surgery, Box ________, c/o SUR, 515 N State St, Chicago, IL 60610.

CANCELLATIONS/CHANGES

Cancellations/changes must be received in writing at least 25 days prior to the date of the issue. In order to expedite, please fax to 312-464-5909 to the attention of your account representative.

GENERAL INFORMATION

To contact a Classified Advertising account representative, call 312-464-2475/2490/2491/4485 or 800-AMA-2260. Or fax your insertion order to 312-464-5909. Mail your materials to AMA Classified Advertising, 12th Floor, 515 N State St, Chicago, IL 60610.

ACADEMIC/FACULTY

THE UNIVERISTY OF CALIFORNIA, IRVINE, SCHOOL OF MEDICINE, DEPARTMENT OF SURGERY: seeks full-time academic surgeons for tenure-track positions at the Assistant Professor level (Transplantation; Cardiothoracic Surgery). Candidates must be Board Certified in General Surgery/area of specialty. California license is required. Candidates must have demonstrated a strong interest in teaching, clinical care and have an active research program. Interested candidates should submit a curriculum vitae along with five names and addresses of referees by March 1, 1999, to Samuel Eric Wilson, MD, Professor and Chair, Department of Surgery, University of California, Irvine Medical Center, 101 The City Drive, Orange, CA 92868. UCI: Rooted in Education, Enriched by Diversity.

LEGAL SERVICES

MALPRACTICE CASE EVALUATION

Board-certified medical experts needed. All specialties. All locations. Defense and plaintiff cases. Excellent remuneration. Send CVs to:

Barry Gustin, MD, MPH, FACEP
AMERICAN MEDICAL FORENSIC SPECIALISTS, Inc
2991 Shattuck Ave, Ste 302
Berkeley, CA 94705

LOCUM TENENS WANTED

HKA LOCUM TENENS is looking for quality surgical specialty physicians to do Locum Tenens. We have opportunities coast-to-coast. We furnish Occurrence Malpractice Insurance (no tail necessary). Please call **HKA LOCUM TENENS** at (800) 226-6347, Extension AM7.1.

SURGERY: GENERAL

FOX RIVER VALLEY, WI: Town of 14,000 (draw 50,000) thirty minutes from Green Bay. Join another surgeon in 14-physician group, proven caseload. Endoscopy, laparoscopy required, C-sections preferred, vascular a plus. For consideration, call Kari Donovan, 800-765-3055, ID#6378AR, Fax: 314-726-3009, e-mail: kdonovan@cejka.com Visit our website: www.cejka.com

GENERAL SURGEON OREGON: Seeking BC/BE General Surgeon to join a 40-physician Multi-specialty Group located in Salem, Oregon. Vascular and laparoscopic skills required. Salem Clinic offers a comprehensive benefit package and competitive income guarantee with opportunity for rapid incorporation into production formula. 1:4 call. Single hospital town. Salem is the capital city located in the heart of the beautiful Willamette Valley, between the Oregon Coast and the Cascade Mountains, with recreational and cultural activities locally and nearby. Those interested mail or Fax your CV and references to Ms Sherry Krog, Salem Clinic, PC, 2020 Capitol St NE, Salem, OR 97303. 503-399-2470, Fax: 503-375-7429.

OPPORTUNITY IN NORTHEASTERN OKLAHOMA LAKE COUNTRY: Strong 70 bed JCAHO accredited not-for-profit hospital has an opportunity for 1 general surgeon. General surgery service area of 60,000+. 12 BC physicians on staff including an anesthesiologist. 40 minutes from Tulsa. Negotiable financial arrangements. Call Stan Schuermann at INTEGRIS Baptist Medical Center at 800-332-8663.

OPPORTUNITY FOR SEASONED, progressive, BC/BE general surgeon to immediately join busy, well established, private surgical practice. Located in Northern Michigan on the Great Lakes. Spectacular four season recreation, safe, caring, family oriented community. Supportive and friendly hospital and professional staff with over forty referring physicians and excellent ER, ICU, and diagnostic imaging support. Efficient, state-of-the-art office suite in new medical office building connected to hospital. Competitive salary with full benefits. Send cover letter and curriculum vitae to T. M. Burandt, DO & Associates, PC, 810 South Main Street, Suite#1, Cheboygan, MI 49721, Facsimile: 616-627-7758, E-mail: tburandt@cdimed.com

SOUTH CAROLINA - GENERAL SURGEON: BC/BE to join two person surgical practice in upstate SC, in metropolitan area. Respond with CV to Box 1099. c/o SUR, 515 N State St, 12th Fl, Chicago, IL 60610.

WELL ESTABLISHED BUSY SURGICAL PRACTICE: Seeking Board Eligible/Board Certified General Surgeon with Vascular Surgery experience to join a four surgeon General/Vascular/Trauma practice. Opportunity for partnership. Practice located approximately one and one-half hours drive from Baltimore/Washington area in Western Maryland. Appalachian Trail, Potomac River and ski resorts in local area. Position available July 1999. For more information, contact or send Curriculum Vitae to Hagerstown Surgical Clinic, 11110 Medical Campus Road, Suite 100, Hagerstown, MD 21742. Telephone: 301-714-4325, Fax: 301-714-4326.

WILLAMETTE VALLEY, OREGON: Opportunity available for BC/BE General Surgeon. Join a 3-member department within large physician-owned multi-specialty group. Corvallis is home to Oregon State University, town of 45,000, located in heart of beautiful Willamette Valley wine country; one hour from coast, two hours from Cascade Mountains ski and recreation areas. Guaranteed salary, incentive bonus, and excellent benefits. Position is available April 1999. Send CV and cover letter to Medical Director, The Corvallis Clinic, PC, 444 NW Elks Dr, Corvallis, OR 97330, Fax: 541-757-1847.

THE UNIVERSITY OF NEW MEXICO: Health Sciences Center, Department of Surgery and the Veterans Affairs Medical Center in Albuquerque, NM are seeking applications for a BE/BC General Surgeon eligible for appointment at the Instructor or Assistant Professor level. This position will be primarily based at the Albuquerque Veterans Affairs Medical Center. Applicants will be expected to be proficient with all aspects of general surgery including laparoscopy and gastrointestinal endoscopy. Applicants will also be expected to participate fully in educational and research missions of the University of New Mexico and the VAMC. Send a cover letter, curriculum vitae, and the names of three references to Angela Hannan, Recruitment Coordinator, University of New Mexico Health Sciences Center, Department of Surgery, ACC - 2nd Floor, Albuquerque, NM 87131-5341. This position will remain open until filled. This position is subject to drug testing. For further information on this position contact David Pitcher, MD, Chief of Surgical Services, VAMC, Albuquerque at 505-265-1711, ext 4250. The University of New Mexico and the Veterans Affairs Medical Center are Affirmative Action/Equal Opportunity Educators and Employers.

SURGERY: ORTHOPEDIC

OPPORTUNITY IN NORTHEASTERN OKLAHOMA LAKE COUNTRY: Strong not-for-profit hospital has an opportunity for 1 orthopedic surgeon. Orthopedic surgery service area of 60,000+. 70 bed JCAHO accredited hospital with 12 BC physicians on staff including an anesthesiologist. 40 minutes from Tulsa. Negotiable financial arrangements. Call Stan Schuermann at INTEGRIS Baptist Medical Center at 800-332-8663.

SURGERY: SURGICAL SPECIALTIES

BC/BE SURGEON every fourth night for Indian Health Service facility with state of the art laparoscopic and endoscopic equipment. College town 1 hour from metro area. Ideally located at base of Ozark Mountains with abundant four season recreational opportunities. Salary negotiable, excellent benefits, loan repayment. We are an equal opportunity employer. Contact Lisa Spry at 918-458-3360.

HOUSTON, TX: MacGregor Medical Association, a multispecialty group practice with over 40 years of experience in quality care, is seeking a Board Certified Colo-Rectal Surgeon with a minimum of 3 years experience. MMA is a group of more than 200 physicians serving over 180,000 patients. Our diverse patient population is comprised of 90% managed care and 10% fee for service clients. Houston is a diverse city that offers a wide array of cultural and recreational pursuits. Texas has no state income tax! MacGregor offers a competitive salary and excellent benefit package. For more information you may call us at 800-716-6060. You may also fax/mail your CV to MacGregor Medical Association, Medical Staff Services, 2550 Holly Hall Houston, TX 77054, 713-746-5441 http://medjobs.macgregor.com/

SOUTH CAROLINA-GENERAL/THORACIC/VASCULAR: Exceptional practice opportunities exist for experienced Surgeons and graduating residents/fellows. The Surgeons selected would join an established, highly successful private practice group in the process of a major expansion at a 300 bed Medical Center located in a town of 50,000 and within an hour's drive of numerous recreational and cultural attractions, multiple colleges, two medical schools and two major cities. Relocation assistance/incentives are available. For further information, contact Dr Chermol, The Regional Medical Center, 800-866-6045.

TWO-SURGEON PRACTICE, located in central New York, seeks general surgeon with laparoscopic, vascular, and/or thoracic capabilities. Recent fellowship training desirable. Based in the scenic and cosmopolitan home of Cornell University. The practice serves two progressive medical centers. Excellent lifestyle opportunities abound in housing, education, and recreation. Reply to Box 323, c/o SUR, 515 N State St, 12th Fl, Chicago, IL 60610.

SURGERY: THORACIC

LONG ISLAND - THORACIC SURGEON: BC/BE Thoracic Surgeon to join a busy 7 surgeon group practicing thoracic/vascular/general surgery 45 minutes from Manhattan. Send CV to Long Island Thoracic Surgeon, Ste 26, 375 E Main St, Bay Shore, NY 11706.

SURGERY: VASCULAR

VASCULAR SURGEON: Beautiful Central Florida. Easy access to Orlando and Tampa. Moss-draped oak trees line hundred year old streets in our beautiful city. Practice vascular surgery and some general surgery as the third surgeon in a busy practice. Affiliate with two hospitals with more than 550 beds in the community. Call Robert Estes at 800-321-2460. FAX CV to 407-253-9055.

WEST VIRGINIA UNIVERSITY

SURGERY CHAIR

The West Virginia University (WVU) School of Medicine is seeking a Chair of the Department of Surgery at the Robert C. Byrd Health Sciences Center. The position requires an individual with strong leadership skills, experience in academic medicine and administration, and a commitment to service, teaching, and research. He/She must have a vision for the future of medical education in the context of a changing health care delivery system. Applicants should send a curriculum vitae and the names and addresses of three references. These materials should provide evidence of qualifications as noted above. Review of applications will begin after February 15, 1999. The position will remain open until filled. Applications should be directed to:

Stephen Wetmore, MD
Chair, Surgery Chair Search Committee
Professor and Chairman of Otolaryngology
WVU School of Medicine
PO Box 9200
Morgantown, WV 26506-9200

WVU is an Equal Opportunity/Affirmative Action Employer. Women and minorities are encouraged to apply.

Index of Advertisers

CLASSIFIED ADVERTISING 225-228
http://www.ama-assn.org

ETHICON INC
Suture Assist .... Cover 2

PFIZER, US PHARMACEUTICAL GROUP
http://www.pfizer.com
Trovan .... Cover 3-Cover 4

While every precaution is taken to ensure accuracy, we cannot guarantee against the possibility of an occasional change or omission in the preparation of this index.

TROVAN® Tablets (trovafloxacin mesylate)
TROVAN® I.V. (alatrofloxacin mesylate injection)
For Intravenous Infusion
BRIEF SUMMARY

The following is a brief summary only. Before prescribing, see complete prescribing information for Trovan Tablets and Injection.

CONTRAINDICATIONS

TROVAN is contraindicated in persons with a history of hypersensitivity to trovafloxacin, alatrofloxacin, quinolone antimicrobial agents or any other components of these products.

WARNINGS

THE SAFETY AND EFFECTIVENESS OF TROVAFLOXACIN IN PEDIATRIC PATIENTS AND ADOLESCENTS LESS THAN 18 YEARS OF AGE, PREGNANT WOMEN, AND NURSING WOMEN HAVE NOT BEEN ESTABLISHED. (See **PRECAUTIONS: Pediatric Use, Pregnancy,** and **Nursing Mothers** subsections.)

As with other members of the quinolone class, trovafloxacin has caused arthropathy and/or chondrodysplasia in immature rats and dogs. The significance of these findings to humans is unknown.

Convulsions, increased intracranial pressure and psychosis have been reported in patients receiving quinolones. Quinolones may also cause central nervous system stimulation which may lead to tremors, restlessness, lightheadedness, confusion, hallucinations, paranoia, depression, nightmares and insomnia. These reactions may occur following the first dose. If these reactions occur in patients receiving trovafloxacin or alatrofloxacin, the drug should be discontinued and appropriate measures instituted. (See **PRECAUTIONS: General, Information for Patients, Drug Interactions** and **ADVERSE REACTIONS.**)

As with other quinolones, TROVAN should be used with caution in patients with known or suspected CNS disorders, such as severe cerebral atherosclerosis, epilepsy, and other factors that predispose to seizures. (See **ADVERSE REACTIONS.**)

Serious and occasionally fatal hypersensitivity and/or anaphylactic reactions have been reported in patients receiving therapy with quinolones. These reactions may occur following the first dose. Some reactions have been accompanied by cardiovascular collapse, hypotension/shock, seizure, loss of consciousness, tingling, angioedema (including tongue, laryngeal, throat or facial edema/swelling), airway obstruction (including bronchospasm, shortness of breath and acute respiratory distress), dyspnea, urticaria, itching and other serious skin reactions.

TROVAN should be discontinued at the first appearance of a skin rash or any other sign of hypersensitivity. Serious acute hypersensitivity reactions may require treatment with epinephrine and other resuscitative measures, including oxygen, intravenous fluids, antihistamines, corticosteroids, pressor amines and airway management, as clinically indicated. (See **PRECAUTIONS** and **ADVERSE REACTIONS.**)

Serious and sometimes fatal events, some due to hypersensitivity and some due to uncertain etiology, have been reported in patients receiving therapy with all antibiotics. These events may be severe and generally occur following the administration of multiple doses. Clinical manifestations may include one or more of the following: fever, rash or severe dermatologic reactions (e.g., toxic epidermal necrolysis, Stevens-Johnson Syndrome); vasculitis, arthralgia, myalgia, serum sickness; allergic pneumonitis, interstitial nephritis; acute renal insufficiency or failure; hepatitis, jaundice, acute hepatic necrosis or failure; anemia, including hemolytic and aplastic; thrombocytopenia, including thrombotic thrombocytopenic purpura; leukopenia; agranulocytosis; pancytopenia; and/or other hematologic abnormalities.

Pseudomembranous colitis has been reported with nearly all antibacterial agents, including TROVAN, and may range in severity from mild to life-threatening. Therefore, it is important to consider this diagnosis in patients who present with diarrhea subsequent to the administration of any antibacterial agent.

Treatment with antibacterial agents alters the flora of the colon and may permit overgrowth of clostridia. Studies indicate that a toxin produced by *Clostridium difficile* is the primary cause of "antibiotic-associated colitis."

After the diagnosis of pseudomembranous colitis has been established, therapeutic measures should be initiated. Mild cases of pseudomembranous colitis usually respond to drug discontinuation alone. In moderate to severe cases, consideration should be given to management with fluids and electrolytes, protein supplementation, and treatment with an antibacterial drug clinically effective against *C. difficile* colitis. (See **ADVERSE REACTIONS.**)

Although not seen in TROVAN clinical trials, ruptures of the shoulder, hand, and Achilles tendons that required surgical repair or resulted in prolonged disability have been reported in patients receiving quinolones. TROVAN should be discontinued if the patient experiences pain, inflammation or rupture of a tendon. Patients should rest and refrain from exercise until the diagnosis of tendinitis or tendon rupture has been confidently excluded. Tendon rupture can occur during or after therapy with quinolones.

Trovafloxacin has not been shown to be effective in the treatment of syphilis. Antimicrobial agents used in high doses for short periods of time to treat gonorrhea may mask or delay the symptoms of incubating syphilis. All patients with gonorrhea should have a serologic test for syphilis at the time of diagnosis.

PRECAUTIONS

General:

The safety and efficacy of TROVAN given for >4 weeks have not been studied. (See **ADVERSE REACTIONS.**)

Moderate to severe phototoxicity reactions have been observed in patients who are exposed to direct sunlight while receiving some drugs in this class. Therapy should be discontinued if phototoxicity (e.g., a skin eruption, etc.) occurs.

The safety and efficacy of TROVAN in patients with severe cirrhosis (Child-Pugh Class C) have not been studied.

During the post-marketing period, Trovan-associated liver enzyme abnormalities and/or symptomatic hepatitis have occurred during short-term or long-term therapy. Liver enzyme abnormalities have been reported in both men and women. Liver failure (including acute hepatic necrosis with eosinophilic infiltration) has also been reported rarely. Symptomatic pancreatitis has been reported on therapy. Clinicians should monitor liver function tests and pancreatic tests in patients who develop symptoms consistent with hepatitis and/or pancreatitis as clinically indicated.

Information for Patients:

Patients should be advised: that TROVAN Tablets may be taken without regard to meals; that vitamins or minerals containing iron, aluminum-, magnesium- or base antacids containing citric acid buffered with sodium citrate, or sucralfate or Videx®, (Didanosine), chewable/buffered tablets or the pediatric powder for oral solution, should be taken at least two hours before or two hours after taking TROVAN Tablets. (See **PRECAUTIONS: Drug Interactions.**); that TROVAN may cause lightheadedness and/or dizziness. Dizziness and/or lightheadedness was the most common adverse reaction reported, and for females under 45 years, it was reported significantly more frequently than in other groups. The incidence of dizziness may be substantially reduced if TROVAN Tablets are taken at bedtime or with food. Patients should know how they react to trovafloxacin before they operate an automobile or machinery or engage in activities requiring mental alertness and coordination; to discontinue treatment and inform their physician if they experience pain, inflammation or rupture of a tendon, and to rest and refrain from exercise until the diagnosis of tendinitis or tendon rupture has been confidently excluded; that TROVAN may be associated with hypersensitivity reactions, even following the first dose, and to discontinue the drug at the first sign of a skin rash, hives or other skin reactions, difficulty in swallowing or breathing, any swelling suggesting angioedema (e.g., swelling of the lips, tongue, face, tightness of the throat, hoarseness), or other symptoms of an allergic reaction. (See **WARNINGS** and **ADVERSE REACTIONS.**); to avoid excessive sunlight or artificial ultraviolet light (e.g., tanning beds) while taking TROVAN and to discontinue therapy if phototoxicity (e.g., sunburn-like reaction or skin eruption) occurs.

Drug Interactions:

No significant interactions with theophylline, cimetidine, digoxin, warfarin, or cyclosporine have been observed with TROVAN Tablets.

Minor pharmacokinetic interactions without clinical significance have been observed with co-administration of TROVAN Tablets with caffeine, omeprazole and calcium carbonate.

Antacids, Sucralfate, and Iron: The absorption of oral trovafloxacin is significantly reduced by the concomitant administration of some antacids containing magnesium or aluminum, citric acid/sodium citrate (Bicitra®), as well as sucralfate and iron (as ferrous ions). These agents as well as formulations containing divalent and trivalent cations such as Videx®, (Didanosine), chewable/buffered tablets or the pediatric powder for oral solution, should be taken at least two hours before or two hours after oral trovafloxacin administration.

Morphine: Co-administration of intravenous morphine significantly reduces the absorption of oral trovafloxacin. Intravenous morphine should be administered at least 2 hours after oral TROVAN dosing in the fasted state and at least 4 hours after oral TROVAN is taken with food. Trovafloxacin administration had no effect on the pharmacokinetics of morphine or its metabolite, morphine-6-β-glucuronide.

Alatrofloxacin should not be co-administered with any solution containing multivalent cations, e.g., magnesium, through the same intravenous line.

Laboratory Test Interactions: There are no reported laboratory test interactions.

Carcinogenesis, Mutagenesis, Impairment of Fertility:

TROVAN did not shorten the time to development of UV-induced skin tumors in hairless albino (Skh-1) mice; thus, it was not photo co-carcinogenic in this model. These mice received oral trovafloxacin and concurrent irradiation with simulated sunlight 5 days per week for 40 weeks followed by a 12-week treatment-free observation period. The daily dose of UV radiation used in this study was approximately 30% of the minimal dose of UV radiation that would induce erythema in Caucasian humans. The median time to the development of skin tumors in the hairless mice (42-43 weeks) was similar in the vehicle control group and those given 10 or 30 mg/kg of trovafloxacin daily. At a dose level of 30 mg/kg/day, the mice had skin trovafloxacin concentrations of approximately 7 mg/g. Following multiple 200 mg daily doses of trovafloxacin, the amount in human skin is estimated to be about 3 mg/g, based upon plasma concentrations measured at this dose level.

Trovafloxacin was not mutagenic in the Ames Salmonella reversion assay or CHO/HGPRT mammalian cell gene mutation assay and it was not clastogenic in mitogen-stimulated human lymphocytes or mouse bone marrow cells. A mouse micronucleus test conducted with alatrofloxacin was also negative. The positive response observed in the *E. coli* bacterial mutagenicity assay may be due to the inhibition of DNA gyrase by trovafloxacin.

Trovafloxacin and alatrofloxacin did not affect the fertility of male or female rats at oral and I.V. doses of 75 mg/kg/day and 50 mg/kg/day, respectively. These doses are 15 and 10 times the recommended maximum human dose based on mg/kg or approximately 2 times based on mg/m^2. However, oral doses of trovafloxacin at 200 mg/kg/day (40 times the recommended maximum human dose based on mg/kg or about 6 times based on mg/m^2) were associated with increased preimplantation loss in rats.

Pregnancy: Teratogenic Effects. Pregnancy Category C:

An increase in skeletal variations was observed in rat fetuses after daily oral 75 mg/kg maternal doses of trovafloxacin (approximately 15 times the highest recommended human dose based on mg/kg or two times based upon body surface area) were administered during organogenesis. However, fetal skeletal variations were not observed in rats dosed orally with 15 mg/kg trovafloxacin. Evidence of fetotoxicity (increased perinatal mortality and decreased body weights) was also observed in rats at 75 mg/kg. Daily oral doses of trovafloxacin at 45 mg/kg (approximately 9 times the highest recommended human dose based on mg/kg or 2.7 times based upon body surface area) in the rabbit were not associated with an increased incidence of fetal skeletal variations or malformations.

An increase in skeletal variations and malformations was observed in rat fetuses after daily intravenous doses of alatrofloxacin at ≥20 mg/kg/day (approximately 4 times the highest recommended human dose based on mg/kg or 0.6 times based upon body surface area) were administered to dams during organogenesis. In the rabbit, an increase in fetal skeletal malformations was also observed when 20 mg/kg/day (approximately equal to the highest recommended human dose based upon body surface area) of alatrofloxacin was given intravenously during the period of organogenesis. Intravenous dosing of alatrofloxacin at 6.5 mg/kg in the rat or rabbit was not associated with an increased incidence of skeletal variations or malformations. Fetotoxicity and fetal skeletal malformations have been associated with other quinolones.

Oral doses of trovafloxacin >5 mg/kg were associated with an increased gestation time in rats, and several dams at 75 mg/kg experienced uterine dystocia.

There are no adequate and well-controlled studies in pregnant women. TROVAN should be used during pregnancy only if the potential benefit justifies the potential risk to the fetus. (See **WARNINGS.**)

Nursing Mothers:

Trovafloxacin is excreted in human milk and was found in measurable concentrations in the breast milk of lactating subjects.

Because of the potential for unknown effects from trovafloxacin in nursing infants from mothers taking trovafloxacin, a decision should be made either to discontinue nursing or to discontinue the drug, taking into account the importance of the drug to the mother.

Pediatric Use:

The safety and effectiveness of trovafloxacin in pediatric patients and adolescents less than 18 years of age have not been established. Quinolones, including trovafloxacin, cause arthropathy and osteochondrosis in juvenile animals of several species. (See **WARNINGS.**)

Geriatric Use:

In multiple-dose clinical trials of trovafloxacin, 27% of patients were ≥ 65 years of age and 12% of patients were ≥75 years of age. The overall incidence of drug-related adverse reactions, including central nervous system and gastrointestinal side effects, was less in the ≥ 65 year group than the other age groups.

ADVERSE REACTIONS

Over 6000 patients have been treated with TROVAN in multidose clinical efficacy trials worldwide.

In TROVAN studies the majority of adverse reactions were described as mild in nature (over 90% were described as mild or moderate). TROVAN was discontinued for adverse events thought related to drug in 5% of patients (dizziness 2.4%, nausea 1.9%, headache 1.1%, and vomiting 1.0%).

TROVAN Drug-Related Adverse Reactions (frequency ≥1%) in Multiple-Dose Clinical Trials

	100 mg oral qd (N=1536)	200 mg oral qd (N=3259)	200 mg I.V.→ 200 mg oral qd (N=634)	300 mg I.V.→ 200 mg oral qd (N=623)
Dizziness	3%	11%	2%	2%
Lightheadedness	2%	4%	2%	<1%
Nausea	4%	8%	5%	4%
Headache	4%	5%	5%	1%
Vomiting	<1%	3%	1%	3%
Diarrhea	2%	2%	2%	2%
Abdominal pain	<1%	1%	1%	0%
Application/ injection/ insertion site reaction	n/a	n/a	5%	2%
Vaginitis	2%	2%	2%	<1%
Pruritus	<1%	<1%	2%	2%
Rash	<1%	<1%	2%	2%

Dizziness/lightheadedness on TROVAN is generally mild, lasts for a few hours following a dose, and in most cases, resolves with continued dosing. The incidence of dizziness and lightheadedness in TROVAN patients over 65 years is 3.1% and 0.6%, respectively. (See **PRECAUTIONS: Information for Patients.**)

TROVAN appears to have a low potential for phototoxicity. In clinical trials with TROVAN, only mild, treatment-related phototoxicity was observed in less than 0.03% (2/7096) of patients.

Additional reported drug-related events in clinical trials (remotely, possibly, probably or unknown) that occurred in <1% of TROVAN-treated patients are: **APPLICATION/INJECTION/INSERTION SITE:** Application/injection/insertion site device complications, inflammation, pain, edema **AUTONOMIC NERVOUS:** flushing, increased sweating, dry mouth, cold clammy skin, increased saliva **CARDIOVASCULAR:** peripheral edema, chest pain, thrombophlebitis, hypotension, palpitation, periorbital edema, hypertension, syncope, tachycardia, angina pectoris, bradycardia, peripheral ischemia, edema, dizziness postural **CENTRAL & PERIPHERAL NERVOUS SYSTEM:** confusion, paresthesia, vertigo, hypoesthesia, ataxia, convulsions, dysphonia, hypertonia, migraine, involuntary muscle contractions, speech disorder, encephalopathy, abnormal gait, hyperkinesia, hypokinesia, tongue paralysis, abnormal coordination, tremor, dyskinesia **GASTROINTESTINAL:** abdominal pain, altered bowel habit, constipation, diarrhea-*Clostridium difficile*, dyspepsia, flatulence, loose stools, gastritis, dysphagia, increased appetite, gastroenteritis, rectal disorder, colitis, pseudomembranous colitis, enteritis, eructation, gastrointestinal disorder, melena, hiccup **ORAL CAVITY:** gingivitis, stomatitis, altered saliva, tongue disorder, tongue edema, tooth disorder, chelitis, halitosis **GENERAL/OTHER:** fever, fatigue, pain, asthenia, moniliasis, hot flushes, back pain, chills, infection (bacterial, fungal), malaise, sepsis, alcohol intolerance, allergic reaction, anaphylactoid reaction, drug (other) toxicity/reaction, weight increase, weight decrease **HEMATOPOIETIC:** anemia, granulocytopenia, hemorrhage unspecified, leukopenia, prothrombin decreased, thrombocythemia, thrombocytopenia **LIVER/BILIARY:** increased hepatic enzymes, hepatic function abnormal, bilirubinemia, discolored feces, jaundice **METABOLIC/NUTRITIONAL:** hyperglycemia, thirst **MUSCULOSKELETAL:** arthralgia, muscle cramps, myalgia, muscle weakness, skeletal pain, tendinitis, arthropathy **PSYCHIATRIC:** anxiety, anorexia, agitation, nervousness, somnolence, insomnia, depression, amnesia, concentration impaired, depersonalization, dreaming abnormal, emotional lability, euphoria, hallucination, impotence, libido decreased-male, paroniria, thinking abnormal **REPRODUCTIVE:** Female: leukorrhea, menstrual disorder; Male: balanoposthitis **RESPIRATORY:** dyspnea, rhinitis, sinusitis, bronchospasm, coughing, epistaxis, respiratory insufficiency, upper respiratory tract infection, respiratory disorder, asthma, hemoptysis, hypoxia, stridor **SKIN/APPENDAGES:** pruritus ani, skin disorder, skin ulceration, angioedema, dermatitis, dermatitis fungal, photosensitivity skin reaction, seborrhea, skin exfoliation, urticaria **SPECIAL SENSES:** taste perversion, eye pain, abnormal vision, conjunctivitis, photophobia, conjunctival hemorrhage, hyperacusis, scotoma, tinnitus, visual field defect, diplopia, xerophthalmia **URINARY SYSTEM:** dysuria, face edema, micturition frequency, interstitial nephritis, renal failure acute, renal function abnormal, urinary incontinence **LABORATORY CHANGES:** Changes in laboratory parameters, without regard to drug relationship, occurring in ≥1% of TROVAN-treated patients were: decreased hemoglobin and hematocrit; increased platelets; decreased and increased WBC; eosinophilia; increased ALT (SGPT), AST (SGOT), and alkaline phosphatase; decreased protein and albumin; increased BUN and creatinine; decreased sodium; and bicarbonate. It is not known whether these abnormalities were caused by the drug or the underlying condition being treated.

The incidence and magnitude of liver function abnormalities with TROVAN were the same as comparator agents except in the only study in which oral TROVAN was administered for 28 days. In this study (chronic bacterial prostatitis) nine percent (13/140) of TROVAN-treated patients experienced elevations of serum transaminases (AST and/or ALT) of ≥ 3 times the upper limit of normal. These liver function test abnormalities generally developed at the end of, or following completion of, the planned 28-day course of therapy, but were not associated with concurrent elevations of related laboratory measures of hepatic function (such as serum bilirubin, alkaline phosphatase, or lactate dehydrogenase). Patients were asymptomatic with these abnormalities, which generally returned to normal within 1-2 months after discontinuation of therapy. (See **ADVERSE REACTIONS: POST-MARKETING EXPERIENCE** subsection.) **POST-MARKETING EXPERIENCE:** Adverse reactions reported with TROVAN during the post-marketing period include: anaphylaxis, symptomatic hepatitis (some patients experienced an associated peripheral eosinophilia), liver failure (including acute hepatic necrosis with eosinophilic infiltration), Stevens-Johnson Syndrome, and symptomatic pancreatitis.

During the post-marketing period, TROVAN-associated liver enzyme abnormalities and/or symptomatic hepatitis have occurred during short-term or long-term therapy. (See **PRECAUTIONS.**)

OVERDOSAGE

Trovafloxacin has a low order of acute toxicity. The minimum lethal oral dose in mice and rats was 2000 mg/kg or greater. The minimum lethal I.V. dose for the prodrug, alatrofloxacin, was 50-125 mg/kg for mice and greater than 75 mg/kg for rats. Clinical signs observed included decreased activity and respiration, ataxia, ptosis, tremors and convulsions.

In the event of acute oral overdosage, the stomach should be emptied by inducing vomiting or by gastric lavage. The patient should be carefully observed and given symptomatic and supportive treatment. Adequate hydration should be maintained. Trovafloxacin is not efficiently removed from the body by hemodialysis.

70-5328-00-2 Revised October 1998

KC427A98 Printed in USA January 1999 Pfizer U.S. Pharmaceuticals

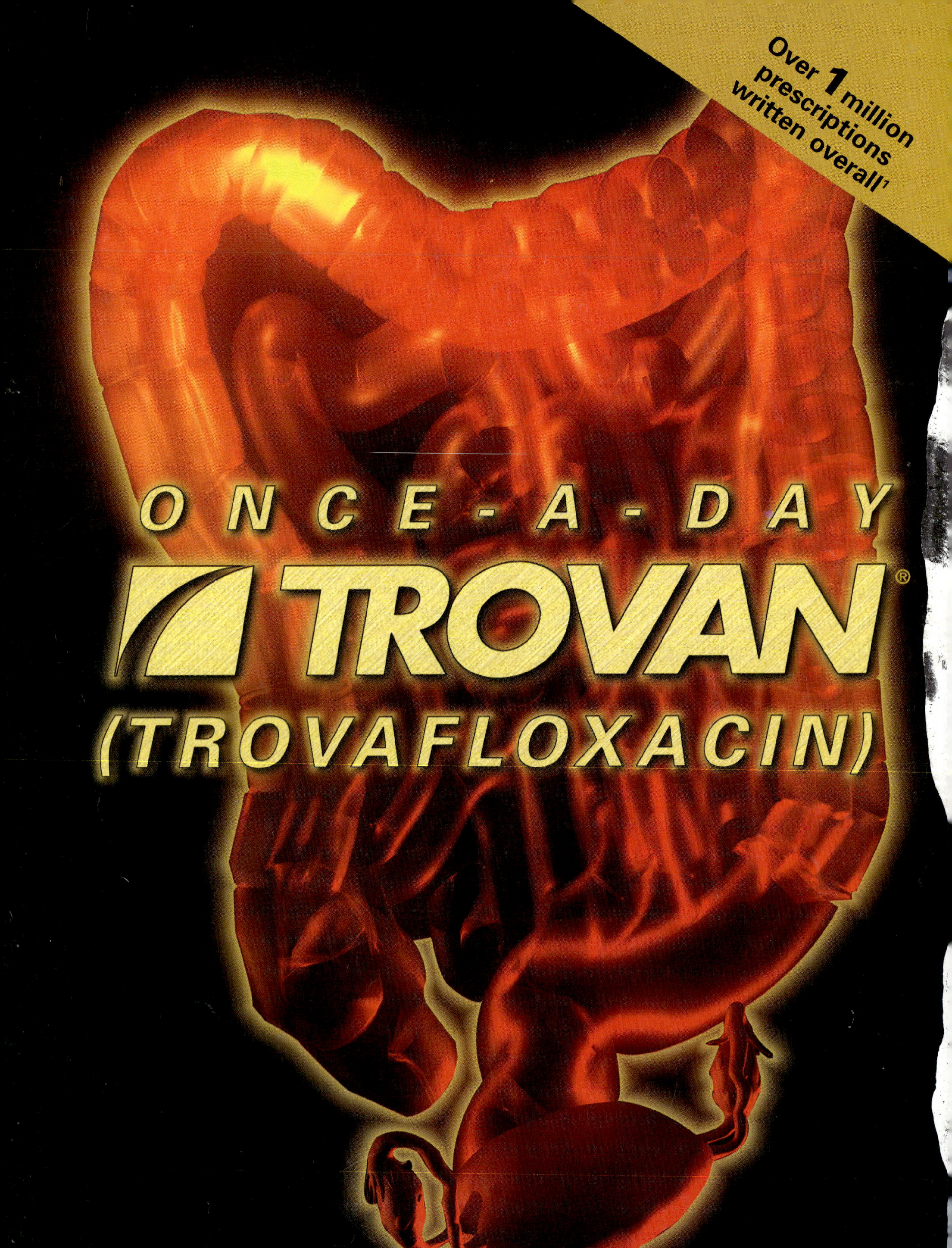
Over 1 million prescriptions written overall[1]
ONCE-A-DAY
TROVAN®
(TROVAFLOXACIN)

ARCHIVES OF SURGERY

MARCH 1999

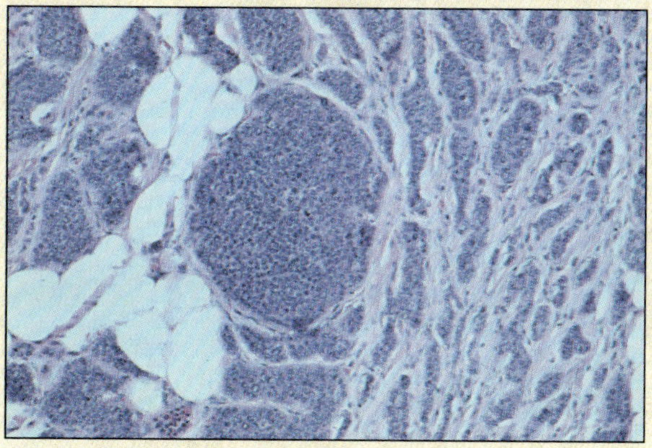

Intestinal carcinoid with subserosal invasion.

FUNCTIONAL OUTCOME AFTER LAPAROSCOPIC OR OPEN NISSEN FUNDOPLICATION

ASSOCIATION OF INCREASED IMMUNOSTAINING FOR iNOS AND NITROTYROSINE WITH FGF TRANSFORMATION IN PANCREATIC CANCER

TIKHOFF-LINBERG PROCEDURE FOR BONE AND SOFT TISSUE TUMORS OF THE SHOULDER GIRDLE

PARATHYROID AUTOTRANSPLANTATION DURING THYROIDECTOMY: IS FROZEN SECTION NECESSARY?

EXPANDABLE METALLIC STENTS VS CONVENTIONAL METHODS IN INTRAHEPATIC BILIARY STRICTURES WITH RECURRENT HEPATOLITHIASIS

TRANSITION FROM OPEN TO LAPAROSCOPIC FUNDOPLICATION: THE LEARNING CURVE

COMPLETE TABLE OF CONTENTS INSIDE

American Medical Association
Physicians dedicated to the health of America
www.ama-assn.org/surgery

Once-daily dosing for a wide range of patients

Indication	Loading dose	Daily therapy
Oropharyngeal candidiasis	**200 mg**	100 mg
Esophageal candidiasis	**200 mg**	100 mg*
Candidal UTI and peritonitis	†	50 to 200 mg‡
Systemic candidal Infections†	†	up to 400 mg
Cryptococcal meningitis (acute)§	**400 mg**	200 mg*
Cryptococcal meningitis (maintenance to prevent relapse)		200 mg
Bone marrow transplant prophylaxis‖		400 mg

*Doses up to 400 mg/day may be used, based on medical judgment of the patient's response to therapy.

†In general, a loading dose of twice the daily dose is recommended on the first day of therapy to result in plasma concentrations close to steady-state by the second day of therapy.

‡Including candidemia, disseminated candidiasis, and pneumonia.

§Three risk factors that may predict a negative outcome for AIDS patients with cryptococcal meningitis are abnormal mental status, CSF with antigen titer >1:1024, and CSF WBC <20 cells per cubic millimeter.

‖Therapy should be continued for 7 days after neutrophil count rises above 1000 cells/mm^3. Patients who are anticipated to have severe granulocytopenia (<500 neutrophils/mm^3) should start Diflucan prophylaxis several days before the anticipated onset of neutropenia and continue for 7 days after the neutrophil count rises above 1000 cells per cubic millimeter.

Pediatric patient dose conversion

Pediatric patients	Adults
3 mg/kg	100 mg
6 mg/kg	200 mg
12 mg/kg‖	400 mg

‖Some older children may have clearances similar to that of adults. Absolute doses exceeding 600 mg/day are not recommended.

References: 1. Data available on request from Roerig. **2.** Laine L, Dretler RH, Conteas CN, et al. Fluconazole compared with ketoconazole for the treatment of candida esophagitis in AIDS: a randomized trial. *Ann Intern Med.* 1992;117:655-660. **3.** Powderly WG, Saag MS, Cloud GA, et al. A controlled trial of fluconazole or amphotericin B to prevent relapse of cryptococcal meningitis in patients with the acquired immunodeficiency syndrome. *N Engl J Med.* 1992;326:793-798. **4.** Saag MS, Powderly WG, Cloud GA, et al. Comparison of amphotericin B with fluconazole in the treatment of acute AIDS-associated cryptococcal meningitis. *N Engl J Med.* 1992;326:83-89.

Diflucan® (fluconazole)

100/150/200 mg Tablets, 10/40 mg/mL Oral Suspension, 200/400 mg IV Injection

BRIEF SUMMARY

INDICATIONS AND USAGE

DIFLUCAN (fluconazole) is indicated for the treatment of:

1. Vaginal candidiasis (vaginal yeast infections due to *Candida*).
2. Oropharyngeal and esophageal candidiasis. In open noncomparative studies of relatively small numbers of patients, DIFLUCAN was also effective for the treatment of *Candida* urinary tract infections, peritonitis, and systemic *Candida* infections including candidemia, disseminated candidiasis, and pneumonia.
3. Cryptococcal meningitis. Before prescribing DIFLUCAN for AIDS patients with cryptococcal meningitis, please see CLINICAL STUDIES section (in full prescribing information). Studies comparing DIFLUCAN to amphotericin B in non-HIV infected patients have not been conducted.

Prophylaxis. DIFLUCAN is also indicated to decrease the incidence of candidiasis in patients undergoing bone marrow transplantation who receive cytotoxic chemotherapy and/or radiation therapy.

Specimens for fungal culture and other relevant laboratory studies (serology, histopathology) should be obtained prior to therapy to isolate and identify causative organisms. Therapy may be instituted before the results of the cultures and other laboratory studies are known; however, once these results become available, anti-infective therapy should be adjusted accordingly.

CONTRAINDICATIONS

DIFLUCAN is contraindicated in patients who have shown hypersensitivity to fluconazole or to any of its excipients. There is no information regarding cross-hypersensitivity between fluconazole and other azole antifungal agents. Caution should be used in prescribing DIFLUCAN to patients with hypersensitivity to other azoles. Coadministration of terfenadine is contraindicated in patients receiving DIFLUCAN at multiple doses of 400 mg or higher based upon results of a multiple dose interaction study. Coadministration of cisapride is contraindicated in patients receiving DIFLUCAN. (See PRECAUTIONS below.)

WARNINGS

(1) Hepatic injury: DIFLUCAN has been associated with rare cases of serious hepatic toxicity, including fatalities primarily in patients with serious underlying medical conditions. In cases of DIFLUCAN-associated hepatotoxicity, no obvious relationship to total daily dose, duration of therapy, sex or age of the patient has been observed. DIFLUCAN hepatotoxicity has usually, but not always, been reversible on discontinuation of therapy. Patients who develop abnormal liver function tests during DIFLUCAN therapy should be monitored for the development of more severe hepatic injury. DIFLUCAN should be discontinued if clinical signs and symptoms consistent with liver disease develop that may be attributable to DIFLUCAN.

(2) Anaphylaxis: In rare cases, anaphylaxis has been reported.

(3) Dermatologic: Patients have rarely developed exfoliative skin disorders during treatment with DIFLUCAN. In patients with serious underlying diseases (predominantly AIDS and malignancy) these have rarely resulted in a fatal outcome. Patients who develop rashes during treatment with DIFLUCAN should be monitored closely and the drug discontinued if lesions progress.

PRECAUTIONS

General: Single Dose. The convenience and efficacy of the single dose oral tablet of fluconazole regimen for the treatment of vaginal yeast infections should be weighed against the acceptability of a higher incidence of drug related adverse events with DIFLUCAN (26%) versus intravaginal agents (16%) in U.S. comparative clinical studies. (See ADVERSE REACTIONS.)

Drug Interactions: Clinically or potentially significant drug interactions between DIFLUCAN and the following agents/classes have been observed. These are described in greater detail below: Oral hypoglycemics, coumarin-type anticoagulants, phenytoin, cyclosporine, rifampin, theophylline, terfenadine, cisapride, astemizole, rifabutin, tacrolimus.

Oral hypoglycemics: Clinically significant hypoglycemia may be precipitated by the use of DIFLUCAN with oral hypoglycemic agents; one fatality has been reported from hypoglycemia in association with combined DIFLUCAN and glyburide use. DIFLUCAN reduces the metabolism of tolbutamide, glyburide, and glipizide and increases the plasma concentration of these agents. When DIFLUCAN is used concomitantly with these or other sulfonylurea oral hypoglycemic agents, blood glucose concentrations should be carefully monitored and the dose of the sulfonylurea should be adjusted as necessary.

Coumarin-type anticoagulants: Prothrombin time may be increased in patients receiving concomitant DIFLUCAN and coumarin-type anticoagulants. Careful monitoring of prothrombin time in patients receiving DIFLUCAN and coumarin-type anticoagulants is recommended.

Phenytoin: DIFLUCAN increases the plasma concentrations of phenytoin. Careful monitoring of phenytoin concentrations in patients receiving DIFLUCAN and phenytoin is recommended.

Cyclosporine: DIFLUCAN may significantly increase cyclosporine levels in renal transplant patients with or without renal impairment. Careful monitoring of cyclosporine concentrations and serum creatinine is recommended in patients receiving DIFLUCAN and cyclosporine.

Rifampin: Rifampin enhances the metabolism of concurrently administered DIFLUCAN. Depending on clinical circumstances, consideration should be given to increasing the dose of DIFLUCAN when it is administered with rifampin.

Theophylline: DIFLUCAN increases the serum concentrations of theophylline. Careful monitoring of serum theophylline concentrations in patients receiving DIFLUCAN and theophylline is recommended.

Terfenadine: Because of the occurrence of serious cardiac dysrhythmias secondary to prolongation of the QTc interval in patients receiving azole antifungals in conjunction with terfenadine, interaction studies have been performed. One study at a 200-mg daily dose of fluconazole failed to demonstrate a prolongation of QTc interval. Another study at a 400-mg and 800-mg daily dose of fluconazole demonstrated that DIFLUCAN taken in doses of 400 mg per day or greater significantly increases plasma levels of terfenadine when taken concomitantly. The combined use of fluconazole at doses of 400 mg or greater with terfenadine is contraindicated. (See CONTRAINDICATIONS.) The coadministration of fluconazole at doses lower than 400 mg/day with terfenadine should be carefully monitored.

Cisapride: There have been reports of cardiac events, including torsade de pointes in patients to whom fluconazole and cisapride were coadministered. The combined use of fluconazole and cisapride is contraindicated. (See CONTRAINDICATIONS.)

Astemizole: The use of fluconazole in patients concurrently taking astemizole or other drugs metabolized by the cytochrome P450 system may be associated with elevations in serum levels of these drugs. In the absence of definitive information, caution should be used when coadministering fluconazole. Patients should be carefully monitored.

Rifabutin: There have been reports of uveitis in patients to whom fluconazole and rifabutin were coadministered. Patients receiving rifabutin and fluconazole concomitantly should be carefully monitored.

Tacrolimus: There have been reports of nephrotoxicity in patients to whom fluconazole and tacrolimus were coadministered. Patients receiving tacrolimus and fluconazole concomitantly should be carefully monitored.

Fluconazole tablets coadministered with ethinyl estradiol-and levonorgestrel-containing oral contraceptives produced an overall mean increase in ethinyl estradiol and levonorgestrel levels; however, in some patients there were decreases up to 47% and 33% of ethinyl estradiol and levonorgestrel levels. The data presently available indicate that the decreases in some individual ethinyl estradiol and levonorgestrel AUC values with fluconazole treatment are likely the result of random variation. While there is evidence that fluconazole can inhibit the metabolism of ethinyl estradiol and levonorgestrel, there is no evidence that fluconazole is a net inducer of ethinyl estradiol or levonorgestrel metabolism. The clinical significance of these effects is presently unknown.

Physicians should be aware that interaction studies with medications other than those listed in the CLINICAL PHARMACOLOGY section (in full prescribing information) have not been conducted, but such interactions may occur.

Carcinogenesis, Mutagenesis and Impairment of Fertility: Fluconazole showed no evidence of carcinogenic potential in mice and rats treated orally for 24 months at doses of 2.5, 5 or 10 mg/kg/day (approximately 2-7x the recommended human dose). Male rats treated with 5 and 10 mg/kg/day had an increased incidence of hepatocellular adenomas.

Fluconazole, with or without metabolic activation, was negative in tests for mutagenicity in 4 strains of *S. typhimurium*, and in the mouse lymphoma L5178Y system. Cytogenetic studies *in vivo* (murine bone marrow cells, following oral administration of fluconazole) and *in vitro* (human lymphocytes exposed to fluconazole at 1000 µg/mL) showed no evidence of chromosomal mutations.

Fluconazole did not affect the fertility of male or female rats treated orally with daily doses of 5, 10 or 20 mg/kg or with parenteral doses of 5, 25 or 75 mg/kg, although the onset of parturition was slightly delayed at 20 mg/kg PO. In an intravenous perinatal study in rats at 5, 20 and 40 mg/kg, dystocia and prolongation of parturition were observed in a few dams at 20 mg/kg (approximately 5-15x the recommended human dose) and 40 mg/kg, but not at 5 mg/kg. The disturbances in parturition were reflected by a slight increase in the number of still-born pups and decrease of neonatal survival at these dose levels. The effects on parturition in rats are consistent with the species specific estrogen-lowering property produced by high doses of fluconazole. Such a hormone change has not been observed in women treated with fluconazole.

Pregnancy: Teratogenic Effects. Pregnancy Category C: Fluconazole was administered orally to pregnant rabbits during organogenesis in two studies, at 5, 10 and 20 mg/kg, and at 5, 25, and 75 mg/kg respectively. Maternal weight gain was impaired at all dose levels, and abortions occurred at 75 mg/kg (approximately 20-60x the recommended human dose); no adverse fetal effects were detected. In several studies in which pregnant rats were treated orally with fluconazole during organogenesis, maternal weight gain was impaired and placental weights were increased at 25 mg/kg. There were no fetal effects at 5 or 10 mg/kg; increases in fetal anatomical variants (supernumerary ribs, renal pelvis dilation) and delays in ossification were observed at 25 and 50 mg/kg and higher doses. At doses ranging from 80 mg/kg (approximately 20-60x the recommended human dose) to 320 mg/kg embryolethality in rats was increased and fetal abnormalities included wavy ribs, cleft palate and abnormal cranio-facial ossification. These effects are consistent with the inhibition of estrogen synthesis in rats and may be a result of known effects of lowered estrogen on pregnancy, organogenesis and parturition.

There are no adequate and well controlled studies in pregnant women. There have been reports of multiple congenital abnormalities in infants whose mothers were being treated for 3 or more months with high dose (400-800 mg/day) fluconazole therapy for coccidioidomycosis (an unindicated use). The relationship between fluconazole use and these events is unclear. DIFLUCAN® (fluconazole) should be used in pregnancy only if the potential benefit justifies the possible risk to the fetus.

Nursing Mothers: Fluconazole is secreted in human milk at concentrations similar to plasma. Therefore, the use of DIFLUCAN in nursing mothers is not recommended.

Pediatric Use: An open-label, randomized, controlled trial has shown DIFLUCAN to be effective in the treatment of oropharyngeal candidiasis in children 6 months to 13 years of age.

The use of DIFLUCAN in children with cryptococcal meningitis, *Candida* esophagitis, or systemic *Candida* infections is supported by the efficacy shown for these indications in adults and by the results from several small noncomparative pediatric clinical studies. In addition, pharmacokinetic studies in children have established a dose proportionality between children and adults. (See DOSING.)

In a noncomparative study of children with serious systemic fungal infections, most of which were candidemia, the effectiveness of DIFLUCAN was similar to that reported for the treatment of candidemia in adults. Of 17 subjects with culture-confirmed candidemia, 11 of 14 (79%) with baseline symptoms (3 were asymptomatic) had a clinical cure; 13/15 (87%) of evaluable patients had a mycologic cure at the end of treatment but two of these patients relapsed at 10 and 18 days, respectively, following cessation of therapy.

The efficacy of DIFLUCAN for the suppression of cryptococcal meningitis was successful in 4 of 5 children treated in a compassionate-use study of fluconazole for the treatment of life-threatening or serious mycosis. There is no information regarding the efficacy of fluconazole for primary treatment of cryptococcal meningitis in children.

The safety profile of DIFLUCAN in children has been studied in 577 children ages 1 day to 17 years who received doses ranging from 1 to 15 mg/kg/day for 1 to 1,616 days. (See ADVERSE REACTIONS.)

Efficacy of DIFLUCAN has not been established in infants less than 6 months of age. A small number of patients (29) ranging in age from 1 day to 6 months have been treated safely with DIFLUCAN.

ADVERSE REACTIONS

In Patients Receiving a Single Dose for Vaginal Candidiasis: During comparative clinical studies conducted in the United States, 448 patients with vaginal candidiasis were treated with DIFLUCAN, 150 mg single dose. The overall incidence of side effects possibly related to DIFLUCAN was 26%. In 422 patients receiving active comparative agents, the incidence was 16%. The most common treatment-related adverse events reported in the patients who received 150 mg single dose fluconazole for vaginitis were headache (13%), nausea (7%), and abdominal pain (6%). Other side effects reported with an incidence equal to or greater than 1% included diarrhea (3%), dyspepsia (1%), dizziness (1%), and taste perversion (1%). Most of the reported side effects were mild to moderate in severity. Rarely, angioedema and anaphylactic reaction have been reported in marketing experience.

In patients receiving multiple doses for other infections: Sixteen percent of over 4000 patients treated with DIFLUCAN in clinical trials of 7 days or more experienced adverse events. Treatment was discontinued in 1.5% of patients due to adverse clinical events and in 1.3% of patients due to laboratory test abnormalities.

Clinical adverse events were reported more frequently in HIV infected patients (21%) than in non-HIV infected patients (13%); however, the patterns in HIV infected and non-HIV infected patients were similar. The proportions of patients discontinuing therapy due to clinical adverse events were similar in the two groups (1.5%).

The following treatment-related clinical adverse events occurred at an incidence of 1% or greater in 4048 patients receiving DIFLUCAN for 7 or more days in clinical trials: nausea 3.7%, headache 1.9%, skin rash 1.8%, vomiting 1.7%, abdominal pain 1.7%, and diarrhea, 1.5%.

The following adverse events have occurred under conditions where a causal association is probable: *Hepatobiliary:* In combined clinical trials and marketing experience, there have been rare cases of serious hepatic reactions during treatment with DIFLUCAN. (See WARNINGS.) The spectrum of these hepatic reactions has ranged from mild transient elevations in transaminases to clinical hepatitis, cholestasis and fulminant hepatic failure, including fatalities. Instances of fatal hepatic reactions were noted to occur primarily in patients with serious underlying medical conditions (predominantly AIDS or malignancy) and often while taking multiple concomitant medications. Transient hepatic reactions, including hepatitis and jaundice have occurred among patients with no other identifiable risk factors. In each of these cases, liver function returned to baseline on discontinuation of DIFLUCAN.

In two comparative trials evaluating the efficacy of DIFLUCAN for the suppression of relapse of cryptococcal meningitis, a statistically significant increase was observed in median AST (SGOT) levels from a baseline value of 30 IU/L to 41 IU/L in one trial and 34 IU/L to 66 IU/L in the other. The overall rate of serum transaminase elevations of more than 8 times the upper limit of normal was approximately 1% in fluconazole-treated patients in clinical trials. These elevations occurred in patients with severe underlying disease, predominantly AIDS or malignancies, most of whom were receiving multiple concomitant medications, including many known to be hepatotoxic. The incidence of abnormally elevated serum transaminases was greater in patients taking DIFLUCAN concomitantly with one or more of the following medications: rifampin, phenytoin, isoniazid, valproic acid, or oral sulfonylurea hypoglycemic agents.

Immunologic: In rare cases, anaphylaxis has been reported.

The following adverse events have occurred under conditions where a causal association is uncertain: *Central Nervous System:* seizures. *Dermatologic:* Exfoliative skin disorders including Stevens-Johnson Syndrome and toxic epidermal necrolysis (see WARNINGS), alopecia. *Hematopoietic and Lymphatic:* leukopenia, including neutropenia and agranulocytosis, thrombocytopenia. *Metabolic:* hypercholesterolemia, hypertriglyceridemia, hypokalemia.

Adverse Reactions in Children: In Phase II/III clinical trials conducted in the United States and in Europe, 577 pediatric patients, ages 1 day to 17 years were treated with DIFLUCAN at doses of up to 15 mg/kg/day for up to 1,616 days. Thirteen percent of children experienced treatment-related adverse events. The most commonly reported events were vomiting (5%), abdominal pain (3%), nausea (2%), and diarrhea (2%). Treatment was discontinued in 2.3% of patients due to adverse clinical events and in 1.4% of patients due to laboratory test abnormalities. The majority of treatment-related laboratory abnormalities were elevations of transaminases or alkaline phosphatase.

Percentage of Patients With Treatment-Related Side Effects

	Fluconazole (N=577)	**Comparative Agents (N=451)**
With any side effect	13.0	9.3
Vomiting	5.4	5.1
Abdominal pain	2.8	1.6
Nausea	2.3	1.6
Diarrhea	2.1	2.2

U.S. Pharmaceuticals

FC255A98

Rev. October 1998

OVERWHELMING ANTIFUNGAL SUCCESS

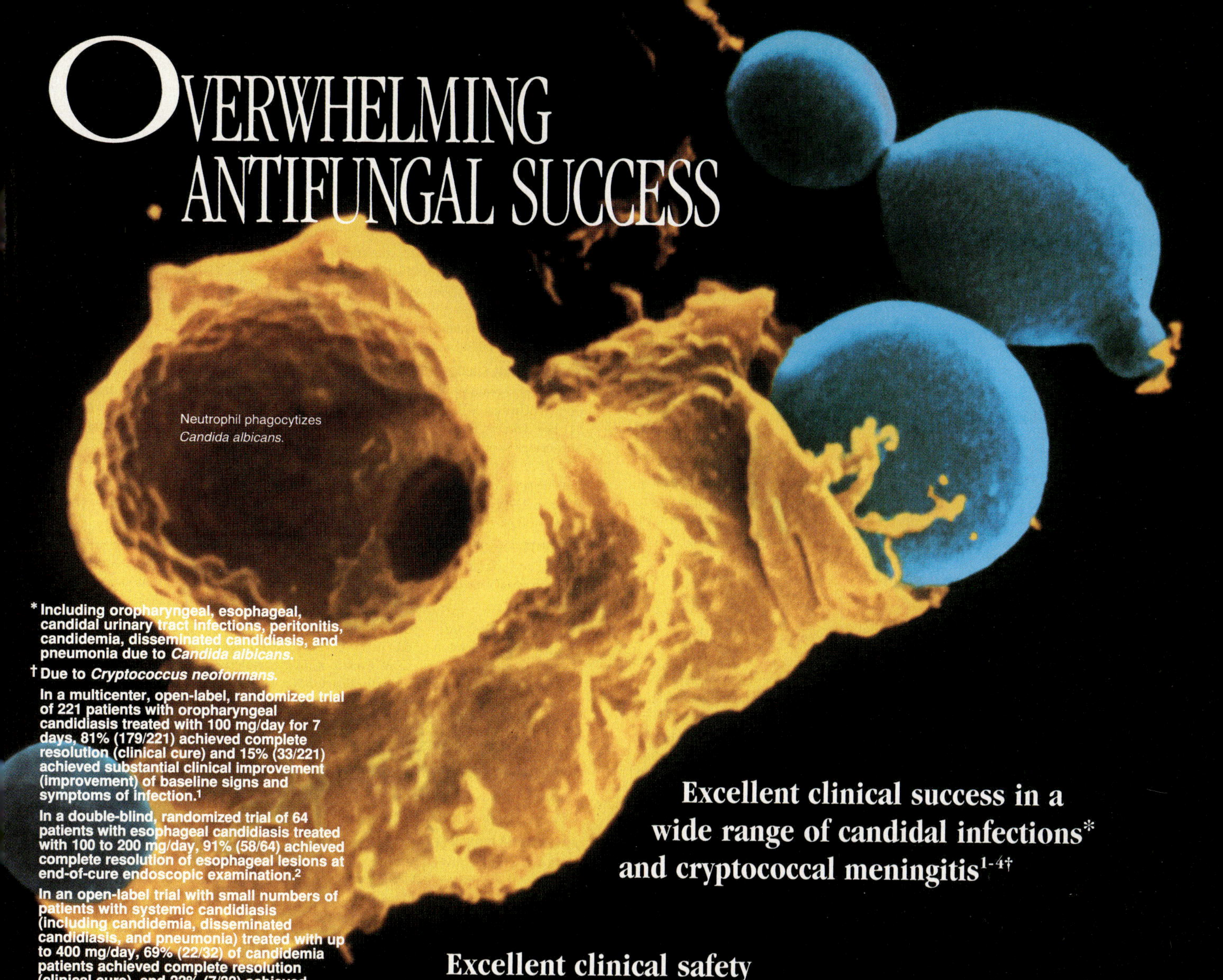

Neutrophil phagocytizes *Candida albicans.*

Excellent clinical success in a wide range of candidal infections* and cryptococcal meningitis[1-4†]

* Including oropharyngeal, esophageal, candidal urinary tract infections, peritonitis, candidemia, disseminated candidiasis, and pneumonia due to *Candida albicans.*

† Due to *Cryptococcus neoformans.*

In a multicenter, open-label, randomized trial of 221 patients with oropharyngeal candidiasis treated with 100 mg/day for 7 days, 81% (179/221) achieved complete resolution (clinical cure) and 15% (33/221) achieved substantial clinical improvement (improvement) of baseline signs and symptoms of infection.[1]

In a double-blind, randomized trial of 64 patients with esophageal candidiasis treated with 100 to 200 mg/day, 91% (58/64) achieved complete resolution of esophageal lesions at end-of-cure endoscopic examination.[2]

In an open-label trial with small numbers of patients with systemic candidiasis (including candidemia, disseminated candidiasis, and pneumonia) treated with up to 400 mg/day, 69% (22/32) of candidemia patients achieved complete resolution (clinical cure), and 22% (7/32) achieved substantial clinical improvement (improvement) of baseline signs and symptoms of infection. In patients with disseminated candidiasis, 52% (16/31) achieved complete resolution (clinical cure), and 19% (6/31) achieved substantial clinical improvement (improvement) of baseline signs and symptoms of infection. In patients with pneumonia, 58% (11/19) achieved complete resolution (clinical cure), and 37% (7/19) achieved substantial clinical improvement (improvement) of baseline signs and symptoms of infection.

In an open-label trial with small numbers of patients with candidal urinary tract infections (UTI) and peritonitis treated with doses of 50 mg to 200 mg/day, 53% (20/38) of those with candidal UTI achieved complete resolution (clinical cure), and 26% (10/38) achieved substantial clinical improvement (improvement) of baseline signs and symptoms of infection. In peritonitis patients, 66% (23/35) achieved complete resolution (clinical cure), and 25% (9/35) achieved substantial clinical improvement (improvement) of baseline signs and symptoms of infection.

In a multicenter comparative study of 111 patients treated with 200 mg/day for suppression of relapse of cryptococcal meningitis, 93% (103/111) achieved successful maintenance without culture-confirmed relapse and without toxicity necessitating discontinuance. Three risk factors which may predict a negative outcome for AIDS patients with cryptococcal meningitis are: abnormal mental status, CSF with antigen titer>1:1024, and CSF WBC<20 cells per cubic millimeter.[3]

In a multicenter, open-label, 10-week trial of 131 AIDS patients treated with 200 mg/day for culture-confirmed acute cryptococcal meningitis, an overall response rate (cure and quiescent disease) of 60% (78/131) was achieved.[4]

Excellent clinical safety

In more than 4,000 patients who received Diflucan for at least 7 days, the most common adverse events were nausea (3.7%), headache (1.9%), skin rash (1.8%), vomiting (1.7%), abdominal pain (1.7%), and diarrhea (1.5%).[1]

Diflucan has been associated with rare cases of serious hepatotoxicity. Patients have rarely developed exfoliative skin disorders during treatment with Diflucan.

ONCE-A-DAY **Diflucan**® (fluconazole) ORAL IV

100/200 mg Tablets, 10/40 mg/mL Oral Suspension, 200/400 mg IV Injection

Overwhelming antifungal success

Please see brief summary of prescribing information on adjacent page of this advertisement.

ARCHIVES OF SURGERY

The ARCHIVES OF SURGERY is a member of the consortium of AMA journals listed below. The complete text of all AMA journals is available online from Dialog Information Services and Information Access Company.

The Journal of the American Medical Association (JAMA)
Archives of Dermatology
Archives of Facial Plastic Surgery
Archives of Family Medicine
Archives of General Psychiatry
Archives of Internal Medicine
Archives of Neurology
Archives of Ophthalmology
Archives of Otolaryngology–Head & Neck Surgery
Archives of Pathology & Laboratory Medicine
Archives of Pediatrics & Adolescent Medicine
Archives of Surgery

The ARCHIVES OF SURGERY (ISSN 0004-0010) is published monthly by the American Medical Association, 515 N State St, Chicago, IL 60610, and is an official publication of the Association. The ARCHIVES OF SURGERY reaches more than 19 000 readers in over 69 countries each month. Periodicals postage paid at Chicago, IL, and at additional mailing offices. GST registration number 12622 5556 RT. Canada Post International Publications Mail (Canadian Distribution) Sales Agreement No. 319309.

Printed in the USA.

Official Publication of the New England Surgical Society, Pacific Coast Surgical Association, Surgical Infection Society, Western Surgical Association.

SUBSCRIPTION RATES—The personal subscription rates for the ARCHIVES OF SURGERY are $145 for 1 year (12 issues) in the United States and US possessions; $195 in the Americas; £125 outside the Americas. The institution rates for 1 year are $245 in the US; $345 in the Americas; £195 outside the Americas. Special rates for residents and medical students are available. Address all subscription communications to: Subscriber Services Center, American Medical Association, PO Box 10946, Chicago, IL 60610-0946. Phone: (800) 262-2350. Fax: (312) 464-5831. E-mail: ama-subs@ama-assn.org. For mailing addresses outside the United States and US possessions, see International Subscription Information.

CHANGE OF ADDRESS—POSTMASTER, send all address changes to ARCHIVES OF SURGERY, c/o Subscriber Services, American Medical Association, 515 N State St, Chicago, IL 60610. Please notify us of address change at least 6 weeks in advance to ensure uninterrupted service. Include both old and new addresses, a recent mailing label, and new ZIP code. For mailing addresses outside the United States and US possessions, see International Subscription Information.

SUBSCRIBER SERVICES—For information about subscribing to any of the AMA publications, change of address, missing issues, or purchasing back issues, please contact Subscriber Services Center, American Medical Association, PO Box 10946, Chicago, IL 60610-0946, or call (800) 262-2350 or (312) 670-SUBS (670-7827) between 8:30 AM and 4:30 PM CST. Fax: (312) 464-5831. E-mail: ama-subs@ama-assn.org. For mailing addresses outside the United States and US possessions, see International Subscription Information.

INTERNATIONAL SUBSCRIPTION INFORMATION—Subscriptions outside the United States and US possessions are served according to geographic region. Please address correspondence to the following 2 offices based on delivery address: (1) For delivery in North America, Central America, and South America, contact Subscriber Services, AMA, PO Box 10946, Chicago, IL 60610-0946. Phone: (312) 670-7827. Fax: (312) 464-5831. E-mail: ama-subs@ama-assn.org. (2) For delivery outside the Americas contact JAMA & Archives Journals, Reader Services Centre, PO Box 299, London WC1H 9TD, England. Phone: +44 (0)171-383-6270. Fax: +44 (0)171-383-6402. E-mail: jama-archives@dial.pipex.com.

REPRINTS—Authors place their reprint order at the time the edited typescript is reviewed and should allow 4 to 6 weeks for delivery following publication. Requests for individual reprints should be sent directly to the author at the address shown in the article.

For bulk reprint orders for distribution by commercial organizations, please contact Wanda Bartolotta, 500 Fifth Ave, #2210, New York, NY 10110. Phone: (212) 354-0050. Fax: (212) 354-1169. E-mail: wanda_bartolotta@ama-assn.org. For reprint orders in limited quantities for distribution by educational organizations and for author reprints, please contact Reprint Coordinator, 515 N State St, Chicago, IL 60610. Phone: (312) 464-4594. Fax: (312) 464-4849.

WORLD WIDE WEB ADDRESS—http://www.ama-assn.org.

SURGERY HOME PAGE—http://www.ama-assn.org/surgery.

PERMISSIONS—Contact Rhonda Bailey, Permissions Assistant, 515 N State St, Chicago, IL 60610. Phone: (312) 464-2513.

ADVERTISING PRINCIPLES—Each advertisement in this issue has been reviewed and complies with the principles governing advertising in AMA scientific publications. A copy of these principles is available on request. The appearance of advertising in AMA publications is not an AMA guarantee or endorsement of the product or the claims made for the product by the manufacturer.

ARCHIVES OF SURGERY

www.ama-assn.org/surgery

VOL 134 NO. 3, MARCH 1999

MISSION STATEMENT

To promote the art and science of surgery by publishing relevant peer-reviewed clinical and basic science information to assist the surgeon in optimizing patient care. The *Archives of Surgery* will also serve as a forum for the discussion of issues that involve ethics, teaching, surgical history, and socioeconomic concerns.

*Approved by the Editorial Board, *Archives of Surgery*, July 19, 1996.

EDITORIAL

***JAMA* and Editorial Independence** 238
JAMA Editors and Editorial Board Members

ORIGINAL ARTICLES

Functional Outcome After Laparoscopic or Open Nissen Fundoplication: A Follow-up Study 240
Tuomo K. Rantanen, MD; Jarmo A. Salo, MD; Jukka T. Salminen, MD; Ilmo H. Kellokumpu, MD

Association of Increased Immunostaining for Inducible Nitric Oxide Synthase and Nitrotyrosine With Fibroblast Growth Factor Transformation in Pancreatic Cancer 245
Selwyn M. Vickers, MD; Lee Ann MacMillan-Crow, PhD; Mary Green, BA; Chris Ellis, BA; John A. Thompson, PhD

Tikhoff-Linberg Procedure for Bone and Soft Tissue Tumors of the Shoulder Girdle 252
Gregor Voggenreiter, MD; Stefan Assenmacher, MD; Klaus-Peter Schmit-Neuerburg, MD

Parathyroid Autotransplantation During Thyroidectomy: Is Frozen Section Necessary? 258
Chung-yau Lo, FRCS(Edin); King-yin Lam, FRCPA

Association of Preoperative Biliary Stenting With Increased Postoperative Infectious Complications in Proximal Cholangiocarcinoma 261
Steven N. Hochwald, MD; Edmund C. Burke, MD; William R. Jarnagin, MD; Yuman Fong, MD; Leslie H. Blumgart, MD

American Medical Association
Physicians dedicated to the health of America

All articles published, including editorials, letters, and book reviews, represent the opinions of the authors and do not reflect the policy of the American Medical Association, the Editorial Board, or the institution with which the author is affiliated, unless this is clearly specified.

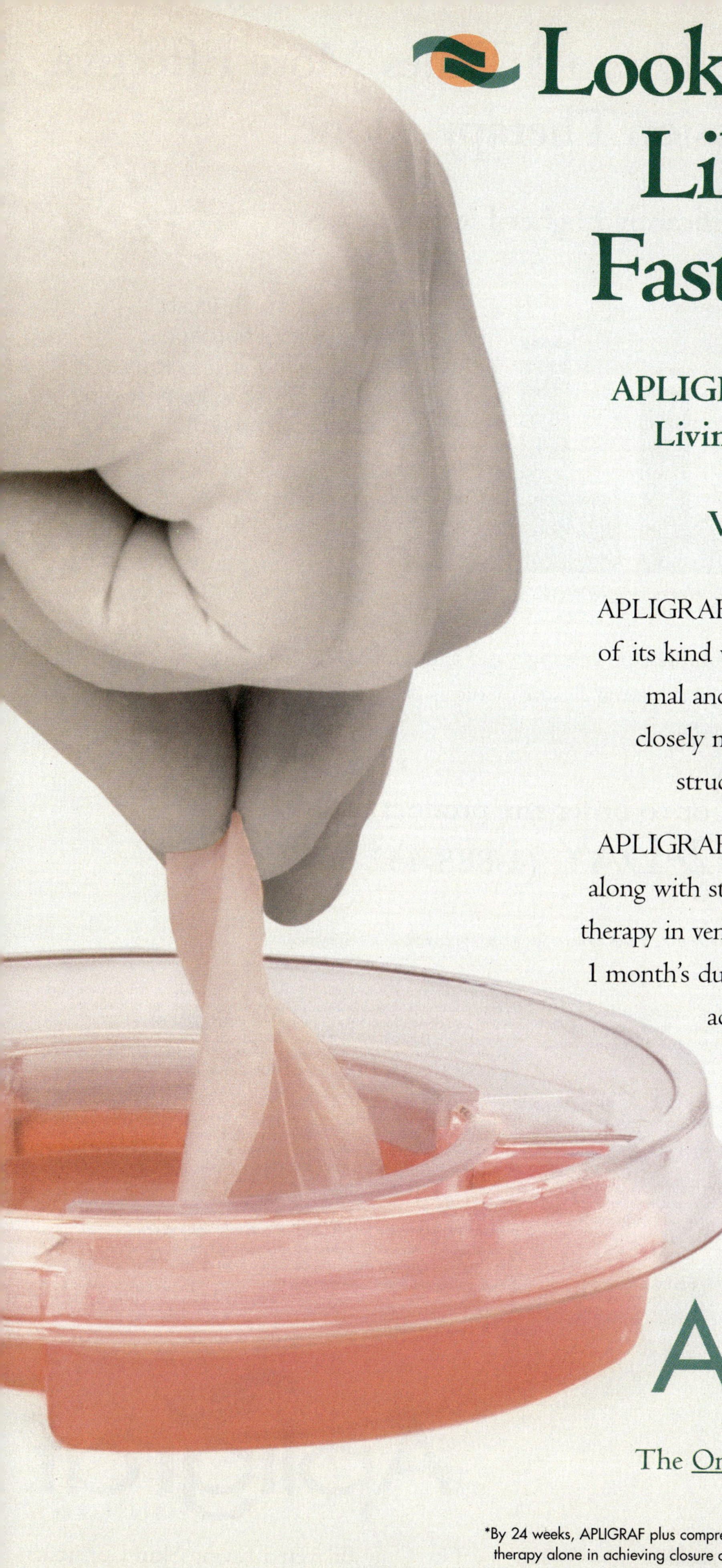

Looks and Feels Like Skin for Faster Healing

APLIGRAF®—The Only Bilayered Living Skin Construct Proven to Close More Hard-to-Heal Venous Ulcers in Less Time*

APLIGRAF is the only product of its kind with both an epidermal and a dermal layer—to closely mimic human skin in structure and function.[1,2]

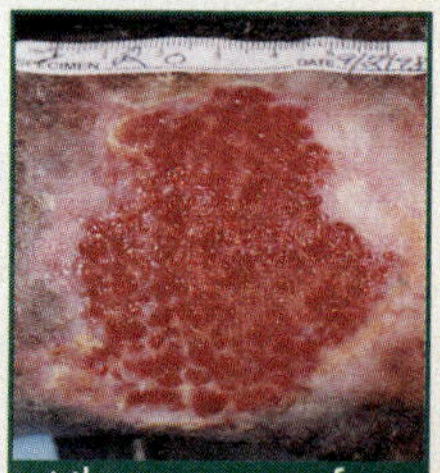

Ulcer present for 13 months before APLIGRAF

APLIGRAF is indicated for use along with standard compression therapy in venous ulcers of at least 1 month's duration that have not adequately responded to conventional ulcer therapy.

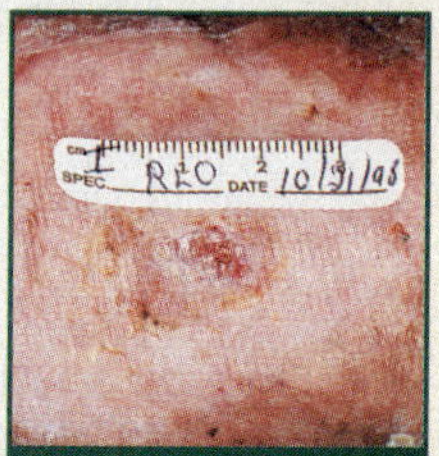

Ulcer healing at week 7 after APLIGRAF

Apligraf®
(Graftskin)

The <u>Only</u> Bilayered Living Skin Construct

*By 24 weeks, APLIGRAF plus compression therapy was more than twice as effective as compression therapy alone in achieving closure of ulcers >1 year's duration (47% vs 19%, respectively; *P*=.002).

Are Expandable Metallic Stents Better Than Conventional Methods for Treating Difficult Intrahepatic Biliary Strictures With Recurrent Hepatolithiasis? **267**
Kuo-Shyang Jeng, MD; I-Shyan Sheen, MD; Fi-Sh Yang, MD

Insulin's Anabolic Effect Is Influenced by Route of Administration of Nutrients **274**
Ronald H. Clements, MD; Clint A. Hayes, MD; E. Rickey Gibbs, MD; John Geiger; Henry L. Laws, MD; Calvin L. Long, PhD

Transition From Open to Laparoscopic Fundoplication: The Learning Curve **278**
Scott J. Soot, MD; Nihnam Eshraghi, MD; Mehrdad Farahmand, MD; Brett C. Sheppard, MD; Clifford W. Deveney, MD

Invited Critique **282**
James C. Rosser, Jr, MD

Growth Hormone Attenuates Tumor Necrosis Factor α in Burned Children **283**
Minas T. Chrysopoulo, MD; Marc G. Jeschke, MD; Roque J. Ramirez, MD; Robert E. Barrow, PhD; David N. Herndon, MD

Enteral Nutrition Prevents Bacterial Translocation but Does Not Improve Survival During Acute Pancreatitis **287**
Joji Kotani, MD; Makoto Usami, MD; Hideaki Nomura, MD; Atsunori Iso, MD; Hiroshi Kasahara, MD; Yoshikazu Kuroda, MD; Harumasa Oyanagi, MD; Yoichi Saitoh, MD

Nitric Oxide and Thromboxane A_2–Mediated Pulmonary Microvascular Dysfunction **293**
Joseph K. Wright, MD; Lawrence T. Kim, MD; Tom E. Rogers, MD; Hao Nguyen, PhD; Richard H. Turnage, MD

A Refined Approach to the Repair of Postcholecystectomy Bile Duct Strictures **299**
Francis Sutherland, MD, FRCSC; Bernard Launois, MD, FACS; Mihail Stanescu, MD; Jean Pierre Campion, MD; Yorgos Spiliopoulos, MD; Christian Stasik, MD

ARCHIVES OF SURGERY

ARCHIVES OF SURGERY

Hyperthermic Isolated Limb Perfusion With Tumor Necrosis Factor α, Interferon Gamma, and Melphalan for Locally Advanced Nonmelanoma Skin Tumors of the Extremities: A Multicenter Study 303
Annette F. T. Olieman, MD, PhD; Danielle Liénard, MD; Alexander M. M. Eggermont, MD, PhD; Bin B. R. Kroon, MD, PhD; Ferdy J. Lejeune, MD, PhD; Harald J. Hoekstra, MD, PhD; Heimen Schraffordt Koops, MD, PhD

Minicholecystectomy: A Safe, Cost-effective Day Surgery Procedure 308
A. Kent Seale, MD; Walter P. Ledet, Jr, MD

Invited Critique 310
Hector Orozco, MD; Miguel Angel Mercado, MD

Recurrent Pancreatitis in Gardner Variant Familial Polyposis: Etiology, Diagnostic Approach, and Interventional Results 311
B. E. Wright, MD; R. A. Kozarek, MD; L. W. Traverso, MD; D. Wechter, MD; R. Thirlby, MD; S. L. Raltz, RN

Reoperation for Severe Pancreatitis: A 10-Year Experience in a Tertiary Care Center 316
François Paye, MD; Pascal Frileux, MD; Paul Lehman, MD; Jean-Marie Ollivier, MD; Jean Christophe Vaillant, MD; Rolland Parc, MD, FACS

Invited Critique 321
Edward L. Bradley III, MD

SURGICAL REMINISCENCES

A Medical Student's Meeting With Two Giants 322
Clifford W. Deveney, MD

SPECIAL ARTICLE

Surgery in the Philippines 323
Antonio A. Limson, MD; Jose Luis J. Danguilan, MD; Romeo R. Gutierrez, MD; Ramon S. de Jesus, MD; Armando C. Crisostomo, MD; Alberto M. Roxas, MD

SURGICAL TECHNIQUE

Management of Acute Mesenteric Ischemia 328
M. Ashraf Mansour, MD

Invited Critique 331
Bruce L. Gewertz, MD

MOMENTS IN SURGICAL HISTORY

***A Treatise on the Malformation, Injuries, and Diseases of the Rectum and Anus*: America's First Textbook on Colorectal Surgery** 332
Ira M. Rutkow, MD, MPH, DrPH

DEPARTMENTS

Surgical Anatomy 282

Calendar 335

Products & Services 338

Classified Advertising 339

Index to Advertisers 343

Instructions for Authors—
See January 1999 issue, page 107, or visit the Web site at http://www.ama-assn.org/surgery.

Editor's Note: The Lundberg era as vice president for Scientific Communications of the American Medical Association will have a prolonged and affirmative impact on medical journalism and health care. George Lundberg brought a distinguished career as an academic pathologist to this position. As editor of *JAMA*, his initiatives and involvement with all phases of the health care community were needed, are now legendary, and have established this journal as a leader. The termination of this distinguished editor appears more as a result of sophomoric management than substance. There were no winners. Adlai Stevenson at Princeton University in the mid-1950s remarked that all progress in society results from the actions of unreasonable men.

Dr Lundberg internationalized the editorial board of *JAMA*, broadened its readership base, and involved THE JOURNAL in relevant issues. He tolerated and encouraged dissent, often enjoying such discussions. The quality of the journal, its substance, variety, and research grew geometrically. The theme issues were eminently successful, including such topics as the underinsured and uninsured, alternative medicine, violence, tobacco, gun control, boxing, communicable diseases, all of which have a profound effect on the quality of life worldwide.

His interaction with the *Archives* journals' editors was always spirited. Lundberg respected and supported the integrity of the *Archives*' editors and their editorial freedom. He practiced what he preached! This interaction with Dr Lundberg will be missed. I suspect, however, that he will not ride away into the sunset. History will be kind to his editorship of *JAMA*. In Proverbs it is said that "iron sharpens iron, therefore one man sharpens another." I have benefited from my association with George Lundberg.

Claude H. Organ, Jr, MD

JAMA and Editorial Independence

On January 15, 1999, George D. Lundberg, MD, was dismissed as Editor of *JAMA* and Editor-in-Chief of AMA's Scientific Information and Multimedia. In a written statement, AMA Executive Vice President E. Ratcliffe Anderson, Jr, MD, said that Dr Lundberg "threatened the historic tradition and integrity of the *Journal of the American Medical Association* by inappropriately and inexcusably interjecting *JAMA* into a major political debate that has nothing to do with science or medicine."[1]

The article in question[2] surveyed college students regarding their perceptions of whether certain sexual practices constituted having "had sex." The study was conducted by leading researchers, was not solicited by *JAMA*, and underwent peer review and editorial scrutiny.

The dismissal of Dr Lundberg has prompted widespread concern within the medical and scientific publishing communities. Innumerable commentators worldwide have interpreted Dr Lundberg's dismissal as a serious challenge to *JAMA*'s editorial freedom and a direct threat to THE JOURNAL's historic tradition and integrity.

During his 17-year tenure, Dr Lundberg demanded and maintained THE JOURNAL's editorial independence,[3] a position affirmed several times by AMA's Board of Trustees and policy-making House of Delegates.[4,5] Under his editorship, *JAMA* has become a world-class scientific publication. Dr Lundberg has been an international leader in the development of a scientifically and ethically sound peer-review process. He has also bridged the gap between clinical researchers and health services researchers by focusing on issues of public policy that directly or indirectly touch the health care and health of the American people. His efforts developed a respected, successful medical journal and family of *Archives* journals that publish important, high-quality articles that advance medical science, improve patient care, protect public health, and inform health policy.

The Key and Critical Objectives of *JAMA*[4,5]

Key Objective: To promote the science and art of medicine and the betterment of the public health

Critical Objectives:

1. To publish original, important, well-documented, peer-reviewed clinical and laboratory articles on a diverse range of medical topics
2. To provide physicians with continuing education in basic and clinical science to support informed clinical decisions
3. To enable physicians to remain informed in multiple areas of medicine, including developments in fields other than their own
4. To improve public health internationally by elevating the quality of medical care, disease prevention, and research provided by an informed readership
5. To foster responsible and balanced debate on controversial issues that affect medicine and health care
6. To forecast important issues and trends in medicine and health care
7. To inform readers about nonclinical aspects of medicine and public health, including the political, philosophic, ethical, legal, environmental, economic, historical, and cultural
8. To recognize that, in addition to these specific objectives, THE JOURNAL has a social responsibility to improve the total human condition and to promote the integrity of science
9. To report American Medical Association policy, as appropriate, while maintaining editorial independence, objectivity, and responsibility
10. To achieve the highest level of ethical medical journalism and to produce a publication that is timely, credible, and enjoyable to read

While we acknowledge Dr Anderson's administrative authority to act as he did, we, the Editors of *JAMA* and AMA *Archives* journals and members of the *JAMA* Editorial Board, strongly disagree with the decision to summarily dismiss Dr Lundberg.

Editorial independence is the lifeblood of THE JOURNAL. The editorial independence that *JAMA* has enjoyed has been the essential foundation on which the publication built its current prestige and, in the process, lent so much prestige to the AMA in the biomedical and health-services research community. For the world-class status of *JAMA* to continue, its editorial independence must be preserved by the AMA, even if some of the AMA's leadership or its members may disagree about the scientific merit or propriety of particular articles, as inevitably they will, from time to time. Dr Anderson stated that "*JAMA*'s hard-earned reputation is based on its editorial independence and integrity, and we intend to keep it that way."[1] We wholeheartedly agree and endorse this pledge.

We, the undersigned, reaffirm and recommit ourselves to upholding the values, goals, and objectives of THE JOURNAL (**Table**). We hope that all who value what Dr Lundberg, many of us, and so many others have built will stand by THE JOURNAL and support its foundation of editorial independence as key to its mission of promoting the science and art of medicine and the betterment of the public health.

JAMA Editors: *Richard M. Glass, MD; Phil B. Fontanarosa, MD; Drummond Rennie, MD; Margaret A. Winker, MD; M. Therese Southgate, MD; Charles B. Clayman, MD; Helene M. Cole, MD; Thomas B. Cole, MD, MPH; David S. Cooper, MD; David H. Mark, MD, MPH; Harriet S. Meyer, MD; Carin M. Olson, MD; Ronna Henry Siegel, MD; Jeanette M. Smith, MD; Jody W. Zylke, MD; Robert A. Clark, MD; Deborah J. Cook, MD; Naomi Vaisrub, PhD; Annette Flanagin; Charlene Breedlove; Roxanne K. Young; Thomas C. Jefferson, MD; William M. Silberg; Marsha Goldsmith; Cheryl Iverson; Elaine Williams.*

AMA Archives *Journals Editors:* *Daniel M. Albert, MD; Kenneth A. Arndt, MD; Jack D. Barchas, MD; Marjorie A. Bowman, MD, MPA; James E. Dalen, MD; Catherine D. DeAngelis, MD; Michael E. Johns, MD; Wayne F. Larrabee, Jr, MD; Claude H. Organ, Jr, MD; Roger N. Rosenberg, MD.*

JAMA *Editorial Board Members:* *H. David Banta, MD; Michael Berger, MD; Robert J. Blendon, ScD; Iain Chalmers, MBBS, MSc; Lois DeBakey, PhD; Ronald G. Evens, MD; Colin I. Johnston, MB,BS; Donald A. B. Lindberg, MD; Hervé Maisonneuve, MD; C. David Naylor, MD, DPhil; Edmund D. Pellegrino, MD; Reed E. Pyeritz, MD, PhD; Uwe E. Reinhardt, PhD; Povl Riis, MD, DSCI, DHC; William L. Roper, MD, MPH; Masaaki Terada, MD.*

Author Affiliations: See JAMA *masthead for author affiliations.*

Reprinted from JAMA. *1999;281:460.*

REFERENCES

1. Anderson ER. American Medical Association statement; Jan 15, 1999; Chicago, Ill.
2. Sanders SA, Reinisch JM. Would you say you had sex if . . . ? *JAMA.* 1999;281: 275-277.
3. Lundberg GD. Editorial freedom and integrity. *JAMA.* 1988;281:2563.
4. American Medical Association. *JAMA* editorial freedom. Board Report Resolution 904, I-92 adopted by the House of Delegates; June 1993.
5. Lundberg GD. House of Delegates reaffirms *JAMA*'s editorial independence. *JAMA.* 1993;270:1248-1249.

ORIGINAL ARTICLE

Functional Outcome After Laparoscopic or Open Nissen Fundoplication

A Follow-up Study

Tuomo K. Rantanen, MD; Jarmo A. Salo, MD; Jukka T. Salminen, MD; Ilmo H. Kellokumpu, MD

Objective: To compare the results of open and laparoscopic fundoplication.

Design: Nonrandomized controlled study with a 3-year follow-up.

Patients and Methods: Fifty-seven consecutive patients with erosive reflux esophagitis underwent laparoscopic (30 patients) or open (27 patients) fundoplication.

Interventions: Interview by an independent person. In addition, 52 patients (91%) underwent postoperative endoscopy, and 38 patients (67%) underwent esophageal 24-hour pH recording.

Results: Temporary dysphagia was reported by 20 patients (67%) after laparoscopic and by 11 (41%) after open fundoplication ($P = .05$). There were no differences between groups concerning incidence of persistent dysphagia (20% vs 18%, respectively) and mild to no reflux symptoms (97% vs 100%, respectively). In addition, bloating (50% vs 63%, respectively) and increased flatus (77% vs 78%, respectively) were equally common. Visual analog scale scores for dysphagia, bloating, and increased flatus were 0.6, 2.4, and 4.3, respectively, in the laparoscopic and 0.6, 3.5, and 3.4, respectively, in the open groups. Normal belching ability was reported by 12 patients (40%) after laparoscopic and by 20 (74%) after open fundoplication ($P = .01$). Visick grade 1 or 2 was reported by 21 patients (70%) after laparoscopic and by 24 (89%) after open fundoplication ($P = .08$). Defective fundic wrap was detected in 4 patients (13%) in the laparoscopic and in none in the open group. In addition, abnormal results of 24-hour pH recording were found in 4 patients (22%) after laparoscopic and in 2 (10.5%) after open fundoplication.

Conclusion: From a functional point of view, both techniques were equally effective except concerning belching ability and temporary dysphagia.

Arch Surg. 1999;134:240-244

SHORT-TERM RESULTS after laparoscopic Nissen fundoplication have been promising, but long-term outcomes are still missing. However, there have been drawbacks to this technique, including more early reoperations than after an open technique.[1] The causes for failure can be several, but one reason can be that the laparoscopic technique is used in almost every case instead of patient-related tailored approach as has been proposed.[2]

To be chosen as the standard method in antireflux surgery, laparoscopic Nissen fundoplication should have at least as good results as open fundoplication. However, there have been few studies comparing the results of open and laparoscopic Nissen fundoplication.[3-8] According to these studies, both techniques were similar concerning reflux control, but in 1 study, there were some differences concerning functional outcomes that favored the open technique.[8] However, there were many shortcomings in these studies, including short follow-up, historical comparisons,[3,8] and lack of objective postoperative evaluation.[4]

Our aim was to compare functional outcome of laparoscopic and open Nissen fundoplication in the management of severe symptomatic gastroesophageal reflux disease with adequate follow-up. Therefore, we used objective and subjective analytical methods.

RESULTS

LAPAROSCOPIC GROUP

Temporary postoperative dysphagia was reported by 20 patients (67%), and it lasted on average 118 days (range, 2-540 days).

Twenty-three patients (77%) had no reflux symptoms at follow-up, whereas 6 patients (20%) had mild and 1 patient (3%)

From the Department of Surgery, Helsinki University Central Hospital, Helsinki, Finland.

PATIENTS AND METHODS

The study group consisted of 57 consecutive patients who underwent primary laparoscopic or open Nissen fundoplication for severe symptomatic gastroesophageal reflux disease and fulfilled our inclusion criteria from January 1, 1993, to May 31, 1995. All operations were performed or directly supervised by two of us (laparoscopic fundoplication, I.H.K.; open fundoplication, J.A.S.) in Helsinki University Central Hospital, Helsinki, Finland. We excluded the first 12 patients to obtain adequate experience. All those surgeons who performed laparoscopic fundoplication in our study were otherwise experienced laparoscopic surgeons before starting to perform fundoplication.

In every case, long-term conservative treatment with histamine blockers or proton pump inhibitors had failed, or patients were dependent on these medicines and requested operative treatment. Inclusion criteria consisted of erosive esophagitis detected at preoperative endoscopy and pathological results of esophageal 24-hour pH recording.[9-11] Those patients who underwent some other abdominal procedure simultaneously were excluded, as were also the patients with Barrett esophagus and esophageal stricture. In addition, we excluded all patients undergoing laparoscopy that had to be converted to an open procedure. There were no statistical differences between groups concerning the severity of gastroesophageal reflux disease, risk factors (severe concomitant diseases, previous laparotomy), and follow-up.

All interviews were performed by one of us (T.K.R.) who had not been involved previously in the patients' care. All patients were interviewed according to standard formula, and incidence of heartburn, regurgitation, and dysphagia were recorded using the DeMeester-Johnson Reflux Scale.[9,10] Postoperative ability to belch and vomit was assessed by the patients as none, with some difficulties, or restored to preoperative ability. The Visick grading system[12] was used for estimation of patient satisfaction. Postfundoplication increase of flatus and bloating was assessed by the patients as none, mild, moderate, or severe. In addition, a Visual Analog Scale (VAS)[13] was used to assess dysphagia, flatus, and bloating, where 0 indicates none and 10 very troublesome symptoms. Savary-Miller grading[14] of the reflux esophagitis was used, and Barrett esophagus was defined when intestinal metaplasia in biopsy samples taken in tubular esophagus was detected.[15] The state of fundic wrap was verified with retroflexed endoscope. Slipping was registered when there was a distinct gastric pouch above the narrowing caused by the folds of the wrap, and disruption implied no visible folds or only distorted, loose folds at the esophagogastric junction. Abnormal reflux was defined using previously presented criteria.[9-11]

During follow-up, repeated fundoplication had to be performed for 2 patients in the laparoscopic group.

STATISTICAL ANALYSIS

The χ^2 2-tailed test, Fisher exact 2-tailed test, and the Mann-Whitney *U* test were used for statistical comparisons. A probability of .05 was accepted as significant.

LAPAROSCOPIC GROUP

Thirty patients underwent laproscopic fundoplication. Fundic mobilization was performed in 24 patients (80%) and hiatoplasty in 28 (93%). Length of fundic wrap was 2 cm, and it was anchored to the esophagus in 8 patients (27%), gastric cardia in 2 (7%), and neither in 20 (67%). Nonabsorbable sutures were used in all patients, and patch where sutures are secured with Teflon pledgets[16] was used in fundic wrap in 17 patients (57%). Nasogastric tubes (18F) and bougies (35F) were used with fundic wrap in all cases. Fundic mobilization and hiatal repair were not performed in every patient if it was otherwise possible to construct loose fundic wrap and if hiatal opening was not large. Preoperative clinical data are shown in **Table 1**.

All 30 patients consented to undergo at least postoperative endoscopy, but esophageal 24-hour pH recording was refused by 12 patients (40%). Manometry was performed in 4 patients. The mean follow-up time was 33 months (range, 12-44 months), and it was at least 24 months among those 28 patients who did not undergo reoperation.

OPEN GROUP

Standard technique was used in all 27 patients. It consisted of fundic mobilization, hiatoplasty, and 2-cm-long fundic wrap that was anchored to cardia in every case. In addition, patch where nonabsorbable suture was secured with Teflon pledgets[16] was used in performing hiatal repair and in fundic wrap. Preoperative clinical data are shown in Table 1.

Postoperative endoscopy was refused by 5 patients (18%) and esophageal 24-hour pH recording by 7 (26%). In 1 patient, pH recording was technically unsuccessful. Postoperative endoscopy or successful esophageal 24-hour pH recording was performed in 23 patients (85%). Esophageal manometry was performed in 11 patients (41%). The mean follow-up time was 33 months (range, 24-45 months).

This study was approved by the Ethics Committee of the Department of Surgery, Helsinki University Central Hospital.

had moderate symptoms. Persistent dysphagia was reported by 6 patients (20%). Dysphagia decreased or disappeared postoperatively in 5 patients, was unchanged in 1 patient, and began postoperatively in 2 patients.

Fifteen patients (50%) had postoperative bloating. It was mild in 8 patients, moderate in 6 patients, and severe in 1 patient. Twenty-three patients (77%) reported increased postoperative flatus. It was mild in 7 patients, moderate in 12, and severe in 4. Preoperatively, 16 patients (53%) had had bloating and 19 (63%) had had increased flatus. Preoperative and postoperative VAS scores are shown in **Table 2**.

Postoperative ability to belch was assessed as none by 7 patients (23%), with some difficulties by 11 (37%), and restored to preoperative ability by 12 (40%). Eleven of those who could belch could not say the exact time when it first occurred; for the others, it happened on average 145 days after operation (range, 0-540 days).

Sixteen patients (53%) had no ability to vomit, whereas 7 (23%) had no need for vomiting postopera-

Table 1. Preoperative Clinical Data

	Operation Type	
	Laparoscopic (n = 30)	Open (n = 27)
Mean age, y (range)	46 (29-66)	47 (22-67)
Sex, No. male-female	22:8	17:10
Mean body mass index, kg/m² (range)	26.9 (22.3-37.2)	26.5 (20.3-33.6)
Previous laparotomy, No. (%)	3 (10)	2 (7)
Esophagitis, No. (%)		
Grade 1	9 (30)	10 (37)
Grade 2	20 (67)	14 (52)
Grade 3	0 (0)	2 (7)
Grade 4	1 (3)	1 (4)
Mean total reflux time, % (range)	13.8 (4-51)	25.5 (2.2-92.5)

Table 2. Preoperative and Postoperative VAS Scores*

	Operation Type	
	Laparoscopic	Open
Increased flatus		
Preoperative	3.3	0.7
Postoperative	4.3	3.4
Bloating		
Preoperative	2.4	2.1
Postoperative	2.4	3.5
Dysphagia		
Preoperative	1.5	1.1
Postoperative	0.6	0.6

VAS indicates Visual Analog Scale.[13] Scoring and the VAS are described in the "Patients and Methods" section of the text.

tively. Only 5 patients (17%) could vomit normally, and 2 (7%) could with some difficulties.

Visick grade 1 was reported by 14 patients (47%), grade 2 by 7 patients (23%), grade 3 by 8 patients (27%), and grade 4 by 1 patient (3%).

Twenty-eight patients (93%) said that they would be willing to have the same operation again with the same symptoms. Postoperative functional results are shown in **Table 3**.

At postoperative endoscopies, fundic wrap was normal in 26 patients (87%). In 4 patients, it was defective, including slipped fundoplication in 1 patient, disrupted fundic wrap in 1, intrathoracic fundic wrap in 1, and paraesophageal herniation in 1. Results of 4 (22%) of the 18 esophageal 24-hour pH recordings were abnormal. The mean and median values when pH was below 4 were 5.5% (range, 0%-31.5%) and 1.0%, respectively. Defective fundic wrap or abnormal esophageal 24-hour pH recording provided objective verification of recurrence of reflux in 6 patients (20%). Four of these had a pathological postoperative 24-hour pH measurement (<4 in 31.0%, 27.0%, 13.3%, and 10.0% of the registration time), and the other 2 had defective fundic wrap at endoscopy with reflux esophagitis. Two reoperations (7%) have been performed during the observation period due to slipped fundoplication with recurrent esophagitis in 1 patient and due to symptomatic paraesophageal herniation in 1.

Table 3. Functional Results and Patient Satisfaction After Laparoscopic and Open Fundoplication

	Operation Type, No. (%) of Patients		
	Laparoscopic	Open	P*
Temporary dysphagia	20 (67)	11 (41)	.05
Persistent dysphagia	6 (20)	5 (18)	NS
Mild or no reflux symptoms	29 (97)	27 (100)	NS
Inability to belch	7 (23)	4 (15)	NS
Normal ability to belch	12 (40)	20 (74)	.01
Inability to vomit	16 (53)	9 (33)	NS†
No need for vomiting	7 (23)	12 (44)	NS†
Normal ability to vomit	5 (17)	4 (15)	NS†
Visick grade 1-2	21 (70)	24 (89)	.08
Willing to undergo surgery again	28 (93)	26 (96)	NS

**NS indicates not significant.*
†Indicates whole scale of vomiting ability.

OPEN GROUP

Temporary postoperative dysphagia was reported by 11 patients (41%), and it lasted on average 96 days (range, 7-360 days).

Twenty-three patients (85%) had no and 4 (15%) had mild reflux symptoms on follow-up. Persistent dysphagia was reported by 5 patients (18%). Dysphagia decreased or disappeared postoperatively in 8 patients, was unchanged in 2, and began in 2. Seventeen patients (63%) had postoperative bloating, which was mild in 7, moderate in 7, and severe in 3. Increased flatus was reported by 21 patients (78%), which was mild in 8, moderate in 11, and severe in 2. Preoperatively, 13 patients (48%) had had bloating and 12 (44%) had had increased flatus. Preoperative and postoperative VAS scores are shown in Table 2.

Postoperative ability to belch was assessed as none by 4 patients (15%), with some difficulties by 3 (11%), and restored to preoperative ability by 20 (74%). Two patients could not say the exact time when they could belch the first time; to the others, it happened on average 79 days after operation (range, 0-360 days).

Nine patients (33%) had no ability to vomit, whereas 12 (44%) had no need for vomiting postoperatively. Only 4 patients (15%) had normal ability to vomit, and 2 (7%) could do it with some difficulties.

Visick grade 1 was reported by 16 patients (59%), grade 2 by 8 (30%), and grade 3 by 3 (11%).

Twenty-six patients (96%) expressed willingness to have the same operation again with the same symptoms. Postoperative functional results are shown in Table 3.

No reoperation was performed during the observation period in this group. At postoperative endoscopies, fundic wrap was normal in every case, and no recurrent esophagitis was detected. Results of 2 (10%) of the 19 esophageal 24-hour pH recordings were pathological. One patient had pH of less than 4 in 6.1% and another in 9.1% at the registration time. However, both patients were asymptomatic, and the endoscopic findings were normal. The mean and median values when pH was below 4 were 2.1% (range, 0%-9.1%) and 1.1%, respectively.

In this group, 2 postoperative incisional hernias (7%) have been found. The patient with the symptomatic hernia has undergone operation.

COMMENT

According to Ollyo et al,[17] 23% of patients with reflux esophagitis receiving nonsurgical therapy progressed steadily to more severe forms of esophagitis. It is well-known that the results of antireflux surgery among patients with end-stage disease are no better than those in patients with milder forms of reflux disease. Therefore, those patients with gastroesophageal reflux disease who are thought to have a risk for progressive disease should be offered surgical treatment as soon as this possibility has been noticed. Guidelines for the increased risk for progressive disease are low pressure of the lower esophageal sphincter and massive acid reflux detected in esophageal 24-hour pH recording. When Nissen fundoplication is performed at this time, success rates have been reported to be 80% to 90%.[16,18]

Our success rates concerning reflux control in both groups are comparable with those presented earlier, 97% and 100% of the patients having no or mild reflux symptoms. In addition, our incidence of persistent dysphagia (20% and 18%) compares favorably with other reports and is equally common in both groups. Instead, we found a higher incidence of postoperative increased flatus (77% and 78%) and bloating (50% and 63%) than in most of the studies, as can be seen from the VAS scores. In addition, many of our patients had these symptoms preoperatively. Luostarinen et al[19] and Blomqvist et al[8] found that many of their patients had these symptoms preoperatively. However, their patients were satisfied with the postoperative situation of not having reflux symptoms any more, even if they quite often had bloating and increased flatus. This was also the case among our patients.

Herniation of the stomach into the chest may be the cause of unsatisfactory long-term results.[20] This complication was present in 2 patients (7%) in the laparoscopic group, whereas none in the open group had the same complication.

However, there were also significant differences between open and laparoscopic fundoplication in our study. Temporary dysphagia was more common ($P = .05$) and normal ability to belch was less frequent ($P = .01$) after laparoscopic technique. Similar findings have been reported previously.[8,21-23] Reasons for these differences remain unknown. In 1 report, esophageal clearance was slower after laparoscopic than after open fundoplication.[23] This might be 1 reason for higher incidence of temporary dysphagia after laparoscopic technique, occurring in all patients in the study of Anvari and Allen.[24] The causes of temporary dysphagia after open Nissen fundoplication were thought to be esophageal stretching[25] and local edema.[20] Maybe there is more esophageal stretching after laparoscopic technique. This speculation is supported by Peters et al,[3] who thought that there might be less fundic mobilization in laparoscopic than in open fundoplication and that this causes more lateral stretching in the fundic region. In open fundoplication, it has been proposed to make a large posterior hiatal window.[16,20] The posterior hiatal window might be smaller in laparoscopic than in open surgery, because video can cause misrepresentation when evaluating size, and the created window can seem bigger than it is. This also can be 1 reason for the higher incidence of temporary dysphagia seen in laparoscopic antireflux surgery. In open fundoplication, 60F bougie, shortening of fundic wrap, and fundic mobilization have been shown to lessen temporary dysphagia.[16] A 60F bougie should be used also in laparoscopic fundoplication; in our patients, it might have diminished the occurrence of postoperative dysphagia. Instead, concerning laparoscopic operation, there have been conflicting reports about the effect of fundic mobilization on temporary dysphagia. In 1 report, fundic mobilization caused less temporary dysphagia[26]; in the other report,[27] it had no effect on it. Also, the incidence of subjectively normal belching ability was more common after open fundoplication (74% vs 40%; $P = .01$) in our study. The subjective evaluation of belching ability has many sources of errors, including difficulties in distinguishing gastric and esophageal belching. However, we think that patients can say reliably if changes have occurred in their ability to belch postoperatively. Thus, subjective evaluation can be used to indicate postoperative changes in belching ability. Also, Blomqvist et al[8] found that inability to belch was more frequent after the laparoscopic procedure. However, some of their open procedures were partial Toupet fundoplications. Reasons for the difference in normal ability to belch after laparoscopic and open fundoplication remain unknown. In 1 study,[3] lower esophageal sphincter pressure was higher and lower esophageal sphincter relaxation occurred less frequently after laparoscopic fundoplication. After open Nissen fundoplication, the subjective ability to belch has been somehow better after floppy fundoplications.[19,28,29] Instead, after laparoscopic operations, inability to belch was more common after fundic mobilization in 1 study.[27] In our study, fundic mobilization was used in every patient in the open group and in 80% in the laparoscopic group.

According to previously presented studies, there were no differences between open and laparoscopic techniques concerning patient satisfaction,[4] or it was better after open fundoplication.[8] In our study, there were no differences in willingness to have surgery again (93% vs 96%). Instead, there were more patients in the laparoscopic group who had Visick grade 3 or 4, even if the difference did not reach statistical significance ($P = .08$). Larger incision had no effect on patient satisfaction, but the final result of surgery is the most important thing to a patient.

Some reports indicated that there would be more early reoperations after laparoscopic surgery.[30] In our study, 4 patients undergoing laparoscopy had defective wrap at follow-up endoscopy, whereas the wrap was intact after open fundoplication in all patients. The reasons may be obscure, but 1 explanation may be that all sutures of the wrap were secured with Teflon pledgets in open fundoplication, whereas the pledgets were used only in 17 patients (57%) in the laparoscopic group. The second explanation may be the more demanding laparoscopic technique. In our study, there have been 2 reoperations (7%) in the laparoscopic group and none in the open group. According to Watson et al,[31] reoperations were more common when a single surgeon had performed fewer than 5 operations or the overall group in same institute had performed fewer than 20 operations. Surgeon experience had no effect on functional outcome and patient satisfaction in our study; we found no recurrences among patients who underwent operation under these circumstances.

Contrary to many other reports where postoperative interviews have been performed by operating surgeons, which may have influenced the results, the same surgeon who had not participated in the patients' care performed our interviews. In addition, we had adequate follow-ups in both groups of at least 2 years (average, 33 months). The longest follow-up after laparoscopic fundoplication that we found was in the study of Anvari and Allen.[24] In their study, 260 (68.2%) of the 381 patients undergoing operation underwent 6-month follow-up studies, and 108 (28.3%) underwent 2-year follow-up studies. Results were good concerning reflux symptoms, persistent dysphagia, and recurrences. However, functional outcomes were not mentioned.

Our study shows that open and laparoscopic Nissen fundoplication were effective in reflux control after almost 3 years of follow-up. However, temporary dysphagia and more disturbed belching ability may lessen advantages of laparoscopic technique.

We thank Yvonne Sundström for her skillful technical and secretarial assistance.

Reprints: Jarmo A. Salo, MD, Department of Surgery, Helsinki University Central Hospital, Haartmaninkatu 4, FIN-00290 Helsinki, Finland (e-mail: jarmo.salo@huch.fi).

REFERENCES

1. Watson DI, Jamieson GG, DeVitt PG, et al. Changing strategies in the performance of laparoscopic Nissen fundoplication as a result of experience with 230 operations. *Surg Endosc.* 1995;9:961-966.
2. Kauer WK, Peters JH, DeMeester TR, Heimbucher J, Ireland AP, Bremner CG. A tailored approach to antireflux surgery. *J Thorac Cardiovasc Surg.* 1995;110: 141-147.
3. Peters JH, Heimbucher J, Kauer WK, Incarbone R, Bremner CG, DeMeester TR. Clinical and physiologic comparison of laparoscopic and open Nissen fundoplication. *J Am Coll Surg.* 1995;380:385-393.
4. Rattner DW, Brooks DC. Patient satisfaction following laparoscopic and open antireflux surgery. *Arch Surg.* 1995;130:289-294.
5. Frantzides CT, Carlson MA. Laparoscopic versus conventional fundoplication. *J Laparosc Surg.* 1995;3:137-143.
6. Incarbone R, Peters JH, Heimbucher J, Dvorak D, Bremner CG, DeMeester TR. A contemporaneous comparison of hospital charges for laparoscopic and open Nissen fundoplication. *Surg Endosc.* 1995;9:151-155.
7. Richards KF, Fisher KS, Flores JH, Christensen BJ. Laparoscopic Nissen fundoplication: cost, morbidity, and outcome compared with open surgery. *Surg Laparosc Endosc.* 1996;6:140-143.
8. Blomqvist A, Lönnroth H, Dalenbäck J, Ruth M, Wiklund I, Lundell L. Quality of life assessment after laparoscopic and open fundoplication. *Scand J Gastroenterol.* 1996;31:1052-1058.
9. DeMeester TR, Johnson LF, Joseph GJ, Toscano MS, Hall AW, Skinner DB. Patterns of gastroesophageal reflux in health and disease. *Ann Surg.* 1976;184:459-470.
10. DeMeester TR, Johnson LF. The evaluation of objective measurements of gastroesophageal reflux and their contribution to patient management. *Surg Clin North Am.* 1976;56:39-53.
11. Salminen JT, Salo JA, Tuominen J, Rämö OJ, Färkkilä M, Mattila S. pH-metric analysis after successful antireflux surgery: comparison of 24-hour pH profiles in patients undergoing floppy fundoplication or Roux-en-Y duodenal diversion. *J Gastrointest Surg.* 1997;1:494-498.
12. Visick A. Measured radical gastrectomy: review of 505 operations for peptic ulcer. *Lancet.* 1948;1:505-510.
13. Reading AE. Testing pain mechanisms in persons in pain. In: Wall P, Melzack R, eds. *Textbook of Pain.* 2nd ed. New York, NY: Churchill Livingstone Inc; 1989: 269-280.
14. Savary M, Miller G. *Der Oesophagus, Lehrbuch und endoskopischer Atlas.* Solothurn, Switzerland: Gassmann; 1977.
15. Salo JA, Kiviluoto T, Kivilaakso E, Virtanen I. Cytokeratin profile suggests metaplastic epithelial transformation in Barrett's esophagus. *Ann Med.* 1996;28:305-309.
16. DeMeester TR, Bonavina L, Albertolucci M. Nissen fundoplication for gastroesophageal reflux disease: evaluation of primary repair in 100 consecutive patients. *Ann Surg.* 1986;204:9-20.
17. Ollyo JB, Monnier P, Fontolliet C, Savary M. The natural history, prevalence and incidence of reflux oesophagitis. *Gullet.* 1993;3(suppl):3-10.
18. Negre JB, Markkula HT, Keyriläinen O, Matikainen M. Nissen fundoplication: results at 10-year follow-up. *Am J Surg.* 1983;146:635-638.
19. Luostarinen M, Koskinen M, Reinikainen P, Karvonen J, Isolauri J. Two antireflux operations: floppy versus standard Nissen fundoplication. *Ann Med.* 1995; 27:199-205.
20. Polk H. Fundoplication for reflux esophagitis: misadventures with the operation of choice. *Ann Surg.* 1976;6:645-650.
21. Perdikis G, Hinder R, Lund R, Raiser F, Katada N. Laparoscopic Nissen fundoplication: where do we stand? *Surg Laparosc Endosc.* 1997;1:17-21.
22. Collard J, Gheldere C, deKock M, Otte J, Kestens P. Laparoscopic antireflux surgery: what is real progress? *Ann Surg.* 1994;2:146-154.
23. Luostarinen M, Koskinen M, Matikainen M, Isolauri J. Esophageal clearance and dysphagia after open or laparoscopic nissen fundoplication. In: Abstracts of the Annual Meeting of The Finnish Surgical Society [in Finnish]; November 13-14, 1997; Helsinki, Finland.
24. Anvari M, Allen C. Laparoscopic Nissen fundoplication: two-year comprehensive follow-up of a technique of minimal paraesophageal dissection. *Ann Surg.* 1998;1:25-32.
25. DeMeester TR, Johnson LF. Evaluation of the Nissen antireflux procedure by esophageal manometry and twenty-four hour pH monitoring. *Am J Surg.* 1975;129: 94-100.
26. Hunter J, Swanström LL, Waring P. Dysphagia after laparoscopic antireflux surgery: the impact of operative technique. *Ann Surg.* 1996;1:51-57.
27. Watson DI, Pike G, Baigrie R, et al. Prospective double-blind randomized trial of laparoscopic Nissen fundoplication with division and without division of short gastric vessels. *Ann Surg.* 1997;5:642-652.
28. Luostarinen M. Nissen fundoplication for gastroesophageal reflux disease: long-term results and functional effects. In: Kirjapaino V, ed. *Thesis, Acta Universitatis Tamperensis.* Vammala, Finland: Vammalan Kirjapaino; 1996 series A;481.
29. Donahue PE, Samuelson S, Nyhus LM, Bombeck CT. The floppy Nissen fundoplication: effective long-term control of pathologic reflux. *Arch Surg.* 1985;120: 663-668.
30. Dallemagne B, Weerts J, Jehaes C, Markiewitz S, Lombard R. Laparoscopic Nissen fundoplication: preliminary report. *Surg Laparosc Endosc.* 1991;1:138-143.
31. Watson DJ, Baigrie R, Jamieson GG. A learning curve for laparoscopic fundoplication: definable, avoidable, or a waste of time? *Ann Surg.* 1996;2:198-203.

ORIGINAL ARTICLE

Association of Increased Immunostaining for Inducible Nitric Oxide Synthase and Nitrotyrosine With Fibroblast Growth Factor Transformation in Pancreatic Cancer

Selwyn M. Vickers, MD; Lee Ann MacMillan-Crow, PhD; Mary Green, BA; Chris Ellis, BA; John A. Thompson, PhD

Background: Despite recognition of the devastating malignant potential of pancreatic cancer, the exact pathophysiological events contributing to tumor growth, vascular invasiveness, and hepatic metastasis remain to be elucidated.

Methods: Twelve human pancreatic adenocarcinomas were evaluated using immunohistochemical and in situ hybridization techniques for the appearance of the angiogenic and neurogenic growth factors, acidic fibroblast (FGF-1) and basic fibroblast growth factor (FGF-2), and their high-affinity receptors. Since FGF biological processes appear to be regulated by oxidant stress, tumors were examined further for the immunoappearance of inducible nitric oxide synthase (iNOS) and nitrotyrosine.

Results: Compared with normal human pancreatic tissue, tumor specimens exhibited varying levels of enhanced staining for FGF ligands and receptors. The increased appearance of FGF-1 and FGF-2 proteins was accompanied by increased detection of messenger RNA encoding each growth factor. In addition, these pancreatic tumors demonstrated the overexpression of iNOS and immunostaining of nitrotyrosine compared with normal pancreatic tissue.

Conclusions: The enhanced expression of FGF and FGF receptors suggests that these polypeptide mitogens may serve as important mediators of growth and of angiogenic and metastatic responses associated with pancreatic tumors, not seen in normal pancreatic tissue. Furthermore, we provide the first indication of increased expression of iNOS and protein tyrosine nitration, thereby predicting the potential involvement of oxidant stress during development and progression of pancreatic adenocarcinoma.

Arch Surg. 1999;134:245-251

HUMAN PANCREATIC adenocarcinoma remains one of the most difficult cancers to treat, as evidenced by little improvement in survival even with the addition of chemotherapy or radiation therapy. During the past 15 years, significant progress has occurred in the clinical management of pancreatic cancer due to increased early diagnosis and improved statistics on operative mortality (25% in the 1960s vs ≤5% more recently). However, the 1997 cancer statistics show that little improvement in overall patient survival has transpired from such progress. Specifically, in 1997 there were 27 600 new cases of pancreatic cancer with 28 100 deaths due to pancreatic cancer, with an overall 5-year survival of less than 5%.[1,2] The simple conclusion is that current detection and therapy are not satisfactory solutions to the unremitting problem of pancreatic cancer.

Recent advances in molecular biology have advanced our understanding of the pathogenesis of neoplasia. Collectively, these efforts have established potential molecular mechanisms associated with tumor development and progression that provide a rational basis for early detection techniques and interventional treatment. Proposed pathophysiological mechanisms associated with pancreatic adenocarcinoma have suggested an important role for numerous polypeptide growth factors and cytokines competent to induce pancreatic cell responses during development, physiologic processes, and tumorigenesis.[3-5] For instance, several recent studies have suggested a role for acidic fibroblast (FGF-1) and basic fibroblast growth factor (FGF-2) during progression of pancreatic adenocarcinoma.[6-9]

Both growth factors are prototypical members of a family of 10 structurally related polypeptides that serve as potent mitogens for neuroectoderm-, ectoderm-, and mesoderm-derived cells in vitro and as hormonal inducers of neurogenic, angiogenic, and wound repair mechanisms in

From the Department of Surgery, School of Medicine, University of Alabama at Birmingham.

MATERIALS AND METHODS

TISSUE SPECIMENS

We analyzed pancreatic cancers from 12 patients who underwent pancreaticoduodenectomy for biliary obstruction or pancreatic adenocarcinoma. Three samples of healthy pancreas obtained from heart-beating donors deemed unsuitable for transplantation were used as control samples.

IMMUNOLOCALIZATION

Thin sections (5 μm) of each formalin-fixed, paraffin-embedded tissue were cut onto commercially available slides (Superfrost/plus; Fisher Scientific, Pittsburgh, Pa), deparaffinized (45 minutes at 55°C), and cleansed through a series of xylene and alcohol washes. Dehydrated sections were examined using light microscopy, after hematoxylin-eosin staining. After exhaustion (3 minutes) of endogenous peroxidase activity with 3% (volume-volume ratio) hydrogen peroxide in methanol and blocking (20 minutes) in 1% (weight-volume ratio) bovine serum albumin, tissues were incubated with polyclonal antibodies (Santa Cruz Labs, Santa Cruz, Calif) directed against FGFR-1 (1:50) and FGFR-2 (1:50). According to the manufacturer, both of these polyclonals were raised against a unique peptide sequence and demonstrated no crossreactivity with other members of the FGFR family. In addition, preincubation (16 hours at 4°C) of the individual antibodies with 100-fold molar excess of the specific peptides (Santa Cruz Labs) completely blocked immunostaining. Fixed sections also were incubated with affinity-purified anti–FGF-1 and anti–FGF-2 (5 μg/mL), as described previously.[46-48] As a control for FGF-1 and FGF-2 monospecificity, the affinity-purified antibodies were preincubated (16 hours at 4°C) with 100-fold molar excess of recombinant FGF-1[46] or FGF-2,[49] a process that completely abrogated immunostaining. The involvement of oxidant stress was characterized using commercially available monoclonal anti-iNOS (1:250) (Upstate Biotechnology, Inc, Lake Placid, NY) and polyclonal anti-nitrotyrosine (1:450) (a generous gift from J. Beckman, PhD, University of Alabama at Birmingham). The specificity of protein tyrosine nitration was demonstrated by preincubating (30 minutes at 25°C) the polyclonal antibody with 10-mmol/L 3-nitrotyrosine (Sigma-Aldrich Corp, St Louis, Mo), which prevented all immunostaining.

All primary antibodies were incubated (45 minutes at 37°C) in a humidified chamber. Negative controls included incubation of fixed sections with preimmune serum and deletion of the primary antibody, a process that completely prevented immunostaining. Antibody binding was detected with a Quick Staining Kit (Dako Corp, Carpinteria, Calif) using swine anti-rabbit or swine anti-mouse horseradish peroxidase–conjugated secondary antibodies. Peroxidase-stained sections were developed with 0.5-mg/mL 3,3′-diaminobenzidine and counterstained with Mayer hematoxylin stain (Sigma-Aldrich Corp). Following chromogenic development of stained samples, slides were dehydrated, coverslips were applied using Permount (Fisher Scientific, Fairlawn, NJ), and positive brown staining was evaluated using light microscopy.

All sections were examined and immunohistochemical staining was assessed by 4 independent investigators (S.M.V., M.G., C.E., and J.A.T.) unaware of control vs cancer specimens. The following scores were assigned to each specimen according to the intensity of staining: 3+ (intense), 2+ (moderate), 1+ (minimal), and 0 (none). Five separate areas for each specimen were evaluated, and the total cumulative score was divided by 12 to obtain an average grade.

IN SITU HYBRIDIZATION

Detection of endogenous FGF-1 and FGF-2 messenger RNA (mRNA) was performed on routine paraffin sections essentially as described.[46-48, 50] Briefly, DNA restriction fragments containing the complete human complementary DNA sequence encoding FGF-1[46] or FGF-2[49] were subcloned into the pBluescript SK+ phagemid (Stratagene, La Jolla, Calif). Endogenous labeling of sense and antisense riboprobes was achieved in the presence of digoxigenin-11-2′-deoxyuridine 5′-triphosphate during in vitro transcription reactions performed according to manufacturer's recommendations (Boehringer Mannheim, Indianapolis, Ind). Fixed sections were permeabilized (30 minutes at 37°C) with proteinase K (10 μg/mL) and hybridized (16 hours at 50°C) with the digoxigenin-labeled antisense riboprobe (4 μg/mL). After extensive washing (20°C) and RNAse A treatment (60 minutes at 37°C), digoxigenin was reacted immunologically (3 hours at 20°C) with a 1:500 dilution of alkaline phosphatase–conjugated sheep anti-digoxigenin antiserum (Boehringer Mannheim). Alkaline phosphatase was detected (18 hours at 4°C) using nitroblue tetrazolium and 5-bromo-4-chloro-3-indoyl phosphate. Phosphatase-stained sections were visualized for the appearance of a dark blue color using light microscopy. Specificity of the riboprobe and staining protocol included hybridization reactions performed in the absence of added riboprobe or in the presence of the sense riboprobe, 2 processes that failed to exhibit alkaline phosphatase activity.

vivo.[10-14] The biological potential of these FGF prototypes is consistent with the histological appearance of pancreatic tumors, characterized by atypical hyperplasia of ductal epithelium, periductal angiogenesis and neurogenesis, invasion of cellular infiltrate, and nonneoplastic stromal cell remodeling and fibrosis.[15] Numerous studies have established that the biological activity of FGF requires extracellular heparin sulfate proteoglycan–dependent cell surface interactions with specific high-affinity receptors, including FGFR-1(flg) and FGFR-2 (bek), to induce responding signal transduction cascades.[16-22] However, these prototypical FGFs differ from the FGF oncoproteins by the absence of a signal peptide sequence to participate in conventional secretory processes.

Ongoing efforts[16,23-25] have established that cellular release of the FGF prototypes involves an endoplasmic reticulum-independent pathway in response to biological stress. Tissue injury and biological stress in a variety of pathologic conditions (eg, tumorigenesis[26-30]) include excess production of reactive oxygen and nitrogen species, including superoxide and nitric oxide (NO).

The limited reactivity of superoxide with many biological molecules has raised questions about its toxic effects,[31] which has led to more recent suggestions that NO is a critical target of superoxide. Nitric oxide has gained general acceptance as a necessary mediator of diverse physiologic functions, and a role for this reactive nitrogen species during pathophysiological processes, such as tumorigenesis,[30,32-34] atherosclerosis,[35] arthritis,[36] and transplant rejection,[32,37] has been described. This paradoxical role for NO may be linked to local levels of NO generated by differential expression of NO synthase (NOS) isoforms. Production of NO is linked to a multitude of cell types[38,39] and involves 3 separate NOS gene products, which are calcium dependent and constitutively expressed (eNOS, type III; nNOS, type I) or calcium independent and cytokine inducible (iNOS, type II). Once activated, iNOS can produce 1000-fold more NO for a longer duration than eNOS.[39] At these concentrations, NO will produce the powerful biological oxidant, peroxynitrite, through a diffusion-limited reaction with superoxide.[40]

Peroxynitrite attacks many biological targets, including metal-catalyzed formation of nitrotyrosine, a permanent modification that can be detected immunologically using anti-nitrotyrosine antibodies.[41] Nitrotyrosine and FGF have been detected immunologically in several human pathologic conditions, including atherosclerosis, arthritis, and renal transplant dysfunction.[41-48] Whereas the involvement of the FGF prototypes and NO in tumorigenesis has been suggested,[6-9,30,32-34] the participation of peroxynitrite during this pathophysiological condition has not been reported. We examined this issue and designed our study to explore correlation between competent FGF-transforming pathways and the presence of NO production and reactivity in pancreatic adenocarcinoma. These experimental results provide a first indication that FGF transformation and oxidant stress induced by reactive nitrogen species participate in the pathophysiological processes of human pancreatic cancer.

RESULTS

This retrospective study included analyses of 12 pancreatic adenocarcinomas, 6 from stage I and II lesions (less than 2 cm, no positive nodes, no metastasis) and 6 from stage III and IV lesions (greater than 2 cm, at least 1 positive node, 3 with metastasis) recovered from patients surviving longer than 3 years or less than 6 months, respectively. In each specimen, pancreatic tumor was located primarily in the head of the pancreas and, where evident (T3 and T4), metastasis was observed in the lymph node and liver. Results of routine histological analyses of control pancreas were unremarkable. In contrast, results of microscopic examination of pancreatic tumors under hematoxylin-eosin staining demonstrated the existence of irregularly shaped ductal structures with distinct lumens. Examination of the ductal epithelium revealed several layers of cells with marked atypical nuclei and general loss of polarity. Nonneoplastic periductal regions demonstrated the appearance of fibrosis, cellular infiltrate, perineural invasion, and angiogenesis.

Immunohistochemical analysis of FGF-1 and FGF-2 in controls was not readily apparent (**Figure 1**, A and C). In contrast, increased immunostaining for FGF-1 and FGF-2 was observed in the hyperplastic ductal epithelium and the periductal cellular infiltrate surrounding the tumor (Figure 1, B and D). Moderate or intense staining for FGF-1 and FGF-2 was seen in 58% and 66%, respectively, when compared with controls (**Table**). In situ hybridization analysis of control tissue (**Figure 2**, A and D) failed to demonstrate significant expression of FGF-1 or FGF-2 mRNA. In contrast, detectable levels of FGF-1 and FGF-2 mRNA were readily apparent in tumor specimens (Figure 2, B and C) with immunostaining associated with hyperplastic ductal epithelium and surrounding cellular infiltrate. Hybridization reactions performed in the presence of sense riboprobe failed to exhibit alkaline phosphatase activity (data not shown). Of the 2 high-affinity FGF receptors analyzed in controls, staining for FGFR-1 and FGFR-2 was restricted to characteristic islands of islet cells (Figure 1, E and G). Moderate or intense staining was observed in 90% of the tumors for FGFR-1 and in 75% of the tumors for FGFR-2 in pancreatic tumors (when compared with controls), primarily in the epithelium lining of irregularly shaped ductal cells of the tumors (Figure 1, F and H) (Table).

Pancreatic tumor specimens routinely demonstrated exaggerated staining in greater than 90% of the tumors for iNOS and nitrotyrosine (when compared with controls) (**Figure 3**, B and D), primarily localized to hyperplastic ductal epithelium and acinar cells with minimal to no staining of the inflammatory infiltrate and surrounding connective tissue. In controls, no staining for iNOS was detected (Figure 3, A), whereas moderate staining for nitrotyrosine was restricted to islands of islet cells (Figure 3, C). Intense immunostaining for both of these markers of reactive nitrogen species was completely abolished in deletion controls. Blocking the polyclonal anti-nitrotyrosine with 10-mmol/L 3-nitrotyrosine totally abrogated immunostaining (data not shown).

A composite summary of immunohistochemical staining intensity for FGF ligands, FGFRs, and markers of reactive nitrogen species is presented in the Table. Differential levels of increased staining for these markers could not be attributed significantly to any aspect of clinical or pathological stage or growth of tumor associated with patients harboring pancreatic adenocarcinoma. However, the sample size within specific categories may not be sufficient to appreciate potential correlations. The principle consistent observation derived from these immunohistochemical analyses demonstrates that increased expression of FGF-1, FGF-2, and FGFRs in hyperplastic ductal epithelium is associated with an environment of oxidative stress, such as that provided by increased production of NO and one of its reaction products, peroxynitrite. Finally, serial sections prohibited direct comparison of tumor sample stains for markers of oxidant stress (iNOS and nitrotyrosine) and FGF-1, FGF-2, and FGFR, which is desirable. This often requires double staining with immunofluorescence. However, as the Table depicts, most tumors stained strongly (≥3+) for the receptor and markers of oxidant stress (iNOS and nitrotyrosine), giving credence to a strong association

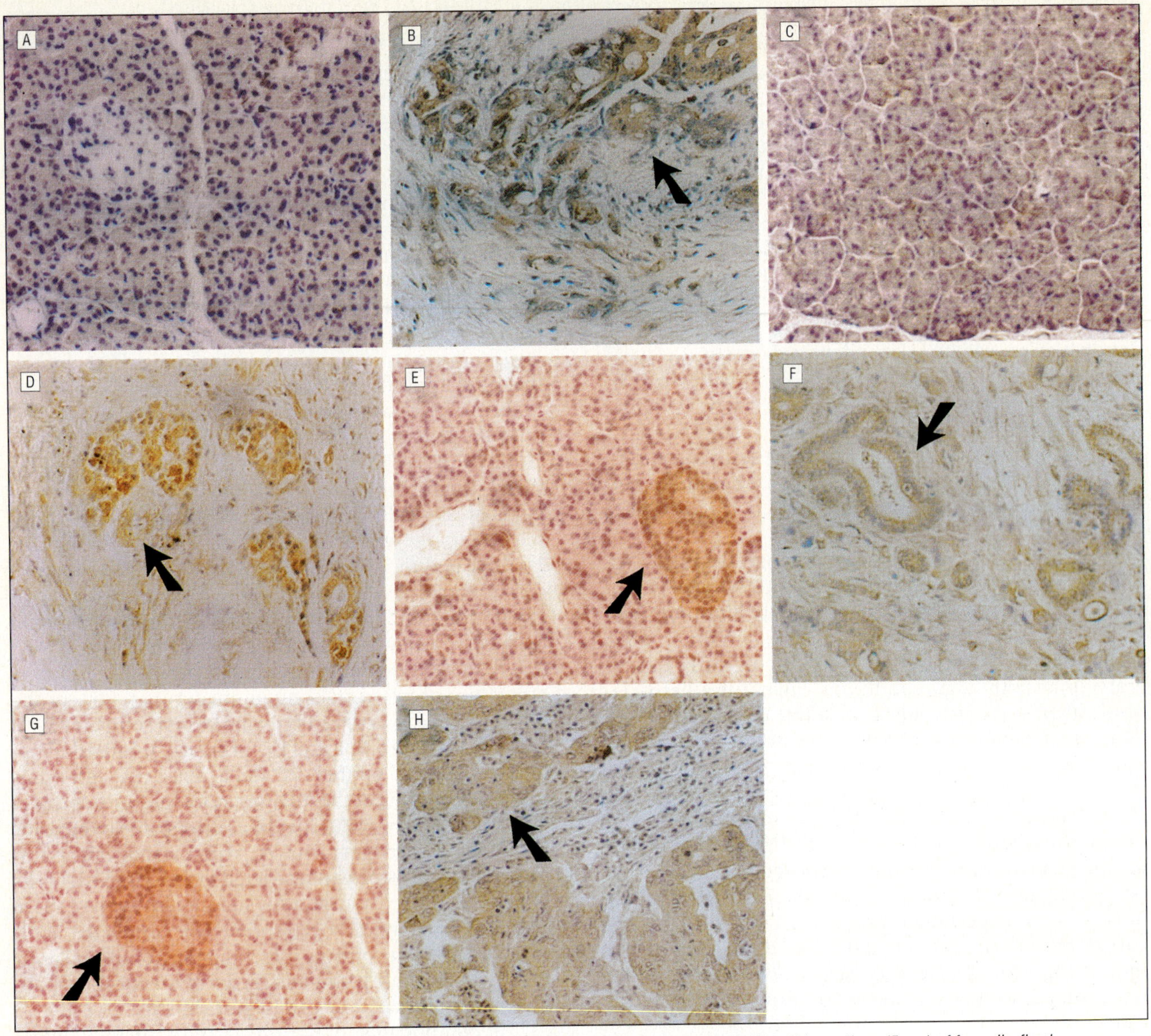

Figure 1. *Immunohistochemical analysis of human pancreas for prototypical fibroblast growth factors (FGFs). Thin sections (5 μm) of formalin-fixed, paraffin-embedded pancreatic tissue from nontransplant donors (controls) (A, C, E, and G) or patients with pancreatic adenocarcinoma were prepared and examined using microscopy after staining with specific antibodies against acidic FGFs (FGF-1; A and B), basic FGFs (FGF-2; C and D), and their high-affinity receptors (FGFR-1 [E and F] and FGFR-2 [G and H], respectively) (original magnification ×200). Arrows on panels B, D, F, and H identify staining of pancreatic ductal cells. Arrows on panels E and G identify staining of islet cells.*

between this growth family of ligands and receptors and oxidant stress.

COMMENT

The in situ hybridization and immunohistochemical studies reported herein demonstrated minimal expression of FGF-1 and FGF-2 mRNA and protein in the ductal epithelium of normal human pancreas. The near absence of detectable FGF ligand expression predicts that normal pancreatic ductal epithelium contains a quiescent cell population, which is supported by the absence of immunostaining for FGFR-1 and FGFR-2. The absence of a local growth response would be consistent with the relatively low cellular turnover occurring in the pancreatic duct under normal conditions.[51-53] In contrast, periductal areas in pancreatic adenocarcinoma tissue demonstrated increased expression of FGF-1 and FGF-2 mRNA and protein. Immunostaining for the FGF proteins correlated well with the appearance of the FGF mRNAs, both of which were associated with resident cellular infiltrate. Since inflammatory cells are a rich source of FGF,[47] and since the involvement of inflammation in pancreatic adenocarcinoma has been described,[15] our observations provide a potential mechanism for delivery of FGF capable of inducing characteristic angiogenic, neurogenic, and stromal remodeling responses.[10,11]

In addition to inflammatory-mediated synthesis and delivery of the prototypical FGFs, results provided herein also demonstrate the exaggerated appearance of intracellular FGF-1 and FGF-2 protein and mRNA in the ductal epithelium associated with pancreatic adenocarcinoma. This observation is consistent with a response to injury, wherein damaged ductal epithelial cells induce

Summary of Immunohistochemical Staining Intensity for Specific Markers Associated With Healthy Pancreatic Tissue and Pancreatic Ductal Adenocarcinomas*

	Healthy Tissue (n = 3)				Adenocarcinomas (n = 12)			
	0	1+	2+	3+	0	1+	2+	3+
FGF-1	3	0	0	0	0	5	3	4
FGF-2	3	0	0	0	0	4	4	4
FGFR-1	0	0	0	3 (islets)	0	1	3	8
FGFR-2	0	0	0	3 (islets)	0	3	1	8
iNOS	3	0	0	0	0	1	0	11
NT	0	3 (islets)	0	0	0	1	0	11

**Data represent the total number of samples in this study that received the representative average grade of staining. Levels of staining intensity are described in the "Immunolocalization" subsection of the "Materials and Methods" section. FGF-1 indicates acidic fibroblast growth factor; FGF-2, basic FGF; FGFR-1 and FGFR-2, their respective high-affinity receptors; iNOS, inducible nitric oxide synthase; and NT, nitrotyrosine.*

expression of FGF-1 and FGF-2 competent to function as a survival factor and promote local growth responses.[54,55] Completion of this potential autocrine-paracrine transforming loop demands expression of specific high-affinity receptors to activate signal transduction processes. Indeed, compared with control specimens, immunostaining for FGFR-1 and FGFR-2 was detected readily in the ductal epithelium of pancreatic adenocarcinoma. Consequently, a local growth response is anticipated by receptor-positive cells exposed to the presence of competent mitogens, a prediction consistent with the appearance of hyperplastic ductal structures.

Several observations in our study provide insight into a potential mechanism regulating the pathologic consequences of increased intrinsic FGF expression beyond that previously reported.[6,8,56] For instance, intracellularly sequestered FGF-1, which lacks a classic signal sequence for secretion, is not available to mediate its bio-

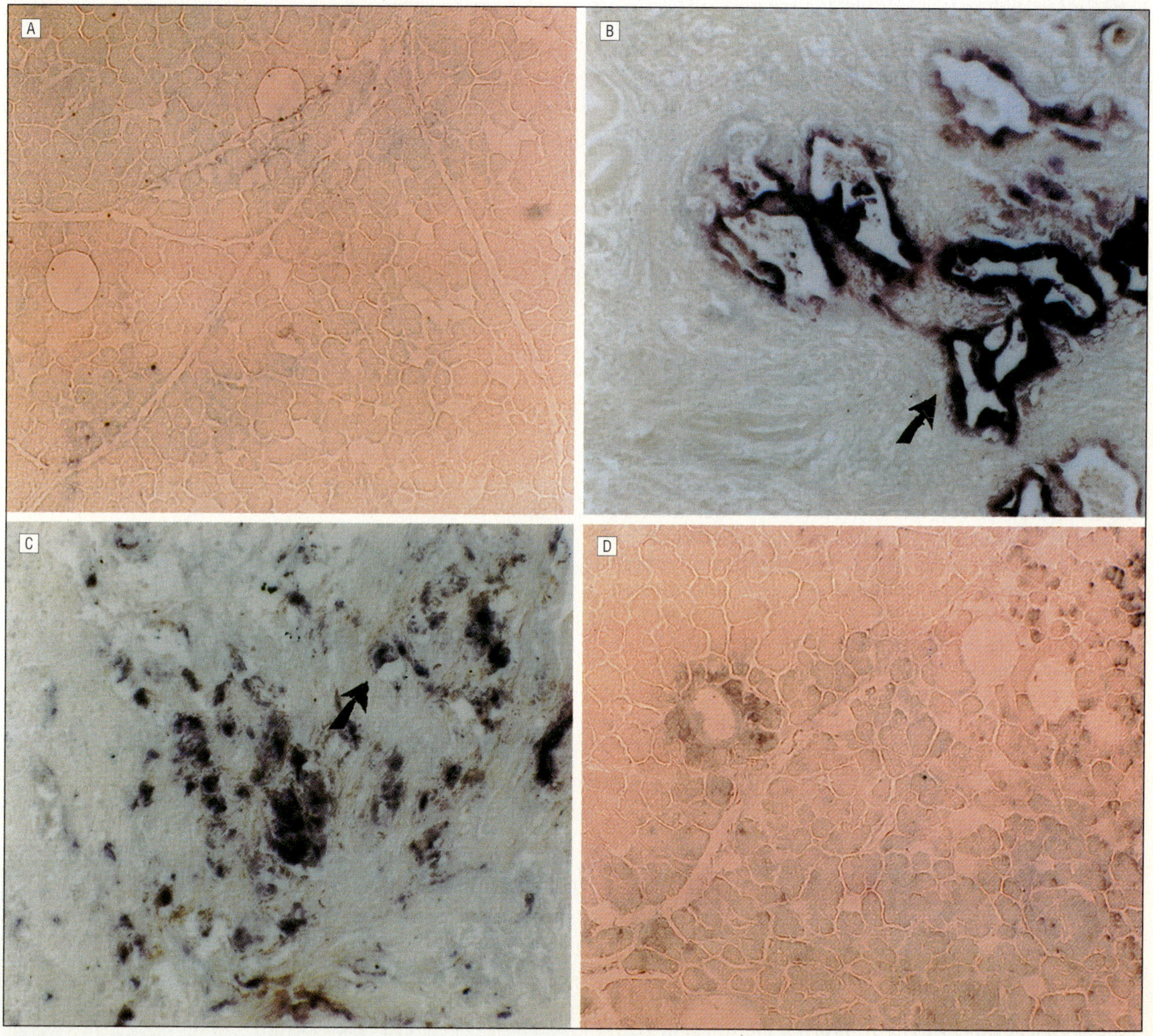

Figure 2. *In situ hybridization analysis of human pancreas for acidic fibroblast (FGF-1) and basic fibroblast growth factor (FGF-2) messenger RNA (mRNA). Thin sections (5 mm) of formalin-fixed, paraffin-embedded pancreatic tissue obtained from nontransplant donors (controls) (A and D) or patients with pancreatic tumors (B and C) were prepared and examined using light microscopy after hybridization with antisense probes against FGF-1 (A and B) and FGF-2 (C and D) mRNA (original magnification ×200). Arrows on panels B and C identify staining of pancreatic ductal cells. Abbreviations are given in the legend to Figure 1.*

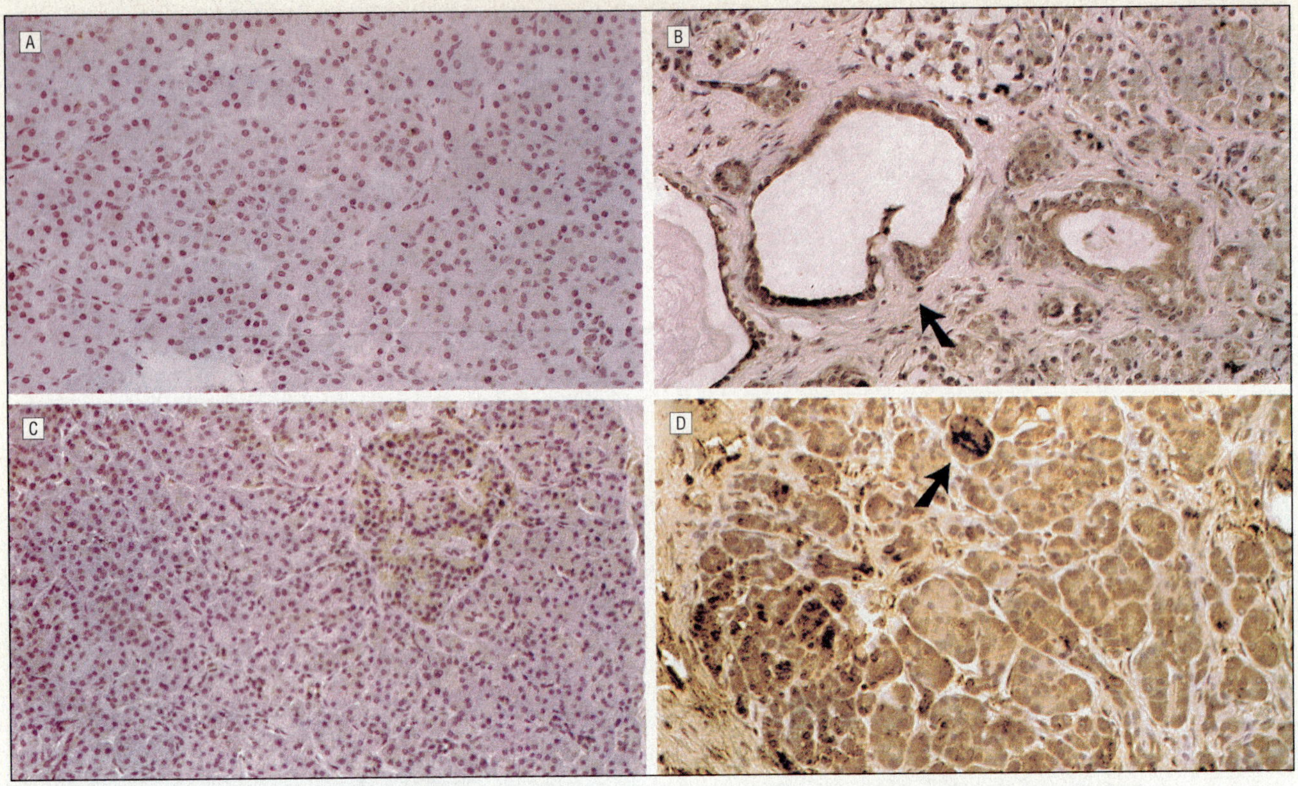

Figure 3. *Immunohistochemical analysis of human pancreas for indicators of reactive nitrogen species. Thin sections (5 mm) of formalin-fixed, paraffin-embedded pancreatic tissue from nontransplant donors (controls) (A and D) or patients with pancreatic tumors (B and C) were examined using light microscopy after staining with specific antibodies against inducible nitric oxide synthase (A and B) and nitrotyrosine (C and D) (original magnification ×200). Arrows on panels B and D identify staining of pancreatic ductal cells.*

logical effects on cell growth.[23] Previous in vitro studies have demonstrated that FGF-1 is released from cells in response to oxidative stress,[16,23,24] a pathologic condition that may involve inflammatory-mediated production of reactive oxygen-nitrogen species.[39,57,58] Our results demonstrate the increased immunoappearance of iNOS and nitrotyrosine in the ductal epithelium of pancreatic tumor tissue. This observation predicts that endogenous production of reactive nitrogen species, as evidenced by markers for NO and peroxynitrite, induces oxidative stress in the ductal epithelium of pancreatic adenocarcinoma. The secretion of FGF-1 in response to this biological stress may be responsible for inducing an extracellular autocrine-paracrine transforming loop in pancreatic tumors. Consequently, hyperplasia of the ductal epithelium during pancreatic adenocarcinoma is consistent with an extracellular FGF pathway and may represent a normal regenerative response of these structures to oxidant stress. Although the enhanced and correlated appearance of FGF and oxidant stress in the ductal epithelium supports a mechanistic transforming role for these agents during development of pancreatic lesions associated with tumorigenesis, additional efforts will be required to establish a direct cause-and-effect relationship beyond that suggested in a limited retrospective analysis.

This work was supported by grants HL45990 and DK51629 from the National Institutes of Health, Bethesda, Md (Dr Thompson); a grant from the Robert Wood Johnson Foundation, Princeton, NJ (Dr Vickers); and a fellowship from the National Kidney Foundation, New York, NY (Dr MacMillan-Crow).

We thank K. L. Luo and Q. Ding for excellent technical assistance.

Corresponding author: Selwyn M. Vickers, MD, University of Alabama at Birmingham, 1922 Seventh Ave S, KB405, Birmingham, AL 35294-0007 (e-mail: smv@uab.edu).

REFERENCES

1. Cameron JL, Crist DW, Sitzmann JV, et al. Factors influencing survival after pancreaticoduodenectomy for pancreatic cancer. *Am J Surg.* 1991;161:120-125.
2. Cameron JL, Pitt HA, Yeo CJ, et al. One hundred and forty-five consecutive pancreaticoduodenectomies without mortality. *Ann Surg.* 1993;217:430-438.
3. Gonzalez AM, Buscaglia M, Ong M, et al. Distribution of basic fibroblast growth factor in the 18-day rat fetus: localization in the basement membranes of diverse tissues. *J Cell Biol.* 1990;110:753-765.
4. de Iongh RU, Lovicu FJ, Chamberlain CG, et al. Differential expression of fibroblast growth factor receptors during rat lens morphogenesis and growth. *Invest Ophthalmol Vis Sci.* 1997;38:1688-1699.
5. Wilkie AO. Craniosynostosis: genes and mechanisms. *Hum Mol Genet.* 1997;6:1647-1656.
6. De Vries L, Tahiri T, Jouti N, et al. Regulation of proliferation by fibroblast growth factor in a pancreatic cancer cell line. *Digestion.* 1990;46:162-165.
7. Estival A, Louvel D, Coudere B, et al. Morphological and biological modifications induced in a rat pancreatic acinar cancer cell line (AR4-2J) by unscheduled expression of basic fibroblast growth factors. *Cancer Res.* 1993;53:1182-1187.
8. Hasegawa Y, Takada M, Yamamoto M, et al. The gradient of basic fibroblast growth factor concentration in human pancreatic cancer cell invasion. *Biochem Biophys Res Commun.* 1994;200:1435-1439.
9. Yamanaka Y, Friess H, Buchler M, et al. Overexpression of acidic and basic fibroblast growth factors in human pancreatic cancer correlates with advanced tumor stage. *Cancer Res.* 1993;53:5289-5296.

10. Thompson JA, Anderson KD, DiPietro JM, et al. Site-directed neovessel formation in vivo. *Science.* 1988;241:1349-1352.
11. Thompson JA, Haudenschild CC, Anderson KD, et al. Heparin-binding growth factor 1 induces the formation of organoid neovascular structures in vivo. *Proc Natl Acad Sci U S A.* 1989;86:7928-7932.
12. Folkman J, Klagsbrun M. Angiogenic factors. *Science.* 1987;235:442-447.
13. Burgess WH, Maciag T. The heparin-binding (fibroblast) growth factor family of proteins. *Annu Rev Biochem.* 1989;58:575-606.
14. Baird A. Fibroblast growth factors: activities and significance of non-neurotrophin neurotrophic factors. *Curr Opin Neurobiol.* 1994;4:78-86.
15. Solcia E, Capella C, Kloppel G. Tumors of the pancreas. In: *Atlas of Tumor Pathology.* Vol 3. Washington, DC: Armed Forces Institute of Pathology; 1995:80-81.
16. Opalenik SR, Shin JT, Wehby JN, et al. The HIV-1 TAT protein induces the expression and extracellular appearance of acidic fibroblast growth factor. *J Biol Chem.* 1995;270:17 457-17 468.
17. Rogelj S, Weinberg RA, Fanning P, et al. Basic fibroblast growth factor fused to a signal peptide transforms cells. *Nature.* 1988;331:173-175.
18. Blam SB, Mitchell R, Tischer E, et al. Addition of growth hormone secretion signal to basic fibroblast growth factor results in cell transformation and secretion of aberrant forms of the protein. *Oncogene.* 1988;129:136-140.
19. Forough R, Xi Z, MacPhee M, et al. Differential transforming abilities of non-secreted and secreted forms of human fibroblast growth factor-1. *J Biol Chem.* 1993;268:2960-2968.
20. Jouanneau J, Gavrilovic J, Caruelle D, et al. Secreted or non-secreted forms of acidic fibroblast growth factor produced by transfected epithelial cells influence cell morphology, motility and invasive potential. *Proc Natl Acad Sci U S A.* 1991; 88:2893-2897.
21. Ornitz DM, Xu J, Colvin JS, et al. Receptor specificity of the fibroblast growth factor family. *J Biol Chem.* 1996;271:15 292-15 297.
22. Jaye M, Schlessinger J, Dionne CA. Fibroblast growth factor receptor tyrosine kinases: molecular analysis and signal transduction. *Biochim Biophys Acta.* 1992; 1135:185-199.
23. Shin JT, Opalenik SR, Wehby JN, et al. Serum-starvation induces the extracellular appearance of FGF-1. *Biochim Biophys Acta.* 1996;1312:27-38.
24. Opalenik SR, Ding Q, Maller SR, et al. Glutathione depletion associated with the HIV-1 TAT protein and the extracellular appearance of FGF-1. *Arch Biochem Biophys.* 1998;351:17-26.
25. Jackson A, Friedman S, Zhan X, et al. Heat shock induces the release of fibroblast growth factor 1 from HIH 3T3 cells. *Proc Natl Acad Sci U S A.* 1992;89: 10 691-10 695.
26. Cendan JC, Souba WW, Copeland EM III, et al. Increased L-arginine transport in a nitric oxide-producing metastatic colon cancer cell line. *Ann Surg Oncol.* 1996; 3:501-508.
27. Chhatwal VJS, Ngoi SS, Chan STF, et al. Aberrant expression of nitric oxide synthase in human polyps, neoplastic colonic mucosa and surrounding peritumoral normal mucosa. *Carcinogenesis.* 1994;15:2081-2085.
28. Deliconstantinos G, Villiotou V, Stavrides JC, et al. Nitric oxide and peroxynitrite production by human erythrocytes: a causative factor of toxic anemia in breast cancer patients. *Anticancer Res.* 1995;15:1435-1446.
29. Farias-Eisner R, Sherman MP, Aeberhard E, et al. Nitric oxide is an important mediator for tumoricidal activity in vivo. *Proc Natl Acad Sci U S A.* 1994;91: 9407-9411.
30. Parkins CS, Dennis MF, Stratford MRL, et al. Ischemia reperfusion injury in tumors: the role of oxygen radicals and nitric oxide. *Cancer Res.* 1995;55:6026-6029.
31. Sawyer DT, Valentine JS. How super is superoxide? *Act Chem Res.* 1981;14: 393-400.
32. Kerby JD, Verran D, Luo KL, et al. Immunolocalization of FGF-1 and human renal allograft vasculopathy associated with chronic rejection. *Transplantation.* 1996; 62:467-475.
33. Ambs S, Hussain SP, Harris CC. Interactive effects of nitric oxide and the p53 tumor suppressor gene in carcinogenesis and tumor progression. *FASEB J.* 1997; 11:443-448.
34. Calmels S, Hainaut P, Ohshima H. Nitric oxide induces conformational and functional modifications of wild-type p53 tumor suppressor protein. *Cancer Res.* 1997; 57:3365-3369.
35. Minor RL, Myers PR, Guerra R, et al. Diet-induced atherosclerosis increases the release of nitrogen oxides from rabbit aorta. *J Clin Invest.* 1990;86:2109-2116.
36. Farrell AJ, Blake DR, Palmer RM, et al. Increased concentrations of nitrite in synovial fluid and serum samples suggest increased nitric oxide synthesis in rheumatic diseases. *Ann Rheum Dis.* 1992;51:1219-1222.
37. Worrall NK, Lazenby WD, Misko TP, et al. Modulation of in vivo alloreactivity by inhibition of inducible nitric oxide synthase. *J Exp Med.* 1995;181:63-70.
38. Moncada S, Higga EA. Endogenous nitric oxide: physiology, pathology and clinical relevance. *Eur J Clin Invest.* 1991;21:361-374.
39. Clancy RM, Abramson SB. Nitric oxide: a novel mediator of inflammation. *Proc Soc Exp Biol Med.* 1995;210:93-101.
40. Huie RE, Padmaja S. The reaction rate of nitric oxide with superoxide. *Free Rad Res Commun.* 1993;18:195-199.
41. Beckman JS, Ye YZ, Anderson P, et al. Extensive nitration of protein tyrosines observed in human atherosclerosis by immunohistochemistry. *Biol Chem Hoppe-Seyler.* 1994;375:81-88.
42. MacMillan-Crow LA, Crow JP, Kerby JD, et al. Nitration and inactivation of manganese superoxide dismutase in chronic rejection of human renal allografts. *Proc Natl Acad Sci U S A.* 1996;93:11 853-11 858.
43. Kaur H, Halliwell B. Evidence for nitric oxide-mediated oxidative damage in chronic inflammation: nitrotyrosine in serum and synovial fluid from rheumatoid patients. *FEBS Lett.* 1994;350:9-12.
44. Brogi E, Winkles JA, Underwood R, et al. Distinct patterns of expression of fibroblast growth factors and their receptors in human atheroma and nonatherosclerotic arteries. *J Clin Invest.* 1993;92:2408-2418.
45. Sano H, Forough R, Maier J, et al. Detection of high levels of heparin binding growth factor-1 (acidic fibroblast growth factor) in inflammatory arthritic joints. *J Cell Biol.* 1990;110:1417-1426.
46. Kerby JD, Luo KL, Ding Q, et al. Immunolocalization of acidic fibroblast growth factor and receptors in the tubointerstitial compartment of chronically rejected human renal allografts. *Transplantation.* 1997;63:988-995.
47. Kerby JD, Verran DJ, Luo KL, et al. Immunolocalization of FGF-1 and receptors in glomerular lesions associated with chronic human renal allograft rejection. *Transplantation.* 1996;62:190-200.
48. Kerby JD, Luo KL, Ding Q, et al. Immunolocalization of acidic FGF-1 and receptors in the tubulointerstitial compartment of chronically rejected human renal allografts. *Transplantation.* 1997;63:988-995.
49. Imamura T, Friedman SA, Gamble S, et al. Molecular shuffling between fibroblast growth factor (FGF)-1 and FGF-2 identifies the heparin-dependence domain for FGF-1 mitogenic activity. *Biochim Biophys Acta.* 1995;1266:124-130.
50. Forough R, Engleka K, Thompson JA, et al. Differential expression in *Escherichia coli* of the alpha and beta forms of heparin-binding acidic fibroblast growth factor-1: potential role of RNA secondary structure. *Biochim Biophys Acta.* 1991; 1090:293-298.
51. Fitzgerald PJ, Herman L, Carol B, et al. Pancreatic acinar cell regeneration, I: cytologic, cytochemical and pancreatic weight changes. *Am J Pathol.* 1968;52: 983-1011.
52. Solomon TE. Regulation of exocrine pancreatic cell proliferation and enzyme synthesis. In: John LR, ed. *Physiology of the Gastrointestinal Tract.* New York, NY: Raven Press; 1981:837-892.
53. Loser C, Nustede R, Becker HJ, et al. Effect of neurotensin on pancreatic growth and pancreatic polyamine metabolism in rats. *Int J Pancreatol.* 1995;18:107-115.
54. Jouanneau J, Gavrilovic J, Caruelle D, et al. Secreted or nonsecreted forms of acidic fibroblast growth factor produced by transfected epithelial cells influence cell morphology, motility and invasive potential. *Proc Natl Acad Sci U S A.* 1991; 88:2893-2897.
55. Tamm I, Kikuchi T, Zychlinsky A. Acidic and basic fibroblast growth factors are survival factors with distinctive activity in quiescent BALB/c 3T3 murine fibroblasts. *Proc Natl Acad Sci U S A.* 1991;88:3372-3376.
56. Friess H, Korc M, Buchler MW. Molecular biology of pancreatic cancer overexpression of fibroblast growth factors. *Chirurg.* 1994;65:604-610.
57. Hamvas A, Palazzo R, Kaiser L, et al. Inflammation and oxygen free radical formation during pulmonary ischemia-reperfusion injury. *J Appl Physiol.* 1992;72: 621-628.
58. Morel D, DiCorleto P, Chisolm G. Endothelial and smooth muscle cells after low density lipoprotein in vitro for free radical oxidation. *Arteriosclerosis.* 1984;4: 357-364.

ORIGINAL ARTICLE

Tikhoff-Linberg Procedure for Bone and Soft Tissue Tumors of the Shoulder Girdle

Gregor Voggenreiter, MD; Stefan Assenmacher, MD; Klaus-Peter Schmit-Neuerburg, MD

Objective: To evaluate complications and the oncological and intermediate-term functional results in patients with bone and soft tissue tumors of the shoulder girdle who were managed with interscapulothoracic resection (Tikhoff-Linberg procedure).

Design: Case series of 19 consecutive patients during a 10-year period at a mean follow-up of 6.3 years (range, 1-11 years).

Setting: University hospital; referral center for musculoskeletal tumor surgery.

Patients: The initial diagnosis in this consecutive series of patients with shoulder girdle tumors requiring the Tikhoff-Linberg procedure was chondrosarcoma in 7 patients, Ewing sarcoma in 3 patients, malignant fibrous histiocytoma in 3 patients, solitary metastasis of thyroid carcinoma in 2 patients, osteosarcoma, synovial sarcoma, angiosarcoma, and neurofibrosarcoma in 1 patient each. According to the Musculoskeletal Tumor Society staging system, there were 6 in surgical stage IB, 10 in stage IIB, and 3 in stage III. Nine tumors involved the proximal humerus, 8 were located in the scapula or surrounding soft tissues, 1 in the lateral clavicle, and 1 in the acromioclavicular joint.

Interventions: For reconstruction of the proximal humerus after en bloc tumor resection an isoelastic cemented shoulder tumor prosthesis was inserted in every patient to restore arm length.

Main Outcome Measures: Complications, and oncological and intermediate-term functional results.

Results: Twelve patients were alive with no evidence of disease. One of these patients died of nontumorous disease 2 years after surgery. One patient is alive with pulmonary metastases after 12 months. Six patients died of metastases at a mean (SD) interval of 18 months (range, 3-35 months) postoperatively. Two of these patients had additional local recurrence. A deep infection necessitated the explantation of the prosthesis in 1 patient. The mean functional score and SD according to the rating system of the Musculoskeletal Tumor Society was 72% ± 14% (range, 33%-87%) for the 12 surviving patients evaluated. Major complications (1 infection and 2 local recurrences) that may be attributed to the procedure occurred in 3 of the 19 patients.

Conclusion: Despite an overall complication rate of 74% the Tikhoff-Linberg procedure proved to be a valuable surgical procedure for extended tumors of the shoulder girdle for functional and oncological outcome and is superior to forequarter amputation.

Arch Surg. 1999;134:252-257

THE TREATMENT of many musculoskeletal neoplasms has changed from radical ablative surgery toward limb salvage. Tumors of the shoulder girdle are challenging the surgeon to preserve function and cosmesis without compromising local tumor control. The reconstruction of skeletal defects created by resection of the proximal humerus includes arthrodesis, prosthetic replacement, osteoarticular allografts, and autogenous grafts.[1]

The en bloc upper humeral interscapulothoracic resection, known as the *Tikhoff-Linberg procedure*, is, in properly selected cases of tumors of the shoulder girdle, an alternative treatment to forequarter amputation.[2-9] The Tikhoff-Linberg procedure is indicated in tumors of the scapula, proximal humerus, lateral clavicle, or of the periscapular soft tissue where tumor invasion of the subchondral bone, the joint capsule, synovial membrane, or the entire joint is evident on preoperative studies. Prerequisites for the procedure are that the tumor does not extend to the axillary neurovascular bundle, to the chest wall, or the lymph nodes. Additional indications are palliation of malignant lesions where amputation is not justified because of chest wall involve-

From the Department of Trauma Surgery, University Hospital Essen, Essen, Germany.

PATIENTS AND METHODS

Between 1986 and 1996 nineteen interscapulothoracic resections were performed (approximately 2 patients per year). There were 15 male and 4 female patients, whose mean age at operation was 49.0 years (age range, 12-83 years). The follow-up period of patients surviving free of disease ranged from 1 to 11 years (mean, 6.3 years). Eleven lesions were primary malignant bone tumors, 6 were malignant soft tissue tumors, and 2 were solitary metastases. According to the Musculoskeletal Tumor Society (MSTS) staging system[11] there were 6 in surgical stage IB, 10 in stage IIB, and 3 in stage III (**Table**). Nine tumors involved the proximal humerus, 8 were located in the scapula or surrounding soft tissues, 1 in the lateral clavicle, and 1 in the acromioclavicular joint. Eight patients were operated on for tumor recurrence after local resections before they were referred to our unit. Imaging studies include plain radiograms, bone scanning, computed tomographic scan of the chest and shoulder girdle, and magnetic resonance imaging. An incisional biopsy was performed to establish the diagnosis.

After the initial staging and diagnosis the patients with Ewing sarcoma (n = 3), osteosarcoma (n = 1), and synovial sarcoma (n = 1) received preoperative and postoperative chemotherapy. Three patients with malignant fibrous histiocytoma received postoperative radiotherapy and 2 patients with solitary metastases of thyroid carcinoma preoperative and postoperative radioactive iodine 131 treatment. After a patient had been managed with neoadjuvant chemotherapy, the tumor was restaged using a computed tomographic scan of the chest and local magnetic resonance imaging of the shoulder girdle. In 1 patient (case 9) pulmonary metastases were detected on the computed tomographic scan before initiating preoperative chemotherapy. After chemotherapy he was free of pulmonary disease on computed tomographic scan and he was referred for operation. The patients who had chondrosarcoma were managed without adjuvant therapy. The operative technique of the classic Tikhoff-Linberg procedure and of modifications has been described in detail in several publications.[2,7]

According to the classification system for shoulder girdle resections of Malawer et al,[7] 11 were type V resections (modified Tikhoff-Linberg resection with osteotomy of the neck of the scapula) and 8 were type VI resections (classic Tikhoff-Linberg resection). After considering the size of the tumor and its anatomic location, the resection of bone and soft tissue was adapted to each patient to achieve the widest margins of resection and greatest preservation of tissue. One patient with infection of a solitary metastasis of a thyroid carcinoma underwent a 2-step procedure. In the first step the tumor was resected and polymethyl methacrylate chains were implanted. Four weeks later after healing of the infection the prosthesis was inserted (**Figure 1**) (second step).

A complication was defined as any condition that led to additional treatment after the initial reconstruction. It was related to the operative procedure, the reconstruction, or tumor recurrence.

In 12 surviving patients function was assessed according to the MSTS functional evaluation system.[12] This system is based on the analysis of the following 6 factors: pain, functional activities, emotional acceptance, position of the hand, manual dexterity, and lifting ability. For each of the 6 factors values of 0 to 5 are assigned. The result is expressed as the proportion of expected normal function for the patient. The patients' occupation and whether the patient was collecting a disability pension was recorded.

ment or distant spread and, in rare cases, in nonmalignant inflammatory lesions around the shoulder.[7,8]

The classic resection consisted of en bloc removal of the whole scapula with the muscles connecting the shoulder, the lateral clavicle, and the proximal humerus.[4] With time a multitude of modifications have been made. Different amounts of scapula, clavicle, humerus, and adjactent soft tissue are removed.[6] A major modification is the removal of only the lateral part of the scapula whenever possible and the prosthetic reconstruction of a proximal humerus to the remaining scapula and clavicle to provide better aesthetic and functional results.[2]

Besides case reports and small case series, the results of 4 large case series were published since 1968. The Russian surgeon Machson[5] reported 19 cases; Marcrove et al[8] 17 cases in 1977; the Bologna, Italy, group of the Instituto Ortopedico Rizzoli (Guerra et al)[10] 21 cases in 1985 and on 41 cases in 1990 (Capanna et al)[2]; and Malawer et al[6] 17 cases of 2 orthopedic oncologic centers in 1991.

This article reviews our experience with 19 Tikhoff-Linberg procedures within the past 10 years that, to our knowledge, is the second largest series of a single institution. Complications and the oncological and intermediate-term functional results were emphasized.

RESULTS

ONCOLOGICAL OUTCOME

Histological margins were free of disease in all patients. Of 19 patients who underwent the Tikhoff-Linberg procedure, 12 were alive with no evidence of disease at a mean follow-up of 6.3 years (range, 1-11 years).[1-11] One patient (case 15) died of nontumorous disease 2 years after surgery. One patient (case 5) is alive with pulmonary metastases and local recurrence after 12 months. The remaining 6 patients died of pulmonary (n = 5) or intracerebral (n = 1) metastases postoperatively at a mean interval of 18 months (range, 3-35 months). All patients with oncological complications had high-grade malignant extracompartmental lesions (6 in stage IIB and 1 in stage III). Two of these patients developed additional local recurrence 5 (case 13) and 11 months (case 5), respectively, after surgery. Four of 8 patients with tumor complications had interscapulothoracic resection for tumor recurrence after previous surgery was performed at another institution. The overall disease free survival rate in stage IB was 6 of 6 patients and 4 of 10 patients in stage IIB.

Local resection performed at another institution had no adverse effects on outcome. Five of 10 patients

Clinical Data on 19 Patients

Patient No./Sex/Age at Diagnosis, y	Type of Tumor	Stage*	Treatment Elsewhere	Type of Resection†	Secondary Procedure/Complication
1/M/60	Solitary metastasis of thyroid carcinoma	III	None	V	Resection of infected tumor and implantation of polymethyl methacrylate chains, implantation of prosthesis at 4 wk; and 2 revisions for seroma at 4 y
2/M/27	Chondrosarcoma	IIB	None	V	None
3/M/27	Chondrosarcoma	IB	None	V	Internal plate fixation and corticocancellous allograft for humeral shaft fracture at 5 y; revision for seroma at 9 y
4/M/12	Angiosarcoma	IIB	None	VI	None
5/M/42	Chondrosarcoma	IIB	None	V	2 Revisions for lymphoid fistula at 4 and 10 wk
6/F/16	Ewing sarcoma	IIB	Local resection with local recurrence	VI	None
7/M/28	Chondrosarcoma	IB	None	V	Transient palsy of median nerve
8/F/52	Chondrosarcoma	IB	None	V	Fracture of prosthesis at 9 y and exchange of prosthesis
9/M/19	Ewing sarcoma	III	None, complete regression of pulmonary metastases with preoperative chemotherapy	VI	None
10/M/20	Synovial sarcoma	IIB	None	VI	Rupture of Trevira tape at 4 mo
11/M/60	Chondrosarcoma	IB	None	V	None
12/M/43	Ewing sarcoma	IIB	Local resection with local recurrence	V	None
13/M/35	Osteosarcoma	IIB	None	V	None
14/M/49	Neurofibrosarcoma	IB	2 Local resections with recurrence	VI	Palsy of brachial plexus; revision for seroma at 2 wk, and explantation of prosthesis at 4 wk due to deep infection
15/M/77	Malignant fibrous histiocytoma	IIB	9 Local resections with recurrence	VI	None
16/M/83	Malignant fibrous histiocytoma	IIB	2 Local resections with recurrence	VI	None
17/F/66	Malignant fibrous histiocytoma	IIB	Local resection with recurrence	VI	None
18/M/69	Solitary metastasis of thyroid carcinoma	III	Local resection with recurrence	V	None
19/F/38	Chondrosarcoma	IB	None	V	None

**According to the Musculoskeletal Tumor Society staging system.[11]*
†According to the staging system for shoulder girdle resections.[6]
‡NED indicates no evidence of disease.
§NA indicates not available for death of patient.

with stage IIB tumors had local resection prior to the Tikhoff-Linberg procedure; 5 had not. In each group pulmonary metastases developed in 3 patients. The 2 patients with local recurrence had not undergone a previous operation.

FUNCTIONAL OUTCOME

The functional range of motion of the hand was unaffected in all but 1 (case 14, patient with palsy of brachial plexus) of 12 surviving patients although strength was slightly diminished. Shoulder abduction was absent in 1 patient (case 14) requiring explantation of the prosthesis for deep infection. In the remaining patients abduction ranged from 30° to 45°.

According to the MSTS evaluation system the mean rating was 72% ± 14% (range, 33%-87%) of normal function (**Figure 2**). There was nothing to suggest that the scores deteriorated with time. The patient with neurologic deficit due to plexus brachialis lesion (case 14) was the only one reporting intermittent pain. The rating for function determined by restriction of activities was 2.9 ± 0.8 points (range, 2 to 4 points) indicating recreational restriction, although one patient continued playing tennis after the operation (case 4). The emotional acceptance of the Tikhoff-Linberg procedure was excellent (3.9 ± 0.8 point; range, 3-5 points). The rating for hand positioning revealed 3.1 ± 1.2 points (range, 1-5 points). The value for manual dexterity determined by the patient's ability to perform complex functions with the hand was 4.0 ± 1.0 points (range, 1-5 points), reflecting almost unaffected dexterity and sensibility. The patient's ability to actively lift objects and place them unaffected was possible for minor loads (2.9 ± 1.0 points; range, 0-4 points). Ten of 11 patients who remained free of disease were able to return to their previous employment. Only one patient (case 8) collected a disability pension. The patient (case 14) with the lowest score (33%) was able to return to his job as a lawyer.

Status at Latest Follow-up‡	Functional Outcome, %§	Length of Follow-up, y
NED, retired	63	6
NED, student	77	3
NED, teacher	73	10
NED, student	77	7
Alive with pulmonary metastasis and local recurrence with involvement of chest wall at 11 mo, disabled	87	1
NED, teacher	80	11
NED, technician	73	11
NED, disability pension	70	9
Death with pulmonary metastases	NA	1
Death due to pulmonary metastases	NA	2
NED, technician	77	4
Death due to osseous and cerebral metastases	NA	2
Local recurrence, interscapulothoracic amputation, and death due to pulmonary metastases	NA	3 mo
NED, lawyer	33	9
NED, death due to cardiopulmonary disease	NA	2
Death due to pulmonary metastases	NA	3 mo
Death due to systemic metastases	NA	2
NED, retired	63	1
NED, resection of pulmonary metastasis after 1 y, housewife	80	4

NONTUMOROUS COMPLICATIONS

Postoperative nontumorous complications due to the operation occurred in 9 of 19 patients. Four of these patients required more than one surgical revision after initial surgery (cases 1, 3, 5, and 14). Early postoperative seroma requiring operative revision developed in 3 patients (cases 1, 3, and 5). One patient (case 3) underwent internal plate fixation for a fracture of the humeral shaft distal of the tip of the prosthesis and allogeneic corticocancellous bone grafting 5 years after surgery. In another patient (case 8) the prosthesis fractured at its tip 9 years after surgery requiring exchange of the prosthesis. In 2 patients (cases 1 and 10) the Trevira tape securing the prosthesis to the scapula and clavicula ruptured. Neurologic complications developed in 2 patients (cases 7 and 14). The same patient (case 14) required the removal of the prosthesis due to a deep infection 4 weeks after surgery. The infection healed after a second surgical revision. No patients had vascular problems or necrosis of skin flaps.

COMMENT

Most sarcomas of the shoulder girdle involving the proximal humerus can be managed with reconstruction of the created defect under preservation of the shoulder joint.[1,12] The interscapulothoracic resection is suitable in extracompartmental high-grade malignant neoplasms of the proximal humerus or scapula involving the shoulder joint. In the series of Malawer et al[6] 3 patients and in the case series of Capanna et al[2] 5 patients undergoing the Tikhoff-Linberg procedure had stage IB tumors. This indicates that resection of the shoulder joint may be necessary in cases of low-grade malignant neoplasms with extensive local disease. Six patients with stage IB tumors were included in our case series. All 5 patients with chondrosarcoma had tumor invasion of the joint capsule and extensive infiltration of the deltoid muscle. Another patient (case 14) had 2 local recurrences of neurofibrosarcoma of the scapula after previous resections elsewhere. If the tumor is located in the proximal humerus and does not involve the glenoid a modified technique with resection of the glenoid lateral to the coracoid provides better functional and aesthetic results.[2]

Jensen and Johnston[1] reported a case series of 19 proximal humeral resections with prosthetic reconstruction. In their case series all 8 patients with stage IIB tumors had resection with preservation of the glenoid (type I resection). Two of these patients had local recurrence. Meller et al[9] had 1 local recurrence of 10 after Tikhoff-Linberg resection and conclude that type I resections in stage IIB tumors might be too dangerous for local tumor control. We observed local recurrence in 2 of 10 patients with stage IIB disease after modified (type V) Tikhoff-Linberg resections. The 2 patients developing local recurrence had extensive local disease preoperatively with tumor diameters of more than 10 cm. A local recurrence rate of 10% compares favorably with other reports of limb salvage when the MSTS staging of the patients is compared.[1,12]

The results of our small case series confirm the observations of Ueda et al[13] that local recurrence after inadequate surgery does not adversely affect outcome. Five of 10 patients with stage IIB tumors had local resection prior to the Tikhoff-Linberg procedure; 5 had not. In each group pulmonary metastases developed in 3 patients. In contrast local recurrence after the Tikhoff-Linberg procedure was associated with pulmonary metastases in 2 cases. In the series of Capanna et al[2] 1 of 24 patients had local recurrence with concomitant pulmonary metastases and 14 of 24 were free of disease after a mean follow-up of 22.5 months.

In our study, the most severe and frequent complications were metastases and local recurrence. Although the stage IIB tumors were managed with adjuvant therapy (with the exception of chondrosarcoma), this rate of metastatic disease (6 of 10 patients) at the time of intermediate-term follow-up evaluation is troubling but reflects the biology of the disease more than the operative approach.

Despite a careful selection of patients for interscapulothoracic resection the postoperative nontumorous complication rate in our series was high (9 of 19) but comparable to other studies.[2,7,8] Capanna et al[2] observed deep

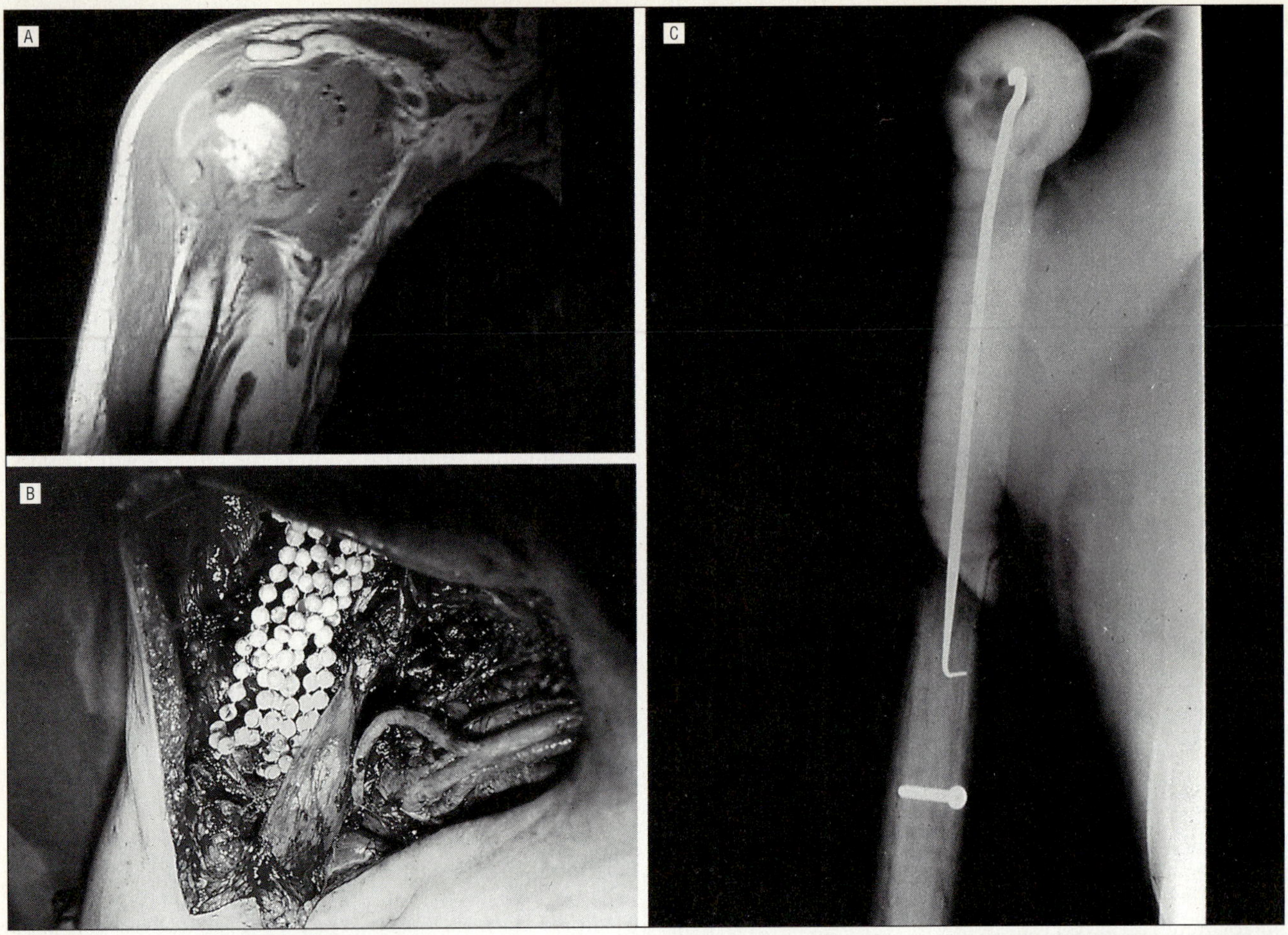

Figure 1. *A, Magnetic resonance image showing solitary metastasis of a thyroid carcinoma with tumor invasion and inflammation of surrounding soft tissue. B, Type V resection, dissection of the neurovascular bundle and temporary insertion of gentamycin sulfate–coated polymethyl methylacrylate chains. C, Implantation of an isoelastic tumor prosthesis 4 weeks later.*

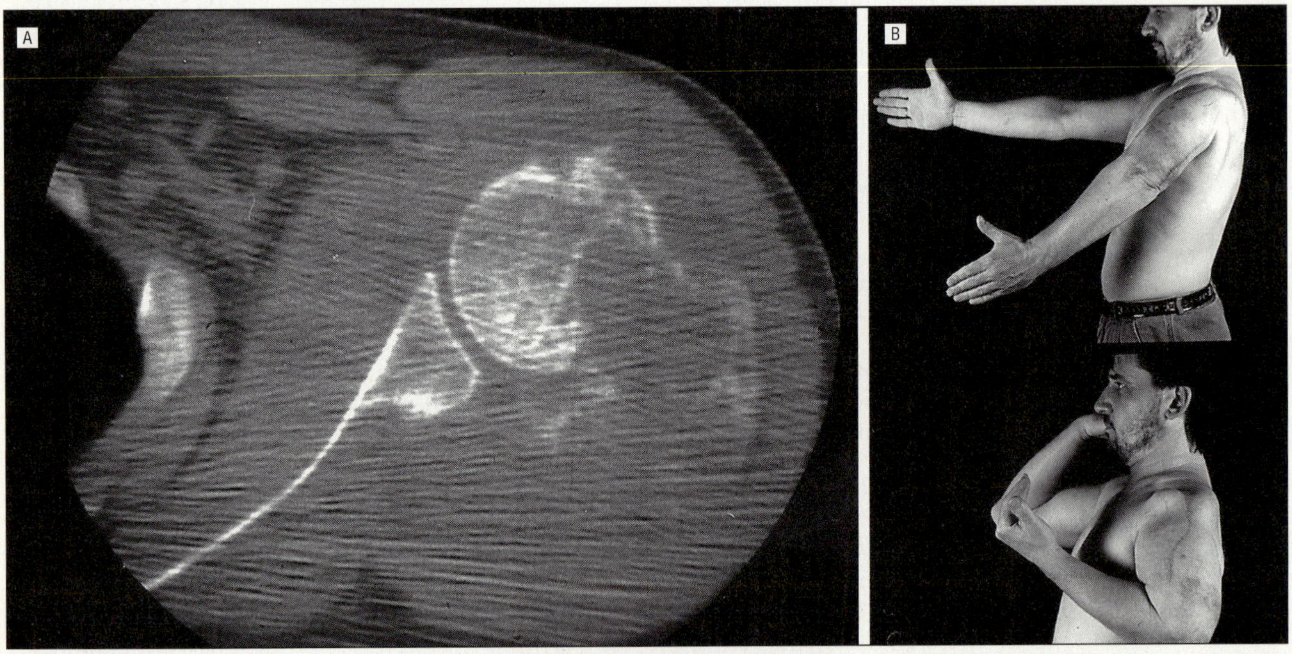

Figure 2. *A, Computed tomographic scan showing chondrosarcoma of the left humeral head with extensive invasion of the shoulder joint and of muscles of the rotator cuff. Implantation of an isoelastic humeral tumor prosthesis after en bloc tumor resection. Functional outcome (active range of motion) with Musculoskeletal Tumor Society staging system[11] score of 73%. B, Notice shortening of the extremity that allows better soft tissue covering.*

infection with removal of the prostheses in 3 of 24 patients.

The limiting factor in functional outcome is the resection of the abductor mechanism to ensure wide margins of resection. Abduction is dependent on contraction of trapezius muscle and sliding of the remaining scapula over the dorsal chest wall. The overall functional result based on the analysis of factors pertinent to the patient as a whole and factors specific to the upper limb revealed a mean rating of 72% of normal function. During the field trail conducted by the MSTS, 87 patients were evaluated after various resections for tumors of the upper limb.[14] The mean rating in their series was 68%. These results are comparable to the findings of Meller et al[9] who reported a rating of 72% after 10 Tikhoff-Linberg resections. The functional results after Tikhoff-Linberg resections are also comparable to the functional outcome reported by Gibbons et al[15] after subtotal scapulectomy (mean MSTS score of 71.6). All but one patient were able to return to their previous employment. We are convinced that the functional results after Tikhoff-Linberg resections based on activity, pain, and subjective psychological factors are clearly superior to amputation. Application of the functional rating system to patients after a forequarter amputation would give uniformly low scores, as a score of 0 would have been given for 3 of 6 items that were directly attributed to function of the hand (position of the hand, manual dexterity, and lifting ability). Even the patient with the worst score in our series (33%) had a score that was probably better than it would have been if a forequarter amputation had been performed. He stated that he accepts the procedure and would do it again.

The importance of reconstruction of the proximal humerus and preservation of major nerves is demonstrated for poor function in one patient in our series requiring early explantation of the prosthesis for deep infection. No abduction or elevation of the arm is possible. Unfortunately a lesion of the brachial plexus occurred in the same patient revealing major sensory and dexterity loss.

The Tikhoff-Linberg procedure proved to be a valuable operation for extended tumors of the shoulder girdle for functional and oncological outcome for local recurrence. However patients must be informed that there are substantial complications. The functional result in consideration of the patient as a whole is almost comparable to less extensive surgery for tumors of the proximal humerus treated by prosthetic replacement and preservation of the shoulder joint.

The Tikhoff-Linberg procedure is associated with substantial complications but is clearly superior to forequarter amputation. Under consideration of the indications of the Tikhoff-Linberg procedure, forequarter amputation should no longer be regarded as an alternative treatment. Forequarter amputation should have a role only in tumors invading the axillary neurovascular bundle. It is imperative that patients with malignant tumors of the shoulder girdle should be referred to specialized institutions.

Corresponding author: Gregor Voggenreiter, MD, Department of Trauma Surgery, University Hospital Essen, 45122 Essen, Germany.

REFERENCES

1. Jensen KL, Johnston JO. Proximal humeral reconstruction after excision of a primary sarcoma. *Clin Orthop.*1995;331:164-175.
2. Capanna R, van Horn JR, Biagini R, Ruggieri P, Ferruzzi A, Campanacci M.The Tikhoff-Linberg procedure for bone tumors of the proximal humerus: the classical "extensive" technique versus a modified "transglenoid" resection. *Arch Orthop Trauma Surg.* 1990;109:63-67.
3. Kumar VP, Satku SK, Mitra AK, Pho RWH. Function following limb salvage for primary tumors of the shoulder girdle. *Acta Orthop Scand.* 1994;65:55-61.
4. Linberg BE. Interscapulo-thoracic resection for malignant tumors of the shoulder joint region. *J Bone Joint Surg.* 1928;10:344-349.
5. Machson NJ. Modifikation der resectio interscapulo-thoracalis. *Beitr Orthop.* 1968; 15:87-88.
6. Malawer MM, Meller I, Dunham WK.. A new surgical classification system for shoulder-girdle resections. *Clin Orthop.* 1991;33-44.
7. Malawer MM, Sugarbaker PH, Lampert M, Baker AR, Gerber NL. The Tikhoff-Linberg procedure: report of ten patients and presentation of a modified technique for tumors of the proximal humers. *Surgery.* 1985;97:518-528.
8. Marcrove RC, Lewis MM, Huvos AG. En bloc upper humeral interscapulo-thoracic resection. *Clin Orthop.* 1977;124:219-228.
9. Meller I, Bickels J, Kollender Y, Ovadia D, Oren R, Mozes M. Malignant bone and soft tissue tumors of the shoulder girdle. *Acta Orthop Scand.* 1997;68:374-380.
10. Guerra A, Capanna R, Biagini R, Ruggieri P, Campanacci M. Resezione extraarticolare della spalla (Tikhoff-Linberg). *G Ital Ortop Traumatol.* 1985;11: 157-163.
11. Enneking WF, Spanier SS, Goodman MA. A system for the surgical staging of musculoskeletal sarcoma. *Clin Orthop.* 1980;153:106-120.
12. Gebhardt MC, Roth YF, Mankin HJ. Osteoarticular allografts for reconstruction in the proximal part of the humerus after excision of a musculoskeletal tumor. *J Bone Joint Surg Am.* 1990;72A:334-345.
13. Ueda T, Yoshikawa H, Mori S, et al. Influence of local recurrence on the prognosis of soft-tissue sarcomas. *J Bone Joint Surg Br.* 1997;79B:553-557.
14. Enneking WF, Dunham W, Gebhardt MC, Malawer M, Pritchard DJ. A system for the functional evaluation of reconstructive procedures after surgical treatment of tumors of the musculoskeletal system. *Clin Orthop.* 1993;286:241-246.
15. Gibbons CLMH, Bell RS, Wunder JS, et al. Function after subtotal scapulectomy for neoplasm of bone and soft tissue. *J Bone Joint Surg Br.* 1998;80B:38-42.

Announcement

The *Archives of Surgery* will give priority review and early publication to seminal works. This policy will include basic science advancements in surgery and critically performed clinical research.

ORIGINAL ARTICLE

Parathyroid Autotransplantation During Thyroidectomy

Is Frozen Section Necessary?

Chung-yau Lo, FRCS(Edin); King-yin Lam, FRCPA

Objective: To evaluate the accuracy of parathyroid gland identification and the need for routine frozen section examination before parathyroid autotransplantation during thyroidectomy.

Design: A prospective case series.

Setting: An endocrine surgical unit.

Patients: From January 1, 1995, to December 31, 1997, parathyroid autotransplantation was attempted for devascularized or inadvertently removed glands in 152 (33.7%) of 450 patients during thyroidectomy. Before autotransplantation, a biopsy specimen of the transplanted tissue was sent for histological examination without frozen section confirmation.

Main Outcome Measures: Positive identification of parathyroid tissue in microscopic examination.

Results: Of 179 attempted autotransplantations of parathyroid glands, parathyroid tissue was confirmed in 167 biopsy specimens (93.3%). Incorrect identification of parathyroid gland occurred in 12 instances. The tissue mistaken as parathyroid gland included fat in 6 cases, thyroid tissue in 4 cases, lymph node in 1 case, and thymus in 1 case. Transplantation of at least 1 parathyroid gland (range, 1-3) was confirmed in 144 patients. For patients with confirmed parathyroid autotransplantation at risk of hypoparathyroidism (n = 112), postoperative transient hypocalcemia occurred in 22 (19.6%), while no patient developed any permanent hypocalcemia during a median follow-up of 6 months.

Conclusions: Devascularized or inadvertently removed parathyroid glands can be identified expeditiously without routine frozen section during thyroid surgery. Immediate autotransplantation should be performed and permanent hypoparathyroidism can be avoided with this measure.

Arch Surg. 1999;134:258-260

THE FIRST successful parathyroid autotransplantation was performed by Lahey[1] in 1926 in patients undergoing partial thyroidectomy. Although the practice of implanting parathyroid glands has a long surgical tradition, not until the past 20 years has indication for parathyroid autotransplantation extended to radical head and neck surgery, including total thyroidectomy.[2-4] Parathyroid autotransplantation has been increasingly performed to prevent permanent hypoparathyroidism during total, subtotal, or completion thyroidectomy for benign or malignant conditions of the thyroid.[5-11]

Although the technique of parathyroid autotransplantation varies, parathyroid identity is routinely confirmed intraoperatively by frozen section before autotransplantation.[5-8] In fact, in an addenum to his 1926 report, Lahey stated that 19 of 26 specimens autotransplanted were subsequently identified histologically as lymph nodes, rather than parathyroid glands.[1] This emphasizes the difficulty of correct identification of normal parathyroid glands for autotransplantation. The present study aims at documenting the accuracy of parathyroid gland identification and evaluating the need for routine frozen section examination before autotransplantation during thyroidectomy.

RESULTS

Parathyroid autotransplantation was attempted in 152 patients (33.7%). There were 26 males and 126 females whose ages ranged from 15 to 75 years (median, 42 years).

Types of operative procedures included total or near-total thyroidectomy in 64 patients, bilateral subtotal thyroid-

From the Departments of Surgery (Dr Lo) and Pathology (Dr Lam), University of Hong Kong Medical Centre, Queen Mary Hospital, Hong Kong, China.

PATIENTS AND METHODS

From January 1, 1995, to December 31, 1997, 450 patients underwent thyroidectomy for treatment of various thyroid diseases by a single surgeon or by senior surgical residents operating in conjunction with that surgeon. Any devascularized or inadvertently removed parathyroid gland was identified for autotransplantation, even for patients who underwent unilateral thyroid lobectomy. The suspected parathyroid gland was minced into small (0.5-mm) pieces of which 1 was sent for microscopic examination to confirm its histological identity. The remaining tissue was immediately implanted into a muscle pocket fashioned in the ipsilateral sternocleidomastoid muscle. Routine frozen section examination was not performed.

The accuracy of parathyroid gland identification and removal for autotransplantation is expressed herein as the numbers of positive biopsy specimens divided by the numbers of attempted parathyroid autotransplantations. The resected thyroid specimens were examined histologically, and the incidence of serendipitiously identified glands during histological examination is expressed as the percentage of glands at risk. Replacement therapy with calcium supplement (calcium carbonate, 2-3 g/d) or calcitriol (Rocaltrol, 0.25-0.5 µg/d) or both was commenced in the presence of symptomatic hypocalcemia or a serum calcium level of 1.70 mmol/L or less (≤6.8 mg/dL) (reference range, 2.10-2.55 mmol/L [8.4-10.2 mg/dL]). Medications were gradually discontinued during 1 to 6 months of follow-up in the presence of normal serum calcium levels.[11]

ectomy in 34, unilateral lobectomy in 33, ipsilateral total and contralateral subtotal thyroidectomy in 14, and completion total thyroidectomy by unilateral lobectomy in 7. The indications for surgery are listed in **Table 1**.

Of the 179 attempted parathyroid autotransplantations performed in 152 patients, 167 parathyroid glands (93.3%) were subsequently confirmed to be normal parathyroid tissue during histological examination of the biopsy specimens. One to 3 (median, 1) parathyroid glands were autotransplanted in 144 patients (94.7%): 1 gland in 123 (85.4%), 2 glands in 19 (13.2%), and 3 glands in 2 (1.4%). The final histological findings in the 12 biopsy specimens that did not confirm parathyroid tissue included fat (n = 6), thyroid (n = 4), lymphatic (n = 1), and thymic (n = 1) tissues. The accuracy of identification of parathyroid glands in relation to their position is shown in **Table 2**. Incorrect identification of parathyroid glands occurred during thyroidectomy for diffuse toxic goiter (n = 7) and nodular goiter (n = 5).

For the 119 patients who were at risk of developing postoperative hypocalcemia after bilateral or completion total thyroidectomy, parathyroid tissue reimplantation was confirmed in 112 patients. Twenty-two patients (19.6%) developed postoperative hypocalcemia requiring calcium or calcitriol supplements or both. During a median follow-up of 6 months (range, 6 weeks to 30 months), all patients reverted to normocalcemia without the need for medications. Of the 264 lobes of thyroid gland examined histologically, 11 parathyroid tissue fragments were identified attached to the resected thyroid lobe (**Figure**). The incidence of serendipitiously discovered parathyroid glands in resected thyroid specimens was 2.1%.

Table 1. Indications for Surgery in 152 Patients With Attempted Parathyroid Autotransplantation

Primary Disease	No. (%)
Nodular goiter*	82 (54)
Graves disease*	32 (21)
Papillary carcinoma	19 (12)
Follicular adenoma	12 (8)
Follicular carcinoma	4 (3)
Miscellaneous†	3 (2)
Total	**152 (100)**

**Occult papillary carcinoma in 6 patients (3.9%).*
†Anaplastic carcinoma (n = 2) and lymphoma of thyroid gland (n = 1).

Table 2. Position of Parathyroid Glands in Relation to Accuracy of Parathyroid Identification

	Position			
	Right		Left	
	Upper	Lower	Upper	Lower
No. transplanted (n = 179)	37	51	35	56
No. confirmed (n = 167)	33	48	35	51
Accuracy, %	89	94	100	91

COMMENT

Permanent hypoparathyroidism is a recognized complication of thyroidectomy and is of sufficient concern that surgeons may refrain from performing radical thyroid surgery, particularly for malignant neoplasms of the thyroid. Parathyroid autotransplantation has been shown to prevent permanent hypoparathyroidism during radical thyroidectomy. Investigators who selectively or routinely use parathyroid autotransplantation reported a low incidence of permanent hypoparathyroidism,[8,9] with more recent series reporting an incidence of less than 2%.[5-7,10,11] One earlier report[12] showed unfavorable results after parathyroid autotransplantation, with a permanent hypoparathyroidism rate of 43%. That report represents an exception to the uniform success, and the poor result was attributed to transplantation of insufficient parathyroid tissue.[5]

The technique of parathyroid autotransplantation differs for different series. Thin sectioning, mincing, and homogenization into a paste form have been described.[2,9,13] In general, a frozen section biopsy specimen is obtained to confirm that it is parathyroid tissue before reimplantation is performed.[5-8] In the case of sur-

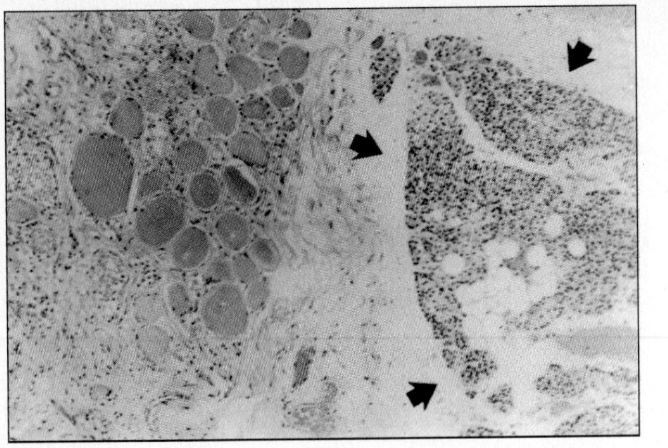

Photomicrograph showing a parathyroid gland (arrows) attached to the resected thyroid specimen at a subcapsular position (hematoxylin-eosin, original magnification ×10).

gery for malignant disease, frozen section examination can also disclose the presence of malignant involvement of the parathyroid gland and avoid the reimplantation of tumor cells.[5] Cervical exploration for primary hyperparathyroidism by experienced surgeons has been shown to be the best localization tool to detect abnormal parathyroid gland, with a success rate of 95% to 99%.[14,15] There is no doubt that enlarged parathyroid glands can be identified expeditiously in their normal or ectopic sites by experienced surgeons. However, it is generally agreed that the identification of normal parathyroid glands can be difficult. The ability of surgeons to identify and preserve parathyroid glands during thyroid surgery has not been well documented and is indirectly reflected by the incidence of permanent hypocalcemia. Routine biopsy of all normal glands is not necessary and should not be recommended. In addition, extensive dissection to identify normal glands should be avoided because of potential devascularization and damage to normal glands. A prospective study to assess the accuracy of correct identification of all parathyroid glands during thyroidectomy would be impractical or unethical.

Intraoperative frozen section confirmation was routinely performed and only patients with confirmed parathyroid tissue reimplantation were included in previous reports.[5-8] As a result, the ability of the surgeons to identify devascularized or inadvertently removed parathyroid glands for autotransplantation has not been documented. Salander and Tisell[8] reported on 86 of 97 patients with well-differentiated thyroid carcinoma who had parathyroid tissue implanted during total thyroidectomy. Biopsy specimens were taken from 132 of the 183 implanted parathyroid glands. The reason for not taking specimens in all cases was the fact that some glands were unquestionable on their macroscopic appearance and the ambition to save a maximal amount of parathyroid tissue.[8] Some parathyroid glands were implanted even before the result of the frozen section biopsy was known.

Parathyroid autotransplantation is advocated because it is simple and effective in preventing permanent hypoparathyroidism by preserving functions of damaged parathyroid glands. Frozen section examination adds additional cost and time to the operation. This is particularly true when inadvertently removed glands are identified at the end of the operation when the resected thyroid lobe is examined. Various sites of autotransplantation have been described,[2,13] although the neck remains an ideal site for patients during thyroidectomy except in surgery for medullary carcinoma in patients with multiple endocrine neoplasia type 2.[5]

Our results showed that devascularized or inadvertently removed glands can be accurately identified before autotransplantation. Most thyroidectomies were performed for benign thyroid conditions, and the risk of reimplantation of malignant tissue should be negligible. The fact that only 1 of the 12 incorrectly identified tissues was confirmed to be lymphoid in origin suggests that implantation of lymph node or metastasis is unlikely. Immediate autotransplantation of suspected devascularized or inadvertently removed glands should be attempted without the need for routine frozen section confirmation. Not only can a maximal amount of parathyroid tissue and operative time be saved, but ischemic damage to the transplanted parathyroid tissue can be reduced.

Reprints: Chung-yau Lo, FRCS(Edin), Division of Endocrine Surgery, Department of Surgery, University of Hong Kong Medical Centre, Queen Mary Hospital, Pokfulam, Hong Kong, China (e-mail: cylo@hkucc.hku.hk).

REFERENCES

1. Lahey FH. The transplantation of parathyroids in partial thyroidectomy. *Surg Gynecol Obstet.* 1926;62:508-509.
2. Wells SA, Ross AJ, Dale JK, Gray RS. Transplantation of the parathyroid glands: current status. *Surg Clin North Am.* 1979;59:167-177.
3. Saxe A. Parathyroid transplantation: a review. *Surgery.* 1984;95:507-526.
4. Baumann DS, Wells SA Jr. Parathyroid autotransplantation. *Surgery.* 1993;113:130-133.
5. Olson JA Jr, DeBenedetti MK, Baumann DS, Wells SA Jr. Parathyroid autotransplantation during thyroidectomy: results of long-term follow-up. *Ann Surg.* 1996;223:472-480.
6. Shaha AR, Burnett C, Jaffe BM. Parathyroid autotransplantation during thyroid surgery. *J Surg Oncol.* 1991;46:21-24.
7. Walker RP, Paloyan E, Keley TF, et al. Parathyroid autotransplantation in patients undergoing a total thyroidectomy: a review of 261 patients. *Otolaryngol Head Neck Surg.* 1994;111:258-264.
8. Salander H, Tisell LE. Incidence of hypoparathyroidism after radical surgery for thyroid carcinoma and autotransplantation of parathyroid glands. *Am J Surg.* 1977;134:358-362.
9. Paloyan E, Lawrence AM, Paloyan D. Successful autotransplantation of the parathyroid glands during total thyroidectomy for carcinoma. *Surg Gynecol Obstet.* 1977;145:364-368.
10. Smith MA, Jarosz H, Hessel P, Lawrence AM, Paloyan E. Parathyroid autotransplantation in total thyroidectomy. *Am Surg.* 1990;56:404-406.
11. Lo CY, Lam KY. Postoperative hypocalcemia in patients who did or did not undergo parathyroid autotransplantation during thyroidectomy: a comparative study. *Surgery.* 1998;124:1081-1087.
12. Ohman V, Granberg P, Lindell B. Function of the parathyroid glands after total thyroidectomy. *Surg Gynecol Obstet.* 1978;146:773-778.
13. Funahasi H, Sutoh Y, Imai T, et al. Our technique of parathyroid autotransplantation in operation for papillary thyroid carcinoma. *Surgery.* 1993;114:92-96.
14. Kaplan EL, Yashiro T, Salti G. Primary hyperparathyroidism in the 1990s: choice of surgical procedures for this disease. *Ann Surg.* 1992;215:300-317.
15. Van Heerden JA, Grant CS. Surgical treatment of primary hyperparathyroidism: an institutional perspective. *World J Surg.* 1991;15:688-692.

A Study of Slippage Rates in Manually Tied and Mechanically Tied Laparoscopic Sutures

Vincent A. Pellegrini, M.D.

Coordinator of Medical Education in Reproductive Endocrinology and Infertility, Reading Hospital and Medical Center

Clinical Associate Professor in OB/GYN, University of Pennsylvania Medical School

Paul A. Prior, M.D.

Ashland, Kentucky

ETHICON ENDO-SURGERY, INC.
a Johnson & Johnson company

INTRODUCTION

Properly tied knots are a cornerstone of the art of surgery. Improperly tied knots can lead to hernia formation, wound dehiscence, hemorrhage, or exsanguination.

The strength and stability of a surgical knot is determined by several factors: the suture material itself (its coefficient of friction, diameter, coating, moisture, and tensile strength); the knot geometry; and knot-tying technique.

Knots may fail by slipping or breaking. Slippage is generally caused by improper knot geometry ("granny" or slip knots) or by improper tying techniques that result in fraying or shearing. Some sources suggest that many board-certified surgeons tie inadequate knots[1,2,3].

Laparoscopic procedures add another layer of complexity to the task of tying a secure knot. Mechanical feedback is diminished, manipulation of the suture is more difficult, and the available range of motion is often smaller.

A number of different knots and techniques for laparoscopic knot tying have been proposed and studied in the past. The present study attempted to answer three questions: 1) How do standard square knots tied by surgeons in our department perform; 2) How do laparoscopic knots tied by the same surgeons perform; and 3) How do both of these compare with knots created by a new laparoscopic knot-tying device, the Suture Assistant, developed by Ethicon Endo-Surgery, Inc.

Over the course of three days, a procedure for studying suture tying was developed at The Reading Hospital and Medical Center. The goal of this study was the evaluation of the open suture-tying abilities of various surgeons, OB/GYN staff and residents.

The "gold standard" was taken to be five alternating half-hitches tied using the traditional technique employed in open surgery. Laparoscopic extracorporeal knots with the same standard five alternating half-hitches were studied, along with knots tied by the Suture Assistant. The three knots were then compared. It was assumed that the openly tied square knot would be of high quality; that is, it would be unlikely to fail by reason of knot slippage, nor would the suture be damaged

Additional goals of this study were to compare the various groups of physicians to each other, and to provide an educational experience through an objective knot tying evaluation.

The study incorporated a computerized data collection device (Instron Instruments, Canton, MA) that evaluated knot and suture integrity. ETHIBOND EXCEL suture was tied in the three different fashions by 32 attending physicians (six resident physicians were also tested, but were not included in the data analysis). Each physician tied an open knot over a 1-inch diameter fixture and a laparoscopic extracorporeal knot using a pelvic trainer and a video laparoscope. The Suture Assistant knot device was deployed using the same pelvic trainer and video laparoscope. Each knotted suture was then tested on the automated testing device. An increasing load was placed on the suture, and the distraction (the displacement of the tensiometer hooks holding the knot) was graphed against the load placed.

Three patterns were developed and evaluated: 1) knot breakage, 2) suture breakage, and 3) knot slippage. The laparoscopic knot tying skills of the various physicians were variable. The study utilized only the data obtained from each participant's first knot attempt at each tying station.

RESULTS

As noted in the box plot at the end of this study, the open knot (SO) had a 34.4% knot slip rate. In other words, 34.4% of all openly tied knots opened up at a load less than that required to break the suture or knot. This knot slippage was considered a knot failure since a properly tied knot would have minimal slippage.

The laparoscopic extracorporeally (LE) tied knot had a slippage of 43.8%. There is no statistical difference between this failure rate and the failure rate of an openly tied square knot. Finally, the Ethicon Endo-Surgery Suture Assistant device (SA) had a slip rate of 3.1%.

Knot failure was almost exclusively found to be related to knot slippage. There were very few knot breaks, implying no undue shearing of suture during the knot-tying procedure. There were also very minimal premature suture breaks that occurred before the known tensile strength of the ETHIBOND EXCEL suture had been reached. The failures were "all or none"; the knot either held until the tensile strength of the suture was reached and the suture broke at the knot, or the knot slipped and fell apart.

DISCUSSION

The technical difficulty of tying laparoscopic knots has proven to be a limiting factor for many surgeons, deterring them from performing certain procedures. Anything that might overcome this technical hurdle would be welcomed.

The clinical significance of knot slippage is sometimes difficult to ascertain. It would certainly not be the experience of the surgeons involved that 43.8% of their patients suffered clinical difficulties due to knot slippage. But the fact that many of these confidently tied knots did indeed slip might have some subclinical implications. This paper, however, did not address the clinical aspects of knot slippage.

One interesting note: Several surgeons tied repetitive knots that failed every time, although their technique appeared perfect to observers, and they tied their knots quite meticulously.

This study did not address various types of suture; only ETHIBOND EXCEL was used.

CONCLUSION

Using a controlled measurement apparatus, we have demonstrated that the security of standard square knots was significantly less than expected by the surgeons tying them. This agrees with previous studies. Most of those participating in this trial were quite surprised to learn that their knots were flawed, supporting the concept that most surgeons are unaware of weaknesses in their technique. Failures were spread across all departments, suggesting not a training or institutional failure, but rather the notion that familiarity does indeed breed contempt.

The clinical significance of these failures is beyond the scope of this study, and the majority of patients do well despite such inadequacies in knot construction. We believe, however, that this should serve as a reminder that attention to detail and to the fundamentals of surgical technique are as important as they ever were.

In our institution, the knots constructed with the Ethicon Endo-Surgery Suture Assistant device demonstrated significantly lower failure rates, even with first-time users. This device appears to offer the laparoscopic surgeon the ability to easily construct knots superior to those that most of them could tie extracorporeally, or even by open hand-tying. Such a device may offer the laparoscopic surgeon better means to complete advanced procedures, and allow him or her to consider a wider range of procedures. This device would be anticipated to facilitate a better outcome in procedures that need exact tissue plane alignment, such as vaginal reparative surgery.

We would respectfully submit, in conclusion, that institutions consider the methods we have described as a method for teaching knot tying to residents and students. Based on our data and the data of those reporting previously, we would expect that many of those reading this paper might be just as surprised as our surgeons were when they saw their knots fall apart under pressure.

1. Thacker JG, Rodeheaver G, Kurz L et al. Mechanical performance of sutures in surgery. Am J Surg 1977;133:713

2. Trimbos JB. Security of various knots commonly used in surgical practice. Obstet Gynecol 1984;64:274

3. Batra EK, Taylor PT, Franz DA et al. A portable tensiometer for assessing surgeon's knot tying technique. Gynecol Oncology 1993;48:114

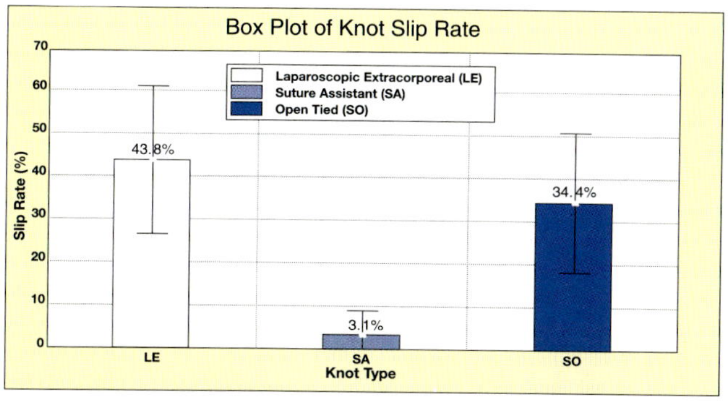

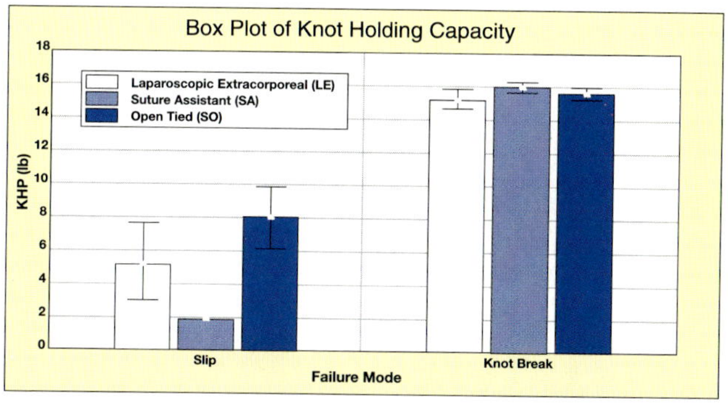

Data on file at Ethicon Endo-Surgery

ETHICON ENDO-SURGERY, INC.
a Johnson & Johnson company

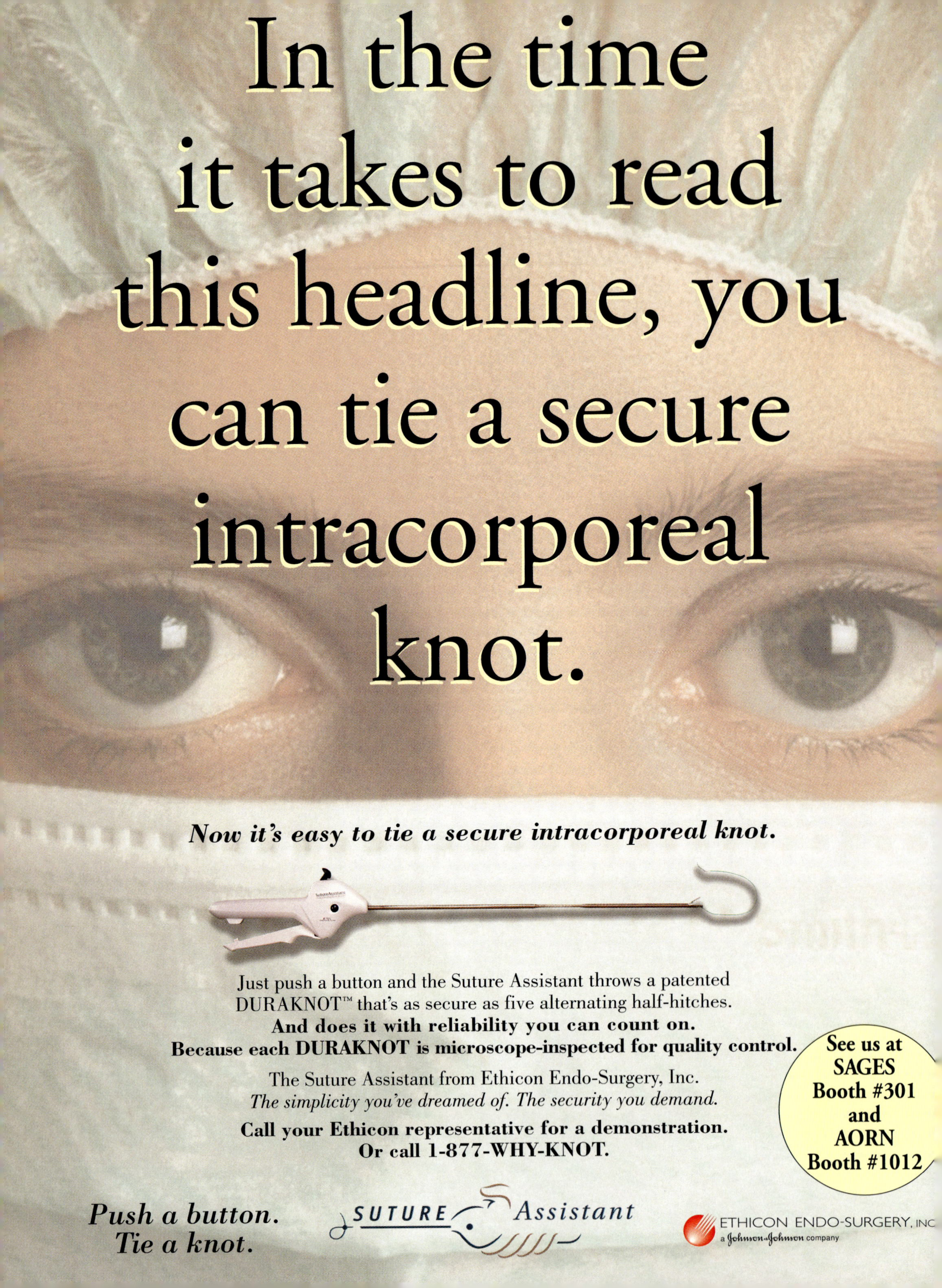
In the time it takes to read this headline, you can tie a secure intracorporeal knot.
Now it's easy to tie a secure intracorporeal knot.
Just push a button and the Suture Assistant throws a patented DURAKNOT™ that's as secure as five alternating half-hitches.
And does it with reliability you can count on.
Because each DURAKNOT is microscope-inspected for quality control.
The Suture Assistant from Ethicon Endo-Surgery, Inc.
The simplicity you've dreamed of. The security you demand.
Call your Ethicon representative for a demonstration.
Or call 1-877-WHY-KNOT.
See us at SAGES Booth #301 and AORN Booth #1012
Push a button. Tie a knot.
SUTURE Assistant
ETHICON ENDO-SURGERY, INC
a Johnson & Johnson company

ORIGINAL ARTICLE

Association of Preoperative Biliary Stenting With Increased Postoperative Infectious Complications in Proximal Cholangiocarcinoma

Steven N. Hochwald, MD; Edmund C. Burke, MD; William R. Jarnagin, MD; Yuman Fong, MD; Leslie H. Blumgart, MD

Background: The indications for preoperative biliary stenting in patients with obstructive jaundice are controversial. We evaluated the effect of preoperative biliary stenting on bacterobilia and infectious complications following surgical treatment of proximal cholangiocarcinoma.

Design: A retrospective review was performed of all patients undergoing surgical treatment of proximal cholangiocarcinoma.

Setting: A metropolitan cancer surgery service.

Patients and Methods: Seventy-one patients underwent palliative biliary bypass or curative resection of proximal cholangiocarcinoma from March 1, 1991, to April 1, 1997, and were entered into a prospective database. Forty-one patients underwent preoperative biliary intubation and stent placement. We analyzed patient, nutritional, laboratory, and operating room factors. Statistical evaluation was performed using Student *t* test and χ^2 analysis.

Main Outcome Measure: Data were recorded for a history of cholangitis, operative time, amount of blood loss, incidence of intraoperative bacterobilia, proportion of patients with postoperative infectious and noninfectious complications, and length of hospital stay.

Results: All patients (n = 14) with a history of preoperative cholangitis had been subjected to previous endoscopic retrograde cholangiopancreatography and/or percutaneous transhepatic biliary drainage. Groups were equivalent for risk for comorbidity, proportion undergoing curative vs palliative procedures, time spent in the operating room, and amount of blood loss. Patients with stents had a significantly lower bilirubin level ($P = .005$). Patients with stents had a significantly increased risk for bacterobilia ($P = .001$) and infectious complications ($P = .03$). Bacterobilia was present in 11 (100%) of 11 patients undergoing endoscopic stenting and in 15 (65%) of 23 patients undergoing percutaneous stenting. There was no increased risk for noninfectious complications, length of hospital stay, or mortality in patients with stents. In 10 (59%) of 17 patients with postoperative infectious complications and positive findings of intraoperative bile culture, the organism was synonymous.

Conclusions: Preoperative biliary stenting in proximal cholangiocarcinoma increases the incidence of contaminated bile and postoperative infectious complications. Endoscopic stents frequently do not relieve jaundice in high biliary obstruction and are rarely indicated, especially in light of their high contamination rate.

Arch Surg. 1999;134:261-266

THERE ARE approximately 4500 new cases of cholangiocarcinoma per year in the United States.[1] Proximal cholangiocarcinomas constitute 30% to 60% of these tumors. The prognosis is poor in these patients, with untreated patients having a median survival of 3 months.[2] In almost all series, rates of resection are low at patient presentation; yet surgery remains the mainstay of treatment.[3-6] Surgical options for proximal cholangiocarcinoma include curative resection or a palliative biliary-enteric bypass.

Despite recent technical advances and improved perioperative care, treatment of patients with proximal cholangiocarcinoma is still challenging. In recent series, whereas mortality rates have decreased significantly over the last several years, morbidity rates remain high.[7,8] A number of studies have indicated that surgery for severe obstructive jaundice is associated with increased risk for complications.[9-12] Due to this high risk, investigators have studied the role of biliary drainage for preoperative preparation. These studies often have included heterogeneous groups with respect to cause of bile duct obstruction. Patients with benign and malignant causes of proximal and distal bile duct obstruction have been grouped

From the Department of Surgery, Memorial Sloan-Kettering Cancer Center, New York, NY. Dr Burke is now with the Department of Surgery, Kaiser Permanente Medical Center, Honolulu, Hawaii.

PATIENTS AND METHODS

From March 1, 1991, to April 1, 1997, 90 patients with proximal cholangiocarcinoma underwent evaluation by the Hepatobiliary Surgical Division at Memorial Sloan-Kettering Cancer Center, New York, NY, and were entered in a prospective database. Proximal cholangiocarcinoma was defined as tumors originating in the common, right, or left hepatic duct. Of these 90 patients, 10 underwent nonoperative palliation, 9 underwent exploration and biopsy alone, and 71 underwent a curvative resection or palliative biliary bypass. Of these 71 patients who form the basis for our study, 42 had a stent in the preoperative period, whereas 29 did not. All patients were admitted to the hospital and underwent preoperative history, physical examination, and laboratory analyses, including determination of serum bilirubin concentration.

Preoperative biliary stents were defined as endoscopic, percutaneous transhepatic, nasobiliary, or T-tube stents that crossed the tumor and/or the ampulla of Vater. Of the 42 patients with stents, 23 underwent percutaneous transhepatic intubation; 13, endoscopic intubation; and 3, T-tube placement. One patient had a nasobiliary drain; another, percutaneous transhepatic and endoscopic stents; and another, endoscopic and nasobiliary stents.

Careful analysis of factors associated with perioperative morbidity was undertaken. Patient factors analyzed were age, preoperative episode of cholangitis, and comorbidity. Comorbidity was defined as the presence of diabetes mellitus, coronary artery disease, or hypertension.

Nutritional factors analyzed included percentage of weight loss and serum albumin concentrations. In addition, biochemical studies included serum urea nitrogen, serum creatinine, and total bilirubin levels.

All but 3 of the operations were performed by 2 surgeons (Y.F. and L.H.B.). Of the 42 patients with preoperative stents, 18 (43%) had curative surgery and 24 (57%) had a palliative biliary bypass. In the 29 patients without stents, 12 (41%) had curative operation and 17 (59%) had a palliative bypass. Of those patients undergoing curative resection, 22 (73%) underwent liver resection. Of those patients undergoing palliative biliary bypass, 38 (93%) underwent bypass to the right sectoral hepatic duct or segment III duct or hepaticojejunostomy. Operating room factors analyzed were the time under anesthesia, operating room blood loss, and results of routine intraoperative bile cultures. Blood transfusion data included the percentage of patients who received a transfusion during their hospital stay and the median number of units transfused. Other factors compared included length of stay, which was tabulated as total hospital stay and time from the date of operation until discharge home. Reoperation and mortality rates were also determined for both groups.

Complications were retrospectively recorded by evaluation of the prospective database, hospital records, and chart review. These were grouped as infectious and noninfectious in nature. Infectious complications recorded were wound infection, intra-abdominal abscess, pneumonia, cholangitis, *Clostridium difficile* colitis, and *Candida* esophagitis. Wound infections were defined as a superficial or deep infection that required antibiotics and/or wound drainage. Intra-abdominal abscesses were defined as an intra-abdominal collection associated with fever and/or leukocytosis that required drainage, culture of which yielded positive findings. Pneumonia was defined as an infiltrate on chest radiogram requiring antibiotic treatment. Cholangitis was defined as positive findings of a bile culture associated with fever. Noninfectious complications included hemorrhage, anastomotic leak, liver necrosis, fascial dehiscence, biloma, biliary fistula, renal failure, cardiac arrhythmia, prolonged ileus, severe ascites, and pancreatitis.

Statistical analyses were performed using χ^2 for categorical variables and Student *t* test for continuous variables. Significance was defined as $P<.05$. Unless otherwise indicated, data are given as mean ± SEM.

together.[13-17] Controversy continues concerning the role of preoperative biliary stenting in malignant bile duct obstruction.

We performed this study to determine if preoperative biliary intubation and stenting increased operative difficulty, rate of complications, and length of hospital stay after operation for proximal cholangiocarcinoma. The study poplulation was a relatively homogeneous group of patients accumulated during a short time.

RESULTS

DEMOGRAPHICS

Seventy-one patients underwent operative treatment during the 6 years studied. Demographic data are listed in **Table 1**. There was no significant difference in age, sex distribution, history of cholangitis, or comorbidity between groups. A history of cholangitis was present in 24% of patients (n = 10) who had a previous stent, compared with 14% (n = 4) in those without a previous stent ($P = .30$).

NUTRITIONAL AND BIOCHEMICAL MEASUREMENTS

Nutritional and biochemical measurements are listed in **Table 2**. The average weight loss was 6% ± 1% in the no stent group vs 8% ± 1% in the stent group ($P = .17$). There were no significant differences in preoperative albumin, serum urea nitrogen, and creatinine levels. As expected, in the no stent group, the mean preoperative bilirubin level (222.3 ± 46.2 μmol/L [13.0 ± 2.7 mg/dL]) was significantly higher than in the stent group (95.8 ± 15.4 μmol/L [5.6 ± 0.9 mg/dL]) ($P = .005$).

OPERATIVE FACTORS

In an effort to evaluate the potential additional operative difficulty with the inflammation that commonly

Table 1. Demographics and Comorbidity

Characteristic	Group* No Stent (n = 29)	Stent (n = 42)	P
Median age, y	64	65	.91
Sex, M:F	13:16	27:15	.10
Cholangitis†	4 (14)	10 (24)	.30
Comorbidity, No. of patients	**12**	**11**	.18
Hypertension	8 (28)	6 (14)	
Diabetes	1 (3)	4 (10)	
Coronary artery disease	3 (10)	1 (2)	

*Groups are described in the "Patients and Methods" section. Unless otherwise indicated, data are given as number (percentage).
†Indicates history of cholangitis in preoperative period.

Table 2. Nutritional and Biochemical Measurements

	Group* No Stent (n = 29)	Stent (n = 42)	P
Weight loss, %	6 ± 1	8 ± 1	.17
Albumin, g/L	37 ± 1	36 ± 1	.14
Serum urea nitrogen, mmol/L (mg/dL)	5.4 ± 0.4 (15 ± 1)	4.6 ± 0.4 (13 ± 1)	.26
Creatinine, μmol/L (mg/dL)	88.4 ± 5.3 (1.0 ± 0.06)	97.2 ± 4.4 (1.1 ± 0.05)	.52
Total bilirubin, μmol/L (mg/dL)	222.3 ± 46.2 (13.0 ± 2.7)	95.8 ± 15.4 (5.6 ± 0.9)	.005

*Groups are described in the "Patients and Methods" section. Data are given as mean ± SEM.

Table 3. Operating Room and Transfusion Measurements

	Group* No Stent (n = 29)	Stent (n = 42)	P
Operating room			
Surgery time, min	253 ± 20	273 ± 16	.42
Operating room blood loss, mL	1083 ± 194	855 ± 191	.42
Type of procedure, %			
Curative	41	43	.80
Palliative	59	57	.70
Blood data			
Hospital transfusion, %	48	38	.43
Median units transfused	2	3	.12

*Groups are described in the "Patients and Methods" section. Data are given as mean ± SEM, unless otherwise specified.

accompanies stent placement, operating room and blood transfusion factors were analyzed (**Table 3**). There were no significant differences in the time under anesthesia (no stent group, 253 ± 20 minutes; stent group, 273 ± 16 minutes; *P* = .42), operating room blood loss (no stent group, 1083 ± 194 mL; stent group, 855 ± 191 mL; *P* = .42) or type of operation. In addition, the percentage of patients who received a blood transfusion during their hospital stay (48% vs 38%; *P* = .43) and the median number of units of blood transfused (2 vs 3 U; *P* = .12) was similar between groups (no stent vs stent, respectively).

Table 4. Infectious Complications

Type	Group* No Stent (n = 29)	Stent (n = 42)	P
Wound infection	4	12	.10
Intra-abdominal abscess	4	5	.81
Pneumonia	1	3	.64
Cholangitis	0	4	.14
Clostridium difficile	1	4	.64
Candida esophagitis	1	0	.41
Total†	**11**	**28**	.03
Total, %‡	28	52	<.05

*Groups are described in the "Patients and Methods" section. Unless otherwise indicated, data are given as number of patients.
†Patients can be listed in more than 1 category if more than 1 complication occurred.
‡Indicates percentage of patients with an infectious complication.

Table 5. Noninfectious Complications

Type	Group* No Stent (n = 29)	Stent (n = 42)	P
Hemorrhage	3	4	.71
Anastomotic leak	3	2	.39
Hepatic infarct	2	1	.56
Biloma	1	2	.79
Wound dehiscence	1	2	.79
Other†	2	6	.46
Total‡	**12**	**17**	.94
Total, %§	33	38	.80

*Groups are described in the "Patients and Methods" section. Unless otherwise indicated, data are given as number of patients.
†Includes biliary fistula, renal failure, cardiac arrhythmia, prolonged ileus, severe ascites, and pancreatitis.
‡Patients can be listed in more than 1 category if more than 1 complication occurred.
§Indicates percentage of patients with a noninfectious complication.

COMPLICATIONS

Complications were recorded as total number of complications and percentage of patients with a complication and were divided into infectious and noninfectious categories (**Table 4** and **Table 5**). The number of noninfectious complications was similar in the stent group (n = 17) and the no stent group (n = 12; *P* = .85). However, there were significantly more infectious complications in the stent group (n = 28) compared with the no stent group (n = 11; *P* = .03). Some patients had more than 1 complication, and if expressed as percentage with a complication, patients with stents had a 52% chance (22 of 42 patients) of having an infection compared with a 28% chance (8 of 29 patients) in patients without stents (*P* = .05). The percentage of patients with a noninfectious complication was similar between groups (stent vs no stent group, 38% [11/29] vs 33% [14/42]; *P* = .80). There was no significant increase in any 1 complication

Table 6. Preoperative Intervention and Bacterobilia*

Preoperative Intervention (No. of Patients)	Intraoperative Bile Cultures, % With Positive Findings	P
No ERCP (19)	37	.20
ERCP (42)†	55	
No stent group (22)	14	.001
Stent group (39)‡	69	
Percutaneous (23)	65	.03
Endoscopic (11)	100	

*Intraoperative bile culture data were available in 61 of 71 patients. ERCP indicates endoscopic retrograde cholangiopancreatography. Groups are described in the "Patients and Methods" section.

†Diagnostic ERCP was performed in the preoperative period.

‡Bile culture data were available in 39 patients. Five patients had a nasobiliary stent, T-tube, or a percutaneous stent and endoprosthesis and were not included.

between groups, but the largest difference was seen in wound infections, with 12 patients in the stent group compared with 4 in the no stent group ($P = .10$).

BACTEROBILIA

Contamination of bile has been associated with biliary tract manipulation, and therefore we examined intraoperative bile culture data (**Table 6**). Bile culture results from intraoperative cultures were available in 61 (86%) of 71 patients. Since a large number of patients underwent preoperative diagnostic endoscopic retrograde cholangiopancreatography (ERCP), we evaluated the incidence of bacterobilia in patients subjected to this procedure. Intraoperative bile cultures yielded positive findings in 7 (37%) of 19 patients who did not undergo preoperative diagnostic ERCP, whereas these cultures were positive in 23 (55%) of 42 patients who did undergo preoperative ERCP ($P = .20$). There was a significant increase in bile cultures that yielded positive findings in patients in the stent group (69%, n = 27) vs those in the no stent group (14%, n = 3; $P = .001$). In addition, there was a significantly increased incidence of bacterobilia in patients who had an endoscopic stent compared with those who had a percutaneous transhepatic stent (100% [11/11] vs 65% [15/23], respectively; $P = .03$). Finally, we found that the time that a stent was in place was associated with a significantly greater incidence of positive findings of intraoperative bile cultures. Those stents that were in place for less than 28 days were associated with a 53% incidence (10 of 19 patients) of bacterobilia, compared with an 89% incidence (16 of 18 patients) of bacterobilia in stents in place for longer than 28 days ($P = .02$).

BILE CULTURES VS CULTURES FROM INFECTIOUS COMPLICATIONS

There were 31 intraoperative bile cultures that yielded negative and 30 that yielded positive findings (data not available for 10 patients). In those patients with positive findings, postoperative infectious complications were seen in 17 (ie, wound infection [n = 7], intra-abdominal abscess [n = 5], pneumonia [n = 2], cholangitis [n = 2], and *Clostridium difficile* colitis [n = 1]). At least 1 organism in the intraoperative bile culture was similar to the organism(s) that grew from the postoperative infectious complication culture in 10 (59%) of the 17 patients. The greatest similarity was seen in findings of intraoperative bile and wound cultures, where there was some agreement in 6 of the 7 patients. The types of organisms obtained from intraoperative bile cultures are shown in the following tabulation:

Organism	No. of Cultures
Enterococcus species	21
Candida species	7
Klebsiella pneumoniae	7
Streptococcus viridans	5
Staphylococcus epidermidis	5
Enterobacter aerogenes	4
Pseudomonas species	3
Enterobacter coli	3
Serratia marcescens	1
Bacteroides fragilis	1
Clostridium difficile	1

In some cultures, more than 1 organism was present.

LENGTH OF HOSPITAL STAY

There was no significant difference in hospital stay (stent group, 17 ± 8 days; no stent group, 16 ± 7 days), postoperative stay (stent group, 14 ± 5 days; no stent group, 14 ± 7 days), reoperation rate (stent group, 10%; no stent group, 12%), or mortality (stent group, 5%; no stent group, 14%).

COMMENT

Our retrospective study compares 2 homogeneous groups of patients with proximal cholangiocarcinoma. The patients were well matched with respect to age, history of cholangitis, comorbidity, and weight loss. The major difference is the presence of a biliary stent with associated improvement in serum bilirubin level in the stent group. We have shown that the presence of a preoperative biliary stent before curative or palliative surgery for hilar cholangiocarcinoma is significantly associated with increased infectious complications. Patients with preoperative stents had 28 infectious complications compared with 11 infectious complications in those patients without stents ($P = .03$). Routine placement of biliary stents in patients with potentially resectable tumors cannot be endorsed.

The role of preoperative biliary drainage has been examined previously. The difference in most of these studies compared with ours is mainly that the previous trials enrolled patients with lesions at varying locations in the biliary tree and some patients with benign disease.

McPherson et al[14] randomized 65 patients with low and high malignant bile duct obstruction to preoperative percutaneous transhepatic biliary drainage followed by laparotomy vs laparotomy alone. Drainage reduced the serum bilirubin level as expected, but there was no difference in overall postoperative morbidity or mortality. Therefore, it was concluded that there was no proven place for preoperative percutaneous transhepatic biliary drainage in the management of malignant obstructive jaundice. In a randomized trial by Hatfield et al[13] a similar conclusion was made after studying patients with benign and malignant obstructive jaundice.

In a study evaluating the effect of preoperative endoscopic biliary drainage, Lai et al[16] randomized 87 patients with high and low malignant biliary obstruction to undergo laparotomy or endoscopic biliary drainage followed by exploration. There was a significant reduction of serum bilirubin concentrations in the stent group but no difference in morbidity or mortality between groups.

The only prospective, randomized study that has shown a benefit with preoperative biliary drainage included patients with low bile duct obstruction and endoscopically placed drains. There were fewer complications in the patients undergoing preoperative drainage. That study has been criticized due to the high incidence of cholangitis in the group without preoperative drains, and the presence of clear signs of infection without drainage before operation is the likely reason for the increased rate of complications in that group.[17]

In our study, patients who had a preoperative stent placed had a 69% incidence of positive results of bile cultures, compared with 14% incidence in patients without a preoperative stent ($P = .001$). Also, there was a significantly higher incidence of positive findings in bile cultures in patients who had an endoscopic stent (100%), compared with patients with a percutaneous stent (65%; $P = .03$). The bile infection rate in our study is similar to that in other studies. Investigators have reported that infected bile occurred in 61% to 95% of patients with percutaneous drains, with the figures varying with the position of the catheter tip.[18,19] In addition, Karsten et al[20] demonstrated that in patients undergoing pancreatic resection, bile cultures in the presence of a biliary endoprosthesis showed bacterial growth in 94%, compared with a 62% incidence in patients with percutaneous drains ($P = .01$). The cause of the increased infection rate with an endoprosthesis may be due to contamination when the stent is inserted or ascent of microorganisms from the open passage to the duodenum and subsequent reflux of duodenal contents. Nonetheless, it is clear that in our study and others,[20] in the absence of a biliary stent, that bile contamination is much less frequent.

In our study, stents that were in place for longer than 28 days were associated with a significantly higher bile infection rate (89%), compared with stents in place for less than 28 days (53%; $P = .02$). Various factors predispose to infections in the presence of biliary drains. Bacterial β-D-glucuronidase has been shown to lead to biliary sludge formation and colonization of bacteria on drains. Surface defects on drains may contribute to the process of bacterial adhesion and colonization. In addition, the presence of side holes in drains is thought to cause an accumulation of debris and sludge and to create surface irregularities that allow for bacterial attachment.[21] The longer a stent is in place, the greater the likelihood that these mechanisms will be in effect.

Controversy still exists concerning the implications of infected bile in biliary tract surgery. Most investigators have shown that patients undergoing biliary tract operations are at a higher risk for development of postoperative sepsis if bacteria are present in their bile at the time of operation.[22-26] In an experimental model of cholestasis in dogs, distal bile duct obstruction followed by biliary drainage resulted in infected bile. Subsequent construction of a biliary-digestive tract anastomosis was associated with an increase in the incidence of postoperative infective complications.[27]

We found 17 infectious complications in the 30 patients with positive findings of bile cultures. There was a correlation between organisms cultured from infectious complications and bile in 10 of these 17 patients. Comparisons of bacteria between those found in bile and in cultures from infectious complications have frequently indicated close similarity in the types of organisms isolated. In a prospective evaluation of 644 patients undergoing biliary tract surgery, Wells et al[25] found that organisms cultured from 27 wound infections correlated with organisms isolated from the bile in 17 (63%) of these patients. Others have shown a close correlation in bacteria between positive findings of postoperative blood cultures and bile culture data.[26]

Whereas mortality rates from curative resection of hilar cholangiocarcinoma have decreased significantly in the last several years, morbidity remains a significant problem.[5,7] Patterns of morbidity have not been well reported in this disease. Our analysis clearly indicates that infectious complications were the greatest source of postoperative morbidity. The use of preoperative biliary stents was associated with increased infectious complications in our series. Judicious use of biliary stents should be the rule in this disease, since prospective trials have not demonstrated their benefit, and since retrospective data document their potential harm. At present, an analysis of bile bacteria may help predict bacteria present in infectious complications after surgery for hilar cholangiocarcinoma. To help guide patient treatment, a knowledge of bile bacterial isolates may direct appropriate early antiobiotic therapy before results are available from cultures taken from infectious complications.

Presented at the 51st Annual Meeting of the Society of Surgical Oncology, San Diego, Calif, March 27, 1998.

Reprints: Leslie H. Blumgart, MD, Department of Surgery, 1275 York Ave, New York, NY 10021 (e-mail: blumgarl@mskcc.org).

REFERENCES

1. Longmire WP. Tumors of the extrahepatic biliary radicals. *Curr Probl Cancer.* 1976;1:1-45.
2. Kuwayti K, Baggenstoss AH, Stauffer MH, et al. Carcinoma of the major intrahepatic and the extrahepatic bile ducts exclusive of the papilla of Vater. *Surg Gynecol Obstet.* 1957;104:357-366.

3. Evander A, Fredlund P, Hoevels J, et al. Evaluation of aggressive surgery for carcinoma of the extrahepatic bile ducts. *Ann Surg.* 1980;191:23-29.
4. Cameron JL, Pitt HA, Zinner MJ, Kaufman SL, Coleman J. Management of proximal cholangiocarcinomas by surgical resection and radiotherapy. *Am J Surg.* 1990;159:91-98.
5. Bismuth H, Nakache R, Diamond T. Management strategies in resection for hilar cholangiocarcinoma. *Ann Surg.* 1992;215:31-38.
6. Fortner JG, Vitelli CE, Maclean BJ. Proximal extrahepatic bile duct tumors: analysis of a series of 52 consecutive patients treated over a period of 13 years. *Arch Surg.* 1989;124:1275-1279.
7. Pichlmayr R, Weimann A, Klempnauer J, et al. Surgical treatment in proximal bile duct cancer. *Ann Surg.* 1996;224:628-638.
8. Burke EC, Jarnigan WR, Hochwald SN, Pisters PWT, Fong Y, Blumgart LH. Hilar cholangiocarcinoma: patterns of spread, the importance of hepatic resection for curative operation, and a preoperative clinical staging system. *Ann Surg.* 1998; 228:385-394.
9. Pitt HA, Cameron JL, Postier RG, Gadacz TR. Factors affecting mortality in biliary tract surgery. *Am J Surg.* 1981;141:66-72.
10. Blamey SL, Fearon KCH, Gilmour WH, et al. Predictors of risk in biliary surgery. *Br J Surg.* 1983;70:535-539.
11. Dixon JM, Armstrong CP, Duffy SW, Davies GC. Factors affecting morbidity and mortality after surgery for obstructive jaundice: a review of 373 patients. *Gut.* 1983;24:845-852.
12. Hunt DR. The identification of risk factors and their application to the management of obstructive jaundice. *Aust N Z J Surg.* 1980;50:476-480.
13. Hatfield ARW, Terblanche J, Fataar S, et al. Preoperative external biliary drainage in obstructive jaundice. *Lancet.* 1982;2:896-899.
14. McPherson GAD, Benjamin IS, Hodgson HJF, Bowley NB, Allison DJ, Blumgart LH. Pre-operative percutaneous transhepatic biliary drainage: the results of a controlled trial. *Br J Surg.* 1984;71:371-375.
15. Pitt HA, Gomes AS, Lois JF, Mann LL, Deutsch LS, Longmire WP. Does preoperative percutaneous biliary drainage reduce operative risk or increase hospital cost? *Ann Surg.* 1985;201:545-553.
16. Lai EC, Mok FP, Fan ST, et al. Preoperative endoscopic drainage for malignant obstructive jaundice. *Br J Surg.* 1994;81:1195-1198.
17. Lygidakis NJ, van der Heyde MN, Lubbers MJ. Evaluation of preoperative biliary drainage in the surgical management of pancreatic head carcinoma. *Acta Chir Scand.* 1987;153:665-668.
18. Nilsson U, Evander A, Ihse I, Lunderquist A, Mocibob A. Percutaneous transhepatic cholangiography and drainage. *Acta Radiol.* 1983;24:433-439.
19. Keighley MRB, Lister DM, Jacobs SI, Giles GR. Hazards of surgical treatment due to microorganisms in the bile. *Surgery.* 1974;75:578-583.
20. Karsten TM, Allema JH, Reinders M, et al. Preoperative biliary drainage, colonisation of bile and postoperative complications in patients with tumors of the pancreatic head: a retrospective analysis of 241 consecutive patients. *Eur J Surg.* 1996;162:881-888.
21. Yu JL, Ljungh A. Infections associated with biliary drains. *Scand J Gastroenterol.* 1996;31:625-630.
22. Robson MC, Bogart JN, Heggers JP. An endogenous source for wound infections based on quantitative bacteriology of the biliary tract. *Surgery.* 1970;68:471-476.
23. Chetlin SH, Elliott DW. Biliary bacteremia. *Arch Surg.* 1971;102:303-307.
24. McPherson GAD, Benjamin IS, Habib NA, Bowley NB, Blumgart LH. Percutaneous transhepatic drainage in obstructive jaundice: advantages and problems. *Br J Surg.* 1982;69:261-264.
25. Wells GR, Taylor EW, Lindsay G, Morton L. Relationship between bile colonization, high-risk factors and postoperative sepsis in patients undergoing biliary tract operations while receiving a prophylactic antibiotic. *Br J Surg.* 1989;76:374-377.
26. Reiss R, Eliashiv A, Deutsch AA. Septic complications and bile cultures in 800 consecutive cholecystectomies. *World J Surg.* 1982;6:195-199.
27. Karsten TM, Davids PHP, Van Gulik TM, et al. Effects of biliary endoprosthesis on the extrahepatic bile ducts in relation to subsequent operation of the biliary tract. *J Am Coll Surg.* 1994;178:343-352.

Are Expandable Metallic Stents Better Than Conventional Methods for Treating Difficult Intrahepatic Biliary Strictures With Recurrent Hepatolithiasis?

Kuo-Shyang Jeng, MD; I-Shyan Sheen, MD; Fi-Sh Yang, MD

Background: Conventional methods for treating patients with recurrent hepatolithiasis associated with complicated intrahepatic biliary strictures include balloon dilatation of the intrahepatic biliary strictures, lithotripsy, and the clearance of difficult stones as completely as possible, with the placement of an external-internal stent for at least 6 months. After these modalities are used, symptomatic refractory strictures remain. Recently we used internal Gianturco-Rosch metallic Z stents to treat patients who had refractory strictures.

Objective: To compare therapeutic results and complications of an internal expandable metallic Z stent with those of repeated external-internal stent placement.

Study Design: Case-control study.

Setting: A referral center.

Patients: From January 1992 to December 1996, 18 patients with recurrent hepatolithiasis and complicated intrahepatic biliary strictures underwent percutaneous dilatation of stricture and transhepatic percutaneous cholangioscopic lithotomy for recurrent stones. After their stones were completely cleared, their biliary strictures failed to dilate satisfactorily. The patients were randomly enrolled into 2 groups: group A (7 patients), who received an expandable metallic Z stent, and group B (11 patients), who had repeated placement of external-internal stents.

Interventions: Percutaneous stricture dilatation, electrohydraulic lithotripsy, balloon dilatation, percutaneous transhepatic cholangioscopic lithotomy, and biliary stenting by a Silastic external-internal catheter or a modified Gianturco-Rosch expandable metallic Z stent (for an internal stent).

Main Outcome Measures: The number of procedures, days in hospital, procedure-related complications, incidents of stone recurrence and recurrence of cholangitis, readmissions to the hospital, treatment sessions required, and mortality rate. Patients' limitations in ordinary activities were also compared.

Results: The follow-up period ranged from 28 to 60 (40.7 ± 12.7 [mean ± SD]) months in group A and from 28 to 49 (36.0 ± 7.2) months in group B. Fewer group A patients (3 [43%]) than group B patients (8 [73%]) tended to have recurrent cholangitis and to require readmission to the hospital, but this was not statistically significant ($P = .33$). When their cumulative probability of a first episode of cholangitis during follow-up was compared, however, it was significantly lower in patients treated with a metallic stent ($P = .04$). Compared with group B patients, group A patients had less frequent recurrence of stones (0% vs 64%; $P = .01$), fewer procedures for the clearance of biliary stones or sludge (1.7 ± 2.2 vs 6.4 ± 4.3; $P = .03$), and shorter hospital stays (8.0 ± 11.5 days vs 17.0 ± 12.0 days; $P = .07$). No patients in group A experienced limitation in ordinary activities, whereas 7 patients in group B did ($P < .02$).

Conclusions: Compared with the repeated placement of external-internal stents, the use of a metallic internal stent effectively decreases stone recurrence, simplifies further procedures, and is more convenient. Its use is suggested as an alternative choice in the treatment of recurrent hepatolithiasis with refractory intrahepatic biliary strictures.

Arch Surg. 1999;134:267-273

From the Departments of Surgery (Dr Jeng) and Radiology (Dr Yang), Mackay Memorial Hospital, and the Liver Research Unit, Chang-Gung Memorial Hospital (Dr Sheen), Taipei, Taiwan.

HEPATOLITHIASIS IS a challenging problem for surgeons in Taiwan and other East Asian countries, where it is particularly prevalent.[1-8] The most difficult aspect of treatment is the association of hepatolithiasis with intrahepatic biliary stricture, which may limit the eradication of stones and pose a propensity for stones to recur.[1-16] Recurrent hepatolithiasis, which may be complicated by recurrent suppurative cholangitis, septicemia, and possible multiorgan failure, is a distinct disease. When repeated treatments fail to remove a stone completely or to eliminate the factors contributing to stone recurrence, severe acute cholangitis and

PATIENTS AND METHODS

One hundred fifteen patients were seen with recurrent hepatolithiasis from January 1989 to December 1996. Recurrent hepatolithiasis was defined as a history of having previous surgical or biliary procedures for hepatolithiasis and no residual stones found on computed tomographic scan or endoscopic retrograde cholangiography, percutaneous transhepatic cholangiography (PTC), or T-tube cholangiography at the end of the previous treatment. Patients with an incomplete study, treatment, or follow-up were not included. Those who had cholangiocarcinoma diagnosed during the treatment or follow-up period also were excluded. Among these 115 patients, 38 patients underwent repeated surgical intervention, and 77 patients underwent PSD and PTCSL. Twenty-five patients received external-internal stenting therapy after the complete clearance of recurrent stones. They were observed at an outpatient clinic and had follow-up PTC once a month. At the end of 6 or more months, a cholangiogram showed persistent strictures in 18 patients. All these patients had evidence of cholangitis, including intermittent episodes of right upper quadrant pain (n = 18), fever (n = 18), jaundice (n = 9), and leukocytosis (n = 12). They were admitted to the hospital for treatment and entered into this study. Follow-up cholangiography through the external-internal stent showed a persistent biliary stricture without stone recurrence. External drainage of infected bile by opening the external cap of the stent and parenteral antibiotic therapy for 1 week lessened the cholangitis. The patients were then randomly assigned to 2 treatment modalities. We planned to enroll 12 patients in each group in 5 years. At the end of 5 years, however, only 18 patients were eligible for this study.

Group A consisted of 7 patients (2 men and 5 women, ranging in age from 32-60 years) who received a modified Gianturco-Rosch expandable metallic wire Z stent (Wilson-Cook Medical Inc, Bloomington, Ind) for the internal stent. We introduced a Z stent into the intrahepatic stenotic bile duct in the following stepwise procedures. Under fluoroscopic guidance, an 8-mm balloon dilator catheter was first inserted into the dilated percutaneous bile duct (PTBD) tract. Then a 12F to 14F Teflon sheath with an introducing catheter inside was inserted. The stent was loaded over a guide wire, introduced into the sheath, and pushed to the end by a pusher. The marked end of the sheath was carefully positioned just distal to the stenotic lesion. The stent was deployed at the long stenotic segment by withdrawing the sheath while holding the stent in position with a pusher (**Figure 1**). A fiberoptic cholangioscope was then inserted through the PTBD tract to evaluate the location of the stent. If the stent is in place at the stenotic site, the wire skirts are usually clearly seen (Figure 1), and the result is regarded as satisfactory. Oral antibiotics were given for 3 days. The external drainage tube was then removed.

Group B consisted of 11 patients (3 men and 8 women, ranging in age from 35-73 years) who had continued external-internal stenting for 6 months more with a Yokohama cholangioscopic catheter (a Cliny Silastic cholangioenterography tube biliary stent with an 8F to 12F catheter [Create Medic, Yokohama, Japan]) introduced by the percutaneous transhepatic route under fluoroscopy. The tip of the stent extended over the stenotic duct, and the external part was closed by a cap. Oral antibiotics were given for 3 days after the stent exchange, and the patient was then discharged from the hospital.

After treatment, patients of both groups were observed monthly at Mackay Memorial Hospital, Taipei, Taiwan, for any symptoms and signs of cholangitis. Liver function tests and abdominal ultrasonography were performed every 3 to 4 months during the first 3 years and every 6 months thereafter. An upper abdominal computed tomographic scan was obtained every 6 months to detect the recurrence of stones. In addition, group A patients had plain abdominal radiography every 3 months to check the location and any migration of the stent (**Figure 2**). Group B patients had follow-up PTC every month to detect occlusion or migration of the stent, and the stent catheter was replaced with a new one.

The sex and age proportions and the number of previous biliary operations and previous biliary dilatation therapy, admissions to the hospital, and in-hospital days of the 2 groups were compared. During follow-up, a patient was admitted to the hospital when there was possible recurrent cholangitis (as evidenced by fever, chills, right upper abdominal pain, or jaundice) and received PTCSL to remove stones or sludge through a PTBD tract. Differentiating between calculi and soft sludge in the stenotic duct on ultrasonography and computed tomographic scan is sometimes difficult. The extracted or drained material was carefully analyzed to differentiate between stones and sludge. During readmissions to the hospital, evidence of septicemia, bacteremia (positive results from blood cultures), or cholangitis (positive results from bile cultures) in each patient was recorded. Complications and the 1-month postprocedure mortality rate due to the entry treatments; the recurrence rate of stones, sludge, and cholangitis; the number and length of further hospital admissions; and the number of repeated biliary procedures were compared. Questionnaires about the degree of pain, the level of satisfaction, and limitations in ordinary activities were sent to both groups of patients at the end of the first 6 months of treatment. Their answers were evaluated and compared.

The Mann-Whitney *U* test, Student *t* test, Fisher exact test, Kaplan-Meier method, and log-rank test were used for statistical analyses.

sepsis will supervene. In addition, recurrent infections may lead to other sequelae such as liver abscess, biliary cirrhosis with portal hypertension, bleeding varices, hepatic failure, and cholangiocarcinoma.[6,9,17-25]

In Taiwan, surgeons have had extensive experience in the treatment of intrahepatic biliary strictures because as many as 85% patients with hepatolithiasis have biliary strictures.[1-7] We have adopted a systematic approach to manage these patients. Recurrent hepatolithiasis is difficult to treat because extensive adhesions, the distortion of the normal anatomy, and scarring of the choledochus due to previous operations make repeated surgical procedures difficult. Patients who have had 1 or more biliary operations or procedures may decline to have more operations. Furthermore, poor liver reserve from prolonged disease and repeated cholangitis may increase the risks of general anesthesia and a major operation. Therefore, we initiated a new policy to treat patients with re-

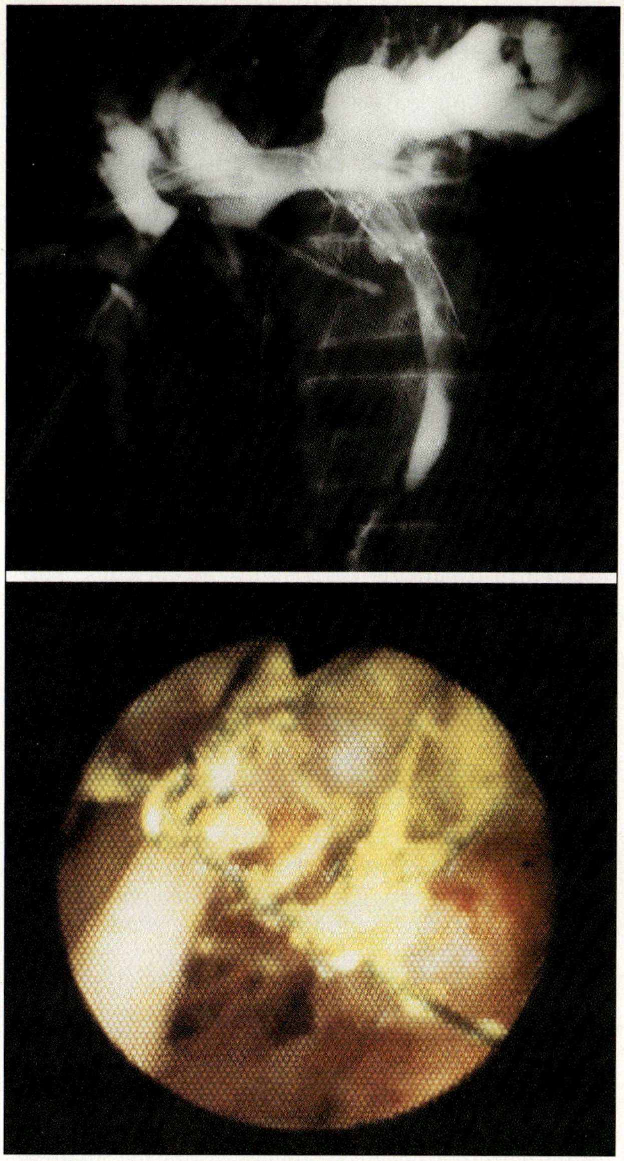

Figure 1. *Top, A metallic Z stent placed by the transhepatic percutaneous route to a long-segment stricture in the right intrahepatic duct. Bottom, Cholangioscopy showing the stent with wire skirts in proper position.*

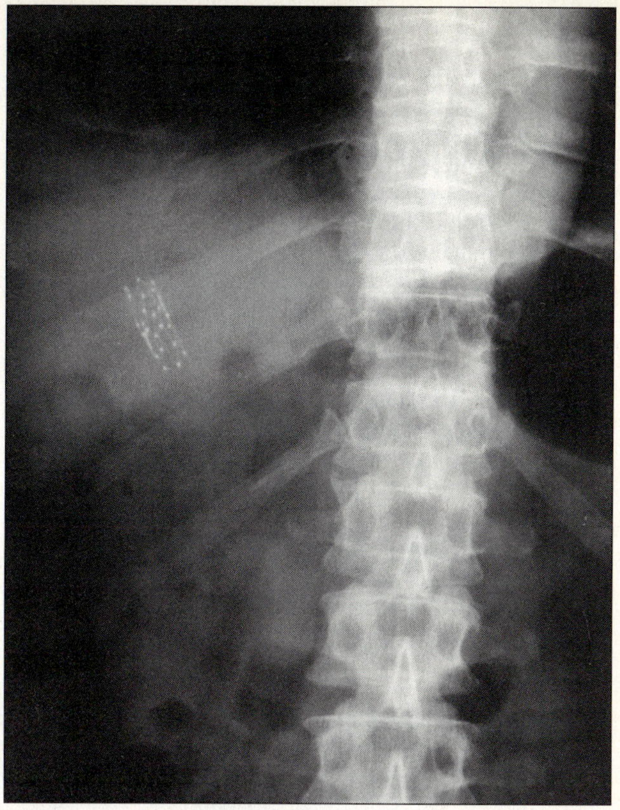

Figure 2. *The stent seen on plain abdominal radiograph.*

current hepatolithiasis and biliary strictures.[1-5] With percutaneous transhepatic manipulations, including percutaneous stricture dilatation (PSD) and subsequent percutaneous transhepatic cholangioscopic lithotomy (PTCSL),[26-30] major surgical procedures are usually avoided. After balloon dilatation therapy for the strictures and repeated clearance of the stones, biliary stenting therapy is necessary for some patients with difficult strictures to maintain the ductal lumen at a minimum diameter because of the high potential for stricture recurrence.[1-5] Following 6 months of stenting, a challenging problem arises when the stenotic duct fails to improve.

Self-expandable metallic stents are being used increasingly in the treatment of both benign and malignant strictures.[31-41] These metallic stents capably improve our treatment of strictures in nearly all realms, such as vascular, tracheobronchial, urogenital, gastrointestinal, pancreatic, and biliary areas. In general, their use is not advisable in patients with benign conditions unless they fail to respond to other treatments. In the past 10 years, most benign biliary disorders in which metallic stents were used have been common bile (or hepatic) ductal strictures from previous operations or chronic pancreatitis. Since 1992, we have incorporated 2 options for the further treatment of these complicated cases. One is to continue using the external-internal stenting for a further 6 months. The other is to place an internal metallic stent. To our knowledge, metallic stents for benign biliary strictures in hepatolithiasis have not been applied in a large number of patients or discussed in detail.[1,2,4,42] The aim of this study was to evaluate this new treatment and to compare its use with that of conventional stenting.

RESULTS

Shortly after entry, patients in both groups were retreated successfully with stricture dilatation therapy through the PTBD tract and repeated sessions of stone extraction by PTCSL. Then either a metallic stent or an internal-external stent was placed. The procedure was successful in all 18 patients, and no 1-month fatality occurred in either group. Patients in both groups had similar baseline conditions (**Table 1**). The site of difficult biliary stricture was mainly on the right side because most left-sided strictures had been resected according to our strategy. One patient who had a difficult stricture at the common hepatic duct with extension to the right hepatic bile duct was entered in group A for the placement of a Z stent.

In group A, 7 patients have had Z internal stenting for 28 to 60 (40.7 ± 12.7 [mean ± SD]) months. During follow-up, 3 patients (43%) needed readmission to the hospital because of acute cholangitis (**Table 2**). One patient was a 58-year-old woman whose Z stent was placed between the proximal common hepatic duct and the right hepatic duct. A recurrence of cholangitis was found at the end of 6 months. She underwent the reestablishment of a PTBD. Percutaneous transhepatic cholangiography showed sludge in multiple radicles of the right intrahepatic bile ducts. Parenteral antibiotic therapy for 7 days and 4 sessions of PTCSL eradicated all the sludge. The sludge was soft, muddy, and easily removed by cholangioscopic basket catheter extraction with irrigation with an isotonic sodium chloride solution. All symptoms and signs of cholangitis subsided after treatment, she was discharged from the hospital, and has been symptom free.

A 35-year-old man with a stent in the right intrahepatic duct had been unavailable for follow-up for 12 months. Jaundice and acute cholangitis recurred 30 months after Z stent placement, and the patient was readmitted to the hospital. We quickly reestablished his PTBD. Sludge was unexpectedly found in the lumen of the stent (**Figure 3**). Four sessions of PTCSL with irrigation with isotonic sodium chloride solution led to satisfactory results, and he was discharged 30 days later.

The third patient was a 57-year-old woman in whom acute cholangitis developed 7 months following Z stent placement. A PTBD was set up, and sludge without definite stones was found. The sludge was cleared after 2 sessions of PTCSL within 10 days. No migration or occlusion of stents was observed during follow-up. No clinical evidence of recurrent cholangitis or stones has been found during further follow-up.

In group B patients, who had external-internal stenting, 3 (27%) of 11 patients had stent dislodgement (**Table 3**). One patient experienced dislodgement of the stent 5 times in 3 months while the other 2 had only 1 dislodgement. We quickly reinserted the stent into the correct position under fluoroscopic guidance. During follow-up (28-49 [36.0 ± 7.2] months), recurrent cholangitis developed in 8 patients (73%) with 14 episodes. Those incidents of cholangitis did not occur within 7 days after PTC, however. Patients with cholangitis were all admitted to the hospital and had redilatation of the PTBD tract, along with Sumitomo catheter decompression, the drainage of purulent bile, and parenteral antibiotic therapy. Stones in 7 patients and sludge in 1 patient were suggested by computed tomographic scans and PTC. These 8 patients had PTCSL, and all recurrent stones or sludge were cleared completely. Afterward, 3 patients refused to have repeated external-internal stents. All of them had recurrent cholangitis during follow-up. The other 5 patients continued with Sumitomo catheter retention for a further 6 months. The stents were then removed, and the ductal stricture abated. They have been observed in the outpatient clinic, and 3 of these 5 patients had recurrent cholangitis.

Group A patients tended to have fewer episodes of recurrent cholangitis and readmission to the hospital than group B patients, but this was not statistically significant (**Table 4**). When their cumulative probability of having a first episode of cholangitis during follow-up was compared, it was lower in patients treated with a metallic stent ($P = .04$) (**Figure 4**). In group A patients, stones

Table 1. Demographic Data of Patients Receiving a Metallic Internal Stent or Repeated External-Internal Stenting*

Demographics	Group A (n=7)	Group B (n=11)
Median age, y	54	56
Sex, M/F	2:5	3:8
Site of stricture		
Right intrahepatic duct	4	8
Left intrahepatic duct	2	3
Common hepatic duct	1	0
History, No. (median)		
Previous biliary operations	1 to 3 (2)	1 to 4 (2)
Previous biliary dilatations	1 to 3 (2)	0 to 4 (2)
Previous hospitalizations	3 to 5 (3)	2 to 6 (2)
Previous days in hospital	79 to 180 (110)	70 to 201 (112)
Patients with evidence of septicemia, bacteremia, or cholangitis, No. (%)	7 (100)	11 (100)

**No statistically significant difference between the groups.*

Table 2. Group A Patients Before and After Metallic Stenting

Before Entry						After Metallic Stent		
						Cholangitis		
Operations, No.	Dilatations, No.	Hospital Admissions, No.	External-Internal Stent, mo	Metallic Stent Site*	Follow-up, mo†	Time Lapse, mo‡	Patients, No.	Sludge/Stones§
3	2	3	9	Rt	60	0	0	–/–
2	3	3	12	Rt	52	30	1	+/–
1	2	2	6	Lt	48	0	0	–/–
2	3	5	6	Rt	38	0	0	–/–
1	1	3	6	Lt	30	0	0	–/–
1	2	4	12	Rt	29	7	1	+/–
2	3	4	6	CHD	28	6	1	+/–

**Rt indicates right intrahepatic duct; Lt, left intrahepatic duct; and CHD, common hepatic duct.*
†The metallic stenting is continuing.
‡Time to the first attack of cholangitis after entry in the study.
§Minus sign indicates absent; plus sign, present.

recurred less frequently ($P = .01$), fewer procedures for the clearance of biliary stones or sludge were needed ($P = .03$), and the hospital stays were shorter ($P = .07$). According to the answers on the questionnaire, no group A patients experienced limitation in ordinary activities, but 7 group B patients did ($P < .02$). Of note, no cholangiocarcinoma has been found in these 18 patients.

COMMENT

Our results showed that cholangitis and stones recurred less frequently in patients treated with metallic stents, and they were managed more easily in at least a 2-year follow-up.

An internal stent is more convenient to use than an external-internal stent. Seven (64%) of our group B patients felt that the external-internal stent limited their working and ordinary activities for fear of dislodgement. Psychological burdens persisted until the stent was removed. Those with an internal metallic stent all returned to work and did well. In addition, various complications from the long-term use of external-internal stents, such as bile leakage; inflammation or infection of the skin around the tube; cholangitis; hemobilia; intrahepatic liver abscess; and clogging, dislodgement, or migration of the stent, are well known. A better opportunity for sludge deposition and bacterial adherence on its surface possibly results from the wall of the Yokohama stent, and its Silastic material is not as inert as the metallic material. For patients with external-internal stents, it is necessary to perform follow-up cholangiography to accurately determine the position of the internal part of the stent and to replace it with a new tube every month to prevent tube occlusion with thick bile or sludge. In contrast, no stent replacement is necessary for metallic stents, and PTC is indicated only if cholangitis recurs.

Metallic stents[13-25] are composed of a thin stainless-steel wire that has been shaped into either a mesh tube (Wallstent) or zigzag bands with the ends soldered to form a cylinder (Z stent). After release from a relatively small catheter (8F-12F), they assume their final shape and achieve a large internal lumen by constant outward radial force. A skilled surgeon can place the stent easily, which minimizes discomfort and inconvenience for the patient. This Z stent has wire skirts without a true stent wall. The small surface area of the metallic stents might decrease the likelihood of bacteria adherence and other secondary depositions on its wall, which possibly decreases the risk of cholangitis. The low occlusion rate from the large lumen and low likelihood of debris deposition further decrease the risk of sepsis.

In the literature, some major (8%) postprocedural complications have been reported, such as biliary pleuritis, peritonitis, hepatic artery aneurysm, intrahepatic artery bleeding, right subphrenic abscess, and sepsis. No procedure-related deaths occurred. In our series, no pro-

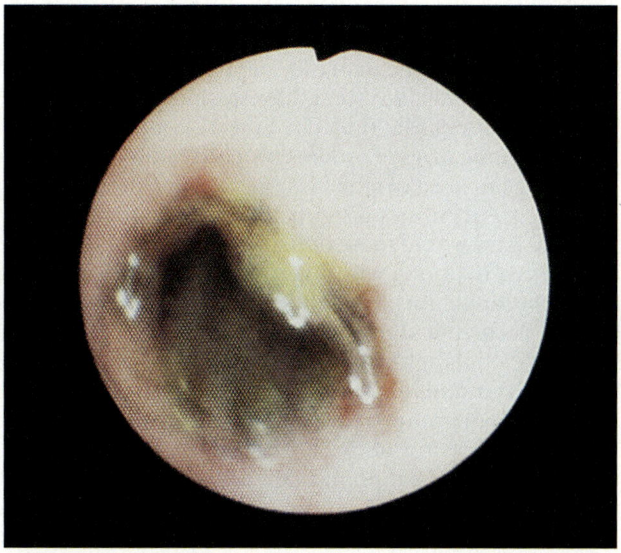

Figure 3. *Sludges noted in the metallic Z stent by cholangioscopy through the percutaneous bile duct route.*

Table 3. Group B Patients Before and After 6 Months of External-Internal Metallic Stenting

Before Entry				Continuing External-Internal Stenting				
						Cholangitis		
Operations, No.	Dilatations, No.	Hospital Admissions, No.	External-Internal Stent, mo	Site*	Follow-up, mo†	Time Lapse, mo‡	Patients, No.	Sludge/Stones§
2	3	3	6	Rt	31	4	2	+/−
2	1	2	8	Rt	33	3	2	−/+
3	2	4	8	Lt	35	0	0	−/−
1	1	2	6	Rt	37	6	1	−/+
2	1	2	6	Rt	29	4	2	−/+
1	1	2	7	Lt	30	0	0	−/−
2	0	2	6	Rt	49	4	2	−/+
2	2	3	9	Rt	45	3	2	−/+
1	2	2	10	Rt	34	5	1	−/+
4	4	6	6	Lt	28	0	0	−/−
1	2	2	6	Rt	45	5	2	−/+

*Rt indicates right intrahepatic bile duct; Lt, left intrahepatic bile duct.
†The 6 months of external-internal stenting was included in the total period of follow-up.
‡Time to the first attack of cholangitis after entry in the study.
§Plus sign indicates present; minus sign, absent.

Table 4. Outcome of the 2 Groups After Entry in the Study*

Outcome	Group A (n=7)	Group B (n=11)	P
Treatment morbidity	0	3 (27)	.24
Recurrence of cholangitis	3 (43)	8 (73)	.33
Sludge	3 (43)	1 (9)	.24
Stone	0	7 (64)	.01
Further hospitalization	3 (43)	8 (73)	.33
Hospital days, mean ± SD	8.0 ± 11.5	17.0 ± 12.0	.07
Percutaneous procedures (sessions), mean ± SD	1.7 ± 2.2	6.4 ± 4.3	.03
Limitations of ordinary activity	0	7 (64)	.01

Except where noted, data are given as number (percentage) of patients.

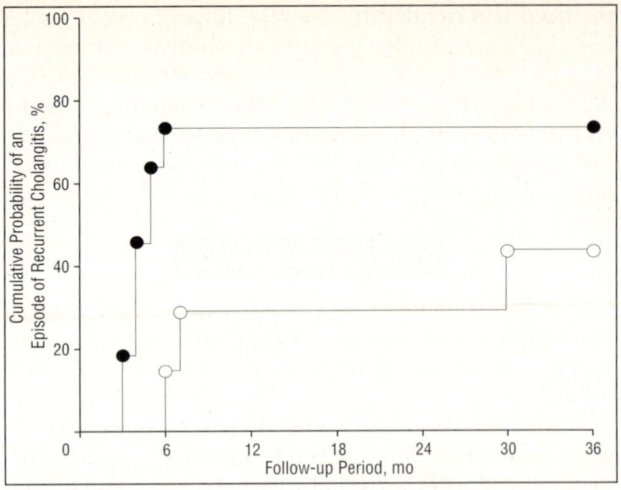

Figure 4. *Cumulative probability of a first episode of recurrent cholangitis (P = .04).*

cedure-related complications were encountered. The long-term effects of metallic stents on the biliary wall are still unclear. Relatively mild reactive inflammatory changes observed in the wall of the bile ducts suggest that they could be used safely to relieve biliary obstruction.[41] Epithelialization over the filament follows the firm anchorage of the stent to the ductal wall. Using at distal common bile duct stricture caused by chronic pancreatitis, a 90% patency rate at 3 years was observed. Only 2 incidents of occlusion occurred 1 month after the placement from excessive epithelial hyperplasia of bile duct mucosa.[36] Of note, the occurrence of occlusion did not increase with longer follow-up. In patients with pyogenic cholangitis, however, Yoon et al[42] reported only 62% and 27% patency rates for intrahepatic ducts and extrahepatic ducts, respectively, at 3 years. The most common causes of stent occlusion were recurrent stone or sludge and epithelial hyperplasia. They suggested that metallic stent is not an effective long-term treatment of benign biliary stricture associated with recurrent pyogenic cholangitis.

The criteria of our patients selected for metallic stents was stricter than those of Yoon et al. They all had failure of a previous dilating-stenting therapy. Four (57%) of our patients had good function of their metallic stents at 5 years , a rate that is similar to that noted by Yoon et al, and the cause of cholangitis was the presence of sludge in 2 patients and stones in 1 patient. Only 3 patients (27%) with external-internal stents had good function at 3 years, however, and the cause of cholangitis was sludge in 1 patient and stones in 7 patients. Although a metallic stent cannot keep an excellent long-term patency, the external-internal stent gave a worse result. Furthermore, it is easier to clear sludge than to clear stones.

Our series showed substantially higher stone recurrence in the group with external-internal stents, but the rate of recurrent stone and sludge did not reach a significant difference compared with that in the group with metallic stents. Interestingly, sludge was more likely to recur than stone in the group with a metallic stent, in contrast to more stone than sludge recurring in the group with external-internal stents. Biliary sludge is bile in a gel form that contains numerous crystals of calcium bilirubinate, cholesterol, and glycoproteins. Its presence implies that the nucleation of bile solute has occurred, and concrete stones may develop later.[43,44] A bigger dilated lumen, inert metallic material, and the small contact surface area of a metallic stent allow a smoother and more constant flow of bile than does the Yokohama stent. So the lithogenic disease process proceeds slowly, and biliary sludge instead of stone is observed in patients with a metallic stent. Stones differ from sludge in that they are formed, harder, and more difficult to remove. The muddy sludge easily drains with bile flow after PTBD and isotonic sodium chloride irrigation with PTCSL. Similar to stones, recurrent sludge may retard bile flow and result in severe cholangitis or even septicemia. Substantially fewer percutaneous procedures were needed to treat cholangitis in group A patients than in group B patients, which supports the above observations.

Two additional points should be addressed. In the literature, 10% to 15% of patients with recurrent pyogenic cholangitis have cholangiocarcinoma. None of the patients in this study have been found to have cholangiocarcinoma. This might be due to the small number of patients and because patients with malignant lesions were excluded from the study. Group B patients had PTC every month to detect occlusion or migration of the stent, and the stent catheter was replaced with a new one. We did not consider that the cholangitis in group B was partly due to contamination of the biliary system from PTC and stent replacement because cholangitis did not occur within 1 week after the procedures. We could not definitely exclude their minor contribution to the occurrence of cholangitis, however. As to the causes of recurrent hepatolithiasis, to our knowledge, no correlation of PTC and stone formation has been found. Although PTC did not appear to be associated with more cholangitis and stone recurrence in group B patients, a decreased need for invasive procedures in group A patients (with metallic stents) is a remarkable benefit.

The firm anchorage of metallic stents to the bile duct wall and epithelialization over the mesh make stent migration almost impossible, but little chance of endoscopic removal make the use of metallic stents in patients with benign disorders debatable. Their use in refractory benign diseases, however, is increasing. Recently, Gorich et al[40] reported that they successfully extracted displaced metallic stents transhepatically with no complications. This challenges the previous concept of removal only by resection.

From this preliminary controlled study, the use of an expandable metallic internal stent in the management of intrahepatic biliary strictures cannot completely avoid the possibility of the recurrence of biliary sludge, stone, and cholangitis. It can effectively decrease the recurrence of cholangitis and stones, simplify further necessary treatment, and result in less limitation of ordinary activities. Therefore, its use is suggested as an alternative for the treatment of refractory recurrent hepatolithiasis with difficult strictures.

Reprints: Kuo-Shyang Jeng, MD, Department of Surgery, Mackay Memorial Hospital, No. 92, Section 2, Chung-Shan North Road, Taipei, Taiwan, Republic of China.

REFERENCES

1. Jeng KS, Ohta I, Yang FS. Reappraisal of the systematic management of complicated hepatolithiasis with bilateral intrahepatic biliary strictures. *Arch Surg.* 1996;131:141-147.
2. Jeng KS. Treatment of intrahepatic biliary stricture associated with hepatolithiasis. *Hepatogastroenterology.* 1997;44:342-351.
3. Jeng KS, Ohta I, Yang FS, et al. Coexisting sharp ductal angulation with intrahepatic biliary strictures in right hepatolithiasis. *Arch Surg.* 1994;129:1097-1102.
4. Jeng KS, Yang FS, Chiang HJ, Ohta I. Bile duct stents in the management of hepatolithiasis with long-segment intrahepatic biliary strictures. *Br J Surg.* 1992;79:663-666.
5. Jeng KS, Yang FS, Ohta I, Chiang HJ. Dilatation of intrahepatic biliary strictures in patients with hepatolithiasis. *World J Surg.* 1990;14:587-593.
6. Jeng KS, Shih SC, Chiang HJ, Chen BF. Secondary biliary cirrhosis: a limiting factor in the treatment of hepatolithiasis. *Arch Surg.* 1989;124:1301-1305.
7. Jeng KS, Chiang HJ, Shih SC. Limitations of percutaneous transhepatic cholangioscopy in the removal of complicated biliary calculi. *World J Surg.* 1989;13:603-610.
8. Nakayama F, Soloway RD, Nakama T, et al. Hepatolithiasis in East Asia: a retrospective study. *Dig Dis Sci.* 1986;31:21-26.
9. Fan ST, Wong J. Complications of hepatolithiasis. *J Gastroenterol Hepatol.* 1992;7:324-327.
10. Fan ST, Choi TK, Le CM, Mok FPT, Lai ECS, Wong J. Treatment of hepatolithiasis: improvement of result by a systemic approach. *Surgery.* 1991;109:474-480.
11. Nakayama F, Koga A. Hepatolithiasis: present status. *World J Surg.* 1984;8:9-14.
12. Nakayama F. Hepatolithiasis: an update. *J Gastroenterol Hepatol.* 1988;3:279-285.
13. Fan ST, Lai ECS, Wong J. Hepatic resection for hepatolithiasis. *Arch Surg.* 1993;128:1070-1074.
14. Choi TK, Wong J, Ong GB. The surgical management of primary intrahepatic stones. *Br J Surg.* 1982;69:86-90.
15. Koga A, Miyazaki K, Ichimiya H, Nakayama F. Choice of treatment for hepatolithiasis based on pathological findings. *World J Surg.* 1984;8:36-40.
16. Matsumoto Y, Fujii H, Yoshioka M, et al. Biliary strictures as a cause of primary intrahepatic bile duct stones. *World J Surg.* 1986;10:867-875.
17. Ohta T, Nagakawa T, Konishi I, et al. Clinical experience of intrahepatic cholangiocarcinoma associated with hepatolithiasis. *Jpn J Surg.* 1988;18:47-53.
18. Chen MF, Jan YY, Wang CS, Jeng LB, Hwang TL, Chen SC. Intrahepatic stones associated with cholangiocarcinoma. *Am J Gastroenterol.* 1989;84:391-395.
19. Rossi RL, Silverman ML, Braasch JW, Munson JL, Remine SG. Carcinomas arising in cystic conditions of the bile ducts: a clinical and pathologic study. *Ann Surg.* 1987;205:377-384.
20. Nakanuma Y, Terada T, Tanaka Y, Ohta G. Are hepatolithiasis and cholangiocarcinoma aetiologically related? *Virchows Arch.* 1985;405:45-48.
21. Chen HH, Zhang WH, Wang SS, Caruana JA. Twenty-two year experience with the diagnosis and treatment of intrahepatic calculi. *Surg Gynecol Obstet.* 1984;159:519-524.
22. Akiyama T, Nagakawa T, Kayahara M, et al. Recurrence of intrahepatic stones after an end-to-side choledochojejunostomy. *Surg Today.* 1994;24:599-605.
23. Takeda T, Yasuda H, Uchiyama K, Hasegawa H, Shikata J, Kuniyasu Y. The relationship between a subcutaneously placed afferent jejunal loop in a hepaticojejunostomy and postoperative cholangitis. *Int Surg.* 1989;74:167-170.
24. Fan ST, Mok F, Zheng SS, Lai ECS, Lo CM, Wong J. Appraisal of hepaticocutaneous jejunostomy in the management of hepatolithiasis. *Am J Surg.* 1993;165:332-335.
25. Fan ST, Lai ECS, Mok FPT, Choi TK, Wong J. Acute cholangitis secondary to hepatolithiasis. *Arch Surg.* 1991;126:1027-1031.
26. Burhenne HJ. Garland lecture: percutaneous extraction of retained biliary tract stones: 661 patients. *AJR Am J Roentgenol.* 1980;134:889-898.
27. Park JH, Choi BI, Han MC, Sung KB, Choo IW, Kim CW. Percutaneous removal of residual intrahepatic stones. *Radiology.* 1987;163:619-623.
28. Mueller PR, van Sonnenberg E, Ferrucci JT Jr, et al. Biliary stricture dilatation: multicenter review of clinical management in 73 patients. *Radiology.* 1986;160:17-22.
29. Little JM, Wong KP, Simmons K. Percutaneous transhepatic dilatation in the management of bile duct strictures. *Aust N Z J Surg.* 1986;56:697-700.
30. Casarella WJ. Percutaneous transhepatic dilatation of intrahepatic biliary strictures. *AJR Am J Roentgenol.* 1980;135:837-840.
31. Ferro C, Perona F, Ambrogi C, Barile A, Cianni R. Malignant biliary obstruction treated by Wallstents and Strecker tantalum stents: a retrospective review. *Cardiovasc Intervent Radiol.* 1995;18:25-29.
32. Rieber A, Brambs HJ. Metallic stents in malignant biliary obstruction. *Cardiovasc Intervent Radiol.* 1997;20:43-49.
33. Hausegger KA, Mischinger HJ, Karaic R, et al. Percutaneous cholangioscopy in obstructed biliary metal stents. *Cardiovasc Intervent Radiol.* 1997;20:191-196.
34. Barrioz T, Ingrand P, Besson I, de Ledinghen V, Silvain C, Beauchant M. Randomised trial of prevention of biliary stent occlusion by ursodeoxycholic acid plus norfloxacin. *Lancet.* 1994;344:581-582.
35. Bonnel DH, Liguory CL, Lefebvre JF, Cornud FE. Placement of metallic stents for treatment of postoperative biliary strictures: long-term outcome in 25 patients. *AJR Am J Roentgenol.* 1997;169:1517-1522.
36. Deviere J, Cremer M, Baize M, Love J, Sugai B, Vandermeeren A. Management of common bile duct stricture caused by chronic pancreatitis with metal mesh self expandable stents. *Gut.* 1994;35:122-126.
37. Smits ME, Rauws EAJ, van Gulik TM, Gouma DJ, Tytgat GNJ, Huibregtse K. Long-term results of endoscopic stenting and surgical drainage for biliary stricture due to chronic pancreatitis. *Br J Surg.* 1996;83:764-768.
38. Seibert DG. Biliary stricture measurement and stent selection. *Am J Gastroenterol.* 1997;92:1510-1514.
39. Esterl RM Jr, St Laurent M, Bay MK, Speeg KV, Halff GA. Endoscopic biliary stent migration with small bowel perforation in a liver transplant recipient. *J Clin Gastroenterol.* 1997;24:106-110.
40. Gorich J, Rilinger N, Kramer S, et al. Displaced metallic biliary stents: technique and rationale for interventional radiologic retrieval. *AJR Am J Roentgenol.* 1997;169:1529-1533.
41. Alvarado R, Palmaz JC, Garcia OJ, Tio FO, Rees CR. Evaluation of polymer-coated balloon-expandable stents in bile ducts. *Radiology.* 1989;170:975-978.
42. Yoon HK, Sung KB, Song HY, et al. Benign biliary strictures associated with recurrent pyogenic cholangitis: treatment with expandable metallic stents. *AJR Am J Roentgenol.* 1997;169:1523-1527.
43. Lee SP, Maher K, Nicholls J. Origin and fate of biliary sludge. *Gastroenterology.* 1988;94:170-176.
44. Carey MC, Cahalane MJ. Whither biliary sludge? *Gastroenterology.* 1988;95:508-523.

Insulin's Anabolic Effect Is Influenced by Route of Administration of Nutrients

Ronald H. Clements, MD; Clint A. Hayes, MD; E. Rickey Gibbs, MD; John Geiger; Henry L. Laws, MD; Calvin L. Long, PhD

Objective: To determine if the anabolic effects of intravenous insulin on protein kinetics could be exploited in the enterally fed trauma victim.

Design: Randomized, crossover control protocol.

Setting: Level I trauma center.

Patients: Ten trauma patients with an Injury Severity Score higher than 20. Exclusion criteria included diabetes mellitus, pregnancy, steroid use, and aged younger than 18 years or older than 65 years.

Interventions: Within the first 24 hours of admission to the intensive care unit, each patient had a transpyloric feeding tube inserted radiographically. Enteral nutrition was provided with a protein supplement (Ensure, Ross Laboratories, Columbus, Ohio) and Promod, supplemented with protein powder to supply 1.5 g/kg per day of protein and 156.9 kJ/kg per day. Intravenous insulin was provided at 0.043 U/kg per hour beginning on the second or fourth day.

Main Outcome Measures: Urinary nitrogen balance and 3-methylhistidine excretion rates were measured at the end of the third and fifth days. Plasma glucose, insulin, and C-peptide levels were obtained at these same times.

Results: Urinary nitrogen balance was not significantly different with or without the administration of insulin (−4.58 ± 50.1 mg/kg per day vs −9.38 ± 50.9 mg/kg per day, respectively). 3-Methylhistidine excretion rates did not change significantly with or without the administration of insulin (5.77 ± 0.67 µmol/kg per day vs 6.15 ± 0.43 µmol/kg per day, respectively). Serum insulin levels did not differ significantly when exogenous infusions were added (57.8 ± 17.9 µU/mL vs 82.1 ± 44.9 µU/mL), but serum C-peptide levels did decrease significantly when exogenous insulin was added (5.11 ± 3.2 µU/mL vs 10.28 ± 3.5 µU/mL; $P = .04$). Serum glucose levels decreased significantly when insulin was administered (5.8 ± 0.4 mmol/L [104.6 ± 7.2 mg/dL] vs 7.7 ± 0.4 mmol/L [138.1 ± 7.4 mg/dL]; $P = .004$).

Conclusion: The anabolic effect of intravenous insulin on protein kinetics is not evident when nutrition is provided enterally in the trauma victim.

Arch Surg. 1999;134:274-277

EARLY NUTRITIONAL support is an integral part of the care of the acutely injured patient. Enteral feeding is the preferred method of providing nutrition to the victims of major trauma because it maintains the integrity of the gut mucosal barrier by directly providing the enterocyte with necessary nutrients. Equally important, early nutritional support provides the necessary components for wound healing and for ameliorating muscle wasting during convalescence. Providing more protein to the catabolic patient to attain a more favorable nitrogen balance has its advantages. However, there should be concern as to the effect of high protein intake on renal function. Therefore, until the body becomes more efficient in the retention of protein during the convalescent period, the use of anabolic hormones should be contemplated to stimulate nitrogen assimilation.

Insulin has been shown to increase skeletal muscle protein synthesis and to decrease it degradation in numerous in vitro and in vivo studies when amino acids are provided intravenously,[1-3] but to our knowledge, no studies have been published regarding its effect when nutrition is provided enterally. Using human skeletal muscle in vitro, Lundholm and Schers[4] demonstrated a decrease in protein degradation and an increase in protein synthesis. Human in vivo studies across a muscle bed have produced conflicting re-

From the Departments of Surgery, Carraway Methodist Medical Center and the Norwood Clinic Inc, Birmingham, Ala.

sults[5-8] Fukagawa et al[9] showed a reduction in proteolysis when studying insulin's effect on whole-body protein kinetics. We have previously demonstrated a reduction in myofibrillar protein breakdown and an increase in protein synthesis leading to positive nitrogen balance as a result of infusing insulin and total parenteral nutrition (TPN) in the trauma victim.[10] To date we are not aware of any reported studies of the effect of insulin on protein synthesis and breakdown from nutrients provided by the preferred enteral route in the trauma victim. Knowing insulin's anabolic effect, and to determine if the benefit of enteral nutrition and hormonal manipulation with insulin could be combined, we investigated the effect of intravenous insulin on nitrogen balance and muscle protein breakdown in the enterally fed trauma victim.

PATIENTS, MATERIALS, AND METHODS

After obtaining informed consent, 10 victims of blunt trauma were enrolled in this randomized, crossover controlled protocol that had been approved by our institutional review board. Patients aged 18 to 65 years were eligible, and diabetes mellitus, pregnancy, steroid administration, or an Injury Severity Score (ISS) of less than 20 were exclusion criteria. Each patient underwent standard evaluation and treatment at our level I trauma center and was admitted to the intensive care unit (ICU). Within 24 hours of admission to the ICU, each patient was administered enteral nutrition through a radiographically placed transpyloric feeding tube. Nutrition consisted of Ensure (Ross Laboratories, Columbus, Ohio) supplemented with Promod protein powder (Ross Labortories) to provide 1.5 g/kg per day of protein and 156.9 kJ/kg per day. After 1 day of incrementally increasing the rate to the desired level, each patient was maintained at this rate for 4 additional days. Beginning on either the second or fourth day of the protocol, each patient was given intravenous regular insulin at 0.043 U/kg per hour. After 48 hours of insulin infusion, the patient was crossed over into the other limb of the protocol, either to receive insulin or to discontinue its use.

Twenty-four–hour urine collections from the third and fifth days of the protocol were analyzed for total urinary nitrogen levels using a nitrogen analyzer (Antek Nitrogen Analyzer; Antek, Houston, Tex) and for 3-methylhistidine (3-MH) excretion using an amino acid analyzer (Beckman Automatic Amino Acid Analyzer; Beckman Instruments, Palo Alto, Calif). Serum samples were analyzed for glucose using the glucose oxidase method, and serum insulin and C-peptide levels were determined by Labcorp (Birmingham, Ala) after each 48-hour study period. Results were analyzed using the paired Student *t* test and are expressed as mean ± SEM. Significance was determined at $P = .05$.

RESULTS

The demographics and injuries of the 10 patients in this study are given in the **Table**. There were 6 male and 4 female patients, with an average age of 31.4 years (age range, 21-64 years). The mean ISS was 33.3 (range, 27-50). The mean weight of this group was 73.0 kg (range, 61-103 kg), and height averaged 176 cm (range, 160-185 cm). There was no mortality during the study period and no morbidity (diarrhea or hypoglycemia) related to the protocol.

Urinary nitrogen balance was not significantly different whether or not insulin was administered (−4.58 ± 50.1 mg/kg per day vs −9.38 ± 50.9 mg/kg per day, respectively). Similarly, urinary 3-MH excretion was not significantly different with or without insulin infusion (5.77 ± 0.67 µmol/kg per day vs 6.15 ± 0.43 µmol/kg per day, respectively). Serum glucose was significantly lower when insulin was administered (5.8 ± 0.4 mmol/L [104.6 ± 7.2 mg/dL] vs 7.7 ± 0.4 mmol/L [138.1 ± 7.4 mg/dL]; $P = .004$). Serum insulin levels did not differ significantly when exogenous infusions were added (415 ± 128 pmol/L vs 589 ± 322 pmol/L), but serum C-peptide levels did decrease significantly when exogenous insulin was added (5.11 ± 3.2 µU/mL vs 10.28 ± 3.5 µU/mL; $P = .04$). Serum glucose values decreased significantly when insulin was administered (5.8 ± 0.4 mmol/L [104.6 ± 7.2 mg/dL] vs 7.7 ± 0.4 mmol/L [138.1 ± 7.4 mg/dL]; $P = .004$).

COMMENT

Following injury, there are hypercatabolic and hypermetabolic responses that may last for days depending on the severity of the traumatic episode.[11] The negative nitrogen balance due to protein catabolism seen in patients who have suffered severe trauma is detrimental in several ways, including longer recovery time, increased morbidity and mortality, decreased wound healing, and inhibition of the immune response. Nutritional intervention during convalescence has proved beneficial in decreasing muscle wasting. Although the provision of energy intake and nitrogen does have an impact on improving nitrogen balance, a positive nitrogen balance is difficult, if not impossible, to attain at the peak of the catabolic response. The catabolic response to injury is thought to be mediated by the increase in catacholamines, cortisol, and glucagon values and by the increased resistance to insulin.

That insulin plays a major role in protein metabolism is well known. Numerous in vitro studies have shown that insulin inhibits protein breakdown and increases protein synthesis.[2,12,13] Fukagawa et al[9] have demonstrated insulin's ability to decrease protein breakdown in a dose-dependent manner in vivo. The availability of amino acid substrates is also vital for maximization of the anabolic effect of insulin to be maximized.[14] In patients who had undergone a major operative procedure, Valarini et al[15] showed that insulin further improved the positive nitrogen balance achieved with a TPN solution that contained 0.25 g/kg of nitrogen and an energy-nitrogen ratio of 150:1 but not with 0.5 g/kg of nitrogen and an energy-nitrogen ratio of 75:1, suggesting that the effect

Patient Demographics and Injury Severity Score*

Patient No./ Sex/Age, y	Weight, kg/ Height, cm	ISS	Diagnosis
1/F/37	53/160	29	MVA, rib Fx, acetabular Fx, femur Fx, and CHT
2/M/35	86/183	34	Crush injury, diaphragm rupture, colon injury, pelvic Fx, clavicle Fx, and hemothorax
3/F/24	53/165	29	MVA, clavicle Fx, tibia Fx, liver laceration, nasal Fx, and splenectomy
4/M/21	83/183	34	MVA, rib Fx, ankle Fx, radius Fx, ulna Fx, humerus Fx, orbital Fx, and liver laceration
5/F/29	61/170	45	MVA, ruptured pulmonary artery, liver laceration, clavicle Fx, pneumothorax, and CHT
6/M/40	103/185	34	MVA, hemothorax, rib Fx, splenectomy, ulna Fx, acetabular Fx, and CHT
7/M/33	66/175	27	MVA, CHT, thoracic vertebrae 11 through 12 Fx, clavicle Fx, bladder rupture, scalp laceration, and pneumothorax
8/M/34	84/183	34	MVA, tibia-fibula Fx, femur Fx, pelvic Fx, acetabular Fx, renal contusion, and splenectomy
9/F/64	67/173	34	MVA, bladder rupture, nasal Fx, facial Fx, clavicle Fx, and pelvic Fx
10/M/35	71/183	50	MVA, hemopneumothorax, diaphragm rupture, kidney laceration, and splenectomy

**ISS indicates Injury Severity Score; MVA, mitral valve area; Fx, fracture; and CHT, closed head trauma.*

of amino acids on the improvement of nitrogen balance is saturable. Inculet et al,[16] using an isolated forearm skeletal muscle model, showed a decrease in nitrogen balance and 3-MH excretion in patients who were given insulin and TPN after surgery. We have recently demonstrated that intravenous insulin and TPN produced a positive nitrogen balance, decreased 3-MH excretion, and facilitated whole-body protein synthesis within 5 days of major trauma.[10] These findings prompted us to perform the present protocol to determine if the anabolic effect of insulin could be combined with the advantages of enteral nutrition.

In our study, intravenous insulin produced no change in either urinary nitrogen balance or the excretion of 3-MH when given as a supplement to enteral nutrition. A possible explanation for a lack of effect is that the amino acids underwent modification by the liver before reaching the muscles. Some of the amino acids may have been incorporated into acute-phase reactants whose synthesis is increased after trauma. The anabolic effect of insulin has been previously evaluated mainly using an intravenous amino acid infusion model. It may be assumed that the provision of amino acids by either route would be equivalent in terms of protein synthesis. However, amino acids provided by the enteral route are first processed through the liver where it is known that this organ temporarily stores a part of the ingested amino acids as proteins, modifies the amino acid flux to muscle, and deaminates and oxidizes others as shown by McMenamy et al[17] with use of a dog model. They showed a wide range in the portion of added amino acids taken up by the liver, from 90% for tryptophan and phenylalanine to approximately 20% for threonine, valine, leucine, and isoleucine. This remodeling of amino acids presented to the muscle might negate the effect of insulin that requires or favors a more appropriate blend of amino acids for protein synthesis as is present in TPN based on requirements as proposed by Rose.[18] Increasing the amount of protein administered in the tube feedings to a level that could overcome the hepatic effect would likely produce undesirable side effects such as diarrhea, azotemia, and impaired renal function.

The intent of nitrogen losses should be reflected during the first 2 days of the protocol since the target rate of the enteral infusion was achieved within the first 24 hours. There should be no question that the third and fifth days are comparable to a steady nutritional state. This short equilibration time is supported by Cerra et al[19] who showed urinary nitrogen losses on a constant elemental feeding to be 11.4 g of nitrogen on day 1, 12.2 g of nitrogen on day 3, and 10.6 g of nitrogen on day 7. Shronts et al[20] showed nitrogen losses on a standard elemental infusion formula to be 16.0 g of nitrogen on day 1 and 18.2 g of nitrogen on day 3. On a modified enteral formula, losses were 15.8 g of nitrogen on day 1 and 18.9 g of nitrogen on day 3. Additionally, Watters et al[21] began full-strength feeding via jejunostomy tubes within 6 hours of major operations and increased to the target rate of either 125% of preoperative energy expenditure or 2500 mL/d (whichever was the lesser) on the second postoperative day. Urine losses were 8.5 g of nitrogen on day 1, 8.9 g of nitrogen on day 2, and 9.3 g of nitrogen on day 3. These data also support the fact that a steady state of nitrogen dynamics is attained by day 2 and certainly by day 3 of this randomized, blinded study even when bypassing the small gastric component of digestion.

In conclusion, the route of administration of nutrition does affect insulin's anabolic effect. Although we had previously demonstrated insulin's ability to produce positive nitrogen balance, increase protein synthesis, and decrease protein breakdown using TPN, this effect could not be achieved with enteral feeding. We believe this is owing to the modification and use of amino acid substrates by the liver before they can reach the skeletal muscle tissue.

Presented as a poster at the Southeastern Surgical Congress, Atlanta, Ga, February 4, 1998.

Reprints: Ronald H. Clements, MD, Surgical Education, 1600 Carraway Blvd, Birmingham, AL 35234.

REFERENCES

1. Garlick PJ, Fern M, Preedy VR. The effect of insulin infusion and food intake on muscle protein synthesis in postabsorptive rats. *Biochem J.* 1983;210:669-676.
2. Fulks RM, Goldberg AL. Effects on insulin, glucose, and amino acids on protein turnover in rat diaphragm. *J Biol Chem.* 1975;250:290-298.

3. Jefferson LS, Li JB, Rannels SR. Regulation by insulin of amino acid release and protein turnover in the perfused rat hemicorpus. *J Biol Chem.* 1977;252:1476-1483.
4. Lundholm K, Schers T. Determination in vitro of the rate of protein synthesis and degradation in human-skeletal-muscle tissue. *Eur J Biochem.* 1975;60: 1-6.
5. Louard RJ, Fryburg DA, Gelfand RA, Barrett EJ. Insulin sensitivity of protein and glucose metabolism in human forearm skeletal muscle. *J Clin Invest.* 1992;90: 2348-2354.
6. Gelfand RA, Barrett EJ. Effect of physiologic hyperinsulinemia on skeletal muscle protein synthesis and breakdown in man. *J Clin Invest.* 1987;80:1-6.
7. Biolo G, Fleming RYD, Wolfe RR. Physiologic hyperinsulinemia stimulates protein synthesis and enhances transport of selected amino acids in human skeletal muscle. *J Clin Invest.* 1995;95:811-819.
8. Newman E, Heslin MJ, Wolf RF, Pisters PWT, Brennan MF. The effect of systemic hyperinsulinemia with concomitant amino acid infusion on skeletal muscle protein turnover in the human forearm. *Metabolism.* 1994;43:70-78.
9. Fukagawa NK, Minaker KL, Rowe JW, et al. Insulin-mediated reduction of whole body protein breakdown. *J Clin Invest.* 1985;76:2306-2311.
10. Clements R, Pinson T, Borghesi L, Laws H, Long C. Nitrogen balance is achieved and myofibrillar protein catabolism is inhibited by insulin and total parenteral nutrition in trauma patients. *Surg Forum.* 1996;47:147-148.
11. Long CL, Schaffel N, Geiger JW, Schiller WR, Blakemore WS. Metabolic response to injury and illness: estimation of energy and protein needs for indirect calorimetry and nitrogen balance. *JPEN J Parenter Enteral Nutr.* 1979;3:452-456.
12. Abumrad NN, Jefferson LS, Rannels SR, Williams PE, Cherrington AD, Lacy WW. Role of insulin in the regulation of leucine kinetics in the conscious dog. *J Clin Invest.* 1982;70:1031-1041.
13. Jefferson LS. Role of insulin in the regulation of protein synthesis. *Diabetes.* 1980; 29:487-495.
14. Flakoll PJ, Kulayalt M, Frexes-Steed M, et al. Amino acids augment insulin's suppression of whole body proteolysis. *Am J Physiol.* 1989;257:E839-E847.
15. Valarini R, Sousa MF, Kalil R, Abumrad NN, Riella MC. Anabolic effects of insulin and amino acids in promoting nitrogen accretion in postoperative patients. *JPEN J Parenter Enteral Nutr.* 1994;18:214-218.
16. Inculet RI, Finley RJ, Duff JH, et al. Insulin decreases muscle protein loss after operative trauma in man. *Surgery.* 1986;99:752-758.
17. McMenamy RH, Shoemaker WC, Richmond JE, Elwyn D. Uptake and metabolism of amino acids by the dog liver perfused in situ. *Am J Physiol.* 1962;202: 407-414.
18. Rose WC. The amino acid requirements of adult men. *Nutr Abstr Rev.* 1957;27: 631.
19. Cerra FB, Shronts EP, Konstantinides NN, et al. Enteral feeding in sepsi: a prospective, randomized, double-blind trial. *Surgery.* 1985;98:632-638.
20. Shronts EP, Konstantinides NN, Teasley KM, Lysne J, Konstantinides FN, Cerra FB. Modified amino acid support in metabolic stree: enteral vs parenteral. *Nutr Suppl Serv.* 1987;7:12-17.
21. Watters JM, Kirkpatrick SM, Norris SB, Shamji FM, Wells GA. Immediate postoperative enteral feeding results in impaired respiratory mechanics and decreased mobility. *Ann Surg.* 1997;226:369-380.

IN OTHER AMA JOURNALS

ARCHIVES OF INTERNAL MEDICINE

Depression and Risk of Coronary Heart Disease in Elderly Men and Women

Carlos F. Mendes de Leon, PhD; Harlan M. Krumholz, MD; Teresa S. Seeman, PhD; Viola Vaccarino, MD, PhD; Christina S. Williams, MPH; Stanislav V. Kasl, PhD; Lisa F. Berkman, PhD

Background: Results of several recent studies suggest that depression is predictive of incident coronary disease. However, few studies have examined this relationship in the elderly, the age at which most coronary heart disease (CHD) becomes clinically manifest.

Methods and Results: Data are from the New Haven, Conn, cohort (N = 2812) of the Established Populations for the Epidemiologic Studies of the Elderly project. Baseline information on depressive symptoms and CHD risk factors was collected during an in-person interview in 1982. Nonfatal myocardial infarctions were identified through monitoring of admissions to local hospitals and were validated by medical chart review. Cause of death was obained from death certificates for all deceased participants. Outcomes were defined as CHD deaths (n = 255) and total incident CHD events (n = 391) between January 1, 1982, and December 31, 1991. There was no association between depressive symptoms and CHD outcomes in men. Among women, depressive symptoms were associated with an age-adjusted relative risk of 1.03 (per unit increase on the symptom scale) for CHD mortality ($P = .001$) and total CHD incidence ($P = .002$). These associations were largely unaffected by adjustment for established CHD risk factors but were reduced to nonsignificant levels after additional adjustment for impaired physical function. Additional analysis showed a significant association for depressive symptoms among women who had no physical function impairments or who survived at least 3 years without an event.

Conclusion: Depressive symptoms may not be independent risk factors for CHD outcomes in elderly populations in general but may increase risk among relatively healthy older women. *(1998;2341-2348)*

Reprints: Carlos F. Mendes de Leon, PhD, Rush Institute for Healthy Aging, 1645 W Jackson Blvd, Suite 675,Chicago, IL 60612 (e-mail: cmendes@rush.edu).

ORIGINAL ARTICLE

Transition From Open to Laparoscopic Fundoplication

The Learning Curve

Scott J. Soot, MD; Nihnam Eshraghi, MD; Mehrdad Farahmand, MD; Brett C. Sheppard, MD; Clifford W. Deveney, MD

Background: Two of us (B.C.S. and C.W.D.) began performing laparoscopic fundoplication in 1992. We have always designated the resident as the operating surgeon.

Objective: To determine the time necessary for both experienced surgeons and residents to become proficient in laparoscopic fundoplication.

Design: The medical records of 241 consecutive patients undergoing laparoscopic fundoplication were reviewed. This period started with the implementation of the procedure in January 1992 and ended in March 1998. For 3 consecutive years, residents were given a questionnaire regarding their confidence in performing laparoscopic fundoplication.

Results: Laparoscopic fundoplication was attempted in 241 patients and completed in 203 patients (84%). Comparing the first 25 attempted laparoscopic fundoplications with the second 25, there were 14 conversions (56%) vs 4 conversions (16%) ($P<.01$). Average operative times decreased from 236 to 199 minutes ($P<.05$), and the intraoperative complication rates were 5 (20%) and 1 (4%), respectively. Subsequently, the conversion rate stabilized at 2%. The operative time continued to decline to an average of 99 minutes for the last 25 laparoscopies. Senior residents and recent graduates returning the questionnaire performed an average of 112 laparoscopic procedures, including 15.7 laparoscopic fundoplications. They felt comfortable with the procdure after performing an average of 10.6 operations.

Conclusions: The learning curve is very steep for the first 25 laparoscopic fundoplications for experienced surgeons. However, improvements, as judged by decreases in operative time, conversion rate, and intraoperative complications, continue to occur after 100 cases. Under supervision, residents can become comfortable with this procedure after about 10 to 15 procedures.

Arch Surg. 1999;134:278-281

GASTROESOPHAGEAL reflux disease is a very common condition for which most patients are treated medically with proton pump inhibitors and prokinetic agents. However, 20% of patients who develop complications or experience recurrent symptoms after discontinuing medical therapy require surgical treatment.[1,2]

See Invited Critique at end of article

Conventional surgical management of gastroesophageal reflux disease with fundoplication is effective, durable, and in some aspects superior to medical therapy.[3-6] The ability to perform this procedure laparoscopically may further expand the applications of this treatment. Laparoscopic fundoplication has been shown to be safe and as effective as open fundoplication, and has become the preferred surgical option.[2,7-9]

The prevalence of gastroesophageal reflux disease and the many patients who benefit from surgical treatment prompted us to evaluate our experience with operative management and to examine how surgeons learn this procedure in a supervised environment. This experience was in a time of transition from the era of open fundoplications to laparoscopic fundoplications, with 2 surgeons (B.C.S. and C.W.D.) who were accustomed to performing open fundoplications. It was our aim to determine the time necessary for experienced surgeons and residents to become proficient in laparoscopic fundoplication.

From the Department of Surgery, Oregon Health Sciences University, and the Portland Veterans Administration Medical Center, Portland, Ore.

PATIENTS AND METHODS

The medical records of 241 patients who had an antireflux procedure initiated laparoscopically at the Oregon Health Sciences University (Portland) and the Portland Veterans Administration Medical Center were reviewed. Patients with achalasia were excluded from the review. The operations were performed with at least 1 staff surgeon present (B.C.S. or C.W.D.), but with the surgical resident as the operating surgeon.

Indications for antireflux surgery did not change during the study and consisted of symptoms refractory to medical management, complicated gastroesophageal reflux disease, and willingness of patients to discontinue medical therapy and undergo surgical treatment. Twenty patients had undergone previous antireflux procedure. A 360° fundoplication was performed on all patients, with 2 exceptions. A partial wrap was performed on 1 patient with scleroderma and in 1 with severe hypomotility of the esophagus. Twenty-eight percent of the patients were obese, 10% had chronic obstructive pulmonary disease, and 8.4% had cardiac disease as comorbid conditions.

A questionnaire was sent to the residents and recent graduates. They were asked which parts of the operation they found difficult and if they could perform the operation alone. We separated the operation into 3 steps on the questionnaire: (1) dissection of the right and left crus and the retroesophageal window, (2) division of the short gastric vessels and mobilization of the fundus, and (3) performing the wrap.

Patient information, presenting symptoms, preoperative studies, and operative records were collected prospectively and entered into an electronic database from which they could subsequently be analyzed. Statistical analysis was performed using the χ^2 test or analysis of variance and confirmed with the Scheffé test when appropriate.

We assessed the learning curve for the operation by examining conversion rate, intraoperative complications, and operative times in sequential groups of 25 patients.

RESULTS

Laparoscopic fundoplication was attempted in 241 patients and completed in 203 patients (84%), 154 men and 87 women. The mean (±SD) age of the patients was 47 ± 14 years. Mean body mass index ([BMI or Quetelet index]: calculated as weight in kilograms divided by the square of the height in meters: weight [kg]/[height (m)]^2) was 29 kg/m^2 (range, 16-47).

There was no mortality in this series and the long-term outcomes for gastroesophageal reflux disease were similar to those of 114 patients who had had an open fundoplication performed at our institution by 2 surgeons (B.C.S. and C.W.D.) between 1989 and 1992.[10]

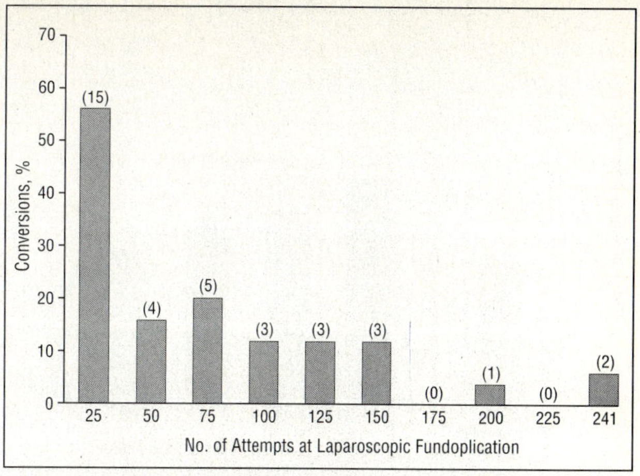

Figure 1. *Conversions to open fundoplication per 25 attempts at laparoscopic fundoplication, given as percentages. Numbers in parentheses are the corresponding actual number of conversions. There was a significant decrease in conversion from the first to the second set of 25 cases (*P<.01*).*

Intraoperative Complications With Open Fundoplication vs Laparoscopic Fundoplication

Intraoperative Complication	Open Fundoplication	Attempts at Laparoscopic Fundoplication: 25	26-50	51-75	76-100	101-241
Splenectomy	6	0	1	0	0	0
Esophageal perforation	1	1	1	0	0	0
Enterotomy	0	0	0	0	0	1
Gastrotomy	2	1	0	0	0	0
Hemorrhage	0	2	0	1	1	2
Pneumothorax	0	0	1	0	0	2
Total	**9**	**4**	**3**	**1**	**1**	**5**
No. of patients	114	25	25	25	25	141
Percentage with complications	8	16	12	4	4	4

CONVERSION RATE

Conversion rates declined progressively, with the sharpest drop between the first and second 25 cases. The conversion rate leveled off at 2% for the last 75 cases (**Figure 1**).

Initially, most cases were converted to open fundoplications because of difficulty in dissecting posterior to the esophagus and in identifying the left diaphragmatic crus and seeing the gastric fundus. Later in the series, a hemorrhage obscuring the view of structures was the major reason for conversion.

INTRAOPERATIVE COMPLICATIONS

In the first 50 cases, there were 4 potentially life-threatening intraoperative complications, 3 perforations of abdominal viscus, and 1 episode of hemorrhage requiring splenectomy. Subsequently, the intraoperative complications have been less serious (ie, pneumothorax or hemorrhage requiring conversion to open fundoplication). Intraoperative complications have decreased to 3% in the last 100 cases. The intraoperative complications are listed in the **Table**. Although many of the

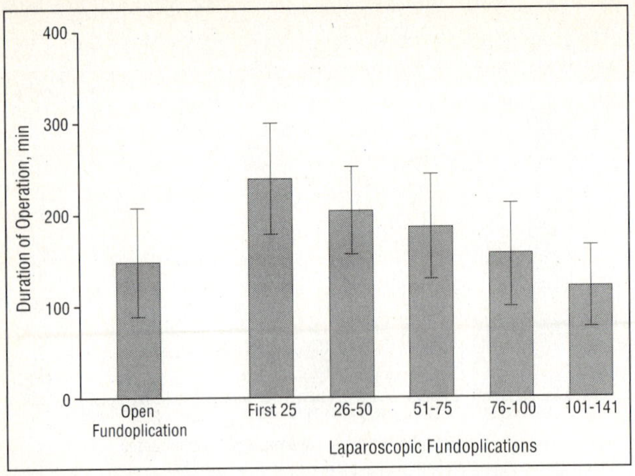

Figure 2. *The first column includes the average time for all open fundoplications. The remaining columns include the average time for all laparoscopic fundoplications in increments. The average duration of laparoscopic fundoplications 101 through 141 is significantly shorter than the average for open fundoplications (P<.01).*

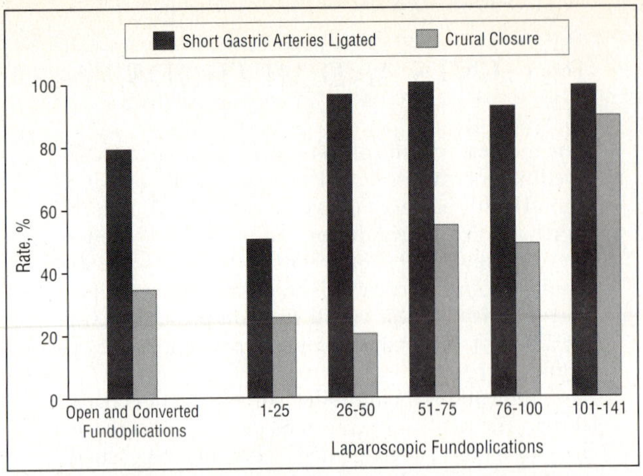

Figure 3. *After the first 25 attempts at laparoscopic fundoplication, there were no significant differences in rates of ligation of short gastric vessels (P<.03). Crural closure rates differed when compared with open fundoplications after 100 cases (P<.01).*

intraoperative complications caused conversion to open fundoplication, none resulted in serious morbidity or death.

OPERATIVE TIME

Operative time is also a measure of the expertise of the operating surgeon. Operative times per 25 patients are shown in **Figure 2**. There was a gradual decrease in operative times in the first 100 cases. Our operative times reached a plateau of 90 to 110 minutes by the end of the study. The resident performing the operation seemed to be the major factor affecting operative times. As shown in Figure 2, the operative time for laparoscopic fundoplication was shorter than for open fundoplication at the end of the study. Our experience with the open fundoplication consisted of 114 cases, also performed by the same 2 staff surgeons (B.C.S. and C.W.D) between 1989 and 1992.

TECHNICAL ASPECTS OF OPERATION

For the open fundoplications, the rates of ligation of the short gastric vessels and closure of diaphragmatic crura were 79% and 34%, respectively. As we performed more laparoscopic fundoplications, we found that fundal mobilization and division of the short gastric vessels greatly facilitated making a loose wrap and that closure of the diaphragm was important in preventing herniation of the wrap into the mediastinum. We now close the crura and divide the short gastric vessels on virtually all patients (**Figure 3**).

A questionnaire was sent out to all residents and returned by 8 of 20 senior and chief residents and 9 practicing surgeons. They each performed an average of 112 laparoscopic procedures and 15.7 laparoscopic fundoplications, and felt comfortable performing a laparoscopic fundoplication alone after being supervised in 10.6 cases. Thirteen of the respondents felt they would be competent with the laparoscopic fundoplication after completion of residency. Retroesophageal dissection of the left crus was considered difficult by 76% of the respondents. Ligation of the short gastric vessels was considered difficult by 59% of the respondents. Wrap development was considered difficult by 35% of the respondents. Seven of 9 former residents performing general surgery who were trained between 1993 and 1998 now perform laparoscopic fundoplication in their practices.

COMMENT

Enthusiasm for fundoplication as treatment of gastroesophageal reflux disease has increased markedly with the advent of minimally invasive techniques. The introduction and refinement of laparoscopic fundoplication has occurred in the past 6 years. Our center, with 2 surgeons who were able to serve as their own controls during the transition from open to laparoscopic fundoplications, provided a unique opportunity to evaluate this process and compare results. Our experience, which was similar to many other studies, shows that the number of fundoplications is increasing.[10] Laparoscopic fundoplication represents most of this increase and has become the operation of choice for gastroesophageal reflux disease.[11,12] Laparoscopic fundoplication requires the ability to perform an operation in multiple planes within a 2-dimensional environment. The acquisition of this skill, along with the need to acquire facility with new instruments, suturing techniques, and new technological devices are challenges in performing safe and effective operations. A learning curve of 20 procedures per surgeon and 50 procedures per institution has been previously established for laparoscopic fundoplication,[11] although it is recognized that individuals may progress at different rates.

Important indicators on the learning curve for laparoscopic surgery are the conversion rate and operative complications. In our experience, the greatest decline in conversion rate was between the first and second 25 cases. Most conversions during this period were for technical reasons; eg, our ability to adequately dissect the posterior "window" behind the esophagus required learning techniques of retraction and new anatomical landmarks or surgical planes. Only a small percentage of all conversions were for potentially life-threatening complications such as esophageal or gastric perforation or hemorrhage. Our conversion rates in the first 25 cases were similar to rates reported by others.[12,13] Other technical challenges were the division of the short gastric vessels and fundal mobilization, closure of the diaphragmatic crura, and suture of the fundoplication. Once these steps were learned, conversion rates remained extremely low (2%-5%). Although the largest decrease in intraoperative complications, conversion rates, and operating times occurred between the first and second set of 25 patients, these factors continued to decrease after 100 cases.

During the second and third set of 25 cases, the harmonic scissors and the endostitch were introduced. These technical devices aided in division of the short gastric vessels and in suturing the wrap and must have also contributed to decreased operative times, but we are unable to quantify this effect. Our overall mean operative time of 140 minutes for the laparoscopic fundoplications compares with operative times for open fundoplications and is well within the range of the large laparoscopic series of fundoplications.[7,8,14,15] The last 50 laparoscopic fundoplications were performed more quickly than open fundoplications (99 vs 142 minutes, $P<.05$).

Initially, we experienced some potentially serious complications. There were 2 esophageal perforations and 1 gastric perforation. All perforations occurred posteriorly and emphasized the potential for problems in the retroesophageal dissection with identification of the left diaphragmatic crus and creation of the window. However, we did not experience this complication after 50 cases. These perforations were recognized, handled properly, and did not result in any long-term morbidity. We also experienced 1 splenic injury requiring splenectomy in the second 25 cases, but none afterward. Our experience compares favorably to other reported series.[16] Certainly, splenic injury occurs much less frequently after laparoscopic fundoplication compared with open fundoplication.

After the first 25 cases, there were no major intraoperative complications and, although there were some episodes of hemorrhage requiring conversion to open fundoplication, they did not require transfusion or splenectomy and were converted because the amount of bleeding obscured the laparoscopic field.

It seems that the bulk of learning occurred during the first 25 cases, since we experienced large decreases in conversion rate and intraoperative complications during this time period. However, in a supervised setting, the residents seem to become proficient in about 12 cases. The most difficult part of this procedure for both staff and residents was the retroesophageal dissection and identification of the left crus, and this is where most supervision is necessary. Residents are able to learn this procedure during their residency and subsequently perform it in their practices.

Accepted for publication October 25, 1998.

Presented at the Society of Veterans Administration Surgeons, Baltimore, Md, April 29, 1998.

Corresponding author: Clifford W. Deveney, MD, Veterans Administration Medical Center P-8-SURG, 3710 SW US Veterans Hospital Rd, Portland, OR 97201 (e-mail: deveney .clifford@portland.va.gov).

REFERENCES

1. Anvari M, Allen C, Borm A. Laparoscopic Nissen fundoplication is a satisfactory alternative to long-term omeprazole therapy. *Br J Surg.* 1995;82:938-942.
2. Mckenzie D, Grayson T, Polk HC. The impact of omeprazole and laparoscopy upon hiatal hernia and reflux esophagitis. *J Am Coll Surg.* 1996;183:413-418.
3. Spechler SJ. Comparison of medical and surgical therapy for complicated gastroesophageal reflux disease in veterans. *N Engl J Med.* 1992;326:786-792.
4. DeMeester TR, Bonavina L, Albertucci M. Nissen fundoplication for gastroesophageal reflux disease: evaluation of primary repair in 100 consecutive patients. *Ann Surg.* 1986;204:9-20.
5. Ortiz A, Martinez de Haro LF, Parrilla P, et al. Conservative treatment versus antireflux surgery in Barrett's oesophagus: long-term results of a prospective study. *Br J Surg.* 1996;83:274-278.
6. Luostarinen M, Isolauri J, Laitinen J, et al. Fate of Nissen fundoplication after 20 years: a clinical, endoscopical, and functional analysis. *Gut.* 1993;34:1015-1020.
7. Hinder RA, Filipi CJ, Wetscher G, Neary P, DeMeester TR, Perdikis G. Laparoscopic Nissen fundoplication is an effective treatment for gastroesophageal reflux disease. *Ann Surg.* 1994;220:472-483.
8. Hunter JG, Trus TL, Branum GD, Waring JP, Wood WC. A physiologic approach to laparoscopic fundoplication for gastroesophageal reflux disease. *Ann Surg.* 1996;223:673-687.
9. Peters JH, Heimbucher J, Kauer WK, Incarbone R, Bremner CG, DeMeester TR. Clinical and physiologic comparison of laparoscopic and open Nissen fundoplication (see "Comments"). *J Am Coll Surg.* 1995;180:385-393.
10. Eshrahgi N, Farahmand M, Soot SJ, Rand-Luby L, Deveney CW, Sheppard BC. Comparison of outcomes of open versus laparoscopic Nissen fundoplication performed in a single practice. *Am J Surg.* 1998;175:371-374.
11. Watson DI, Baigrie RJ, Jamieson GG. A learning curve for laparoscopic fundoplication: definable, avoidable, or a waste of time? *Ann Surg.* 1996;224:198-203.
12. Deschamps C, Allen MS, Trastek VF, Johnson JO, Pairolero PC. Early experience and learning curve associated with laparoscopic Nissen fundoplication. *J Thorac Cardiovasc Surg.* 1998;115:281-285.
13. Meehan JJ, Georgeson KE. The learning curve associated with laparoscopic antireflux surgery in infants and children. *J Ped Surg.* 1997;32:426-429.
14. Gotley DC, Smithers BM, Rhodes M, Menzies B, Branicki FJ, Nathanson L. Laparoscopic Nissen fundoplication: 200 consecutive cases. *Gut.* 1996;38:487-491.
15. Watson DI, Jamieson GG, Baigrie RJ, et al. Laparoscopic surgery for gastro-oesophageal reflux: beyond the learning curve. *Br J Surg.* 1996;83:1284-1287.
16. Munro W, Brancatisano R, Adams IP, Falk GL. Complications of laparoscopic fundoplication: the first 100 patients. *Surg Laparosc Endosc.* 1996;6:421-423.

Invited Critique

This article is an excellent overview of the results of the introduction of laparoscopic fundoplication to university and Veterans Affairs academic programs. It is always encouraging to see advanced procedures practiced, taught, and evaluated in these settings. This introduction contrasts sharply with the introduction of laparoscopic cholecystectomy, which was mainly championed by community-based surgical pioneers, while academics were slow to recognize its potential dramatic effect on the practice of surgery. The authors must be commended for their heroic efforts to establish resident proficiency in performing this procedure. Unfortunately, this level of commitment and implementation has not been observed universally.

The article provided answers about the authors' experience as the result of their approach to introducing laparoscopic antireflux procedures into their institution. But the review raises more questions than answers about the learning curve they encountered. First of all, whose learning curve is being assessed, that of the residents or that of the attending surgeons? The article does not provide enough detailed information about the experience of individual participants to make a valid conclusion about the learning curve. This is in sharp contrast to the work of Waston et al,[1,2] as referenced by the authors. In addition, the sample size of responses to the questionnaires was small; therefore, the authors' conclusions may be incorrect.

Previous experience was shown by the authors in open fundoplication, but was not documented by the attending surgeons in laparoscopic fundoplication. No mention is made of the use of proctors during the initial procedures. There is no information given on cognitive instruction, suturing and advanced skill development, or laboratory experience with live animals prior to embarking on initial cases. If the attending surgeons proceeded with only their initial open experience as a guide and allowed the resident to be first surgeon on all of the cases, I am not surprised at the early results. A conversion rate of 56% and a major complication rate of 16% to 20% suggest that the aforementioned preparatory instructional way stations were not established. I take issue with the authors' suggestion that these numbers are within the norm for the initial (first 25) experiences with these procedures. Many references demonstrate better initial results and the 2 references cited may be the result of the same training deficiencies. However, I must note that after the first 100 cases, results similar to those of other series were documented. This experience reinforces suggestions that have been made by others concerning the establishment of advanced, minimally invasive procedures. Optimally, initial cases are accompanied by maximal skill development and cognitive preparation along with experienced proctoring to achieve early success and patient safety.

James C. Rosser, Jr, MD
New Haven, Conn

1. Watson DI, Baigrie RJ, Jamieson GG. A learning curve for laparoscopic fundoplication: definable, avoidable, or a waste of time? *Ann Surg.* 1996;224:198-203.
2. Watson DI, Jamieson GG, Baigrie RJ, et al. Laparoscopic surgery for gastro-oesophageal reflux: beyond the learning curve. *Br J Surg.* 1996;83:1284-1287.

Surgical Anatomy

The **left recurrent laryngeal nerve** loops around the aorta at the level of the ligamentum arteriosum and then extends up posterior to the inferior thyroid artery. **The right recurrent laryngeal nerve** branches off the vagus, loops around the right subclavian artery, and courses posterior to the inferior thyroid artery.

1. Blackbourne LH, Fleischer KJ. *Advanced Surgical Recall.* Baltimore, Md: Williams & Wilkins; 1997;576-577.

ORIGINAL ARTICLE

Growth Hormone Attenuates Tumor Necrosis Factor α in Burned Children

Minas T. Chrysopoulo, MD; Marc G. Jeschke, MD; Roque J. Ramirez, MD; Robert E. Barrow, PhD; David N. Herndon, MD

Background: Recombinant human growth hormone (rhGH) has been shown to favorably modulate the acute-phase response and may improve the clinical outcome.

Objective: To examine whether rhGH attenuates the elevated tumor necrosis factor α (TNF-α) levels that correlate with increased multiorgan failure and mortality in burned adults and children.

Design: Twenty children with burns of greater than 40% of the total body surface area were randomly divided into 2 groups to receive placebo (n = 10) or rhGH, 0.2 mg/kg per day intramuscularly (n = 10).

Setting: Pediatric burn hospital.

Main Outcome Measure: Serum TNF-α levels by enzyme-linked immunoassay at baseline (day 0) and at 21 and 42 days after injury. For statistical analysis, we used the Kruskal-Wallis and Friedman tests.

Results: No significant differences in age (mean ± SD, 6.2 ± 1.6 vs 5.0 ± 1.2 years) or percentage of total body surface area burn (mean ± SD, 65.1% ± 8.2% vs 57.1% ± 5.2%) could be shown between the groups given rhGH and placebo. Baseline TNF-α levels were elevated from reference values in both groups. Twenty-one and 42 days after rhGH administration, serum TNF-α levels were significantly decreased from those at baseline ($P<.05$). No significant decrease in TNF-α levels was observed in the placebo group ($P = .5$).

Conclusions: Recombinant human growth hormone significantly lowers serum TNF-α levels after burn injury. This is consistent with the beneficial effect that rhGH has on the acute-phase response.

Arch Surg. 1999;134:283-286

From the Shriners Hospitals for Children, Galveston Burns Institute and the Department of Surgery, University of Texas Medical Branch, Galveston.

AN ACUTE hypercatabolic state is often observed following major illness or trauma, such as a severe burn. Increases in catecholamine, glucagon, and cortisol levels raise the energy requirements, and protein-degradation products (amino acids) are used for fuel. Most of these amino acids are supplied by muscle. The resultant muscle wasting and nitrogen imbalance are not improved by early aggressive nutritional supplementation. Extracellular to intracellular glucose-transport mechanisms are changed, as evidenced by the development of postinjury insulin resistance. Futile substrate cycling of glucose and triglycerides yields no net conversion of substrate to product for fuel. These changes are typical of the hypermetabolic response to a thermal injury.

One of the main components of this response is the alteration in serum concentrations of a large number of plasma proteins known as the acute-phase proteins.[1] One of the principal mediators of these acute-phase proteins is tumor necrosis factor α (TNF-α). Indeed, altered body composition has been associated with elevated serum levels of TNF-α, and TNF-α has been shown to induce anorexia, weight loss, and an acute-phase response.[2,3] Studies of animals have shown that TNF-α may be responsible for the tissue wasting associated with malignancy,[4] and increased serum levels have been found in many patients with chronic diseases such as rheumatoid arthritis.[5] Elevated levels also have been found in the serum of burned patients with sepsis.[6] Yamada et al[7] showed that serum levels of TNF-α were elevated following a thermal injury and correlated this with an increase in the incidence of sepsis and mortality and sepsis-induced muscle proteolysis.[8]

PATIENTS AND METHODS

Twenty children with acute burn injury were entered into a randomized, double-blind study to receive either placebo (n = 10) or rhGH, 0.2 mg/kg per day (n = 10). Randomization was performed by computer random number selection. Inclusion criteria for these studies were age 1 to 18 years, admission to our burn hospital within 3 days of injury, burn size of more than 40% of total body surface area, with a third-degree burn of more than 10% requiring a minimum of 1 donor-site harvest. The rhGH was dissolved in isotonic sodium chloride solution and given intramuscularly each day for 6 weeks. Serum specimens were taken on admission before treatment (day 0) and on days 21 and 42 after the burn.

Serum TNF-α concentrations were determined using a TNF-α human enzyme-linked immunosorbent assay (Endogen, Inc, Woburn, Mass). A 3-step technique was used. Standard curves for quantifying human TNF-α were obtained. The standard curve observed was linear from 0 to 1000 pg/mL on a logarithmic scale. Absorbance was measured at 450 nm.

Patient records were reviewed for the development of organ failure and sepsis and for mortality. Acute renal failure was defined as oliguria for at least 36 hours (urine output <0.5 mL · kg^{-1} · h^{-1}), a serum urea nitrogen-to-creatinine ratio of less than 20, a serum creatinine level of greater than 177 μmol/L (>2 mg/dL), or any combination of these criteria. We determined whether burned children required ventilatory support and the duration of support. Cardiac function was examined, with cardiac failure defined as a cardiac arrest requiring pediatric advanced life support. Sepsis was defined as having a blood culture positive for pathogenic bacteria or fungus either during the clinical course or at autopsy.

Statistical analysis was performed using the Kruskal-Wallis test to determine differences in treatment and the Friedman test to determine differences in time. The paired *t* test with the Bonferroni correction was used post hoc to determine differences within groups. Data are expressed as the mean ± SD. Significance was accepted at $P<.05$.

In addition to elevated levels of stress hormones, a reduction in anabolic hormones, including growth hormone (GH) and insulinlike growth factor type I (IGF-I) is observed after a thermal injury.

The purpose of this study was to determine whether treatment with recombinant human growth hormone (rhGH) affects TNF-α serum levels in burned children.

Patient Demographics*

Treatment Group	Age, y	Sex, M:F	TBSA Burn, %	Third-degree Burn, %
Growth hormone (n = 10)	6.2 ± 1.6	6:4	64 ± 19	56 ± 14
Placebo (n = 10)	5.0 ± 1.2	7:3	61 ± 18	47 ± 9

**All values are expressed as mean ± SD. TBSA indicates total body surface area.*

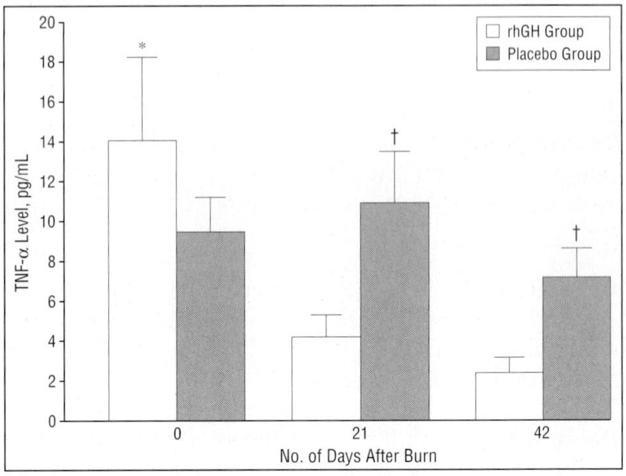

Figure 1. *Mean ± SEM values for serum tumor necrosis factor α (TNF-α) after drug treatment. Asterisk indicates a significant difference between levels before treatment (day 0) and those 21 and 42 days after the burn (P<.05); dagger, a significant difference between the group receiving recombinant human growth hormone (rhGH) and the placebo group (P<.05).*

RESULTS

No differences in age, sex, burn size, or depth of burn between the group receiving rhGH and the placebo group could be demonstrated (**Table**). Before treatment (day 0), TNF-α levels in both groups were significantly elevated compared with reference values (14.0 ± 13.4 pg/mL in the group receiving rhGH and 9.4 ± 5.9 pg/mL in the placebo group; $P<.06$). Twenty-one and 42 days after therapy, TNF-α levels were significantly decreased in patients receiving rhGH compared with baseline (4.2 ± 3.4 pg/mL and 2.3 ± 2.9 pg/mL, respectively; $P<.05$). Serum TNF-α levels did not change with time in the placebo group (**Figure 1**). **Figure 2** shows the change in individual serum TNF-α levels with time in the group receiving rhGH and the placebo group. No significant differences in mortality or incidence of renal failure, cardiac arrest, or sepsis could be shown between patients receiving rhGH and those receiving placebo ($P>.05$). No significant difference could be shown in the number of patients requiring mechanical ventilatory support ($P>.05$). Patients receiving rhGH had a greater increase in body weight than those receiving placebo (4.6% ± 4.3% vs −1.1% ± 3.9%; $P<.05$), but no differences in energy intake or protein and fat intake between the groups could be shown during the 6 weeks.

COMMENT

The beneficial effects of rhGH on metabolism in patients with burn injury have been described in some detail.[9-13] Herndon et al[14] showed that rhGH shortened

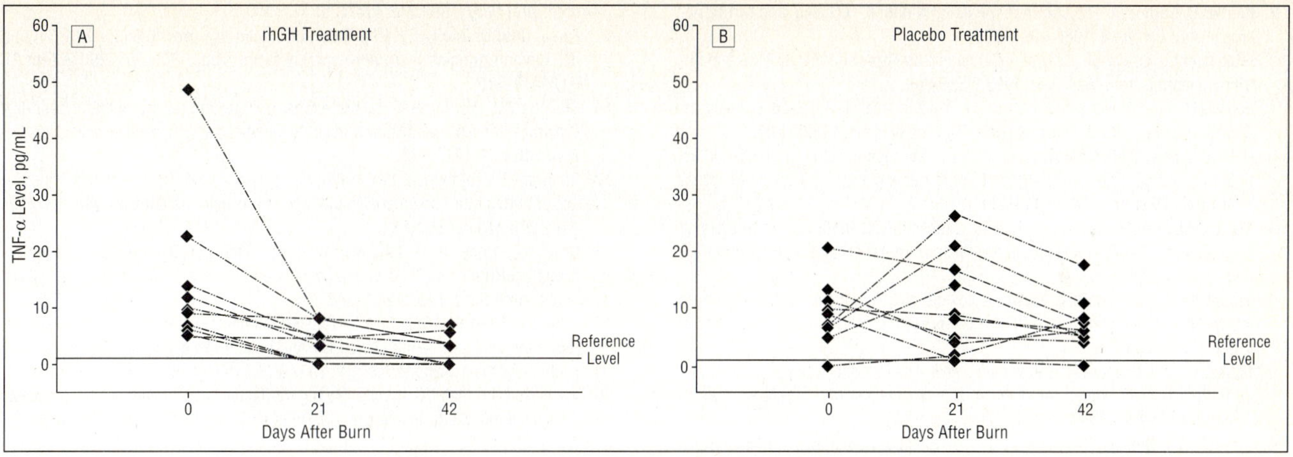

Figure 2. *A schematic showing the individual changes in serum tumor necrosis factor α (TNF-α) levels during the study in burned children receiving (A) recombinant human growth hormone (rhGH) (n = 10) and (B) placebo (n = 10). The mean ± SD reference serum TNF-α level is 1.4 ± 0.2 pg/mL (from Petersen et al[1]).*

donor site healing times and subsequently decreased the length of hospital stays. These shorter wound healing times were associated with elevated levels of serum IGF-I. Growth hormone has been suggested to act primarily in the liver, both directly and indirectly through IGF-I production.[15-17] Protein anabolism is 1 outcome of GH administration that has been studied in an extensive randomized, double-blind clinical trial[11] in which the administration of GH was shown to increase protein turnover as a result of elevated protein synthesis and breakdown. Protein synthesis, however, was increased by a greater degree than protein breakdown in severely burned patients.[18] The net result was a reduction in protein loss of as much as 50% and a reduction in weight loss. In the present study, burned patients receiving rhGH gained substantially more weight than those receiving placebo.

Tumor necrosis factor α has been previously shown to directly inhibit the basal level of protein synthesis and IGF-I– and serum-stimulated protein synthesis in myoblasts and myotubules.[19] This action of TNF-α is similar to that observed in the skeletal muscle of animals with sepsis.[20] Exposing myoblasts to TNF-α for 10 minutes inhibited the stimulation of protein synthesis by serum and IGF-I for as long as 48 hours after administration. This suggests that TNF-α acts rapidly and that even transient exposures to this cytokine may decrease protein synthesis long after its disappearance from the circulation.[19] Increased serum levels of TNF-α due to inflammatory states can persist for up to several days.[21] Our study indicates higher serum levels in children for as long as 6 weeks after a burn.

Fan et al[21] analyzed changes in circulating and tissue concentrations of IGF-I and selected IGF-I–binding proteins in rats after the infusion of TNF-α at various rates. Their study showed that TNF-α is an important regulator of the GH-insulinlike growth factor axis in vivo. Substantially reduced plasma levels of GH and IGF-I were detected even in the lowest TNF-α infusion rates.[21] In similar studies,[22-24] levels of IGF-I were decreased following burns, trauma, surgical therapy, and the administration of lipopolysaccharides. It has been postulated that this decrease in plasma IGF-I levels is partly caused by a reduction in the synthesis and release of IGF-I by the liver. This theory emerged because the liver is the major source of IGF-I entering the circulation,[25] and TNF-α has been shown to decrease IGF-I concentrations in the liver, muscles, and pituitary gland.[21] These TNF-α–induced reductions may be mediated by the concomitant decrease in plasma GH levels.[25,26]

Frost et al[19] reported that the exposure of human myoblasts to TNF-α does not change IGF-I–receptor binding characteristics. This suggests that the cytokine acts on a component of the IGF-I signal transduction pathway that lies distal to the receptor and to the autophosphorylation processes. Tumor necrosis factor α has not been shown to impair IGF-I– or serum-stimulated thymidine uptake, which implies that TNF-α acts specifically on the part of the signaling transduction pathway involved in the stimulation of protein synthesis.[19] By impairing this process, together with other components of the IGF-I signaling pathway, TNF-α may inhibit protein synthesis.

The decrease in serum TNF-α levels observed in burned children receiving rhGH may be one mechanism by which rhGH exerts its favorable modulation on protein metabolism and the acute-phase response.

This study was supported by grant 8040 from the Shriners Hospitals for Children, Galveston, Tex.

Presented as a poster at the 18th Annual Meeting of the Surgical Infection Society, New York, NY, May 1-2, 1998.

Corresponding author: Robert E. Barrow, PhD, Shriners Hospitals for Children, 815 Market St, Room 718, Galveston, TX 77550.

REFERENCES

1. Petersen SR, Jeevanandam M, Shahbazian LM, Holaday NJ. Reprioritization of liver protein synthesis resulting from recombinant human growth hormone supplementation in parenterally fed trauma patients: the effect of growth hormone on the acute-phase response. *J Trauma.* 1997;42:987-996.

2. Beutler B, Cerami A. The common mediator of shock, cachexia, and tumor necrosis. *Adv Immunol.* 1988;42:213-231.
3. Moldawer LL, Lowry SF, Cerami A. Cachectin: its impact on metabolism and nutritional status. *Annu Rev Nutr.* 1988;8:585-609.
4. Balkwill FR. Tumor necrosis factor and lymphotoxin. In: Balkwill FR, ed. *Cytokines in Cancer Therapy.* Oxford, England: Oxford University Press; 1989:54-87.
5. Rall LC, Rosen CJ, Dolnikowski G, et al. Protein metabolism in rheumatoid arthritis and aging: effects of muscle strength training and tumor necrosis factor α. *Arthritis Rheum.* 1996;39:1115-1124.
6. Marano M, Fong Y, Moldawer LL, et al. Cachectin/TNF in the serum of ICU and burn patients. Paper presented at: American Burn Association Annual Proceedings; 1988;20:18.
7. Yamada Y, Endo S, Inada K. Plasma cytokine levels in patients with severe burn injury—with reference to the relationship between infection and prognosis. *Burns.* 1996;22:587-593.
8. Balteskard L, Unneberg K, Halvorsen D, et al. The influence of growth hormone on tumour necrosis factor and neutrophil leukocyte function in sepsis. *Scand J Infect Dis.* 1997;29:393-399.
9. Liljedahl SO, Gemzell CA, Plantin LO, et al. Effect of human growth hormone in patients with severe burns. *Acta Chir Scand.* 1961;22:1-14.
10. Soroff HS, Rozin RR, Mooty J, Lister J, Raben MS. Role of human growth hormone in the response to trauma, I: metabolic effects following burns. *Ann Surg.* 1967;166:739-752.
11. Muller MJ, Gilpin DA, Herndon DN. Modulation of wound healing and the postburn response. In: Herndon DN, ed: *Total Burn Care.* Philadelphia, Pa: WB Saunders Co; 1996:223-236.
12. Wilmore DW, Moylan JA Jr, Bristow BF, Mason AD Jr, Pruitt BA Jr. Anabolic effects of growth hormone and high caloric feedings following thermal injury. *Surg Gynecol Obstet.* 1974;138:875-884.
13. Soroff HS, Pearson E, Green NL, et al. The effect of growth hormone on nitrogen balance at various levels of intake in burned patients. *Surg Gynecol Obstet.* 1960; 111:875-884.
14. Herndon DN, Barrow RE, Kunkel KR, Broemeling L, Rutan RL. Effects of recombinant human growth hormone on donor site healing in severely burned children. *Ann Surg.* 1990;212:424-429.
15. Fan J, Char D, Bagby GJ. Regulation of insulin-like growth factor-I (IGF-I) and IGF-binding proteins by tumor necrosis factor. *Am J Physiol.* 1995;269(pt 2): R1204-R1212.
16. Chwans WJ, Bistrian BR. Role of exogenous growth hormone and insulin-like growth factor-I in malnutrition and acute metabolic stress: a hypothesis. *Crit Care Med.* 1991;19:1317-1322.
17. Boulware SD, Tamborlane WV, Matthews LS, Sherwin RS. Diverse effects of insulin-like growth factor I on glucose, lipid, and amino acid metabolism. *Am J Physiol.* 1992;262(pt 1):E130-E133.
18. Gore DC, Honeycutt D, Jahoor F, Wolfe RR, Herndon DN. Effect of exogenous growth hormone on whole-body and isolated-limb protein kinetics in burned patients. *Arch Surg.* 1991;126:38-43.
19. Frost RA, Lang CH, Gelato MC. Transient exposure of human myoblasts to tumor necrosis factor-α inhibits serum and insulin-like growth factor I stimulated protein synthesis. *Endocrinology.* 1997;138:4153-4159.
20. Jurasinski CV, Vary TC. Insulin-like growth factor I accelerates protein synthesis in skeletal muscle during sepsis. *Am J Physiol.* 1995;269(pt 1):E977-E981.
21. Fan J, Molina PE, Gelato MC, Lang CH. Differential tissue regulation of insulin-like growth factor-I content and binding proteins after endotoxin. *Endocrinology.* 1994;134:1685-1692.
22. Davies SC, Wass JAH, Ross RJM, et al. The induction of a specific protease for insulin-like growth factor binding protein-3 in the circulation during severe illness. *J Endocrinol.* 1991;130:469-473.
23. Ghahary A, Fu S, Shen YJ, Shankowsky HA, Tredget EE. Differential effects of thermal injury on circulating insulin-like growth factor binding proteins in burn patients. *Mol Cell Biochem.* 1994;135:171-180.
24. Wojnar MM, Fan J, Frost RA, Lang CH. Alterations in the insulin-like growth factor system in trauma patients. *Am J Physiol.* 1995;268(pt 2):R970-R977.
25. Schwander JC, Hauri C, Zapf J, Froesch ER. Synthesis and secretion of insulin-like growth factor and its binding protein by the perfused rat liver: dependence on growth hormone status. *Endocrinology.* 1983;113:297-305.
26. Underwood LE, D'Ercole AJ, Van Wyk JJ. Somatomedin C and the assessment of growth. *Pediatr Clin North Am.* 1980;27:771-782.

Enteral Nutrition Prevents Bacterial Translocation but Does Not Improve Survival During Acute Pancreatitis

Joji Kotani, MD; Makoto Usami, MD; Hideaki Nomura, MD; Atsunori Iso, MD; Hiroshi Kasahara, MD; Yoshikazu Kuroda, MD; Harumasa Oyanagi, MD; Yoichi Saitoh, MD

Objective: To evaluate the effect of enteral nutrition (EN) in attenuating bacterial and/or endotoxin translocation, maintaining immune responsiveness, and improving outcome in early acute pancreatitis (AP) in Wistar male rats.

Design: Acute pancreatitis was induced in rats receiving total parenteral nutrition (TPN) (AP/TPN group) (n=34) and EN (AP/EN group) (n=35) by pressure injection of 1% deoxycholate into the biliopancreatic duct (0.6 mg/kg of body weight). Rats in the sham/TPN and sham/EN groups (n=10 each) underwent laparotomy without induction of AP. Catheters for TPN and EN were placed into the external jugular vein and jejunum, respectively. Rats were infused with Ringer lactate solution for 48 hours followed by TPN in the AP/TPN and sham/TPN groups, and EN in the AP/EN and sham/EN groups until day 7. The fluid volume and energy (calories) intake were similar in all groups.

Setting: Medical school research laboratory.

Main Outcome Measures: Survival, blood endotoxin level, villus height, 5-bromo-2'-deoxyuridine (BrdU) uptake in the jejunum and ileum, bacterial culture of mesenteric lymph nodes, and CD4/CD8 ratio of T cells in mesenteric lymph nodes, spleen, and peripheral blood.

Results: There was no difference in survival and pancreatic healing between the AP/TPN and AP/EN groups. Colony-forming units of the mesenteric lymph nodes and the endotoxin level were significantly lower in the AP/EN group than in the AP/TPN group ($P<.05$). Villus height and BrdU intake was significantly higher in the AP/EN group than in the AP/TPN group ($P<.05$). The CD4/CD8 ratio of T cells in spleen and peripheral blood was higher in the AP/EN group than in the AP/TPN group ($P<.05$), whereas there was no difference in mesenteric lymph nodes.

Conclusions: Jejunal administration of EN is well tolerated in early AP, maintains immune responsiveness and gut integrity, and reduces bacterial and/or endotoxin translocation. However, compared with TPN, EN does not improve outcome. These results suggest that factors other than bacterial and/or endotoxin translocation may be responsible for mortality in this rat model of early AP. However, additional studies of both early bacterial and/or endotoxin translocation and late assessment of outcome are indicated.

Arch Surg. 1999;134:287-292

From the First Department of Surgery, Kobe University School of Medicine, Kobe, Japan (Drs Kotani, Usami, Iso, Kasahara, Kuroda, and Saitoh); Department of Surgery, University of Medicine and Dentistry of New Jersey–Robert Wood Johnson Medical School, New Brunswick (Dr Kotani); and Second Department of Surgery, Kinki University School of Medicine, Osaka, Japan (Drs Nomura and Oyanagi).

INFECTIOUS COMPLICATIONS account for more than 80% of mortality in human acute pancreatitis (AP).[1,2] Although the pathogenesis of infection in AP is unclear, it is known that the microorganisms that cause pancreatic infection and sepsis in patients with AP are generally common enteric bacteria.[2,3] This suggests that these bacteria may originate from the gastrointestinal tract. In fact, recent work on animals in AP has demonstrated that there is a loss of gut mucosal integrity with subsequent bacterial and/or endotoxin translocation (BET) from the gut lumen to other organs.[4,5] However, few reports have demonstrated that BET per se has deleterious consequences for the host in experimental models of AP.

Extensive studies have demonstrated 3 major mechanisms that promote BET and secondary infections. These are disruption of the indigenous intestinal microflora, damage to the intestinal mucosa causing increased permeability, and impairment of host immunity.[6-10] Further, compared with total parenteral nutrition (TPN), enteral nutrition (EN) attenuates cecal bacterial overgrowth,[11] maintains gut mucosal integrity[12] and permeability,[13] and maintains immune responsiveness of the host.[8,14,15]

Since BET is thought to be deleterious to the host and the route of nutrition can modulate BET, the purpose of this study was to compare the effect of TPN and EN on gut and immune system integrity and outcome in AP in Wistar male rats.

MATERIALS AND METHODS

ANIMALS

The experiments conducted were approved by the Kobe (Japan) University of Medicine Animal Care and Use Committee. All animals were maintained according to the recommendations of the National Institutes of Health Guide for Care and Use of Laboratory Animals and handled under the Guideline for Animal Experiments of the Kobe University School of Medicine. Animals were anesthetized with ether (Wako Pure Chemical Industries Ltd, Osaka, Japan). Laparotomy was performed though a midline incision, and the abdomen was closed in 2 layers. All procedures were performed using aseptic techniques.

EXPERIMENTAL GROUPS

Eighty-nine adult male Wistar rats weighing 230 to 250 g were studied in 4 groups: 34 rats underwent laparotomy with induction of AP and received TPN (AP/TPN group) and 35 rats underwent laparotomy with induction of AP and received EN (AP/EN group). The remaining 20 rats underwent laparotomy without induction of AP and received TPN (sham/TPN group; n=10) or EN (sham/EN group; n=10).

INDUCTION OF AP

Acute pancreatitis was induced in the AP/TPN and AP/EN groups as follows. A microaneurysm clip was placed on the biliary duct close to the liver. An incision was made, and a sterilized polyethylene catheter (inner diameter, 0.28 mm; outer diamter, 0.38 mm; Becton Dickinson and Co, Franklin Lakes, NJ) was inserted into the common biliopancreatic duct, introduced into the duodenum through the ampulla of Vater, and then the end of the catheter was taken out of a small antimesenteric duodenotomy on the opposite site of ampulla of Vater and attached to a 0.5-mL syringe (1/2 cc U-100 insulin syringe; Becton Dickinson and Co, Rutherford, NJ). The other end of the catheter was also introduced into the common biliopancreatic duct, and fixed above and below the incision by ligation with 3-0 silk sutures.Then, 0.6 mL/kg of 1% deoxycholate (Wako Pure Chemical Industries Ltd) was injected into the common biliopancreatic duct under steady manual pressure. Once the injection was finished, the microclip was removed.

PLACEMENT OF TPN AND EN CATHETER

In all animals, a silicon catheter (inner diameter, 0.6 mm; outer diameter, 1.0 mm; Imamura Co, Tokyo, Japan) was surgically inserted into the external jugular vein for TPN, and a silicon catheter (inner diameter, 1.0 mm; outer diameter, 2.0 mm; Imamura Co) was surgically placed into the jejunum via a gastrostomy for EN using standard techniques. The feeding catheters were tunneled subcutaneously and brought out in the suprascapular region. The catheters were passed through a stainless protective coil and attached to a swivel apparatus allowing mobility. Sterile polyethylene tubing was connected from the swivel apparatus through a microtube pump (Tokyo Rikakikai Co, Tokyo) to the sterile nutritional source.

NUTRITIONAL SUPPORT

All animals were placed in metabolic cages, and infused intravenously with Ringer lactate solution at the rate of 400 mL/kg per day for the first 24 hours, and then 300 mL/kg for the next 24 hours. Then, the intravenously fed animals (AP/TPN and sham/TPN groups) or intrajejunally fed animals (AP/EN and sham/EN groups) were infused with a commercially available TPN solution (TAB; Otsuka Pharmacy Co, Osaka, Japan) via the TPN tube or with a commercially available EN solution (Enterued; Terumo Co, Tokyo) via the EN tube, respectively, at the rate of 264 mL/kg per day by day 7.

The TPN solution (glucose, 111.1 g/L; xylitol, 27.8 g/L; fructose, 55.6 g/L; amino acids, 33.3 g/L) was diluted to 1:2 on day 3 or 1:1.3 on day 4 with water. The EN solution (dextrin, 161.3 g/L; protein hydrolysate, 41.2 g/L; fat, 11.2 g/L; pH 6.5-7.5; osmoral pressure, 510-550 mOsm/kg) was diluted similarly with isotonic sodium chloride solution. On days 5 to 7, undiluted solutions were given for both TPN and EN. The administered energy intake per day was 502 kJ/kg (120 kcal/kg) on day 3, 753 kJ/kg (180 kcal/kg) on day 4, and 1004 kJ/kg (240 kcal/kg) on days 5 to 7 in all animals.

LABORATORY TESTS

All animals were reanesthetized with ether inhalation on day 7. After careful skin disinfection and draping, the abdominal cavity was opened through a wide midline

RESULTS

SURVIVAL

The survival rate was 85% (29/34)for the AP/TPN group and 74% (26/35) for the AP/EN group (**Figure 1**). There was no statistically significant difference in survival between these 2 groups. No rats died in the sham roups.

PANCREATIC PATHOLOGY

At the killing of the rats on day 7, the pancreas in the AP/TPN and AP/EN groups appeared slightly enlarged and swollen without visible areas of parenchymal or fat necrosis. No ascites were found in any rats in either group. Histological examination revealed a mixed finding of pancreatic collapse and healing fibrosis with mononuclear leukocytic infiltration of the stroma in both the AP/TPN group and the AP/EN group (**Figure 2**). There was no difference in pancreatic healing between these 2 groups. No ascites were found at the time the rats were killed, and the pancreas was grossly and histologically normal in the 2 sham groups.

TOTAL PROTEIN, ALBUMIN, AMYLASE, AND LIPASE LEVELS

Serum amylase and lipase levels were significantly lower in the AP/EN group than in the AP/TPN group (**Table 1**). There was no difference in serum total protein and albumin levels between the 2 AP groups, although they tended to be lower in the AP/EN group compared with the AP/TPN group.

laparotomy, and then blood was drawn from the aorta for determination of serum total protein, albumin, amylase, lipase, and plasma endotoxin levels. An Auto Analyzer 7170 (Hitachi Ltd, Tokyo) was used for the total protein, albumin, amylase, and lipase assays. Plasma endotoxin level was measured by means of an endotoxin-specific limulus amebocyte lysate assay (Endospecy; Seikagaku, Tokyo)[16] after pretreatment of the plasma with a conventional perchloric acid method.[17]

TISSUE HISTOLOGY

The pancreas was excised, fixed in 10% formalin, and stained with hematoxylin-eosin for histological evaluation. A 5-cm segment of the ileum, beginning 5 cm before the ileocecal junction, was also harvested, fixed in 10% formalin, and stained with hematoxylin-eosin for histological measurement of villus height. The mucosal thickness from the top of the villus to the basal level of lamina muscularis was measured with an eyepiece micrometer for 200 villi per sample and the mean value was evaluated as ileum villus height in each animal.

BrdU UPTAKE BY EPITHELIUM IN JEJUNUM

A total of 20 mg/kg of 5-bromo-2′-deoxyuridine (BrdU) (Sigma Chemical Co, St Louis, Mo) was injected intraperitoneally 1 hour before the AP-induced rats were humanely killed. At the time the animals were killed, a 5-cm segment of jejunum, beginning 5 cm beyond the pyloroduodenal junction, was taken, fixed in 70% ethanol, stained with rabbit anti-BrdU antibody (Becton Dickinson and Co, Sandy, Utah) followed by peroxidase conjugate anti-rabbit IgG (Dako Co, Carpinteria, Calif). The number of BrdU-positive epithelial cells from the bottom of the crypt to the top of the villus was measured in 200 villi in each sample, and the mean value was evaluated as BrdU uptake per crypt in the jejunum of each animal.

LYMPHOCYTE ANALYSIS WITH MONOCLONAL ANTIBODIES AND FLOW CYTOMETRY

The spleen and mesenteric lymph nodes (MLN) were teased through fine stainless steel screens into 5 mL of RPMI 1640 (Gibco, Ground Island, NY), and the heparinized peripherial blood was incubated with 100 µL of lysing solution (Cyto-Lyse; Cytec, Fremont, Calif) for 10 minutes at room temperature followed by 1 mL of distilled water to lyse red blood cells. These cell suspensions were incubated with fluorescein isothiocyanate–conjugated anti-rat CD4 antibody (W3/25) (Serotec Ltd, Kidlington, England) and phycoerythrin-conjugated anti-rat CD8 antibody (OX8) (Serotec Ltd) for 30 minutes at room temperature and analyzed using a fluorescence-activated cell sorter (FACS 440; Becton Dickinson and Co, San Jose, Calif).

BACTERIAL TRANSLOCATION TO MLN

The MLN complex from the ileocecal area to the root of the mesentery were collected into a sterile plastic bag (Organo Co, Tokyo), weighed, and homogenized with a stomacher (Tekmar, Cincinnati, Ohio) in 1 mL of sterile phosphate-buffered saline. The inoculums (100 L) of the homogenates were spread and incubated on blood agar (Becton Dickinson and Co, Cockeysville, Md) and cystin-lactose-electrolyte-deficient (CLED) agar plates (Nissui Pharmaceutical Co, Tokyo) under aerobic conditions, or on Gifu anaerobic medium agar plates (Nissui Pharmaceutical Co) under anaerobic conditions at 35°C for 48 hours, and then examined for bacterial growth. The bacterial count was calculated as log number of colony-forming units per milligram of tissue.

BACTERIAL IDENTIFICATION

Gram-negative rods were identified using the Auto-scan 4 system (Dade Behring Co Ltd, Deerfield, Ill). Gram-positive cocci and rods were identified at the genus level using standard microbiologic methods.

STATISTICAL ANALYSIS

Probability of cumulative survival were assessed by the Kaplan-Meier method, and differences were compared using the log-rank test. All laboratory data were evaluated by analysis of variance and Fisher protected least significant difference method as post hoc test using a statistical software program (StatView-J 4.5; Abacus Concepts Inc, Berkeley, Calif) with a Macintosh computer 6500/250 (Apple Computer Inc, Cupertino, Calif). Probabilities less than .05 were considered significant.

ILEUM VILLUS HEIGHT AND JEJUNUM BrdU INTAKE

Ileum villus height was significantly higher in the EN groups compared with the TPN groups for both AP and sham rats (Table 1). Furthermore, villus height was not different between AP and sham rats in either EN or TPN group. Jejunum BrdU intake, an index of enterocyte proliferation, was significantly higher in the AP/EN group than in the AP/TPN group.

CD4/CD8 RATIO

In both sham and AP rats, the CD4/CD8 ratio of T cells of spleen cells was significantly higher in the EN groups than in the TPN groups (Table 1). Although the CD4/CD8 ratio was lower in the AP/TPN group than in the sham/TPN group, there was no significant difference between AP/EN and sham/EN groups. Similar results for this ratio were seen in MLN and peripheral blood, except for MLN of rats in the AP/TPN group, which had a mean ratio as high as that in MLN of the AP/EN group.

MAGNITUDE OF BACTERIAL TRANSLOCATION IN MLN

Intravenous feeding induced bacterial translocation to MLN in the sham/TPN group, whereas no positive culture was found in the sham/EN group (**Figure 3**, top). Furthermore, AP induced a significantly greater bacterial translocation to MLN. However, the magnitude was significantly lower in the AP/EN group than in the AP/TPN group, indicating that enteral feeding prevented AP-induced bacterial translocation compared with intravenous feeding.

BACTERIAL SPECIES ISOLATED FROM MLN

Species of bacteria isolated from MLN were not different between the AP/TPN and AP/EN groups. Bacterial species were all common enteric bacteria and mostly gram-negative bacteria (**Table 2**).

PLASMA ENDOTOXIN LEVEL

The plasma endotoxin level was significantly higher in the AP/TPN group than in the AP/EN group, in which it was as low as both sham groups (Figure 3, bottom). In other words, EN prevented AP-induced endotoxin translocation from the gut to the systemic circulation.

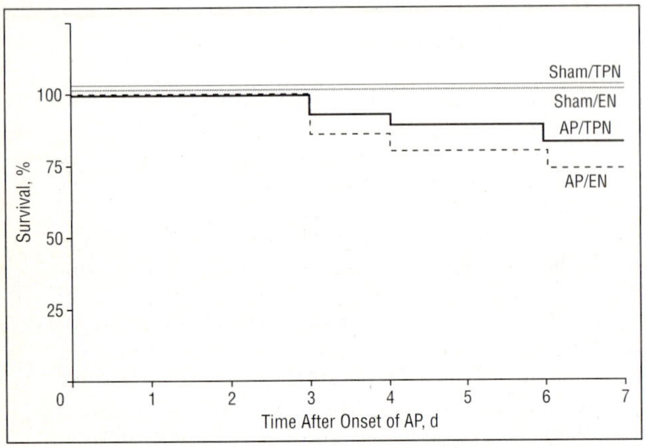

Figure 1. *Kaplan-Meier plots of overall survival in rats after onset of acute pancreatitis (AP) followed by total parenteral nutrition (TPN) (AP/TPN group) or enteral nutrition (EN) (AP/EN group), and sham operation followed by TPN (sham/TPN group) or EN (sham/EN group).*

COMMENT

Recent work in animal models has demonstrated that there is a loss of gut mucosal integrity with subsequent BET from the gut lumen to other organs in AP.[4,5] Likewise, in this study, the overall incidence of AP-induced translocation of enteric bacteria to the MLN was 100% in both AP groups, and blood endotoxin levels were significantly higher in the AP/TPN group than in the control rats (sham groups). However, few reports have demonstrated the contribution of BET to deleterious consequences for the host in experimental AP. Isaji et al[18] reported experimental data showing the effect of oral antibiotics on the prognosis and incidence of infections in diet-induced hemorrhagic AP of mice. The data suggested that reduction of the intestinal flora inhibits secondary infection caused by bacterial translocation and improves survival. However, as the authors pointed out, there is the pos-

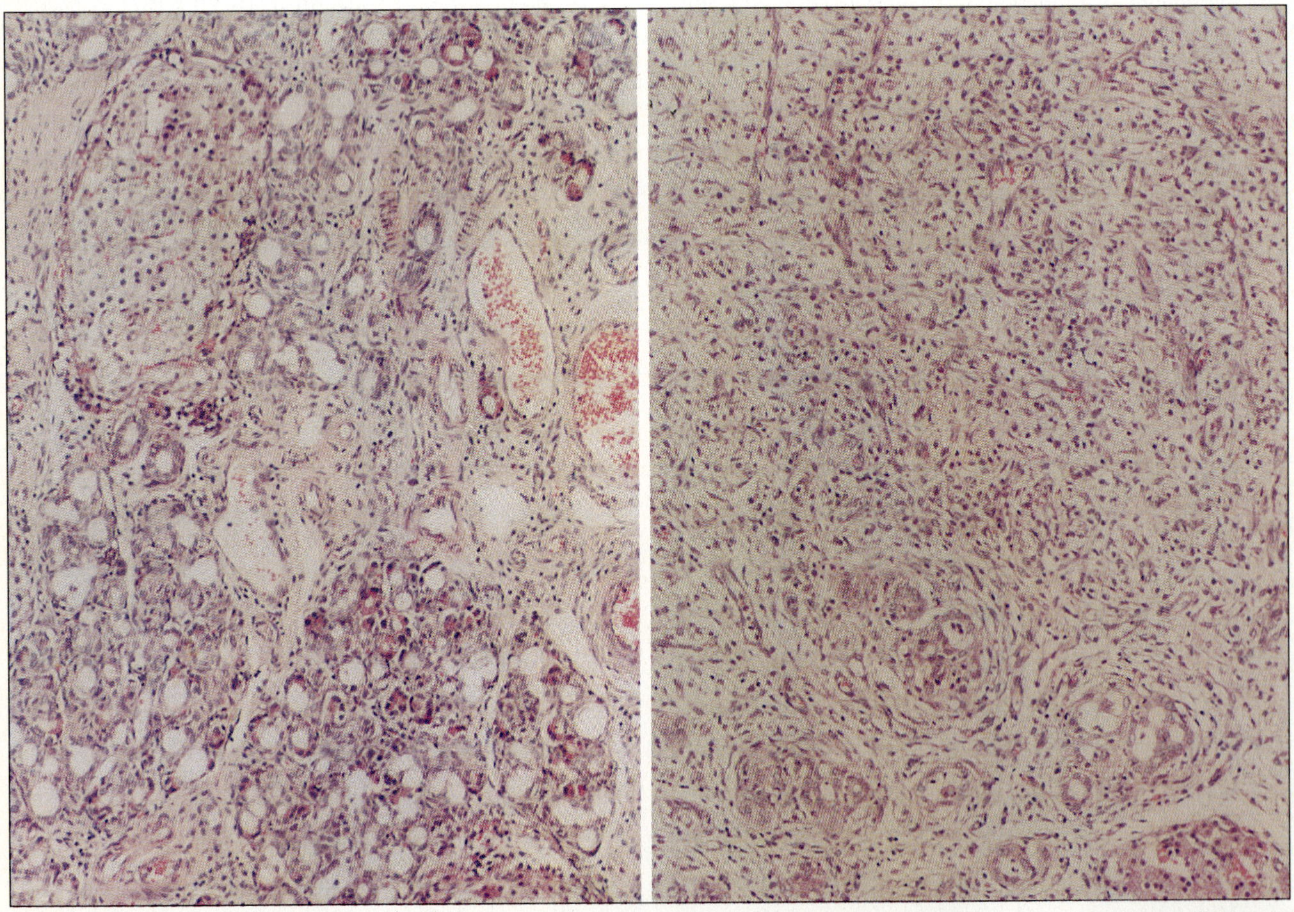

Figure 2. *Histological findings of pancreas in a rat induced with acute pancreatitis (AP) followed by total parenteral nutrition (left) and a rat induced with AP followed by enteral nutrition (right) on day 7 after AP induction (hematoxylin-eosin, magnification ×200).*

Table 1. Effect of Feeding Route and Acute Pancreatitis on Liver, Intestine, and Immune Parameters*

Parameter	Sham/TPN	Sham/EN	AP/TPN	AP/EN
Amylase, IU/L	5125 ± 71	3688 ± 423‡	4490 ± 148	3103 ± 162§
Lipase, IU/L	8.6 ± 0.5	9.7 ± 0.5	41.0 ± 9.5‡	10.0 ± 4.1§
Total protein, g/L	54 ± 3.8	56 ± 0.3	53 ± 0.9	48 ± 2.4
Albumin, g/L	40 ± 0.1	46 ± 0.5‡	39 ± 0.7	36 ± 0.1‖
Villus height of ileum, mm	0.342 ± 0.022	0.487 ± 0.024‡	0.418 ± 0.022	0.531 ± 0.016§
Jejunum BrdU (per crypt)	No data	No data	16.4 ± 0.84	21.9 ± 0.71§
CD4/CD8 ratio				
Spleen†	1.81 ± 0.023	2.62 ± 0.17‡	1.42 ± 0.07‡	2.31 ± 0.30§
Mesenteric lymph nodes†	2.94 ± 0.13	3.7 ± 0.12‡	3.76 ± 0.13‡	3.72 ± 0.31
Peripheral blood†	2.47 ± 0.04	2.51 ± 0.09	1.77 ± 0.13‡	2.81 ± 0.16§

*Data are mean ± SEM. TPN indicates total parenteral nutrition; EN, enteral nutrition; AP, acute pancreatitis; and BrdU, 5-bromo-2′-deoxyuridine.
†T cells of spleen cells, T cells of mesenteric lymph node cells, and T cells of peripheral blood cells.
‡P<.05 vs sham/TPN group.
§P<.05 vs AP/TPN group.
‖P<.05 vs sham/EN group.

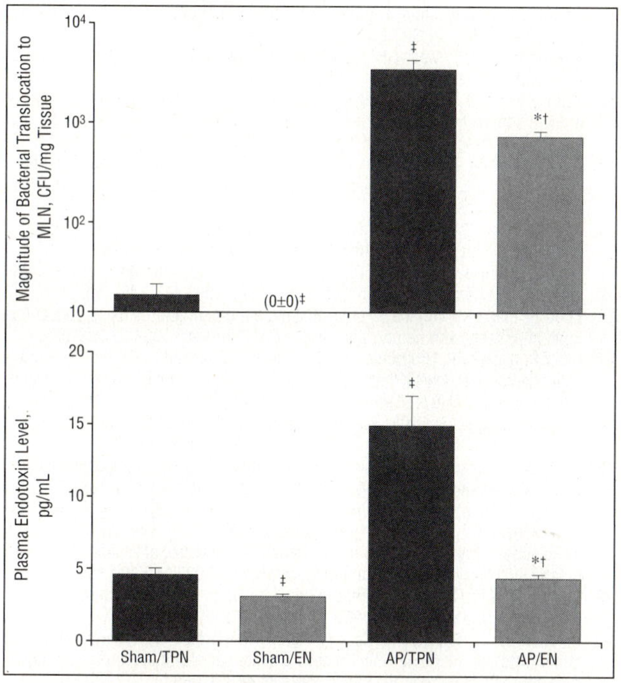

Figure 3. *Magnitude of bacterial translocation to mesenteric lymph nodes (MLN) (top) and plasma endotoxin level (bottom) in rats induced with acute pancreatitis (AP) followed by total parenteral nutrition (TPN) and enteral nutrition (EN) and rats without AP induction receiving TPN (sham/TPN) and EN (sham/EN). Asterisk indicates P<.05 vs AP/TPN group; dagger, P<.05 vs sham/EN group; and double dagger, P<.05 vs sham/TPN group. Data represent mean ± SEM. CFU indicates colony-forming unit.*

sibility that oral antibiotics might improve the survival by diminishing the severity of injury to the pancreas as a result of decreased absorption of ethionine rather than reduced translocation of bacteria from the gut.

In the present study, all bacterial species isolated from MLN were common enteric bacteria, suggesting a process whereby intestinal microflora relocated to this site. In addition, the lower magnitude of recovery of bacteria from the MLN in the AP/EN group compared with the AP/TPN group on day 7 suggests that enteral feeding (1) induced more rapid clearance of bacteria in MLN, (2) prevented continuing translocation from the intestine to MLN, and/or (3) did not permit a persistent infection in

Table 2. Rats With Bacterial Translocation to Mesenteric Lymph Nodes According to Bacterial Species Isolated*

Bacteria	AP/TPN Group (N=29)	AP/EN Group (N=26)
Escherichia coli	29 (100)	18 (69)
Enterococcus faecalis	21 (72)	26 (100)
Klebsiella pneumonia	17 (59)	5 (19)
Enterobacter aerogenes	17 (59)	5 (19)
Morganella morganii	17 (59)	3 (12)
Clostridium	4 (14)	5 (19)

*Data are number (percentage) of rats. AP/TPN indicates acute pancreatitis and total parenteral nutrition; AP/EN, acute pancreatitis and enteral nutrition.

MLN following temporary translocation from the intestine to MLN.[19] Despite the significantly lower magnitude of bacterial translocation and significantly lower blood endotoxin levels on day 7 in the AP/EN group than in the AP/TPN group, the survival rate was not different between these 2 groups. These results suggest that the presence of live bacteria in MLN does not play a decisive role for a deleterious outcome at least up to day 7 in this AP rat model. However, it is still possible that BET early after onset of AP may be responsible for the similar mortality in both groups because it is assumed that BET occurred to the same extent in both groups before EN or TPN was initiated. Furthermore, it is also possible that BET may influence the subsequent outcome after day 7. In fact, in human AP, the development of a bacterial infection has emerged as a major determinant affecting survival in patients with necrotizing pancreatitis surviving longer than 1 week,[1] although bacterial contamination in pancreatic necrosis could be detected as early as the first week.[3]

In humans, the most severe complication of AP is pancreatic infection.[3] The finding that the microorganisms causing pancreatic infection are comon enteric bacteria implies that the bacterial translocation from intestinal tract to pancreas may play a role in the pathogenesis of pancreatitis-induced sepsis, However, consistent pancreatic infection is rarely observed in experimental AP models in animals.[4,5,18,20] This was confirmed in the present study in that no organisms were found in the pancreas of rats in the AP/TPN or AP/EN groups on day 7 (data not shown). Because pancreatic infection is related to the extent of pancreatic necrosis in human[3] and animal AP,[21] one explanation for the lack of infection in this model of AP is that pancreatic necrosis was seen only after 24 hours (data not shown), but not seen on day 7 in either of the AP groups. One may thus expect pancreatitis with necrosis in a more severe and/or sustained model of pancreatitis.

Enteral feedings reportedly have several noteworthy advantages over TPN other than for the prevention of BET. In a number of disease states, such as AP, burns, trauma, and sepsis, EN decreases risk of nosocomial infection, multiple-organ failure, and length of hospitalization,[22-26] and lowers cost[27] when compared with TPN. These advantages of EN might be due to restoration of defective macrophage function,[15] attenuation of both the counterregulatory hormone and enhanced proinflammatory cytokine responses,[27] down-regulation of coagulation,[28] and normalization of the tumor necrosis factor receptor systems.[29] Recent evidence in both animal and human studies suggests that elemental or semi-elemental small peptide formulas are well tolerated, and efficiently absorbed in the gut lumen with little or no pancreatic enzyme secretion.[30-32] Previous studies have shown that jejunal feeding results in negligible increases in pancreatic enzyme, bicarbonate, and volume output from the pancreas.[33,34] Similarly, the present study showed that jejunal administration of small peptide formulas was well tolerated in AP-induced rats. Furthermore, compared with TPN, early EN not only maintained normal intestinal structure, which is probably implicated in increased enterocyte proliferation, but also restored the depressed CD4/CD8 ratio of T cells, suggesting that early EN can potentially maintain immune system integrity during AP. Further studies regarding the safety and efficacy of EN via jejunal feeding in AP are needed.

In summary, jejunal administration of EN was well tolerated in early AP, maintained immune responsiveness and gut integrity, and reduced BET. However, compared with TPN, EN did not improve outcome. These results suggest that BET to MLN is not associated with deleterious consequences for the host during the early period of experimental AP in rats. Finally, factors other than BET may be responsible for mortality in the rat AP model.

This study was supported by a research grant from Otsuka Pharmaceutical Factory Inc, Naruto, Tokushima, Japan, and Alpha Therapeutic Corporation, Los Angeles, Calif.

Presented at the 18th Annual Meeting of the Surgical Infection Society, New York, NY, May 1, 1998.

We thank Steve E. Calvano, PhD, and Edward Lin, DO, for help with preparation of the manuscript. We acknowledge the help of Syohiro Kinoshita, BS, Hiroomi Yokoyama, PhD, Yoshiyuki Shinagawa, BS, Seiichiro Kano, BS, and Keiichi Okamoto, BS, in the development of this project.

Reprints: Joji Kotani, MD, Department of Surgery, University of Medicine and Dentistry of New Jersey–Robert Wood Johnson Medical School, Surgical Science, CAB, Room 7076, 125 Patterson St, New Brunswick, NJ 08903-0019 (e-mail: kotani4@ibm.net).

REFERENCES

1. Renner IG, Savage WT III, Pantoja JL, Renner VJ. Death due to acute pancreatitis: a retrospective analysis of 405 autopsy cases. *Dig Dis Sci.* 1985;30:1005-1018.
2. Lumsden A, Bradley EL III. Secondary pancreatic infection: abscess, infected necrosis, and infected pseudocyst. *Surg Gynecol Obstet.* 1990;170:459-467.
3. Beger HG, Bittner R, Block S, Buchler M. Bacterial contamination of pancreatic necrosis: a prospective clinical study. *Gastroenterology.* 1986;91:433-438.
4. Runkel NS, Moody FG, Smith GS, et al. The role of the gut in the development of sepsis in acute pancreatitis. *J Surg Res.* 1991;51:18-23.
5. Liu Q, Djuricin G, Nathan C, Gattuso P, Weinstein RA, Prinz RA. The effect of epidermal growth factor on the septic complications of acute pancreatitis. *J Surg Res.* 1997;69:171-177.
6. Deitch EA. The role of intestinal failure and bacterial translocation in the development of systemic infection and multiple organ failure. *Arch Surg.* 1990;125:403-404.
7. Berg RD. Bacterial translocation from the gastrointestinal tract. *J Med.* 1992;23:217-214.
8. Maddaus MA, Wells CL, Platt JL, Condie RM, Simmons RL. Effect on T cell modulation on the translocation of bacteria from the gut and mesenteric lymph node. *Ann Surg.* 1988;207:387-398.
9. Williams RC, Gibbons RJ. Inhibition of bacterial adherence by secretory immunoglobin: a mechanisms of antigen disposal. *Science.* 1972;177:697-699.
10. Barber AE, Jones WG II, Minei JP, Fahey TJ III, Lowry SF, Shires GT. Bacterial overgrowth and intestinal atrophy in the etiology of gut barrier failure in the rat. *Am J Surg.* 1991;161:300-304.
11. Alverdy JC, Aoys E, Moss GS. Total parenteral nutrition promotes bacterial translocation from the gut. *Surgery.* 1988;104:185-190.
12. Saito H, Trocki O, Alexander JW, Kopcha R, Heyd T, Joffe SN. The effect of route of nutrient administration on the nutritional state, catabolic hormone secretion, and gut mucosal integrity after burn injury. *JPEN J Parenter Enteral Nutr.* 1987;11:1-7.
13. Illig KA, Ryan CK, Hardry DJ, Rhodes J, Locke W, Sax HL. Total parenteral nutrition-induced changes in gut mucosal function: atrophy alone is not the issue. *Surgery.* 1992;112:631-637.
14. Alverdy J, Chi HS, Sheldon GF. The effect of parenteral nutrition on gastrointestinal immunity: the importance of enteral stimulation. *Ann Surg.* 1985;202:681-684.
15. Shou J, Lappin J, Minnard EA, Daly JM. Total parenteral nutrition, bacterial translocation, and host immune function. *Am J Surg.* 1994;167:145-150.
16. Endo S, Inada K, Yamada Y, et al. Plasma endotoxin and cytokine concentrations in patients with hemorragic shock. *Crit Care Med.* 1994;22:949-955.
17. Ditter B, Becker KP, Urbascheck R, Urbasheck B. Quantitative endotoxin determination: automated kinetic limulus amebocyte lysate microtiter test with measurement of sample related interference. *Arzneimittelforschung.* 1983;22:681-687.
18. Isaji S, Suzuki M, Frey CF, Ruebner B, Carlson J. Role of bacterial infection in diet-induced acute pancreatitis in mice. *Int J Pancreatol.* 1992;11:49-57.
19. Wells CL, Maddaus MA, Jechorek RP, Simmons RL. Ability of intestinal *Escherichia coli* to survive within mesenteric lymph nodes. *Infect Immun.* 1987;55:2834.
20. Runkel NS, Rodriguez LF, Moody FG. Mechanisms of sepsis in acute pancreatitis in opossums. *Am J Surg.* 1995;169:227-232.
21. Widdison AL, Karanjia ND, Alvarez C, Reber HA. Influence of levamisole on pancreatic infection in acute pancreatitis. *Am J Surg.* 1992;163:100-104.
22. Zaloga GP, MacGregor DA. What to consider when choosing enteral or parenteral nutrition. *J Crit Illness.* 1990;5:1180-1200.
23. Kalfarentzos F, Kehagias J, Mead N, Kokkinis K, Gogos CA, Enteral nutrition is superior to parenteral nutrition in severe acute pancreatitis: results of a randomozed prospective trial. *Br J Surg.* 1997;84:1665-1669.
24. Moore EE, Moore FA. Immediate enteral nutrition following multi-system trauma: a decade perspective. *J Am Coll Nutr.* 1991;10:633-648.
25. Kudsk KA, Croce MA, Fabian TC, et al. Enteral versus parenteral feeding: effects on septic morbidity after blunt and penetrating abdominal trauma. *Ann Surg.* 1992;215:503-511.
26. McClave SA, Greene LM, Snider HL, et al. Comparison of the safety of early enteral vs parenteral nutrition in mild acute pancreatitis. *JPEN J Parenter Enteral Nutr.* 1997;21:14-20.
27. Fong YM, Marano MA, Barber A, et al. Total parenteral nutrition and bowel rest modify the metabolic response to endotoxin in humans. *Ann Surg.* 1989;210:449-457.
28. van der Poll T, Levi M, Braxton CC, et al. Parenteral nutrition facilitates activation of coaglation but not of fibrinolysis during human endotoxemia. *J Infect Dis.* 1998;177:793-795.
29. Braxton CC, Coyle SM, Montegut WJ, et al. Parenteral nutrition alters monocyte TNF receptor activity. *J Surg Res.* 1995;59:23-28.
31. Imondi AR, Stradley RP. Utilization of enzymatically hydrolyzed soybean protein and crystalline amino acid diets by rats with exocrine pancreatic insufficiency. *J Nutr.* 1974;104:793-801.
32. Milla PJ, Kilby A, Rassam UB, Ersser R, Harries JT. Small intestinal absorption of aminoacids and a dipeptide in pancreatic insufficiency. *Gut.* 1983;24:818-824.
33. Vison N, Hecketsweiler P, Butel J, Bernier JJ. Effect of continuous jejunal perfusion of elemental and complex nutritional solutions on pancreatic enzyme secretion in human subjects. *Gut.* 1978;19:194-198.
34. Ragins H, Levenson SM, Signer R, Stamford W, Seifter E. Intrajejunal administration of an elemental diet at neutral pH avoids pancreatic stimulation. *Am J Surg.* 1973;126:606-614.

ORIGINAL ARTICLE

Nitric Oxide and Thromboxane A_2–Mediated Pulmonary Microvascular Dysfunction

Joseph K. Wright, MD; Lawrence T. Kim, MD; Tom E. Rogers, MD; Hao Nguyen, PhD; Richard H. Turnage, MD

Objectives: To examine whether the lung releases nitric oxide (NO) in response to thromboxane A_2 and to examine the local release of NO as a protective compensatory mechanism by which the lung responds to the proinflammatory and vasoactive effects of thromboxane A_2.

Design: The lungs of anesthetized Sprague-Dawley rats were perfused in vitro with Krebs-Henseleit buffer that contained an inhibitor of NO synthase (nitroglycerine-nitro-L-arginine methyl ester [L-NAME]) (10^{-4} mol/L), an NO donor (sodium nitroprusside) (10^{-8} mol/L), or perfusate alone. Following equilibration, the thromboxane A_2 receptor agonist 9,11-dideoxy-11α, 9α-epoxymethanoprostaglandin $F_{2\alpha}$ (U-46 619) (7.1×10^{-8} mol/L) was added to the perfusate. Fifteen minutes later, the capillary filtration coefficient, pulmonary arterial pressure, and vascular resistance were measured. Pulmonary NO release was assessed by quantitating the release of cyclic guanosine monophosphate into the perfusate.

Results: The capillary filtration coefficient of lungs exposed to U-46 619 was 3.5 times greater than that of lungs perfused with buffer alone ($P<.05$). The addition of sodium nitroprusside reduced the increase in capillary filtration coefficient associated with U-46 619 by 50% ($P<.05$) whereas L-NAME had no effect. The addition of U-46 619 to the perfused lung caused a 3.0 ± 0.4 mm Hg increase in pulmonary artery pressure ($P<.01$) with a corresponding rise in total vascular resistance ($P<.05$). This effect was exacerbated by L-NAME ($P<.05$) and inhibited by sodium nitroprusside ($P<.05$). Exposure of the isolated lungs to U-46 619 caused a 4-fold increase in cyclic guanosine monophosphate levels within the perfusate.

Conclusion: These data are consistent with the hypothesis that NO release may be an important protective mechanism by which the lung responds to thromboxane A_2.

Arch Surg. 1999;134:293-298

THROMBOXANE A_2 (TXA_2) has important proinflammatory effects on the pulmonary microvasculature that include vasoconstriction, enhanced permeability, and neutrophil and platelet activation. It has been incriminated in the pathogenesis of acute lung injury following remote organ reperfusion,[1] pulmonary ischemia-reperfusion injury,[2] and endotoxemia.[3] Clinically, TXA_2 is thought to be involved in the pathogenesis of adult respiratory distress syndrome and primary and secondary pulmonary hypertension.[4]

In each of these inflammatory states, the lungs release substances possessing anti-inflammatory and vasodilatory effects. These agents may serve to limit or abrogate the potentially injurious effects of TXA_2 and other proinflammatory mediators. The constitutive release of nitric oxide (NO) by the vascular endothelium likely serves a particularly important function. The release of picomolar quantities of NO by the vascular endothelium has been shown to maintain normal microvascular permeability,[5] inhibit neutrophil-endothelial cell adherence,[6] and maintain normal tissue perfusion through its role as a potent and important vasodilator.[7] Our series of experiments examine the role of NO in counteracting the proinflammatory and vasoactive effects of TXA_2. In particular, we examine whether the lungs generate NO in response to TXA_2 exposure and whether this is one of the protective mechanisms by which the lungs compensate for the vasoactive and proinflammatory effects of TXA_2.

RESULTS

EFFECT OF TXA_2 RECEPTOR ACTIVATION ON PULMONARY cGMP RELEASE

The addition of U-46 619 to the perfusate of the isolated, perfused lung caused a 4-fold increase in cGMP release. This increase was totally prevented by the presence of L-NAME within the perfusate. The concentration of cGMP within the perfusate of lungs exposed to U-46 619 was 0.43 ± 0.03 pmol/mL per gram of lung

From the Departments of Surgery (Drs Wright, Kim, Nguyen, and Turnage) and Pathology (Dr Rogers), University of Texas Southwestern Medical School and Dallas Veterans Affairs Medical Center, Dallas.

MATERIALS AND METHODS

ISOLATED, PERFUSED LUNG MODEL

Pathogen-free Sprague-Dawley rats (weight, 250-350 g) were anesthetized with pentobarbital sodium (40 mg/kg, intraperitoneally). The pulmonary arterial trunk and left atrium were cannulated via the right and left ventricles, respectively, and the heart and lungs excised en bloc. The lungs were suspended by a ligature from a force transducer (TSD 125C; Biopac Systems Inc, Santa Barbara, Calif) for continuous measurement of lung weight. The lungs were perfused with Krebs-Henseleit buffer that contained 3% bovine serum albumin at 0.04 mL · gram body weight^{-1} · minute^{-1} and ventilated with room air at a rate of 60 strokes per minute. Pulmonary arterial (PA) and left venous (PV) pressures were continuously measured with pressure transducers (TSD 104A; Biopac Systems Inc) with 0 reference at the level of the apex of the lung. These measurements were continuously recorded by a data acquisition unit (MP100 Manager version 3.2.3; hardware version 1.1f, Biopac Systems Inc) interfaced with a personal computer (Dell Computer Corp, Austin, Tex). The perfusate was maintained in a 37°C water bath. The first 75 mL of perfusate was discarded to remove blood elements from the vascular space; the perfusate was recirculated after that. Pulmonary venous pressure was maintained at 2 to 3 mm Hg and all lungs were perfused under zone 3 conditions with PA > PV > PAIRWAY. The lungs were isogravimetric throughout the experiment.

EXPERIMENTAL PROTOCOL

The experimental protocol is shown in **Figure 1**. The lungs were perfused with Krebs-Henseleit buffer either alone (10^{-8} mol/L) or containing the NO donor sodium nitroprusside (SNP) (10^{-10} mol/L) or the NO synthase inhibitor nitroglycerine-nitro-L-arginine-methyl ester (L-NAME) (Sigma-Aldrich Co, St Louis, Mo) (10^{-4} mol/L and 10^{-2} mol/L). These doses of SNP have been previously demonstrated to induce vasodilatation in a similar experimental protocol using the isolated, perfused lung model.[8] The dose of L-NAME has been shown to inhibit NO formation by nearly 100% in cultured endothelial cells[9] and has been previously used in similar experiments with the isolated, perfused lung model.[10,11] Following a 15-minute period of equilibration, baseline measurements of PA and PV were obtained, from which pulmonary vascular resistance (R_t) was calculated. The TXA_2 receptor agonist 9,11-dideoxy-11α, 9α-epoxymethanoprostaglandin $F_{2\alpha}$ (U-46 619) (7.1×10^{-8} mol/L) was then added to the perfusate. Fifteen minutes later, PA and PV pressures were recorded and the capillary filtration coefficient (K_f) and R_t determined. This dose of U-46 619 is similar to that used by other investigators in this experimental system[12] and induces an increase in pulmonary microvascular permeability similar to that of several in vivo injury models, including intestinal reperfusion injury.[1] In preliminary experiments, a dose-response relationship was demonstrated between increases in U-46 619 concentrations (10^{-11} to 10^{-7} mol/L) and increases in K_f. Furthermore, this increase in K_f was totally prevented by the TXA_2 receptor antagonist SQ-29 548 (data not shown). Perfusate was collected for the measurement of cyclic guanosine monophosphate (cGMP) concentration.

MEASUREMENT OF PULMONARY MICROVASCULAR DYSFUNCTION

Capillary Filtration Coefficient

Pulmonary microvascular permeability was quantitated by determining the K_f as described by Drake et al.[13] Fifteen minutes after the addition of U-46 619, the capillary pressure was measured using the double occlusion technique.[14] Pulmonary venous pressure was then elevated from

weight. This was significantly greater than that of lungs perfused with Krebs-Henseleit buffer alone (0.10 ± 0.01 pmol/mL per gram of lung weight, $P<.001$). The concentration of cGMP within the perfusate of lungs exposed to U-46 619 and L-NAME was 85% less than that of lungs exposed to U-46 619 alone ($P<.001$).

EFFECT OF TXA_2 RECEPTOR ACTIVATION ON PULMONARY MICROVASCULAR FUNCTION

Capillary Filtration Coefficient

The addition of U-46 619 to the isolated, perfused lung model resulted in a 3-fold increase in K_f when compared with lungs perfused with buffer alone ($P<.01$). This is illustrated in **Figure 2**. The K_f of lungs perfused with U-46 619 (7.1×10^{-8} mol/L) and SQ-29 548 (2 μmol/L) was 0.006 ± 0.002 g · minute^{-1} · millimeters of mercury^{-1} · 100 g body weight^{-1}. This was not different than that of lungs exposed to Krebs-Henseleit buffer alone (0.007 ± 0.001 g · minute^{-1} · millimeters of mercury^{-1} · 100 g of body weight^{-1}). These data suggest that the effects of U-46 619 are mediated through activation of the TXA_2 receptor and not a toxic or nonspecific effect.

Pulmonary Vascular Resistance

The addition of U-46 619 to the isolated, perfused lung model resulted in prompt vasoconstriction, with an average increase in PA of 3.0 ± 0.3 mm Hg over baseline measurements ($P<.01$). These data are shown in **Figure 3**. As expected, U-46 619 altered R_t in a manner similar to PA. These data are shown in **Figure 4**.

EFFECT OF NO ON TXA_2-MEDIATED CHANGES IN PULMONARY MICROVASCULAR FUNCTION

Capillary Filtration Coefficient

Inhibition of NO release with L-NAME (10^{-4} mol/L) had no effect on U-46 619–induced changes in K_f. These data are shown in Figure 2. Even a 100-fold increase in the dose of L-NAME (10^{-2} mol/L) did not significantly alter the effect of U-46 619 on K_f (0.019 ± 0.003 g · minute^{-1} · millimeters of mercury^{-1} · 100 g of body weight^{-1}). The addition of SNP (10^{-8} mol/L) to the perfusate reduced U-46 619–induced changes in K_f by 50% ($P<.01$). A 100-fold decrease in the concentration of SNP (10^{-10} mol/L) had a similar

8 to 10 mm Hg by raising the height of the venous reservoir. This resulted in a 2-component weight gain consisting of an initial rapid increase related primarily to recruitment and distention of the vascular bed (minutes 0-1) and a second slow, constant weight increase due to fluid filtration across the microvasculature (minutes 1-5). After 5 minutes of partial venous occlusion, capillary pressure was again measured (prior to releasing the partial outflow occlusion). The K_f was calculated:

$$K_f = (\Delta W/\Delta T)/\Delta P,$$

where ΔW is the change in lung weight between minutes 1 and 5 of partial venous outflow occlusion; ΔT is the duration of partial outflow occlusion during which ΔW is measured; and ΔP is the difference between the partial outflow occlusion and the capillary pressure. The K_f is normalized to body weight and expressed as gram · minute^{-1} · millimeters of mercury^{-1} · 100 g body weight^{-1}.

Pulmonary Vascular Resistance

Immediately prior to the addition of U-46 619, PA and PV pressures were recorded and compared with measurements obtained 15 minutes after the addition of U-46 619. The total R_t was calculated as the total pressure drop across the lung:

$$R_t = (PA-PV)/Q,$$

where Q is the flow through the isolated perfused lung. The calculation of pulmonary vascular resistance was normalized for body weight and expressed as the difference before and after treatment with U-46 619 (millimeters of mercury · milliliters^{-1} · minute^{-1} · 100 g body weight^{-1}).

REAGENTS

Krebs-Henseleit buffer was made fresh daily from a stock solution. The pH of the solution was 7.4 to 7.5 and remained stable throughout the perfusion. Bovine serum albumin (3 g/100 mL; Sigma-Aldrich Co) was added to the perfusate immediately prior to use. Sodium nitroprusside (Gensia Pharmaceuticals Inc, Irvine, Calif) was suspended in sterile water and then diluted in the perfusate daily for a working solution. Nitroglycerine-nitro-L-arginine-methyl ester (Sigma-Aldrich Co) was suspended in perfusate daily prior to use. The U-46 619 (Cayman Chemical Co, Ann Arbor, Mich) was supplied as a stock solution in methyl acetate and diluted in perfusate daily for a final concentration of 7.1×10^{-8} mol/L. In one experiment, the specificity of U-46 619 was examined by adding the TXA_2 antagonist SQ-29 548 (2 μmol/L) (Cayman Chemical Co) to the perfusate of the isolated, perfused lung apparatus. This agent was suspended in ethanol and then diluted in perfusate for a concentration of 200 mol/L prior to use.

MEASUREMENT OF NO RELEASE

A 1-mL aliquot of perfusate was obtained from the venous port of the isolated, perfused lung at the conclusion of the experiment. This was frozen at −20°C until assayed for cGMP by a commercially available enzyme immunoassay (Cayman Chemical Co). Nitric oxide activates soluble guanylyl cyclase, converting GMP to cGMP. Increased concentrations of cGMP are thought to reflect endogenous NO generation.[12]

STATISTICAL ANALYSIS

All data are expressed as mean ± SEM. Analysis of unpaired data from 2 groups was performed using a 2-tailed, unpaired Student t test. Data from multiple groups were compared by analysis of variance with a Fisher post hoc test (StatView R 4.0; Abacus Concepts, Berkeley, Calif). Statistical significance was considered for a type I error of less than 5%. All experiments have been approved by the Committee on the Care and Use of Animals at the University of Texas Southwestern Medical School and Dallas Veterans Affairs Medical Center.

effect on U-46 619–induced changes in K_f (0.006 ± 0.001 g · minute^{-1} · millimeters of mercury^{-1} · 100 g body weight^{-1}). In the absence of U-46 619, the addition of SNP or L-NAME had no effect on the K_f of Krebs-Henseleit buffer–perfused lungs.

Pulmonary Vascular Resistance

The effect of L-NAME and SNP on U-46 619–induced vasoconstriction is shown in Figures 3 and 4. In contrast to its effect on K_f, the presence of L-NAME in the perfusate of the isolated, perfused lung notably enhanced the vasoconstrictive effects of U-46 619. The change in PA induced by U-46 619 in the presence of L-NAME was twice that induced by U-46 619 alone ($P<.01$). The change in R_t of lungs exposed to L-NAME and U-46 619 was about 60% greater than that of lungs treated with U-46 619 alone ($P = .06$). The addition of the 10-mmol/L concentration of L-NAME to the isolated, perfused lung did not result in greater vasoconstriction than that induced by the 100-μmol/L concentration. The addition of SNP (10^{-8} and 10^{-10} mol/L) to the perfusate completely abolished the vasoconstrictive effects of U-46 619 with or without L-NAME. The addition of L-NAME or SNP to the perfusate of the isolated, perfused lung in the absence of U-46619 had no effect on PA or R_t.

COMMENT

These experiments are consistent with the hypothesis that the lungs release NO as a protective, compensatory mechanism in response to TXA_2. Evidence is provided by the observations that (1) cGMP is released by the lungs in response to TXA_2 receptor activation; (2) inhibition of the constitutive release of NO by the lungs exacerbates the vasoconstrictive effects of U-46 619; and (3) the provision of exogenous NO attenuates the vasoconstriction and increased capillary permeability that characterizes TXA_2-mediated microvascular dysfunction.

Thromboxane A_2 has been incriminated in the pathogenesis of pulmonary microvascular dysfunction in adult respiratory distress syndrome[4] and in a plethora of animal models of acute lung injury.[1-3] The U-46 619 binds and activates TXA_2 receptor and is a useful tool for studying its effects on microvascular function.[15] The principal effects of the activation of TXA_2 receptor on the mi-

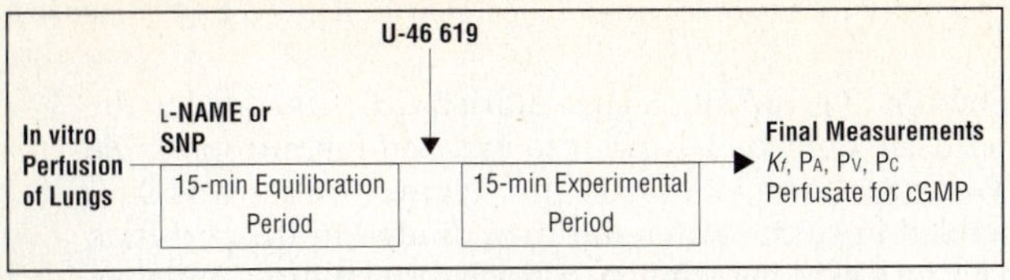

Figure 1. *In the experimental protocol, normal rat lungs were perfused with Krebs-Henseleit buffer (10^{-4} mol/L) with or without the nitric oxide synthase inhibitor nitroglycerine-nitro-L-arginine methyl ester (L-NAME) (10^{-10} mol/L) or the nitric oxide donor sodium nitroprusside (SNP) (10^{-4} and 10^{-2} mol/L). The thromboxane A_2 receptor agonist 9,11-dideoxy-11α,9α-epoxymethanoprostaglandin $F_{2\alpha}$ (U-46 619) (7.1×10^{-8} mol/L) was added to the perfusate. Pulmonary microvascular dysfunction was then quantitated by measuring the capillary filtration coefficient (K_f) and pulmonary artery (PA), venous (PV), and capillary (PC) pressures. Perfusate was also sampled for measurement of cyclic guanosine monophosphate (cGMP) concentrations as an index of nitric oxide release.*

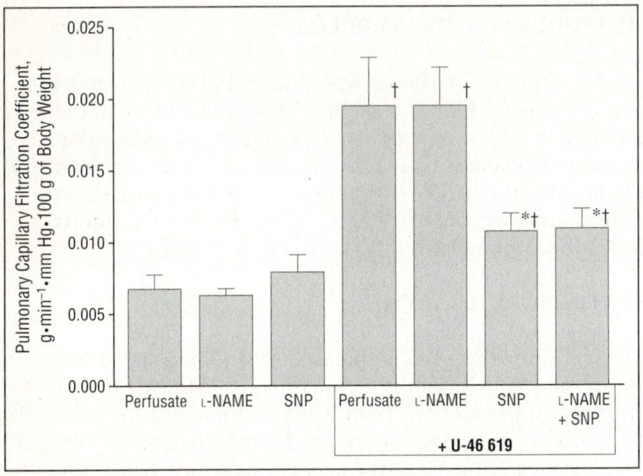

Figure 2. *The effect of the thromboxane A_2 receptor agonist 9,11-dideoxy-11α,9α-epoxymethanoprostoglandin $F_{2\alpha}$ (U-46 619) (7.1×10^{-8} mol/L) on the pulmonary capillary filtration coefficient (K_f) of isolated, perfused lungs exposed to nitroglycerine-nitro-L-arginine methyl ester (L-NAME) (10^{-4} mol/L) and sodium nitroprusside (SNP) (10^{-8} mol/L). The K_f is expressed as grams · minutes^{-1} · millimeters of mercury^{-1} · 100 g body weight^{-1} (asterisk indicates $P<.05$ vs perfusate alone; dagger, $P<.05$ vs perfusate + U-46 619).*

crovasculature include vasoconstriction that results in increased capillary hydrostatic pressure and enhanced permeability to fluid and solutes. Together, these phenomena contribute to the development of pulmonary edema during systemic inflammatory states.

Our study demonstrates that within 15 minutes of TXA_2 receptor activation there is a 4-fold increase in pulmonary NO release. These findings are similar to those of Wilson et al[12,16] using a similar experimental model. Many investigators have implicated increased vascular shear stress as an important signal for endothelial NO release.[12,16-18] Vascular shear stress is proportional to the flow rate and viscosity of the perfusate and inversely proportional to the diameter of the vessel. Hence, vasoconstrictors such as U-46 619 should increase the shear forces in vessels perfused at a constant flow rate such as in our study. Wilson et al[12] demonstrated that the addition of U-46 619 to lungs perfused at a constant rate increased NO release; this effect was not observed with those perfused at a constant pressure. Other investigators have related NO release in isolated lung models to increasing perfusate viscosity[16] and flow rates.[19]

Our study also suggests that the constitutive re-

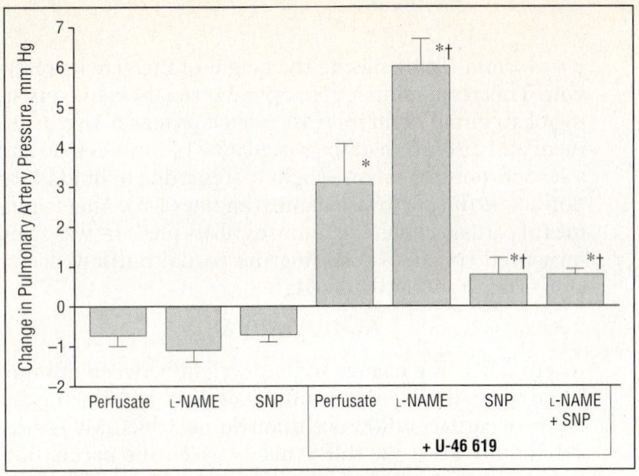

Figure 3. *The effect of thromboxane A_2 receptor agonist 9,11-dideoxy-11α,9α-epoxymethanoprostaglandin $F_{2\alpha}$ (U-46 619) (7.1×10^{-8} mol/L) on the pulmonary artery pressure of Krebs-Henseleit buffer–perfused lungs exposed to nitroglycerine-nitro-L-arginine methyl ester (L-NAME) (10^{-4} mol/L) and sodium nitroprusside (SNP) (10^{-8} mol/L). These data are expressed as the difference in pulmonary artery pressure before and 15 minutes after the addition of U-46 619 to the perfusate (asterisk indicates $P<.01$ vs perfusate alone; dagger, $P<.01$ vs U-46 619 alone).*

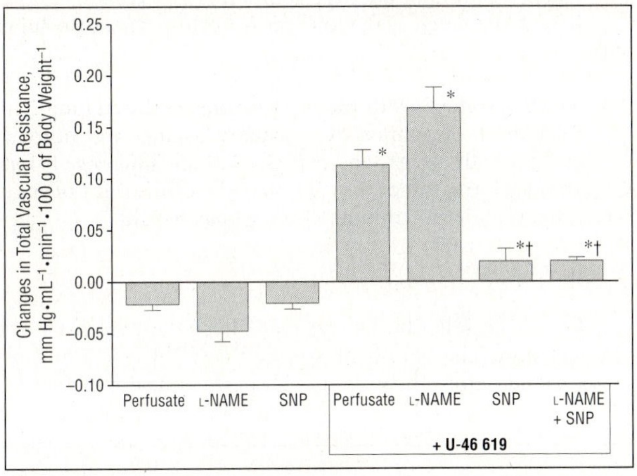

Figure 4. *The effect of thromboxane A_2 receptor agonist 9,11-dideoxy-11α,9α-epoxymethanoprostaglandin $F_{2\alpha}$ (U-46 619) (7.1×10^{-8} mol/L) on the total vascular resistance of Krebs-Henseleit buffer–perfused lungs exposed to nitroglycerine-nitro-L-arginine methyl ester (L-NAME) (10^{-4} mol/L) and sodium nitroprusside (SNP) (10^{-8} mol/L). These data are expressed as the difference in vascular resistance before and 15 minutes after the addition of U-46 619 to the perfusate and as millimeters of mercury · milliliters^{-1} · minutes^{-1} · 100 g of body weight^{-1} (asterisk indicates $P<.01$ vs perfusate alone; dagger, $P<.01$ vs U-46 619 alone).*

lease of NO by the pulmonary vascular endothelium attenuates the vasoconstrictive effects of TXA_2. Evidence is provided by the observations that L-NAME enhances and SNP prevents U-46 619–induced pulmonary vasoconstriction. Similar results have been reported by other investigators using the isolated, perfused lung model in which U-46 619–induced vasoconstriction was found to be augmented by the NO synthase inhibitor N^{ω}-methyl-L-arginine and the soluble, guanylyl cyclase inhibitor 6-anilino-5,8-quinolinodione (LY 83583).[12] In other in vivo and in vitro models of acute lung injury, NO administered by inhalation or intravascular NO donors attenuates the vasoconstrictive effects of oxidants,[10,20] remote organ injury,[21,22] and endotoxemia[23]; agents that inhibit NO release enhance the vasoconstrictive effects of these injuries.[10,20,21,23] The therapeutic potential of these findings has been realized with the use of inhaled NO in the management of patients with adult respiratory distress syndrome and other disease states in which pulmonary hypertension is a important component.[24,25]

It is less clear whether endothelial-derived NO protects the lung from TXA_2-mediated changes in microvascular permeability. This conclusion is based principally on the observation that inhibiting NO release with L-NAME had no effect on U-46 619–induced changes in K_f; however, the NO donor SNP attenuated U-46 619–induced changes in permeability. One would have anticipated that if endogenous NO release protects the pulmonary microvasculature from TXA_2-mediated changes in permeability, inhibition of NO synthesis would exaggerate the changes in K_f associated with U-46 619.

These results may have been related to the neutrophil-depleted nature of this experimental model. Investigators using similar buffer-perfused lung models have demonstrated that inhibition of NO synthase does not affect microvascular permeability in either normal or acutely injured lungs.[10,11] In contrast, the provision of even small quantities of NO has been shown to protect the lung from TXA_2-mediated microvascular dysfunction and dysfunction associated with oxidant exposure,[10] pulmonary ischemia-reperfusion injury,[11] and remote tissue reperfusion injury.[21,22,26] Interestingly, in vivo models of acute lung injury show that inhibition of NO synthase with L-NAME notably increased the extravasation of plasma proteins into the lung.[21,26] In each of these models, L-NAME–induced increases in pulmonary microvascular permeability have been associated with increases in neutrophil sequestration within the lung, a phenomenon prevented by NO donors. These data are consistent with the findings of Kurose et al,[27] who attributed, at least in part, L-NAME–induced increases in intestinal microvascular permeability to neutrophil recruitment and to neutrophil-mediated tissue injury. In these and subsequent studies, inhibition of NO synthesis with L-NAME has been shown to up-regulate the expression of many endothelial adhesion glycoproteins, including P-selectin and intracellular adhesion molecule–1, suggesting an important functional relationship between endothelial-derived NO production and the expression of various endothelial adhesion molecules.[27,28]

There are several potential mechanisms by which exogenously administered NO may have attenuated TXA_2-mediated changes in microvascular permeability. One of these mechanisms is a direct effect on the endothelial cytoskeleton along with stress fiber disassembly and expansion of intercellular junctions.[29-31] Nitric oxide has been postulated to maintain normal microvascular permeability by preserving endothelial cytoskeletal integrity and normal intercellular junctions,[27,32] although the mechanisms by which this might occur are poorly defined.

Given the neutrophil-depleted nature of the isolated, perfused lung system used in our study, it would seem unlikely that the primary effector of TXA_2-mediated changes in microvascular function is the neutrophil. Nevertheless, Siebert et al[33] have suggested that neutrophils sequestered within the pulmonary microvasculature during harvesting of the lungs may contribute to the microvascular dysfunction in this experimental model. This may be particularly relevant given the previously described relationship between the constitutive release of NO and neutrophil-mediated tissue injury.[21,26-28]

Last, the release of NO by the vascular endothelium may also serve to limit oxygen-free, radical-mediated endothelial injury. Nitric oxide inhibits neutrophil superoxide anion production by a direct effect on nicotinamide adenine dinucleotide phosphate oxidase.[34] Furthermore, many investigators have presented evidence that NO released constitutively by the endothelium scavenges superoxide radical and prevents oxidant-mediated tissue injury.[35,36] In addition, NO may also induce the synthesis and activity of other antioxidants such as heme oxygenase.[37]

Many laboratory studies and a handful of clinical studies have sparked tremendous enthusiasm for the development of therapeutic regimens that either augment NO delivery to the microvasculature or inhibit its exaggerated production. Dysfunction of NO formation by the vascular endothelium has been implicated in the pathogenesis of diseases as diverse as hypertension, hypercholesterolemia, diabetes mellitus, ischemia reperfusion injury, angina pectoris, and various forms of circulatory shock.[38-43] Several investigators have suggested that the administration of NO by inhalation may be associated with notable improvement in pulmonary function in patients with adult respiratory distress syndrome.[24,25] Our study suggests that the beneficial effect of exogenous administration of NO may be due to the restoration of normal pulmonary microvascular permeability and reduction of pulmonary capillary hydrostatic pressure. Other studies have related the hemodynamic "collapse" associated with septic shock to the overproduction of NO. These investigators postulated that inhibition of this exaggerated NO release will prevent or attenuate the hypotension associated with septic shock.[44-46] The observations in our study are consistent with those of other investigators,[47,48] suggesting that the pharmacologic inhibition of endothelially derived NO (eg, that which occurs following treatment with nonselective NO synthase inhibitors such as L-NAME or nitroglycerine-monomethyl-L-arginine) may in fact be detrimental. In patients with acute lung injury, the nonselective inhibition of NO release may actually worsen pulmonary hypertension, ventilation-perfusion mismatch, and oxygen delivery in these already critically ill patients.

This work is supported in part by a merit review grant from the Department of Veterans Affairs, Dallas, Tex (Dr Turnage) and a research grant from the American Lung Association of Texas, Austin (Dr Turnage).

Presented in part at the 18th Annual Meeting of the Surgical Infection Society, New York, NY, May 2, 1998.

Corresponding author: Richard H. Turnage, MD, Department of Surgery, University of Texas Southwestern Medical Center, 5323 Harry Hines Blvd, Dallas, TX 75235-0156 (e-mail: Turnage.Richard_H@Dallas.VA.GOV).

REFERENCES

1. Turnage RH, LaNoue JL, Kadesky KM, Meng Y, Myers SI. Thromboxane A_2 mediates increased pulmonary microvascular permeability after intestinal reperfusion. *J Appl Physiol.* 1997;82:592-598.
2. Zamora CA, Baron DA, Heffner JE. Thromboxane contributes to pulmonary hypertension in ischemia-reperfusion lung injury. *J Appl Physiol.* 1993;74:224-229.
3. Schumacher WA, Adams HD, Ogletree ML. Effect of the thromboxane A_2-receptor antagonists, SQ-29,548 and SQ 28,668, on the pulmonary hypertensive response to endotoxemia in swine. *Pharmacology.* 1987;34:301-308.
4. Christman BW, McPherson CD, Newman JH, et al. An imbalance between the excretion of thromboxane and prostacyclin metabolites in pulmonary hypertension. *N Engl J Med.* 1992;327:70-75.
5. Kubes P, Granger DN. Nitric oxide modulates microvascular permeability. *Am J Physiol.* 1992;262:H611-H615.
6. Kubes P, Suzuki M, Granger DN. Nitric oxide: an endogenous modulator of leukocyte adhesion. *Proc Natl Acad Sci U S A.* 1991;88:4651-4655.
7. Furchott RF, Vanhoutte PM. Endothelium derived relaxing and contracting factors. *FASEB J.* 1989;3:2007-2018.
8. Farhat MY, Cunard TG, Cole E, Myers AK, Ramwell PW. Vasodilatory property of *N*-alpha benzoyl-L-arginine ethyl ester in the rat isolated pulmonary artery and perfused lung. *J Pharmacol Exp Ther.* 1990;254:289-293.
9. Rees DD, Palmer RMJ, Schulz R, Hodson HF, Moncada S. Characterization of three inhibitors of endothelial nitric oxide synthase in vitro and in vivo. *Br J Pharmacol.* 1990;101:746-752.
10. Kavanagh BP, Mouchawar A, Goldsmith J, Pearl RG. Effects of inhaled NO and inhibition of endogenous NO synthesis in oxidant-induced acute lung injury. *J Appl Physiol.* 1994;76:1324-1329.
11. Moore TM, Khimenko PL, Wilson PS, Taylor AE. Role of nitric oxide in lung ischemia and reperfusion injury. *Am J Physiol.* 1996;271:H1970-H1977.
12. Wilson PS, Thompson WJ, Moore TM, Khimenko PL, Taylor AE. Vasoconstriction increases pulmonary nitric oxide synthesis and circulating cyclic GMP. *J Surg Res.* 1997;70:75-83.
13. Drake R, Garr KA, Taylor AE. Estimation of the filtration coefficient of pulmonary exchange vessels. *Am J Physiol.* 1978;234:H266-H274.
14. Townsley MI, Korthuis RJ, Rippe B, Parker JC, Taylor AE. Validation of double vascular occlusion method for Pc,i in lung and skeletal muscle. *J Appl Physiol.* 1986;61:127-132.
15. Folger WH, Lawson D, Wilcox CS, Mehta JL. Response of rat thoracic aortic rings to thromboxane minetic U-46619: roles of endothelium-derived relaxing factor and thromboxane A_2 release. *J Pharmacol Exp Ther.* 1991;258:669-675.
16. Wilson PS, Khimenko PL, Moore TM, Taylor AE. Perfusate viscosity and hematocrit determine pulmonary vascular responsiveness to NO synthase inhibitors. *Am J Physiol.* 1996;270:H1757-H1765.
17. Koller A, Sun D, Huang A, Kaley G. Corelease of nitric oxide and prostaglandins mediate flow-dependent dilation of rat gracilis muscle arterioles. *Am J Physiol.* 1994;267:H326-H332.
18. Pohl U, Herlan K, Huang A, Bassenge E. EDRF-mediated shear-induced dilation opposes myogenic vasoconstriction in small rabbit arteries. *Am J Physiol.* 1991;261:H2016-H2023.
19. Barnard JW, Wilson PS, Moore TM, Thompson WJ, Taylor AE. Effect of nitric oxide and cyclooxygenase products on vascular resistance in dog and rat lungs. *J Appl Physiol.* 1993;74:2940-2948.
20. Rimar S, Gillis CN. Pulmonary vasodilation by inhaled nitric oxide after endothelial injury. *J Appl Physiol.* 1992;73:2179-2183.
21. Terada LS, Mahr NN, Jacobson ED. Nitric oxide decreases lung injury after intestinal ischemia. *J Appl Physiol.* 1996;81:2456-2460.
22. Turnage RH, Wright JK, Iglesias J, et al. Intestinal reperfusion induced pulmonary edema is related to increased pulmonary inducible nitric oxide synthase activity. *Surgery.* 1998;124:457-462.
23. Weitzberg E, Rudehill A, Alving K, Lundberg JM. Nitric oxide inhalation selectively attenuates pulmonary hypertension and arterial hypoxia in porcine endotoxin shock. *Acta Physiol Scand.* 1991;143:451-452.
24. Rossaint R, Falke KJ, Lopez F, Slama K, Pison U, Zapol WM. Inhaled nitric oxide for the adult respiratory distress syndrome. *N Engl J Med.* 1993;328:399-405.
25. Pepke-Zaba J, Higebottam TW, Dinh-Xuan AT, Stone D, Wallwork J. Inhaled nitric oxide as a cause of selective pulmonary vasodilation in pulmonary hypertension. *Lancet.* 1991;38:1173-1174.
26. Abdih H, Kelly CJ, Bouchier-Hayes D, et al. Nitric oxide (endothelium-derived relaxing factor) attenuates revascularization-induced lung injury. *J Surg Res.* 1994;57:39-43.
27. Kurose I, Kubes P, Wolf R, et al. Inhibition of nitric oxide production: mechanisms of vascular albumin leakage. *Circ Res.* 1993;73:164-171.
28. Davenpeck KL, Gauthier TW, Lefer AM. Inhibition of endothelial-derived nitric oxide promotes P-selectin expression and actions in the rat microcirculation. *Gastroenterology.* 1994;107:1050-1058.
29. Welles SL, Shepro D, Hechtman HB. Eicosanoid modulation of stress fibers in cultured bovine aortic endothelial cells. *Inflammation.* 1988;9:439-450.
30. Alexander JS, Hechtman HB, Shepro D. Phalloidin enhances endothelial barrier function and reduces inflammatory permeability in vitro. *Microvasc Res.* 1988;35:308-315.
31. Korthuis RJ, Carden DL, Kvietys PR, Shepro D, Fuseler J. Phalloidin attenuates postischemic neutrophil infiltration and increased microvascular permeability. *J Appl Physiol.* 1991;71:1261-1269.
32. Oliver JA. Endothelium-derived relaxing factor contributes to the regulation of endothelial permeability. *J Cell Physiol.* 1992;151:506-511.
33. Siebert AF, Haynes J, Taylor A. Ischemia-reperfusion injury in the isolated rat lung: role of flow and endogenous leukocytes. *Am Rev Respir Dis.* 1993;147:270-275.
34. Clancy RM, Leszczynska-Piziak J, Abramson SB. Nitric oxide, an endothelial cell relaxation factor, inhibits neutrophil superoxide anion production via a direct action on the NADPH oxidase. *J Clin Invest.* 1992;90:1116-1121.
35. Payne D, Kubes P. Nitric oxide donors reduce the rise in reperfusion-induced intestinal mucosal permeability. *Am J Physiol.* 1993;265:G189-G195.
36. Rubanyi GM, Ho EH, Cantor EH, Lumma WC, Parker Botelho LH. Cytoprotective function of nitric oxide: inactivation of superoxide radicals produced by human leukocytes. *Biochem Biophys Res Commun.* 1991;181:1392-1397.
37. Motterlini R, Foresti R, Intaglietta M, Winslow RM. NO-mediated activation of heme oxygenase: endogenous cytoprotection against oxidative stress to endothelium. *Am J Physiol.* 1996;270:H170-H114.
38. Bucala R, Tracey KJ, Cerami A. Advanced glycosylation products quench nitric oxide and mediate defective endothelium-dependent vasodilation in experimental diabetes. *J Clin Invest.* 1991;87:432-438.
39. Szabo C, Farago M, Horvath I, Lohinai Z, Kovach AG. Hemorrhagic hypotension impairs endothelium-dependent relaxations in the renal artery of the cat. *Circ Shock.* 1992;36:238-241.
40. Parker JL, Adams HR. Selective inhibition of endothelium-dependent vasodilator capacity by *Escherichia coli* endotoxemia. *Circ Res.* 1993;72:539-551.
41. Dinerman JL, Lowenstein CJ, Snyder SH. Molecular mechanisms of nitric oxide regulation. Potential relevance to cardiovascular disease. *Circ Res.* 1993;73:217-222.
42. Calver A, Collier J, Vallance P. Nitric oxide and cardiovascular control. *Exp Physiol.* 1993;78:303-326.
43. Lowenstein CJ, Dinerman JL, Snyder SH. Nitric oxide: a physiologic messenger. *Ann Intern Med.* 1994;120:227-237.
44. Thiemermann C, Vane J. Inhibition of nitric oxide synthesis reduces the hypotension induced by bacterial lipopolysaccharides in the rat in vivo. *Eur J Pharmacol.* 1990;182:591-595.
45. Nava E, Palmer RM, Moncada S. The role of nitric oxide in endotoxic shock: effects of NG-monomethyl-L-arginine. *J Cardiovasc Pharmacol.* 1992;20(suppl 12):S132-S134.
46. Szabo C. Alterations in nitric oxide production in various forms of circulatory shock. *New Horiz.* 1995;3:2-32.
47. Kilbourn RG, Szabo C, Traber DL. Beneficial versus detrimental effects of nitric oxide synthase inhibitors in circulatory shock: lessons learned from experimental and clinical studies. *Shock.* 1997;7:235-246.
48. Szabo C, Southan GJ, Thiemermann C. Beneficial effects and improved survival in rodent models of septic shock with S-methylisothiourea sulfate, a potent and selective inhibitor of inducible nitric oxide synthase. *Proc Natl Acad Sci U S A.* 1994;91:12472-12476.

ORIGINAL ARTICLE

A Refined Approach to the Repair of Postcholecystectomy Bile Duct Strictures

Francis Sutherland, MD, FRCSC; Bernard Launois, MD, FACS; Mihail Stanescu, MD; Jean Pierre Campion, MD; Yorgos Spiliopoulos, MD; Christian Stasik, MD

Objective: To assess the results of a refined approach to repair of postcholecystectomy bile duct strictures.

Design: An 11-year retrospective review of patients who had surgical repair of bile duct strictures developing late after cholecystectomy.

Setting: A major university teaching hospital in France.

Patients and Interventions: During an 11-year period from 1987 to 1997, 22 patients (mean [±SD] age, 55 ± 15 years) were operated on for bile duct strictures after cholecystectomy (11 after laparoscopic surgery and 11 after open surgery). Thirteen (59%) of the 22 patients had previous repair. Most patients had episodic cholangitis (14 patients [64%]) and biochemical evidence of cholestasis (20 patients [91%]). There were 5 Bismuth type 1 strictures; 4, type 2; 7, type 3; 5, type 4; and 1, type 5. The average (±SD) time from initial surgery to repair was 6.3 ± 9.6 years. Intraoperative cholangiography was used to plan the repair in 18 patients (82%). Fifteen patients (68%) were repaired with high Hepp-Couinaud hepaticojejunostomies. The last 4 patients had the hilum exteriorized by the posterior approach to improve access.

Results: There was 1 intraoperative complication (bleeding) and 4 postoperative complications (biloma, fistula, and 2 cholangitis). There were no deaths; mean (±SD) length of stay was 12.8 ± 5.8 days; and mean (±SD) follow-up was 4.8 ± 3.3 years (range, 1-10.7 years). Three patients were reoperated on, 1 with an obstructed Roux-en-Y limb and the 2 others for incisional hernias. Eighteen patients remain well, 3 had sporadic recurrent cholangitis after surgery that resolved spontaneously, and 1 patient remains unwell requiring antibiotics to control cholangitis.

Conclusions: Hepp-Couinaud hepaticojejunostomy without stenting remains a reliable repair of postcholecystectomy strictures. Intraoperative cholangiography and exteriorizing the hilum by the posterior approach are useful adjuncts to this technique.

Arch Surg. 1999;134:299-302

IN THEIR definitive paper in 1956 Hepp and Couinaud[1] outlined the technique for repair of high bile duct strictures by lowering the hilar plate and hepaticojejunostomy to the left hepatic duct. While the wisdom of this high anastomosis to healthy bile duct mucosa is clear, the various approaches to preoperative and postoperative care remain the subject of much debate. Hepp and Couinaud used intraoperative cholangiography to define the anatomy and stented their anastomoses in the 2 patients they described. Today many authors[2-4] recommend extensive preoperative investigations to identify anatomy, and many place endoscopic or percutaneous stents in these patients prior to surgery. Repairs are often stented postoperatively for periods of up to 3 years.[5] Other authors report using minimal preoperative investigations and do not stent their anastomoses.[6] Recent studies have suggested that stenting may be a source of clinically significant complications.[6,7]

The nonoperative approach to benign bile duct strictures with either transhepatic or endoscopic dilatation and stenting recently has gained popularity.[8] Long-term results are variable but are always inferior to surgical repair.[2] The affect of repeated dilation, stent changes, and episodic cholangitis on the patient's quality of life are also a concern.

In patients with postcholecystectomy bile duct strictures we have followed a surgical approach that seeks only to establish the diagnosis preoperatively and then relies on good intrahepatic exposure and intraoperative cholangiography to define the bile duct anatomy. Repair is accomplished without relying on stents before, during, or after surgery.

From the Clinique Chirurgicale et Unité de Transplantation,Hôpital Pontchaillou, Rennes, France. Dr Sutherland is now with the Department of Surgery, University of Calgary, Peter Lougheed Centre, Calgary, Alberta.

This article is also available on our Web site: www.ama-assn.org/surgery.

PATIENTS AND METHODS

Twenty-two patients with strictures developing after cholecystectomy were treated surgically at Pontchaillou Hôpital, Rennes, France, between 1987 and 1997. There were 15 female and 7 male patients, with a mean (±SD) age of 55 ± 14 years. The patient's hospital records were reviewed and long-term follow up was obtained by mailed questionnaires. Further follow up was obtained by telephone with the patient and/or the referring physician, if required. Mean (±SD) length of follow up was 4.8 ± 3.3 years (range, 1-10.7 years). Results are expressed as mean ± SD. Unpaired *t* tests were performed using Stata Quest software (Release 2; Stata Corporation, Los Angeles, Calif).

Eleven patients received their injury at laparoscopic cholecystectomy, 5 of whom were converted to open cholecystectomy. The other 11 sustained their injury during open cholecystectomy. In 4 patients the injury may have resulted from an open common bile duct exploration. One patient had Mirizzi type 2 syndrome diagnosed at initial surgery that was repaired with suture over a T tube. One patient had a low hepaticojejunostomy at the initial procedure for a completely severed bile duct. There was immediate repair of only 2 other patients (suture over T tube). Thirteen patients (59%) were reoperated on after the initial surgery: 8 had hepaticojejunostomies, 3 had drainage procedures, 1 had an end-to-end anastomosis; and 1 had dilation of a stricture. Two of these patients had 2 previous attempts at repair. Two of the patients had their initial cholecystectomy at Pontchaillou Hôpital; the remainder were referred from outside institutions.

Patients presented in 4 basic patterns. Two patients had a persistent biliary fistula more than 6 months after cholecystectomy and 2 patients only had pain. Four patients had jaundice; the remaining 14 patients suffered repeated episodes of cholangitis with findings of fluctuating elevations in their liver function test results. There was biochemical evidence of cholestasis in 20 (91%) of the 22 patients at the preoperative assessment.

All patients had an initial abdominal ultrasonographic and biochemical evaluations. Patients without previous intestinal derivation were subjected to an endoscopic retrograde cholangiopancreatogram (13 patients [59%]) to establish the diagnosis and rule out retained common bile duct stones or papillary stenosis. Patients who underwent previous bypass surgery had various procedures: 4 had transhepatic cholangiography, and 2 underwent computed tomography. One patient had a magnetic resonance imaging cholangiogram and 1 had a hepato-iminodiacetic acid scan. Both patients with fistulae underwent fistulograms. The ERCP investigations were successful in establishing the lower limits of the stricture in all 13 patients; 1 had a retained stone removed below the stricture. There were 2 episodes of post-ERCP pancreatitis requiring hospitalization of the patients. Two of the 4 transhepatic cholangiographic investigations adequately demonstrated the proximal anatomy. All patients received antibiotics at the time of their investigation; no preoperative stents were placed.

At surgery, the technique was as follows: A midline incision was preferred. The adhesions surrounding the hilum were taken down. If a previous hepaticojejunostomy had been performed, the Roux-en-Y limb was dissected up to the anastomosis. A loop cholangiogram was then performed by placing a clamp across the distal limb and inserting an angiocatheter into the bowel lumen and securing it with a pursestring suture. Radiocontrast medium was then injected into the bowel lumen and the roentgenogram taken (7 patients). Five of these patients had the anastomosis assessed by endoscopy through a small enterotomy in the Roux-en-Y limb using the rigid choledococoscope. Patients without previous bowel anastomosis were approached by dissecting above the stricture. The bile duct was found by needle aspiration and intraoperative cholangiography was performed through the needle to delineate the proximal anatomy.

To expose the proximal bile duct adequately required varying degrees of surgery. Four patients had low strictures that were easily found; these patients did not have intraoperative cholangiography. The remainder required dissection high in the hilum to take down the hilar plate exposing the left hepatic duct. In all cases the intraoperative cholangiography was successful in showing the proximal anatomy. As a rule, the sclerosed hilum was not dissected and instead healthy bile ducts well above the stricture were exposed for a wide anastomosis, usually across the convergence.

Four patients had the left and right intrahepatic ducts exposed by exteriorizing the entire hepatic hilum using the posterior approach. This approach has been previously described.[9] In short, the anterior hilar plate dissection is extended by making a posterior incision in the caudate process to dissect the posterior part of the plate and then completely detaching the hilum from liver parenchyma. The hilum was then encircled with tapes and brought from its interior position to an exterior location providing very adequate exposure to the left and right hepatic ducts.

The proximal levels of bile duct strictures and operative procedures are listed in **Table 1**. Low hepaticojejunostomies were defined as below the level of the bifurcation. High hepaticojejunostomies were anastomoses that required an incision in either the right or the left hepatic ducts. Two patients with mild stenosis had dilation and reconstruction of their Roux-en-Y limbs. Extensive destruction of the convergence required separate segmental ductal anastomoses in 2 patients. The anastomoses were performed with interrupted 5.0 to 7.0 polydioxanone sutures (Ethicon Inc, Somerville, NJ) using loop magnification. Full-thickness bile duct wall was sutured to jejunal submucosa, and seromuscular layers with the posterior wall knots tied on the inside. Jejunal mucosa was not included in the suture. Temporary extracorporeal stents were used in 1 patient where multiple anastomoses to small segmental ducts were done.

RESULTS

Intraoperative assessment revealed 8 patients with proximal ducts dilated more than 1.5 cm. In the remaining 14 patients the ducts were less than 1.5 cm in diameter, of which 4 were described as normal and 3 were described as fine. In 2 patients excluded ducts from a previously created hepaticojejunostomy were found. In 3 other patients, problems with the previously created Roux-en-Y limb were believed to contribute to the cholangitis: 2

Table 1. Bismuth Level of Stricture and Operative Procedure

Bismuth Type	No. (%) of Patients	Operative Procedure*
1	5 (23)	Low HJ (n = 3) and dilation (n = 2)
2	4 (18)	Low HJ (n = 1) and high HJ (n = 3)
3	7 (32)	High HJ
4	5 (23)	High HJ†
5	1 (4)	Low HJ

*HJ indicates hepaticojejunostomy.
†Two patients had right-sided hepatectomy and left-sided hepaticojejunostomy for associated vascular injuries and hepatic ischemia.

Table 2. Preoperative and Postoperative Liver Biochemistry Study Results

Factor	Before Surgery	After Surgery	*P*
Total bilirubin, μmol/L (mg/dL)	56 ± 79 (5.6 ± 7.9)	21 ± 19 (2.1 ± 1.7)	.08
Alkaline phosphatase, U/L	370 ± 321	210 ± 122	.07
Alanine aminotransferase, U/L	93.8 ± 61.2	60.5 ± 84.4	.18
τ-Glutamyltransferase, U/L*	542 ± 547	164 ± 142	.007

*Indicates a significant difference.

Roux-en-Y limbs were very short (<40 cm) and the other had adhesions blocking the Roux-en-Y limb.

There was 1 intraoperative complication: bleeding (14 U of packed red blood cells were transfused) in a patient with a biliocutaneous fistula and an extensive inflammatory reaction at the hilum. There were 4 postoperative complications, 1 biloma that was drained percutaneously without the development of a fistula. One fistula did occur postoperatively and this closed after 2 weeks of observation. Three patients underwent reoperation, 2 for incisional hernias and the other for obstruction of the Roux-en-Y limb. The average length of hospital stay was 12.8 ± 5.8 days. There were no deaths.

The results of preoperative and postoperative liver biochemistry studies are given in **Table 2**. There was a decline in all factors in the immediate postoperative period. Three patients had persistent elevation of their serum alkaline phosphatase levels at the most recent follow up (2 are asymptomatic).

Fourteen (64%) of the 22 patients had a liver biopsy at the time of surgery. In no case was the liver biopsy specimen normal. Six patients had results described as mild: fibrosis confined to the portal area and mild proliferative and inflammatory changes. Six patients had moderate changes: bridging fibrosis and/or moderate inflammatory changes. There were 2 patients whose biopsy specimens were reported as showing extensive bridging fibrosis with regenerative nodules/cirrhosis.

Long-term results were categorized according to the system of clinical grading suggested by Terblanche[10]: grade 1, no biliary symptoms and normal liver function; grade 2, transitory symptoms–currently no symptoms and normal liver function; grade 3, clear-cut related symptoms at follow-up visit and/or deteriorating liver function; and grade 4, recurrent strictures requiring correction or therapy. Normal liver function implies normal bilirubin and liver transaminase levels. A mildly elevated level of serum alkaline phosphatase was accepted as normal provided the level had decreased from the preoperative level. Eighteen patients were entirely well (Terblanche grade 1). Three had sporadic episodes of cholangitis postoperatively that resolved completely after receiving short courses of antibiotics (Terblanche grade 2). One patient remains unwell, requiring prolonged antibiotic therapy to control symptoms of cholangitis (Terblanche grade 3). There have been no reoperations or stenting for bile duct strictures.

COMMENT

This article demonstrates excellent long-term results of bile duct stricture repair after cholecystectomy. The approach used was to establish the diagnosis and then proceed to surgery without extensive investigations or temporary extracorporeal stenting. The precise proximal anatomy was determined by intraoperative cholangiography, followed by careful hepaticojejunostomy to healthy bile ducts well above the injury. This technique was facilitated by lowering the hilar plate and/or using the posterior approach to exteriorize the hilum. Patients with devascularized lobes underwent resections and postoperative temporary extracorporeal stenting was used in only 1 patient.

The anatomy of the bile ducts above the convergence is extremely variable. Couinaud has suggested that in 30% of persons the anatomy of the left hepatic duct may not be suitable for these high repairs by simply taking down the hilar plate.[11] The main problem is the variability in the position of the duct to segment IV. This duct may enter posteriorly very close to the convergence or may divide the drainage of the left lobe into a segment IV/III duct and a segment I/II duct. Thus, the use of just the anteriorly placed duct for the repair will drain only half of the left lobe. Furthermore, when the left ductal system is split so also is the right ductal system, creating a confusing situation where there is neither a right nor a left hepatic duct proper (17% of cases).[11]

French surgeons have stressed that intraoperative cholangiography is necessary to appreciate intrahepatic bile duct anatomy.[11-13] Failure to appreciate this anatomy may result in the complete or partial exclusion of segmental ducts and result in recurrent cholangitis in the face of a seemingly wide open anastomosis.[14] Two of our patients were found to have excluded ducts that may have contributed to their cholangitis. Patients with devascularized livers,[15] found in 2 patients in this series, or Roux-en-Y limb obstruction[16] (3 patients) can also present with recurrent cholangitis. Often, it is very difficult to uncover bile ducts in the scarred hepatic pedicle. Finding the duct by needle aspiration and then performing a cholangiogram instantly shows the surgeon the position of the bile ducts and creates a "road map for repair." This approach also increases the likelihood of finding accessory ducts, high stones, or other strictures. We believe intraoperative cholangiography is more useful than trying to find the bile ducts by feeling for preoperatively placed stents; thick scar tissue and glissonian sheath covering these ducts can make identification of stents difficult.

Hepp and Couinaud[1] established the principles of repairing these lesions 40 years ago. They outlined the technique of exposing the left hepatic duct by "taking down the hilar plate." However, this approach may not always provide adequate exposure, with the left hepatic duct still deep in the liver parenchyma or situated behind the portal vein in 5.6% of cases.[11] In these circumstances' Champeau[17] has suggested opening the umbilical fissure, the main portal fissure, and even the resection of segment IV as possible ways of improving exposure of the left hepatic duct. We prefer to use the posterior approach[9] to encircle the entire intrahepatic hilum and bring it and the bile ducts from their deep position to a more superficial extrahepatic location. The bile ducts are not always dilated as was the case in 7 of our patients. These cases can be particularly difficult and adequate exposure is of paramount importance. Furthermore, the dissection of the ducts on the left side and high on the right side are facilitated for Bismuth type 3 and type 4 stricture repairs. One need not worry about devascularizing these high ducts by separating the glissonian sheath from the liver parenchyma as their blood supply is from within the sheaths and changes from axial to direct once the convergence is reached.[18] This is probably the main reason that the level of the stricture often migrates up to the level of the convergence.[19] The anastomosis to the left hepatic duct should be as wide as possible to reduce the risk of restricture. We often carry the incision across the convergence onto the right hepatic duct to be sure both sides of the liver are adequately drained and any central ducts are included.

Temporary extracorporeal stenting of anastomoses is always a topic of controversy. Proponents of stenting often follow a strict protocol of preoperative and postoperative stenting including various tests and cholangiograms.[2-5,20,21] There is, however, little evidence that stents are necessary as many authors have publishing equivalent or better results without them.[6,13,22-26] To date there is no randomized trial supporting their use and decompression decreases bile duct size making the procedure more difficult.[6] Furthermore, a neglected stent can be the focus of morbidity and even mortality from infection or bleeding.[6] We use stents only to protect difficult anastomoses to small segmental ducts where leakage is likely, as was the case in 1 of our patients. The fact that all patients tested had abnormal liver histologic features and cirrhosis had developed in 2 patients argues in favor of early definitive repair rather than a prolonged temporizing course of stenting. Secondary biliary cirrhosis leading to transplantation can be the result of an inadequate initial repair.

We offer a simplified approach to the difficult problem of postcholecystectomy bile duct strictures that relies on high intrahepatic ductal exposure and intraoperative cholangiography to plan and carry out a satisfactory Hepp-Couinaud hepaticojejunostomy.

Reprints: Francis Sutherland, MD, FRCSC, Department of Surgery, University of Calgary, Peter Lougheed Centre, 3500-26th Ave NE, Calgary, Alberta, Canada T1Y 6J4 (e-mail: Francis.Sutherland@CRHA-Health.ab.ca).

REFERENCES

1. Hepp J, Couinaud C. L'Abord et l'utilisation du canal hepatique gauche dans les reparations de la voie biliare principale. *Presse Med.* 1956;64:947-948.
2. Pitt HA, Kaufman SL, Coleman J, et al. Benign postoperative biliary strictures: operate or dilate? *Ann Surg.* 1989;210:417-427.
3. Blumgart LH, Kelley CJ, Benjamin IS. Benign bile duct stricture following cholecystectomy: critical factors in management. *Br J Surg.* 1984;71:836-843.
4. Crist DW, Kadir S, Cameron JL. The value of perioperatively placed percutaneous biliary catheters in reconstruction of the proximal part of the biliary tract. *Surg Gynecol Ostet.* 1987;165:421-424.
5. Braasch JW, Bolton JS, Rossi RL. A technique of biliary tract reconstruction with complete follow-up in 44 consecutive cases. *Ann Surg.* 1981;194:636-638.
6. Lewis WD, Cady B, Rohrer RJ, et al. Avoidance of transhepatic drainage prior to hepaticojejunostomy for obstruction of the biliary tract. *Surg Gynecol Obstet.* 1987;165:381-386.
7. Heslin MJ, Brooks AD, Hochwald SN, et al. A preoperative biliary stent is associated with increased complications after pancreatodoudenodenectomy. *Arch Surg.* 1998;133:149-154.
8. Moore AV, Illescas FF, Mills SR, et al. Percutaneous dilation of benign biliary strictures. *Radiology.* 1987;163:625-628.
9. Launois B, Jamieson GG. The posterior intrahepatic approach for hepatectomy or removal of segments of the liver. *Surg Gynecol Obstet.* 1992;174:155-158.
10. Terblanche J, Worthley CS, Spence RAJ, Kringe JE. High or low hepaticojejunostomy for bile duct strictures? *Surgery.* 1990;108:828-834.
11. Couinaud C. Exposure of the left hepatic duct through the hilum or in the umbilical of the liver: anatomic limitations. *Surgery.* 1989;105:21-27.
12. Bismuth H, Franco D, Corlette MB. Long-term results of Roux-en-Y hepaticojejunostomy. *Surg Obstet Gynecol.* 1978;146:161-167.
13. Hepp J. Hepaticojejunostomy using the left biliary trunk for iatrogenic biliary lesions: the French connection. *World J Surg.* 1985;9:507-511.
14. Matthews JB, Baer HU, Schweizer WP, et al. Recurrent cholangitis with and without anastomotic stricture after biliary-enteric bypass. *Arch Surg.* 1993;128: 269-272,
15. Gupta N, Solomon H, Fairchild R, et al. Management and outcome of patients with combined bile duct and hepatic artery injuries. *Arch Surg.* 1998;133: 176-181.
16. Goldman LD, Steer ML, Silen W. Recurrent cholangitis after biliary surgery. *Am J Surg.* 1983;145:450-454.
17. Champeau M. La segmentectomie IV dans l'exposition chirurgicale des voies biliaires. *Mem Acad Chir.* 1966;20:966-970.
18. Northover JMA, Terblanche J. A new look at the arterial supply of the bile duct in man and its surgical implications. *Br J Surg.* 1979;66:379-384.
19. Terblanche J, Allison HF, Northover JMA. An ischemic basis for biliary strictures. *Surgery.* 1983;94:52-57.
20. Nealon WH, Urrutia F. Long-term follow-up after bilioenteric anastomosis for benign bile duct strictures. *Ann Surg.* 1996;223:639-648.
21. Castrini G, Pappalardo G. Iatrogenic strictures of the bile ducts: our experience with 66 cases. *World J Surg.* 1981;5:753-758.
22. Tocchi A, Costa G, Lepre L, et al. The long-term outcome of hepaticojejunostomy in the treatment of benign bile duct strictures. *Ann Surg.* 1996;224: 162-167.
23. Myburgh JA. The Hepp-Couinaud approach to strictures of the bile ducts, I: injuries, choledocal cysts, and pancreatitis. *Ann Surg.* 1993;218:615-620.
24. Innes JT, Ferrara JJ, Carey LC. Biliary reconstruction without transanastomotic stenting. *Am Surgeon.* 1988;54:27-30.
25. Hatfield ARW, Terblanche J, Fataar S, et al. Preoperative external biliary drainage in obstructive jaundice: a prospective controlled trial. *Lancet.* 1982;2:896-899.
26. McPherson GAD, Benjamin IS, Hodgson HJF, et al. Preoperative percutaneous biliary drainage: the results of a controlled trial. *Br J Surg.* 1984;71:371-375.

Hyperthermic Isolated Limb Perfusion With Tumor Necrosis Factor α, Interferon Gamma, and Melphalan for Locally Advanced Nonmelanoma Skin Tumors of the Extremities

A Multicenter Study

Annette F. T. Olieman, MD, PhD; Danielle Liénard, MD; Alexander M. M. Eggermont, MD, PhD; Bin B. R. Kroon, MD, PhD; Ferdy J. Lejeune, MD, PhD; Harald J. Hoekstra, MD, PhD; Heimen Schraffordt Koops, MD, PhD

Background: Hyperthermic isolated limb perfusion (HILP) with tumor necrosis factor α (TNF-α), interferon gamma, and melphalan has proved to be useful in the treatment of recurrent malignant melanoma and of locally advanced soft tissue sarcomas of the extremities.

Objective: To determine whether this modality is also effective in the treatment of locally advanced nonmelanoma skin tumors of the extremities.

Patients and Methods: Fifteen patients with locally advanced primary, recurrent, or metastatic skin tumors of the extremities (12 with squamous cell carcinoma and 3 with Merkel cell carcinoma) underwent HILP with TNF-α, interferon gamma, and melphalan. Six tumors were localized in the upper extremity (40%), and 9 in the lower extremity (60%). Treatment-related complications, limb salvage rate, local recurrence, and regional and distant metastases were scored during a median follow-up of 20 months.

Results: After HILP, 9 patients (60%) showed a complete response (with histopathological confirmation). Four patients (27%) showed a partial response (with histopathological confirmation in 1 patient), and 2 patients (13%) showed no change (with histopathological confirmation in 1 patient and with clinical evidence in 1 patient). Two patients (13%) showed treatment-related complications. The limb salvage was achieved in 12 patients (80%), and the local recurrences developed in 4 patients (27%). During follow-up, regional lymph node metastases were observed in 2 patients (13%) and distant metastases in 2 patients (13%).

Conclusion: Based on our results, HILP with TNF-α, interferon gamma, and melphalan should be considered as a limb-saving treatment modality in patients with locally advanced nonmelanoma skin tumors of the extremities who would otherwise be candidates for ablative surgery.

Arch Surg. 1999;134:303-307

From the Departments of Surgical Oncology, University Hospital Groningen, Groningen (Drs Olieman, Hoekstra, and Koops), University Hospital–Daniel den Hoed Cancer Centre Rotterdam, Rotterdam (Dr Eggermont), and Netherlands Cancer Institute Antoni van Leeuwenhoek ziekenhuis, Amsterdam (Dr Kroon), the Netherlands; and the Centre Pluridisciplinaire d'Oncologie, Centre Hospitalier Universitaire Vaudois, Lausanne, Switzerland (Drs Liénard and Lejeune).

AFTER CREECH et al[1] introduced the technique of hyperthermic isolated limb perfusion (HILP) in 1957, it has most commonly been used in patients with recurrent malignant melanoma of the extremities, satellitosis, and in-transit metastases.[1-4] The standard cytotoxic drug in HILP for melanoma is melphalan.[5] In HILP for soft tissue sarcoma (STS) of the extremities, melphalan and various other cytotoxic agents did not improve treatment results, compared with previously described combined-treatment modalities of surgery and radiotherapy.[6,7] After the addition of high-dose tumor necrosis factor α (TNF-α), the results improved dramatically. Meanwhile, HILP with TNF-α and melphalan has proved to be a promising limb-saving treatment modality for patients with locally advanced STS of the extremities.[8-10]

The treatment of locally advanced carcinomas of the skin, other than malignant melanoma, also can be a major problem for the surgical oncologist. It may be impossible to resect the tumor curatively without losing or causing severe functional impairment of the extremity. At present, there is no standard therapy for this group of patients. The promising results of HILP with TNF-α, interferon gamma, and melphalan, under circumstances of mild (39°C-40°C) hyperthermia, in patients with melanoma and STS prompted us to investigate this treatment modality in patients with locally advanced nonmelanoma skin tumors of the extremities who otherwise cannot undergo curative resection. We evaluated the efficacy of HILP with TNF-α, interferon gamma, and melphalan and the treatment-related complications in patients with locally advanced

PATIENTS AND METHODS

Fifteen patients (11 male and 4 female; median age, 71 years; range, 31-78 years) underwent HILP with TNF-α, interferon gamma, and melphalan for primary, recurrent, or metastatic squamous and Merkel cell carcinoma localized in the extremities. Patients were treated at 1 of the 4 institutes involved in this multicenter study (University Hospital Groningen, Groningen, University Hospital–Daniel den Hoed Cancer Centre Rotterdam, Rotterdam, Netherlands Cancer Institute Antoni van Leeuwenhoek ziekenhuis, Amsterdam, the Netherlands; and the Centre Pluridisciplinaire d'Oncologie, Centre Hospitalier Universitaire Vaudois, Lausanne, Switzerland). In 6 patients (40%), the tumor was localized in the upper extremity; in 9 patients (60%), in the lower extremity. Tumor size varied from 3 × 3 to 15 × 12 cm (median, 52 cm^2). Owing to the size and/or the location, curative resection of these tumors was impossible without causing severe mutilation of the extremity or impairment of function. Two patients (13%) had local recurrence after surgical resection and external beam radiotherapy (patients 6 and 9), 2 patients (13%) had metastatic lesions in the soft tissues of the extremity (13%), 1 patient (7%) was treated for a primary tumor and a metastasis in the same extremity (patient 3), and 1 patient (7%) was treated for tumor recurrence (after surgery) and a metastasis of that tumor in the same extremity (patient 10). Characteristics of patients and tumors are provided in the **Table**.

Before HILP, an incisional biopsy was performed to obtain the definitive histopathological diagnosis. Twelve patients were treated for squamous cell carcinoma, and 3 patients were treated for Merkel cell carcinoma. Besides incisional biopsy, preoperative work-up consisted of magnetic resonance imaging or computed tomographic scan (patients treated in Lausanne), selective angiography of the affected extremity, chest x-ray and computed tomographic scan of the lungs. After informed consent was obtained, the patients were treated in a phase 2 study consisting of HILP with TNF-α, interferon gamma, and melphalan.

The perfusion technique has previously been described extensively.[11,12] Before HILP, the patients received 0.2-mg recombinant interferon gamma (Boehringer Ingelheim, Ingelheim/Rhein, Germany) subcutaneously once a day for 2 days. Isolation of the blood circulation of the limb was achieved by clamping the major artery and vein after heparinization. After inserting the cannulae, the patient was connected to a heart-lung machine. Collateral vessels were ligated, and a tourniquet was applied to compress the remaining minor vessels. Leakage of the drugs from the perfusion circuit to the systemic circulation was measured using human serum albumin with radioactive iodine and technetium.[13,14] The extremities were perfused for 90 minutes under mild hyperthermic conditions (39°C-40°C) with 0.2 mg of interferon gamma, 3 (arm) to 4 (leg) mg of TNF-α (Boehringer Ingelheim), and 10 (limb volume, leg) to 13 (limb volume, arm) mg/L of melphalan (L-phenylalanine mustard; Glaxo-Wellcome, London, England). After perfusion, patients were admitted to the intensive care unit to monitor the clinical toxic effects of HILP.

Six to eight weeks after perfusion, the patients underwent restaging with magnetic resonance imaging or computed tomographic scan and angiography. Tumor resection, if possible, was performed 6 to 8 weeks after perfusion. The histopathological response to HILP was standardized, based on results of the histopathological examination and scored with the following criteria: complete histopathological response, indicated by no viable tumor cells; partial histopathological response, indicated by more than 50% necrosis; and no change, indicated by less than 50% necrosis.[9] Treatment results are summarized in the Table.

All patients participated in an intensive physical therapy rehabilitation program to improve functional morbidity. During follow-up, we scored treatment-related complications, limb salvage rate, local recurrence, local progression, regional recurrence, and distant metastases. Survival curves were calculated according to the Kaplan-Meier method.

Patient, Treatment, and Follow-up Characteristics*

Patient No./ Sex/Age, y	Tumor Localization (Size, cm)	Tumor Histological Characteristics	Synchronous Metastases at Time of HILP	Artery Used for HILP	Resection	Histopathological Response
1/M/44	Foot (3 × 3)	Primary squamous cell	No	Popliteal	Yes	Complete
2/M/72	Elbow region (6 × 8)	Primary squamous cell	No	Brachial	Yes	Partial
3/M/74	Hand and wrist (15 × 12); forearm (0.5 × 0.5)	Primary squamous cell; metastatic squamous cell	No	Axillary	No	No change
4/M/58	Hand (13 × 11)	Recurrent squamous cell	No	Axillary	Yes	Complete
5/M/61	Lower leg (7 × 5)	Recurrent squamous cell	No	Iliac	Yes	Complete
6/F/71	Lower leg (10 × 4)	Recurrent squamous cell	No	Iliac	Yes	Complete
7/M/62	Lower leg (15 × 12)	Recurrent squamous cell	No	Femoral	Yes	Complete
8/M/78	Lower leg (15 × 10)	Recurrent squamous cell	No	Femoral	No	Partial
9/M/58	Lower leg (8 × 10)	Recurrent squamous cell	No	Femoral	Yes	Complete
10/F/77	Forearm (7 × 3); upper arm (5 × 3)	Recurrent squamous cell; metastatic squamous cell	No	Axillary	Yes	Complete
11/F/71	Foot (8 × 7)	Metastatic squamous cell	Inguinal lymph nodes	Femoral	No	Partial
12/M/73	Lower leg (5 × 5)	Metastatic squamous cell	Lung	Popliteal	Yes	Complete
13/M/31	Hand (5 × 2)	Primary Merkel cell	Axillary lymph nodes	Axillary	Yes	No change
14/F/78	Lower leg (multiple)	Recurrent Merkel cell	No	Femoral	Yes	Complete
15/M/73	Elbow (9 × 7)	Recurrent Merkel cell	Axillary lymph nodes	Axillary	No	Partial

**HILP indicates hyperthermic isolated limb perfusion; NED, no evidence of disease; MOF, multiple organ failure; DRT, death related to treatment; AWD, alive with disease; DND, death not related to malignant lesion; and DOD, death due to disease.*

squamous cell carcinoma or Merkel cell carcinoma localized in the extremities.

RESULTS

The median follow-up was 20 months (range, 1-65 months). Resection of the residual tumor mass following HILP was performed in 11 of the 15 patients. In these patients, the histopathological response of the tumor to HILP with TNF-α, interferon gamma, and melphalan was evaluated microscopically, whereas in the other 4 patients, the response was assessed clinically. Reasons for not performing tumor resection were death due to other causes before biopsy or resection (patient 11) and deterioration of the general condition of the patient due to metastatic disease (patient 15). In patients 3 and 8, a complete resection of the tumor after HILP was not possible, so an amputation was performed after 2 and 5 months, respectively. After HILP, the tumors showed completed histopathological response in 8 patients with squamous cell carcinoma and 1 patient with Merkel cell carcinoma (60%, with confirmation in all), partial response in 3 patients with squamous cell carcinoma and 1 patient with Merkel cell carcinoma (27%, with histopathological confirmation in 1), and no change in 2 patients (13%, squamous cell carcinoma without histopathological confirmation in 1 patient, and Merkel cell carcinoma with histopathological confirmation in 1). **Figure 1** demonstrates the effect of HILP in patient 4, who was treated for an unresectable squamous cell carcinoma, localized on the hand.

Limb salvage could be achieved in 12 patients (80%; 9 with squamous cell carcinoma and 3 with Merkel cell carcinoma). Reasons for ablative surgery were deep infection of the tumor bed shortly after perfusion in 1 patient (patient 5) and local progression during follow-up in 2 patients (patients 3 and 8). Complications occurred in 2 patients (13%). After HILP, a distributive shock with multiple organ failure developed in patient 5, followed by a deep infection of the tumor bed that necessitated amputation. He died of septic shock in the postoperative period. A superficial wound infection developed in patient 11. Altogether, treatment-related mortality was 7% (1 patient).

During follow-up, local recurrence was observed in 2 patients (patients 10 and 13), 6 and 8 months after HILP, respectively, after a complete histopathological response of a squamous cell carcinoma in 1 patient and after no histopathological change of a Merkel cell carcinoma in the other. In the latter patient (patient 13), amputation was not performed due to the development of fulminant disseminated disease. In 2 patients in whom resection of the residual tumor mass was not performed, local progressive disease developed 2 and 5 months after HILP (patients 3 and 8, respectively). Thus, a total of 4 patients (27%; 3 patients with squamous cell carcinoma and 1 patient with Merkel cell carcinoma) suffered local recurrence or local progressive disease.

Regional lymph node metastases developed during follow-up in 2 patients (13%), 1 patient treated for squamous cell carcinoma and 1 patient treated for Merkel cell carcinoma (patients 3 and 14, respectively). In 2 patients treated for Merkel cell carcinoma (13%), distant metastases developed during follow-up (patients 13 and 15). Both patients died during follow-up due to metastatic disease, 16 and 7 months, respectively, after HILP. One patient with multiple metastases from a squamous cell carcinoma at the time of HILP died 8 months following HILP, due to progressive metastatic disease (patient 12). The 2 other deaths (13%) during follow-up were due to suicide (patient 11) and sepsis as described in patient 5. The overall survival and the local and regional recurrence in patients are presented in **Figure 2**.

Complications	Limb Salvage	Treatment Failure (mo)	Overall Survival (mo)
No	Yes	No	NED (34)
No	Yes	No	NED (52)
No	No	Local (2); regional (2)	Unavailable for follow-up
No	Yes	No	NED (15)
Shock, MOF, infection of tumor bed	No	No	DRT (1)
No	Yes	No	NED (65)
No	Yes	No	NED (20)
No	No	Local (5)	NED (11)
No	Yes	No	NED (60)
No	Yes	Local (6)	AWD (28)
Wound infection	Yes	No	DND (1)
No	Yes	No	DOD (8)
No	Yes	Local (8); distant (1)	DOD (16)
No	Yes	Regional (12)	NED (37)
No	Yes	Distant (3)	DOD (7)

COMMENT

Maximum locoregional control with minimum treatment-related morbidity was the primary goal of our study. The incidence of local recurrence and (functional) morbidity after HILP could therefore be used to measure these criteria.[12] As a considerable number of patients with locally advanced malignant neoplasms of the extremities will die of distant metastases, limb-sparing treatment modalities now are considered preferable for a significant number of musculoskeletal tumors.[15,16] In this respect, HILP with TNF-α, interferon gamma, and melphalan has meant a breakthrough in the limb-saving treatment of locally advanced STS of the extremities.[8,9] Treatment with TNF-α causes early and selective changes in tumor-associated endothelial cells of human tumors, which can lead to necrosis of the tumor.[17-19] Disappearance of all tumor-associated vessels has been described within 7 to 14 days after HILP with TNF-α, interferon gamma, and melphalan, whereas other vessels remained unchanged.[20,21] Even with palliative intent, HILP with TNF-α, interferon gamma, and melphalan can be an effective treatment modality to control local disease, alleviate pain, and avoid ablative surgery.[8,10,22-24]

All patients treated in our study had locally advanced disease or local recurrence after previous treat-

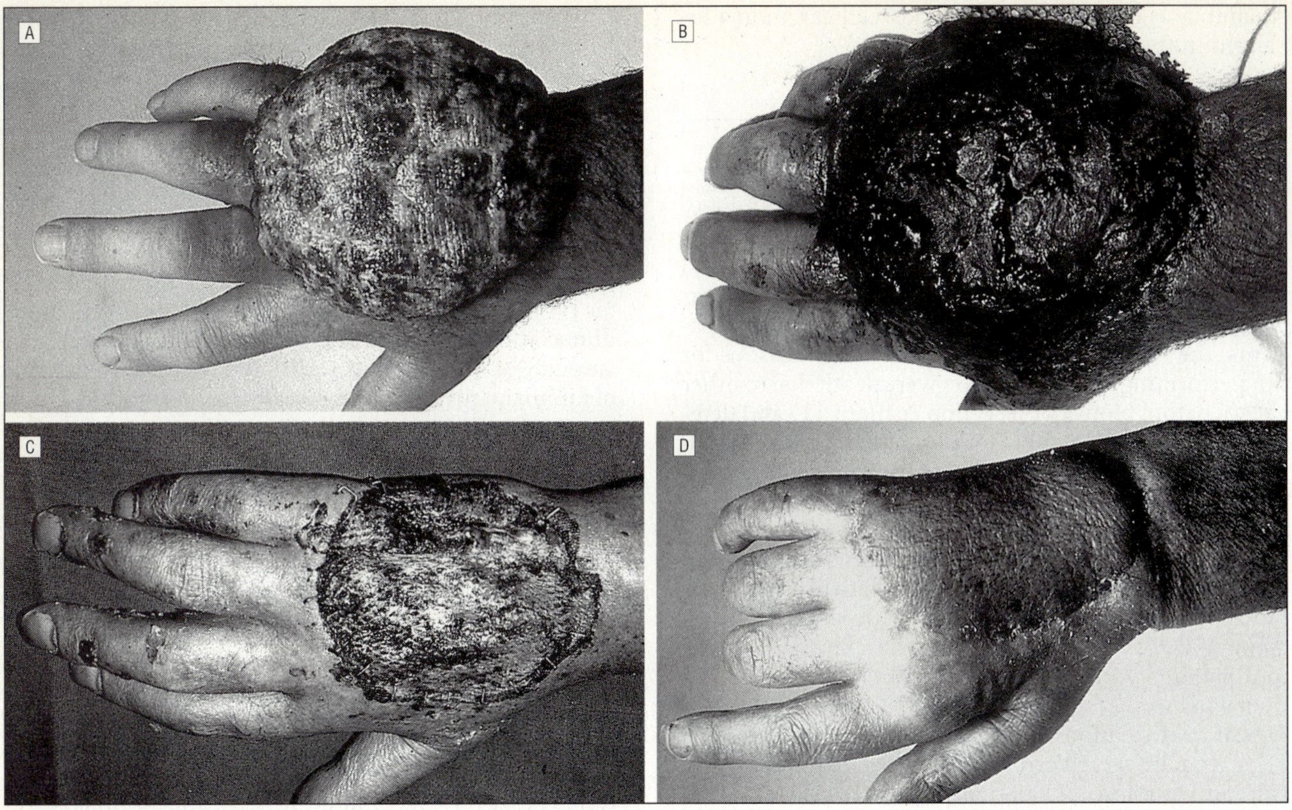

Figure 1. *Patient 4 before hyperthermic isolated limb perfusion (HILP) (A), 10 days following HILP (B), after tumor-resection with splitskin graft (C), and with full-thickness graft (D).*

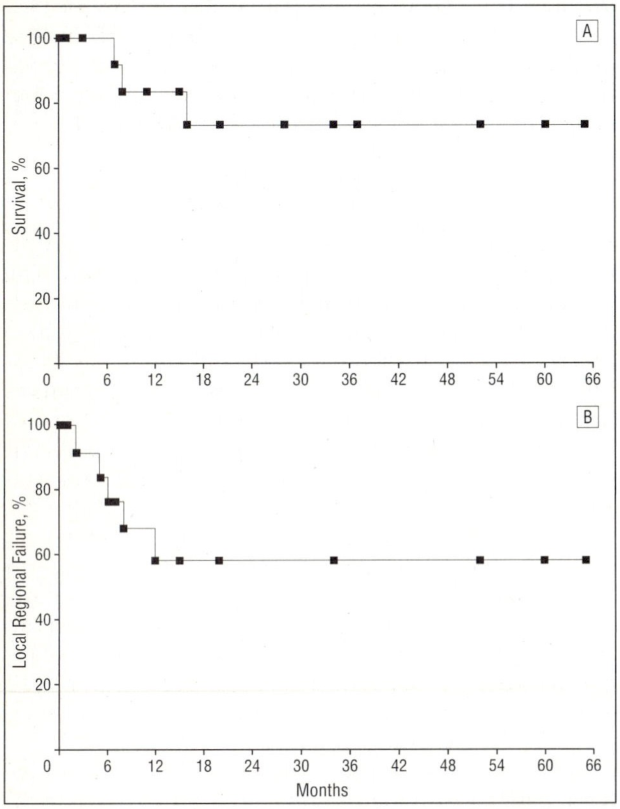

Figure 2. *Kaplan-Meier life tables depicting overall survival (A) and local and regional recurrence (B) after hyperthermic isolated limb perfusion with tumor necrosis factor α, interferon gamma, and melphalan in patients treated for locally advanced squamous cell carcinoma and Merkel cell carcinoma of the extremities.*

ment and were considered candidates for ablative surgery. In the selection of a treatment modality for squamous cell carcinoma, factors such as size and localization of the lesion, depth of infiltration, age of the patient, and desired cosmetic result all play a role. Tumor resection with adequate margins and radiotherapy are the most frequently used therapies, whereas radiotherapy or chemotherapy may be used for local or distant metastases.[25] In the past, isolated limb perfusion with methotrexate has been described as a limb-saving treatment modality in 2 patients with locally advanced squamous cell carcinoma of the lower extremities. However, both perfusions were performed under true hyperthermia (>41°C), which may lead to serious local toxic side effects.[26]

On the basis of our results, we can conclude that the limb salvage rate and the local control rate in patients treated with HILP consisting of TNF-α, interferon gamma, and melphalan followed by tumor resection for squamous cell carcinoma correspond with those in patients treated with the same modality for locally advanced STS of the extremities.[9]

In our study, 1 patient had major treatment-related complications (patient 5), leading to the death of this patient. Preoperatively, this patient had severe lymphedema. Lymphedema may lead to retention of TNF-α and thereby to distributive shock and multiple organ failure. Therefore, lymphedema must be an exclusion criteria in the TNF-α–based protocols.

Merkel cell carcinomas are known to have a high incidence of locoregional recurrences, regional lymph node involvement, and distant metastases, resulting in a very poor prognosis after surgical treatment.[27] In the 3 patients we treated with this condition, however, limb salvage was achieved.

We conclude that in patients with locally advanced nonmelanoma skin tumors of the extremities who cannot be treated curatively with conventional treatment modalities, HILP with TNF-α, interferon gamma, and melphalan is a promising limb-saving treatment modality mostly without major treatment-related morbidity.

Corresponding author: H. Schraffordt Koops, MD, PhD, Department of Surgical Oncology, University Hospital Groningen, PO Box 30.001, 9700 RB Groningen, the Netherlands.

REFERENCES

1. Creech OJ, Krementz ET, Ryan RF, Winblad JN. Chemotherapy of cancer: regional perfusion utilizing an extracorporeal circuit. *Ann Surg.* 1958;148:616-632.
2. Baas PC, Schraffordt Koops H, Hoekstra HJ, Oosterhuis JW, van der Weele LT, Oldhoff J. Isolated regional perfusion in the treatment of local recurrence, satellitosis and in transit metastasis of the extremities. *Reg Cancer Treat.* 1988;1:33-36.
3. Franklin HR, Schraffordt Koops H, Oldhoff J, et al. To perfuse or not to perfuse? a retrospective comparative study to evaluate the effect of adjuvant isolated regional perfusion in patients with stage I extremity melanoma with a thickness of 1.5 mm or greater. *J Clin Oncol.* 1988;6:701-708.
4. Stehlin JS Jr. Hyperthermic perfusion with chemotherapy for cancer of the extremities. *Surg Gynecol Obstet.* 1969;129:305-308.
5. Thompson JF, Giatoutsos MP. Isolated perfusion for melanoma: effectiveness and toxicity of cisplatin compared with that of melphalan and other drugs. *World J Surg.* 1992;61:227-233.
6. Hoekstra HJ, Schraffordt Koops H, Molenaar WM, et al. A combination of intraarterial chemotherapy, preoperative and postoperative radiotherapy, and surgery as limb saving treatment of primarily unresectable high-grade soft tissue sarcomas of the extremities. *Cancer.* 1989;63:59-62.
7. Klaase JM, Kroon BBR, Benckhuijsen C, Van Geel AN, Albus-Lutter ChE, Wieberdink J. Results of regional isolation perfusion with cytostatics in patients with soft tissue tumors of the extremities. *Cancer.* 1989;64:616-621.
8. Lienard D, Ewalenko P, Delmotte JJ, Renard N, Lejeune FJ. High-dose recombinant tumour necrosis factor-alpha in combination with interferon gamma and melphalan in isolation perfusion of the limbs for melanoma and sarcoma. *J Clin Oncol.* 1992;10:52-60.
9. Eggermont AMM, Schraffordt Koops H, Lienard D, et al. Isolated limb perfusion with high-dose tumor necrosis factor-α—in combination with interferon-γ—and melphalan for nonresectable extremity soft tissue sarcomas: a multicenter trial. *J Clin Oncol.* 1996;14:2653-2665.
10. Gutman M, Inbar M, Lev-Shlush D, et al. High dose tumor necrosis factor-α and melphalan administered via isolated limb perfusion for advanced limb soft tissue sarcoma results in a >90% response rate and limb preservation. *Cancer.* 1997;79:1129-1137.
11. Schraffordt Koops H, Oldhoff J, Oosterhuis JW, Beekhuis J. Isolated regional perfusion in malignant melanoma of the extremities. *World J Surg.* 1987;11:527-533.
12. Olieman AFT, Pras E, van Ginkel RJ, Molenaar WM, Schraffordt Koops H, Hoekstra HJ. Feasibility and efficacy of external beam radiotherapy after hyperthermic isolated limb perfusion with TNF-α, IFN-γ and melphalan for limb saving treatment in locally advanced extremity soft tissue sarcoma. *Int J Radiat Oncol Biol Phys.* 1998;40:807-814.
13. Hoekstra HJ, Naujocks T, Schraffordt Koops H, et al. Continuous leakage monitoring during hyperthermic isolated regional perfusion of the lower limb: technique and results. *Reg Cancer Treat.* 1992;4:301-304.
14. Klaase JM, Kroon BBR, van Geel AN, Eggermont AMM, Franklin HR. Systemic leakage during isolated limb perfusion for melanoma. *Br J Surg.* 1993;80:1124-1126.
15. Hoekstra HJ, Schraffordt Koops H, Oldhoff J. Soft tissue sarcoma of the extremity. *Eur J Surg Oncol.* 1994;20:3-6.
16. Mazanet R, Antman KH. Sarcomas of soft tissue and bone. *Cancer.* 1991;68:463-473.
17. Carswell EA, Old LJ, Kassel RL, Green S, Fiore N, Williamson B. An endotoxin-induced serum factor that causes necrosis of tumours. *Proc Natl Acad Sci U S A.* 1975;72:3666-3670.
18. Renard N, Lienard D, Lespagnard L, Eggermont A, Heiman R, Lejeune F. Early endothelium activation and polymorphonuclear cell invasion precede specific necrosis of human melanoma and sarcoma treated by intravascular high-dose tumour necrosis factor alpha (rTNFα). *Int J Cancer.* 1994;57:656-663.
19. Pan M, Wasa M, Lind S, Gertler J, Abbott W, Suoba W. TNF-stimulated arginine transport by human endothelium requires activation of protein kinase C. *Ann Surg.* 1995;221:590-601.
20. Eggermont AMM, Lienard D, Schraffordt Koops H, Rosenkaimer F, Lejeune FJ. Treatment of irresectable soft-tissue sarcomas of the limbs by isolation perfusion with high-dose TNFα in combination with interferon-γ and melphalan. In: Fiers W, Buurman W, eds. *Tumor Necrosis Factor: Molecular and Cellular Biology and Clinical Relevance.* Farmington, Conn: S Karger AG; 1993:239-243.
21. Olieman AFT, van Ginkel RJ, Hoekstra HJ, et al. The angiographic response of locally advanced soft tissue sarcoma following hyperthermic isolated limb perfusion with tumor necrosis factor. *Ann Surg Oncol.* 1997;4:64-69.
22. Lienard D, Eggermont AMM, Schrafford Koops H, et al. Isolated perfusion of the limb with high-dose TNFα, IFNγ and melphalan for melanoma stage III: results of a multicentric pilot study. *Melanoma Res.* 1994;4:21-26.
23. Eggermont AMM, Schraffordt Koops H, Klausner J, et al. Isolated limb perfusion with tumour necrosis factor and melphalan for limb salvage in 186 patients with locally advanced soft tissue extremity sarcomas: the cumulative multicenter European experience. *Ann Surg.* 1996;224:756-765.
24. Olieman AFT, van Ginkel RJ, Molenaar WM, Schraffordt Koops H, Hoekstra HJ. Hyperthermic isolated limb perfusion with TNF-α and melphalan as palliative limb-saving treatment in patients with locally advanced soft tissue sarcomas of the extremities with regional or distant metastases: is it worthwhile? *Arch Orthop Trauma Surg.* 1998;118:70-74.
25. Robinson JK. What are adequate treatment and follow-up care for nonmelanoma cutaneous cancer? *Arch Dermatol.* 1987;123:331-333.
26. Vaglini M, Andreola S, Attili A, et al. Limb-salvage procedure in two patients with spindle cell carcinoma of the lower extremities using isolation perfusion. *Tumori.* 1985;71:271-275.
27. Fenig E, Brenner B, Katz A, Rakovsky E, Hana MB, Sulkes A. The role of radiation therapy and chemotherapy in the treatment of Merkel cell carcinoma. *Cancer.* 1997;80:881-885.

Minicholecystectomy

A Safe, Cost-effective Day Surgery Procedure

A. Kent Seale, MD; Walter P. Ledet, Jr, MD

Objective: To document effectiveness of minicholecystectomy as a safe, cost-effective day surgery procedure with rapid return to work.

Design: Review of medical records.

Setting: Small community hospital.

Patients: A total of 1207 patients who underwent minicholecystectomies from January 1, 1986, through December 31, 1997.

Intervention: Minicholecystectomy.

Main Outcome Measures: Complications, length of hospital stay, cost, and time until return to work.

Results: Of the 1207 patients who underwent minicholecystectomy, 74% were admitted for day surgery, 88% of whom were discharged in less than 12 hours, 9.3% in 24 hours or less, and 1.7% in greater than 24 hours; 0.3% were readmitted within 2 weeks. The complication rate was 0.2%; 2 cases required laparotomy, with no common duct injuries. The cost of the procedure was $435; the average time it took working patients to return to work was 11.4 days.

Conclusions: Minicholecystectomy is a safe, inexpensive day surgery method of cholecystectomy with minimal time off work after surgery.

Arch Surg. 1999;134:308-310

HISTORICALLY, cholecystectomy has been done through an 8- to 12-cm incision that cuts the majority of the rectus muscle. The introduction of laparoscopic cholecystectomy in 1989 by Dubois et al[1] decreased both inpatient time and the time until return to work, but a significant number of complications resulted. In a review of 77 604 cases, Deziel et al[2] reported a 1.2% instance of complications requiring laparotomy (0.6% rate of common duct injury). Fullertin and Bell[3] showed complications requiring laparotomy in 2.4% of cases (0.6% bile duct injuries).

By decreasing the incision size to 4 to 7 cm, preserving the rectus muscle, and using headlights, we have reduced our operative morbidity at no increased risk to the patient. We refer to this procedure as a "minicholecystectomy." Adding local anesthesia and long-acting dexamethasone acetate further improved patient tolerance, and we were able to begin day surgery cholecystectomies in 1986. Today, with the use of minicholecystectomy techniques, the majority of our cholecystectomies are done as day surgery, with patients returning to work in 12 to 14 days. Minicholecystectomy is also very economical, costing $435 per procedure in our hospital. In this study, we report our experience with minicholecystectomy from 1986 through 1997.

Drs Seale and Ledet are in private practice in Sulphur, La.

RESULTS

Of 1207 cholecystectomies performed (**Table 1**), 898 (74.4%) were in patients admitted for day surgery; 88.9% were discharged within 12 hours, 9.3% were discharged between 12 and 24 hours, and 1.8% were discharged more than 24 hours after surgery (**Table 2**). Three hundred nine patients underwent surgery as inpatients. Of these, 36.9% were discharged within 24 hours, and 63.1% were discharged more than 24 hours after surgery (**Table 3**).

See Invited Critique at end of article

All cholecystectomies, acute or elective, inpatient or outpatient, were done by 1 of the 2 of us by means of the minicholecystectomy technique. We had no procedures that required incisions greater than 7 cm. None of our patients had sufficient blood loss to require transfusions. There were no intra-abdominal abscesses. Only patients who had common duct exploration underwent drainage. We had 2 com-

PATIENTS AND METHODS

We reviewed the records of all minicholecystectomies performed at West Calcasieu Cameron Hospital, Sulphur, La, between January 1, 1986, and December 31, 1997. We evaluated complications and length of stay in all cases. In procedures performed from January 1, 1991, through January 1, 1998, we also studied the time from surgery until the patient returned to work.

We perform minicholecystectomy much like an open cholecystectomy, except that we make a small incision, substituting retractors for hands, and preserve as much rectus muscle as possible. The surgery is done through a 4- to 7-cm incision. Essential tools for the surgery are retractors (Harrington-Pemberton 1.9- or 6.4-cm; Allegiance Healthcare Corp, Deerfield, Ill, and Deaver 2.5-cm; Allegiance Healthcare Corp), a headlight, ×2.5 magnification loops, metal tonsil sucker, cautery (with extension), and 20 mg of long-acting dexamethasone acetate in 0.25% bupivacine hydrochloride with epinephrine (1 mL/kg).

A transverse incision is used 2 to 3 fingers below the xiphoid process. The gallbladder is visualized, and laparotomy sponges (Medical Action Industries, Inc, Asheville, NC) are introduced to isolate the area. Harrington retractors are then introduced, placing the wide ends (1) superolaterally to elevate the liver off of Calot triangle, (2) superomedially to create traction across the common duct, and (3) in Morrison pouch to create traction along the length of the common duct. In very obese patients, the incision is extended to 7 cm to accommodate 6.4-cm Harrington retractors. Ninety-eight percent of the dissection is done with the cautery (coagulation mode) by means of a touch and push technique. If the gallbladder is distended, it is aspirated. The Calot triangular area is dissected, with identification of the cystic artery and the cystic duct. Unless there is questionable anatomy, the cystic artery is ligated and cut. The gallbladder is then taken down from the liver bed and the cystic duct is traced down to its juncture with the common duct. If the gallbladder is inflamed and no dissection plane can be developed between the gallbladder and the liver, the gallbladder is opened. The bile and stones are removed. The margins of the gallbladder are excised at the junction of the gallbladder bed and liver, leaving the gallbladder wall in the liver. The mucosa remaining in the liver bed is cauterized. If a cholangiogram is not indicated, the cystic duct is clipped 0.5 cm from its juncture with the common duct and the gallbladder is removed. Bupivacaine with dexamethasone is introduced into the area of the surgery and meticulously injected into the wound margins.

The current average cost per procedure was determined for minicholecystectomies.

plications requiring reoperation. One patient had acute onset of abdominal pain 5 days postoperatively. She was returned to the operating room, where a leak at the site of the cystic and common duct juncture was noted. There was no residual cystic duct or clip present. A T-tube was positioned and eventually removed. The patient did well. The second patient developed pain 24 hours postoperatively. She was returned to surgery, and a similar bile duct leak was found. The site of the previous connection of the cystic duct to the common duct was sutured with two 3-0 chromic sutures. This patient also did well.

We compiled statistics on the time until the patient returned to work for patients treated since 1991. During this period there were 278 patients who worked regularly. The average time off work was 11.4 days (**Table 4**). The time it took for patients who performed heavy manual work to return to work was less than the time for nonmanual workers, which may indicate that desire and incentive are of equal importance or more important than surgical technique.

Table 1. Overview of Minicholecystectomies Performed

Type of Procedure	No. of Patients: Men	Women	Total	% of All Minicholecystectomies
Day surgery	315	583	**898**	74
Inpatient	99	210	**309**	26
Total	**414**	**793**	**1207**	**100**

Table 2. Minicholecystectomy: Day Surgeries

	No. (%)	Comments
Admitted as day surgery	898 (100.0)	None
Discharged <12 h	798 (88.9)	None
Discharged 12-24 h	84 (9.3)	None
Discharged >24 h	16 (1.8)	Combined surgeries: 2 hiatal hernia repairs; remainder: nausea or pain, no attendant at home
Readmitted within 2 wk	3 (0.3)	2 Bile leaks, 1 hypertension

Table 3. Minicholecystectomy: Inpatient Length of Stay

	No. of Patients: Men	Women	Total	% of All Inpatient Minicholecystectomies
Inpatient consultations	**99**	**210**	**309**	**100.0**
Discharge ≤24 h	42	72	**114**	36.9
Discharge >24 h	57	138	**195**	63.1

COMMENT

Our results confirm that the majority of minicholecystectomies can be done as outpatient surgeries. Operating room costs for laparoscopic cholecystectomy at Lake Charles Memorial Hospital averaged $1600. Those charges do not include the equipment necessary to perform laparoscopic surgery, such as scopes and cameras. Low operating room cost ($435 per procedure) for minicholecystectomy, with no increased hospital stay, results in a $1165 saving when compared to laparoscopic cholecystectomy. Our complication rate requiring laparotomy of 0.2% was significantly better than those reported by Deziel

Table 4. Time Until Return to Work by Age*

Type of Work	10-19	20-29	30-39	40-49	50-59	60-69	70-79	Total
	Age, y							
Nonmanual								
No. of patients	0	10	25	20	9	3	4	**71**
Average time off work, d	0.0	14.5	12.0	12.5	14.5	12.5	10.5	12.8
Light manual								
No. of patients	1	14	29	36	34	3	1	**118**
Average time off work, d	12.0	17.5	14.0	12.0	13.0	8.5	4.0	11.6
Heavy manual								
No. of patients	0	4	17	35	26	7	0	**89**
Average time off work, d	0.0	8.0	7.0	17.0	11.5	8.5	0.0	10.4

Total number of patients working, 278; average time off, 11.4 days.

et al[2] (1.2%) and Fullertin and Bell[3] (2.4%). We had no common duct injuries and no deaths.

The majority of articles in the literature promote laparoscopic cholecystectomy as being cost-effective because of short hospital stay and earlier return to work. Since the hospital stay cannot be shorter than that for day surgery, and our average return to work was 11 days, the benefits of laparoscopic cholecystectomy are questionable. Complication rates and costs of laparoscopic cholecystectomy are also higher than those in our series of minicholecystectomy.

Companies that produce laparoscopic equipment market the laparoscopic technique as the newest and the best for the general population. We, as surgeons, should question why we have rushed to embrace a procedure that eliminates depth perception. Minicholecystectomy is safe, effective, and inexpensive, and should be considered for all cholecystectomies.

Reprints: A. Kent Seale, MD, 914 Cypress St, Sulphur, LA 70663.

REFERENCES

1. Dubois F, Berthelot G, Levard H. Cholecystectomie par coeliospie [Cholecystectomy by coelioscopy]. *Presse Med.* 1989;18:980-982.
2. Deziel DJ, Millikan KW, Economou SG, Doolas A, Ko ST, Airan MC. Complication of laparoscopic cholecystectomy: a national survey of 4,292 hospitals and an analysis of 77,604 cases. *Am J Surg.* 1993;165:9-14.
3. Fullertin GM, Bell G. Prospective audit of the introduction of laparoscopic cholecystectomy in the west of Scotland: West of Scotland Laparoscopic Cholecystectomy Audit Group. *Gut.* 1994;35:1121-1126.

Invited Critique

Laparoscopic cholecystectomy has become the standard criterion for treatment of symptomatic gallbladder lithiasis in developed countries. No doubt about its advantages has been raised, and although biliary tract injuries are higher when compared with the open approach, they have no statistical significance. For developing countries (ie, most of the countries of the world), there is no information available whether cholecystectomies are always done through the laparoscopic route.

Seale and Ledet report their results with minicholecystectomy and explain its advantage, as a safe, cost-effective, day surgical procedure. A large series of cases is performed with virtually no complications and no common duct injuries, challenging and even surpassing all the results reported with the laparoscopic approach. Should this be the preferred approach for both rich and poor countries? Given the results reported, there can be no doubt that the surgical community worldwide could benefit from this kind of approach.

To demonstrate the advantage of one procedure over the other, prospective, controlled, randomized trials should be done. It is the only way to validate results and to convince the surgical community. Some of these studies have been conducted and their findings published, showing no differences between the laparoscopic and open approach. Nevertheless, regarding rehabilitation and postoperative outcome, the laparoscopic approach has always shown a slight advantage.

Whether the results obtained by Seale and Ledet are reproducible is another concern. Worldwide, there is an average incidence of biliary duct injury, a complication that cannot be overlooked. Every hospital has these kinds of risks. According to expectancy, no center can expect such impressive results. The same can also be addressed for their low frequency of common duct exploration (very low incidence of common duct stones), the very low frequency of abdominal wall infections, and also gallbladders with acute processes.

Results that are only valid and reproducible in one hospital of the world cannot be generalized in the surgical community. Seale and Ledet have to be congratulated and admired for their excellent results and skills in their personal series, but no recommendation and generalization of their results can be done, even for poor countries. Minicholecystectomy is an alternate choice for surgeons with special skills. However, if compared in prospective controlled randomized trials with laparoscopic and classical open cholecystectomy, probably no advantages would be shown.

Hector Orozco, MD
Miguel Angel Mercado, MD
Mexico City, Mexico

Recurrent Pancreatitis in Gardner Variant Familial Polyposis

Etiology, Diagnostic Approach, and Interventional Results

B. E. Wright, MD; R. A. Kozarek, MD; L. W. Traverso, MD; D. Wechter, MD; R. Thirlby, MD; S. L. Raltz, RN

Hypothesis: Pancreatitis arising from an obstructing ampullary neoplasm in patients with Gardner variant familial polyposis is an infrequently described clinical entity. We reviewed all patients with Gardner variant polyposis presenting with pancreatitis during a 12-year period in our institution, hoping to better define etiology and the appropriate diagnostic and interventional approach.

Methods: A retrospective record review (1986-1998) defined patient demographics, presenting features, initial and subsequent endoscopic retrograde cholangiopancreatography (ERCP) findings, subsequent treatments, and both immediate and long-term outcomes. Particular consideration was given to initial post-ERCP diagnosis and to endoscopic interventions undertaken at that time. We also looked at those patients who eventually required surgical intervention after long-term failure of medical and endoscopic therapy, the indications for surgery, final pathological characteristics, and follow-up results.

Results: Eight patients (6 women and 2 men), with a mean age of 42 years at initial presentation, were found. Each patient was known to have Gardner variant familial polyposis at the time of the initial bout of pancreatitis. All had undergone prior colectomy and 4 of 8 had undergone prior cholecystectomy. None were known to be taking medications or ingesting pancreatoxic substances. Five of 8 patients had obstructing focal or diffuse adenomatous disease involving the ampulla. Two of 8 patients had pancreatitis attributed to other causes (divisum, stones) and a single patient had no clear etiology. Three of 5 patients with ampullary adenomatous disease underwent pancreaticoduodenectomy for recurrent adenomatous encroachment and ampullary stenosis, despite repetitive snare resection and papillotomy. All of these patients had ampullary and other duodenal adenomas, and none had malignant disease.

Conclusions: Patients presenting with pancreatitis in the setting of Gardner variant familial polyposis will frequently have an obstructing ampullary neoplasm, although additional etiologies should be sought. Initial endoscopic therapy affords transient relief but may not be definitive. The abnormal scarring and fibrosis (keloid formation, desmoid reaction) that characterize this disease likely play a large role in endoscopic or subsequent surgical failure. A significant number of these patients will go on to require surgical referral and intervention.

Arch Surg. 1999;134:311-315

From the Sections of Gastroenterology and Surgery, Virginia Mason Medical Center, Seattle, Wash.

GARDNER SYNDROME was initially described as one of the familial polyposis syndromes; however, it also has extensive extracolonic manifestations. These include osteomas of the skull, jaw, and other bones as well as desmoid tumors and other soft tissue lesions.[1,2] Also well described are gastric and small-bowel polyps.[3-5] This syndrome is now known to be an expressional variant of the same dominant, autosomally inherited gene mutation that characterizes familial adenomatous polyposis. Frequently mentioned in the discussion of upper gastrointestinal tract polyps is their malignant potential, reported to be as high as 12% in some series.[6,7] Less often discussed, and found in the literature only as sporadic case reports, are the obstructive problems these neoplasms can create in the region of the ampulla—specifically, obstructive pancreatitis. Our review of the literature to date revealed only several single-case reports of obstructive pancreatitis secondary to ampullary neoplasm and prompt surgical intervention was undertaken in most cases.[8-10] We reviewed our own experience to help define the frequency of obstructing lesions in this setting and to establish the role of endoscopic and surgical treatments.

RESULTS

Eight patients (6 women and 2 men), with a mean age of 42 years, were found. All had GV familial polyposis at the onset of

PATIENTS AND METHODS

We retrospectively reviewed all admissions for pancreatitis during a 12-year period that included a diagnosis of gastrointestinal tract tumor at the time of discharge or preexisting at the time of admission. We found 8 patients who had a diagnosis of Gardner variant (GV) familial polyposis that preceeded the diagnosis of pancreatitis. In each case, midepigastric abdominal pain and tenderness, an elevated amylase level, and abdominal ultrasonography and computed tomography of the abdomen established the diagnosis. All patients ultimately underwent diagnostic endoscopic retrograde cholangiopancreatography (ERCP). The results of these initial studies were reviewed and findings confirmed the etiology of the pancreatitis. Patients found to have obstructive ampullary adenomas were noted to have either a focal or diffuse pattern of disease.

Endoscopic interventions were then reviewed and outcomes noted by status of symptoms after treatment. For those patients who underwent initial endoscopic sphincterotomy, we noted the type (biliary vs pancreatic) and presence or absence of stenosis at these sites on repeated ERCP.

Follow-up endoscopic findings, particularly in the setting of pancreatitis recurrence, were also noted. We looked at those cases that eventually required surgery, the indications for that surgery, and long-term outcomes. No statistical analysis was attempted given the small number of patients involved.

initial pancreatitis. All had undergone previous colectomy and 4 of 8 patients had undergone prior cholecystectomy. No patients were taking medications or ingesting substances known to be pancreatoxic and all noninvasive abdominal imaging procedures were negative for stones or tumor. All patients underwent ERCP by a single endoscopist at the time of initial presentation. Findings and treatment results are summarized in the **Table**. Five of 8 patients were found to have obstructive ampullary adenomatous disease at ERCP. Two of the 8 patients had other ERCP findings thought responsible for their presentation (stones and divisum) and a final patient had no abnormalities noted at ERCP.

Of the 5 patients noted to have obstructive adenomatous disease, 4 had diffuse adenomatous changes and 1 had a focal adenoma compressing the ampulla. An example of each is shown in **Figure 1** and **Figure 2**. Four of the 5 patients with ampullary adenomatous disease underwent initial biopsy with snare resection and biliary sphincterotomy. Resection was by piecemeal snare cautery and sphincterotomy was done using a blended current 30-mm wire sphincterotome. Initial resolution of symptoms was observed. The final patient had adenomatous changes high within the ampulla and underwent initial stenting only. On final pathological examination, malignant disease or carcinoma in situ was not found, although several patients were noted to have adenomatous hyperplasia with mild atypia.

The 2 patients with nonadenomatous etiologies (stones, divisum) underwent biliary sphincterotomy with stone extraction and endoscopic dorsal pancreatic duct sphincterotomy, respectively. The patient with no endoscopic abnormalities other than a mildly dilated pancreatic duct (upper-limit normal) was thought by exclusion to have probable major papillary sphincter dysfunction and underwent major pancreatic duct sphincterotomy.

All 3 of the patients with nonadenomatous etiologies improved initially. The patient who underwent common bile duct stone extraction had lasting relief with no recurrence to date. The other 2 patients had recurrent pancreatitis within 3 months and underwent repeated ERCP and repeated pancreatic duct sphincterotomy at stenosed sphincterotomy sites. Both again experienced symptomatic relief for 3 to 6 months but ultimately had recurrence of symptoms. Each underwent eventual pancreaticoduodenectomy for recurrent sphincterotomy stenosis and recurrent pancreatitis. One of these patients had desmoid reaction pathologically. The patient with divisum continues to have chronic pain problems and has been diagnosed with recurrent pancreatitis at an outside institution. The final patient in this group has undergone 2 pancreaticojejunostomy revisions for stenosis heralded by relapses of pancreatitis and is now symptom free.

The patients with ampullary adenomatous disease who underwent biliary sphincterotomy and snare resection also had initial resolution of symptoms, followed by attacks of recurrent pancreaitis within 6 months of initial endoscopy. The single case of focal adenomatous disease had further encroachment and obstruction requiring 2 more endoscopic sessions of snare piecemeal resection, followed by complete and lasting resolution of symptoms. The patient who had only a stent placed at initial ERCP had a questionable filling defect in the distal common bile duct and brush cytological test results consistent with a malignant stricture, which prompted surgical referral in the absence of a recurrent attack. This patient underwent transduodenal sphincteroplasty and choledochoscopy. Diffuse ampullary adenomatous hyperplasia was noted, no neoplasm was found, and pancreatitis has not recurred.

The 3 other patients with a diffuse pattern of disease had varying degrees of stenosis and scarring at the previous sphincterotomy site. Some progression of the adenomatous disease at the ampulla had also occurred, and further snare resection, along with pancreatic duct sphincterotomy and extension of biliary sphincterotomy, was carried out (**Figure 3**). These 3 patients, 1 of whom had a minor papilla adenoma and cystic dilation of the duct of Santorini (**Figure 4**), continued to have recurrent bouts of pancreatitis, and went on to surgical referral and eventual pancreaticoduodenectomy. One of these patients had initial transduodenal sphincteroplasty with recurrent stenosis despite multiple revisions and a second had a desmoplastic reaction in the resected specimen. All of these patients have denied recurrent pancreatitis since surgery with a mean follow-up time of 3 years (range, 1-4 years). Characteristics of pathology specimens obtained at operation remained benign and consistent with endoscopic biopsy specimens in all cases. Of note, sphincter manometrics were

Summary of Endoscopic Findings, Interventions, Results, and Subsequent Surgical Referrals*

Patient No.	Etiology	Endoscopic Therapy	Pancreatitis Relief	Recurrence	Etiology of Recurrence	Surgical Therapy	Long-Term Relief
1	DAA	ES/SR†	Yes	Yes	ST/AE	PD	Yes
2	FAA	ES/SR†	Yes	Yes	AE	NA	Yes
3	DAA	ES/SR†	Yes	Yes	ST/AE	TDDS, PD‡	Yes
4	DAA	ES/SR†	Yes	Yes	ST/AE	PD	Yes
5	DAA	Stent	Yes	No	NA	TDDS	Yes
6	Pdiv	ES†	Yes	Yes	ST	TDDS, PD‡	No
7	Stones	ES	Yes	No	NA	NA	Yes
8	UNK	ES†	Yes	Yes	ST	PD	No§

**DAA indicates diffuse ampullary adenoma; ES, endoscopic sphincterotomy (biliary, pancreatic, or both); SR, snare resection; ST, stenosis; AE, adenoma encroachment; PD, pancreaticoduodenectomy; FAA, focal ampullary adenoma; NA, not applicable; TDDS, transduodenal sphincteroplasty; Pdiv, pancreatic divisum; and UNK, unknown.*

† Multiple times.

‡ In both cases transduodenal sphincteroplasty failed and was followed by pancreaticoduodenectomy.

§ Patient underwent multiple revisions of pancreaticojejunostomy due to recurrent stenosis.

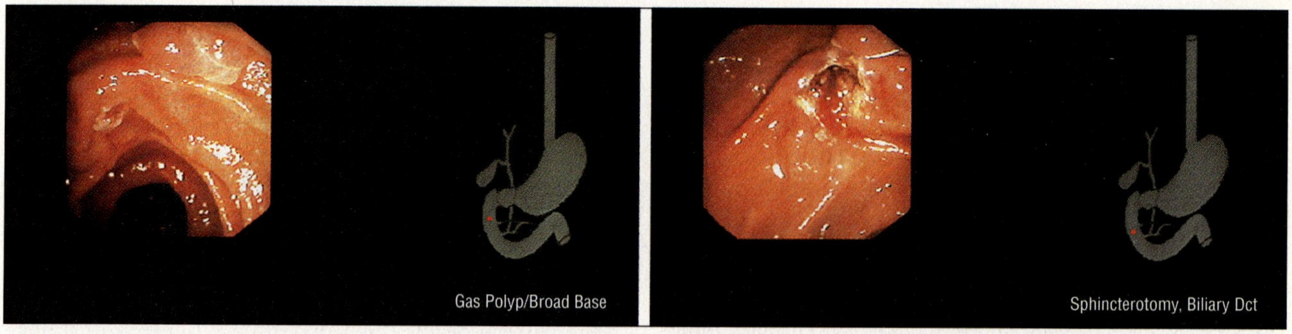

Figure 1. *A single large periampullary adenoma in a patient with a focal pattern of disease (left). This patient responded to initial sphincterotomy and repetitive snare resection alone (right).*

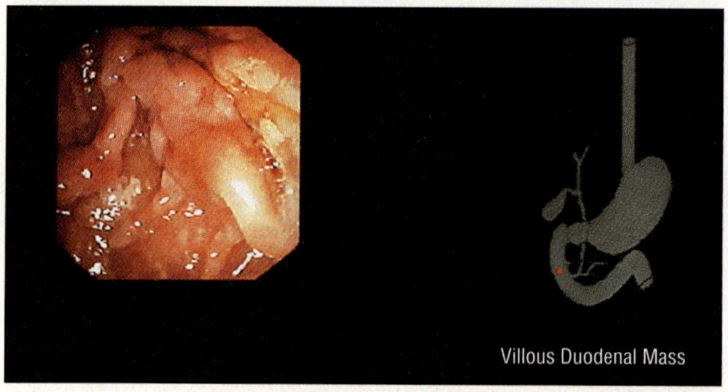

Figure 2. *Diffuse adenomatous disease completely encasing and obstructing the ampulla.*

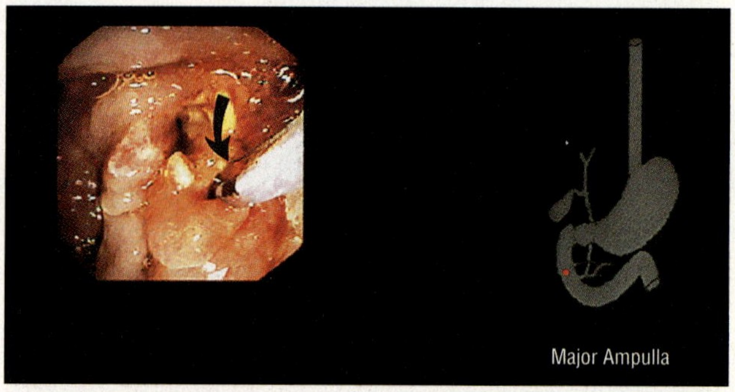

Figure 3. *At repeated endoscopic retrograde cholangiopancreatography after recurrent pancreatitis, a patient with diffuse adenomatous disease and stenosis at prior sphincterotomy site undergoes extension of biliary sphincterotomy with pancreatic duct sphincterotomy (arrow) as well.*

not uniformly performed at initial or subsequent ERCP. When recorded (1 patient), readings were below 20 mm Hg and no sphincter dysfunction was noted. To summarize, 6 of 8 patients underwent surgical referral and intervention. Of those 6 patients, 5 underwent eventual pancreaticoduodenectomy without major complications and 3 of those 5 are free of recurrence, with a mean follow-up time of 36 months.

COMMENT

A marked increase in the frequency of upper gastrointestinal tract neoplasms, forming in the stomach, duodenum, and even more distal small bowel, is well known as one of the extracolonic manifestations of familial polyposis.[3-5] The much heralded increased risk of malignant neoplasms, generally considered to range between 2% and 10%, has resulted in widespread recommendation for frequent endoscopic surveillance and biopsy to detect malignancy early.[6,7,11] Medications such as sulindac have been routinely used in hopes of halting progression of C-loop adenomas to invasive cancer, but data supporting its efficacy are sparse.[12,13]

Less frequently described are the potential nonmalignant complications of adenomatous disease in the periampullary region. Pancreatitis in the specific setting of GV familial polyposis is distinctly uncommon. However, when it does occur, obstructive ampullary adenomatous disease may be the cause. In fact, pancreatitis may be the presenting manifestation of upper gastrointestinal tract neoplasm in these patients.[8-10,14] Also additional and unrelated etiologies, such as gallstones or ana-

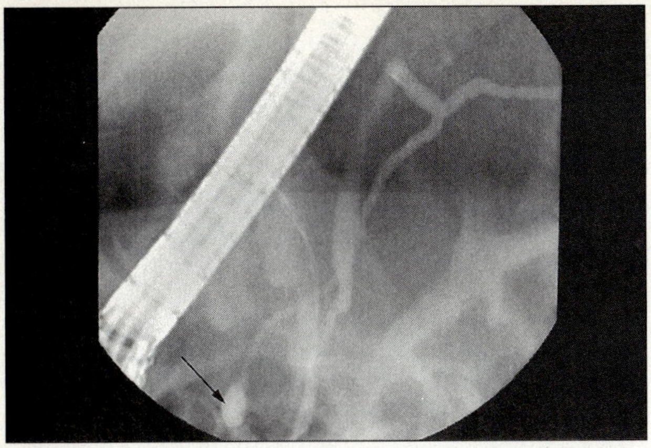
Figure 4. *Cystic dilatation of the accessory duct of Santorini (arrow) from obstructive ampullary adenomatous disease involving both the major and minor papilli. This patient ultimately underwent pancreaticduodenectomy.*

tomical ductal abnormalities, may be causative in these patients and should be ruled out early in the workup.

As noted earlier, endoscopic intervention in these patients has not been previously described. The few case reports in the literature generally discuss endoscopic biopsy and prompt surgical referral.[8,9] Our review demonstrates that patients can often be palliated with piecemeal resection and sphincterotomy but that relief will be temporary, will require close endoscopic follow-up, and will be somewhat dependent on the pattern of disease. The single patient who was "definitively" treated with serial snare resection had a single, large, obstructing ampullary mass rather than diffuse adenomatous disease, a pattern that frequently extends up and into the ampulla, making it difficult to resect. This group has a near 100% eventual failure rate of endoscopic sphincterotomy alone. Stenosis of the biliary sphincterotomy orifice outside of this patient subset has a much lower incidence (1%-5% in most published series) but does seem to be higher for pancreatic sphincterotomy.[15,16] For example, we have previously reported a 14% incidence of stenosis with pancreatic sphincterotomy in this institution.[17]

A question might be raised regarding the evidence that ampullary adenomas are the cause of pancreatitis in the 5 patients reviewed here. While we acknowledge that the evidence is somewhat indirect, we maintain that ampullary tumors as a cause of obstructing pancreatitis is reasonably well established in the literature and has been described not only in patients with familial polyposis but in the general population as well.[18] A single patient in this series had curative therapy with snare resection and debulking of a solitary ampullary adenoma. Another patient with a diffuse pattern of ampullary disease, involving not only the ampulla but the accessory duct as well, was found to have cystic dilatation of the duct of Santorini (Santorinicele), a finding indicative of obstruction (Figure 4).

The extracolonic manifestations classically described with GV familial polyposis, keloid reaction and fibromas in the form of desmoid tumors and osteomas, bely the abnormal scarring and fibroblast activity of these patients.[1,2] Unusual in the general population, desmoid tumors are seen in many patients with GV familial polyposis and desmoplastic reactions were noted in 2 of the patients in the current series. The latter are typically found intra-abdominally in areas of previous surgery or trauma and can be thought of as a marker of defective fibroblast control.[19,20] This may account for the failure of conventional sphincterotomy techniques in this setting. The patient in this series who failed transduodenal sphincteroplasty because of recurrent stenosis, despite several revisions, and the patient who required repetitive pancreaticojejunostomy revision, emphasize this. Some debate exists regarding the ability of sulindac to induce regression of C-loop adenomas,[12,13] but both sulindac and the antiestrogen analogue, tamoxifen, have been shown to limit desmoid growth and recurrence in patients with GV familial polyposis.[21-24] Although not used in the current series, it seems reasonable to extrapolate that one or both of these agents might have a similarly protective effect on scarring and stenosis at the sphincterotomy site if dosage and timing are appropriate for the initial procedure.

Despite the fact that no patient in this series was found to have malignant adenomatous disease, 60% of patients with obstructive adenomas ultimately underwent pancreaticoduodenectomy. The indication in all cases was recurrent or chronic pancreatitis plus failure of endoscopic sphincterotomy. Mean follow-up, to date, is 36 months with full symptom resolution. The question is whether these patients should be immediately referred for surgical evaluation. The patients with a diffuse pattern of adenomatous disease likely would have benefited from earlier surgical consideration. However, the diagnostic and, at least, temporizing role of initial ERCP in these patients is clear. Early relief with snare resection and sphincterotomy is common and could be particularly useful in a sick patient. Longer-lasting results may or may not be observed with the use of either sulindac or tamoxifen. Patients with large, focal, periampullary adenomas may also do well with therapeutic ERCP maneuvers alone, as may other patients with nonadenomatous etiologies, such as the sole patient with choledocholithiasis in this series. However, the need for surgical intervention may be inevitable in most of these patients. The results of pancreaticoduodenectomy have been superior in this series and it would clearly be the operation of choice for malignant disease. Surgical sphincteroplasty can be successful but does not remove the long-term risk of progression to malignant disease or prevent cicatrization from progressive desmoid reaction.

In conclusion, pancreatitis occurring secondary to obstructive adenomatous disease in the patient with known familial polyposis is relatively uncommon. Despite the small body of information in the literature, some clear management recommendations can be made. Careful questioning into patient background and medications, along with the use of noninvasive imaging modalities (such as ultrasonography and computed tomography), should always be done to rule out other common causes of pancreatitis. These patients should all undergo upper endoscopy and ERCP. If obstructive ampullary adenomas are found, then biopsy specimens should be obtained and snare resection with sphincterotomy considered. We advocate snare resection at initial ERCP if the lesion is low in the ampulla and not part of a diffuse adenomatous hyperplasia. We also recommend sphincterotomy at initial ERCP unless the endoscopist believes the obstructive lesion is extra-ampullary and amenable to snare resection alone. A postinstrumentation regimen of sulindac should be considered. For patients with malignant disease at biopsy or diffuse adenomatous disease involving the ampulla with recurrent encroachment and stenosis at the sphincterotomy site, prompt surgical referral should be strongly considered.

Presented at the annual meeting of the American College of Surgeons, Washington State Chapter, Chelan, Wash, June 15, 1998.

Reprints: R. A. Kozarek, MD, Section of Gastroenterology, Virginia Mason Medical Center, 1100 Ninth Ave, PO Box (CS-GAS), Seattle, WA 98111.

REFERENCES

1. Gardner EJ, Richards RC. Multiple cutaneous and subcutaneous lesions occurring simultaneously with hereditary polyposis and osteomatosis. *Am J Hum Genet.* 1953;5:139-147.
2. Schuchardt WA, Ponsky JL. Familial polyposis and Gardner's syndrome. *Surg Gynecol Obstet.* 1979;148:97-103.
3. Burt RW, Berenson MM, Lee RG, Tolman KG, Freston JW, Gardner EJ. Upper gastrointestinal polyps in Gardner's syndrome. *Gastroenterology.* 1984;86:295-301.
4. Jarvinen H, Nyberg M, Peltokallio P. Upper gastrointestinal tract polyps in familial adenomatosis coli. *Gut.* 1983;24:333-339.
5. Goedde TA, Rodriguez-Bigas MA, Herrera L, Petrelli NJ. Gastroduodenal polyps in familial adenomatous polyposis. *Surg Oncol.* 1992;1:357-361.
6. Offerhaus GJ, Giardiello FM, Krush AJ. The risk of upper gastrointestinal cancer in familial adenomatous polyposis. *Gastroenterology.* 1991;102:1980-1982.
7. Beckwith PS, Van Heerden JA, Dozois RR. Prognosis of syptomatic duodenal adenomas in familial adenomatous polyposis. *Arch Surg.* 1991;126:825-828.
8. Burt RW, Rikkers LF, Gardner EJ, Lee RG, Tolman KG. Villous adenoma of the duodenal papilla presenting as necrotizing pancreatitis in a patient with Gardner's syndrome. *Gastroenterology.* 1987;92:532-535.
9. Berk T, Freidman LS, Goldstein SG, Marks GP, Rosato FE. Relapsing acute pancreatitis as the presenting manifestation of an ampullary neoplasm in a patient with familial polyposis coli. *Am J Gastroenterol.* 1985;80:627-629.
10. Clarke DN, Norman JN, Smith JAR. Pancreatitis and duodenal obstruction due to periampullary carcinoma associated with familial polyposis coli. *Postgrad Med.* 1978;54:418-420.
11. Bleau BL, Gostout CJ. Endoscopic treatment of ampullary adenomas in familial adenomatous polyposis. *J Clin Gastroenterol.* 1996;22:237-241.
12. Giardiello FM. NSAID-induced polyp regression in familial adenomatous polyposis patients. *Gastroenterol Clin North Am.* 1996;25:349-359.
13. Nugent KP, Farmer KCR, Spigelman AD. Randomized controlled clinical trial of sulindac on intestinal polyposis in FAP. *Br J Surg.* 1993;80:1618-1619.
14. Sener SF, Miller HH, DeCosse JJ. The spectrum of polyposis. *Surg Gynecol Obstet.* 1984;159:525-532.
15. Prat F, Malak NA, Pelletier G, et al. Biliary symptoms and complications more than 8 years after endoscopic sphincterotomy for choledocholithiasis. *Gastroenterology.* 1996;110:894-899.
16. Watanapa P, Williamson RCN. Pancreatic sphincterotomy and sphincteroplasty. *Gut.* 1992;33:865-867.
17. Kozarek RA, Ball TJ, Patterson DJ, Brandabur JJ, Traverso LW, Raltz S. Endoscopic pancreatic duct sphincterotomy: indications, technique, and analysis of results. *Gastrointest Endosc.* 1994;40:592-598.
18. Norton ID, Sorbi D, Geller A, Petersen BT, Gostout CJ. Endoscopic management of sporadic periampullary adenomas [abstract]. *Gastrointest Endosc.* 1998;47:258.
19. Hizawa K, Iida M, Mibu R, Aoyagi K, Yao T, Fujishima M. Desmoid tumors in familial adenomatous polyposis/Gardner's syndrome. *J Clin Gastroenterol.* 1997;25:334-337.
20. Khorsand J, Karakousis CP. Desmoid tumors and their management. *Am J Surg.* 1985;149:215-218.
21. Tsukada K, Church JM, Jagelman DG, et al. Noncytotoxic drug therapy for intra-abdominal desmoid tumor in patients with familial adenomatous polyposis. *Dis Colon Rectum.* 1992;35:29-33.
22. Sportiello DJ, Hoogerland DL. A recurrent pelvic desmoid tumor successfully treated with tamoxifen. *Cancer.* 1991;67:1443-1446.
23. Belliveau P, Graham AM. Mesenteric desmoid tumor in Gardner's syndrome treated by sulindac. *Dis Colon Rectum.* 1984;27:53-54.
24. Waddell WR, Gerner RE, Reich MP. Non-steroidal anti-inflammatory drugs and tamoxifen for desmoid tumors and carcinoma of the stomach. *J Surg Oncol.* 1983;22:197-211.

IN OTHER AMA JOURNALS

JAMA

Aspirin and Risk of Hemorrhagic Stroke: A Meta-analysis of Randomized Controlled Trials

Jiang He, MD, PhD; Paul K. Whelton, MD, MSc; Brian Vu, BA; Michael J. Klag, MD, MPH

Context.—Aspirin has been widely used to prevent myocardial infarction and ischemic stroke but some studies have suggested it increases risk of hemorrhagic stroke.
Objective.—To estimate the risk of hemorrhagic stroke associated with aspirin treatment.
Data Sources.—Studies were retrieved using MEDLINE (search terms, *aspirin*, *cerebrovascular disorders*, and *stroke*), bibliographies of the articles retrieved, and the authors' reference files.
Study Selection.—All trials published in English-language journals before July 1997 in which participants were randomized to aspirin or a control treatment for at least 1 month and in which the incidence of stroke subtype was reported.
Data Extraction.—Information on country of origin, sample size, duration, study design, aspirin dosage, participant characteristics, and outcomes was abstracted independently by 2 authors who used a standardized protocol.
Data Synthesis.—Data from 16 trials with 55 462 participants and 108 hemorrhagic stroke cases were analyzed. The mean dosage of aspirin was 273 mg/d and mean duration of treatment was 37 months. Aspirin use was associated with an absolute risk reduction in myocardial infarction of 137 events per 10 000 persons (95% confidence interval [CI], 107-167; $P<.001$) and in ischemic stroke, a reduction of 39 events per 10 000 persons (95% CI, 17-61; $P<.001$). However, aspirin treatment was also associated with an absolute risk increase in hemorrhagic stroke of 12 events per 10 000 persons (95% CI, 5-20; $P<.001$). This risk did not differ by participant or study design characteristics.
Conclusions.—These results indicate that aspirin therapy increases the risk of hemorrhagic stroke. However, the overall benefit of aspirin use on myocardial infarction and ischemic stroke may outweigh its adverse effects on risk of hemorrhagic stroke in most populations. (*1998;280:1930-1935*)

Reprints: Jiang He, MD, PhD, Department of Biostatistics and Epidemiology, Tulane University School of Public Health and Tropical Medicine, 1430 Tulane Ave, SL 18, New Orleans, LA 70112 (e-mail: jhe@mailhost.tcs.tulane.edu).

Reoperation for Severe Pancreatitis

A 10-Year Experience in a Tertiary Care Center

François Paye, MD; Pascal Frileux, MD; Paul Lehman, MD; Jean-Marie Ollivier, MD; Jean Christophe Vaillant, MD; Rolland Parc, MD, FACS

Objectives: To analyze the specific problems encountered in treating patients previously operated on for necrotizing pancreatitis and to determine the benefit of such a complex and demanding procedure.

Design and Setting: Review of a case series in an academic tertiary care referral center.

Patients: Forty-four consecutive patients referred and reoperated on in 10 years.

Interventions: Reiterative laparotomy with complete debridment of all necrotic sites, followed by Mikulicz packing. Mikulicz packs were replaced by removable drains allowing both local prolonged lavage and open drainage of large solid necrotic debris. Enteral nutrition was performed through a feeding jejunostomy. Associated gastrointestinal tract lesions were simultaneously treated.

Main Outcome Measures: Operative findings, bacteriological status of necrosis, in-hospital mortality, length of hospitalization, and surgical complications and their management.

Results: Necrosis was infected in 36 (82%) of the 44 cases and associated gastrointestinal tract lesions were found in 20 (45%) of these patients. Mortality was 23%, and was significantly ($P = .03$) related to the preoperative clinical status. Surgical complications occurred in 31 (70%) of the 44 patients necessitating surgical treatment in 18 (41%) of these patients. Mean (± SD) stay in the intensive care unit was 66 ± 8 days for survivors.

Conclusion: This complex and demanding surgical procedure is worthwhile, yielding mortality rates comparable to those observed in de novo severe necrotizing pancreatitis.

Arch Surg. 1999;134:316-320

THE REPORTED mortality rates of severe necrotizing pancreatitis in surgical series still vary today from 8% to 35% despite improvements in intensive care management and imaging techniques.[1-4] Surgical treatment by necrosectomy followed by either local lavage or scheduled relaparotomy has reduced mortality compared with pancreatic resection.[2] The benefit of these complex surgical procedures is accepted in patients of necrotizing pancreatitis with infection but remains debatable in patients of sterile necrosis.[5-7] Today, tertiary care centers frequently are asked to manage patients operated on elsewhere and referred because of deterioration of clinical status. Numerous series including only a few transferred and reoperated on patients reported higher mortality rates than those observed in "first-hand pancreatitis."[3,6,8] To our knowledge, there is no large study to date specifically devoted to this subgroup of patients. Therefore, we have reviewed our experience in the last decade in the management of those patients previously operated on elsewhere, transferred, and then reoperated on in our center, using an original procedure combining necrosectomy, open drainage, and prolonged lavage. The aims of this retrospective work were to analyze the specific problems encountered in treating these patients and to determine the benefit of such a complex and demanding procedure.

See Invited Critique at end of article

RESULTS

On admission to our intesive care unit, 41 patients (93%) received intravenous antibiotics. Peripheral bacteriological samples (drainages or blood cultures) were positive

From the Department of Digestive Surgery, Hôpital Saint-Antoine, University Pierre et Marie Curie, Paris, France.

PATIENTS AND METHODS

From 1986 to 1996, 44 patients with acute pancreatitis previously operated on elsewhere were secondarily referred for clinical deterioration and reoperated on in our unit, using a standardized technique of necrosectomy and drainage followed by continuous irrigation.

This study group consisted of 27 men and 17 women, with a mean (± SD) age of 47 ± 13 years. Acute pancreatitis was due to gallstones in 20 patients, alcohol in 8 patients, abdominal trauma in 6 patients, hypertriglyceridemia in 3 patients, endoscopic sphincterotomy in 1 patient, and idiopathic in 6 patients.

At the initial center, the diagnosis of acute pancreatitis was suspected in only 20 (45%) of the 44 patients before surgery. Ranson score was never assessed properly in the first 48 hours of admission. Acute pancreatitis was confirmed or diagnosed intraoperatively in all patients with necrosis noted in 31 patients (70%). Necrosectomy was performed in 13 patients and 2 patients underwent distal pancreatectomy. Peripancreatic drainage was performed using rubber drains in 27 patients. No patient underwent continuous irrigation of the pancreatic bed. Bacteriological analysis of pancreatic necrosis was unavailable retrospectively in most cases.

Patients were referred to our center with a mean (± SD) delay of 21 ± 14 days after the onset of the pancreatitis. Bacteriological analysis of drained fluids and blood cultures were systematically performed on admission to our intensive care unit.

Abdominal computed tomographic (CT) scan with bolus intravenous infusion of contrast material was performed if the patient's clinical status allowed this examination. Lesions were classified according to the Balthazar scoring system.[9,10] There was no attempt at percutaneous puncture or drainage of the fluid collections found on CT scans.

Reoperations were decided on either because of a surgical complication of the first procedure (evisceration, undrained gastrointestinal (GI) tract fistula, or hemorrage), or because of clinical deterioration with a septic course and evidence of organ failure (hemodynamic shock, acute respiratory distress syndrome, or renal insufficiency) persisting after 48 hour of maximal intensive supporting therapy.

The simplified acute physiologic score (SAPS)[11] was assessed in the 12 hour preceeding reoperation. Clinical findings and biological anomalies considered in our current practice in assessing patient's status[12] were collected. Reoperation was performed by a senior surgeon through the previous incision frequently extended (bilateral subcostal incisions extending to the flanks or xypho-pubic incisions). All potential sites of necrosis and collections were explored. The anterior aspect of the pancreas was exposed through large openings of the gastrocolic ligament and lesser omentum. The posterior aspect of the pancreatic head was exposed by a Kocher maneuver. Mobilization of the right and left colon exposed the right and left pararenal spaces. The peritoneum at the base of the mesentery was divided. Areas of fluid collections and necrosis were sampled for bacteriological analysis. A complete necrosectomy was performed. Mikulicz gauze packs (**Figure 1**) were placed in these necrotic sites and were brought out of the abdomen through the incision (**Figure 2**). The tail of the pancreas was drained by a Mikulicz gauze pack located behind the left colic angle and exteriorized in the left flank. An ileostomy was performed in case of dubious colic viability,[13] while necrotic colon or colic fistula led to segmental colectomy and double stoma. Biliary drainage (cholecystostomy, transcystic drainage, or choledochal T tube) and a feeding jejunostomy were placed.

Continuous enteral nutrition was started as soon as postoperative ileus resolved. Mikulicz gauze packs were removed at the 14th day, leaving large channels giving access to the necrotic sites, into which large bore (36F catheter) 3-channeled soft silicon spiral drains[14] (Figure 1 and **Figure 3**) were inserted. A continuous irrigation with 2 L/d of dialysate added with 20 mL of povidone-iodine per liter of dialysate (Betadine; Asta Medica Laboratory, Merignac, France) and 50 000 UI/L of aprotinin (Trasylol; Bayer Pharma Laboratory, Puteaux, France) was immediately started through these drains. They were temporarily removed daily by the nursing staff for at least 3 weeks to perform local lavage with dialysate under pressure, to dislodge large solid necrotic debris. Antibiotics were adapted to the bacteriological analysis of the necrosis. Somatostatin analogues were not used in these patients.

Numeric results are expressed as mean ± SD. Statistical analysis was performed using the χ^2 test with Yates correction and the Student *t* test where appropriate.

in 23 patients. Abdominal CT scan preceded reoperation in 27 patients. A Balthazar grade E CT scan was noted in 20 patients (74%) and a Balthazar grade D in 7 patients (16%). Lack of enhancement was noted in 13 patients (44%), affecting more than 50% of the gland in 10 patients, and less in 3 patients. Gas bubbles in peripancreatic collections were noted in 11 patients (6 patients had drains in place).

Reoperation was indicated because of continuing sepsis with evidence of organ failure after 48 hour of maximal therapy in 36 patients, sepsis with undrained GI tract fistula in 4 patients, sepsis with evisceration in 3 patients, and massive hemorrage exteriorized through a drain in 1 patient. The description of patient's status prior to reoperation is detailed in **Figure 4**. The mean value of the SAPS was 8.5 ± 3.7.

Parenchymatous necrosis affected more than 50% of the pancreas in 18 patients, was less than 50% in 17 patients, and was absent in 9 patients. Extra pancreatic fat necrosis was always present. Necrosis was infected in 36 patients (82%) and sterile in 8 patients (18%) (**Table 1**). In 14 patients, a fistula of the upper GI tract was found affecting the stomach in 2 patients, the duodenum in 4 patients, the small bowel in 2 patients, and the biliary tract in 5 patients. They were due to traumatic injury by previous drainages, feeding tubes and endoscopic procedures, or the involvement of the viscera by extra pancreatic necrosis. These were treated by intubation or stoma. Nine segmental or subtotal colectomies were performed to treat 3 colic necrosis and 6 colic fistulae. Fifteen loop ileostomies were performed to divert a colon of dubious viability. One splenic injury necessitated a splenectomy. The abdominal wall was closed using an exclusive cutaneous closure in 21 patients with relaxation incisions in 6 patients.[15]

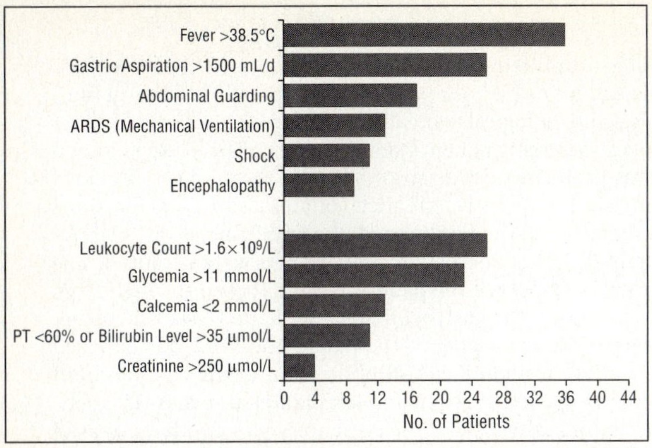

Figure 1. *Patient's status in the 12 hours preceding reoperation. An output of gastric aspiration more than 1500 mL/d reflected gastrointestinal (GI) tract ileus. Shock was defined as a mean arterial pressure of 80 mm Hg or by the necessity to use pressive amines. ARDS indicates adult respiratory distress syndrome; PT, prothrombin time.*

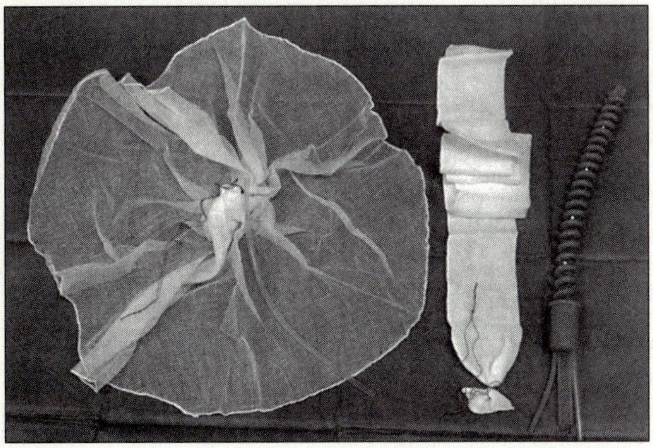

Figure 2. *The Mikulicz gauze packs and the spiral drain. Each Mikulicz drainage system comprises a 60-cm gauze disk filled with 1 to 3 (90 × 7.5-cm) rectangular gauze pieces. At the 14th day, the spiral drain replaces the Mikulicz pack. It is daily removed for local lavage of the necrotic sites with dialysate under pressure. Its large central channel is used for aspiration and 2 fine-bore tubes for continuous irrigation and air circulation.*

Ten patients died postoperatively after a median delay of 48 days (range, 6-250 days), accounting for a mortality rate of 23%. Causes of death were 5 multiple organ failures, 2 noscocomial pneumonias, 1 massive hematemesis, 1 cerebral stroke, and 1 pulmonary embolism. Age, sex ratio, delay of reoperation, bacteriological status of necrosis and associated GI tract lesions did not differ between survivors and nonsurvivors. The SAPS calculated prior to reoperation was significantly higher in patients who ultimately died (SAPS, 10.6 ± 4.2 vs 7.8 ± 3.4; $P = .03$).

Continuous enteral nutrition was started after a delay of 11 ± 1 days and was used during 56 ± 5 days. Continuous irrigation and drainage were maintained to ensure complete evacuation of necrotic debris over 40 ± 6 days. Mechanical ventilation was used for 14 ± 2 days. Forty-one surgical complications affected 31 patients (70%) during postoperative course and were treated either medically or with an iterative surgical procedure (18 patients) (**Table 2**). Pancreatic and GI tract fistulae were the most frequent complications affecting 10 and 7 patients, respectively. One gastric fistula occurred and was due to the reopening of a previous gastric fistula, present and sutured at first reoperation performed in our center. The remaining 6 GI tract fistulae occurred de novo. Iterative necrotic undrained collection justified a second surgical drainage in only 6 patients. No patient required more than 2 surgical drainages The mean stay in the intesive care unit was 66 ± 8 days for survivors. Continuity of the GI tract was restored in all survivors. In 8 patients abdominal wall hernia causing esthetic or functional discomfort has necessitated delayed reparative surgery.

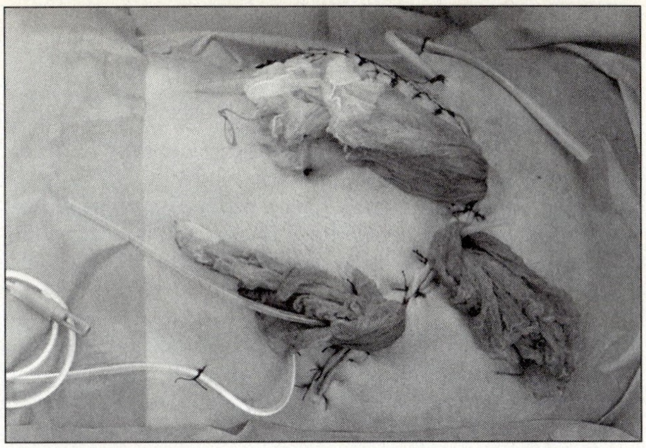

Figure 3. *View of the abdomen at the end of the reoperation. Mikulicz packs are exteriorized through the closed bilateral-subcostal incision. The jejunostomy feeding tube is on the patient's left side and the cholecystostomy tube is on the right side.*

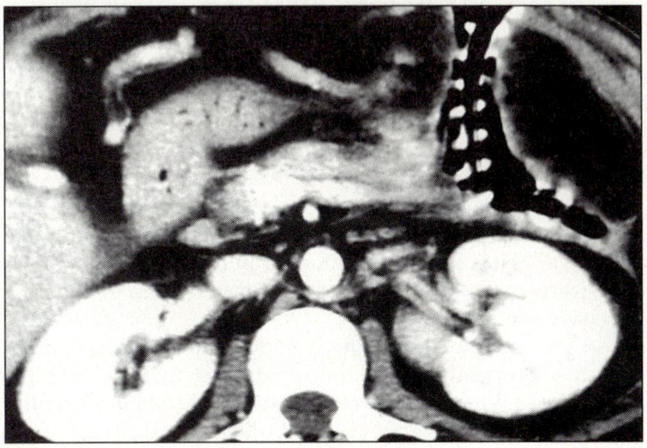

Figure 4. *Computed tomographic scan showing a spiral drain in situ. The shaft leading to the necrotic area is quite visible.*

COMMENT

This case series demonstrates the value of a formal reoperation combining necrosectomy, prolonged irrigation of the pancreatic bed with active debridement of necrosis for patients previously operated on for severe acute pancreatitis and referred in a specialized center for clinical deterioration. Indeed, despite higher rates of superinfection of undrained necrosis and associated GI tract lesions than observed in de novo severe pancreatitis, this procedure yields a 23% in-hospital mortality rate comparable to that reported by specialized surgical teams for patients without operative intervention.[4,6,16]

Table 1. Bacteriological Analysis of Necrosis Collected Before Reoperation*

Gram Staining	Microorganisms	No. of Patients
Aerobes		
Gram-positive	*Staphylococcus* coagulase-positive	2
	Staphylococcus coagulase-negative	3
	Enterococcus species	13
	Escherichia coli	8
	Proteus mirabilis	5
	Klebsiella oxytoca	5
Gram-negative	*Enterobacter* species	4
	Serratia species	2
	Pseudomonas aeruginosa	7
	Acinetobacter species	6
	Xanthomonas maltophilia	1
Anaerobes	*Bacteroides fragilis*	2
Fungi	*Candida albicans*	4

**A single species of microorganism was present in 17 patients, 2 different species were present in 12 patients, and 3 different species were found in 7 patients. Cultures were sterile for 8 patients.*

Table 2. Complications Following Reoperation and Their Treatments

Complications	No. (%) of Patients	Duration of Treatment, d	Treatments
Undrained necrotic collection	6 (14)	5-82	Surgical drainage
Pseudocyst	2 (4)	65-74	Enterocystostomy
Pancreatic fistula	10 (23)	3-195	Distal pancreatectomy (n = 4) Spontaneous closure (n = 6)
GI tract fistula*	7 (16)	3-30	Delayed surgery (n = 6) Spontaneous closure (n = 1)
Biliary fistula	1 (2)	14	Spontaneous closure
Evisceration	1 (2)	1	Spontaneous closure
Upper GI tract bleeding	6 (14)	2-75	Antisecretory drugs and endoscopic sclerosis

**Involving the stomach (1 patient with reopening of a gastric fistula sutured at the initial reoperation), the duodenum (1 patient), the small bowel (2 patients), and the colon (3 patients without diverting ileostomy). GI indicates gastrointestinal.*

Prognostic scores commonly used for acute pancreatitis[17-19] include data collected in the first 48 hour of first admission. These scores were therefore unsuitable for these reoperated on patients. The SAPS, which prognostic value has been established for de novo pancreatitis,[11] seems of comparable prognostic value for these reoperated on patients when it is calculated in the 12 hours prior to reoperation. Its high mean value reflects the severity of pancreatitis in this series.

Most patients were reoperated on because of severe clinical deterioration occurring despite appropriate intensive supportive treatment. We did not preoperatively assess the bacteriological status of necrosis by percutaneous CT-guided fine needle aspiration.[20] This strategy could be criticized by those operating exclusively infected necrosis,[5,4,21,22] but the mortality of severe pancreatitits even with sterile necrosis can reach 38%.[7] Moreover, the bacteriological status of the necrosis has no significant influence on the outcome for patients operated on after the third week of evolution of the pancreatitis[23] and the surgical debridment of symptomatic necrosis seems beneficial irrespective of its bacteriological status.[6] Lastly, infection of necrosis was actually present in most patients, probably favored by previous inadequate prolonged surgical drainage.[24,25]

A poor correlation was found between CT scan and either extra pancreatic necrosis or outcome, consistent with previous findings.[10,26,27] Gas bubbles within necrosis were not reliably attributable to infection in these operated on patients because of previously placed abdominal drains. We did not use the CT-guided percutaneous drainage of necrotic collections because of poor results in pancreatitis,[28] attributable to their inability to drain large solid necrotic debris.[6,24] Since our surgical procedure systematically explores all potential sites of necrotic collections, CT scan was not obtained in hemodynamically unstable patients before reoperation.

The transperitoneal route was preferred to the retroperitoneal approach recently promoted,[24,29] to perform simultaneously complete debridment of all necrotic sites, treatment of associated visceral lesions, and placement of a feeding jejunostomy. The procedure of initial packing followed by insertion of the silicon spiral drains that were removed daily for local lavage, combines the advantages of techniques of repeated necrosectomy, with prolonged evacuation of large solid necrotic debris[4,30,31] with those of the closed irrigation, namely, dilution of toxic compounds, prolonged drainage, closure of the abdominal wall with protection GI tract fistulization, and early use of enteral nutrition.[1,32] The 14% incidence of undrained infected collections necessitating surgical drainage and the 4% incidence of late pseudocyst observed in this series compares favorably with previous reports,[1,6,8] and reflects the efficiency of this drainage procedure.

The 6 de novo GI tract fistulae (14%) observed during the postoperative course were attibutable either to the necrotizing process or more likely to GI tract traumatism by the removal of the Mikulicz gauze packs or by iterative mobilization of the spiral drains. These fistulae are, however, also observed with other techniques.[33] They could be well drained and irrigated by the spiral drains and were closed by delayed simple surgery. Pancreatic fistulae were the most frequent complication but closed spontaneously in 60% of cases. They constitute probably the unavoidable drawback of an efficient necrosectomy and drainage procedure and are observed with comparable frequency by several teams, no matter what surgical technique is used.[4] The prophylactic use of somatostatin analogues may reduce the incidence of these pancreatic fistulae or favor a spontaneous closure.[34]

Mortality of patients transferred from other units for severe acute pancreatitis has been reported to be greater than for direct admission in a specialized unit and to reach 35% to 75%.[3,6,8] Contrary to these previous reports including only a few patients operated on, transferred, and reoperated on in specialized centers,[3,6,8] the 23% mortality rate observed in this series is comparable to the mortality rates reported by us and others[2,6,12,29,35] for de novo necrotizing pancreatitis. The efficiency of our operative approach may be responsible for this difference. Its results argue for the early transfer of such patients in specialized centers and justify this complex and demanding treatment.[36]

We thank John Serius, MD, for his assistance in reading the manuscript.

Corresponding author: Rolland Parc, MD, FACS, Service de Chirurgie Digestive, Hôpital Saint-Antoine, 184 rue du Faubourg Saint-Antoine, 75012 Paris, France.

REFERENCES

1. Beger HG, Buchler M, Bittner R. Necrosectomy and postoperative local lavage in patients with necrotizing pancreatitis: results of a prospective multicenter trial. *World J Surg.* 1988;12:255-262.
2. D'Edigio A, Schein M. Surgical strategies in the treatment of pancreatic necrosis and infection. *Br J Surg.* 1991;78:133-137.
3. De Beaux AC, Palmer KR, Carter DC. Factors influencing morbidity and mortality in acute pancreatitis; an analysis of 279 cases. *Gut.* 1995;37:121-126.
4. Bradley EL. Surgical indications and techniques in acute pancreatitis. In: Bradley EL, ed. *Acute Pancreatitis: Diagnosis and Therapy.* New York, NY: Raven Press; 1994:105-120.
5. Bradley EL, Allen K. A prospective longitudinal study of observation versus surgical intervention in the management of necrotizing pancreatitis. *Am J Surg.* 1991; 161:19-25.
6. Rattner DW, Legermate DA, Lee MJ, Mueller PR, Warshaw AL. Early surgical debridement of symptomatic pancreatic necrosis is beneficial irrespective of infection. *Am J Surg.* 1992;163:105-109.
7. Karimgani I, Porter KA, Langevin E, Banks PA. Prognostic factors in sterile pancreatic necrosis. *Gastroenterology.* 1992;103:1636-1640.
8. Wilson C, McArdle CS, Carter DC, Imrie CW. Surgical treatment of acute necrotizing pancreatitis. *Br J Surg.* 1988;75:1119-1123.
9. Balthazar EJ, Ranson JHC, Naidich DP, Megibow AJ, Caccavale R, Cooper M. Acute pancreatitis: prognostic value of CT. *Radiology.* 1985;156:767-772.
10. Balthazar EJ, Robinson DL, Megibow AJ, Ranson JHC. Acute pancreatitis: value of CT in establishing prognosis. *Radiology.* 1990;174:331-336.
11. Loirat P, Gayraud M, Bonnet F, Rigattieri S, Le Gall JR, Alperovitch A. Comparison of three severity score indices in acute hemorragic pancreatitis. *Intensive Care Med.* 1983;9:236-240.
12. Frileux P, Levy E, Entremont A, Cugnenc PH, Parc R. Necrotizing pancreatitis in France. In: III ELB, ed. *Acute Pancreatitis: Diagnosis and Therapy.* New York, NY: Raven Press, 1994:133-138.
13. Borie D, Frileux P, Tiret E, et al. Colonic complications of acute necrotizing pancreatitis. *Presse Med.* 1992;21:519-523.
14. Frileux P, Cugnenc PH, Fontaine E, et al. Acute necrotizing pancreatitis: surgical management with capillary drainage, long-term lavage, and continuous enteral nutrition. *Acute Pancreatitis.* Berlin, Germany: Springer-Verlag; 1987:231-237.
15. Levy E, Palmer DL, Frileux P, Hannoun L, Nordlinger B, Parc R. Septic necrosis in the middle wound in postoperative peritonitis: successful management by debridment, myocutaneous advancement and primary skin closure. *Ann Surg.* 1988; 207:470-479.
16. Mier J, Luque-de-Leon E, Castillo A, Robledo F, Blanco R. Early versus late necrosectomy in severe necrotizing pancreatitis. *Am J Surg.* 1997;173:71-75.
17. Ranson JC, Rifkindt KM, Roses DF, Fink SD, Eng K, Spencer FC. Prognostic signs and the role of operative management in acute pancreatitis. *Surg Gynecol Obstet.* 1974;139:69-81.
18. Blamey SL, Imrie CV, O'Neill J, Gilmour WH, Carter DC. Prognostic factors in acute pancreatitis. *Gut.* 1984;25:1340-1346.
19. Wilson C, Heath DI, Imrie CW. Prediction of outcome in acute pancreatitis: a comparative study of Apache II, clinical assessment and multiple factor scoring systems. *Br J Surg.* 1990;77:1260-1264.
20. Gerzof SG, Banks PA, Robbins AH, Johnson WC, Spechler SJ, Wetzner SM. Early diagnosis of pancreatic infection by computed tomography-guided aspiration. *Gastroenterology.* 1987;93:1315-1320.
21. Mc Fadden DW, Reber HA. Indications for surgery in severe acute pancreatitis. *Int J Pancreatol.* 1994;15:83-80.
22. Reber HA. Surgical intervention in necrotizing pancreatitis. *Gastroenterology.* 1986; 91:233-237.
23. Beger HG, Bittner R, Block S, Büchler M. Bacterial contamination of pancreatic necrosis. *Gastroenterology.* 1986;91:433-438.
24. Fagniez PL, Rotman N, Kracht M. Direct retroperitoneal approach to necrosis in severe acute pancreatitis. *Br J Surg.* 1989;76:264-267.
25. Saxon A, Reynolds JT, Doolas A. Management of pancreatic abscesses. *Ann Surg.* 1981;194:543-552.
26. Bradley EL. A clinically based classification system for acute pancreatitis. *Arch Surg.* 1993;128:586-590.
27. London NJM, Leese T, Lavelle JM, et al. Rapid-bolus contrast-enhanced dynamic computed tomography in acute pancreatitis: a prospective study. *Br J Surg.* 1991;78:1452-1456.
28. Adams DB, Harvey TS, Anderson MC. Percutaneous catheter drainage of infected pancreatic and peripancreatic fluid collections. *Arch Surg.* 1990;125:1554-1557.
29. Van Vyve EL, Reynaert MS, Lengele BG, Pringot JT, Otte JB, Kestens PJ. Retroperitoneal laparostomy: a surgical treatment of pancreatic abcesses after an acute necrotizing pancreatitis. *Surgery.* 1992;111:369-375.
30. Bradley EL. Management of infected pancreatic necrosis by open drainage. *Ann Surg.* 1987;206:542-550.
31. Pemberton JH, Becker JM, Dozois RR, Nagorney DM, Ilstrup D, Remine WH. Controlled open lesser sac drainage for pancreatic abscess. *Ann Surg.* 1986; 203:600-604.
32. Larvin M, Chalmers AG, Robinson PJ, McMahon MJ. Debridment and closed cavity irrigation for the treatment of pancreatic necrosis. *Br J Surg.* 1989;76:465-471.
33. Tsiotos GG, Smith D, Sarr MG. Incidence and management of pancreatic and enteric fistulas after surgical management of severe necrotizing procedure. *Arch Surg.* 1995;130:48-52.
34. Friess H, Büchler MW. Efficacy of somatostatin and its analogues in pancreatic surgery and pancreatic disorders. *Digestion.* 1996;57(suppl 1):97-102.
35. Sarr MG, Nagorney DM, Mucha P Jr, Farnell MB, Johnson CD. Acute necrotizing pancreatitis: management by planned, staged pancreatic necrosectomy/debridement and delayed primary wound closure over drains. *Br J Surg.* 1991;78:576-581.
36. Fenton-Lee D, Imrie CV. Pancreatic necrosis: assessment of outcome related to quality of life and cost of management. *Br J Surg.* 1993;80:1579-1582.

Invited Critique

The preceding article from our French colleagues focuses on a difficult subgroup of patients with necrotizing pancreatitis in whom an initial surgical exploration failed to control sepsis. Their reoperative approach consisted of extensive debridement of residual necrosis, exteriorized Mikulicz packs, feeding jejunostomy, biliary drainage, and loop ileostomy whenever colon viability was problematic. After 2 weeks, packs were replaced with proprietary silicon drains, which were exchanged daily and continuously irrigated. Since this approach is essentially a modification of lesser sac lavage, it is not surprising that their 23% mortality rate is comparable to traditional lesser sac lavage.[1] Several comments are in order. Infected pancreatic necrosis was present in 82% of these previously surgically explored patients, a significantly greater incidence of infected necrosis than the 20% incidence of infected necrosis in unoperated necrotizing pancreatitis.[2] Surgically induced secondary infection of sterile pancreatic necrosis is a real risk and results in measurable escalation of mortality.[3] When combined with prospective observations that neither mortality nor morbidity is improved by surgical debridement when compared with supportive therapy,[4] the rationale for surgical intervention in sterile necrotizing pancreatitis is, at best, unclear.

From a technical standpoint, the somewhat higher rate of fistula formation in the current series (14%) may have arisen from repetitive tube exchanges. Moreover, the 43% incidence of loop ileostomy in this report may have been the price paid by Paye et al to avoid determination of colonic viability by scheduled surgical reexplorations. Unfortunately, no justification was offered for programmatic biliary drainage by cholecystostomy or choledochotomy, procedures largely abandoned in other pancreatic centers. Despite these minor misgivings, Paye et al are to be congratulated for their excellent results in these salvage cases, results that speak eloquently not only for the skill and dedication of their pancreatic team, but also for early referral of patients with necrotizing pancreatitis to centers of excellence.

Edward L. Bradley III, MD
Buffalo, NY

1. Bradley EL III. Surgical indications and techniques in necrotizing pancreatitis. In: Bradley EL III, ed. *Acute Pancreatitis: Principles and Practice*. New York, NY: Raven Press; 1994:105-115.
2. Uomo G, Visconti M, Manes G, Calise F, Laccetti M, Rabitti PG. Nonsurgical treatment of acute necrotizing pancreatitis. *Pancreas*. 1996;12:142-148.
3. Widdison AL, Alvarez C, Reber HA. Surgical intervention in acute pancreatitis: when and how. *Pancreas*. 1991;6:544-551.
4. Bradley EL III. Debridement is rarely necessary in patients with sterile pancreatic necrosis. *Pancreas*. 1996;13:220-223.

IN OTHER AMA JOURNALS

ARCHIVES OF INTERNAL MEDICINE

The Clinical Diagnosis of Deep Venous Thrombosis

Susan R. Kahn, MD, MSc

Symptoms and clinical signs suggestive of deep venous thrombosis (DVT) are common and have numerous possible causes. Studies have shown that symptoms and clinical signs in themselves are inaccurate for the diagnosis of DVT. However, clinicians have other information at hand, such as data on risk factors for DVT, that may help improve their ability to predict a diagnosis of DVT in the individual patient. Epidemiological data on DVT incidence and risk factors were reviewed, as were published data on the accuracy of clinical diagnosis of DVT, with the use of both symptoms and signs in isolation and symptoms and signs combined with other clinical information in the form of clinical prediction indexes. Symptoms and clinical signs, when combined with other patient information such as the presence or absence of known risk factors for DVT, can improve clinical prediction considerably. Further study is needed to determine whether clinical prediction indexes have a role in improving the diagnostic process in patients with suspected DVT. (*1998;158:2315-2323*)

Corresponding author: Susan R. Kahn, MD, MSc, Center for Clinical Epidemiology and Community Studies, Sir Mortimer B. Davis Jewish General Hospital, 3755 Cote Ste Catherine, Room A118.1, Montreal, Quebec, Canada H3T 1E2 (e-mail: susank@epid.jgh.mcgill.ca).

A Medical Student's Meeting With Two Giants

IN 1967, as a second-year medical student at University of California, San Francisco, I had the fortune or misfortune of diagnosing an arteriovenous malformation in my wife's neck near the base of her skull. After acquiring a bit of knowledge in physical examination and cardiovascular physiology, I came to the conclusion that the "machinery-like" murmur I had heard in her neck might be pathological. I referred my wife to my preceptor in internal medicine, Joe Kaufman, MD, a cardiologist, who told us that my wife had a cirsoid aneurysm off the vertebral artery and that it was serious.

My wife and I were quite distraught and we were referred to Jack Wylie, MD, for possible repair of the aneurysm. An angiogram confirmed that my wife did indeed have an arteriovenous malformation feeding off the right vertebral artery and thyrocervical trunk with connections at the base of the skull. In 1967 there were no angiographic techniques to tackle these fistulae and surgery was proposed. In fact, my wife was scheduled for surgery and her parents flew to San Francisco because the operation was considered risky in terms of blood loss and possible stroke.

The night before the operation I asked to meet with Dr Wylie. As a second-year medical student I did not know how famous this man was or how formidable he could be, so I simply asked to meet with him regarding my wife's surgery. He saw me in his office at about 8 PM the night before surgery and explained that we should try to "shut off" this fistula because it could cause heart failure or deprive her brain of blood and cause a stroke. I asked him about the success rate with such an operation and he said that too few had been done to assess success but that he thought he could fix my wife's fistula—because when he put his finger over the area of the thrill, he could obliterate the bruit. I then asked him if he had ever done one of these operations and he said no. Recall that I was just a second-year medical student, and I was just thinking out loud about someone who was very important to me. I then said to Dr Wylie, "She's not in heart failure presently and she has no evidence of cerebrovascular insufficiency; could we wait on surgery?" He looked at me and cleared his throat ("hhemm!"), as I later learned he was wont to do when he had a message to deliver. He said, "That's not a bad idea, let's wait." He then called his chief resident and told him to cancel the morning operation.

He was very cordial to me during this visit and at the end he said, "I would like you to see another vascular surgeon. He's a little old, but he has great experience and I value his judgment. His name is Emile Holman."

Several days later my wife and I took her x-rays over to the old Stanford University Medical Center in San Francisco to see Dr Holman. Dr Holman, then in his 80s, was as slight as Dr Wylie was imposing. He was a pixielike man with a twinkle in his eyes. During the examination we mentioned to Dr Holman that my wife would be applying to medical school. At the end of the examination my wife, who had been living with this dilemma too long, plaintively asked Dr Holman, "Should I have surgery?" He looked at my wife with a smile on his face. He didn't answer the question. Instead he said, "I think you should go to medical school!" The implication was she would probably live long enough without an operation to become a productive surgeon.

Drs Wylie and Holman, giants of their era, took time to listen to a patient and his wife and alter a planned therapy. When we think of giants of the bygone era, we think of autocrats; but these two were much more than that. In talking with us, they had a humanity and understanding of our problem. Maybe that is part of what made them great.

My wife entered medical school, became a surgeon, and has had a very successful career in academic surgery. Approximately 10 to 15 years after its discovery, the fistula closed spontaneously and remains undetectable. One could say that Dr Wylie successfully treated a cirsoid aneurysm arteriovenous fistula by following the wishes of a second-year medical student. Dr Holman injected a little levity into the situation and enabled us to get on with our lives. For us they will always be giants.

Clifford W. Deveney, MD
Portland, Ore

SPECIAL ARTICLE

Surgery in the Philippines

Antonio A. Limson, MD; Jose Luis J. Danguilan, MD; Romeo R. Gutierrez, MD; Ramon S. de Jesus, MD; Armando C. Crisostomo, MD; Alberto M. Roxas, MD

The Philippines is an archipelago of about 7000 islands, with an area about the size of England, situated just above the equator in Southeast Asia. It has a population of 70 million. The Philippines has had extensive commercial and social contact with Asian neighbors, specifically the Chinese, even before the 377 years of Spanish colonization from 1521 to 1898 and the 48 years of American rule from 1898 to 1946. More than 80% of Filipinos are Catholics; the rest are Muslims and Protestants of various denominations, including those who belong to Filipino church groups. Infectious diseases such as tuberculosis, amoebiasis, typhoid fever, and malaria are still prevalent, and arteriosclerosis, cancer, and stroke are common and on the rise.

Arch Surg. 1999;134:323-327

HISTORY

Before the colonization of the Philippines by Spain in the early 16th century, wounds were treated by application of leaves and bark of trees, a system that is still practiced among indigenous tribes in remote areas that were not colonized. There may have been rudiments of foreign medical practice, since the Philippines engaged in trade with China, India, and successive empires in Southeast Asia. The systematic and purposeful destruction of early Philippine civilization by the Spanish colonizers left little of written accounts of medical practice by early Philippine natives.

Like any colonizing power, Spain took care of her soldiers and her citizens in the Philippines. The first hospital in the Philippines was a military one that was built on the southern island of Cebu in 1565. This was transferred to the walled city of Intramuros in Manila in 1571 and later renamed Sternburg Hospital by the invading Americans in 1898. This hospital was destroyed during World War II. In 1577, another dispensary made of bamboo and thatched material was built by a Spanish Franciscan missionary in Manila. This was destroyed by earthquake or fire several times, but was always rebuilt. This hospital was renamed the Hospital de San Juan de Dios in 1596 and became the teaching hospital of the Royal and Pontifical University of Santo Tomas, one of Asia's oldest universities, until the start of World War II in 1941. The first recorded exploratory laparotomy in the Philippines was performed at the Hospital de San Juan de Dios by the Philippines' finest surgeons in 1900. During this time, surgical instruments were washed and polished with the belief that the brighter and more shiny the instrument, the less danger there was of producing contamination.

During the Spanish possession, surgery was being practiced by Spanish barber surgeons, Chinese physicians, Dutch surgeons, and physicians of various nationalities, although the type of surgery is not known. The Philippines was at the center of a busy trading route in Southeast Asia, even before the Spanish colonization. Mention from written reports of Spanish expeditions was also made of sutured head wounds among the crew of expeditions sent to colonize the Muslims in the southern islands of the Philippines. The

From the Department of Surgery, College of Medicine and Philippine General Hospital, University of the Philippines, Manila.

only abdominal operation performed during the early Spanish regime by Spanish surgeons was a postmortem cesarean section, a practice that was sanctioned by the Catholic Church.

Manila as a city did not seem, in the medical aspect, to be behind other medieval cities of Europe. The University of Santo Tomas was founded before any other academic institution in North America. There were many attempts to establish a medical school in this university, starting in 1682, which was only realized in 1871. There was opposition to establishment of schools of science by the colonizers because of the fear that further education of the natives would make them aware of their rights and therefore they would be difficult to govern. This was proved true during the closing years of Spain's rule. Filipinos educated in Europe, exemplified by the physician and national hero of the Philippines, Dr Jose Rizal, were at the forefront of the insurrection against Spain.

The first medical graduates in 1877 were called licentiates or medicos titulares and these degrees were not invested doctoral degrees; they could only be obtained at the Universidad Central de Madrid. Ether was used as an anesthetic in 1847, 1 year after William T. C. Morton, DDM, described its use in Boston, Mass. Chloroform was used not long after James Young Simpson, MD, used it in Edinburgh in 1847. A list of operations at the Hospital de San Juan de Dios from 1878 to 1879 included trephination, rhinoplasty, cheiloplasty, staphylorrhaphy, operation for squint, cataract extraction, enucleation of the eye, amputation of arm and forearm, disarticulation of shoulders and elbow, and ligation of the common carotid, subclavian, and axillary arteries for aneurysms.

The defeat of the Filipinos by the better-equipped American army at the turn of the century saw the establishment of hospitals in the Philippines by American military surgeons. American influence in Philippine medicine was deep and lasting. In 1904, as part of the American policy of attraction for the ilustrados or Filipino elite, Filipino surgeons were sent to the United States to study and train in American hospitals. Their eventual return to the Philippines marked the beginning of the golden age of Philippine surgery.[1] Thyroidectomies, colon resections, and mastectomies were performed, along with the introduction of low-segment cesarean section,[2] craniotomy,[3] treatment of fractures and burns,[4,5] and open prostatectomy.[6]

MEDICAL SCHOOLS AND UNDERGRADUATE SURGICAL EDUCATION

There are now 30 medical schools in the Philippines; 6 are government owned and the rest are private institutions. The system of medical education is Western oriented, specifically American influenced, whether in curriculum, textbooks, or teaching methods, including postgraduate training. Many of the practicing specialists are trained abroad, usually in American hospitals and university medical centers. A few of the medical schools, particularly the new ones, use problem-based learning.

A 4-year bachelor's degree in preparatory medicine is a requirement for entry into the 4-year medicine proper course. After graduation, graduates undergo 1 year of rotating internship in a hospital of their choice. Only after completion of internship are medical graduates allowed to take the physician licensure examinations, which are given twice a year. A licensed physician usually proceeds to residency training in the Philippines or abroad, goes into general practice, or opts to continue further schooling. At the state-run University of the Philippines, an additional entry point for the top 50 freshmen with inclination to go into medicine is the 7-year integrated arts and medicine curriculum, which includes 2 years of liberal arts, 4 years of medical school, and a year of rotating internship.

During the second year of medical school, students are taught the principles of surgery, followed by general and specialty surgery the third year. Didactic lectures, small group discussions, and preceptorships are the teaching methods used. English is the medium of instruction. In the fourth year, medical students undergo a clinical clerkship rotating through the different clinical departments with a graduated process of increasing responsibilities and expectations. An average of 2300 medical students graduate each year; they then participate in an intern-matching program with 118 accredited hospitals throughout the country. Interns undergo rigorous clinical training, particularly those who choose to work in large urban government-run hospitals.

SURGICAL RESIDENCY TRAINING

The earliest evidence of surgical training in the Philippines was through a royal decree during the Spanish colonial period at the Hospital de San Juan de Dios,[7] the teaching hospital of the Royal and Pontifical University of Santo Tomas. During the American occupation, a Pensionado Law was passed in 1904 that enabled Filipino doctors to train in surgery in the United States. Prior to the 1930s, the apprenticeship method of surgical training predominated. It was basically tutorial, haphazard, but highly personalized. Between 1930 and 1950, there was a gradual shift to the hospital-based type of training as it slowly became evident that those who trained as apprentices were less skilled and competent than their hospital-based colleagues. The influx of US-trained surgeons into the established medical schools from 1950 to 1960 led to the establishment of more formally structured surgical residency training programs that were essentially patterned after the American or Halsted model.

Basically, residency training in general surgery is a 4- to 5-year program designed to develop in the trainee a satisfactory level of clinical maturity, surgical judgment, and technical skill. Basic areas of study include wound healing, hemostasis, oncology, shock, circulatory physiology, gastrointestinal physiology, surgical endocrinology, surgical nutrition, fluids and electrolytes, metabolic response to stress and injury, applied surgical anatomy, surgical pathology, surgical infections, and burns.

General surgical residents are provided opportunities for direct patient management experience with trainees in government and university-based hospitals given a wider latitude. Residents are required to have a work-

Specialty	No. of Training Programs	No. of Graduates per Year*	No. of Certified Practitioners*
General surgery	66	160	1000
Obstetrics-gynecology	73	200	1200
Orthopedics	16	20	300
Urology	9	12	150
Neurosurgery	5	6	50
Plastic surgery	4	4	40
Thoracic and cardiovascular	3	6	65
Pediatric surgery	3	4	32
Colorectal surgery	1	1	22

Philippine Surgical Training Manpower Profile, 1998

*Estimated.

ing knowledge of congenital, degenerative, neoplastic, infectious, and other surgical diseases of the gastrointestinal tract and other abdominal organs, the head and neck, breast, and soft tissues. Residents are also expected to develop surgical expertise from rotations in the management of trauma and surgical intensive care, aside from subspecialty rotations in thoracic and cardiovascular surgery, neurosurgery, plastic and reconstructive surgery, burns, pediatric surgery, urology, gynecology, and orthopedic surgery.

Residents in the specialties need 1 or 2 years of general surgery residency training except for those who go to pediatric surgery and thoracic and cardiovascular surgery, who must be board-eligible in general surgery. In addition, residents are given ample opportunities for research work as well as opportunities to present research papers in special conferences, scientific paper contests, and surgical congresses.

In 1936, the Philippine College of Surgeons (PCS) was organized and in 1969, the Philippine Board of Surgery was formed. In 1975, both organizations started work through the joint committee on accreditation to establish a system of accrediting general surgery training. Similar accreditation procedures for other surgical specialties followed.

The number of accredited training programs in general surgery and other surgical specialties has grown progressively over the last decade (**Table**). For general surgery alone, there are 66 accredited training programs that are classified into private hospitals, government medical centers, and university hospitals. Evaluation of these training programs, however, have pinpointed a number of problems resulting in marked discrepancies in the quality of residency training.[8,9] These include (1) maldistribution—the majority of training programs and resources are in Manila and other highly urbanized centers; (2) lack of resources—most training programs are poorly funded with a poorly compensated faculty; and (3) erratic training program implementation—differences in characteristics such as caseload, operative experience, adequacy of faculty supervision, and quality of teaching activities exist between university-based government and privately owned institutions.

However, several developments over the past few years have given some cause for optimism and possible progress in the area of surgical training. Among them are the formulation of a standard curriculum and evaluation system for residency in general surgery that is constantly being reviewed and streamlined,[10] the formation of an association of training officers in 1992 committed to upgrade the skills of the surgical faculty, and establishment of training programs and upgrading the skills of noncertified surgeons in underdeveloped far-flung areas of the Philippines.

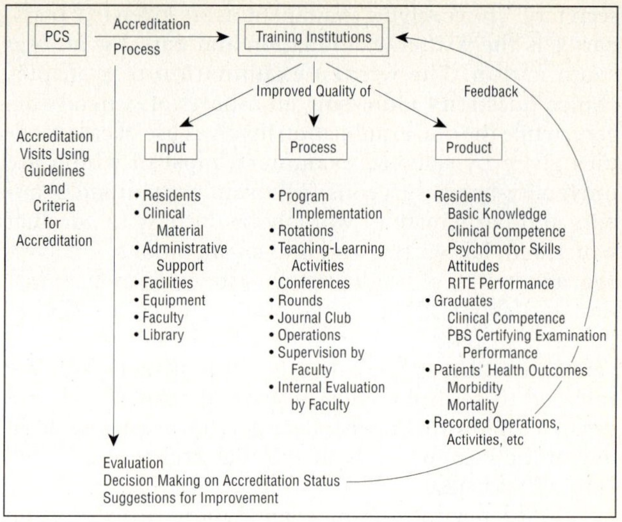

Framework for the accreditation program of the Philippine College of Surgeons (PCS). RITE indicates Residents' In-Training Examinations; PBS, Philippine Board of Surgery.

CERTIFYING PROCESS AND ACCREDITATION OF TRAINING PROGRAMS

The accreditation committee of the PCS evaluates and certifies all general surgery training programs in the Philippines. Its main objective is to upgrade and standardize surgical training programs to ensure graduates who are ethical, safe, and competent. Minimum requirements, policies, and guidelines for accreditation are implemented by all training programs. This committee has 12 members, which is divided into 3 groups for accreditation visits to all surgical training centers nationwide.

The accreditation process focuses on the training center's implementation of a unified competency-based training curriculum and the performance of its residents and graduates. Through the process of internal evaluations, in-training, certifying examinations, and feedback from accreditation visits, surgical departments formulate and design what is needed to improve the quality of their programs (**Figure**). Accredited training programs are evaluated once every 4 years and based on the overall evaluation, the program may be fully accredited, placed on conditional status, warned, or suspended for cause as stipulated in the official guidelines and standards. Only graduates of surgical residency training programs accredited by the PCS can qualify for the certifying written and oral examinations. An average of 150 board-eligible general surgeons graduate from these programs each year.

The Philippine Board of Surgery is the examining arm of the college.[11] It is composed of 11 directors who elect from among themselves a chair, a vice-chair, and a secretary. The certifying examinations are given in 2 parts: part 1 is the written examination and part 2 is an oral examination. The written examination is multiple-choice questions addressing all aspects of general surgery, while the oral examination involves use of case modules given by selected examiners, most of whom are university-based surgeons. All examiners attend seminars and participate in workshops on how to conduct structured, fair written and oral examinations. On average, about 50% of candidates pass the written examination and about 30% pass the oral examination. Candidates who pass both examinations are awarded a certificate of a specialist in general surgery and are referred to as diplomates in general surgery. After 2 years, a diplomate in general surgery may apply as a fellow of the PCS, which is the mother organization of all surgical specialties.

Residency in-training examinations are also given by the Philippine Board of Surgery once a year to evaluate theoretical knowledge of residents at a given level of training. Another role of the Philippine Board of Surgery is to assist training officers in assessing the strengths and weaknesses of the surgical residents who take these examinations by providing the standard scores and percentile rank of their residents compared with the other examinees.

SURGICAL RESEARCH AND TECHNOLOGICAL ADVANCES

Progress and development in surgical research has been slow. Much of this can be attributed to poor economic conditions with a consequent low priority given to research in other areas as well. The *Philippine Journal of Surgical Specialties,* the official publication of the PCS, has been in existence since 1946 along with later journal publications in obstetrics and gynecology, ophthalmology, orthopedics, urology, and thoracic and cardiovascular surgery. Despite these avenues for publication, there remains a lack of institutional direction and support given for surgical research, except for a few selected university training programs. Financial incentives are few and confined to sponsorship of research competitions. Furthermore, there are very few surgeons with full-time careers in research.

Likewise, economic conditions have influenced the influx and development of new surgical technology. Although advances in communications and information technology have made the Filipino surgeon up-to-date with the latest surgical advances, applications of this new technology have been limited to a few, well-financed private medical centers in urban areas.

Open heart surgery was first performed in the Philippines in 1959, with 2 university medical centers performing open correction of congenital heart defects, although ligation of patent ductus arteriosus and closed mitral commisurotomy were being performed a few years earlier.[12] Surgery for abdominal aortic aneurysms using a homograft cadaver aorta was introduced in the Philippines 5 years after Charles DuBost, MD, performed his pioneering operation.[13] The first attempts at kidney transplantation were done in 1968 and 1969; to date, about 1500 kidney transplants have been performed and about 150 transplants are performed annually.[14] Heart, liver, pancreas, bone marrow, and other multiorgan transplantations are done occasionally mainly because of economic reasons. Minimally invasive surgery is part of surgical reality in the Philippines today since the introduction of laparoscopic cholecystectomy in 1991. Video-assisted thoracic surgery is also being used in some tertiary care hospitals. Surgery for the aftermath of tropical diseases such as schistosomiasis and biliary ascariasis is also performed.[15,16]

ECONOMIC IMPACT OF HEALTH MAINTENANCE ORGANIZATIONS

Health maintenance organizations (HMOs) proliferated in the Philippines after the historic 1986 bloodless revolution that toppled the Marcos dictatorship. Its modest rate of growth of 20% annually is commensurate with the slow but steady industrialization of the country. Presently, there are 36 registered HMOs with a total enrollment of more than 2 million. Like its counterpart in the United States, HMOs were introduced in the Philippines as an antidote to the escalating premiums of medical insurance.

A great majority of the population depends on free government primary and tertiary health care. With HMO coverage, about 33% of the population can afford private medical care. The professional fees covered by the HMO are lower than the average fee for service. The hospitals are paid their normal fees with a discount ranging from 5% to 10% based on the volume of business generated. This enables hospitals to have a higher occupancy rate. The percentage of HMO patients admitted in different hospitals at a given time varies form 25% to 70%.

MANPOWER DISTRIBUTION

The population–health manpower ratio for physicians is 1190:1, which is similar to that of Japan.[17] The Philippines has an adequate number of physicians, including surgeons, to handle its medical needs; the problem lies in regional maldistribution. More than 50% of board-certified general surgeons and other surgical specialists are practicing in Manila and its environs. This skew toward the urban centers is primarily because of better financial and professional remuneration. To address this problem, short-term strategies such as offering better compensation packages and incentives for specialists to practice in the provinces have been considered. A long-term strategy is changing the medical curriculum to a community-oriented type. Again, as in most developing countries, this problem can be traced to its economic roots.

We are deeply indebted to the late Porfirio M. Recio, MD, former chair of the Department of Surgery, College of Medicine and Philippine General Hospital, University of the Philippines, Manila, for the data in his unpublished history of surgery in the Philippines, which was used for this article. We thank Benito R. Reverente, MD, president of the Association of Health Maintenance Organizations of the Philippines for the data on HMOs.

Reprints: Antonio A. Limson, MD, Department of Surgery, College of Medicine and Philippine General Hospital, University of the Philippines, Manila, Taft Avenue, Manila, Philippines (e-mail: tessie@pgh.stat.net.ph).

REFERENCES

1. Recio P. Brief history of the department of surgery. *Surg Bull Philippine Gen Hosp.* 1960;1:165-173.
2. Acosta-Sison H. Laparotrachelotomy versus classical caesarean section during labor. *J Philippine Islands Med Assoc.* 1929;9:209-211.
3. Ibay R, Recio P. Dr. Jose Ignacio Abuel y Villasenor: pioneer Filipino neurosurgeon. *Surg Bull Philippine Gen Hosp.* 1961;2:173-176.
4. Vasquez A. The operative treatment of simple fractures. *J Philippine Islands Med Assoc.* 1926;6:245-260.
5. Ramirez A. Burn treatment through the years: a historical perspective. *Philippine J Surg Spec.* 1990;45:55-60.
6. Eduque J. Perineal versus suprapubic prostatectomy. *J Philippine Islands Med Assoc.* 1926;6:287-290.
7. Bantug J. The San Juan de Dios Hospital and the progress of surgery. In: *A Short History of Medicine in the Philippines.* Quezon City: University of the Philippines Press; 1953:51-63.
8. Caballes A. The making of a "perfect chirurgeon": a historical perspective. *Surg Bull Philippine Gen Hosp.* 1990;7:3-4.
9. Eufemio G, Laudico A, Pareja N. Facilities for training surgeons in the Philippines. *Southeast Asian J Surg.* 1979;2:60-64.
10. Crisostomo A, Limson A. Surgical residency training in the Philippines: 1990. *Philippine J Surg Spec.* 1990;45:89-97.
11. Ona E, ed. *The Philippine Board of Surgery 25th Anniversary Commemorative Book.* Manila, Philippines: Philippine Board of Surgery; 1994:36-38.
12. Danguilan JL. Development of thoracic and cardiovascular surgery in the Philippines. *Philippine J Thorac Cardiovasc Surg.* 1994;1:5-11.
13. Garcia G. Resection of aneurysm of the abdominal aorta and restoration of continuity with homograft. *J Philippine Med Assoc.*1956;32:229-235.
14. Ona E. Organ transplantation in the Philippines. *Chimera.* 1995;6:6-8.
15. Garcia G, Limson A. Gastroesophageal decongestion and splenectomy as a method of treatment for bleeding esophageal varices. *Philippine J Surg Spec.* 1969;24:3-11.
16. Horrilleno E, Limbo D, Eufemio G, Silao J Jr, Garcia A. Hepatobiliary ascariasis. *J Philippine Med Assoc.* 1964;40:40-47.
17. *Health Manpower Profile and Market Analysis.* Manila, Philippines: Policy Unit, Development Academy of the Philippines; 1993.

IN OTHER AMA JOURNALS

JAMA

Impact of Hospital Volume on Operative Mortality for Major Cancer Surgery

Colin B. Begg, PhD; Laura D. Cramer, ScM; William J. Hoskins, MD; Murray F. Brennan, MD Mortality for Major Cancer Surgery

Context.—Hospitals that treat a relatively high volume of patients for selected surgical oncology procedures report lower surgical in-hospital mortality rates than hospitals with a low volume of the procedures, but the reports do not take into account length of stay or adjust for case mix.

Objective.—To determine whether hospital volume was inversely associated with 30-day operative mortality, after adjusting for case mix.

Design and Setting.—Retrospective cohort study using the Surveillance, Epidemiology, and End Results (SEER)–Medicare linked database in which the hypothesis was prospectively specified. Surgeons determined in advance the surgical oncology procedures for which the experience of treating a larger volume of patients was most likely to lead to the knowledge or technical expertise that might offset surgical fatalities.

Patients.—All 5013 patients in the SEER registry aged 65 years or older at cancer diagnosis who underwent pancreatectomy, esophagectomy, pneumonectomy, liver resection, or pelvic exenteration, using incident cancers of the pancreas, esophagus, lung, colon, and rectum, and various genitourinary cancers diagnosed between 1984 and 1993.

Main Outcome Measure.—Thirty-day mortality in relation to procedure volume, adjusted for comorbidity, patient age, and cancer stage.

Results.—Higher volume was linked with lower mortality for pancreatectomy ($P = .004$), esophagectomy ($P < .001$), liver resection ($P = .04$), and pelvic exenteration ($P = .04$), but not for pneumonectomy ($P = .32$). The most striking results were for esophagectomy, for which the operative mortality rose to 17.3% in low-volume hospitals, compared with 3.4% in high-volume hospitals, and for pancreatectomy, for which the corresponding rates were 12.9% vs 5.8%. Adjustments for case mix and other patient factors did not change the finding that low volume was strongly associated with excess mortality.

Conclusions.—These data support the hypothesis that when complex surgical oncologic procedures are provided by surgical teams in hospitals with specialty expertise, mortality rates are lower. (*1998;280:1747-1751*)

Corresponding author: Colin B. Begg, PhD, 1275 York Ave, Box 44, New York, NY 10021 (e-mail: beggc@mskcc.org).

Management of Acute Mesenteric Ischemia

M. Ashraf Mansour, MD

Acute mesenteric ischemia is a serious illness requiring prompt surgical attention. The clinical presentation, diagnostic strategy, and management of this disease are reviewed. Options for revascularization are briefly outlined. *Arch Surg. 1999;134:328-330*

Acute mesenteric ischemia (AMI) is a catastrophic surgical illness that, if not promptly treated, will lead to a uniformly poor outcome in most patients. In several large series, the mortality of mesenteric ischemia and bowel infarction ranges between 60% and 100%.[1-4] The gut poorly tolerates hypoxic insults. The cellular damage and the profound metabolic derangement induced by ischemic reperfusion injury often lead to a series of events that culminate in multiple organ dysfunction and death.[3]

See Invited Critique at end of article

Acute mesenteric ischemia occurs when arterial blood and oxygen delivery to the gut is interrupted. There is a wide variety of causes that can lead to AMI, including arterial embolism or thrombosis, strangulation obstruction from mechanical occlusion (eg, adhesive bands), arterial trauma or dissection, mesenteric venous thrombosis, and nonocclusive mesenteric ischemia.[3] In order of frequency, the origin of AMI is embolism in 50%, thrombosis in 25%, and nonocclusive mesenteric ischemia in 20%.[2-4] Mesenteric venous thrombosis and other rare causes occur in 5% of patients.[5-7] This article focuses on the surgical techniques employed in the management of AMI caused by arterial embolism or thrombosis.

CLINICAL PRESENTATION

Patients with AMI complain of severe abdominal pain. The examiner will note that the abdominal pain associated with AMI is frequently out of proportion to the physical findings.[8] Sudden gut emptying, by vomiting and defecation, may also occur. Laboratory investigation reveals leukocytosis in most patients. Other abnormalities in serum analysis include elevated levels of liver enzymes, hyperamylasemia, and metabolic acidosis.[8] The triad of sudden abdominal pain, gut emptying, and a cardiac source of embolization to the superior mesenteric artery (SMA) was first described by Klass in 1951.[9] Two other frequently made observations may be added to the triad: leukocytosis and a history of embolic events.[8]

DIAGNOSIS

The clinical findings in patients with AMI are occasionally confusing because they are nonspecific. The surgeon must decide if any objective tests can be helpful in the overall management of the patient. Any unnecessary delays in the ultimate revascularization may lead to dire consequences.[10] A bedside, abdominal, color-flow duplex scan is a simple, noninvasive test that can help determine whether the mesenteric vessels are patent.[11] The test can be obtained while the patient is being resuscitated and prepared for exploratory laparotomy. Imaging of the celiac axis and the SMA can be very difficult or impossible in an obese or uncooperative patient and in cases where extensive bowel gas overlies the vessels.

Mesenteric angiography is considered the criterion standard for the diagnosis of AMI. Among the many advantages of angiography is the ability to visualize the vessels and define the cause of ischemia. Also, detection of any underlying atherosclerotic disease causing mesenteric stenosis or non-

From the Department of Surgery, Loyola University Medical Center, Maywood, Ill.

occlusive mesenteric ischemia will help the surgeon make a therapeutic decision. In cases of nonocclusive mesenteric ischemia, intra-arterial vasodilators can be given immediately.[6] In select cases, the opportunity to perform mesenteric angioplasty is afforded at the time of angiography.[12] Some authors[3] have advocated the use of intra-arterial thrombolytics under certain conditions. The major drawbacks of angiography are the obligatory delay in obtaining the test, the undesirable side effects of administering contrast media, and the cost. Precious minutes may be lost while angiography is being performed when more effective therapy can be started. Echocardiography is helpful in identifying whether the source of embolization is of cardiac origin. This test will help in the postoperative management, especially if anticoagulation is considered. Plain abdominal films and computed tomographic scans are frequently obtained prior to a formal surgical consultation. Abdominal films help rule out another disease process that may mimic AMI, such as acute small-bowel obstruction or a perforated viscus.[3,8] If the computed tomographic scan is done with intravenous contrast, it may show mesenteric arterial occlusion. Computed tomographic scans are also helpful in identifying mesenteric venous thrombosis that may be treated with anticoagulation.[5]

PREOPERATIVE PREPARATION

Patients with AMI have profound metabolic disturbances that should be corrected prior to laparotomy.[10] Intravenous fluid resuscitation with crystalloids and blood products, if necessary, should be started promptly to correct the volume deficit and acidosis. Prophylactic broad-spectrum antibiotics should be given. A bolus of intravenous heparin sodium should be given as soon as the diagnosis of AMI is suspected to avoid any further thrombus propagation, and adequate intravenous access and an arterial line should be established. The surgeon must decide if central venous access or a pulmonary artery catheter (Swan-Ganz) is required for judicious fluid resuscitation and hemodynamic monitoring in elderly, moribund patients. Nasogastric decompression to avoid aspiration and a Foley indwelling catheter should also be used routinely.[3,10]

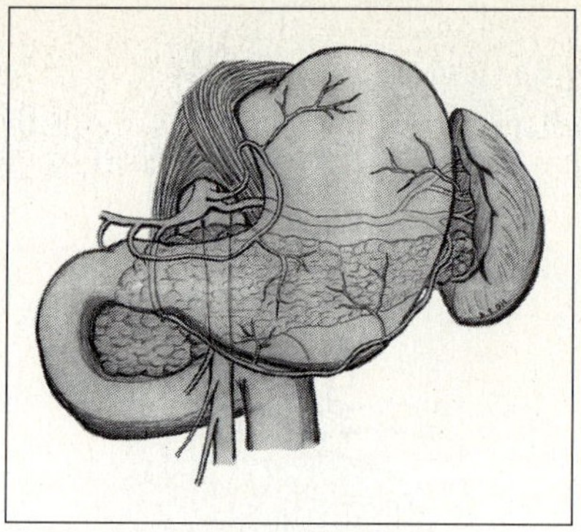

Figure 1. *The location of the superior mesenteric artery in relation to the fourth portion of the duodenum. The celiac axis can be approached through the gastrohepatic ligament and by exposing the crus of the diaphragm.*

OPERATIVE TECHNIQUE

The operating room environment should be warmed to avoid heat loss from the patient during surgical exploration. Cold can induce notable vasospasm and complicate intraoperative assessment of intestinal viability. The use of warm, humidified air in the ventilators and blood warmers should be standard. The skin is prepared from the chest to the mid thighs. A remote site (ankle or arm) for possible vein harvest should also be selected and prepared.

A midline incision provides wide exposure for full exploration. Once the abdomen is entered, a quick survey should provide the clue to the cause of the patient's symptoms and extent of bowel ischemia. The surgeon's primary objective should be to restore mesenteric blood flow expeditiously. The transverse colon is elevated, the ligament of Treitz identified, and the fourth portion of the duodenum mobilized (**Figure 1**). The root of the mesentery is then palpated in search of a SMA pulse. If the origin of AMI is an embolus (the most likely probability), a proximal SMA pulse can be felt. Most SMA emboli are found 3 to 8 cm from the origin of the SMA, usually at a point of bifurcation or at the take off of the middle colic artery.[3,8,10]

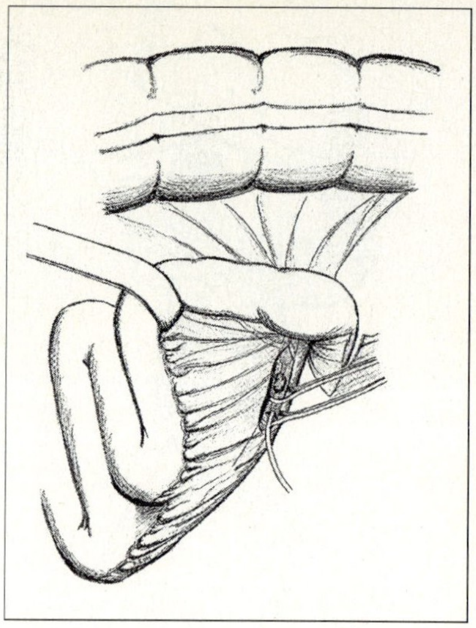

Figure 2. *A transverse arteriotomy is used to insert the No. 3 or No. 4 Fogarty balloon catheter for embolectomy.*

EMBOLECTOMY

The mesentery is opened sharply along the course of the SMA and the vessels are dissected and mobilized. Vascular loops are used for proximal and distal control. Heparin anticoagulation should have already been started by this point. A small transverse arteriotomy in the SMA is made and a No. 3 or No. 4 Fogarty balloon catheter is passed proximally and distally in the artery to retrieve the embolus (**Figure 2**). The surgeon should avoid multiple unnecessary passages with the catheter since there is a potential risk of endothelial damage. A longitudinal arteriotomy may also be used to gain arterial access; however, closure should be performed with a vein patch to avoid narrowing the vessel. Once adequate inflow and back bleeding are established, the vessel is irrigated with heparin saline. Papaverine hydrochloride can be used in the irrigant or dripped directly in the vessel to overcome vasospasm. The arteriotomy is closed with an interrupted monofilament suture (Prolene 6.0; Ethicon Inc, Johnson & Johnson Co, Somerville, NJ). The ischemic bowel is now observed for improvement in perfusion. Many techniques can be used to assess intestinal viability, including continuous-wave Doppler, pulse oximetry, and fluoroscein dye.[13] Frankly necrotic segments of bowel should be resected, but intestinal segments with questionable viability

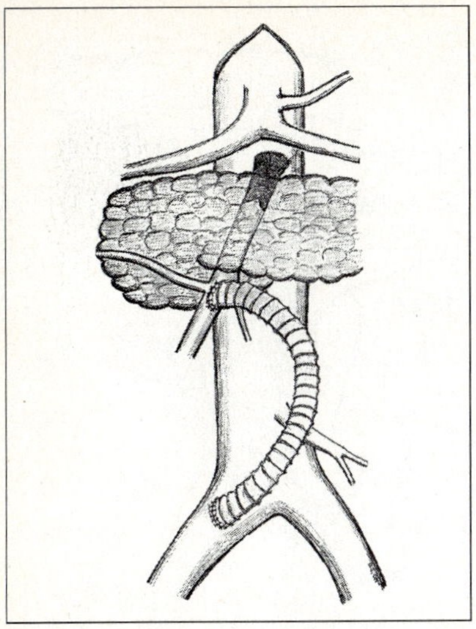

Figure 3. *A retrograde iliac to superior mesenteric artery bypass is made with externally supported polytef (polytetrafluoroethylene).*

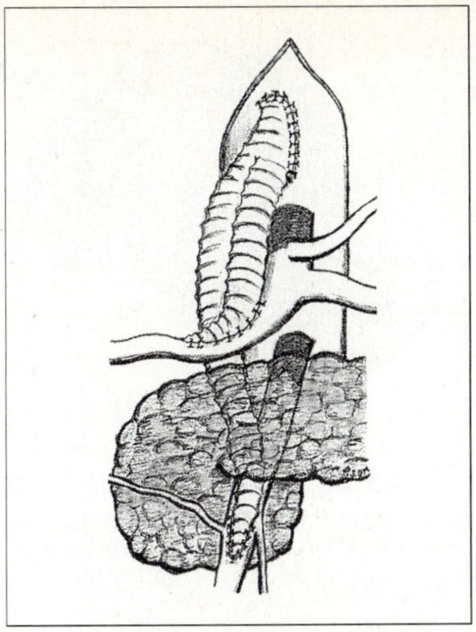

Figure 4. *An antegrade aorta to celiac artery and the superior mesenteric artery–bifurcated Dacron graft for severe stenosis of both the celiac and superior mesenteric arteries.*

should be left in place with the plan to return for a second look in 12 to 24 hours. After resection of dead gut, the most conservative approach regarding the remaining bowel with questionable viability is to avoid primary anastomosis and bring out the ends as stomas. This will permit frequent assessments of intestinal viability and help in setting the time for another operation.[10]

BYPASS

Thrombosis of the proximal 1 to 3 cm of the SMA is the second most likely cause of ischemia.[3,10] In this instance, thrombosis occurs at the site of a diseased artery that is narrowed by notable atherosclerotic plaque. Attempts at thrombectomy will likely fail because the balloon catheter cannot traverse the occlusion. Restoration of SMA blood flow will require a bypass. In some situations, nonpulsatile arterial inflow is established indicating that the thrombus has been removed but the proximal stenosis is still present. A temporary indwelling shunt, such as the Javid carotid shunt, can be inserted to allow restoration of arterial blood during preparation for grafting.[10] In the presence of gross abdominal contamination from a necrotic or perforated bowel, a vein graft is preferable. If no vein is available, polytef, (polytetrafluoroethylene) or Dacron can be used as vein substitutes. The surgeon must decide whether a retrograde or antegrade bypass can be performed (**Figure 3**).[14] Severe calcification of the distal aorta and iliac arteries will preclude a retrograde bypass. In patients with SMA thrombotic occlusion, there may be additional involvement of the celiac axis with atherosclerotic occlusive disease. In a hemodynamically stable patient, careful consideration should be given to a bypass to both the celiac artery and the SMA (**Figure 4**).[15] Care should be taken not to kink or twist the graft. Externally supported polytef grafts may provide a theoretical advantage over vein grafts because they resist kinking.

MESENTERIC ENDARTERECTOMY

An alternative to performing a bypass, especially when no suitable vein is available and there are clear contraindications to using a prosthetic graft, is aortomesenteric endarterectomy.[4] This is technically the most difficult procedure to perform and requires considerable skill and experience in exposing the supraceliac aorta and proximal mesenteric vessels.[10] To gain access to the proximal celiac artery and the SMA, a medial visceral rotation is required together with mobilization of the crus of the diaphragm. A trapdoor incision is made on the aorta after gaining proximal and distal control of the vessels. Endarterectomy is performed and the aortotomy is closed primarily. Supraceliac cross clamping with all its hazards may not be well tolerated in these elderly debilitated individuals.

CONCLUSIONS

Acute mesenteric ischemia is a potentially lethal disease if not recognized and treated early. Once the diagnosis is made, unnecessary delays should be avoided. Clearly, improvement in outcome can be achieved by early recognition, improved perioperative care, and prompt revascularization.

I would like to thank Daniel Oh, BS, for providing the illustrations for this article.

Corresponding author: M. Ashraf Mansour, MD, Department of Surgery, K-352900-3, Loyola University Medical Center, 2160 S First Ave, Maywood, IL 60153-3304 (e-mail: amansou@luc.edu).

REFERENCES

1. Klempnauer J, Grothues F, Bektas H, Pichlmayr R. Long-term results after surgery for acute mesenteric ischemia. *Surgery.* 1997;121:239-243.
2. Montgomery RA, Venbrux AC, Bulkley GB. Mesenteric vascular insufficiency. *Curr Probl Surg.* 1997;34:945-1025.
3. McKinsey JF, Gewertz BL. Acute mesenteric ischemia. *Surg Clin North Am.* 1997;77:307-318.
4. Stoney RJ, Cunningham CG. Acute mesenteric ischemia. *Surgery.* 1993;114:489-490.
5. Rhee RY, Gloviczki P. Mesenteric venous thrombosis. *Surg Clin North Am.* 1997;77:327-338.
6. Bassiouny HS. Nonocclusive mesenteric ischemia. *Surg Clin North Am.* 1997;77:319-326.
7. Krupski WC, Selzman CH, Whitehill TA. Unusual causes of mesenteric ischemia. *Surg Clin North Am.* 1997;77:471-502.
8. Bergan JJ. Diagnosis of acute intestinal ischemia. *Semin Vasc Surg.* 1990;3:143-148.
9. Klass AA. Embolectomy in acute mesenteric ischemia. *Ann Surg.* 1951;134:913-917.
10. Whitehill TA, Rutherford RB. Acute intestinal ischemia caused by arterial occlusions: optimal management to improve survival. *Semin Vasc Surg.* 1990;3:149-156.
11. Nicoloff AD, Williamson WK, Moneta GL, Taylor LM, Porter JM. Duplex ultrasonography in evaluation of splanchnic artery stenosis. *Surg Clin North Am.* 1997;77:339-355.
12. Allen RC, Martin GH, Rees CR, et al. Mesenteric angioplasty in the treatment of chronic intestinal ischemia. *J Vasc Surg.* 1996;24:415-423.
13. Tollefson DFJ, Wright DJ, Reddy DJ, Kintanar EB. Intraoperative determination of intestinal viability by pulse oximetry. *Ann Vasc Surg.* 1995;9:357-360.
14. Johnston KW, Lindsay TF, Wlaker PM, Kalman PG. Mesenteric arterial bypass grafts: early and late results and suggested surgical approach for chronic and acute mesenteric ischemia. *Surgery.* 1995;118:1-7.
15. Kazmers A. Operative management of chronic mesenteric ischemia. *Ann Vasc Surg.* 1998;12:299-308.

Invited Critique

Despite better insights into the pathophysiology of acute mesenteric ischemia, these syndromes remain highly morbid events with reported mortality rates exceeding 60%. The increase in the incidence of these disorders (0.1% of hospital admissions) is secondary to multiple factors, such as heightened awareness for the diagnosis, the advanced mean age of the population, and the increasing number of critically ill patients. Acknowledged risk factors for acute mesenteric ischemia include cardiac arrhythmias, advanced age, low cardiac output states, generalized atherosclerosis, congestive heart failure, severe valvular cardiac disease, recent myocardial infarction, and intra-abdominal malignancy.

Mansour's concise review addresses the proper diagnostic and operative approach to these lethal syndromes. Early and precise diagnosis is key to survival since once bowel infarction has occurred, outcomes are invariably compromised.

To my knowledge, limited information exists regarding the long-term outlook for patients who survive an episode of intestinal ischemia. In a comprehensive report by Klempnauer et al[1] of 90 patients suffering from intestinal ischemia, 31 patients survived and were discharged from the hospital. The cumulative 5-year survival rate was about 50% (16 of 31 patients); the mortality was greatest during the first year after the incident. The worst survival rate (20% at 5 years) was seen in patients who suffered mesenteric arterial thrombosis, while the best survival was seen in patients with embolus or nonocclusive ischemia. Only one patient with previous arterial thrombosis died because of recurrent bowel ischemia. Remarkably, 8 of 15 patients returned to work.

The morbidity and mortality of acute mesenteric ischemia has remained high despite heightened sensitivity to the diagnosis. Since the duration of the ischemic episode is the most important determinant of outcome, an aggressive diagnostic and treatment protocol must be maintained. While this stance may precipitate many negative angiographic studies, such an approach is the only opportunity to save in these critically ill patients.

Bruce L. Gewertz, MD
Chicago, Ill

1. Klempnauer J, Grothues F, Bektas H, Pichlmayr R. Long-term results after surgery for acute mesenteric ischemia. *Surgery*. 1997;121:239-243.

IN OTHER AMA JOURNALS

ARCHIVES OF INTERNAL MEDICINE

Diet and Exercise in the Treatment of Obesity: Effects of 3 Interventions on Insulin Resistance

Ruth S. Weinstock, MD, PhD; Huiliang Dai, MD; Thomas A. Wadden, PhD

Background: In short-term studies, diet and exercise both improve insulin sensitivity.
Objective: To determine the effects of a 48-week supervised diet and exercise program on weight and insulin sensitivity after initial weight loss and weight maintenance, and then subsequent weight regain over 96 weeks.
Methods: Forty-five obese women were randomly assigned to 1 of 3 treatment groups: (1) diet alone, (2) diet and aerobic training, and (3) diet and strength training. All subjects received the same 48-week group behavior modification program and diet (approximately 3879 kJ/d [approximately 925 kcal/d] for the first 16 weeks; approximately 6276 kJ/d [approximately 1500 kcal/d] thereafter). Exercising subjects were provided 3 supervised exercise sessions per week for the first 28 weeks and 2 sessions weekly until week 48. During weeks 48 to 96, subjects were unsupervised. Oral glucose tolerance tests were performed at baseline and weeks 16, 24, 44, and 96.
Results: Subjects across the 3 conditions achieved a mean weight loss of 13.8 kg by week 16, which was associated with decreased insulin levels (61.8% of baseline). There were no significant differences among groups in changes in body mass index, which is a measure of weight in kilograms divided by the square of the height in meters, weight, glucose tolerance, or insulin levels at weeks 16, 24, and 44. No additional beneficial effect of aerobic or strength exercise on insulin resistance, as reflected by serum insulin levels before and after a glucose load, was demonstrated. The 22 subjects who were studied at week 96 maintained a loss of approximately 10% of initial weight. Insulin levels, however, had returned to pretreatment levels.
Conclusions: This study confirms the beneficial effect of weight reduction on hyperinsulinemia in obese individuals. Participation in supervised exercise did not result in additional improvement in weight loss or insulin sensitivity. We also observed a marked increase in insulin levels with only partial weight regain. Determining the amount of sustained weight loss necessary for continued improvement in insulin sensitivity will require further study. *(1998;158:2477-2483)*

Reprints: Ruth S. Weinstock, MD, PhD, SUNY Health Science Center, 750 E Adams St (CWB 353), Syracuse, NY 13210 (e-mail: weinstor@vax.cs.hscsyr.edu).

A Treatise on the Malformation, Injuries, and Diseases of the Rectum and Anus

America's First Textbook on Colorectal Surgery

IT WAS during the 1820s, 30s, and 40s that American surgeons first began to author textbooks and monographs reflective of a growing interest in specialty areas within the whole of surgery. Such examples as George Frick's (1793-1870) *A Treatise on the Diseases of the Eye* (1823), William Dewees' (1768-1841) *A Treatise on the Diseases of Females* (1826), Samuel Gross' (1805-1884) *The Anatomy, Physiology, and Diseases of the Bones and Joints* (1830), Horace Green's (1802-1866) *A Treatise on Diseases of the Air Passages* (1846), and Homer Bostwick's (?-1862) *A Complete Practical Work on the Nature and Treatment of Venereal Diseases, and Other Affections of the Genito-Urinary Organs of the Male and Female* (1848) represent the rudimentary beginnings of "surgical specialization." Joining this esteemed list is George Macartney Bushe's (1793-1836) *A Treatise on the Malformations, Injuries, and Diseases of the Rectum and Anus* (1837). Considered the first textbook on colon and rectal surgery to be published in the United States, the work is unique in the annals of American medicine in that it is the only 19th-century surgical monograph to be issued with a separate atlas of lithograph plates (in this case 9 illustrations, 7 of which are hand-colored), a practice already well-established in Europe.

Bushe notes in the "Preface" that he was

> induced to pay particular attention to the diseases of the rectum and anus, in consequence of their frequency, and the diversity of opinion which prevailed in relation to their nature and treatment. My opportunities for investigating them have been ample, and I may safely say, that I spared neither time, trouble, nor expense, in endeavouring to arrive at just conclusions.

Among the 26 chapters are "Malformations of the Rectum and Anus," "Neuralgia of the Extremity of the Rectum," "Spasmodic Contraction of the Sphincter Ani," "Affections Called Hemorrhoidal," "Itching of the Anus," "Excrescences About the Anus," and "Carcinomatous Degeneration of the Rectum."

Bushe was born in Ireland and received his medical and surgical education and training in Europe. He came to America in 1818, at the request of the recently formed faculty from Rutgers Medical College in New York City, to serve as professor of anatomy and physiology. Widely regarded as a surgeon, Bushe gave daily office lectures on various surgical topics for almost 3 years until the political demise of the medical school. He decided to remain in America and in 1831 founded a periodical, the *New York Medico-Chirurgical Bulletin*. However, it remained in publication only until mid 1832. Bushe also authored various case reports, including surgical treatment of phymosis and hypospadias (1831), the country's third known common iliac artery ligation (1832), and the treatment of cleft palate (1835). Unfortunately, Bushe died of tuberculosis shortly after completing his colorectal surgery text but prior to its being published. He was buried in a now unmarked grave in Jersey City, NJ.

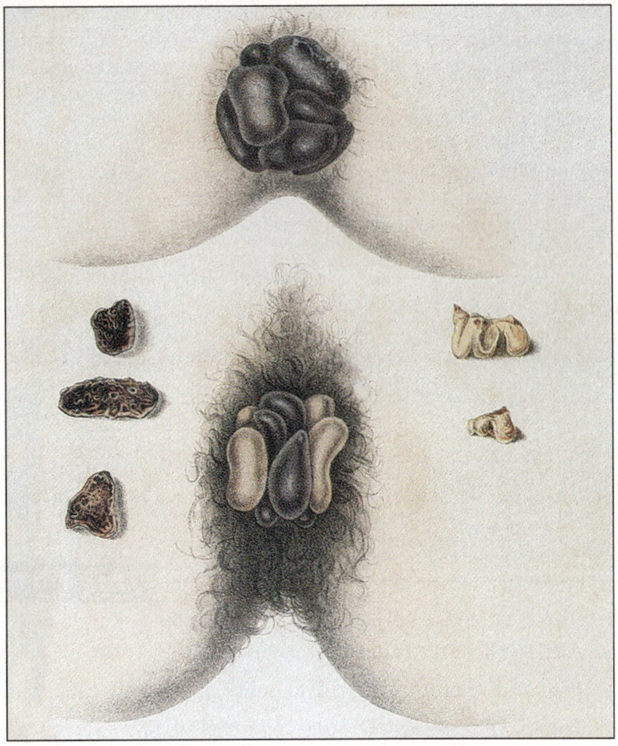

Plate II from Bushe's treatise shows various views of internal hemorrhoids, including those from 2 patients on whom he had previously operated.

Ira M. Rutkow, MD, MPH, DrPH

for prevention of postoperative nausea and vomiting

Zofran® ODT™

ondansetron Orally Disintegrating Tablets

NEW

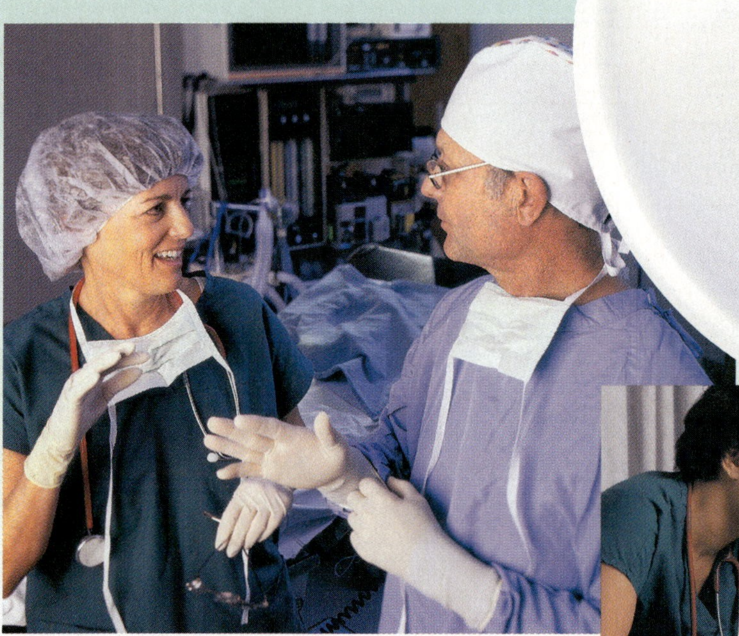

Delivers the 24-hour efficacy You demand

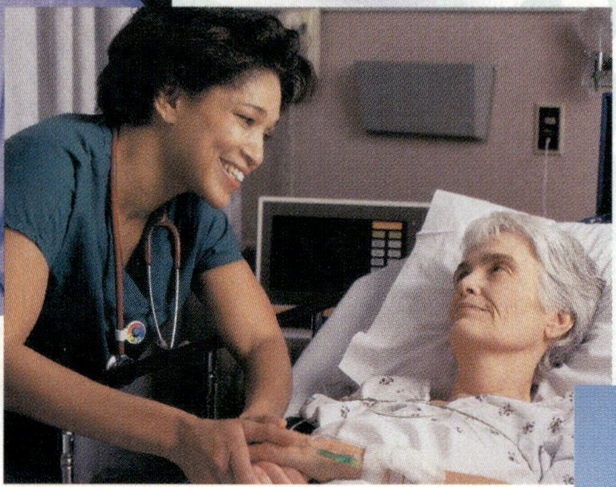

Delivers nonsedation in the PACU – A major benefit in day surgery

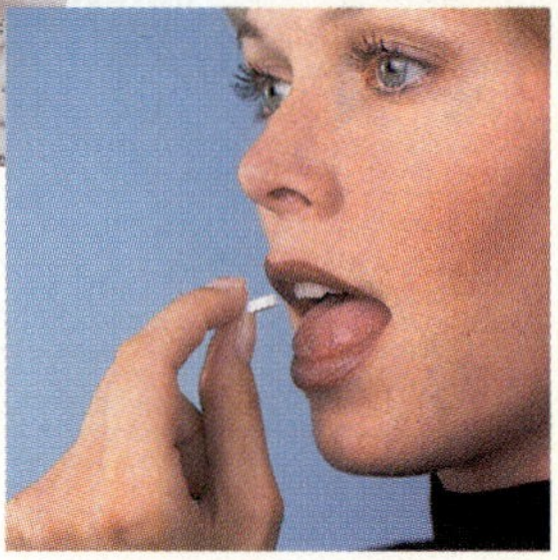

Delivers flexibility—take ODT anywhere; dissolves instantly on the tongue – without water

Choose

ZOFRAN –

Your partner for patient satisfaction

The most commonly reported adverse events in patients receiving ZOFRAN in clinical trials were headache (5% to 27%), diarrhea (<1% to 16%), constipation (<1% to 9%), fever (<1% to 8%), and malaise/fatigue (0% to 13%).*

*Data on file, Glaxo Wellcome, Inc.

Please see Brief Summary of Prescribing Information on next page.

GlaxoWellcome

ZOFRAN®
(ondansetron hydrochloride)
Injection

BRIEF SUMMARY

ZOFRAN®
(ondansetron hydrochloride)
Injection Premixed

ZOFRAN® ODT™
(ondansetron)
Orally Disintegrating Tablets

ZOFRAN®
(ondansetron hydrochloride)
Tablets

ZOFRAN®
(ondansetron hydrochloride)
Oral Solution

The following is a brief summary only; see full prescribing information for complete product information.

CONTRAINDICATIONS: ZOFRAN Injection, ZOFRAN Injection Premixed, ZOFRAN Tablets, ZOFRAN ODT Orally Disintegrating Tablets, and ZOFRAN Oral Solution are contraindicated for patients known to have hypersensitivity to the drug.

WARNINGS: Hypersensitivity reactions have been reported in patients who have exhibited hypersensitivity to other selective 5-HT_3 receptor antagonists.

PRECAUTIONS: Ondansetron is not a drug that stimulates gastric or intestinal peristalsis. It should not be used instead of nasogastric suction. The use of ondansetron in patients following abdominal surgery or in patients with chemotherapy-induced nausea and vomiting may mask a progressive ileus and/or gastric distention.
Information for Patients: ***Phenylketonurics:*** Phenylketonuric patients should be informed that ZOFRAN ODT Orally Disintegrating Tablets contain phenylalanine (a component of aspartame). Each 4-mg and 8-mg orally disintegrating tablet contains <0.03 mg phenylalanine.

Patients should be instructed not to remove ZOFRAN ODT Tablets from the blister until just prior to dosing. The tablet should not be pushed through the foil. With dry hands, the blister backing should be peeled completely off the blister. The tablet should be gently removed and immediately placed on the tongue to dissolve and be swallowed with the saliva. Peelable illustrated stickers are affixed to the product carton that can be provided with the prescription to ensure proper use and handling of the product.
Drug Interactions: Ondansetron does not itself appear to induce or inhibit the cytochrome P-450 drug-metabolizing enzyme system of the liver. Because ondansetron is metabolized by hepatic cytochrome P-450 drug-metabolizing enzymes, inducers or inhibitors of these enzymes may change the clearance and, hence, the half-life of ondansetron. On the basis of limited available data, no dosage adjustment is recommended for patients on these drugs. Tumor response to chemotherapy in the P 388 mouse leukemia model is not affected by ondansetron. In humans, carmustine, etoposide, and cisplatin do not affect the pharmacokinetics of ondansetron.
Use in Surgical Patients: The coadministration of ondansetron had no effect on the pharmacokinetics and pharmacodynamics of temazepam.
Carcinogenesis, Mutagenesis, Impairment of Fertility: Carcinogenic effects were not seen in 2-year studies in rats and mice with oral ondansetron doses up to 10 and 30 mg/kg per day, respectively. Ondansetron was not mutagenic in standard tests for mutagenicity. Oral administration of ondansetron up to 15 mg/kg per day did not affect fertility or general reproductive performance of male and female rats.
Pregnancy: ***Teratogenic Effects:*** Pregnancy Category B. Reproduction studies have been performed in pregnant rats and rabbits at IV doses up to 4 mg/kg per day and at daily oral doses up to 15 and 30 mg/kg per day, respectively, and have revealed no evidence of impaired fertility or harm to the fetus due to ondansetron. There are, however, no adequate and well-controlled studies in pregnant women. Because animal reproduction studies are not always predictive of human response, this drug should be used during pregnancy only if clearly needed.
Nursing Mothers: Ondansetron is excreted in the breast milk of rats. It is not known whether ondansetron is excreted in human milk. Because many drugs are excreted in human milk, caution should be exercised when ondansetron is administered to a nursing woman.
Pediatric Use: ***ZOFRAN Injection:*** Little information is available about dosage in pediatric patients under 2 years of age (see DOSAGE AND ADMINISTRATION section of full prescribing information for use in pediatric patients 4 to 18 years of age receiving cancer chemotherapy or for use in pediatric patients 2 to 12 years of age receiving general anesthesia).

ZOFRAN Tablets: Little information is available about dosage in children 4 years of age or younger (see CLINICAL PHARMACOLOGY and DOSAGE AND ADMINISTRATION sections of full prescribing information for use in children 4 to 18 years of age).
Use in Elderly Patients: Dosage adjustment is not needed in patients over the age of 65 (see CLINICAL PHARMACOLOGY section of full prescribing information). Prevention of nausea and vomiting in elderly patients was no different than in younger age-groups.

ADVERSE REACTIONS
ZOFRAN Injection: ***Chemotherapy-Induced Nausea and Vomiting:*** The following adverse events have been reported in individuals receiving ondansetron at a dosage of three 0.15-mg/kg doses or as a single 32-mg dose in clinical trials. These patients were receiving concomitant chemotherapy, primarily cisplatin, and IV fluids. Most were receiving a diuretic.

Table 1: Principal Adverse Events in Comparative Trials

	Number of Patients With Event			
	ZOFRAN Injection 0.15 mg/kg x 3 n = 419	ZOFRAN Injection 32 mg x 1 n = 220	Metoclopramide n = 156	Placebo n = 34
Diarrhea	16%	8%	44%	18%
Headache	17%	25%	7%	15%
Fever	8%	7%	5%	3%
Akathisia	0%	0%	6%	0%
Acute dystonic reactions*	0%	0%	5%	0%

*See Neurological

The following have been reported during controlled clinical trials:
Cardiovascular: Rare cases of angina (chest pain), electrocardiographic alterations, and tachycardia have been reported. In many cases, the relationship to ZOFRAN Injection was unclear.
Gastrointestinal: Constipation has been reported in 11% of chemotherapy patients receiving multiday ondansetron.
Hepatic: In comparative trials in cisplatin chemotherapy patients with normal baseline values of aspartate transaminase (AST) and alanine transaminase (ALT), these enzymes have been reported to exceed twice the upper limit of normal in approximately 5% of patients. The increases were transient and did not appear to be related to dose or duration of therapy. On repeat exposure, similar transient elevations in transaminase values occurred in some courses, but symptomatic hepatic disease did not occur.
Integumentary: Rash has occurred in approximately 1% of patients receiving ondansetron.
Neurological: There have been rare reports consistent with, but not diagnostic of, extrapyramidal reactions in patients receiving ZOFRAN Injection, and rare cases of grand mal seizure. The relationship to ZOFRAN was unclear.
Other: Bronchospasm and rare case of hypokalemia have been reported. The relationship to ZOFRAN Injection was unclear.
Postoperative Nausea and Vomiting: The following adverse events have been reported in ≥2% of adults receiving ondansetron at a dosage of 4 mg IV over 2 to 5 minutes in clinical trials. Rates of these events were not significantly different in the ondansetron and placebo groups. These patients were receiving multiple concomitant perioperative and postoperative medications.

Table 2: Adverse Events in ≥2% of Adults Receiving Ondansetron at a Dosage of 4 Mg IV over 2 to 5 Minutes in Clinical Trials

	ZOFRAN Injection 4 mg IV n = 547 patients	Placebo n = 547 patients
Headache	92 (17%)	77 (14%)
Dizziness	67 (12%)	88 (16%)
Musculoskeletal pain	57 (10%)	59 (11%)
Drowsiness/sedation	44 (8%)	37 (7%)
Shivers	38 (7%)	39 (7%)
Malaise/fatigue	25 (5%)	30 (5%)
Injection site reaction	21 (4%)	18 (3%)
Urinary retention	17 (3%)	15 (3%)
Postoperative CO_2-related pain*	12 (2%)	16 (3%)
Chest pain (unspecified)	12 (2%)	15 (3%)
Anxiety/agitation	11 (2%)	16 (3%)
Dysuria	11 (2%)	9 (2%)
Hypotension	10 (2%)	12 (2%)
Fever	10 (2%)	6 (1%)
Cold sensation	9 (2%)	8 (1%)
Pruritus	9 (2%)	3 (<1%)
Paresthesia	9 (2%)	2 (<1%)

*Sites of pain included abdomen, stomach, joints, rib cage, shoulder.

Pediatric Use: The following were the most commonly reported adverse events in pediatric patients receiving ondansetron (a single 0.1-mg/kg dose for pediatric patients weighing 40 kg or less, or 4 mg for pediatric patients weighing more than 40 kg) administered intravenously over at least 30 seconds. Rates of these events were not significantly different in the ondansetron and placebo groups. These patients were receiving multiple concomitant perioperative and postoperative medications.

Table 3: Frequency of Adverse Events From Controlled Studies

Adverse Event	Ondansetron IV n = 755 Patients	Placebo n = 731 Patients
Wound problem	80 (11%)	86 (12%)
Anxiety/agitation	49 (6%)	47 (6%)
Headache	44 (6%)	43 (6%)
Drowsiness/sedation	41 (5%)	56 (8%)
Pyrexia	32 (4%)	41 (6%)

Observed During Clinical Practice: In addition to adverse events reported from clinical trials, the following events have been identified during post-approval use of intravenous formulations of ZOFRAN. Because they are reported voluntarily from a population of unknown size, estimates of frequency cannot be made. The events have been chosen for inclusion due to a combination of their seriousness, frequency of reporting, or potential causal connection to ZOFRAN.
Cardiovascular: Arrhythmias (including ventricular and supraventricular tachycardia, premature ventricular contractions, and atrial fibrillation, electrocardiographic alterations (including second degree heart block), palpitations, and syncope.
General: Rare cases of hypersensitivity reactions, sometimes severe (e.g., anaphylaxis, bronchospasm, shortness of breath, hypotension, shock, angioedema, urticaria) have also been reported.
Hepatic: Liver failure and death have been reported in patients with cancer receiving concurrent medications including potentially hepatotoxic cytotoxic chemotherapy and antibiotics. The etiology of the liver failure is unclear.
Local Reactions: Pain, redness, and burning at site of injection.
Neurological: Oculogyric crisis, appearing alone, as well as with other dystonic reactions.
Special Senses: Transient blurred vision, in some cases associated with abnormalities of accommodation.

ZOFRAN Tablets: The following have been reported as events in clinical trials or in the routine management of patients treated with ondansetron, the active ingredient of ZOFRAN Tablets. A causal relationship to therapy with ZOFRAN Tablets has been unclear in many cases.
Chemotherapy-Induced Nausea and Vomiting: The following adverse events have been reported in adults receiving either 8 mg of ZOFRAN Tablets two or three times a day for 3 days or placebo in four trials. These patients were receiving concurrent chemotherapy, primarily cyclophosphamide-based regimens.

Table 4: Principal Adverse Events in US Trials: 3 Days of Therapy With ZOFRAN Tablets

Event	Ondansetron 8 mg b.i.d. n = 242	Ondansetron 8 mg t.i.d. n = 415	Placebo n = 262
Headache	58 (24%)	113 (27%)	34 (13%)
Malaise/fatigue	32 (13%)	37 (9%)	6 (2%)
Constipation	22 (9%)	26 (6%)	1 (<1%)
Diarrhea	15 (6%)	16 (4%)	10 (4%)
Dizziness	13 (5%)	18 (4%)	12 (5%)
Abdominal pain	3 (1%)	13 (3%)	1 (<1%)
Xerostomia	5 (2%)	6 (1%)	1 (<1%)
Weakness	0 (0%)	7 (2%)	1 (<1%)

Central Nervous System: There have been rare reports consistent with, but not diagnostic of, extrapyramidal reactions in patients receiving ondansetron.
Hepatic: In 723 patients receiving cyclophosphamide-based chemotherapy in US clinical trials, AST and/or ALT values have been reported to exceed twice the upper limit of normal in approximately 1% to 2% of patients receiving ZOFRAN Tablets. The increases were transient and did not appear to be related to dose or duration of therapy. On repeat exposure, similar transient elevations in transaminase values occurred in some courses, but symptomatic hepatic disease did not occur. The role of cancer chemotherapy in these biochemical changes cannot be clearly determined.

There have been reports of liver failure and death in patients with cancer receiving concurrent medications including potentially hepatotoxic cytotoxic chemotherapy and antibiotics. The etiology of the liver failure is unclear.
Integumentary: Rash has occurred in approximately 1% of patients receiving ondansetron.
Other: Rare cases of anaphylaxis, bronchospasm, tachycardia, angina (chest pain), hypokalemia, electrocardiographic alterations, vascular occlusive events, and grand mal seizures have been reported. Except for bronchospasm and anaphylaxis, the relationship to ZOFRAN was unclear.
Radiation-Induced Nausea and Vomiting: The adverse events reported in patients receiving ZOFRAN Tablets and concurrent radiotherapy were similar to those reported in patients receiving ZOFRAN Tablets and concurrent chemotherapy. The most frequently reported adverse events were headache, constipation, and diarrhea.
Postoperative Nausea and Vomiting: The following adverse events have been reported in ≥5% of patients receiving ZOFRAN Tablets at a dosage of 16 mg orally in clinical trials. With the exception of headache, rates of these events were not significantly different in the ondansetron and placebo groups. These patients were receiving multiple concomitant perioperative and postoperative medications.

Table 5: Frequency of Adverse Events From Controlled Studies with ZOFRAN Tablets

Adverse Event	Ondansetron 16 mg (n = 550)	Placebo (n = 531)
Wound problem	152 (28%)	162 (31%)
Drowsiness/sedation	112 (20%)	122 (23%)
Headache	49 (9%)	27 (5%)
Hypoxia	49 (9%)	35 (7%)
Pyrexia	45 (8%)	34 (6%)
Dizziness	36 (7%)	34 (6%)
Gynecological disorder	36 (7%)	33 (6%)
Anxiety/agitation	33 (6%)	29 (5%)
Bradycardia	32 (6%)	30 (6%)
Shiver(s)	28 (5%)	30 (6%)
Urinary retention	28 (5%)	18 (3%)
Hypotension	27 (5%)	32 (6%)
Pruritus	27 (5%)	20 (4%)

Preliminary observations in a small number of subjects suggest a higher incidence of headache when ZOFRAN ODT Orally Disintegrating Tablets are taken with water, when compared to without water.

DRUG ABUSE AND DEPENDENCE: Animal studies have shown that ondansetron is not discriminated as a benzodiazepine nor does it substitute for benzodiazepines in direct addiction studies.

OVERDOSAGE: There is no specific antidote for ondansetron overdose. Patients should be managed with appropriate supportive therapy. Individual IV doses as large as 145 mg and total daily IV doses (three doses) as large as 252 mg have been inadvertently administered without significant adverse events. These doses are more than 10 times the recommended daily dose.

"Sudden blindness" (amaurosis) of 2 to 3 minutes' duration plus severe constipation occurred in one patient that was administered 72 mg of ondansetron intravenously as a single dose. Hypotension (and faintness) occurred in another patient that took 48 mg of ZOFRAN Tablets. Following infusion of 32 mg over only a 4-minute period, a vasovagal episode with transient second degree heart block was observed. In all instances, the events resolved completely.

US Patent Nos. 4,695,578; 4,753,789; and 5,578,628

GlaxoWellcome
Glaxo Wellcome Inc.
Research Triangle Park, NC 27709

ZOFRAN® Tablets, Oral Solution, and Injection:
Manufactured by Glaxo Wellcome Inc., Research Triangle Park, NC 27709

ZOFRAN® ODT™ Orally Disintegrating Tablets:
Manufactured for Glaxo Wellcome Inc.
Research Triangle Park, NC 27709
by Scherer DDS, Blagrove, Swindon, Wiltshire, UK SN5 8RU

ZOFRAN® Injection Premixed:
Manufactured for Glaxo Wellcome Inc.
Research Triangle Park, NC 27709
by Abbott Laboratories, North Chicago, IL 60064

August 1998/January 1999 RL-611/607

1999

March

4-6	Central Surgical Association, St Louis, Mo
4-7	Society of Surgical Oncology, Orlando, Fla
18-20	Society of Black Academic Surgeons, Louisville, Ky
18-20	Association of Program Directors in Surgery, Orlando, Fla
24-27	American Burn Association, Lake Buena Vista, Fa
24-27	Society of American Gastrointestinal Endoscopic Surgeons (SAGES), San Antonio, Tex
24-28	Society for Clinical Vascular Surgery, Orlando, Fla

April

7-10	Association for Surgical Education, Boston, Mass
15-17	American Surgical Association, San Diego, Calif
17-21	Southwestern Surgical Congress, Coronado, Calif
18-21	American Association for Thoracic Surgery, New Orleans, La
23-28	American Thoracic Society/American Lung Association, San Diego, Calif
25-28	American College of Surgeons' Spring Meeting, New York, NY
29–May 1	Surgical Infection Society, Seattle, Wash

May

1-6	American Society of Colon and Rectal Surgeons, Washington, DC
2-4	American Association of Endocrine Surgeons, New Haven, Conn
8-12	American Association for Head and Neck Surgery, Palm Desert, Calif
9-13	Royal Australasian College of Surgeons Annual Scientific Congress, Auckland, New Zealand
16-19	American Pediatric Surgical Association, Rancho Mirage, Calif
16-19	American Society for Gastrointestinal Endoscopy–Digestive Disease Week, Orlando, Fla
16-19	Society for Surgery of the Alimentary Tract, Orlando, Fla
19-22	American Society of Transplant Surgeons, Chicago, Ill

June

6-9	Society for Vascular Surgery and the North American Chapter, International Society for Cardiovascular Surgery, Washington, DC
9-11	Endovascular Surgery Workshop, Washington, DC
23-26	Western Thoracic Surgical Association, Olympic Valley, Calif

July

15-17	Association of Women Surgeons' Summer Conference, Hershey, Pa

August

8-13	National Medical Association, Las Vegas, NV
15-21	International Association of Endocrine Surgeons, Vienna, Austria
15-21	38th World Congress of Surgery, Vienna, Austria

September

1-4	American Society for Surgery of the Hand, Boston, Mass
12-16	International Society for Cardiovascular Surgery, Melbourne, Australia
24-25	Midwestern Vascular Surgical Society, Chicago, Ill
24-26	New England Surgical Society, Newport, RI

October

1-3	New England Society for Vascular Surgery, Chadham, Mass (Cape Cod)
10-15	American College of Surgeons Annual Clinical Congress, San Francisco, Calif

November

14-17	Western Surgical Association, Santa Fe, NM
18-20	Association for Academic Surgery, Philadelphia, Pa

December

5-8	Southern Surgical Association, Hot Springs, Va

IN OTHER AMA JOURNALS

JAMA

What's the Relative Risk? A Method of Correcting the Odds Ratio in Cohort Studies of Common Outcomes

Jun Zhang, MB, PhD; Kai F. Yu, PhD

Logistic regression is used frequently in cohort studies and clinical trials. When the incidence of an outcome of interest is common in the study population (>10%), the adjusted odds ratio derived from the logistic regression can no longer approximate the risk ratio. The more frequent the outcome, the more the odds ratio overestimates the risk ratio when it is more than 1 or underestimates it when it is less than 1. We propose a simple method to approximate a risk ratio from the adjusted odds ratio and derive an estimate of an association or treatment effect that better represents the true relative risk. *(1998;280:1690-1691)*

Corresponding author: Jun Zhang, MB, PhD, Division of Epidemiology, Statistics and Prevention Research, National Institute of Child Health and Human Development, Bldg 6100, Room 7B03, Bethesda, MD 20892-7510 (e-mail: Jun_Zhang@NIH.GOV).

The information given here is supplied by the companies cited. Publication of these notices does not imply endorsement or warranty by the American Medical Association, publishers of the *Archives of Surgery*.

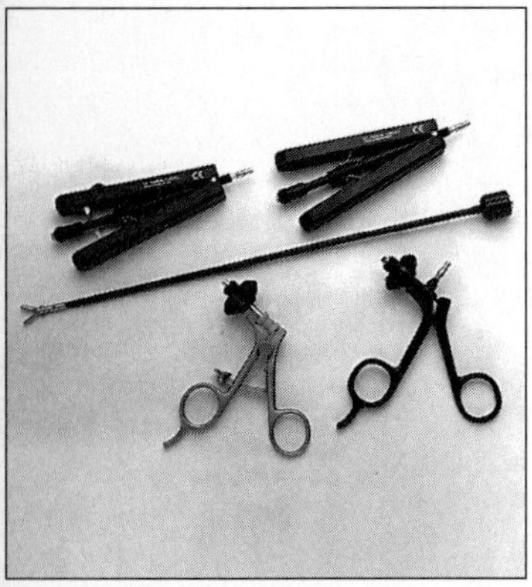

SURGICAL INSTRUMENT —

Aslan Medical Technologies has introduced the VersaLap™ system of instruments for minimally invasive surgery. The modular line includes dozens of interchangeable, reusable tips. For the first time, surgeons can also choose between conventional scissors handles or Aslan's new inline Sensor™ handles.

The system's new Sensor™ handles are available in locking and non-locking styles, with both being insulated and electrocautery-capable. The lightweight handles are made of surgical stainless steel and durable autoclavable ULTEM® for multiple re-use.

For surgeons who prefer a conventional scissors grip, handles are available in locking stainless steel or non-locking insulated electrocautery-capable modes.

Dozens of instrument tips are offered for use with Sensor™ and scissors-grip handles, all with insulation for electrocautery use. All tips can be disassembled for thorough cleaning and sterilization.

Aslan Medical Technologies manufactures a growing line of custom instruments for minimally invasive surgery.

For information write
ASLAN MEDICAL TECHNOLOGIES
4110 South 9th Street
Kalamazoo, MI 49009

Call toll free
800-551-4561

Fax
616-372-9639

Web site
www.aslanmedical.com

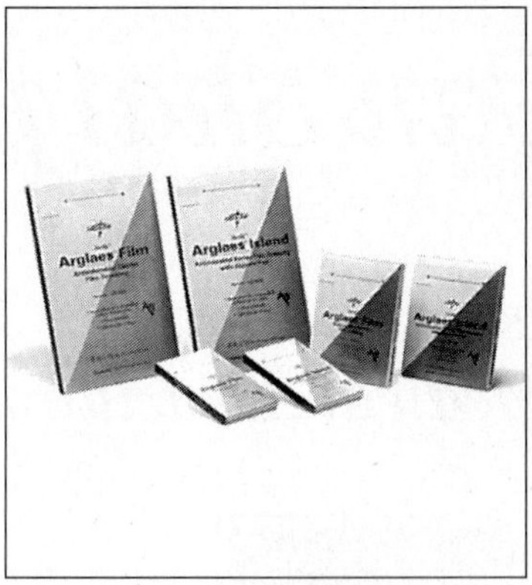

SURGICAL PRODUCT —

Physicians at Chicago's Michael Reese Hospital and Medical Center, the New York University School of Medicine and at other health care facilities across the country are discovering that Arglaes, the newest weapon in the fight against antibiotic resistant bacteria, is having a major impact on their infection control programs. Arglaes has no known resistance and no known major side effects.

Arglaes is a revolutionary new technology that utilizes ionic silver in a patented controlled release polymer film to help prevent infection.

The ionic silver is released at a constant rate onto the wound through controlled-release polymers, which are added to the dressing during the manufacturing process. Arglaes maintains full efficacy for seven days, releasing a constant stream of silver, calcium and sodium ions. The silver ions are released at the same rate in the presence of a microscopic quantity of moisture vapor or a large quantity of fluid.

Arglaes was developed by Maersk Medical, Inc, based in England. Medline Industries, Inc, has the exclusive distribution and marketing rights in the United States.

For information write
MEDLINE INDUSTRIES, INC.
Attn: John J. Marks
One Medline Place
Mundelein, IL 60060-4486

Phone
847-949-3011

Call toll free
800-MEDLINE

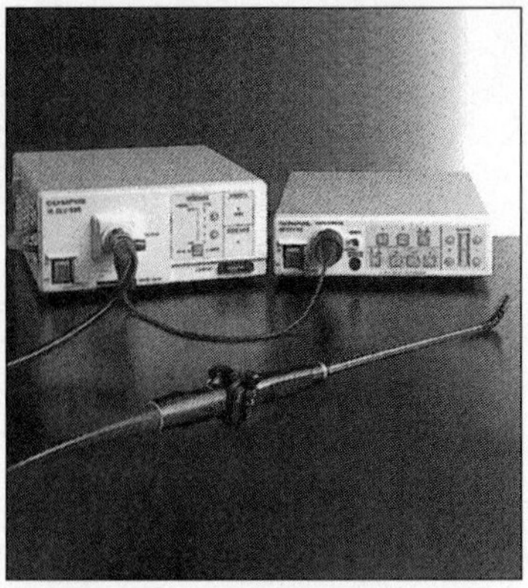

VIDEO EQUIPMENT —

From Olympus-High quality video images and four-way angulation for more advanced thoracic and abdominal procedures. The Olympus LTF-V OES Laparo-Thoraco Videoscope gives you high-quality images you need to perform any procedure easily and efficiently.

Incorporating an ultra-compact high-performance CCD in the tip of the scope, the LTF-V achieves picture quality equivalent to that provided by laparo-thoraco fiberscopes. The built-in-CCD design allows the scope tip to bend freely in four different directions, so you can not only see better, you can see more.

Designed to maximize procedural efficiency and efficacy, the LTF-V also offers a variety of convenient features such as a lens cleaning sheath and valve.

For information write
OLYMPUS AMERICA INC.
Two Corporate Center Drive
Melville, NY 11747-3157

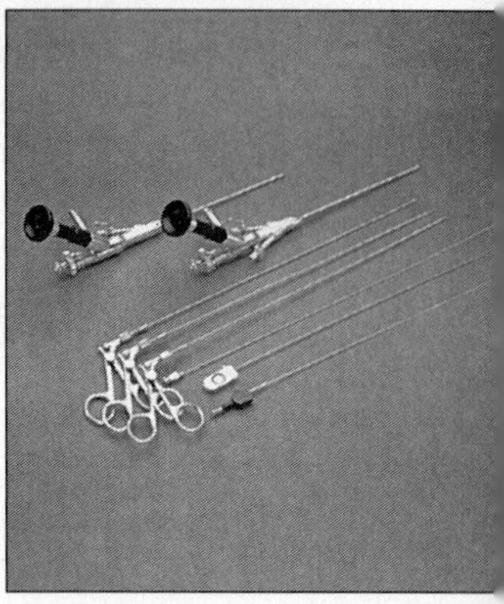

SURGICAL INSTRUMENT —

Karl Storz Endoscopy-America, Inc offers a line of pediatric cystoscopes designed to accommodate the special needs of children. The product line includes autoclavable HOPKINS® neonatal and pediatric telescopes as well as 7.5 Fr. and 1 Fr. operating pediatric cystoscopes

Autoclavable pediatric cystoscopes generate brilliant images with the highest possible resolution thanks to Hopkins® rod lens technology. Fragile neonatal tissue is protecte by a special tip configuration on the neonate sheath, facilitating atraumatic introduction. Each tele scope is available in a range of sizes for the newborn on up.

Karl Storz operating pediatric cyst scopes are available with 7.5 Fr. and 10 Fr. fiberoptic systems. They permit the treatment of posterior urethral valves, uteroceles and ute ral stones in children. Their integr design maximizes ergonomics and working capacity while their atrau matic tips minimize trauma to the delicate tissue of pediatric patient

The pediatric cystoscopes are available with a complete line of working instruments, including hook electrodes, ball electrodes, graspers, biopsy forceps and injection needles.

For information write
KS ENDOSCOPY-AMERICA, INC
600 Corporate Pointe
Culver City, CA 90230-7600

Call toll free
800-421-0837

Web site
www.karlstorz.com

Classified Advertising

Academic/Faculty
Cardiovascular/Thoracic Surgery
CME Corner
Chiefs/Department Heads/Directors
Courses/Symposia/Seminars
Facial Plastic Surgery
Graduate Training/Residencies/Fellowships
Locum Tenens Wanted
Multiple Specialties/Group Practice
Neurosurgery
Notices
Othopedic Surgery
Pediatric Surgery
Plastic Surgery
Practices For Sale
Surgical Specialities
Thoracic Surgery
Vascular Surgery

Sales Information

1999 CLASSIFIED ADVERTISING RATES

Regular	1x 1.65/wd	*3x 1.55/wd
Bold	1x 1.85/wd	*3x 1.75/wd

*In order to receive the 3-time frequency price, the request must be made upon initial placement. The minimum charge is 20 words. A word consists of one or more letters surrounded by space on each side. For information on display advertising and our network buys contact an account representative.

POLICY

Orders for classified advertising must be submitted in writing. Although the American Medical Association believes the classified advertisements in these pages to be from reputable sources, the Association does not investigate the offers made and assumes no liability concerning them. Acceptance of advertising is restricted to professional opportunities, practices for sale, and medical office space available. The Association reserves the right to decline, withdraw, or edit advertisements at its discretion. Every care is taken to avoid mistakes but responsibility cannot be accepted by the Association for clerical or printer's errors.

REPLY BOX SERVICE

Confidential box numbers are available for an additional $25 per issue, plus the words: Box ________, c/o SUR. When responding to a box number, please send to Archives of Surgery, Box ________, c/o SUR, 515 N State St, Chicago, IL 60610.

CANCELLATIONS/CHANGES

Cancellations/changes must be received in writing at least 25 days prior to the date of the issue. In order to expedite, please fax to 312-464-5909 to the attention of your account representative.

GENERAL INFORMATION

To contact a Classified Advertising account representative, call 312-464-2475/2490/2491/4485 or 800-AMA-2260. Or fax your insertion order to 312-464-5909. Mail your materials to AMA Classified Advertising, 12th Floor, 515 N State St, Chicago, IL 60610.

ACADEMIC/FACULTY

BARIATRIC/GI/LAPAROSCOPIC SURGEON: Immediate opening for a full time academic gastrointestinal surgeon specializing in the surgical treatment of obesity at the instructor, assistant or associate professor level at the Beth Israel Deaconess Medical Center, a major teaching hospital of the Harvard Medical School. Candidates must be BE/BC and committed to teaching and research (clinical or laboratory). Expertise in surgical nutrition is essential, and the successful candidate will work closely with the program in obesity and nutrition lead by Dr George Blackburn. Underrepresented minority candidates and women are encouraged to apply. BIDMC is an equal opportunity employer. Send CV to Dr Jeffrey Matthews, Chief, Division of General and Gastrointestinal Surgery, 330 Brookline Ave, Boston, MA 02215.

SURGICAL CRITICAL CARE/TRAUMA. ASSISTANT/ASSOCIATE PROFESSOR: The Department of Surgery at Robert C. Byrd Health Sciences Center of WVU/Charleston Division/Charleston Area Medical Center, is seeking a general surgeon with interest in surgical critical care and trauma. Fellowship training with eligibility or added certification qualifications in Surgical Critical Care required. Charleston Area Medical Center is a State, Level I trauma center with helicopter and ACGME accredited General Surgery Residency. Opportunities for clinical research, resident and student education, and general surgery practice are available. Application Deadline: Position will remain open until filled. Send curriculum vitae to James P. Boland, MD, Professor and Chairman, Department of Surgery, 3110 MacCorkle Ave, SE, Charleston, WV 25304. Phone: 304-347-1233 Fax: 304-347-1343. E-mail: james.boland@camcare.com

SPARTANBURG REGIONAL HEALTHCARE SYSTEM. SURGICAL EDUCATION. SOUTH CAROLINA - GENERAL SURGERY RESIDENCY PROGRAM: An exceptional opportunity for a board-certified Surgeon with an emphasis in general surgery and critical care medicine to join the Surgical Education Faculty at Spartanburg Regional Medical Center. The physician will be responsible for teaching general surgery residents as well as conducting a limited private practice. Affiliated with the Medical University of South Carolina and the University of South Carolina. Exceptional call coverage arrangement. A previous academic appointment will be a plus. Trauma experience is necessary, as Spartanburg Regional Medical Center is one of four Level I Trauma facilities in the state of South Carolina. Outstanding salary based upon background and experience, as well as an excellent comprehensive benefits package including relocation expenses, CME and professional liability insurance. Research opportunities are also available. For confidential consideration please contact Cathy K. Benson, CMSR, Spartanburg Regional Medical Center, 800-890-0138 or Fax your CV: 864-560-7472. Cbenson@srhs.com EOE.

CRITICAL CARE

TRAUMA SURGEON

Exciting opportunity to lead a Trauma Service currently under development at Baptist Medical Center South, in Montgomery, Alabama. Baptist Health, the leading not-for-profit health system in Central Alabama, is seeking a board certified or eligible General Surgeon with fellowship in Critical Care/Trauma. The position offers an attractive compensation and benefits plan. Interested candidates should send a CV to:

Neal Kelley
Director, Medical Staff Development
Baptist Health
PO Box 11010
Montgomery, AL 36111-0010
Fax: 334-273-4529
E-mail: nkelley@bmcmont.hbocvan.com

GRADUATE TRAINING/ RESIDENCIES/FELLOWSHIPS

LAHEY CLINIC: Minimally Invasive Research Fellowship. The Lahey Clinic Division of Surgery is offering a Minimally Invasive Surgical Research Fellowship beginning 7/1/99 - 6/30/00. Basic and Clinical Research. Lahey Clinic is a large multi-specialty group practice 10 miles from Boston. Please send CV and letter to Desmond H. Birkett, MD, Chairman, Department of General Surgery, Lahey Clinic, 41 Mall Rd, Burlington, MA 01805; Fax: 781-744-5636; Or call 781-744-8585. An Equal Opportunity Employer.

LEGAL SERVICES

MALPRACTICE CASE EVALUATION

Board-certified medical experts needed. All specialties. All locations. Defense and plaintiff cases. Excellent remuneration. Send CVs to:

Barry Gustin, MD, MPH, FACEP
AMERICAN MEDICAL FORENSIC SPECIALISTS, Inc
2991 Shattuck Ave, Ste 302
Berkeley, CA 94705

LOCUM TENENS WANTED

HKA LOCUM TENENS is looking for quality surgical specialty physicians to do Locum Tenens. We have opportunities coast-to-coast. We furnish Occurrence Malpractice Insurance (no tail necessary). Please call HKA LOCUM TENENS at (800) 226-6347, Extension AM7.1.

HEMATOLOGY & ONCOLOGY

SPARTANBURG REGIONAL HEALTHCARE SYSTEM. SURGICAL EDUCATION. SURGICAL ONCOLOGIST: South Carolina - General Surgery Residency Program: An exceptional opportunity for a board-certified Surgical Oncologist to join the Surgical Education Faculty at Spartanburg Regional Medical Center. The physician will be responsible for teaching general surgery residents as well as conducting a limited private practice. Affiliated with the Medical University of South Carolina and the University of South Carolina. Exceptional call coverage arrangement. A previous academic appointment will be a plus. Trauma experience is necessary, as Spartanburg Regional Medical Center is one of four Level I Trauma facilities in the state of South Carolina. The system offers a range of specialized healthcare services that is unrivaled in its five-county service region, featuring world-class specialty centers, including the Regional Cancer Center, a 100,000+ square foot state-of-the-art facility scheduled to open in June of 1999. Outstanding salary based upon backgroun and experience, as well as an excellent comprehensive benefits package including relocation expenses, CME and professional liability insurance. Research opportunities are also available. For confidential consideration please contact Cathy K. Benson, CMSR, Spartanburg Regional Medical Center, 800-890-0138 or Fax your CV: 864-560-7472. Cbenson@srhs.com EOE.

PRACTICES FOR SALE

SENIOR SOLO: General Surgeon in Atlanta area wishes to sell practice totally. FAX inquires to 770-739-2803.

SURGERY: GENERAL

FOX RIVER VALLEY, WI: Town of 14,000 (draw 50,000) thirty minutes from Green Bay. Join another surgeon in 14-physician group, proven caseload. Endoscopy, laparoscopy required, C-sections preferred, vascular a plus. For consideration, call Kari Donovan, 800-765-3055, ID#6378AR, fax: 314-726-3009, e-mail: kdonovan@cejka.com Visit our website: www.cejka.com

---

GENERAL SURGERY: Portland, Oregon. Northwest Permanente, PC, a physician-managed multispecialty group serving the members of Kaiser Permanente in the Northwest Division, has two excellent opportunities for BC/BE general and/or vascular surgeons. Our new associate will practice with the 21 general surgeons at Kaiser Permanente's affiliated hospitals in the Portland/Vancouver metropolitan area. The Northwest Division has a total of 24 general surgeons providing quality care to over 435,000 plan members in Oregon and Washington. Ours is a collegial and professionally stimulating practice in one of the most successful managed care programs in the country. In addition to a lifestyle inherent to the beautiful Pacific Northwest, we offer a predictable work schedule, and a competitive salary and benefit package which includes professional liability coverage, a comprehensive pension program, sabbatical leave and more. For additional information please forward CV to A. S. Weiland, MD, Regional Medical Director, NORTHWEST PERMANENTE, PC, 500 NE Multnomah, Ste 100, Portland, OR 97231-2099. EOE.

LOGAN, UTAH: One BE/BC general surgeon needed for an outstanding practice opportunity. Employment position in a multi-specialty clinic within Intermountain Health Care's Physician Division. Practice in an area where many people visit to ski, fish, hike, camp and enjoy the beauty of the area. A low crime rate and family oriented culture makes this an ideal place in which to live. A negotiable salary and generous benefits package are offered with moving costs negotiable. For more information, send/Fax a CV to IHC Physician Services, Attn: Wilf Rudert, 36 S State St, 20th Fl, Salt Lake City, UT 84111. 800-888-3134 #1. Fax: 801-442-2999. E-mail: comdixon@ihc.com Internet: http://www.ihc.com/phys_recruit

---

OHIO - NW - GENERAL SURGEON: Financially strong, community hospital in NW OH needs a full-time Surgeon to take over for retiring physician. Call Doug Page. Lawlor and Associates 800-238-7150; or Fax 610-431-4092; or E-mail: LawlorRctg@aol.com

---

OPPORTUNITY IN NORTHEASTERN OKLAHOMA LAKE COUNTRY: Strong 70 bed JCAHO accredited not-for-profit hospital has an opportunity for 1 general surgeon. General surgery service area of 60,000+. 12 BC physicians on staff including an anesthesiologist. 40 minutes from Tulsa. Negotiable financial arrangements. Call Stan Schuermann at INTEGRIS Baptist Medical Center at 800-332-8663.

OPPORTUNITY FOR SEASONED, progressive, BC/BE general surgeon to immediately join busy, well established, private surgical practice. Located in Northern Michigan on the Great Lakes. Spectacular four season recreation, safe, caring, family oriented community. Supportive and friendly hospital and professional staff with over forty referring physicians and excellent ER, ICU, and diagnostic imaging support. Efficient, state-of-the-art office suite in new medical office building connected to hospital. Competitive salary with full benefits. Send cover letter and curriculum vitae to T. M. Burandt, DO & Associates, PC, 810 South Main Street, Suite#1, Cheboygan, MI 49721, Facsimile: 616-627-7758, E-mail: tburandt@cdimed.com

---

PENNSYLVANIA - NW - GENERAL SURGEON: with established practice in Erie County. Take advantage of what retired physicians have left behind. Located between Pittsburgh, Cleveland and Buffalo with easy access to Lake Erie. Contact David Finney. Lawlor and Associates 800-238-7150; or Fax: 610-431-4092; or E-mail: LawlorRctg@aol.com

---

PIEDMONT NORTH CAROLINA: General Surgeon. Ideal candidate should have a strong vascular interest. You would be co-located with a solo general surgeon who has built a tremendous practice since moving here from residency nearly three years ago. This position will offer a guaranteed salary for the first year and a partnership tract. Candidates should have completed medical school at a LCME-accredited program and residency at an ACGME-accredited program. Safe, family-oriented community enjoys excellent school system, low crime, 97%+ employment, and many recreational activities in the beautiful rolling hills of NC. Mail CV to Randy Mitchell, Randolph Hospital, 364 White Oak St, Asheboro, NC 27203. Or Fax: 336-626-7664. Or call: 336-633-7777. E-mail: rlm@atomic.net Visit our website at www.randolphhospital.org

---

TEXAS: Take over lucrative, highly successful practice with 70-member multispecialty group. Extremely well-managed group with incomes in the top 99th percentile nationwide. 1 in 4 call. Community of 80,000 just over 2 hours from Dallas. Exceptional real estate values, gorgeous homes and country clubs. Contact Todd Dillon, 800-883-7345, ID#6439AR, Fax: 810-603-2942, E-mail: tdillon@cejka.com Visit our website www.cejka.com

---

WILLAMETTE VALLEY, OREGON: Opportunity available for BC/BE General Surgeon. Join a 3-member department within large physician-owned multi-specialty group. Corvallis is home to Oregon State University, town of 45,000, located in heart of beautiful Willamette Valley wine country; one hour from coast, two hours from Cascade Mountains ski and recreation areas. Guaranteed salary, incentive bonus, and excellent benefits. Position is available April 1999. Send CV and cover letter to, Medical Director, The Corvallis Clinic, PC, 444 NW Elks Dr, Corvallis, OR 97330, Fax: 541-757-1847.

GENERAL SURGERY OPPORTUNITY: Opportunity to join a well-established one surgeon practice with one in four on call rotation. The practice is located in beautiful western Massachusetts in an area known as the "Five College Area" with the University of Massachusetts at Amherst, Smith, Mt Holyoke, Amherst and Hampshire Colleges located within a 10 mile radius. These colleges with their large student and faculty populations create a sophisticated urban environment nestled within a rural setting. Enjoy full spectrum general surgery with a busy caseload plus the full support of a strong hospital system and excellent referral base. Send CV and addresses of three references to CDPA, PO Box 911, Northampton, MA 01061 or Fax to 413-582-2951.

SURGERY: ORTHOPEDIC

OPPORTUNITY IN NORTHEASTERN OKLAHOMA LAKE COUNTRY: Strong not-for-profit hospital has an opportunity for 1 orthopedic surgeon. Orthopedic surgery service area of 60,000+. 70 bed JCAHO accredited hospital with 12 BC physicians on staff including an anesthesiologist. 40 minutes from Tulsa. Negotiable financial arrangements. Call Stan Schuermann at INTEGRIS Baptist Medical Center at 800-332-8663.

SURGERY: SURGICAL SPECIALTIES

BC/BE SURGEON every fourth night for Indian Health Service facility with state of the art laparoscopic and endoscopic equipment. College town 1 hour from metro area. Ideally located at base of Ozark Mountains with abundant four season recreational opportunities. Salary negotiable, excellent benefits, loan repayment. We are an equal opportunity employer. Contact Lisa Spry at 918-458-3360.

HOUSTON, TX: MacGregor Medical Association, a multispecialty group practice with over 40 years of experience in quality care, is seeking a Board Certified Colo-Rectal Surgeon with a minimum of 3 years experience. MMA is a group of more than 200 physicians serving over 180,000 patients. Our diverse patient population is comprised of 90% managed care and 10% fee for service clients. Houston is a diverse city that offers a wide array of cultural and recreational pursuits. Texas has no state income tax! MacGregor offers a competitive salary and excellent benefit package. For more information you may call us at 800-716-6060. You may also fax/mail your CV to MacGregor Medical Association, Medical Staff Services, 2550 Holly Hall, Houston, TX 77054, 713-746-5441 http://medjobs.macgregor.com/

TWO-SURGEON PRACTICE, located in central New York, seeks general surgeon with laparoscopic, vascular, and/or thoracic capabilities. Recent fellowship training desirable. Based in the scenic and cosmopolitan home of Cornell University. The practice serves two progressive medical centers. Excellent lifestyle opportunities abound in housing, education, and recreation. Reply to Box 323, c/o SUR, 515 N State St, 12th Fl, Chicago, IL 60610.

SURGERY: THORACIC

LONG ISLAND - THORACIC SURGEON: BC/BE Thoracic Surgeon to join a busy 7 surgeon group practicing thoracic/vascular/general surgery 45 minutes from Manhattan. Send CV to Long Island Thoracic Surgeon, Ste 26, 375 E Main St, Bay Shore, NY 11706.

SURGERY: VASCULAR

SPARTANBURG REGIONAL HEALTHCARE SYSTEM: SURGICAL EDUCATION. VASCULAR SURGEON: South Carolina - General Surgery Residency Program: An Exceptional opportunity for a board-certified Vascular Surgeon to join the Surgical Education Faculty at Spartanburg Regional Medical Center. The physician will be responsible for teaching general surgery residents as well as conducting a limited private practice. Affiliated with the Medical University of South Carolina and the University of South Carolina. Exceptional call coverage arrangement. A previous academic appointment will be a plus. Trauma experience is necessary, as Spartanburg Regional Medical Center is one of four Level I Trauma facilities in the state of South Carolina. The system offers a range of specialized healthcare services that is unrivaled in its five-county service region, featuring world-class specialty centers, including the Regional Heart Center. Outstanding salary based upon background and experience, as well as an excellent comprehensive benefits package including relocation expenses, CME and professional liability insurance. Research opportunities are also available. For confidential consideration please contact Cathy K. Benson, CMSR, Spartanburg Regional Medical Center, 800-890-0138 or Fax your CV: 864-560-7472. Cbenson@srhs.com EOE.

VASCULAR SURGEON: Beautiful Central Florida. Easy access to Orlando and Tampa. Moss-draped oak trees line hundred year old streets in our beautiful city. Practice vascular surgery and some general surgery as the third surgeon in a busy practice. Affiliate with two hospitals with more than 550 beds in the community. Call Robert Estes at 800-321-2460. FAX CV to 407-253-9055.

WISCONSIN: General/vascular surgeon sought for 3-surgeon group. Take over for departing associate. Must be willing to do general and vascular, but fellowship training not required. Community of 100,000 only 1 1/2 hours from Minneapolis/St Paul. Prefer a '99 resident. $160,000 salary, bonus, benefits and partnership. Contact Todd Dillon, 800-883-7345, ID#6338AR, Fax: 810-603-2942, E-mail: tdillon@cejka.com Visit our website: www.cejka.com

THE DEPARTMENT OF SURGERY AT THE UNIVERSITY OF CALIFORNIA, DAVIS, EAST BAY DIVISION, AT THE UNIVERSITY OF CALIFORNIA, DAVIS: is seeking a full-time academic minimally invasive and/or trauma surgeon. The appointment will be at the Assistant or Associate Professor level commensurate with credentials. Applicants must be Board Certified in General Surgery or have successfully completed an ACGME approved program in General Surgery and be eligible for licensure in the State of California. Duties include patient care in both the inpatient and out-patient clinical settings, research, and teaching of medical students, interns, residents, and groups within the community.

A letter outlining research and teaching background, a complete Curriculum Vitae and bibliography, along with the names, addresses (with fax numbers and E-mail addresses) of five references should be forwarded to Claude H. Organ, Jr, MD, Professor & Chair, Department of Surgery, University of California, East Bay Division, 1411 E 31st St, Oakland, CA 94602. **Please refer to Search 2349.** This position will remain open until filled, but no later than **September 30, 1999**. All applications must be received no later than **September 30, 1999**.

The University of California is an Affirmative Action/Equal Opportunity Employer.

The Department of Surgery at the University of California, Davis wishes to recruit, at the Associate or Professor level, a full-time, experienced Vascular Surgeon, who is Board Certified or Board Eligible, as Chief of Vascular Surgery at the Sacramento VA Hospital. The position requires a joint University/VA appointment and will be paid Salary Cost Recovery. As the VA Chief of Vascular Surgery, incumbent is responsible for activities of the Vascular Inpatient Service and Vascular Outpatient Clinic at the Sacramento VA. Duties will also include limited clinical participation and teaching at UCDMC. Incumbent also responsible for vascular outpatient VA clinic activities in Redding and Martinez. Duties include supervising medical students, interns, and residents. Research of the incumbent's choice will be considered as integral part of the assigned duties.

A letter outlining research and teaching background, a complete Curriculum Vitae and the names, addresses, (with fax numbers and E-mail addresses) of three references should be forwarded to F. William Blaisdell, Professor, Department of Surgery, UC Davis Medical Center, 4301 X St, Rm 2310, Sacramento, CA 95817. This position will remain open until filled but no later than **May 31, 1999**. All applications must be received no later than **May 31, 1999**.

The University of California is an Affirmative Action/Equal Opportunity Employer.

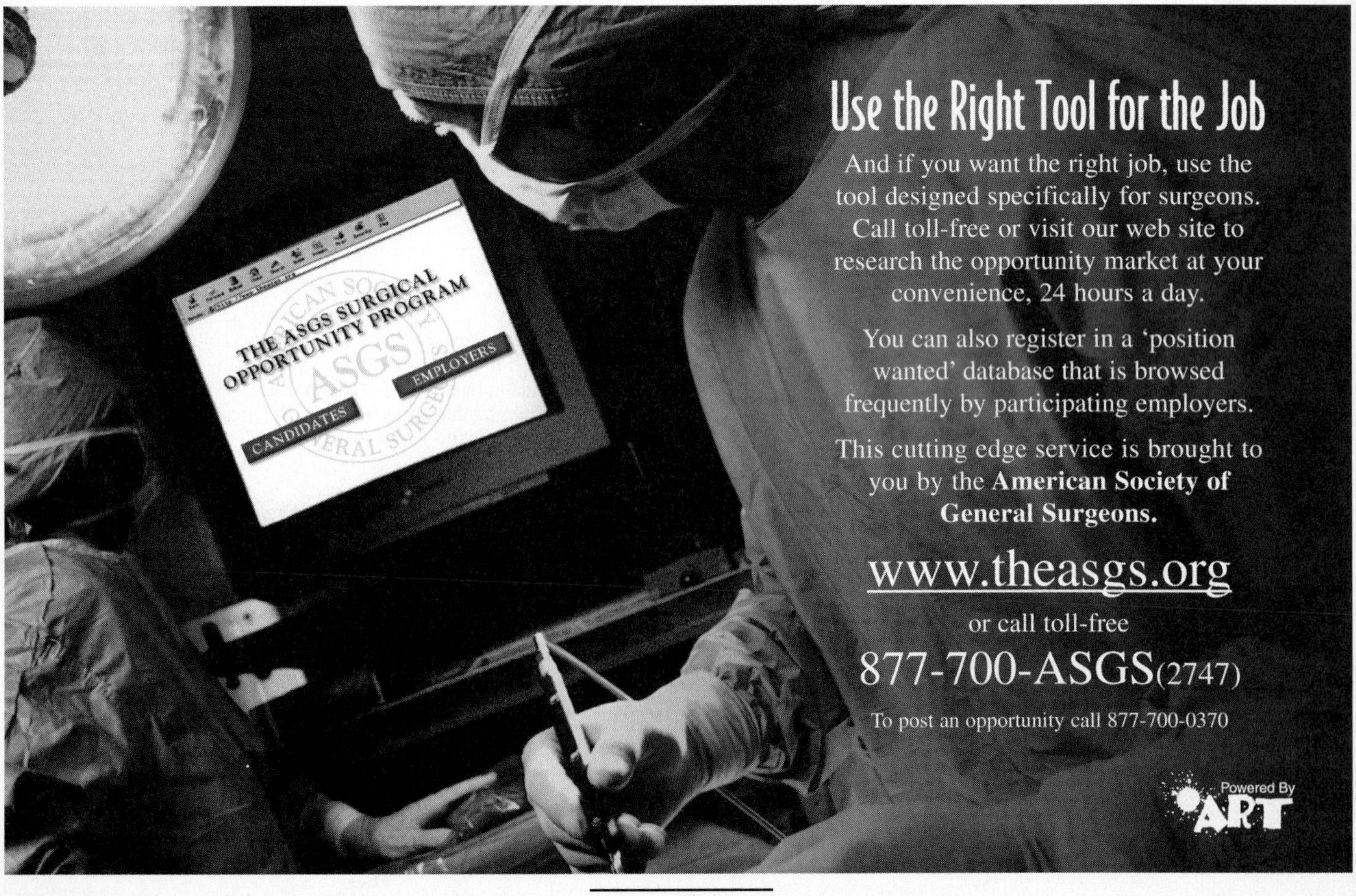

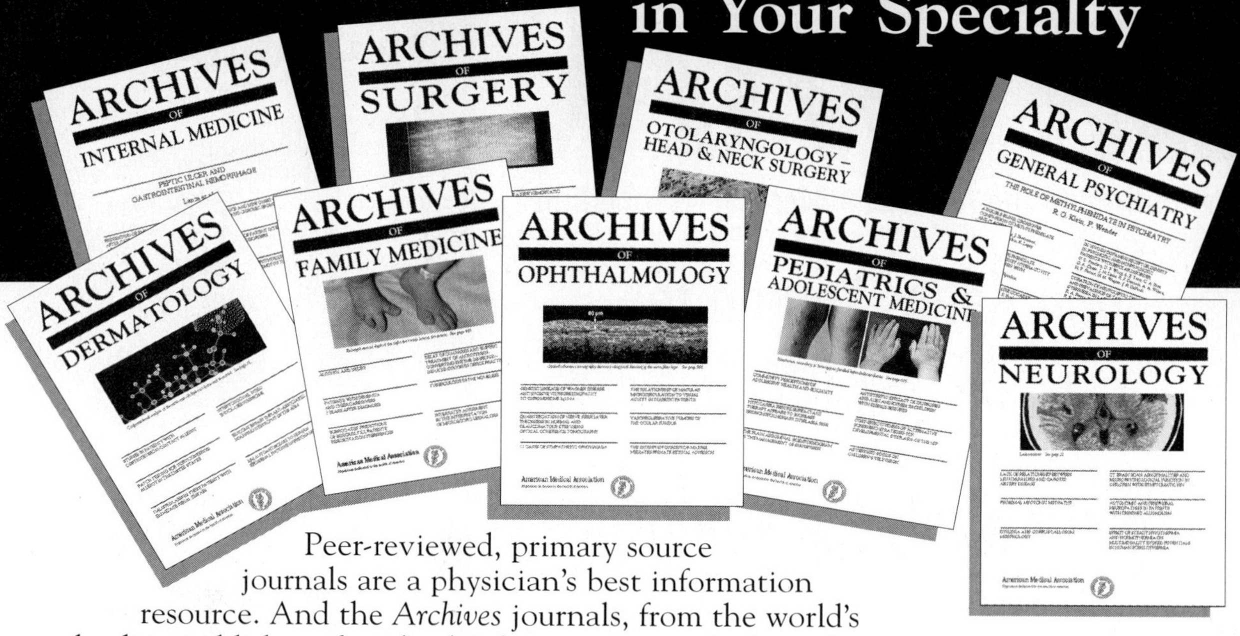

Index of Advertisers

BRAINTREE LABORATORIES
Nulytely .... Cover 4

CLASSIFIED ADVERTISING 339-343
http://www.ama-assn.org

ETHICON INC
Suture Assist 231
Suture Assist 260A-D

GLAXO WELLCOME
Zofran 333-334

NOVARTIS PHARMACEUTICALS CORP
http://www.norvartis.com
Apligraf 233-234

PFIZER, US PHARMACEUTICAL GROUP
http://www.pfizer.com
Diflucan .... Cover 2-229

While every precaution is taken to ensure accuracy, we cannot guarantee against the possibility of an occasional change or omission in the preparation of this index.

Document Delivery Information

UnCover
Tel: 800-787-7979
303-758-3030
Fax: 303-758-5946
URL: http://uncweb.carl.org
E-mail: uncover@carl.org

Institute for Scientific Information (ISI)
Tel: 800-336-4474
215-386-0100
Fax: 215-386-6362
URL: http://www.isinet.com

WOW! ONLY 1 PREP HAS...

52% LESS SALT & NO SODIUM SULFATE

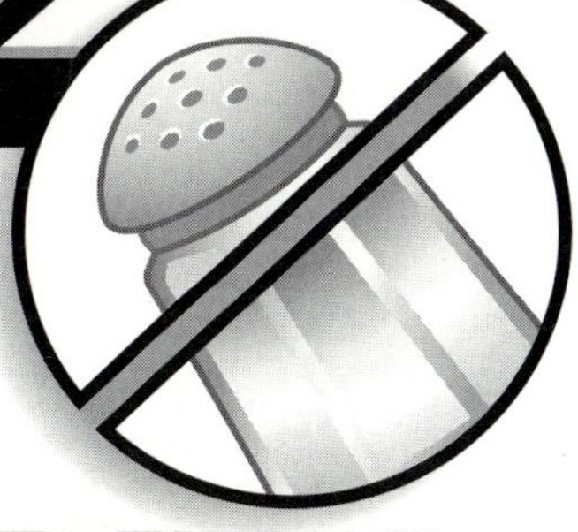

FOR GREAT TASTE

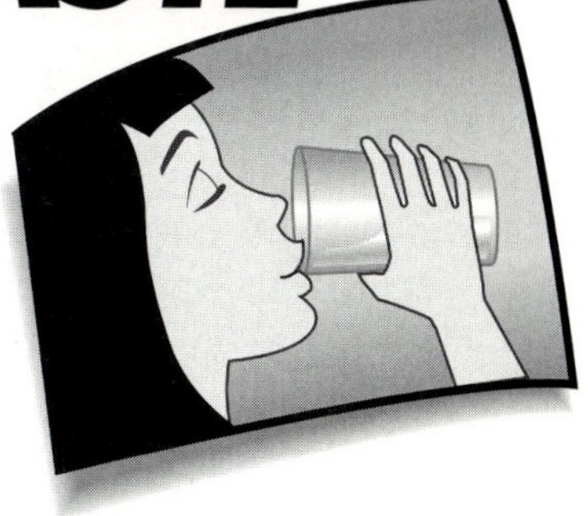

NuLYTELY®

and

CHERRY FLAVOR NuLYTELY®

PEG 3350, Sodium Chloride, Sodium Bicarbonate and Potassium Chloride for Oral Solution

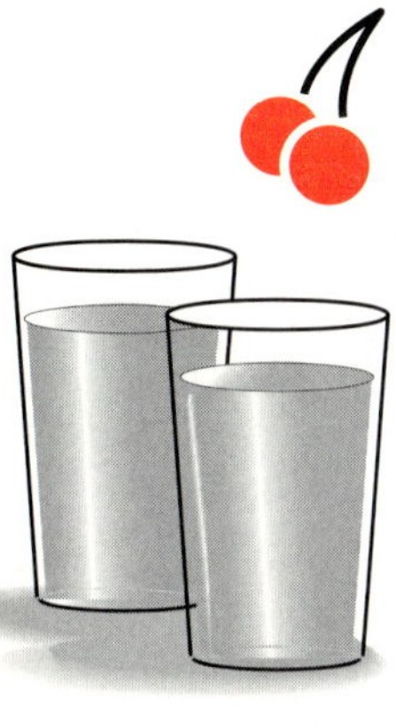

This UNIQUE FORMULA eliminates sodium sulfate and reduces total salt by 52%[1] ... your patients get a bowel prep with improved taste

Patients have a choice: Cherry Flavor NuLYTELY or Regular NuLYTELY with a pleasant mineral-water taste

Cherry Flavor NuLYTELY is the #1 prescribed flavored bowel prep[2]

Contraindicated in patients with gastrointestinal obstruction, gastric retention, bowel perforation, toxic colitis or toxic megacolon

Brief summary: Before prescribing, please see full prescribing information.

Indications and Usage: NuLYTELY is indicated for bowel cleansing prior to colonoscopy. **Contraindications:** NuLYTELY is contraindicated in patients with gastrointestinal obstruction, gastric retention, bowel perforation, toxic colitis or toxic megacolon. **Warnings:** No additional ingredients, e.g. flavoring, should be added to the solution. NuLYTELY should be used with caution in patients with severe ulcerative colitis. Use of NuLYTELY in children younger than 2 years of age should be carefully monitored for occurrence of possible hypoglycemia, as this solution has no caloric substrate. Dehydration has been reported in 1 child and hypokalemia has been reported in 3 children. **Precautions: General:** Patients with impaired gag reflex, unconscious, or semiconscious patients, and patients prone to regurgitation or aspiration should be observed during the administration of NuLYTELY, especially if it is administered via nasogastric tube. If a patient experiences severe bloating, distention or abdominal pain, administration should be slowed or temporarily discontinued until the symptoms abate. If gastrointestinal obstruction or perforation is suspected, appropriate studies should be performed to rule out these conditions before administration of NuLYTELY. **Adverse Reactions:** Nausea, abdominal fullness and bloating are the most common adverse reactions (occurring in up to 50% of patients) to administration of NuLYTELY. Abdominal cramps, vomiting and anal irritation occur less frequently. These adverse reactions are transient and subside rapidly. Isolated cases of urticaria, rhinorrhea, dermatitis and (rarely) anaphylactic reaction have been reported which may represent allergic reactions. **Oral Administration, Pediatric Patients:** (aged 6 months or greater): At a rate of 25 mL/kg/hour, until the rectal effluent is clear or 4 liters are consumed. Rapid drinking of each portion is preferred to drinking small amounts continuously. **Storage:** Store in sealed container at 25°C. When reconstituted, keep solution refrigerated. Use within 48 hours. Discard unused portion. NDC 52268-301-01. ℞ **only.** Distributed by Braintree Laboratories, Inc., Braintree, MA 02185. Revised 9/97

References: 1. Fordtran JS, Santa Ana CA, Cleveland MvB. *Gastroenterology.* 1990;98:11-16. **2.** Data on file, Braintree Laboratories, Inc.

Braintree LABORATORIES · IN

The Leader in Lavage

ARCHIVES OF SURGERY

APRIL 1999

PAPERS PRESENTED AT THE 79TH ANNUAL MEETING OF THE NEW ENGLAND SURGICAL SOCIETY, TORONTO, ONTARIO, SEPTEMBER 25-27, 1998

FAMILIAL PATTERNS OF THORACIC AORTIC ANEURYSMS

THE VALUE OF PHYSICIAN ASSISTANTS TO SURGICAL EDUCATION IN TEACHING HOSPITALS

INTERVAL OR PERMANENT NONOPERATIVE MANAGEMENT OF ACUTE TYPE A AORTIC DISSECTION

SURGERY IN ARGENTINA

DISTAL SPLENORENAL SHUNT: ROLE, INDICATIONS, AND UTILITY IN THE ERA OF LIVER TRANSPLANTATION

MECHANISM OF ADRENAL INSUFFICIENCY FOLLOWING TRAUMA AND SEVERE HEMORRHAGE: ROLE OF HEPATIC 11β-HYDROXYSTEROID DEHYDROGENASE

COMPLETE TABLE OF CONTENTS INSIDE

American Medical Association
Physicians dedicated to the health of America

www.ama-assn.org/surgery

for prevention of postoperative nausea and vomiting

Zofran® ODT™

ondansetron Orally Disintegrating Tablets

NEW

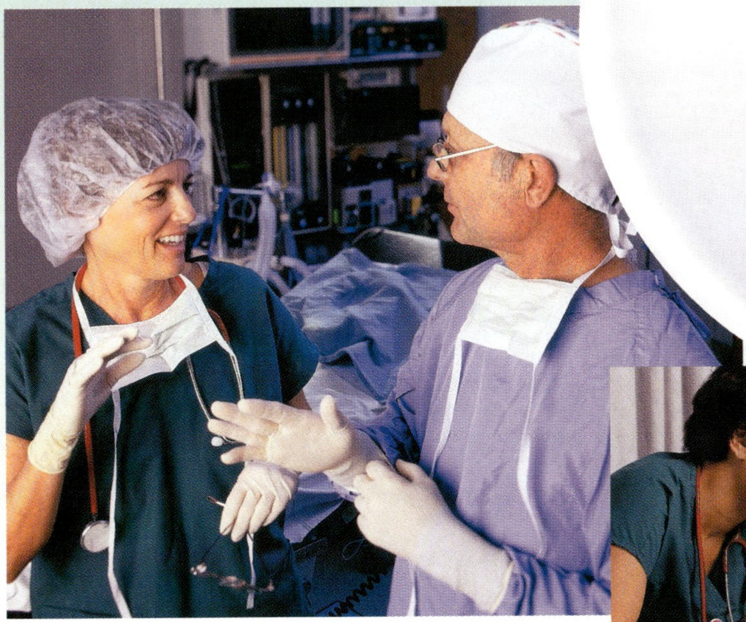

Delivers the 24-hour efficacy You demand

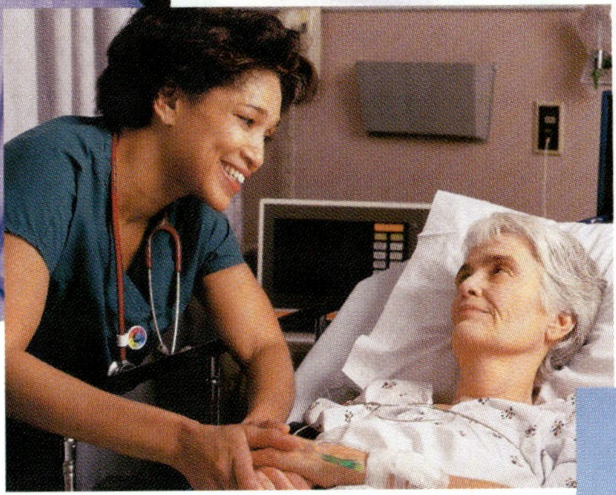

Delivers nonsedation in the PACU – A major benefit in day surgery

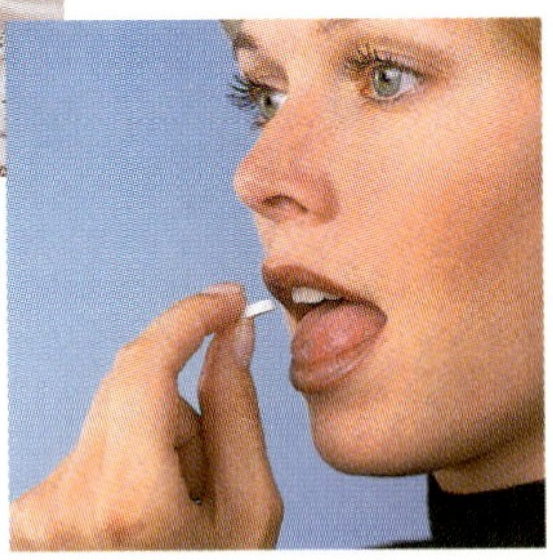

Delivers flexibility—take ODT anywhere; dissolves instantly on the tongue – without water

Choose

ZOFRAN –

Your partner for patient satisfaction

The most commonly reported adverse events in patients receiving ZOFRAN in clinical trials were headache (5% to 27%), diarrhea (<1% to 16%), constipation (<1% to 9%), fever (<1% to 8%), and malaise/fatigue (0% to 13%).*

*Data on file, Glaxo Wellcome, Inc.

Please see Brief Summary of Prescribing Information on next page.

GlaxoWellcome

BRIEF SUMMARY

ZOFRAN®
(ondansetron hydrochloride)
Injection

ZOFRAN®
(ondansetron hydrochloride)
Injection Premixed

ZOFRAN®
(ondansetron hydrochloride)
Tablets

ZOFRAN® ODT™
(ondansetron)
Orally Disintegrating Tablets

ZOFRAN®
(ondansetron hydrochloride)
Oral Solution

The following is a brief summary only; see full prescribing information for complete product information.

CONTRAINDICATIONS: ZOFRAN Injection, ZOFRAN Injection Premixed, ZOFRAN Tablets, ZOFRAN ODT Orally Disintegrating Tablets, and ZOFRAN Oral Solution are contraindicated for patients known to have hypersensitivity to the drug.

WARNINGS: Hypersensitivity reactions have been reported in patients who have exhibited hypersensitivity to other selective 5-HT_3 receptor antagonists.

PRECAUTIONS: Ondansetron is not a drug that stimulates gastric or intestinal peristalsis. It should not be used instead of nasogastric suction. The use of ondansetron in patients following abdominal surgery or in patients with chemotherapy-induced nausea and vomiting may mask a progressive ileus and/or gastric distention.
Information for Patients: ***Phenylketonurics:*** Phenylketonuric patients should be informed that ZOFRAN ODT Orally Disintegrating Tablets contain phenylalanine (a component of aspartame). Each 4-mg and 8-mg orally disintegrating tablet contains <0.03 mg phenylalanine.
Patients should be instructed not to remove ZOFRAN ODT Tablets from the blister until just prior to dosing. The tablet should not be pushed through the foil. With dry hands, the blister backing should be peeled completely off the blister. The tablet should be gently removed and immediately placed on the tongue to dissolve and be swallowed with the saliva. Peelable illustrated stickers are affixed to the product carton that can be provided with the prescription to ensure proper use and handling of the product.
Drug Interactions: Ondansetron does not itself appear to induce or inhibit the cytochrome P-450 drug-metabolizing enzyme system of the liver. Because ondansetron is metabolized by hepatic cytochrome P-450 drug-metabolizing enzymes, inducers or inhibitors of these enzymes may change the clearance and, hence, the half-life of ondansetron. On the basis of limited available data, no dosage adjustment is recommended for patients on these drugs. Tumor response to chemotherapy in the P 388 mouse leukemia model is not affected by ondansetron. In humans, carmustine, etoposide, and cisplatin do not affect the pharmacokinetics of ondansetron.
Use in Surgical Patients: The coadministration of ondansetron had no effect on the pharmacokinetics and pharmacodynamics of temazepam.
Carcinogenesis, Mutagenesis, Impairment of Fertility: Carcinogenic effects were not seen in 2-year studies in rats and mice with oral ondansetron doses up to 10 and 30 mg/kg per day, respectively. Ondansetron was not mutagenic in standard tests for mutagenicity. Oral administration of ondansetron up to 15 mg/kg per day did not affect fertility or general reproductive performance of male and female rats.
Pregnancy: ***Teratogenic Effects:*** Pregnancy Category B. Reproduction studies have been performed in pregnant rats and rabbits at IV doses up to 4 mg/kg per day and at daily oral doses up to 15 and 30 mg/kg per day, respectively, and have revealed no evidence of impaired fertility or harm to the fetus due to ondansetron. There are, however, no adequate and well-controlled studies in pregnant women. Because animal reproduction studies are not always predictive of human response, this drug should be used during pregnancy only if clearly needed.
Nursing Mothers: Ondansetron is excreted in the breast milk of rats. It is not known whether ondansetron is excreted in human milk. Because many drugs are excreted in human milk, caution should be exercised when ondansetron is administered to a nursing woman.
Pediatric Use: ***ZOFRAN Injection:*** Little information is available about dosage in pediatric patients under 2 years of age (see DOSAGE AND ADMINISTRATION section of full prescribing information for use in pediatric patients 4 to 18 years of age receiving cancer chemotherapy or for use in pediatric patients 2 to 12 years of age receiving general anesthesia).
ZOFRAN Tablets: Little information is available about dosage in children 4 years of age or younger (see CLINICAL PHARMACOLOGY and DOSAGE AND ADMINISTRATION sections of full prescribing information for use in children 4 to 18 years of age).
Use in Elderly Patients: Dosage adjustment is not needed in patients over the age of 65 (see CLINICAL PHARMACOLOGY section of full prescribing information). Prevention of nausea and vomiting in elderly patients was no different than in younger age-groups.

ADVERSE REACTIONS
ZOFRAN Injection: ***Chemotherapy-Induced Nausea and Vomiting:*** The following adverse events have been reported in individuals receiving ondansetron at a dosage of three 0.15-mg/kg doses or as a single 32-mg dose in clinical trials. These patients were receiving concomitant chemotherapy, primarily cisplatin, and IV fluids. Most were receiving a diuretic.

Table 1: Principal Adverse Events in Comparative Trials

	Number of Patients With Event			
	ZOFRAN Injection 0.15 mg/kg x 3 n = 419	ZOFRAN Injection 32 mg x 1 n = 220	Metoclopramide n = 156	Placebo n = 34
Diarrhea	16%	8%	44%	18%
Headache	17%	25%	7%	15%
Fever	8%	7%	5%	3%
Akathisia	0%	0%	6%	0%
Acute dystonic reactions*	0%	0%	5%	0%

*See Neurological

The following have been reported during controlled clinical trials:
Cardiovascular: Rare cases of angina (chest pain), electrocardiographic alterations, and tachycardia have been reported. In many cases, the relationship to ZOFRAN Injection was unclear.
Gastrointestinal: Constipation has been reported in 11% of chemotherapy patients receiving multiday ondansetron.
Hepatic: In comparative trials in cisplatin chemotherapy patients with normal baseline values of aspartate transaminase (AST) and alanine transaminase (ALT), these enzymes have been reported to exceed twice the upper limit of normal in approximately 5% of patients. The increases were transient and did not appear to be related to dose or duration of therapy. On repeat exposure, similar transient elevations in transaminase values occurred in some courses, but symptomatic hepatic disease did not occur.
Integumentary: Rash has occurred in approximately 1% of patients receiving ondansetron.
Neurological: There have been rare reports consistent with, but not diagnostic of, extrapyramidal reactions in patients receiving ZOFRAN Injection, and rare cases of grand mal seizure. The relationship to ZOFRAN was unclear.
Other: Bronchospasm and rare case of hypokalemia have been reported. The relationship to ZOFRAN Injection was unclear.
Postoperative Nausea and Vomiting: The following adverse events have been reported in ≥2% of adults receiving ondansetron at a dosage of 4 mg IV over 2 to 5 minutes in clinical trials. Rates of these events were not significantly different in the ondansetron and placebo groups. These patients were receiving multiple concomitant perioperative and postoperative medications.

Table 2: Adverse Events in ≥2% of Adults Receiving Ondansetron at a Dosage of 4 Mg IV over 2 to 5 Minutes in Clinical Trials

	ZOFRAN Injection 4 mg IV n = 547 patients	Placebo n = 547 patients
Headache	92 (17%)	77 (14%)
Dizziness	67 (12%)	88 (16%)
Musculoskeletal pain	57 (10%)	59 (11%)
Drowsiness/sedation	44 (8%)	37 (7%)
Shivers	38 (7%)	39 (7%)
Malaise/fatigue	25 (5%)	30 (5%)
Injection site reaction	21 (4%)	18 (3%)
Urinary retention	17 (3%)	15 (3%)
Postoperative CO_2-related pain*	12 (2%)	16 (3%)
Chest pain (unspecified)	12 (2%)	15 (3%)
Anxiety/agitation	11 (2%)	16 (3%)
Dysuria	11 (2%)	9 (2%)
Hypotension	10 (2%)	12 (2%)
Fever	10 (2%)	6 (1%)
Cold sensation	9 (2%)	8 (1%)
Pruritus	9 (2%)	3 (<1%)
Paresthesia	9 (2%)	2 (<1%)

*Sites of pain included abdomen, stomach, joints, rib cage, shoulder.

Pediatric Use: The following were the most commonly reported adverse events in pediatric patients receiving ondansetron (a single 0.1-mg/kg dose for pediatric patients weighing 40 kg or less, or 4 mg for pediatric patients weighing more than 40 kg) administered intravenously over at least 30 seconds. Rates of these events were not significantly different in the ondansetron and placebo groups. These patients were receiving multiple concomitant perioperative and postoperative medications.

Table 3: Frequency of Adverse Events From Controlled Studies

Adverse Event	Ondansetron IV n = 755 Patients	Placebo n = 731 Patients
Wound problem	80 (11%)	86 (12%)
Anxiety/agitation	49 (6%)	47 (6%)
Headache	44 (6%)	43 (6%)
Drowsiness/sedation	41 (5%)	56 (8%)
Pyrexia	32 (4%)	41 (6%)

Observed During Clinical Practice: In addition to adverse events reported from clinical trials, the following events have been identified during post-approval use of intravenous formulations of ZOFRAN. Because they are reported voluntarily from a population of unknown size, estimates of frequency cannot be made. The events have been chosen for inclusion due to a combination of their seriousness, frequency of reporting, or potential causal connection to ZOFRAN.
Cardiovascular: Arrhythmias (including ventricular and supraventricular tachycardia, premature ventricular contractions, and atrial fibrillation, electrocardiographic alterations (including second degree heart block), palpitations, and syncope.
General: Rare cases of hypersensitivity reactions, sometimes severe (e.g., anaphylaxis, bronchospasm, shortness of breath, hypotension, shock, angioedema, urticaria) have also been reported.
Hepatic: Liver failure and death have been reported in patients with cancer receiving concurrent medications including potentially hepatotoxic cytotoxic chemotherapy and antibiotics. The etiology of the liver failure is unclear.
Local Reactions: Pain, redness, and burning at site of injection.
Neurological: Oculogyric crisis, appearing alone, as well as with other dystonic reactions.
Special Senses: Transient blurred vision, in some cases associated with abnormalities of accommodation.

ZOFRAN Tablets: The following have been reported as events in clinical trials or in the routine management of patients treated with ondansetron, the active ingredient of ZOFRAN Tablets. A causal relationship to therapy with ZOFRAN Tablets has been unclear in many cases.
Chemotherapy-Induced Nausea and Vomiting: The following adverse events have been reported in adults receiving either 8 mg of ZOFRAN Tablets two or three times a day for 3 days or placebo in four trials. These patients were receiving concurrent chemotherapy, primarily cyclophosphamide-based regimens.

Table 4: Principal Adverse Events in US Trials: 3 Days of Therapy With ZOFRAN Tablets

Event	Ondansetron 8 mg b.i.d. n = 242	Ondansetron 8 mg t.i.d. n = 415	Placebo n = 262
Headache	58 (24%)	113 (27%)	34 (13%)
Malaise/fatigue	32 (13%)	37 (9%)	6 (2%)
Constipation	22 (9%)	26 (6%)	1 (<1%)
Diarrhea	15 (6%)	16 (4%)	10 (4%)
Dizziness	13 (5%)	18 (4%)	12 (5%)
Abdominal pain	3 (1%)	13 (3%)	1 (<1%)
Xerostomia	5 (2%)	6 (1%)	1 (<1%)
Weakness	0 (0%)	7 (2%)	1 (<1%)

Central Nervous System: There have been rare reports consistent with, but not diagnostic of, extrapyramidal reactions in patients receiving ondansetron.
Hepatic: In 723 patients receiving cyclophosphamide-based chemotherapy in US clinical trials, AST and/or ALT values have been reported to exceed twice the upper limit of normal in approximately 1% to 2% of patients receiving ZOFRAN Tablets. The increases were transient and did not appear to be related to dose or duration of therapy. On repeat exposure, similar transient elevations in transaminase values occurred in some courses, but symptomatic hepatic disease did not occur. The role of cancer chemotherapy in these biochemical changes cannot be clearly determined.
There have been reports of liver failure and death in patients with cancer receiving concurrent medications including potentially hepatotoxic cytotoxic chemotherapy and antibiotics. The etiology of the liver failure is unclear.
Integumentary: Rash has occurred in approximately 1% of patients receiving ondansetron.
Other: Rare cases of anaphylaxis, bronchospasm, tachycardia, angina (chest pain), hypokalemia, electrocardiographic alterations, vascular occlusive events, and grand mal seizures have been reported. Except for bronchospasm and anaphylaxis, the relationship to ZOFRAN was unclear.
Radiation-Induced Nausea and Vomiting: The adverse events reported in patients receiving ZOFRAN Tablets and concurrent radiotherapy were similar to those reported in patients receiving ZOFRAN Tablets and concurrent chemotherapy. The most frequently reported adverse events were headache, constipation, and diarrhea.
Postoperative Nausea and Vomiting: The following adverse events have been reported in ≥5% of patients receiving ZOFRAN Tablets at a dosage of 16 mg orally in clinical trials. With the exception of headache, rates of these events were not significantly different in the ondansetron and placebo groups. These patients were receiving multiple concomitant perioperative and postoperative medications.

Table 5: Frequency of Adverse Events From Controlled Studies with ZOFRAN Tablets

Adverse Event	Ondansetron 16 mg (n = 550)	Placebo (n = 531)
Wound problem	152 (28%)	162 (31%)
Drowsiness/sedation	112 (20%)	122 (23%)
Headache	49 (9%)	27 (5%)
Hypoxia	49 (9%)	35 (7%)
Pyrexia	45 (8%)	34 (6%)
Dizziness	36 (7%)	34 (6%)
Gynecological disorder	36 (7%)	33 (6%)
Anxiety/agitation	33 (6%)	29 (5%)
Bradycardia	32 (6%)	30 (6%)
Shiver(s)	28 (5%)	30 (6%)
Urinary retention	28 (5%)	18 (3%)
Hypotension	27 (5%)	32 (6%)
Pruritus	27 (5%)	20 (4%)

Preliminary observations in a small number of subjects suggest a higher incidence of headache when ZOFRAN ODT Orally Disintegrating Tablets are taken with water, when compared to without water.

DRUG ABUSE AND DEPENDENCE: Animal studies have shown that ondansetron is not discriminated as a benzodiazepine nor does it substitute for benzodiazepines in direct addiction studies.

OVERDOSAGE: There is no specific antidote for ondansetron overdose. Patients should be managed with appropriate supportive therapy. Individual IV doses as large as 145 mg and total daily IV doses (three doses) as large as 252 mg have been inadvertently administered without significant adverse events. These doses are more than 10 times the recommended daily dose.
"Sudden blindness" (amaurosis) of 2 to 3 minutes' duration plus severe constipation occurred in one patient that was administered 72 mg of ondansetron intravenously as a single dose. Hypotension (and faintness) occurred in another patient that took 48 mg of ZOFRAN Tablets. Following infusion of 32 mg over only a 4-minute period, a vasovagal episode with transient second degree heart block was observed. In all instances, the events resolved completely.

US Patent Nos. 4,695,578; 4,753,789; and 5,578,628

GlaxoWellcome

Glaxo Wellcome Inc.
Research Triangle Park, NC 27709

ZOFRAN® Tablets, Oral Solution, and Injection:
Manufactured by Glaxo Wellcome Inc., Research Triangle Park, NC 27709

ZOFRAN® ODT™ Orally Disintegrating Tablets:
Manufactured for Glaxo Wellcome Inc.
Research Triangle Park, NC 27709
by Scherer DDS, Blagrove, Swindon, Wiltshire, UK SN5 8RU

ZOFRAN® Injection Premixed:
Manufactured for Glaxo Wellcome Inc.
Research Triangle Park, NC 27709
by Abbott Laboratories, North Chicago, IL 60064

August 1998/January 1999 RL-611/607

ARCHIVES OF SURGERY

The ARCHIVES OF SURGERY is a member of the consortium of AMA journals listed below. The complete text of all AMA journals is available online from Dialog Information Services and Information Access Company.

The Journal of the American Medical Association (JAMA)
Archives of Dermatology
Archives of Facial Plastic Surgery
Archives of Family Medicine
Archives of General Psychiatry
Archives of Internal Medicine
Archives of Neurology
Archives of Ophthalmology
Archives of Otolaryngology–Head & Neck Surgery
Archives of Pathology & Laboratory Medicine
Archives of Pediatrics & Adolescent Medicine
Archives of Surgery

The ARCHIVES OF SURGERY (ISSN 0004-0010) is published monthly by the American Medical Association, 515 N State St, Chicago, IL 60610, and is an official publication of the Association. The ARCHIVES OF SURGERY reaches more than 19 000 readers in over 69 countries each month. Periodicals postage paid at Chicago, IL, and at additional mailing offices. GST registration number 12622 5556 RT. Canada Post International Publications Mail (Canadian Distribution) Sales Agreement No. 319309.

Printed in the USA.

Official Publication of the New England Surgical Society, Pacific Coast Surgical Association, Surgical Infection Society, Western Surgical Association.

SUBSCRIPTION RATES—The personal subscription rates for the ARCHIVES OF SURGERY are $145 for 1 year (12 issues) in the United States and US possessions; $195 in the Americas; £125 outside the Americas. The institution rates for 1 year are $245 in the US; $345 in the Americas; £195 outside the Americas. Special rates for residents and medical students are available. Address all subscription communications to: Subscriber Services Center, American Medical Association, PO Box 10946, Chicago, IL 60610-0946. Phone: (800) 262-2350. Fax: (312) 464-5831. E-mail: ama-subs@ama-assn.org. For mailing addresses outside the United States and US possessions, see International Subscription Information.

CHANGE OF ADDRESS—POSTMASTER, send all address changes to ARCHIVES OF SURGERY, c/o Subscriber Services, American Medical Association, 515 N State St, Chicago, IL 60610. Please notify us of address change at least 6 weeks in advance to ensure uninterrupted service. Include both old and new addresses, a recent mailing label, and new ZIP code. For mailing addresses outside the United States and US possessions, see International Subscription Information.

SUBSCRIBER SERVICES—For information about subscribing to any of the AMA publications, change of address, missing issues, or purchasing back issues, please contact Subscriber Services Center, American Medical Association, PO Box 10946, Chicago, IL 60610-0946, or call (800) 262-2350 or (312) 670-SUBS (670-7827) between 8:30 AM and 4:30 PM CST. Fax: (312) 464-5831. E-mail: ama-subs@ama-assn.org. For mailing addresses outside the United States and US possessions, see International Subscription Information.

INTERNATIONAL SUBSCRIPTION INFORMATION—Subscriptions outside the United States and US possessions are served according to geographic region. Please address correspondence to the following 2 offices based on delivery address: (1) For delivery in North America, Central America, and South America, contact Subscriber Services, AMA, PO Box 10946, Chicago, IL 60610-0946. Phone: (312) 670-7827. Fax: (312) 464-5831. E-mail: ama-subs@ama-assn.org. (2) For delivery outside the Americas contact JAMA & Archives Journals, Reader Services Centre, PO Box 299, London WC1H 9TD, England. Phone: +44 (0)171-383-6270. Fax: +44 (0)171-383-6402. E-mail: jama-archives@dial.pipex.com.

REPRINTS—Authors place their reprint order at the time the edited typescript is reviewed and should allow 4 to 6 weeks for delivery following publication. Requests for individual reprints should be sent directly to the author at the address shown in the article.

For bulk reprint orders for distribution by commercial organizations, please contact Wanda Bartolotta, 500 Fifth Ave, #2210, New York, NY 10110. Phone: (212) 354-0050. Fax: (212) 354-1169. E-mail: wanda_bartolotta@ama-assn.org. For reprint orders in limited quantities for distribution by educational organizations and for author reprints, please contact Reprint Coordinator, 515 N State St, Chicago, IL 60610. Phone: (312) 464-4594. Fax: (312) 464-4849.

WORLD WIDE WEB ADDRESS—http://www.ama-assn.org.

SURGERY HOME PAGE—http://www.ama-assn.org/surgery.

PERMISSIONS—Contact Rhonda Bailey, Permissions Assistant, 515 N State St, Chicago, IL 60610. Phone: (312) 464-2513.

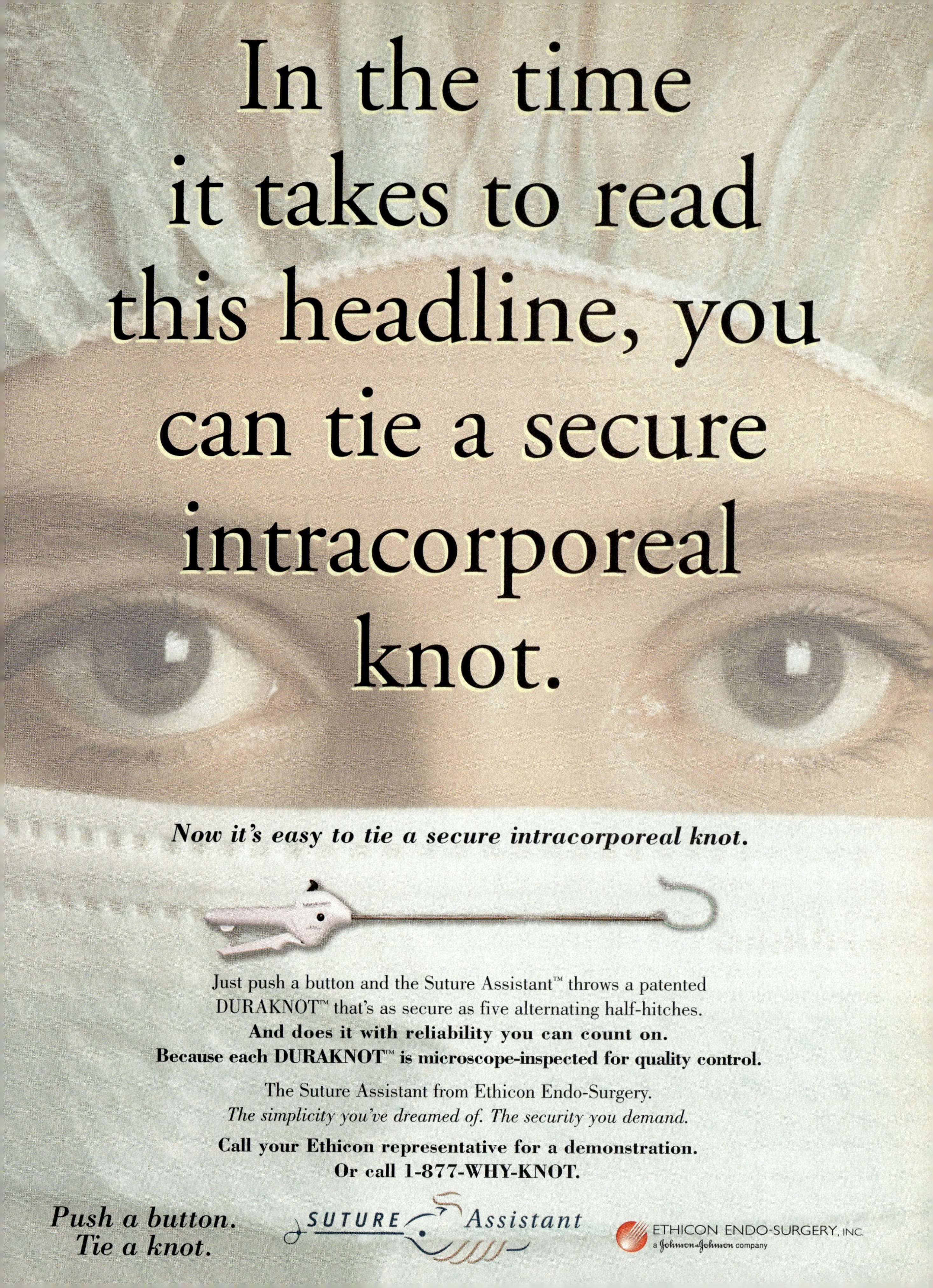
In the time it takes to read this headline, you can tie a secure intracorporeal knot.
Now it's easy to tie a secure intracorporeal knot.
Just push a button and the Suture Assistant™ throws a patented DURAKNOT™ that's as secure as five alternating half-hitches.
And does it with reliability you can count on.
Because each DURAKNOT™ is microscope-inspected for quality control.
The Suture Assistant from Ethicon Endo-Surgery.
The simplicity you've dreamed of. The security you demand.
Call your Ethicon representative for a demonstration.
Or call 1-877-WHY-KNOT.
Push a button.
Tie a knot.
SUTURE Assistant
ETHICON ENDO-SURGERY, INC.
a Johnson&Johnson company

ARCHIVES OF SURGERY

www.ama-assn.org/surgery

VOL 134 NO. 4, APRIL 1999

MISSION STATEMENT

To promote the art and science of surgery by publishing relevant peer-reviewed clinical and basic science information to assist the surgeon in optimizing patient care. The *Archives of Surgery* will also serve as a forum for the discussion of issues that involve ethics, teaching, surgical history, and socioeconomic concerns.

*Approved by the Editorial Board, *Archives of Surgery*, July 19, 1996.

PRESIDENTIAL ADDRESS

Commendably and With a Good Conscience 354
Leslie W. Ottinger, MD

PAPERS

Familial Patterns of Thoracic Aortic Aneurysms 361
Michael A. Coady, MD, MPH; Ryan R. Davies, BA; Michele Roberts, MD, PhD; Lee J. Goldstein, BA; Matthew J. Rogalski, BS; John A. Rizzo, PhD; Graeme L. Hammond, MD; Gary S. Kopf, MD; John A. Elefteriades, MD

Does Uninjured Skin Release Proinflammatory Cytokines Following Trauma and Hemorrhage? 368
Robert A. Catania, MD; Martin G. Schwacha, PhD; William G. Cioffi, MD; Kirby I. Bland, MD; Irshad H. Chaudry, PhD

Extracorporeal Membrane Oxygenation for Nonneonatal Acute Respiratory Failure 375
Peter T. Masiakos, MD; Saleem Islam, MD; Daniel P. Doody, MD; Jay J. Schnitzer, MD, PhD; Daniel P. Ryan, MD

Outcome of Patients With Melanoma and Histologically Negative Sentinel Lymph Nodes 381
Michele A. Gadd, MD; A. Benedict Cosimi, MD; Jeanne Yu, BS; Lyn M. Duncan, MD; Lawrence Yu, MB, BS, FRCPA, Dip RC Path; Thomas J. Flotte, MD; Wiley W. Souba, MD, ScD; Mark J. Ott, MD; Lisa S. Wong, BS; Arthur J. Sober, MD; Martin C. Mihm, MD; Frank G. Haluska, MD, PhD; Kenneth K. Tanabe, MD

Multimodality Management of Merkel Cell Carcinoma 388
Mark J. Ott, MD; Kenneth K. Tanabe, MD; Michele A. Gadd, MD; Paul Stark, MS; Barbara L. Smith, MD, PhD; Dianne M. Finkelstein, PhD; Wiley W. Souba, MD, ScD

American Medical Association

Physicians dedicated to the health of America

All articles published, including editorials, letters, and book reviews, represent the opinions of the authors and do not reflect the policy of the American Medical Association, the Editorial Board, or the institution with which the author is affiliated, unless this is clearly specified.

Mechanism of Adrenal Insufficiency Following Trauma and Severe Hemorrhage: Role of Hepatic 11β-Hydroxysteroid Dehydrogenase 394
Ping Wang, MD; Zheng F. Ba; Doraid Jarrar, MD; William G. Cioffi, MD; Kirby I. Bland, MD; Irshad H. Chaudry, PhD

Interval or Permanent Nonoperative Management of Acute Type A Aortic Dissection 402
Frank G. Scholl, MD; Michael A. Coady, MD, MPH; Ryan Davies; John A. Rizzo, PhD; Graeme L. Hammond, MD; Gary S. Kopf, MD; John A. Elefteriades, MD

Cavernous Hemangioma of the Liver: Anatomic Resection vs Enucleation 407
Roberto Gedaly, MD; James J. Pomposelli, MD, PhD; Elizabeth A. Pomfret, MD, PhD; W. David Lewis, MD; Roger L. Jenkins, MD

Perioperative Strokes After 1001 Consecutive Carotid Endarterectomy Procedures Without an Electroencephalogram: Incidence, Mechanism, and Recovery 412
Allen D. Hamdan, MD; Frank B. Pomposelli, Jr, MD; Gary W. Gibbons, MD; David R. Campbell, MD; Frank W. LoGerfo, MD

Distal Splenorenal Shunt: Role, Indications, and Utility in the Era of Liver Transplantation 416
Roger L. Jenkins, MD; Roberto Gedaly, MD; James J. Pomposelli, MD, PhD; Elizabeth A. Pomfret, MD, PhD; Fredric Gordon, MD; W. David Lewis, MD

Invited Critique 420
J. Michael Henderson, MD

ORIGINAL ARTICLES

Reticuloendothelial System Activity and Organ Failure in Patients With Multiple Injuries 421
Hans-Christoph Pape, MD; Dierk Remmers, MD; Martin Grotz, MD; Jörg Kotzerke, MD; Sabine von Glinski, MD; Martijn van Griensven, PhD; Michael Dahlweid, MD; Susanne Sznidar, MD; Harald Tscherne, MD

Perioperative Immunonutrition in Patients Undergoing Cancer Surgery: Results of a Randomized Double-blind Phase 3 Trial 428
Marco Braga, MD; Luca Gianotti, MD, ScD; Giovanni Radaelli, PhD; Andrea Vignali, MD; Gilberto Mari, MD; Oreste Gentilini, MD; Valerio Di Carlo, MD

ARCHIVES OF SURGERY

ARCHIVES OF SURGERY

BASIC SCIENCE REVIEW

Clinical Implications of Hemoglobin as a Nitric Oxide Carrier 434
Nirmal K. Veeramachaneni, BS; Alden H. Harken, MD; Charles B. Cairns, MD

SPECIAL ARTICLE

Surgery in Argentina 438
Enrique M. Beveraggi, MD

COMMENTARY

The Value of Physician Assistants to Surgical Education in Teaching Hospitals 445
Marvin A. McMillen, MD; Paul West, PA-C

BOOK REVIEWS

Comprehensive Vascular Exposures 448
Edward J. Immelman, FCSSA, FRCSE

Safe Answers for the American Board of Surgery Certifying Exam 448
Brian S. Cain, MD

CORRESPONDENCE AND BRIEF COMMUNICATIONS

An Update of Tumor Metastasis to the Breast Data 450
Suraj Alva, MD; Neetha Shetty-Alva, MD

SURGICAL REMINISCENCES

From Tennis Courts to Transplants 451
Rosemary Hickman, MD

MOMENTS IN SURGICAL HISTORY

Medical Education in Early 19th Century America 453
Ira M. Rutkow, MD, MPH, DrPH

DEPARTMENTS

Surgical Anatomy 374

Products & Services 454

Classified Advertising 455

Index to Advertisers 460

**Instructions for Authors—
See January 1999 issue, page 107, or visit the Web site at http://www.ama-assn.org/surgery.**

Commendably and With a Good Conscience

Leslie W. Ottinger, MD

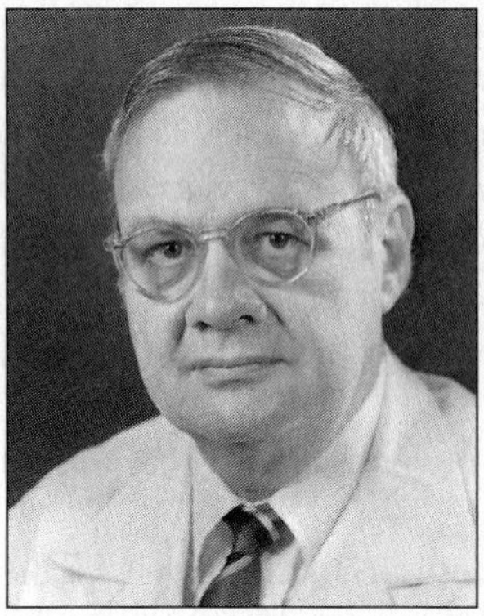

Leslie W. Ottinger, MD

Since its publication in 1913, *An Introduction to the History of Medicine*[1] by Fielding Garrison has been the standard reference book for students and amateur historians with an interest in medical history. In it, I am able to find reference to only four 19th-century New Hampshire surgeons. One is the ubiquitous Nathan Smith, described as "the first all–New England surgeon" in Gordon Donaldson's presidential address to the New England Surgical Society in 1977, who was in fact born in Rehoboth, Mass. Two, Reuben D. Mussey, born in Pelham, NH, and Dixi Crosby, born in Sandwich, NH, followed Smith as distinguished professors of surgery at the Dartmouth Medical School, Hanover, NH. The fourth, Amos Twitchell, was a comparatively obscure physician and surgeon who was born in Dublin, NH, and spent most of his professional life in Keene, NH. The citation about him in Garrison's book reads:

> In connection with the work of Post and Mott, it is proper to mention here some early ligations of arteries by American surgeons in the same field. The primitive carotid artery was successfully ligated for primary hemorrhage by Mason Fitch Cogswell of Connecticut in 1803, and for secondary hemorrhage by Amos Twitchell of New Hampshire, in 1807, 8 months prior to Sir Astley Cooper's case.

Of the surgeons mentioned in the paragraph, Sir Astley Cooper was, of course, by far the best known. A pupil of John Hunter, he was the leading surgeon of at least the English-speaking part of the world in the first decades of the 19th century. Wright Post of Long Island, born in 1766, was the first surgeon in the United States to ligate the femoral artery successfully in the treatment of a popliteal aneurysm, an approach that we attribute to Hunter. Valentine Mott, born in 1785 and also of Long Island, had actually studied under Cooper and was, like him, a great pioneer in vascular surgery, being the first to successfully ligate the innominate artery in 1818 and introducing several other innovations for the management of vascular lesions. Mason Fitch Cogswell, born in 1761, practiced in Hartford, Conn. In addition to his surgical achievement, it is interesting to note that he was offered, but declined, the invitation that eventually brought Nathan Smith to Yale University in 1811.

It is about Amos Twitchell (**Figure**), the southwest New Hampshire country surgeon, that I wish to speak, however, beginning with an event that occurred in October 1807, some 191 years ago, in Temple, NH. Twitchell left Norwich, Vt, only about 1 month before to begin working with his brother-in-law, David Carter, in Marlborough, NH, planning, insofar as it was possible in that day, to devote himself to surgical cases.

By the accounts that have been preserved, October 10, 1807, was one of those

This article is also available on our Web site: www.ama-assn.org/surg.

From the Massachusetts General Hospital, Boston.

bright, clear autumn days that we associate with this season in New England. In Temple, the day had been set aside as a town holiday, perhaps because most of the autumn farmwork was done. In keeping with the customs of the time, there may have been a dancing bear and a puppet show on the common in the center of town. The main activity, though, was several hours of training and maneuvers for the town's militia.

The role of the militia and its importance to the young republic was a plain fact to the townspeople, many of whom had served in the Continental army. And these were worrisome times, with conflict in Europe threatening to spill over to this side of the Atlantic Ocean. Activities of the British navy were already suggesting the possibility of another war with England, and the necessity for a disciplined and organized armed force had been established clearly in the memory of many citizens of the small southern New Hampshire village.

Following a day of close and extended marching and countermarching, and other exercises as described in the drill manuals of the day, a grand mock battle was to conclude the events. A troop of cavalry galloped down Oak Hill and into the muskets of a detachment of infantry kneeling behind a stone wall. Guns were loaded with only powder and wadding, but otherwise nothing was spared to make the charge and clash realistic. It seemed serious training, but also good fun, until John Taggart, a 22-year-old cavalry trooper, fell to the ground, bleeding heavily from a wound on the right side of his neck. John Crombie, the regimental surgeon, was called. Crombie was the town physician, having arrived in 1798. Like most physicians of his time, he had secured his medical education as an apprentice to another village physician. Although he later became known for his diagnostic skills and persistence in the management of chronic medical problems, at the time he had no training and apparently little experience in surgical matters.

Taggart was carried to the inn in the center of town. On examining him, Crombie noted a wound that seemed to have been caused by pistol wadding. It included the right side of the face and neck with penetration into the mouth from an object that had entered from behind. There were burns on the periphery and the external carotid artery and its branches had been destroyed. Crombie did the best he could to stop the bleeding and make the young trooper comfortable. According to the town records, he, being aware of the serious nature of the wound, then said, sadly, "If anybody can save that boy, it's Amos Twitchell." Twitchell, who was apparently either in town or nearby, was sent for and on arrival examined and bandaged the wound with Crombie and agreed to take over the care of the young soldier, despite the 60-mile (96-km) daily round-trip that would be required.

Of course, we have no idea what Crombie knew of Twitchell. Perhaps only that he had worked with Smith, who sometimes traveled into southern New Hampshire and even western Massachusetts to perform operations and who enjoyed a wide reputation for his skill as a surgeon. And perhaps he knew David Carter of Marlborough with whom Twitchell had just come to work. And there is mention of a letter that Twitchell wrote to Carter the year before saying that he might "visit your part of the country and bring

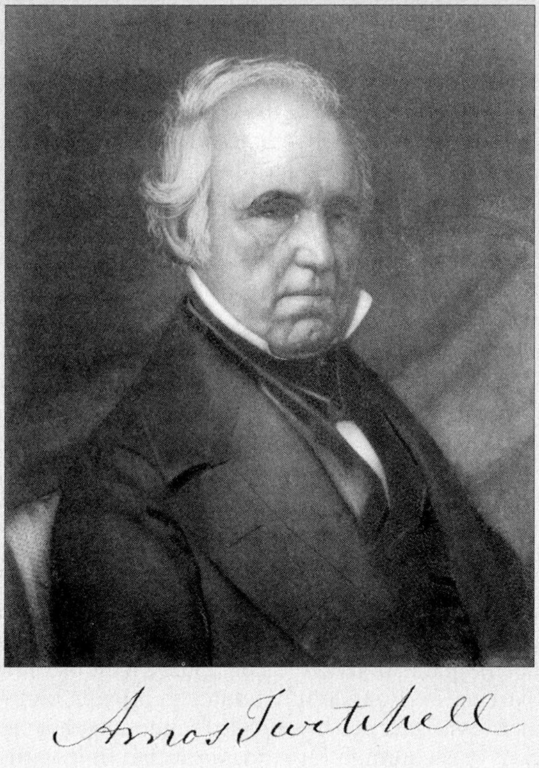

Amos Twitchell. Frontispiece from Memoir of Amos Twitchell *by Henry I. Bowditch.*[2]

my knives," although we do not know whether he did so. After completing work on his medical degree at the Dartmouth Medical School, Twitchell opened a practice across the Connecticut river in Norwich so that he could continue to assist and learn from his mentor, Smith. He found the 2 years of practice in Norwich difficult, writing to his brother-in-law, who supported him financially during his Dartmouth years, "my business, as yet has paid only two-thirds of my expenses." He complained that 2 of the town's 4 resident practitioners were "as malicious as the devil" and that he received little encouragement from the others. At any rate, after 2 years he gave up and moved to Marlborough, perhaps to help Carter and to begin to repay his loans. And, certainly, no physician in southern New Hampshire was actually as qualified as Twitchell for this type of case. Almost every town had a physician, but few of them had any background or training to qualify as a surgeon.

Twitchell was born in Dublin, NH, on April 14, 1781, the seventh of 9 children of Samuel and Alice Wilson Twitchell. His father grew up in Sherburn, Mass, and was one of the earliest settlers of Dublin. He rose to command a company of colonial troops during the revolution and served in Hale's regiment during the Rhode Island campaign of 1778. His farm and mill were near the outlet of Thornton Pond in the southeast corner of Dublin. He is said to have been a substantial farmer and miller. With limited education but an active mind, he served in the state legislature and was instrumental in the establishment and chartering of one of the earliest libraries in the state, the town library of Dublin. He was even known to have at times employed a governess for the children, who all also attended the town school.

Twitchell's mother, Alice Wilson, was also born in Sherburn. A kindly person, she was noted for her abilities in nursing the sick of the community. Amos was a bright child, reading actively by the age of 6 years, and it seems that she was determined early on that he receive a college education. She was, in fact, from a well-educated family, her father having been a physician. The further educational experiences of Amos's siblings are unknown to me, but young Amos, after attending the local school for 4 months a year, was sent at age 14 years to the New Ipswich Academy, New Ipswich, NH, for 7 or 8 months, and then to Townsend, Mass, to prepare himself for college under a Reverend Palmer.

According to an often-repeated story, in August 1798, Amos rode on horseback to Cambridge, Mass, to enroll at Harvard University. Since he had not studied all of the books required for admission, he was denied admission. Without returning home, he rode directly to Hanover, NH, to enroll in the college. At Dartmouth, it seems that Twitchell was a good student, excelling especially in mathematics and the classics. He was assigned the Greek oration as part of the graduation exercises in 1802. On the other hand, his parents were apparently unable to provide him with financial assistance and he struggled continuously with poverty. As was common for students at that time with this problem, he taught for the winter term in village schools in Rockingham, Marlborough, and Dublin, NH, and perhaps elsewhere. Some of his correspondence with his brother-in-law, Dr David Carter, was available to Henry Bowditch, who prepared a little memorial volume about him in 1851,[2] citing a letter from February 1802, in which Twitchell lamented that he had "80 or 90 ignorant scholars in my school in Rockingham." Despite this, he was determined to pursue studies in medicine, a plan he had entertained for several years, and with encouragement and financial help from his brother-in-law, Dr Carter, he enrolled in the medical school on completing the 4-year course of studies.

Only 6 years before, Dr Smith wrote to the board of trustees of the college offering to start a medical school, and then began, at his own expense, to better prepare himself for the enterprise by furthering his own medical education. Previously, this included study with Dr Josiah Goodhue in Putney, Vt, 2 years of practice in Cornish, NH, and completion of the course of study at Harvard Medical School. He planned to spend a good part of his time in Edinburgh, Scotland, and then to take in the medical scene in London, England, before returning to New Hampshire in time to start lectures in November 1797. Thus, 5 years before Twitchell was enrolled, Smith gave an 11-week course of lectures even though actual approval of the plans for the medical school did not come from the trustees until the following August, when the first 2 MB degrees in medicine were awarded.

In 1802, the requirements for a medical degree from Dartmouth included, first, 3 years of study with a reputable practitioner for those with a college degree, or 5 for candidates without a college degree. Second, the candidate must have attended 2 courses of lectures, 1 at Dartmouth Medical School, and must have successfully completed an examination in all medical subjects. These were, at that time, anatomy, surgery, chemistry, materia medica, and the theory and practice of physics, which included the study of physiology and pathology. Finally, a thesis must have been submitted.

Twitchell did his apprenticeship directly under Dr Smith, rooming at his house for at least part of the 3 years and also serving as his assistant. He participated in the preparation of materials for the course of lectures for chemistry and in anatomy demonstrations and courses. In fact, legend has it that he was especially resourceful and active in the obtaining of bodies for dissection. At that time, the study of anatomy in New England was a secret and perilous pursuit. Teachers were forced to obtain material by whatever means possible. The dissection of a human body or possession of one for this purpose was not only a crime but considered especially abhorrent by the general public. By Massachusetts law, passed 10 years later in 1815, anyone who dug up or received any human body for dissection was liable to be imprisoned for up to 1 year or to be fined as much as $1000. Legal provisions for dissection were not formulated in Massachusetts until 1831 and considerably later than that in New Hampshire.

"Raising the dead," illegal or not, was the only recourse for meeting the needs of students in the study of anatomy and one of the duties of Dr Smith's assistant was, it seems, to obtain subjects for the anatomy courses. Twitchell allegedly preferred to work alone, traveling an appropriate distance from Hanover on moonless nights. He is even said to have once been arrested, although he did escape prosecution. His reputation as a daring and effective resurrectionist was known to Bowdich, the Boston physician who wrote his memoir, and to several historians of the New Hampshire Medical Society.

Still in tight financial straits, Twitchell was allowed to defer payment of the required $20 and took the degrees of AM and MB in 1805. At the urging of Smith, he opened up his practice in Norwich and continued to assist his friend and professor, lecturing on anatomy and surgery when Smith was ill. The next year he was able to write to his brother-in-law and chief creditor, "my business has rather exceeded my expenses; yet that is no object to a person so much in debt as I am." He described at the same time his unhappiness that he could not satisfy his ambition to visit the medical institutions in Philadelphia and also to pursue further studies in Europe. All this considered, it is not surprising that he was subject to episodes of severe despondency and that he decided to give up his informal position with Dr Smith and the college. Thus, in October 1807, he joined his sister and her husband, Dr David Carter, in Marlborough, at about the time he received the summons to attend the wounded trooper, Taggart, in Temple.

Twitchell's account of the Taggart case was subsequently published in the *New England Quarterly Journal of Medicine and Surgery*.[3] After a brief mention of the events leading up to the injury, he proceeds to a detailed description of the wound. He writes,

> We found the whole of the right side of the head, face, and neck very much burned; and a large wound penetrating the phar-

ynx and mouth, by which were destroyed, or greatly lacerated, nearly the whole of the parotid gland, the temporal, masseter, and pterygoid muscles; and also parts of the muscles on the anterior neck between the inferior maxillary bone and hyoid bone.

The angle, ramus and coronoid process of the inferior maxillary bone and the pterygoid process of the sphenoid bone were shattered and a finger could be introduced into the antrum. The external carotid artery and its branches had been divided.

The wound was debrided of bone fragments and devitalized soft tissue. After 2 days Taggart began to take a little liquid, at first hampered by swelling and leakage through the wound, and was then able to be moved to the home of his parents in the nearby village of Sharon. Twitchell was seeing him daily or every other day to change his dressings and further debride the wound. We take up his own narrative, beginning on the 10th postinjury day:

The wound had now become cleared of all dead portions of muscle and cellular membrane; and presented a large circular aperture from two to three inches in diameter; at the bottom of which might be distinctly seen the internal carotid artery denuded from near the bifurcation of the common trunk, to where it forms a curve to enter the canal of the petrous portion of the temporal bone. Directly upon this curve of the artery might be seen a dark speck, of a line or two in diameter, which seemed to be a dead portion of cellular membrane adhering to the coats of the vessel. I carefully touched it with a probe; but finding that it adhered, I desisted from the attempt to remove it; and expressed to the patient and his friends my fears of a dangerous if not fatal hemorrhage when that should separate. I applied the usual dressings, left the room, and was about leaving the house, when someone of the family cried out that he was bleeding. I hastened back to his room, and found forcibly, in a large stream, to the distance of three or four feet. With the thumb of my left hand, I instantly compressed the artery against the base of the skull; and thus effectually controlled the hemorrhage. The patient had fainted; and fifteen or twenty minutes had elapsed before he was so much revived that I dared to make any attempt to secure the artery. Then, still keeping the thumb firmly pressed on the orifice, I proceeded to clear the wound from blood; and having done this, I made an incision, with a scalpel, downward, along the course of the artery, to more than an inch below the point where the external branch was given off; which, as stated above, had been destroyed at the time of the injury. Having but one hand at liberty, I depended upon the mother of the patient to separate the sides of the wound; which she did, partly with a hook and occasionally with her fingers. At length, partly by careful dissection and partly by using my fingers and the handle of the scalpel, I succeeded in separating the artery from its attachments; and passing my finger under it, I raised it up sufficiently for my assistant to pass a ligature round it. She tied it with a surgeons knot, as I directed, at about half an inch below the bifurcation.

I removed my thumb and sponged away the blood, not doubting that the hemorrhage was effectually controlled. But to my surprise and disappointment, the blood immediately began to ooze from the rupture in the artery; and in less than ten minutes it flowed with a pulsating jet. I compressed it again with my thumb; and began to despair of saving my patient. What further could I do? It was impossible to apply a ligature above the orifice; compression, then, was the only alternative. How was this to be effected? Should someone sit by the patient and compress the artery constantly with the fingers till adhesion should take place? Possibly that might have been done; but I resolved to make another attempt first. Raising my thumb, I placed a small piece of dry sponge directly over the orifice of the artery; and renewing the compression till a larger piece of sponge could be prepared, I placed that upon the first; and so went on, pressing the gradually enlarged pieces upwards and backwards against the base of the skull, till I had filled the wound with a firm cone of sponge, the base of which projected two or three inches externally. Then I applied a linen roller, in such a manner as to press firmly upon the sponge; passing it in repeated turns, over the head, face and neck.

With local care, the wound rapidly began to close. On the 10th day the carotid artery ligature came away and the last piece of sponge was removed from the site of the rupture 2 days later. When the patient began to eat, the jaw was drawn so much to the left that the teeth did not meet.

Dr Twitchell reports that:

. . . to remedy this inconvenience, I caused an ingenious blacksmith in the neighborhood to make an instrument something like a [hernia] truss; one end of this being fitted to the top of the head, it was brought down, on the right side, under the chin; and the pad on the other end was made to press on the left side of the inferior maxillary bone. He wore this instrument most of the time during the remainder of the treatment; and it effectually answered the purpose.

At the end of 2½ months, the wound was was almost closed and the young man was able to move the jaw and masticate solid food with ease. Twitchell provided no follow-up in his paper. There is, however, in an address commemorative of his life and character, given to the New Hampshire Medical Society 1 year after his death, a firsthand account.[4] The speaker, Albert Smith, was born and practiced medicine in Peterborough, NH, taught at Dartmouth Medical School, and became the president of the New Hampshire Medical Society in 1853. After describing the case, Smith said:

This patient of Dr Twitchell was one of a class of men, formerly well known in my vicinity as horse-jockies, who were nothing less than idle, drinking, worthless vagabonds; and my early recollections of him are those of a thin, spare man, on horseback, full of the spirit of his vocation, always wearing a narrow folded handkerchief, which passed over his head and under his chin, to conceal the great deformity occasioned by the wound. He was ever afterwards known by the title of Pistol John.

Twitchell said:

This case seemed to me at the time highly important and valuable; since it established surgical facts, which as far as my knowledge extended, had not till then been known. The question of the practicality of the safe application of the ligature to the common carotid artery, was, in my opinion, now solved. I had entertained that opinion for some time before; having repeatedly tied the vessels in dogs, and in one instance in a horse, without causing them much inconvenience; but at that time, I had seen no account of its having been attempted on the human subject.

As a matter of fact, respecting the collateral circulation of the brain, Cheselden,[5] in a book Twitchell used while a medical student, speaking first of the 2 cervical arteries, says:

> These two arteries, uniting soon after their entrance [into the skull] they [*sic*] give off branches to the cerebellum, and then passing forward, divide and communicate with the carotids; and the carotid arteries communicating with each other, there is an entire communication between them all; and these communicant branches are so large that every one of these four great vessels, with all their branches, may be easily filled with wax through any one of them.

The first successful ligation of the common carotid artery was for some decades attributed to Sir Astley Cooper, who interrupted the vessel in the treatment of a carotid aneurysm the year after Twitchell's case. It was later discovered that in 1803 a British naval surgeon had tied off the vessel in a servant who had attempted suicide on board the ship. He recovered, and this case ultimately was accorded the distinction of being the first. Nevertheless, at the time of his own operation, Amos Twitchell could have known at most of only a single unsuccessful case reported by John Abernathy, an earlier English surgeon.

The account of the management and recovery of Trooper Taggart that I have been quoting was not published until 1842 and was apparently solicited by one of Twitchell's Boston friends for a new journal, *The New England Quarterly Journal of Medicine and Surgery*.[4] Bowditch quotes a nephew, who had studied with Twitchell, as saying, "His unwillingness this case should be published, with others I had drawn up, was partly for the reason, if I remember rightly, that the operation had in some degree been forced upon him in this instance by the circumstances, which left him no option." This, and a lifelong preference for speaking, but not writing for publication, perhaps accounts for the 35-year delay.

Three years later in 1810, at the age of 29 years, Dr Twitchell left Marlborough and established a practice of surgery in Keene, where he was to remain until his death 40 years later. In June 1815, he married Elizabeth Goodhue, the daughter of the same Dr Josiah Goodhue, who had been Dr Smith's preceptor in 1784. She was a capable and supportive, but somewhat retiring, person. Their marriage was childless. They were, by accounts, a harmonious and devoted couple. She died in 1848, 2 years before her husband, of a lung infection, a loss from which he never fully recovered.

Dr Twitchell had a busy and extensive surgical practice that encompassed much of southern New Hampshire. It was usual for him to travel 30 to 40 miles (48-64 km) a day, first on horseback, and later in a small carriage for which he kept spare horses in several surrounding towns. In the early 1830s, he established a hospital for his surgical patients in a large brick building in Keene and operated it for many years. It was one of the first hospitals in New Hampshire, and as a place for the care of surgical, rather than indigent patients, was a unique institution for the time. Apparently, it was not carried on after his death.

Dr Twitchell was a strong supporter of the medical organizations of the day. He became a member of the New Hampshire Medical Society in 1811 and is said to have rarely missed an annual meeting. He served as censor, counselor, as president from 1827 to 1830, and as orator in 1833. He was elected to represent the Society in the American Medical Association twice and at the convention for the revision of the United States Pharmacopoeia. He was also very active in the Western District medical society, which had a dominant role in medical affairs in his corner of the state.

As his reputation as a surgical practitioner spread, he received overtures from 4 medical schools to become a member of their faculty. These were Dartmouth (Hanover, NH), Bowdoin (Brunswick, Me), Castleton (Castleton, Vt); and Vermont (Burlington). Also, he was strongly urged to move to Boston, where he had become well known for his surgical exploits.

Dr Twitchell performed all the standard and many of the new operations of the day, some, such as the carotid ligation, before it was known that they had been successfully performed by other surgeons. Included were oophorectomies prior to knowledge of Ephraim McDowell's cases, and trephining of the tibia for occult osteomyelitis in 1840, after, but without knowledge, of the report of the diagnosis and technique for treatment by Sir Benjamin Brodie. In 1838, he amputated the arm, scapula, and clavicle in the case of a 23-year-old man with an osteosarcoma of the scapula, in retrospect, the third time this operation is known to have been performed. The patient lived for 2 years after the operation, then died of intra-abdominal metastases. He performed several successful operations for the removal of bladder stones. In short, he brought surgical care to his rural region that could scarcely be matched in the great American centers of the day in Philadelphia, New York, and Boston. One further case report will help us picture the circumstances of his practice and how he confronted them. At an annual meeting of the New Hampshire Medical Society, probably in his presidential address, he described 3 cases of tracheostomy.[6] One was of a 22-month-old child that he was called to visit and found to have symptoms of suffocation. She had been playing with dried beans and, to quote, "I came to the conclusion that a bean was in the trachea, near its bifurcation, and probably lodged on or over the left bronchial tube, as the lung on that side of the chest did not expand on respiration."

He proposed an operation as the only means to rescue the child from immediate danger, but the parents would not consent to it. When he returned to her house after about 3 hours, again to quote from his paper:

> I was met at the door by someone saying "the child is dying." I found her with a livid countenance, tossing herself about in various directions, and gasping for breath. By pressing and rubbing the larynx and trachea, the bean appeared to descend again to its former situation. An operation was no longer objected to, as it was evident that she must have immediate relief, or death would be the consequence. . . . The child was placed upon a table on her back, with a roll of cotton under her neck, and her head bent backward over it, so as to stretch the integument on the fore part of the neck, which was very short and fleshy.

After separating with some difficulty the large thymus from the thyroid gland, a half-inch incision was made in the trachea. The bean was not at first visible but during "some little struggle of the child" it came into view and was seized with forceps and removed. The child was turned face downward to prevent blood entering the trachea and immediately she breathed easily and was soon asleep. The wound was brought together with strips of adhesive plaster and supported with a circumferential bandage.

Dr Twitchell reports, "The next day when I visited the child, [I] found her running about the house, apparently well." In the same report he gives the details of 2 other children, aged 1 and 4 years, who also underwent emergency tracheotomy for removal of beans, likewise with a successful outcome.

Only these and a very few other cases ever found their way into published reports, and even then, it must be observed, usually only at the insistence and sometimes under the authorship of his students and friends. Yet for 4 decades he carried on an active practice, preferring the pace and work and apparently having no ambition for anything more than this and teaching the students who regularly attached themselves to, as his Boston friend, Bowditch, said, "the surgeon who stood literally at the head of the profession throughout that portion of the country."

From the reports that we have, Dr Twitchell was a gregarious, robust, and energetic man of strongly held and defended opinions and with a good sense of humor. He was scrupulously fair and courteous with other physicians, but seldom, if ever, asked for consultations. He met every case with skill, perseverance, and unwearied effort. His knowledge was extensive and current and he was noted for his rapid diagnostic powers. His operations were slow and deliberate and he was never appalled by unforeseen circumstances. He was equally devoted to the poor and rich. He advocated strongly for temperance and against the use of tobacco and worked and spoke out against quackery throughout his career. With respect to this, he said to the New Hampshire Medical Society:

> The most rational, and I presume the only successful, method, for us to combat quackery, will be, in the first place, to avoid it ourselves; and then endeavor to enlighten the common people as much as possible. Let them understand that the principles of the profession are founded upon reason and science, and that we are governed by these principles. We make no pretensions to supernatural powers. Let us banish all technical phraseology from our conversation and prescriptions, if not from our pharmacopoeias. Let us be unwearied in our efforts to investigate the nature and causes of disease, and the effects of remedies. When called to the bed of sickness, let us be very critical in our inquiries and examinations, and patiently investigate every circumstance relating to the case; and after having formed an opinion, let us be candid in stating our views of the case to the patient or his friends, explain to them, if possible, the location and nature of the disease, the indications of cure which are to be pursued, and the remedies we intend to prescribe, with the effect we expect they will produce. If we have any doubt in the case, or think we do not rightly understand it, let us acknowledge it, and call for advice if thought necessary.

Though the intensity diminished, Dr Twitchell continued to practice surgery until the spring of 1850. Then, after a few days of indisposition, he sustained a stroke with hemiparalysis and 6 days later, on Sunday, May 26, at the age of 69 years, he died.

So why do I choose to describe and celebrate Dr Twitchell, this country surgeon who, as his biographer said, left no monument, was no famous man? The title of my address comes from a quotation on the title page of the book *To Work in the Vineyard of Surgery: The Reminiscences of J. Collins Warren*,[7] edited, with appendixes, notes, and comments, by Edward D. Churchill. Churchill was the chairman of the Massachusetts General Hospital, Boston, department of surgery when I started my training there and his presence and ideas still pervade and guide the department and especially the surgical residency program.

The actual quotation is " . . . to labour commendably, and, with a good conscience to work in the Vineyard of Surgery." It comes from a book on the treatment of struma, the enlargement and inflammation of the cervical lymph nodes, a condition that later came to be known as scrofula and to be caused by the tubercle bacillus. The book was published in 1602, and was written by William Clowes who was, among other things, surgeon to the English fleet against the Spanish Armada and physician to Queen Elizabeth. Speaking almost 4 centuries ago, he expresses a concept that seems to characterize the career of Dr Twitchell and is also a useful way to judge the performance of a surgeon today.

I would call attention to the 2 components. To labor commendably carries the requirement to fulfill the expectations and receive the approval of those being served; those committing themselves to the surgeon's hand; the goal of meeting their standard in our performance. A good conscience is another thing entirely—this is to satisfy an internal compulsion to do what we know is right; to hold ourselves to our own high standard. So I wish to celebrate not just Dr Twitchell, but also you, the clinical surgeons here who likewise meet Clowes' 2 conditions and, commendably and with a good conscience, work in the Vineyard of Surgery.

In fact, you have still not heard the full quotation from Clowes' book. The complete sentence is:

> Indeed, it is, I suppose, unpossible [*sic*] in the whole course of a man's life that he is able without great care, study, and much diligence, to labour commendably, and with a good conscience to work in the Vineyard of Surgery; yet I know there be many young students in the Art will be always ready and most willing to discharge their duties in such matters as they shall take upon them to deal in, whether it be in this kind of cure [which refers to the subject of his book], or otherwise.[8]

So, for students and residents, what qualities should you forge and sustain to work commendably and with a good conscience in the Vineyard of Surgery?

First, there is the duty to serve not all patients but, in a singular way, the patient before you; to adopt this as your principal ambition, placing it when necessary before your own personal interests.

Second, to develop self-reliance, for even though assistants are needed, you must learn to work alone, self-possessed and self-critical. To face mistakes and complications and bad results directly, learning from them and moving on with resilience and energy.

Next, to be tenacious and persistent, unyielding and unwearied. Steadfast and single-minded for each patient.

Then, to be calm and steady, unperturbable and unruffled, even in the face of disaster and failure.

And to embrace honesty and fairness and by this to earn and deserve the trust of your patients and the respect of your colleagues.

Next, to go on learning, adopting the new, and giving up the outworn, but always and only to benefit the patient.

And finally, to educate and teach, with skill and patience, students, residents, your peers and, equally important, the patient himself.

My interest in Dr Twitchell turned up few material objects, but some of these may interest you. His picture as a young man hangs in the corridor of the Dean's suite at the Dartmouth Medical School, the gift of his family at an unknown date. A picture of him in old age, which is said to have hung in the Keene Town Hall for many years, I found stored in the attic of the Keene Historical Society. On the back is a handwritten note that says:

> Mr Eldridge Clarke, one of the donors, moved by his long cherished respect and admiration of Dr Amos Twitchell, and for the purpose of preserving a remembrance of the man, caused this picture to be painted by one Wallace, a young artist of Boston, from an old and very small daguerreotype and his recollection of him in life, 38 years after he had passed away.

The Temple Inn is still there, now the Birchwood Inn. A brick, 2-story, 4-room addition was constructed in 1800. The rooms on the first floor were a kitchen and barroom with 2 bedrooms on the second floor. Presumably Trooper Taggart was placed in 1 of these bedrooms. What was the barroom is now a place for dining and you can enjoy a fine meal there, surrounded by the Rufus Porter murals that were added around 1832, having as your predecessor, it is said, no less a personage than Henry David Thoreau.

The site of the Twitchell homestead in Dublin is identifiable only by a few stones from the foundation of the mill. The wonderful early town burying ground, overlooked by Mount Monadnock, contains the headstones of Samuel and Alice Wilson Twitchell and nearby that of the brother-in-law, Dr David Carter.

A small monument and headstones for Amos Twitchell and his wife and sister are to be found in the old Keene cemetery near the center of town. They are in rather poor condition and in need of restoration. His house was torn down to make room for a railroad station and I could not discover the site of his hospital so I do not know if the building still stands.

In closing, I feel pleased to mention to you and acknowledge some of my own teachers and mentors. In medical school, there was Francis Moore who early on converted me to a career in surgery, and Edward A. Edwards, a brilliant surgeon-anatomist and an unparalleled teacher with whom I worked for several years as an instructor in his surgical anatomy course, which I was able to have for my own after his retirement. Then there were the 3 chiefs under whom I trained and worked: Edward D. Churchill, Paul S. Russell, and W. Gerald Austen and the remarkable collection of clinical surgeons during my early years in surgery: Richard Sweet, Frank Wheelock, Wyland Leadbetter, Robert Shaw, Leland McKittrick, Robert Linton, Howard Ulfelder, Oliver Cope, Gordon Scannell, Earle Wilkins, Claude Welch, and Marshall Bartlett, who also gave me a start as a private surgeon. Finally, there were and are my 2 best friends during my 36 years at the Massachusetts General Hospital, Ronald Malt and Ashby Moncure.

It has been a great and unexpected honor to serve as your president this year and for this I express my gratitude.

Presented at the 79th Annual Meeting of the New England Surgical Society, Toronto, Ontario, September 26, 1998.

Reprints: Leslie W. Ottinger, MD, 6 Harbor Terr, Nantucket, MA 02554.

REFERENCES

1. Garrison FH. *An Introduction to the History of Medicine.* 4th ed. Philadelphia, Pa: WB Saunders Co; 1929.
2. Bowditch HI. *Memoir of Amos Twitchell With an Appendix Containing His Addresses, etc.* Boston, Mass: John Wilson & Son; 1851.
3. Twitchell A. Gunshot wound of the face and neck: ligature of the carotid artery. *N Engl Q J Med Surg.* 1842-1843;1:188-193.
4. Smith A. Commerative of the life and character of Amos Twitchell M.D. *N Hampshire J Med.* 1851;1:287-300.
5. Cheselden W. *The Anatomy of the Human Body, Second American Edition.* Boston, Mass: David West; 1806.
6. Twitchell A. Cases of tracheostomy. *N Engl Q J Med Surg.* 1842-1843;1:305-312.
7. Churchill ED. *To Work in the Vineyard of Surgery: The Reminiscences of J. Collins Warren, 1842-1927.* Cambridge, Mass: Harvard University Press; 1958.
8. Clowes W. *A Right Fruteful and Approoved Treatise, for the Artificiall Cure of That Malady Called in Latin Struma, and in English, the Evill, Cured by Kinges and Queenes of England.* London, England: Edward Allde; 1602.

Your best medical information source...

ARCHIVES OF SURGERY

from the
American Medical Association

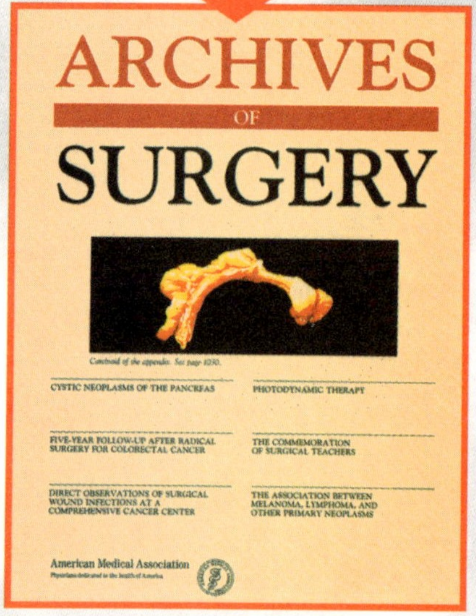

Archives of Surgery is the best read journal representing a full range of specialty interests. Original submissions, the best papers from surgical societies, stringent statistical reviews, invited commentaries and a greater use of illustration set the standard in its field.

Enter a personal subscription — send in a reply card today!

ARCHIVES OF SURGERY

SUBSCRIPTION ORDER FORM

☑ **YES!** Enter my personal subscription to ***Archives of Surgery*** at the special money saving rate checked below:

- ❑ AMA Member rate: One year (12 issues) — $95*.
- ❑ Individual non-member rate: One year (12 issues) — $145*.
- ❑ Corporate/Institutional rate: One year (12 issues) — $245.
- ❑ *My personal check in U.S. $ is enclosed. (Make check payable to *American Medical Association*).
- ❑ Charge my personal credit card: ❑ VISA ❑ MASTERCARD ❑ AMEX ❑ OPTIMA

Card No.__________ Exp. Date__________ Signature__________

Name (Please print) __________

Address __________

City__________ State/Province__________ Zip/Postal Code __________

Phone__________ Fax__________ e-mail __________

IMPORTANT: The individual non-member rate is available in the U.S. and Canada only. Payment must accompany order. Corporate/Institutional checks are not accepted for personal subscriptions. Canada residents add 7% GST. GST # (12622 5556 RT). I9X2DZ

ARCHIVES OF SURGERY

SUBSCRIPTION ORDER FORM

☑ YES! Enter my personal subscription to Archives of Surgery at the special money saving rate checked below:

❑ AMA Member rate: One year (12 issues) — $95*.
❑ Individual non-member rate: One year (12 issues) — $145*.
❑ Corporate/Institutional rate: One year (12 issues) — $245.
❑ *My personal check in U.S. $ is enclosed. (Make check payable to American Medical Association).
❑ Charge my personal credit card: ❑ VISA ❑ MASTERCARD ❑ AMEX ❑ OPTIMA

Card No.__________ Exp. Date__________ Signature__________

Name (Please print) __________

Address __________

City__________ State/Province__________ Zip/Postal Code __________

Phone__________ Fax__________ e-mail __________

IMPORTANT: The individual non-member rate is available in the U.S. and Canada only. Payment must accompany order. Corporate/Institutional checks are not accepted for personal subscriptions. Canada residents add 7% GST. GST # (12622 5556 RT). I9X2DZ

ARCHIVES OF SURGERY

SUBSCRIPTION ORDER FORM

☑ YES! Enter my personal subscription to Archives of Surgery at the special money saving rate checked below:

❑ AMA Member rate: One year (12 issues) — $95*.
❑ Individual non-member rate: One year (12 issues) — $145*.
❑ Corporate/Institutional rate: One year (12 issues) — $245.
❑ *My personal check in U.S. $ is enclosed. (Make check payable to American Medical Association).
❑ Charge my personal credit card: ❑ VISA ❑ MASTERCARD ❑ AMEX ❑ OPTIMA

Card No.__________ Exp. Date__________ Signature__________

Name (Please print) __________

Address __________

City__________ State/Province__________ Zip/Postal Code __________

Phone__________ Fax__________ e-mail __________

IMPORTANT: The individual non-member rate is available in the U.S. and Canada only. Payment must accompany order. Corporate/Institutional checks are not accepted for personal subscriptions. Canada residents add 7% GST. GST # (12622 5556 RT). I9X2DZ

NO POSTAGE NECESSARY IF MAILED IN THE UNITED STATES

BUSINESS REPLY MAIL
FIRST-CLASS MAIL PERMIT NO. 1376 CHICAGO IL

POSTAGE WILL BE PAID BY ADDRESSEE

SUBSCRIBER SERVICES CENTER
AMERICAN MEDICAL ASSOCIATION
PO BOX 10945
CHICAGO IL 60610-9902

NO POSTAGE NECESSARY IF MAILED IN THE UNITED STATES

BUSINESS REPLY MAIL
FIRST-CLASS MAIL PERMIT NO. 1376 CHICAGO IL

POSTAGE WILL BE PAID BY ADDRESSEE

SUBSCRIBER SERVICES CENTER
AMERICAN MEDICAL ASSOCIATION
PO BOX 10945
CHICAGO IL 60610-9902

NO POSTAGE NECESSARY IF MAILED IN THE UNITED STATES

BUSINESS REPLY MAIL
FIRST-CLASS MAIL PERMIT NO. 1376 CHICAGO IL

POSTAGE WILL BE PAID BY ADDRESSEE

SUBSCRIBER SERVICES CENTER
AMERICAN MEDICAL ASSOCIATION
PO BOX 10945
CHICAGO IL 60610-9902

ARCHIVES OF SURGERY

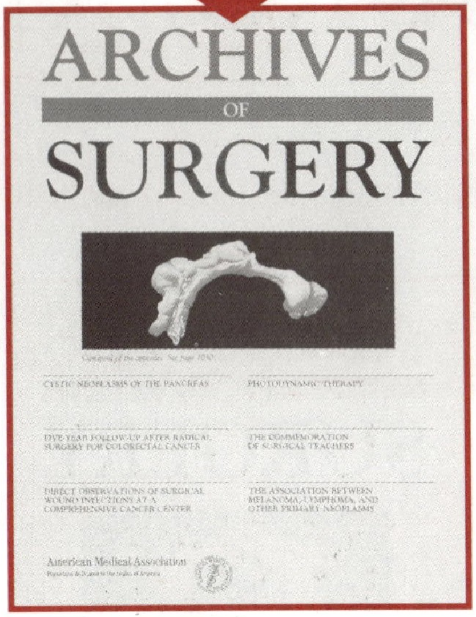

Essential reading to stay on the cutting-edge of clinical developments...

SUBSCRIBE NOW!

NO RISK GUARANTEE:

If you are not completely satisfied with your first issue, you may cancel and receive a full refund of your subscription payment. Or, if at any time, *Archives of Surgery* stops meeting your needs, you may cancel and receive a full refund of all unmailed issues.

PAPER

Familial Patterns of Thoracic Aortic Aneurysms

Michael A. Coady, MD, MPH; Ryan R. Davies, BA; Michele Roberts, MD, PhD; Lee J. Goldstein, BA; Matthew J. Rogalski, BS; John A. Rizzo, PhD; Graeme L. Hammond, MD; Gary S. Kopf, MD; John A. Elefteriades, MD

Hypothesis: To provide evidence that genetic factors contribute to the development of thoracic aortic aneurysms (TAA) by demonstrating familial patterns of the disease.

Design: Retrospective review.

Setting: University hospital.

Patients and Methods: We sought to identify familial patterns of TAA from a database of 598 patients evaluated or treated for TAA at the Yale Center for Thoracic Aortic Disease, New Haven, Conn, from January 1985 to August 1998. Of the 598 patients, 45 patients had a diagnosis of Marfan syndrome and 553 patients had no known history of any collagen vascular disorder. Of the 553 patients in the latter category, 398 patients had confirmed TAA, 66 had TAA with concomitant aortic dissections, and 89 had aortic dissections. From the group of 464 patients with TAA with or without concomitant aortic dissections, 2 interviewers attempted to contact 150 randomly selected patients for telephone screening to determine the presence of familial patterns of aortic disease. Fifteen of these patients were lost to follow-up. Complete medical and family histories of the remaining 135 patients (85 men, 50 women) were reviewed. Of the 135 individuals screened, 26 (18 men, 8 women) (19.3%) were found to belong to multiplex pedigrees. These 26 patients with familial nonsyndromic TAA were compared with the remaining 109 patients with sporadic TAA and the 45 patients with Marfan syndrome–associated TAA.

Main Outcome Measures: Groups were examined for statistical differences in age and aortic size at the time of diagnosis, growth rates of TAA, and rates of concomitant diseases. Nonsyndromic family pedigrees were analyzed and potential modes of inheritance were determined.

Results: The mean age at presentation for patients with familial nonsyndromic TAA (56.8 years) was significantly younger than the mean age of presentation in sporadic cases (64.3 years, $P \leq .03$), and significantly older than that of patients with Marfan syndrome (24.8 years, $P \leq .001$). Patients with a family history of aortic aneurysms had faster growth rates (0.22 cm/y) compared with patients with sporadic TAA (0.03 cm/y) ($P \leq .001$) and patients with Marfan syndrome (0.10 cm/y) ($P \leq .04$). Familial nonsyndromic TAA in patients with a concomitant aortic dissection had a growth rate of 0.33 cm/y, which was greater than that of patients with sporadic TAA (0.10 cm/y) and patients with Marfan syndrome (0.08 cm/y) with associated aortic dissection. This growth of 0.33 cm/y was significantly faster than the overall growth rate estimate of aneurysms in patients with aortic dissection (0.14 cm/y) ($P \leq .05$). Ten pedigrees (38.5%) showed direct father to son transmission, consistent with an autosomal dominant mode of inheritance. Six family pedigrees (23.1%) suggested an autosomal dominant or X-linked mode of inheritance. Seven pedigrees (26.9%) suggested a recessive mode of inheritance; 2 an autosomal recessive mode, and 5 an X-linked recessive or autosomal recessive mode. The remaining 3 pedigrees displayed more complex modes of inheritance.

Conclusions: This study supports the role of genetic factors influencing familial aggregation of TAA. Thoracic aortic aneurysms in association with multiplex pedigrees represent a new risk factor for aneurysm growth. Pedigree analysis suggests genetic heterogeneity. The primary mode of inheritance seems to be autosomal dominant, but X-linked dominant and recessive modes are also evident.

Arch Surg. 1999;134:361-367

From the Department of Surgery (Drs Coady, Hammond, Kopf, and Elefteriades, and Messrs Davies, Goldstein, and Rogalski), Section of Cardiothoracic Surgery, Department of Human Genetics (Dr Roberts), and the Department of Epidemiology and Public Health (Dr Rizzo), Yale University School of Medicine, New Haven, Conn.

THORACIC AORTIC aneurysms (TAA) of any cause involve a structural weakness in the aortic wall, resulting in progressive dilatation in accord with the relationships expressed in LaPlace's law. The manifestations of aneurysmal disease result in considerable morbidity and mortality for affected individuals. Understanding familial aggregation patterns and recognition of high-risk groups may lead to earlier detection and treatment and to the isolation of genetic factors contributing to the development and growth of thoracic aortic aneurysms.

Although abdominal aortic aneurysms (AAA) have been well characterized in terms of familial clustering, risk factors, growth rates, and possible modes of inheritance, less is known about TAA. Aneurysms affecting the thoracic aorta in patients with Marfan syndrome behave more aggressively than TAA in patients without Marfan syndrome; however, the natural history of TAA in patients who do not have Marfan syndrome but who demon-

PATIENTS AND METHODS

Several sources were used for identification of patients with TAA evaluated or treated at Yale University between January 1985 and August 1998. The computerized records of the Yale Center for Thoracic Aortic Disease were searched. This database stores longitudinal information (mean follow-up of 32 months) on 598 patients evaluated or treated for diseases of the thoracic aorta. In addition, the computerized database of the Department of Diagnostic Imaging at Yale University was searched for patients who underwent computed tomography, magnetic resonance imaging, angiography, and ultrasound studies of the thoracic aorta. Records of all patients undergoing operations of the thoracic aorta were reviewed. Autopsy records of all patients who died of aortic disease were examined. These sources identified 598 patients with TAA, and 1529 multiple imaging studies on most patients (computed tomography, magnetic resonance imaging, angiography, transesophageal echocardiography, and transthoracic echocardiography). Data recovered from hospital records and computer files were cross-checked with hospital discharge abstract data monitored by the Connecticut Hospital Association and Connecticut State Mortality Records, Wallingford, Conn.

Of the 598 patients, 45 patients had a diagnosis of Marfan syndrome, and 553 patients had no history of Marfan syndrome or any other collagen vascular disorder. From the 553 patients in the latter category, 398 patients had confirmed TAA, 66 had TAA with concomitant aortic dissections, and 89 had aortic dissections. From the group of 464 patients with TAA with or without concomitant aortic dissections, 2 interviewers (M.A.C. and M.J.R.) attempted to contact 150 randomly selected patients for telephone screening to determine the presence of familial patterns of aortic disease. Fifteen of these patients were lost to follow-up. Complete medical and family histories of the remaining 135 patients (85 men, 50 women) were reviewed. All telephone screening was carried out consistently by 2 trained interviewers. Responses were recorded on standardized forms. Pedigree analysis was performed on families in which more than one member had an aortic aneurysm.

We defined familial nonsyndromic TAA as those occurring in patients having 1 or more first-generation relatives with an aortic aneurysm and no history of Marfan syndrome or any other collagen vascular disorder. Sporadic cases of thoracic aneurysms are defined as those with no family history of aneurysmal disease and no history of Marfan syndrome or any other collagen vascular disorder. Patients with a diagnosis of Marfan syndrome met the revised criteria for the diagnosis outlined by DePaepe et al[2] in 1996.

Risk factors for vascular diseases were assessed (tobacco use, diabetes mellitus, hypertension, lipid profile, cardiac disease, and renal dysfunction), and were graded as mild, moderate, or severe according to the suggested standards for reports pertaining to lower extremity ischemia as formulated by the Ad Hoc Committee on Reporting Standards of the Society of Vascular Surgery and the International Society of Cardiovascular Surgery North America.[3]

Statistical methods were used to compare 3 categories of TAA: familial nonsyndromic TAA, sporadic TAA, and Marfan syndrome–associated TAA. Univariate analyses were performed using a commercial software program (SAS, version 6.12; SAS Institute Inc, Cary, NC). Analysis of variance was performed to compare means between familial nonsyndromic patients, sporadic patients, and patients with Marfan syndrome. The Bonferroni technique was performed to test for differences between means in multiple groups.[4]

Dinsmore et al[5] reported an extremely high correlation among magnetic resonance imaging, computed tomography scans, and ultrasound studies in TAA measurement. In this study, these 3 modalities were used for growth rate measurement. Serial information on aneurysm size was available for 18 patients in the familial nonsyndromic group, 45 patients in the sporadic group, and 39 patients in the Marfan syndrome group. Mean follow-up time for the 3 categories of TAA was 52.9 months (range, 0.07-304 months) for patients with familial nonsyndromic TAA, 31.6 months (range, 0.3-174 months) for sporadic TAA, and 58.3 months (range, 0.03-220 months) for Marfan syndrome–associated TAA.

Once patients underwent surgical repair, their subsequent imaging measurements were excluded from growth rate estimates. Serial imaging studies for the 3 categories of TAA were performed at mean (±SD) intervals of 9.75 ± 14.5 months for patients with familial nonsyndromic TAA, 11.14 ± 16.4 months for sporadic TAA, and 9.06 ± 12.5 months for Marfan syndrome–associated TAA.

Growth rate estimates were performed as we have reported previously, using multivariable regression analysis in which aneurysm growth follows an exponential path.[1,6,7] Specifically, an instrumental variables regression-based estimation technique was employed that is designed to mitigate measurement errors, yielding more stable and less biased estimates of aneurysm growth.[7] This approach correlates the change in aneurysm size with a variable, which, unlike aneurysm size, has little measurement error. The natural logarithm of the last measured size to the first measured size was related to the interval between the 2 tests and interactions between this time variable and risk factors.[8,9] This relationship is then estimated by ordinary least squares regression analysis, yielding an estimate that relates the interval between diagnostic imaging tests to aneurysm growth.[7] Importantly, the estimate will only be correlated with the true variation in aneurysm growth, not with the measurement error terms.

The overall growth rate estimates of aneurysms were calculated by examining all patients in our database for whom serial imaging measurements were available (n = 258). Initial risk factors for aortic growth were analyzed and included chronic dissection, aneurysm location (ascending or arch vs descending or thoracoabdominal), age, smoking history, hypertension (diastolic blood pressure >95 mm Hg), and sex.

strate a family history that is positive for aortic aneurysms has not been not well-described.[1]

We sought to identify familial patterns of TAA from a database of 553 patients evaluated or treated for diseases of the thoracic aorta at the Yale Center for Thoracic Aortic Disease, New Haven, Conn. One hundred thirty-five patients selected at random were interviewed, and both medical and family histories were obtained. Age and sex distributions, risk factors, and aneurysm growth rates are reported. These factors are compared for sporadic, famil-

Table 1. Demographics and Clinical Characteristics of Patients With Familial Nonsyndromic Thoracic Aortic Aneurysms*

Pedigree	Age, y/Sex	Tobacco Use	DM	HTN	Lipid Status	Cardiac Disease	Renal Dysfunction	CT	MRI	TEE	AG	TTE	Initial Aortic Size, cm	Site	Dissection
P007	45/M	Mild	None	Moderate	Mild	Mild	None	+	–	+	–	+	4.2	Desc	–
P027	28/M	None	None	Mild	None	None	None	+	+	–	–	+	5.0	Asc	–
P042	58/M	Severe	None	Moderate	Severe	Mild	None	–	–	–	–	+	3.9	Arch	–
P141	52/M	Mild	None	Mild	Severe	Severe	None	+	+	–	–	–	4.7	Asc	–
P145	33/M	None	None	None	None	None	None	+	–	–	+	+	4.8	Asc	–
P167	57/F	Severe	Mild	Mild	None	None	Mild	+	+	–	–	+	9.8	TA	–
P184	74/F	Moderate	None	Moderate	Severe	Moderate	None	+	–	+	+	+	6.0	Asc	–
P188	59/M	None	None	Mild	None	Moderate	None	+	–	–	+	–	4.5	Asc	–
P271	74/M	Severe	None	None	None	None	None	–	–	–	–	+	4.0	Asc	–
P284	37/M	None	None	None	None	None	None	+	–	–	+	+	6.3	Asc	–
P286	65/F	Severe	Mild	Mild	None	Mild	None	+	–	–	–	+	3.3	TA	–
P330	14/F	None	None	None	None	None	None	–	+	–	–	+	6.0	Asc	–
P422	45/M	Mild	None	Moderate	None	None	None	–	+	–	+	+	4.5	Asc	–
P470	58/M	None	None	Severe	None	Mild	Mild	+	–	–	+	+	4.9	Desc	–
P511	64/M	None	None	None	None	None	None	+	+	+	–	–	3.3	Desc	Type B
P518	78/F	None	None	Mild	Mild	None	None	+	+	–	–	–	5.0	Asc	–
P546	69/M	None	None	Severe	None	None	None	+	–	–	+	–	4.0	Asc	Type A
P547	76/M	Mild	None	Mild	None	Mild	None	+	+	+	–	+	5.5	Asc	–
P557	79/M	None	None	Mild	None	Severe	None	+	+	+	–	+	4.2	Desc	Type B
P563	72/F	None	Mild	Mild	None	Moderate	None	+	–	–	–	–	7.0	Desc	Type B
P565	70/M	None	None	Severe	None	None	None	+	–	–	+	+	4.1	Asc	Type A
P571	75/M	Mild	Mild	Severe	Severe	Moderate	Mild	+	+	–	–	+	5.0	Asc	–
P572	61/M	Mild	None	Mild	None	Mild	None	–	+	–	–	–	3.3	Asc	Type A
P580	46/F	Moderate	None	Mild	None	Mild	None	+	–	–	–	–	4.0	Desc	–
P585	53/F	Moderate	None	None	None	None	Mild	+	–	–	–	–	4.1	Desc	–
P588	49/M	None	None	None	None	None	None	+	–	–	–	–	5.4	Asc	–

DM indicates diabetes mellitus; HTN, hypertension; CT, computed tomography; MRI, magnetic resonance imaging; TEE, transesophageal echocardiography; AG, angiography; TTE, transthoracic echocardiography; +, study was performed for either diagnosis or follow-up; –, study not performed; Desc, descending aorta; Asc, ascending aorta; and TA, thoracoabdominal aorta. Risk factors are graded as per the "Patients and Methods" section.

Table 2. Comparison of Patients With Familial Nonsyndromic, Sporadic, and Marfan Syndrome–Associated Thoracic Aortic Aneurysms*

Variable	Familial Nonsyndromic	Sporadic	Marfan Syndrome Associated
No. of patients (sex)	26 (18 M, 8 F)	109 (67 M, 42 F)	45 (29 M, 16 F)
Age, y	56.8 ± 18.2†‡	64.3 ± 14.0†‡	24.8 ± 17.1‡
Initial aortic diameter, cm	4.87 ± 1.3	5.25 ± 1.3‡	4.02 ± 1.1‡
Associated hypertension, %	73‡	75‡	16‡
Growth rate, cm/y	0.22 (0.14 to 0.31)§‖	0.03 (−0.04 to 0.10)§	0.10 (0.05 to 0.15)‖

Values are given as mean ± SD. The Bonferroni test for differences between means was used in the analysis of variance procedure.
†$P \leq .03$.
‡$P \leq .001$.
§$P \leq .0012$.
‖$P \leq .04$.

ial nonsyndromic, and Marfan syndrome–associated TAA. The prevalence of aortic aneurysms among relatives of patients in our database is evaluated, and possible modes of inheritance are discussed.

RESULTS

DEMOGRAPHICS AND CLINICAL CHARACTERISTICS

One hundred thirty-five patients were interviewed, and information was collected regarding 1014 first-degree relatives, 510 of whom were men (50.3%) and 504 of whom were women (49.7%). Of the 135 patients interviewed, 26 patients (18 men, 8 women) (19.3%) with TAA were found to have at least 1 first-degree relative with an aortic aneurysm; the remaining 109 patients were considered sporadic cases. **Table 1** summarizes the demographic and clinical features of these 26 familial nonsyndromic patients. The mean age at presentation (56.8 years) was significantly younger than the mean age of presentation in sporadic cases (64.3 years, $P \leq .03$), and significantly older than that of patients with Marfan syndrome (24.8 years, $P \leq .001$) (**Table 2**).

Sixteen (61.5%) of 26 patients with TAA and family history positive for nonsyndromic aortic aneurysms had an aneurysm located in the ascending aorta; the remaining 10 patients (38.5%) had an aneurysm located

Table 3. Comparison of Aortic Growth Rate According to Dissection Status in Patients With Familial Nonsyndromic, Sporadic, and Marfan Syndrome–Associated Thoracic Aortic Aneurysms (TAA)*

Type of TAA	Aortic Dissection, cm/y	No Dissection, cm/y
Familial nonsyndromic	0.33 (0.07 to 0.60)† (n = 5)	0.20 (0.10 to 0.30) (n = 8)
Sporadic	0.10 (0.00 to 0.20) (n = 18)	0.01 (−0.01 to −0.10) (n = 13)
Marfan syndrome associated	0.08 (−0.08 to 0.24) (n = 39)	0.09 (0.04 to 0.14) (n = 27)
Overall	0.14 (0.07 to 0.21)† (n = 90)	0.09 (0.06 to 0.13) (n = 168)

Values indicate aortic growth rate based on regression analysis for patients with serial imaging studies, both with and without aortic dissection. They are expressed as mean (±SD).

†*P*<.05.

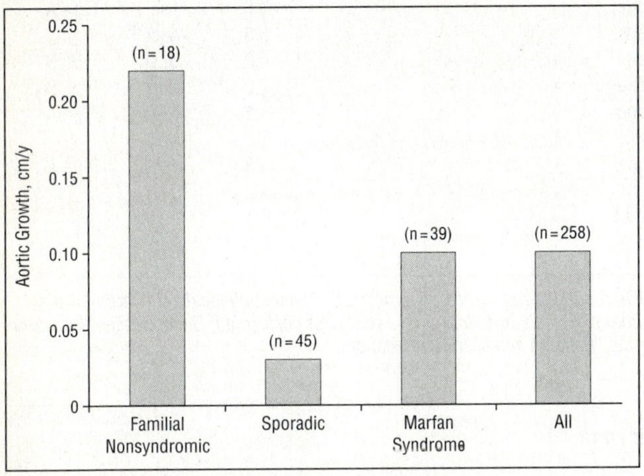

Figure 1. *Mean growth rates for thoracic aortic aneurysms. For the familial nonsyndromic group, P ≤ .04.*

in the descending aorta (Table 1). Six patients (26.0%) had concomitant aortic dissections, 3 in the ascending aorta and 3 in the descending aorta.

Accompanying medical problems were common among the 26 patients (Table 1), particularly, tobacco use (13 patients, 50.0%), diabetes mellitus (4 patients, 15.4%), hypertension (19 patients, 73.1%), hypercholesterolemia (6 patients, 23.1%), cardiac disease (13 patients, 50.0%), and renal dysfunction (4 patients, 15.4%). Hypertension was associated more frequently with patients with familial nonsyndromic TAA and sporadic TAA (73% and 75%, respectively) than with Marfan syndrome–associated TAA (16%) (*P* ≤ .001) (Table 2).

Several different imaging studies were used in the diagnosis of TAA and in the follow-up of these patients (Table 1). One or more methods were used for every patient, and size measurements over time were used in growth rate calculations. Computed tomography, the most commonly used imaging modality, was used in 22 cases (84.6%). In addition, magnetic resonance imaging was performed in 11 patients (42.3%), angiography in 8 patients (30.7%), transesophageal echocardiography in 5 patients (19.2%), and transthoracic echocardiography in 16 patients (61.5%).

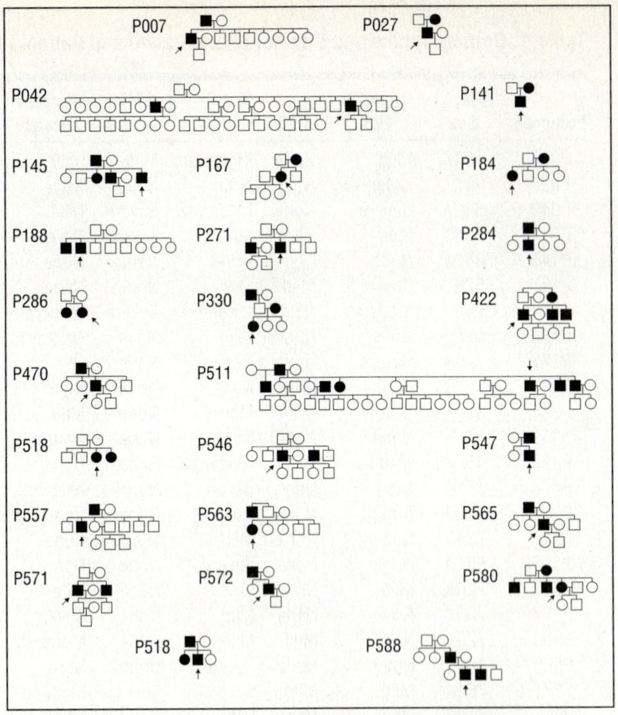

Figure 2. *Nonsyndromic thoracic aortic aneurysm family pedigree. Squares represent the men and circles, the women. An arrow indicates the proband with a thoracic aortic aneurysm. Blackened squares or circles represent affected patients with aortic aneurysms.*

ANEURYSMAL GROWTH RATES

The initial aortic diameter at the time of diagnosis was similar for patients with familial nonsyndromic TAA and patients with sporadic TAA (means, 4.87 cm and 5.25 cm, respectively) (Table 2). Patients with Marfan syndrome–associated TAA tended to have smaller aortic aneurysm diameters at the time of diagnosis (mean ± SD, 4.02 cm ± 1.1 cm) compared with familial cases (4.87 cm ± 1.3 cm), and a statistically significant difference compared with patients with sporadic TAA (5.25 cm ± 1.3 cm) (*P* ≤ .001).

Aortic aneurysm growth rates for familial nonsyndromic, sporadic, and Marfan syndrome–associated TAA are displayed in Table 2 and **Table 3**. Patients with a family history of aortic aneurysms had faster growth rates (0.22 cm/y) compared with patients with sporadic TAA (0.03 cm/y) (*P*≤.001) and patients with Marfan syndrome–associated TAA (0.10 cm/y) (*P*≤.04). This is depicted graphically in **Figure 1**. The presence of a dissection also increased aortic growth. Familial nonsyndromic TAA in patients with a concomitant aortic dissection had a growth rate of 0.33 cm/y, which was greater than in patients with sporadic TAA (0.10 cm/y) and in patients with Marfan syndrome–associated TAA (0.08 cm/y). This growth of 0.33 cm/y was significantly faster than the overall growth rate estimate of aneurysms in patients with aortic dissection (*P*≤.05) (Table 3).

PEDIGREE ANALYSIS

Figure 2 displays the family pedigrees of the 26 patients and their first-order relatives.

Ten pedigrees (38.5%) display direct father to son transmission (P007, P145, P284, P470, P511, P547, P565,

P572, P585, and P588) consistent with an autosomal dominant mode of inheritance. Six family pedigrees (23.1%) suggest an autosomal dominant or X-linked mode of inheritance (P027, P141, P167, P184, P557, and P580). Seven pedigrees (26.9%) suggest a recessive mode of inheritance; 2 autosomal recessive (P286 and P518), and 5 X-linked recessive or autosomal recessive (P042, P188, P271, P546, and P571).

The final 3 pedigrees represent more complex modes of inheritance. In P330, the proband and her mother have an aortic aneurysm and her sister does not have an aneurysm. This situation may represent an autosomal dominant or X-linked dominant transmission. However, the paternal grandfather is also affected. The contribution of this on the proband is unclear.

In P422, the proband and his 2 brothers are affected. The paternal aunt is also affected. If the proband's father were affected and the gene was not penetrant, this might represent an autosomal transmission. Autosomal recessive transmission is less likely.

Finally, in P563 the proband and her paternal aunt are affected. Considerations include autosomal or X-linked dominant transmission with incomplete penetrance.

COMMENT

Most of what is known about the genetic factors involved in aortic aneurysms is derived from studies of patients with AAA. In 1977, Clifton[10] was the first to note a familial aggregation of AAA, describing a family of 3 male siblings who underwent surgery for ruptured aneurysms. Tilson and Seashore[11] later reported on 50 families with 1 or more first-degree relatives with AAA. Studies involving the familial nature of AAA have considered almost every possible genetic model (**Table 4**).[11-14] These studies confirm that AAA is one of the most common familial diseases, with at least 18% of patients with AAA having a first-degree relative with an aortic aneurysm.[15] For most patients, however, the cause of the aortic aneurysm remains unknown.

Although AAA has been studied extensively, less is known regarding TAA. Biddinger et al[16] in 1997 confirmed the familial aggregation of TAA. Similar to that study, our data support a genetic predisposition to the development of TAA in 19% of patients. We have demonstrated that patients with familial nonsyndromic TAA are younger at the time of diagnosis (56.8 years) than are patients with sporadic TAA (64.3 years) ($P \leq .03$), but are older than patients with Marfan syndrome (24.8 years) (Table 2). Ascertainment bias may be a contributing factor in both familial nonsyndromic TAA and Marfan syndrome–associated TAA. Patients who have a close relative with an aneurysm may seek medical attention earlier than patients with sporadic TAA. Patients with Marfan syndrome are screened for asymptomatic aortic disease. The relative contribution of these factors remains to be elucidated.

Our data are similar to data presented by Biddinger et al[16]; hypertension is strongly associated with both familial nonsyndromic and sporadic cases (73% and 75%, respectively) (Table 2). Although it is well known that hypertension is associated with aortic aneurysms, aneurysm formation cannot simply be ascribed to elevated

Table 4. Familial Studies of Abdominal Aortic Aneurysms

Source, y	Proposed Genetic Models
Tilson and Seashore,[11] 1984	X-linked
Tilson and Seashore,[11] 1984	Autosomal dominant
Bowers and Cave,[12] 1985	Autosomal recessive
Tilson and Seashore,[11] 1984	Multifactorial
Powell and Greengalgh,[13] 1987	Multifactorial
Majumder et al,[14] 1991	Autosomal recessive, diallelic locus

blood pressure alone.[16] Interestingly, hypertension was found in only 16% of the patients with Marfan syndrome in our study. Thus, the inherent vessel weakness due to the genetic defect in the fibrillin gene may represent the greatest influence on aneurysm formation in these patients. In addition, patients may have different genetic predispositions to respond to hypertensive stresses imposed on their aortas. This may be reflected by our findings of an increased aneurysmal growth rate in the absence of a disparity in rates of hypertension between familial nonsyndromic and sporadic TAA.

We recently reported the overall growth rate for TAA to be 0.10 cm/y.[6,7] In this study, we have demonstrated that the growth rate of aortic aneurysms in familial nonsyndromic TAA is 0.22 cm/y (Table 2). Thus, the current study defines a new risk factor for aneurysm growth, namely, probands belonging to multiplex pedigrees. The aneurysmal growth rate of 0.22 cm/y is significantly faster than the growth rate of aneurysms in patients belonging to the sporadic (0.03 cm/y, $P \leq .001$) or Marfan syndrome groups (0.10 cm/y, $P \leq .04$) (Table 2, Figure 1).

We have also recently reported that the presence of an aortic dissection significantly increases the aneurysm growth rate.[1] This study demonstrates that patients with familial nonsyndromic aneurysms and superimposed aortic dissections also display a faster rate of aneurysmal growth (0.33 cm/y, $P \leq .05$) when compared with the overall growth rate of aortic dissections alone. The reasons for faster growth rates in patients exhibiting familial patterns and with concomitant aortic dissections are not clear, but may reflect a compounded environmental insult on a genetically weakened aortic wall. There are likely to be additional contributing factors affecting aortic growth that have not been clarified.

Pedigree analysis (Figure 2) demonstrates more than 1 possible mode of transmission of aortic aneurysms. In this study, most seem to be autosomal dominant (38.5%), and an additional 23.1%, autosomal dominant or X-linked dominant. Twenty-seven percent represented a recessive mode of transmission. The current literature supports our findings that there may be more than 1 genetic model (Table 4).[11-14] This suggests that genetic heterogeneity (ie, more than 1 gene causing a single phenotype) may play an important role in aortic aneurysm formation.

One point that warrants discussion is the possibility of noninclusion of asymptomatic aneurysms in our pedigree analysis. It is possible that there are additional family members who have undetected TAA or AAA. Likewise, a relative may have died before an aneurysm developed. It is also possible that there may be undiagnosed familial clustering of aneurysms incorrectly placed in the sporadic category. With the small number of pedigrees and the limited number of generations, our pedigree analysis may be affected by these potential pitfalls. It is also necessary to make a disclaimer for the incomplete accuracy of family history data acquired by interview. Errors including inaccurate or incomplete memory, lack of confirmation of diagnosis, and misinformation may have occurred. We made efforts to maximize consistency during data acquisition by maintaining 2 trained interviewers and confirming diagnoses whenever possible.

To avoid noninclusion of asymptomatic family members, we have begun to screen by ultrasound all first-generation family members of our 26 pedigrees to identify additional patients with previously undetected aneurysms and to confirm or refute absence of aortic disease in other family members. Screening the general population for TAA would not be cost effective. In a theoretical screening model for AAA of a population of 100 000 individuals, it has been proposed that 1500 lives could be saved at a cost of $78 000 per life saved.[17] Most of the aneurysms detected by screening are small, with few aneurysms detected that were 6 cm in diameter or larger. Screening selective populations is far more cost effective. For instance, in 561 patients with peripheral vascular disease, almost all of whom were cigarette smokers, aneurysms 3 cm in diameter or larger were found in 14%.[18] Screening brothers of patients with aneurysms renders an incidence of aneurysms of 20% to 29%.[19] Therefore, we expect that ultrasound screening of the 26 families with familial nonsyndromic TAA will find additional affected patients and permit more accurate pedigree analysis.

The genetic basis of aortic aneurysms was reviewed by Kuivaniemi et al[20] in 1991. The major determining factor in the appearance of aortic aneurysms may be an inborn defect of collagen type III or of another component of the connective tissue matrix. In patients with Ehlers-Danlos syndrome, defects in the type III collagen gene (*COL3A1*) have been implicated.[21] The mutations associated with collagen diseases such as Ehlers-Danlos syndrome and osteogenesis imperfecta are heterogeneous, and a similar situation may exist for aortic aneurysms.[20] The gene for Marfan syndrome has recently been identified, and there is optimism that this will provide a basis for preventative medicine.[22] The gene has been linked to markers in or near the fibrillin-1 gene in chromosome band 15q21.1.[23] Interestingly, the Gly1127Ser mutation in an EGF domain of the fibrilllin-1 gene has been shown to be a risk factor for ascending aortic aneurysms and dissections.[24] A mutation in the *COL3A1* gene resulting in an amino acid substitution was identified in a family with a strong history of AAA.[25] Although this mutation was not detected in any of 140 other patients with AAA, variants of the *COL3A1* gene are thought to predispose to aneurysm formation in the presence of other components of a multifactorial process.[26] Mutations of the *FBN1* and *COL3A1* genes may produce a spectrum of connective-tissue disorders responsible for abnormal or reduced matrix deposition in the aorta and subsequent aneurysm development.

As mentioned previously, we are supplementing the present pedigrees by ultrasound screening of families. Patients are examined and peripheral blood is drawn on both affected and unaffected family members. We are presently employing mutation and linkage analysis in an effort to isolate candidate gene(s) causing TAA. The latter approach employs markers that have been mapped to a particular locus on the genome, and is used to test whether the marker is coinherited with aortic aneurysms in families.[27]

In summary, clarifying the genetic basis for the development of TAA is a complex and challenging endeavor. We have confirmed that familial clustering of TAA does occur. The current study defines a new risk factor for aneurysm growth, namely, probands belonging to multiplex pedigrees. The aneurysmal growth rate of patients with familial nonsyndromic TAA is significantly faster than the growth rate of aneurysms in patients with sporadic or Marfan-associated TAA. In addition, the growth rate of familial TAA with concomitant aortic dissection exceeds both the growth rate for sporadic cases with aortic dissection as well as the overall growth rate for aortic dissection alone. Pedigree analysis demonstrates that the primary mode of inheritance seems to be autosomal dominant, but X-linked dominant and recessive modes are also evident.

This work was funded by Grant-in-Aid CT-BP97-GR-45 from the American Heart Association, Dallas, Tex.

Presented at the 79th Annual Meeting of the New England Surgical Society, Toronto, Ontario, September 25, 1998.

Corresponding author: John A. Elefteriades, MD, Section of Cardiothoracic Surgery, Yale University School of Medicine, 333 Cedar St, New Haven, CT 06510 (e-mail: johnelefteriades@QM.yale.edu).

REFERENCES

1. Coady MA, Rizzo JA, Hammond GL, et al. What is the appropriate size criterion for resection of thoracic aortic aneurysms? *J Thorac Cardiovasc Surg.* 1997; 113:476-91.
2. DePaepe A, Devereux RB, Dietz HC, Mennekam RCM, Pyeritz RE. Revised diagnostic criteria for the Marfan syndrome. *Am J Med Genet.* 1996;62:417-26.
3. Rutherford RB, Flanigan DP, Gupta SK, et al. Suggested standards for reports dealing with lower extremity ischemia. *J Vasc Surg.* 1986;4:80-94.
4. McClave JT, Dietrich FH. Analysis of variance: comparing more than two means. In: *Statistics.* 6th ed. New York, NY: Macmillan Publishing Co Inc; 1994.
5. Dinsmore RE, Liberthson RR, Wismer GL, et al. Magnetic resonance imaging of thoracic aortic aneurysms. *Am J Radiol.* 1986;146:309-314.
6. Coady MA, Rizzo JA, Hammond GL, Kopf GS, Elefteriades JA. Surgical intervention criteria for thoracic aortic aneurysms. *Ann Thorac Surg.* In press.
7. Rizzo JA, Coady MA, Elefteriades JA. Procedures for estimating growth rates in thoracic aortic aneurysms. *J Clin Epidemiol.* 1998;51:747-754.
8. Hirose Y, Hamada S, Takamiya M. Predicting the growth of aortic aneurysms: a comparison of linear vs exponential models. *Angiology.* 1995;46:413-419.
9. Hsiao C. *Analysis of Panel Data.* New York, NY; Cambridge University Press: 1989.
10. Clifton MA. Familial abdominal aortic aneurysms. *Br J Surg.* 1977;64:765.
11. Tilson MD, Seashore MR. Fifty families with abdominal aortic aneurysm in two or more first-order relatives. *Am J Surg.* 1984;147:551-553.
12. Bowers D, Cave WS. Aneurysm of the abdominal aorta: a 20-year study. *J R Soc Med.* 1985;78:812-820.
13. Powell JT, Greengalgh RM. Multifactorial inheritance of abdominal aortic aneurysm. *Eur J Surg.* 1987;1:29-31.
14. Majumder RR, St Jean P, Ferrell RE, Webster MW, Steed DL. On the inheritance of abdominal aortic aneurysm. *Am J Hum Genet.* 1991;48:164-170.
15. Johansen K, Koepsell T. Familial tendency for abdominal aortic aneurysms. *JAMA.* 1986;256;1934-1936.
16. Biddinger A, Rocklin M, Coselli J, Milewicz DM. Familial thoracic aortic dilatations and dissections: a case control study. *J Vasc Surg.* 1997;25:506-511.
17. Quill DS, Colgan MP, Sumner DS. Ultrasonic screening for the detection of abdominal aortic aneurysms. *Surg Clin North Am.* 1989;69:713.
18. Galland RB, Simmons MJ, Torrie EPH. Prevalence of abdominal aortic aneurysm in patients with occlusive peripheral vascular disease. *Br J Surg.* 1991;78:1259.
19. Adamson J, Powell JT, Greenhalgh RM. Selection for screening for familial aortic aneurysms. *Br J Surg.* 1992;79:897.
20. Kuivaniemi H, Tromp G, Prockop DJ. Genetic causes of aortic aneurysms. *J Clin Invest.* 1991;88:1441-1444.

21. Kuivaniemi H, Tromp G, Kuivaniemi H, et al. A mutation in collagen genes: causes of rare and some common diseases in humans. *FASEB J.* 1991;5:2025.
22. Young I. Understanding Marfan syndrome. *Br Med J.* 1991;30:1414-1415.
23. Kainulainen K, Pulkkinen L, Savolainen A, Kaitila I, Peltonen L. Location on chromosome 15 of the gene defect causing Marfan syndrome. *N Engl J Med.* 1990; 323:935-939.
24. Francke U, Berg MA, Tynan K, et al. A Gly1127Ser mutation in an EGF-like domain of the fibrillin-1 gene is a risk factor for ascending aortic aneurysm and dissection. *Am J Hum Genet.* 1995;56:1287-1296.
25. Kontusaari S, Tromp G, Kuivaneimo H, et al. A mutation in the gene for type III collagen (*COL3A1*) in a family with aortic aneurysms. *J Clin Invest.* 1990;86:1465.
26. Prockop DJ. Mutations in collagen genes as a cause of connective tissue diseases. *N Engl J Med.* 1992;326:540.
27. Tromp G, Kuivaniemi. DNA sequencing as a method to identify mutations in patients with familial forms of aneurysms. *J Vasc Surg.* 1992;15:928-930.

DISCUSSION

Richard Cambria, MD, Boston, Mass: Congratulations to Dr Coady on a very nice presentation and we've heard this afternoon the latest installment in a series of enlightening publications referable to thoracic aortic disease from Dr Elefteriades' group at Yale. The authors sought to establish the presence of familial clustering of thoracic aortic aneurysms. This information was previously available in only a single report in the literature for aneurysm disease north of the diaphragm, but as alluded to in the presentation, firmly established for the more commonly encountered AAA. Using telephone inquiry of 150 patients selected at random from their sizable registry, they recorded a 19.3% rate of familial clustering of thoracic aneurysms, that is, patients with a first-blood-order relative afflicted with the disease. In comparing familial with sporadic thoracic aneurysm patients, they noted younger age at treatment and significantly faster growth rates in familial cases. The latter discovery, of course, has potentially important clinical implications. They report a variety of inheritance modes and the frustration they note in attempting to clarify simple or uniform modes of inheritance is exactly paralleled in the literature referable to AAA.

My knowledge of genetics is limited to the fact that I know a fellow named Mendel who grew peas. We do, however, have complete demographic data on some 230 patients treated for thoracoabdominal aortic aneurysm with familial clustering noted in some 10% of these patients. I've recently had the opportunity to review the available data on the natural history of thoracic and thoracoabdominal aneurysms. I can assure you the information we heard today is a valuable addition to the literature.

Approximately 10 years ago, our group, under the leadership of Clem Darling, published a sizable series of 550 abdominal aneurysm repairs designed to answer many of the questions that Dr Coady asked today. Is there familial clustering; if so, are there characteristics of these familial aneurysms that are clinically important?

In this series we noted familial clustering in 15.1% of patients, a figure almost identical to that reported today. While AAA growth rates were not available from our studies since they were all operated cases, we did note that familial aneurysm patients were more likely in women and when such a familial aneurysm occurred in women, there was a significantly increased risk of presentation with rupture. Thus, our data is consistent with that from the Yale group, ie, familial cases seem to be more prone to expansion and rupture. Furthermore, in our vascular registry, the male-female sex ratio for abdominal aneurysms is the typically reported 5 to 6 to 1, but in our thoracoabdominal aneurysm cohort, the sex predilection is 1 to 1. This introduces my first question. Dr Coady, do you have information from your registry on sex distribution for degenerative vs chronic dissection aneurysms in the thoracic aorta?

My other questions relate to the issue of aneurysm growth rates, which the authors have emphasized as among their most important findings. Apparently, part of the significance they've assigned to the growth rates of familial cases relates to the comparison to an extremely low, 0.03 cm/y, rate of expansion assigned to sporadic cases. This latter figure is approximately 10 times lower than my understanding of the available literature on this topic, and indeed lower than the information from your own registry. Could you comment on possible explanations for the apparent minuscule expansion rate in sporadic cases? Is it fair or logical to group growth rates in different regions of the thoracic aorta, namely ascending, arch, descending, and thoracoabdominal together, since the pathology may be different (dissection vs degenerative aneurysm) and it is well known that the lamellar architecture of the aorta is different in the ascending as opposed to the descending aorta.

Michael Coady, MD: Dr Cambria, thank you very much. I'll answer each of your questions in series. The first question addresses the interesting observation by Dr Darling made in 1989 (*J Vasc Surg.* 1989;10:39-43). Dr Darling, in a 9-year prospective study, noted an increased prevalence of female patients in a group of familial abdominal aortic aneurysms. He also studied the association between sex and the risk of aortic rupture. Dr Darling found that those families with AAA and a female member with an aneurysm had a strong correlation with aneurysm rupture. The term "black widow syndrome" was employed to describe the female member belonging to this group of familial AAA, as she served as a marker for families which were at significant risk for having at least 1 member of their family experience an aneurysm rupture. In our present series, we have not observed any sex predilection for aortic aneurysm rupture. Currently, the number of patients who had a ruptured aneurysm in these familial, sporadic, and Marfan groups is too small to make any meaningful observations regarding sex distribution. In our larger aneurysm registry, we have not identified any differences in the sex distribution for degenerative or chronic dissecting aneurysms of the thoracic aorta.

Regarding your second question on the growth rate, our sporadic group had a very small growth rate of 0.03 cm/y. While this is certainly much slower in comparison to the overall growth rate estimate of 0.12 cm/y that we published last year in a larger series, this is the first time we have attempted to segregate the groups of aneurysms into familial nonsyndromic, sporadic, and Marfan syndrome associated. While sample size may be affecting the growth rate estimates in all groups, I suspect that there may be true differences in growth that may directly relate to the genetic defect in the aortic wall. When segregated, familial and Marfan-associated aneurysms grow faster than sporadic aneurysms. Growth rate estimates for these groups have not been well studied. As we increase our sample size we hope to continue to achieve more accurate estimates.

Your last question addresses whether it is logical to analyze growth rates in different regions of the thoracic aorta. Our group has analyzed aneurysm growth rates at various aortic locations because it has been well documented that the growth rate varies by location. Descending and thoracoabdominal aortic aneurysms, for instance, may actually grow faster than ascending and arch aneurysms. Using regression techniques, we have previously shown that descending and thoracoabdominal aortic aneurysms grow 0.29 cm/y (*J Thorac Cardiovasc Surg.* 1997;113:476-491), which closely approximates the growth rate estimates reported by Dapunt et al (*J Thorac Cardiovasc Surg.* 1994;107:1323-1333) for aneurysms in this location. In this study, we have chosen to measure overall growth rates for the 3 groups primarily because the sample size did not permit more sophisticated analysis of aneurysm growth rates by location. As we continue to expand our database, we hope to refine further statistically-based growth rate estimates.

PAPER

Does Uninjured Skin Release Proinflammatory Cytokines Following Trauma and Hemorrhage?

Robert A. Catania, MD; Martin G. Schwacha, PhD; William G. Cioffi, MD; Kirby I. Bland, MD; Irshad H. Chaudry, PhD

Hypothesis: Uninjured skin contributes to the elevation in circulating levels of proinflammatory cytokines seen following severe injury.

Design: Male C3H/HeN mice underwent trauma, trauma-hemorrhage and resuscitation, or closed long-bone fracture. Serum, skin, and liver samples were harvested at designated times after experimental treatment.

Main Outcome Measures: Levels of interleukin (IL) 1β, IL-6, and tumor necrosis factor α (TNF-α) were determined in serum and skin cultures at 1, 8, and 24 hours after trauma-hemorrhage. The RNA was isolated from liver and skin samples at 1, 2, 4, 8, and 24 hours from all 3 experimental groups, and gene expression of the cytokines was determined.

Results: Remote (nontraumatized) skin from trauma-hemorrhage animals released significantly more IL-6 and TNF-α into culture supernatants at 1 and 24 hours and significantly more IL-1β at 1, 8, and 24 hours than did skin from sham animals. Serum levels of all 3 cytokines were significantly elevated at 1 and 24 hours after trauma-hemorrhage relative to sham animals. Gene expression of all 3 cytokines was detected in skin and liver following trauma-hemorrhage. Furthermore, gene expression of all 3 cytokines was detected in uninjured skin after soft tissue trauma and closed long-bone fracture.

Conclusions: Proinflammatory cytokine gene expression is up-regulated in uninjured skin following trauma, trauma-hemorrhage, and long-bone fracture. This increase in gene expression correlates with increased cytokine production by cultured skin as well as increased circulating cytokine levels. These results suggest that uninjured skin may also contribute to the rise in circulating cytokine levels seen after injury.

Arch Surg. 1999;134:368-374

SEVERE INJURY, particularly with concomitant hemorrhagic shock, predisposes patients to the development of infectious complications and multiple organ failure.[1] In particular, hypotension induces a decline in cell-mediated immunity that is more profound in the presence of concurrent soft tissue trauma[2] or long-bone fracture.[3] Our laboratory has previously demonstrated that Kupffer cells are primed following hemorrhagic shock, and that unlike other macrophage populations, they produce increased amounts of proinflammatory cytokines under those conditions.[4] In combination with activation of neutrophils,[5] the systemic release of inflammatory mediators such as interleukin (IL) 1, IL-6, and tumor necrosis factor α (TNF-α) is believed to have a negative impact on the function of many organ systems.[1]

The body's largest immune organ, the skin, is composed of multiple cell types that are also capable of producing cytokines.[6] Specifically, keratinocytes, fibroblasts, dermal endothelial cells, Langerhans cells, dendritic cells, and inflammatory cells infiltrating the skin are able to release cytokines under various conditions.[6,7] Previous investigations have established that thermally injured skin produces detectable levels of several cytokines, including IL-1,[8,9] IL-6,[10,11] and TNF.[10] Since early burn wound excision has been shown to restore the depressed cellular immune response seen after thermal injury,[12] this suggests that skin-derived mediators are capable of modulating systemic immune function. Interestingly, cytokines produced by the skin in response to topical irritants have been shown to be measurable in draining lymph,[13,14] indicating that skin-derived cytokines can reach the systemic circulation.

Direct injury to the skin is known to incite a vigorous immune response associated with wound healing.[15] Furthermore, after the onset of severe shock, the skin is known to be one of the first organs from which blood is shunted to preserve central perfusion.[16] Given the known ability of skin to produce cytokines in response to topical injury, and given the sustained cutaneous hypoperfusion that occurs

From the Center for Surgical Research and Department of Surgery, Brown University School of Medicine and Rhode Island Hospital, Providence.

MATERIALS AND METHODS

EXPERIMENTAL MODEL

We used inbred male C3H/HeN mice (Charles River Laboratories, Wilmington, Mass), 7 weeks of age. Mice in the trauma-hemorrhage groups were lightly anesthetized with methoxyflurane and restrained in a supine position, and a 2.5-cm midline laparotomy (ie, trauma induction) was performed. The incision was then closed aseptically using 6-0 monofilament nylon (Ethilon; Ethicon Inc, Somerville, NJ) sutures. Next, both femoral arteries were aseptically cannulated with polyethylene-10 tubing (Clay-Adams, Parsippany, NJ). Blood pressure was constantly monitored using a commerically available arterial blood pressure analyzer (Digi-Med; Micro-Med Inc, Louisville, Ky). On awakening, the animals were bled rapidly through the other catheter to a mean (±SEM) arterial blood pressure of 35 ± 5 mm Hg (prehemorrhage mean [±SEM] arterial blood pressure, 95 ± 5 mm Hg), which was maintained for 90 minutes. After hemorrhage, the animals were resuscitated with lactated Ringer solution (4 times the shed blood volume for 30 minutes), the catheters were removed, the vessels were ligated, and the groin incisions were closed. Animals undergoing sham operation (sham animals, control group for trauma-hemorrhage) underwent anesthesia and the same groin dissection, which included ligation of both femoral arteries, but no hemorrhage or fluid resuscitation. Mice in the trauma group underwent anesthesia and midline laparotomy as described above; mice in the fracture group underwent anesthesia and had a unilateral closed tibial fracture induced as described previously.[3] In the fracture group, the fractured limb was splinted to prevent further soft tissue injury or conversion to an open fracture. Control animals for the trauma and fracture groups underwent anesthesia and restraint (sham trauma) or splinting (sham fracture). Animals were killed at 1, 2, 4, 8, or 24 hours for RNA isolation or 1, 8, or 24 hours for skin culture.Different groups of animals were used for the experiments involving RNA isolation and skin culture. There was no mortality in any group within the 24 hours. All procedures were performed in accordance with the guidelines set forth in the Animal Welfare Act and the Guide for the Care and Use of Laboratory Animals by the National Institutes of Health. This project was approved by the Institutional Animal Care and Use Committee of Rhode Island Hospital and Brown University, Providence.

RNA ISOLATION

Animals were killed with an overdose of methoxyflurane, and skin and liver samples were harvested. The tissues were homogenized in thiocyanate and phenol in monophase solution (Tri-Reagent; Sigma-Aldrich Corporation, St Louis, Mo) using a Dounce homogenizer. To clarify the samples, they were centrifuged at 10 000g for 10 minutes, and the liquid phase was used. Chloroform was added, and the samples were shaken vigorously for 15 seconds and then allowed to stand at room temperature for 15 minutes. The samples were centrifuged at 12 000g for 15 minutes at 4°C, and the aqueous phase was transferred to a fresh tube to which isopropanol was added. The samples were again shaken and allowed to stand overnight at −20°C. Following centrifugation at 12 000g for 10 minutes at 4°C, the pellets were washed in 75% ethanol. The resultant pellets were resuspended in a minimal volume of diethylpyrocarbonate (DEPC)–treated water. The RNA was run on a 1% agarose gel using morpholinopropanesulfonic (MOPS) running buffer to ensure there was no RNA degradation or contaminating genomic DNA.

REVERSE TRANSCRIPTASE–POLYMERASE CHAIN REACTION

A commercially available kit (RETROscript; Ambion, Austin, Tex) was used for the reverse transcriptase (RT) reaction as described by the manufacturer. Briefly, 2 μg of RNA

Continued on next page

during hemorrhagic shock, it seems plausible that skin contributes to the systemic elevation in proinflammatory cytokines following trauma and hemorrhage. Our aim, therefore, was to determine if proinflammatory cytokine expression was up-regulated after trauma-hemorrhage and resuscitation. Furthermore, the effect of remote soft tissue trauma and fracture on skin cytokine production was investigated.

RESULTS

GENE EXPRESSION FROM UNINJURED SKIN AND LIVER FOLLOWING TRAUMA-HEMORRHAGE

The results shown in **Figure 1** demonstrate expression of IL-1β, IL-6, and TNF-α in uninjured skin and liver samples harvested following trauma-hemorrhage and resuscitation. Skin samples (Figure 1, A) were obtained from dorsal uninjured skin that was remote from the site of laparotomy. Proinflammatory gene expression was also noted in the liver (Figure 1, B).

PROINFLAMMATORY CYTOKINE PRODUCTION IN ISOLATED SKIN

The results presented in **Figure 2** demonstrate release of IL-1β, IL-6, and TNF-α from skin placed in culture media following trauma-hemorrhage and resuscitation. Production of IL-1β by skin was significantly greater in trauma-hemorrhage animals relative to sham animals at all times assayed. Production of IL-6, although greater in trauma-hemorrhage animals at all times, was only found to be elevated to a significant degree at 1 and 24 hours after resuscitation. Production of TNF-α similarly was elevated in trauma-hemorrhage animals relative to sham animals at all times; however, statistically significant increases were seen only at 1 and 24 hours.

CIRCULATING LEVELS OF PROINFLAMMATORY CYTOKINES

Serum levels of IL-1β, IL-6, and TNF-α were elevated in trauma-hemorrhage animals relative to sham animals at 1 and 24 hours. Maximal circulating levels were seen at was added to the supplied deoxynucleotidetriphosphate (dNTP) mix and first-strand primers (Random Decamers; Ambion) in a final volume of 20 mL. The cocktail was heated to 85°C for 3 minutes and placed on ice. To this, 10× RT–polymerase chain reaction (PCR) buffer, placental RNAse inhibitor, and Moloney-murine leukemia virus RT were added and incubated at 42°C for 1 hour. The mixture was incubated at 92°C for 10 minutes to inactivate the RT, and the resultant complementary DNA was used in the PCR. A DNA Taq polymerase kit (SuperTaq; Ambion) was used to perform PCR as described by the manufacturer. Briefly, 4 mL of RT product was added to the reaction master mix (containing 10× reaction buffer and magnesium chloride, dNTP mix, and 5′-, and 3′-primers) in a final volume of 24 mL. The mixture was vortexed and heated to 95°C for 5 minutes, followed by 58°C for 5 minutes. Samples were then placed at 72°C, and 1 mL (0.5 U) of SuperTaq enzyme was added. The samples were run through a 30-cycle amplification on a programmable thermocycler gradient 96 (RoboCycler; Stratagene, La Jolla, Calif) set up as follows: 95°C for 1.5 minutes, 58°C for 2.5 minutes, and 72°C for 3 minutes. The primers for murine IL-1, IL-6, and TNF-α were obtained from Clontech, Palo Alto, Calif, and used according to the manufacturer's specifications. To control for RT activity and ensure uniform sample concentration, a control primer (S15 rRNA) was run with all samples. Resultant amplified DNA was run on a 2% agarose gel containing ethidium bromide, and the gels were photographed using commercially available film (Polaroid ISO 3000/36; Polaroid Corp, Cambridge, Mass). Images were captured using commercially available image analysis software (Mocha; Jandel Scientific, San Rafael, Calif). Results shown represent repeated experiments (n = 4).

SKIN CULTURE

At the appropriate time after the experimental procedure, animals were killed using methoxyflurane overdose. The dorsal surface of the animal was shaved and rinsed with 70% ethanol. A 2 × 2-cm sample of skin was dissected free from the underlying fascia and minced using surgical scissors. The tissue was placed in 2 mL of RPMI 1640 media supplemented with 10% fetal bovine serum, 10-mg/mL gentamycin, and 100-U/mL penicillin. The samples were incubated under standard tissue culture conditions (37°C, 5% carbon dioxide, and 85% humidity) for 8 hours. Following incubation, the supernatants were harvested and centrifuged at 10 000g and frozen at −80°C until assayed for cytokine concentration.

SKIN SUPERNATANT CYTOKINE PRODUCTION

The levels of IL-1β, IL-6, and TNF-α present in skin culture supernatants was determined using commercially available murine enzyme-linked immunosorbent assay (ELISA) kits. Six animals were included for each time. The IL-1β and TNF-α ELISA kits (DuoSet) were obtained from Genzyme Diagnostics (Cambridge, Mass). The IL-6 ELISA kit (OptEIA) was obtained from PharMingen (San Diego, Calif). The kits were used as described by the manufacturer.

CIRCULATING CYTOKINE LEVELS

Whole blood samples were obtained from sham and trauma-hemorrhage groups by cardiac puncture (n = 6) at the appropriate time after experimental treatment and methoxyflurane overdose. The samples were centrifuged at 10 000g for 10 minutes in serum separator tubes (Microtainer; Becton Dickinson, Franklin Lakes, NJ). The serum was removed and frozen at −80°C until assayed for cytokine concentration. Cytokine levels were determined using the ELISA kits described above.

STATISTICS

Differences between experimental groups were considered to be statistically significant if $P<.05$ as determined using 1-way analysis of variance and Tukey test.

1 hour for all 3 cytokines. These results are presented in the **Table**.

GENE EXPRESSION FROM INJURED AND UNINJURED SKIN FOLLOWING SOFT TISSUE TRAUMA

The results in **Figure 3A**, demonstrate that IL-1β, IL-6, and TNF-α gene expression is up-regulated in injured and uninjured skin following laparotomy (ie, soft tissue trauma) alone, in the absence of hemorrhagic shock. Figure 3B, also demonstrates proinflammatory cytokine gene expression in uninjured remote skin following unilateral closed tibial fracture.

COMMENT

Investigators have long sought the mechanisms responsible for the depression in organ function noted after injuries. The discovery and characterization of soluble mediators of inflammation, including cytokines and prostanoids, has greatly facilitated this study. Specifically, the proinflammatory cytokines IL-1β, IL-6, and TNF-α have been implicated in the mediation of organ dysfunction following hemorrhage and/or injury. The prevailing hypothesis regarding cytokine production following trauma and hemorrhage holds that the liver is the organ responsible for elaboration of these mediators. Ayala et al[17] demonstrated that production of Kupffer cell IL-1 and TNF was significantly increased following trauma and hemorrhage. Furthermore, O'Neill et al[18] reported that hepatic Kupffer cells were responsible for IL-6 release following trauma-hemorrhage and resuscitation and that depleting or inhibiting Kupffer cells with gadolinium chloride reduced the circulating levels of IL-6 by 80%. The effect of gadolinium chloride on the skin cytokine expression remains unknown, as does the effect of gadolinium chloride treatment on IL-1 and TNF production; thus it is not clear whether the liver is the sole organ affected by gadolinium chloride treatment. Using a model of hemorrhagic shock in rats, Deitch et al[19] found that portal vein levels of IL-1 and TNF were significantly higher than the concentration of these cytokines in cardiac (ie, systemic) blood, allowing them to conclude that the gut becomes a cytokine-liberating organ following hemorrhagic shock as well.

Our results indicate that proinflammatory gene expression is induced in the liver following trauma and hemorrhage. We also report an increase in IL-1β, IL-6, and TNF-α gene expression in uninjured skin following trauma-hemorrhage and resuscitation. Skin from trauma-hemorrhage animals released significantly more IL-1β, IL-6, and TNF-α at 1 and 24 hours after resuscitation, indicating that the increase in gene expression correlates with an increased elaboration of these cytokines. Since the skin is the largest immune organ in the body, and since it is capable of producing proinflammatory cytokines following trauma-hemorrhage, we suggest that skin may be another important source of circulating cytokines following injury. Evidence supporting the ability of skin to produce systemic elevations in cytokine levels is present in the literature. Skin injured by UV radiation is known to release histamine, kinins, cytokines, and cyclooxygenase- and lipoxygenase-derived products of

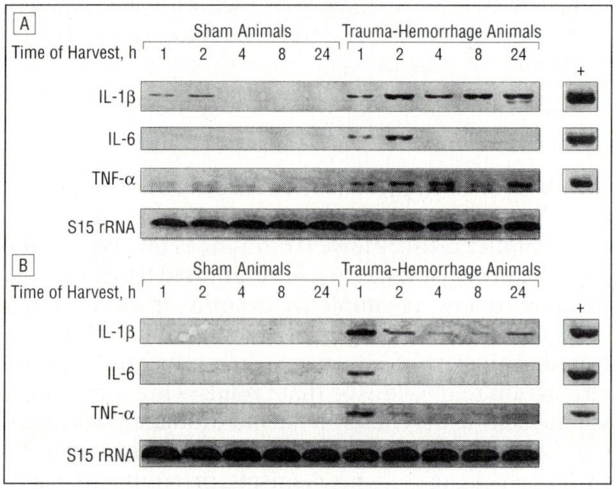

Figure 1. *Proinflammatory cytokine gene expression following trauma-hemorrhage and resuscitation. Expression of interleukin (IL) 1β, IL-6, tumor necrosis factor α (TNF-α), and S15 rRNA (positive control for RNA quality) was determined in animals undergoing sham operation (sham animals) and trauma-hemorrhage (trauma-hemorrhage animals) using reverse transcriptase–polymerase chain reaction with RNA isolated from uninjured skin (A) and liver (B). Samples were harvested 1, 2, 4, 8, or 24 hours after completion of resuscitation. Sham animals underwent anesthesia, groin dissection, and bilateral femoral artery ligation, and the time of harvest was adjusted to be comparable to the time of harvest in the trauma-hemorrhage animals. The lane at the far right (plus sign) is a positive control, indicating molecular weight of the amplified polymerase chain reaction product.*

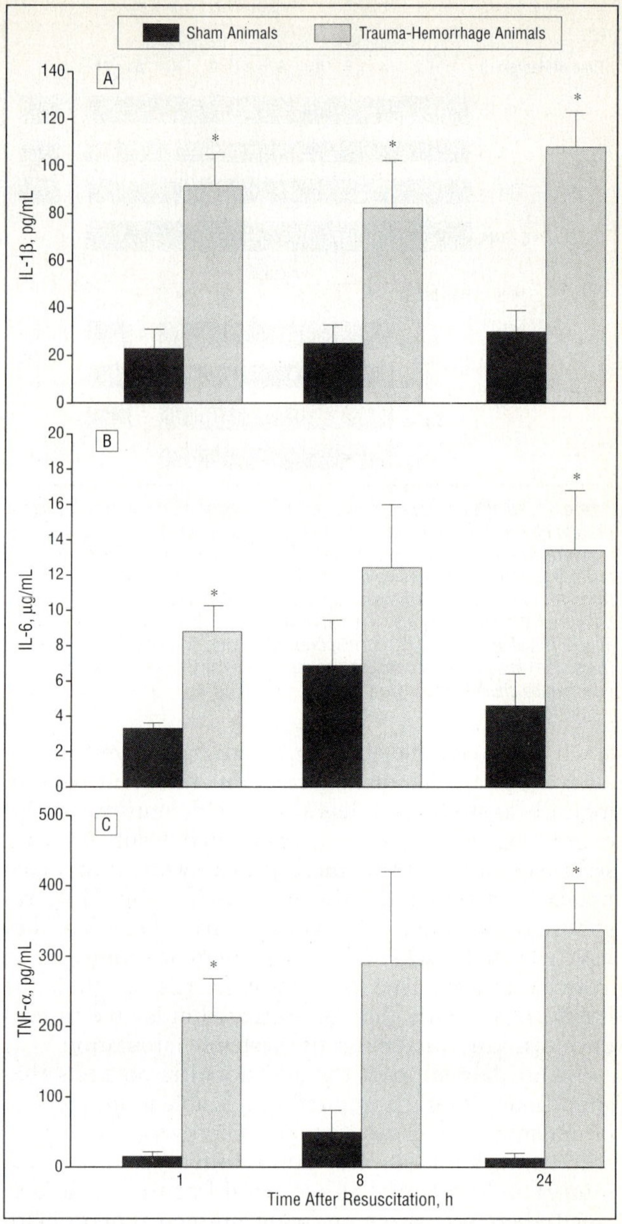

Figure 2. *Proinflammatory cytokine production by cultured skin following trauma-hemorrhage and resuscitation (trauma-hemorrhage animals). Culture supernatant levels of interleukin (IL) 1β (A), IL-6 (B), and tumor necrosis factor α (TNF-α) (C) were determined using enzyme-linked immunosorbent assay at 1, 8, and 24 hours after completion of resuscitation. Data are represented as mean ± SEM and compared using 1-way analysis of variance and Tukey test. Asterisk indicates* P<*.05 compared with animals undergoing sham operation (sham animals).*

Circulating Levels of Proinflammatory Cytokines After Trauma-Hemorrhage and Resuscitation*

Time of Harvest, h	IL-1β, pg/mL Sham	IL-1β, pg/mL Trauma-Hemorrhage	IL-6, pg/mL Sham	IL-6, pg/mL Trauma-Hemorrhage	TNF-α, pg/mL Sham	TNF-α, pg/mL Trauma-Hemorrhage
1	43.6 ± 13.4	129.6 ± 18.4†	16.5 ± 16.5	830.5 ± 150.1†	0	365.9 ± 49.7†
8	38.4 ± 9.3	75.4 ± 27.0	24.8 ± 15.7	172.6 ± 67.9	0	88.8 ± 51.3
24	20.3 ± 9.5	93.6 ± 20.0†	50.8 ± 18.8	457.1 ± 181.2†	8.4 ± 8.4	127.2 ± 59.4†

**IL indicates interleukin; TNF, tumor necrosis factor. Serum levels of IL-1β, IL-6, and TNF-α were determined using enzyme-linked immunosorbent assay at 1, 8, and 24 hours after completion of resuscitation. Data are represented as mean ± SEM and compared using 1-way analysis of variance and Tukey test.*

†P<*.05, animals undergoing trauma-hemorrhage vs animals undergoing sham operation.*

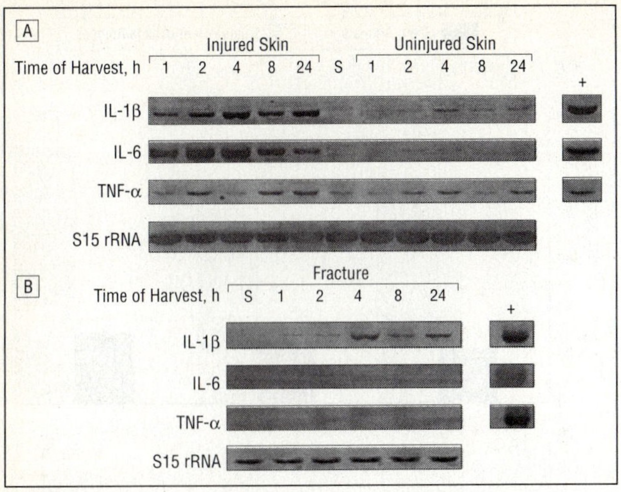

Figure 3. *Proinflammatory cytokine gene expression after soft tissue trauma (A) and closed long-bone fracture (B). Expression of interleukin (IL) 1β, IL-6, tumor necrosis factor α (TNF-α), and S15 rRNA (positive control for RNA quality) was determined using reverse transcriptase–polymerase chain reaction with RNA isolated from injured and uninjured skin (A) or remote, uninjured skin (B). Samples were harvested 1, 2, 4, 8, or 24 hours after injury. The sham control (S) corresponds to 1 hour. The lane at the far right (plus sign) is a positive control indicating molecular weight of the amplified polymerase chain reaction product.*

Statement of Clinical Relevance

Sepsis syndrome and multiple organ failure are the leading causes of death after hemorrhagic shock. The postulated mechanism responsible for this is an uncontrolled systemic inflammatory response. Circulating levels of proinflammatory cytokines are elevated after injury and hemorrhagic shock, and the gut and liver have been postulated to be the organ systems responsible for releasing these soluble mediators. Clinical trials aimed at reducing the systemic inflammatory response using anticytokine antibodies have shown promise in the experimental setting, yet they have been disappointing in human clinical trials. A better understanding of the mechanisms responsible for the up-regulation of proinflammatory cytokine production may allow us to tailor our therapy to prevent their release. Our data indicate that injured and uninjured skin are potential sources of circulating cytokines following hemorrhagic shock and severe injury. Further study aimed at elucidating the signals responsible for up-regulating skin cytokine production may allow us ultimately to block the production of proinflammatory cytokines after hemorrhagic shock, thus reducing the morbidity and mortality associated with severe injury.

arachidonic acid metabolism,[20] with these agents mediating the local inflammatory reaction evident histopathologically as sunburn. It has also been demonstrated that circulating levels of TNF-α are elevated in subjects with severe sunburn.[21] Furthermore, patients with primary cold urticaria, a skin condition in which a shocklike response occurs after cold exposure, have been found to have elevated levels of TNF-α in efferent venous blood from hands immersed in cold water.[22] Clearly, then, the literature supports the notion that skin is able to produce cytokines that enter the systemic circulation.

Our data support the additional hypothesis that after distant injury, uninjured skin is able to up-regulate proinflammatory genes. Cytokine expression was detectable using RT-PCR after laparotomy (ie, soft tissue injury) and unilateral closed tibial fracture. As anticipated, there was also a profound up-regulation of cytokine expression noted in injured skin. Previous investigators have found that following thermal injury, unburned skin produces TNF, IL-6, and IL-8 at the messenger RNA (mRNA) and protein levels.[10] In addition, Wichmann et al[23] have shown immune function to be more compromised after closed bone fracture and hemorrhagic shock than hemorrhage alone, suggesting that bone fracture induces the release of mediators that inhibit immune function. Thus, evidence suggests that soft tissue injury and long-bone fracture induce cytokine production in uninjured skin, and that the ability to induce cytokine gene expression in remote skin may account for the elevation in circulating cytokine levels associated with such injuries.

The mechanism mediating the up-regulation of cytokine gene expression in skin remains unknown. It is tempting to speculate that under conditions of hypoperfusion and regional hypoxia, skin cells respond with the production of proinflammatory cytokines. Previous studies from our laboratory have shown that hypoxemia, in the absence of hypotension or blood loss, is sufficient stimulus to induce the production of IL-1, IL-6, and TNF from Kupffer cells.[24] However, this does not explain the expression of cytokines in truly uninjured tissue (ie, that obtained following simple laparotomy or distant long-bone fracture). We propose that humoral factors are released at the site of injury and then travel through the circulation to the skin, or that impulses are transmitted via the central nervous system and ultimately act to up-regulate proinflammatory cytokine gene expression. To further elucidate these mechanisms, pretreatment of animals with anti-inflammatory drugs or nerve blocks would be illustrative.

Although this study provides evidence that the skin may be an important source of elevated cytokine levels following multiple types of injuries, many questions remain unanswered. We have not demonstrated the cellular source of cytokine expression in skin. As previously noted, skin contains numerous different cell populations known to produce cytokines. We propose that this question may be answered by using the technique of in situ hybridization. Despite the evidence that cytokines are spontaneously released from cultured skin after trauma-hemorrhage, we have not demonstrated that these cytokines in fact reach the circulation. In addition, the time course of gene expression and cytokine release from the tissue differed somewhat. Although IL-1β and TNF-α gene expression was elevated as early as 1 hour and as late as 24 hours after completion of resuscitation, IL-6 gene expression was limited to earlier times (1 and 2 hours). This is in contrast to tissue IL-6 release, which was elevated as late as 24 hours. Finally, circulating levels of IL-6, although elevated 24 hours after injury, were much higher at 1 hour, whereas IL-6 production in tissue culture remained elevated through 24 hours. Taken together, this suggests that skin is not the principal source of circulating IL-6 after injury.

Our study demonstrates that circulating proinflammatory cytokine levels are elevated following trauma-hemorrhage, and that this elevation correlates with enhanced gene expression and tissue culture production of these cytokines from uninjured skin. Furthermore, gene expression of IL-1β, IL-6, and TNF-α are up-regulated in uninjured skin after soft tissue trauma and closed bone fracture. Given the known deleterious effects of circulating proinflammatory cytokines on organ function after severe injury, therapies aimed at reducing or eliminating skin production of cytokines may be beneficial to the care of the trauma patient. Although extrapolation of these results to the human system is premature, given the accessibility of skin, reproduction of this study in humans should be possible.

This investigation was supported by grant R01 GM 37127 from the National Institutes of Health, Bethesda, Md (Dr Chaudry).

Presented at the 79th Annual Meeting of the New England Surgical Society, Toronto, Ontario, September 25, 1998.

Reprints: Irshad H. Chaudry, PhD, Center for Surgical Research, Rhode Island Hospital, Middle House II, 593 Eddy St, Providence, RI 02903 (e-mail: ichaudry@lifespan.org).

REFERENCES

1. Chaudry IH, Ayala A. *Immunological Aspects of Hemorrhage.* Austin, Tex: Medical Intelligence Unit, RG Landes Co; 1992.
2. Zellweger R, Ayala A, DeMaso CM, Chaudry IH. Trauma-hemorrhage causes prolonged depression in cellular immunity. *Shock.* 1995;4:149-153.
3. Narahara H, Johnston JM. Effects of endotoxins and cytokines on the secretion of platelet-activating factor acetylhydrolase by human decidual macrophages. *Am J Obstet Gynecol.* 1993;169:531-537.
4. Ayala A, Perrin MM, Ertel W, Chaudry IH. Differential effects of haemorrhage on Kupffer cells: decreased antigen presentation despite increased inflammatory cytokine (IL-1, IL-6 and TNF) release. *Cytokine.* 1992;4:66-75.
5. Simpson R, Alon R, Kobzik L, Valeri CR, Shepro D, Hechtman HB. Neutrophil and non-neutrophil-mediated injury in intestinal ischemia-reperfusion. *Ann Surg.* 1993;218:444-453.
6. Bos JD. The skin as an organ of immunity. *Clin Exp Immunol.* 1997;107:3-5.
7. Paquet P, Pierard GE. Interleukin-6 and the skin. *Int Arch Allergy Immunol.* 1996; 109:308-317.
8. Gatto H, Viac J, Charveron M, Schmitt D. Effects of thermal shock on interleukin-1 levels and heat shock protein 72 (HSP72) expression in normal human keratinocytes. *Arch Dermatol Res.* 1992;284:414-417.
9. Kupper TS, Deitch EA, Baker CC, Wong WC. The human burn wound as a primary source of interleukin-1 activity. *Surgery.* 1986;100:409-415.
10. Rodriguez JL, Miller CG, Garner WL, et al. Correlation of the local and systemic cytokine response with clinical outcome following thermal injury. *J Trauma.* 1993; 34:684-694.
11. Ohazto H, Monden M, Yoshizaki K, et al. Systemic production of interleukin-6 following acute inflammation. *Biochem Biophys Res Comm.* 1993;197:1556-1562.
12. Cetinkale O, Ulualp KM, Ayan F, Duren M, Cizmeci O, Pusane A. Early wound excision and skin grafting restores cellular immunity after severe burn trauma. *Br J Surg.* 1993;80:1296-1298.
13. Holliday MR, Dearman RJ, Corsini E, Basketter DA, Kimber I. Selective stimulation of cutaneous interleukin 6 expression by skin allergens. *J Appl Toxicol.* 1996; 16:65-70.
14. Hope JC, Dearman RJ, Kimber I, Hopkins SJ. The kinetics of cytokine production by draining lymph node cells following primary exposure of mice to chemical allergens. *Immunology.* 1994;83:250-255.
15. Martin P. Wound healing: aiming for perfect skin regeneration. *Science.* 1997; 276:75-81.
16. Peitzman AB, Billiar TB, Harbrecht BG, Udekwu AO, Kelly E, Simmons RL. Hemorrhagic shock. *Curr Probl Surg.* 1995;32:925-1002.
17. Ayala A, Perrin MM, Wang P, Ertel W, Chaudry IH. Hemorrhage induces enhanced Kupffer cell cytotoxicity while decreasing peritoneal or splenic macrophage capacity: involvement of cell-associated TNF and reactive nitrogen. *J Immunol.* 1991;147:4147-4154.
18. O'Neill PJ, Ayala A, Wang P, et al. Role of Kupffer cells in interleukin-6 release following trauma-hemorrhage and resuscitation. *Shock.* 1994;1:43-47.
19. Deitch EA, Xu D, Franko L, Ayala A, Chaudry IH. Evidence favoring the role of the gut as a cytokine-generating organ in rats subjected to hemorrhagic shock. *Shock.* 1994;1:141-146.
20. Soter NA. Acute effects of ultraviolet radiation on the skin. *Semin Dermatol.* 1990; 9:11-15.
21. Kock A, Schwarz T, Kirnbauer R, et al. Human keratinocytes are a source for tumor necrosis factor α: evidence for synthesis and release upon stimulation with endotoxin or ultraviolet light. *J Exp Med.* 1990;172:1609-1614.
22. Tillie-Leblond I, Gosset P, Janin A, et al. Tumor necrosis factor-α release during systemic reaction in cold urticaria. *J Allergy Clin Immunol.* 1994;93:501-509.
23. Wichmann MW, Zellweger R, DeMaso CM, Ayala A, Williams C, Chaudry IH. Immune function is more compromised after closed bone fracture and hemorrhagic shock than hemorrhage alone. *Arch Surg.* 1996;131:995-1000.
24. Ertel W, Morrison MH, Ayala A, Chaudry IH. Hypoxemia in the absence of blood loss or significant hypotension causes inflammatory cytokine release. *Am J Physiol.* 1995;269:R160-R166.

DISCUSSION

Herbert B. Hechtman, MD, Boston, Mass: These are superb testable hypotheses with crisp data, giving us the nicely presented results. Drs Catania and Chaudry have continued to educate us at these meetings with regard to the mechanisms of inflammation following trauma. The subject matter, that is, cytokines, is in step with their recent emphasis on Kupffer cells that we heard about last year.

There are 3 separate models that are presented, each of which stimulates cytokine production by skin. Following hemorrhage and resuscitation, one might argue that the cytokine response is secondary to the generalized as well as local stimulus of ischemia and reperfusion. Of equal interest is the observation that the so-called sham group, those animals that had only their femoral arteries ligated, also expressed cytokine mRNA.

I had the opportunity of seeing the manuscript and studying the blots which are presented there, but might have escaped your scrutiny during this presentation. This is fascinating to me. Would the authors think that this rise in mRNA could be a remote tissue response to hind-limb ischemia and reperfusion much as occurs remotely in other organs that they've described, such as the liver and the lungs?

Positive findings in another sham group are more perplexing. That a sham incision leads to message expression for TNF-α indicates that multiple variables may be operative. Is there any information available regarding the role of changes in skin temperature on cytokine production?

Your observation of the importance of a simple laparotomy incision in provoking remote cytokine gene expression was really unexpected. It's reminiscent of our experience in patients of prominent systemic prostacycline synthesis accompanied by a slight but significant fall in blood pressure following simple laparotomy. Could you speculate about the mechanism of your observation? You imply that circulating mediators are of primary importance, and I certainly agree.

Dr Catania: There are quite a few questions to answer. In terms of the up-regulation of IL-1 that was evident in the sham group, I agree with you there is something occurring during the sham procedure. Whether it is related to the hind-limb ischemia, which could result from our bilateral catheterization of the femoral arteries, or in the case of shams, tying off the femoral arteries, or whether it is due to the incision itself, I'm not entirely sure. What is clear is that in animals that undergo no surgical procedure, there is no up-regulation of IL-1 in skin, so there is some component to the sham procedure which does elevate gene expression.

In terms of the elevated TNF in sham incisions, TNF was a rather interesting gene to work with, both in the liver and in the skin. We did see TNF expression variably in our sham animals, usually at very low levels. Whether this has something to do with the change in tissue temperature, or whether it has something to do with the actual procedure of anesthesia and restraint which the sham animals all undergo, I'm not exactly sure.

I agree with you that the findings following simple laparotomy were somewhat unexpected. When we designed this experiment, we actually thought that laparotomy would be a negative control. We believed that the main driving force behind cytokine expression in skin following trauma-hemorrhage would be hypotension and tissue hypoxia or hypoperfusion. There are a few experiments we would like to perform to further elucidate the mechanisms responsible for this up-regulation in gene expression. A soluble factor, such as prostanoid, may mediate this effect, and pretreatment with either ibuprofin or indomethacin to block these pathways would be interesting to determine if this is the mechanism which regulates skin gene expression. However, given the fact that this up-regulation occurs so rapidly, I also think that there is a fair chance the central nervous system is playing a role, and as we all know, the skin is very densely innervated. We would like to try to denervate the area where we perform our laparotomy and see if that has any effect on gene expression.

Mark Callery, MD, Worcester, Mass: I'd like you to just talk to us about nature for a second if you would. It seems that nature put 2 of the largest macrophage populations in the body conveniently at an environmental interface, namely, the macrophages of the skin (air) and the macrophages of the liver (gut). So my question to you is whether this response is a protective response that nature has provided, or is it wrong just because you're saying it's producing cytokines in response to an injury?

Dr Catania: I would be hesitant to ever criticize nature on evolution, which seems to have done a pretty good job in most cases. In the case following trauma and hemorrhage, however, I don't know that we were necessarily meant to survive some of the injuries that we now routinely survive, thanks to medical intervention. Whether or not a less vigorous response would be protective in a less significant injury, I can only assume that it would be. This is why we're always hesitant to tinker with the cytokine release, because clearly if it didn't have some beneficial role it would have evolved away. Exactly what constitutes a good response and what constitutes an overactive response remains to be determined.

Brad Patterson, MD, Weybridge, Vt: For those of us who are not very familiar with cytokine levels, could you make some comment about whether these are important at a systemic level, the kind of thing we're used to hearing about as side effects of cytokines?

Dr Catania: I believe most cytokines function in a microenvironment. When we start seeing high levels of cytokines systemically, that's usually when the cytokines are implicated in having a negative role. What the levels of the cytokines are in the microcirculation around the area of injury is probably the important factor in things like wound healing. Clearly the levels of cytokines in a healing wound are well in excess of the systemic levels we see here. However, when systemic cytokines levels do increase significantly, their action becomes less predictable. Their influence on neutrophil function following gut ischemia, for example, has been fairly well described by Dr Hechtman's group. Based on previous research, we presume that systemic elevations in cytokine levels have a detrimental effect.

Surgical Anatomy

The branches of the thyrocervical trunk may be remembered by the acronym, STAT:

S = suprascapular artery
T = transverse cervical artery
A = ascending cervical artery
T = thyroid artery, inferior

1. Blackbourne LH, Fleischer KJ. *Advanced Surgical Recall*. Baltimore, Md: Williams & Wilkins; 1997:34.

PAPER

Extracorporeal Membrane Oxygenation for Nonneonatal Acute Respiratory Failure

Peter T. Masiakos, MD; Saleem Islam, MD; Daniel P. Doody, MD; Jay J. Schnitzer, MD, PhD; Daniel P. Ryan, MD

Hypothesis: Extracorporeal membrane oxygenation (ECMO) is effective in nonneonatal acute respiratory failure under certain circumstances.

Design: Retrospective medical record review.

Setting: The intensive care unit of a tertiary care hospital.

Patients: Thirty-four nonneonatal patients (mean age, 22 years; range, 8 days to 56 years), with ratios of the PaO_2 to the fraction of inspired oxygen persistently below 70, who were treated with ECMO after maximal ventilator therapy had failed (mean time of ventilator therapy, 6.9 days; range, 1-41 days). The mean ECMO duration was 304 hours (range, 56-934 hours). Patients were grouped into 7 categories based on their diagnosis: sepsis or sepsis syndrome (n = 3), bacterial or fungal pneumonia (n = 10), viral pneumonia (n = 5), trauma or burn (n = 2), inhalation injury without burn (n = 1), immunocompromised state (due to transplantation or chemotherapy) (n = 8), and acute respiratory failure of unknown origin (n = 5).

Main Outcome Measure: Survival to hospital discharge following ECMO therapy.

Results: Overall survival was 53% (18 patients). All 6 patients (100%) with viral pneumonias or isolated inhalation injuries survived. Of 13 patients with bacterial pneumonia, sepsis, or sepsis syndrome not complicated by multiorgan failure, 10 (77%) survived. In contrast, all but 1 of the immunocompromised patients died. Survival in patients who were intubated for less than 9 days before ECMO was 64%, whereas survival fell precipitously to 22% for patients who experienced mechanical ventilation for 9 or more days before the implementation of ECMO. Finally, the proportion of patients who died while receiving ECMO therapy was greater when the ECMO duration exceeded 300 hours (62% vs 38%; $P<.05$).

Conclusions: Nonneonatal survival with ECMO therapy is strongly dependent on the diagnosis. Pre-ECMO intubation for less than 9 days had little effect on survival. Survival rates decreased when the length of time of receiving ECMO exceeded 300 hours.

Arch Surg. 1999;134:375-380

Acute respiratory failure (ARF) in nonneonatal patients is an infrequent occurrence with devastating consequences. Although fewer than 2% of all admissions to intensive care units are complicated by severe ARF, mortality rates reported in the pediatric and adult literature[1,2] exceed 80%. Conventional mechanical ventilatory support is designed to improve gas exchange without worsening the underlying lung injury. The support these critically ill patients require, however, often exceeds the supplemental oxygen, positive end-expiratory pressure (PEEP), and positive pressure ventilation limits that have been shown to cause irreversible damage and fibrosis of the lung parenchyma.[3,4]

Extracorporeal membrane oxygenation (ECMO), introduced successfully in 1972,[5] has been most commonly used as a means of cardiopulmonary support for patients with recoverable pulmonary insufficiency in whom maximal conventional therapies were exhausted. Generally accepted as an alternative method of ventilatory support in neonates, it has only recently begun to attract advocates of its use in nonneonatal, noncardiac patients.[6-9] Most recently, in a retrospective review, Green et al[9] showed an ECMO-dependent improvement in survival for 331 pediatric patients aged 13 days to 18 years from 32 hospitals. Still, many critics[10] argue that ECMO remains a futile or expensive technology that extends intensive care unit admissions but offers little more for outcome than current optimal therapies do. The controversy has spurred the users of ECMO technology to review current management schemes frequently and to provide evidence for changing them based on experience. These reviews have also provided further insight into identifying when ECMO has ceased to be beneficial for the subset of patients described here.

From the Department of Surgery, Pediatric Surgical Service, Massachusetts General Hospital, Harvard Medical School, Boston.

PATIENTS AND METHODS

Between February 1, 1990, and April 30, 1998, 34 patients aged 8 days to 56 years with refractory ARF were consecutively treated with venoarterial or venovenous extracorporeal lung support in the neonatal, pediatric, and adult intensive care units at the Massachusetts General Hospital, Boston. Patients were identified retrospectively by reviewing office records from the pediatric surgical service ECMO database. The hospital medical record for each patient was reviewed, and pertinent information was recorded. A favorable outcome was defined as patient survival and discharge from the hospital.

Patients were considered for enrollment using a modification of Extracorporeal Life Support Organization criteria[11]; all patients were treated with ECMO after severe ARF developed and maximal ventilator therapy that required prolonged oxygenation with 100% oxygen failed. The patients had mean ± SD ratios of PaO_2 to the fraction of inspired oxygen of 85.0 ± 22.9 for survivors and 56.9 ± 4.8 (P=.27) for nonsurvivors. They were considered for ECMO therapy only after all septic foci had been drained, pulmonary air leaks were managed with thoracostomy tubes, and all identified infections were treated with appropriate antibiotic therapy.

Patients were separated into 2 groups: survivors (n = 18) and nonsurvivors (n = 16). The characteristics for these patients—age, the duration of ECMO therapy, ventilatory support variables before ECMO therapy, and laboratory values—are shown in **Table 1**.

Ventilator management while receiving ECMO was directed at limiting airway pressures by maintaining peak inspiratory pressures of less than 30 cm H_2O and PEEP between 20 and 24 cm H_2O. Large air leaks were treated with no PEEP and minimal ventilation until they resolved. Anticoagulation maintained activated clotting times at 180 ± 20 (mean ± SD) seconds for all patients.

Statistical analyses on the data presented in Table 1 were performed using the Student *t* test. To determine whether age was a significant predictor of outcome, analysis of variance was performed.

The purpose of this retrospective study is to report the results of the ECMO experience in nonneonatal patients with severe ARF. In addition, the data presented here provide confirmatory evidence that ECMO can be beneficial in this patient population. Finally, this report may aid in the design of more appropriate selection criteria for critically ill patients with ARF for whom conventional therapy has failed.

RESULTS

Thirty-four nonneonatal patients received ECMO support during the 8 years that were reviewed. The male-to-female ratio was 5:9 for the survivors and 13:3 for the nonsurvivors. Of the 34 patients with ARF, 21 (62%) recovered lung function and were weaned from extracorporeal support. Of these, 18 patients (53%) survived and were discharged from the hospital. Of patients who were weaned from ECMO and subsequently died, 1 patient died of complications from an underlying congenital heart lesion, and 2 patients who were previously treated with bleomycin sulfate had gradually progressive respiratory failure. The mean age for the group as a whole was 22 years (range, 8 days to 56 years). The age of the patients in the survivor group ranged from 8 days to 53 years (mean, 19.8 years) compared with the patients in the nonsurvivor group, whose age ranged from 2 months to 56 years (mean, 24.6 years). The mean of the 2 groups did not differ significantly; however, a bimodal distribution was observed when patient age was plotted against the frequency of survival (**Figure 1**). Furthermore, there was a significant increase in survival of patients in the later peak ($P<.05$) as the ECMO experience progressed through the 8 years (**Figure 2**).

The total number of days during which the patients were treated with assisted ventilation before ECMO therapy varied from 1 to 41 days (mean, 6.9 days). The duration of ECMO ranged from 56 to 934 hours (mean, 304 hours). The proportion of patients who died while receiving ECMO was greater when the ECMO duration exceeded 300 hours (8/13 [62%] vs 8/21 [38%]; $P<.05$). Survival by the duration of mechanical ventilation preceding ECMO is shown in **Figure 3**. Patients who received ventilatory support for fewer than 9 days had a significantly better outcome ($P<.05$).

For all categories, differences between the survivors and nonsurvivors were not significant, with the exception of the number of hours that PEEP exceeded 8 cm H_2O and the number of units of packed red blood cells transfused before and during the implementation of ECMO. Patients were grouped into 7 categories based on their primary discharge diagnosis: sepsis or sepsis syndrome (n = 3), bacterial or fungal pneumonia (n = 10), viral pneumonia (n = 5), trauma or burn (n = 2), inhalation injury without burn (n = 1), immunocompromised state (due to transplantation or chemotherapy) (n = 8), and ARF, unknown origin (n = 5). Survival for each group is shown in **Table 2**.

COMMENT

Respiratory insufficiency in nonneonatal patients is usually self-limiting. In the few patients in whom fulminant respiratory failure develops, however, reported mortality exceeds 50%. If pulmonary failure progresses in this group, and conventional management schemes are exhausted, mortality rates approach 90%.[12] Experimental models[3] suggest that the irreversible progression to death in nonneonatal patients is caused in part by the iatrogenic damage of the lung occurring with prolonged positive-pressure mechanical ventilation needed to overcome the ventilation-perfusion mismatches resulting from parenchymal shunting. Management strategies have been designed[13] to improve oxygenation and minimize the mechanical damage associated with high alveolar pressure. These include low-volume and high-frequency ventilation, reversed inhalation to exhalation ratios, pressure-

Table 1. Patient Characteristics, Arterial Blood Gas Values, and Laboratory Values*

Variable	Survivors (n = 18)	Nonsurvivors (n = 16)	*P*
Age, y	19.8 ± 3.9	24.6 ± 4.3	.46
Time on ECMO therapy, h	250.0 ± 42.1	366.0 ± 72.7	.16
Pre-ECMO ventilation			
Ventilatory support, d	4.8 ± 2.5	9.3 ± 0.8	.08
Peak inspiratory pressure (PIP), cm H_2O	46.4 ± 3.0	53.8 ± 4.7	.18
Positive end-expiratory pressure (PEEP), cm H_2O	13.6 ± 1.1	15.8 ± 1.2	.19
FIO_2 >0.9, h	32.3 ± 9.7	74.3 ± 43.8	.33
PIP >40 cm H_2O, h	37.7 ± 9.7	134.5 ± 55.9	.08
PEEP >8 cm H_2O, h	42.7 ± 6.6	177.8 ± 58.4	.02
Pre-ECMO arterial blood gas values			
pH	7.30 ± 0.02	7.32 ± 0.03	.57
PaO_2, mm Hg	78.8 ± 20.4	53.9 ± 3.5	.26
$PaCO_2$, mm Hg	61.4 ± 5.5	60.8 ± 5.7	.94
Alveolar-arterial gradient	531 ± 30	559 ± 21	.46
PaO_2/FIO_2 ratio	85 ± 23	57 ± 5	.27
Laboratory values			
Pre-ECMO PRBC transfusion, U	2.3 ± 0.9	9.6 ± 3.2	.03
PRBC transfusions on ECMO therapy, U	15.5 ± 4.6	41.7 ± 9.6	.02
Pre-ECMO WBC count, × 10^9/L	18.0 ± 1.9	15.7 ± 3.7	.57
Pre-ECMO hematocrit, %	34.0 ± 1.3	33.7 ± 1.6	.87
Pre-ECMO platelet count, × 10^9/L	215 ± 40	170 ± 37	.42
Pre-ECMO serum creatinine, µmol/L (mg/dL)	66.0 ± 8.8 (0.8 ± 0.1)	97.2 ± 17.7 (1.1 ± 0.2)	.09

Data are given as mean ± SEM. ECMO indicates extracorporeal membrane oxygenation; FIO_2, fraction of inspired oxygen; PRBC, packed red blood cell; and WBC, white blood cell.

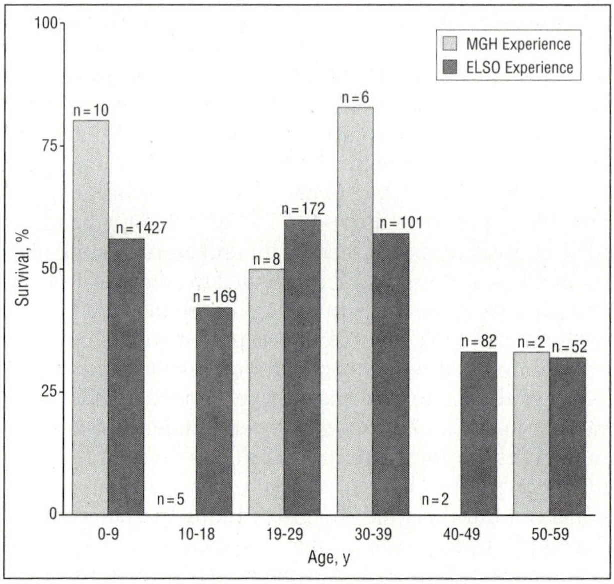

Figure 1. *Patient survival (percentage) by age. The Massachusetts General Hospital (MGH), Boston, experience was compared with the Extracorporeal Life Support Organization (ELSO) database.*

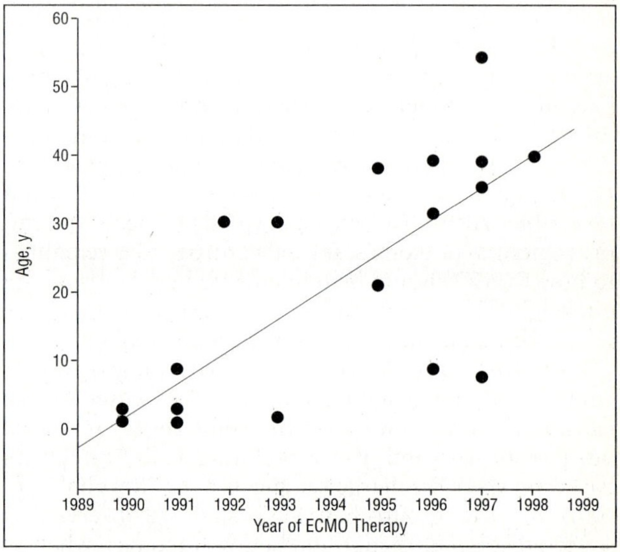

Figure 2. *Survival by year of extracorporeal membrane oxygenation (ECMO) therapy and age of patient. Each circle represents a patient who survived therapy with ECMO and was discharged from the hospital.*

controlled ventilation to maintain peak inspiratory pressures under 40 cm H_2O, permissive hypercapnia, and inhaled nitric oxide. All strategies are designed to promote optimal ventilation and perfusion, to minimize positive pressure–related parenchymal damage, and to afford the greatest capacity for recovery of the already-insulted lung.[14,15] Still, the mortality of the patients not responding to these therapies exceeds 50%, and alternative methods of support have been studied.

Poor survival in adults was initially reported by Zapol et al[16] after an ambitious multicenter, randomized ECMO trial. Subsequently, the application of ECMO in this population was forestalled. At the same time, however, Bartlett et al[17] showed dramatic successes in the treatment of refractory neonatal ARF by ECMO. There is little debate regarding its efficacy in these patients, as it has been shown[18] to improve survival rates to 80% in patients with a predicted mortality of 90%. Soon thereafter, Gattinoni et al[19] reported improved survival for adults with ARF using extracorporeal removal of carbon dioxide. The Extracorporeal Life Support Organization and its registry, as well as others,[8,13,20] have since reported a combined survival for the nonneonatal, noncardiac group of pa-

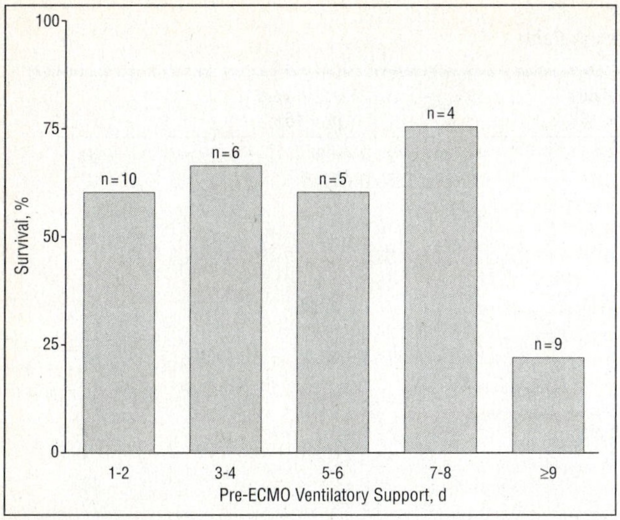

Figure 3. *Patient survival (percentage) by duration of mechanical ventilation. A significant difference (P<.05) in survival after extracorporeal membrane oxygenation (ECMO) therapy was observed when mechanical ventilation before ECMO exceeded 8 days.*

tients of greater than 50%. The growing neonatal experience, together with reports of successes in adults, has led to an expanded use in patients other than neonates. In addition to longer treatment periods, the improvement in survival is thought to have been most influenced by the development of newer technologies, management strategies, and a better understanding of which patients may benefit from these technologies. Guidelines have been established to aid in the selection of patients who would be the most appropriate candidates for ECMO. These were defined as those who had "severe but reversible" ARF.[21] Despite changes in protocols and improvement in outcomes, several controversies remain as to how ECMO should be implemented so that risks are outweighed by benefits and outcomes are better than they would be if conventional therapies were applied.

Recently, several investigators[13] have studied the outcomes for nonneonatal patients with ARF based on the cause of their respiratory failure. Similarly, we reviewed our patient base and placed each into 1 of 7 categories based on their discharge diagnosis (see "Results" section). As other groups have suggested, we observe that several disease states portend better outcomes, whereas the course of others is unchanged by ECMO therapy. Overall survival in our institution was 53% (18 patients). More interestingly, survival in patients presenting with isolated viral pneumonias, isolated inhalation injuries, or with sepsis or sepsis syndrome with ARF but not complicated by multiorgan failure was 100% (9 patients). In contrast, 1 (12%) of the 8 patients who were immunocompromised either as a result of chemotherapy for the treatment of cancer or by immunosuppression for organ transplantation survived to hospital discharge. Although 2 of the 7 nonsurvivors were weaned from extracorporeal support and the cannula removed, they subsequently died of a progressive respiratory failure thought to be related to their past bleomycin therapy. Therefore, as many have thought, these patients may not be suitable candidates for ECMO therapy. Similarly poor

Table 2. Cause of Acute Respiratory Failure and Outcome

Diagnosis	No. of Patients (n = 34)	Survival, No. (%)
Sepsis or sepsis syndrome	3	3 (100)
Bacterial or fungal pneumonia	10	4 (40)
Viral pneumonia	5	5 (100)
Trauma or burn	2	0 (0)
Inhalation injury without burn	1	1 (100)
Immunocompromised state*	8	1 (12)
Unknown etiology	5	4 (80)

**Transplantation or chemotherapy.*

outcomes were seen for patients with ARF complicated by multiorgan failure or precipitated by trauma or burns. In this series, the disease process appeared to be significantly effective in identifying those patients with "reversible" lung injury in whom ECMO may be of benefit.

Most authors agree that limiting lung injury before and during ECMO is of paramount importance when considering whether a patient is capable of survival. Identifying patients earlier in their "reversible" disease progression, and thereby limiting the well-characterized pre-ECMO ventilatory insult, should improve survival. Pranikoff et al[20] showed that pre-ECMO mechanical ventilation exceeding 5 days was a poor prognostic indicator in adults. Our data suggest that there is no significant difference in survival in those patients who had had up to 9 days of pre-ECMO ventilatory support and that a lesser but substantial percentage of patients who receive mechanical ventilation for longer than 9 days will survive to discharge after ECMO therapy.

Early in the ECMO experience, Zapol et al[16] considered the appropriate duration of ECMO therapy in adults to be equivalent to that seen by investigators treating neonates. Most authors at that time failed to take into account any possible differences in the resilience of the damaged lung parenchyma that may be expected in the nonneonates compared with neonates. The results reported by Zapol et al, therefore, as many have come to realize, came early in the ECMO learning curve and underestimated the time necessary for the return of lung function in the nonneonatal group. The centers that participated in the National Institutes of Health–sponsored adult trial allowed only 5 days of ECMO, and if no improvement was seen, it was considered futile and discontinued. Since then, the average time of extracorporeal support in nonneonatal patients has been better defined, the mean ± SD duration of ECMO for these patients now being reported as 10.3 ± 6.8 days.[22] The cannulation time for our patients ranged from 2.3 to 38.9 days (mean, 12.6 days). More important, the difference in the mean cannulation time of the survivors (10.4 days) from that of the nonsurvivors (15.3 days) is apparently not significant. The proportion of patients who died while receiving ECMO, however, was greater when the ECMO duration exceeded 12.5 days (8/13 [62%] vs 8/21 [38%]; *P*<.05). Still, 5 of the 18 patients in the survivor group had ECMO durations exceeding 300 hours.

When considering a patient with ARF of unknown origin, age may prove to be a useful prognostic indicator. When the age of the patients in this series was plotted as a function of survival, a bimodal distribution resulted. The survivors tended to cluster between 8 days and 9 years of age and then again between 29 and 38 years of age (Figure 1). Patients who were older than 38 years had poorer outcomes. Meyer and Jepson[6] made a similar observation for their group of patients. We first thought that this phenomenon was a reflection of the small number of patients in our series. When all available data from the Extracorporeal Life Support Organization database for the nonneonatal, noncardiac patients was accumulated and plotted in the same way, however, this distribution was confirmed (Figure 1). Although we cannot conclusively identify the reason for this observation, a likely explanation may be, as Meyer and Jepson suggest, that diseases (viral or bacterial pneumonias) that cluster in certain age groups may result in more easily reversible pulmonary dysfunction. The Extracorporal Life Support Organization database should be reviewed to compare the underlying diseases in the various age groups.

CONCLUSIONS

Improvements in ECMO technology and the reevaluation of criteria for patient selection for extracorporeal support have greatly improved survival. We provide additional data that may be helpful when deciding whether a patient with ARF might benefit from the lung rest that is afforded by ECMO. Still, many questions remain unanswered. A multicenter, randomized trial would be appropriate to better define the population of patients who would most benefit by this therapeutic option.

Presented at the 79th Annual Meeting of the New England Surgical Society, Toronto, Ontario, September 26, 1998.

We would like to thank the respiratory therapists; neonatal, pediatric, and adult intensive care unit nursing staff; and our colleagues in pediatric and adult intensive care medicine who cared for these patients during their most critical hours. We also thank Steve Conrad, MD, PhD, of Louisiana State University, Baton Rouge, and Peter Rycus, MPH, of the University of Michigan, Ann Arbor, and the Extracorporeal Life Support Organization registry for generously providing us with the current registry data.

Corresponding author: Daniel P. Ryan, MD, Department of Surgery, Pediatric Surgical Service, Massachusetts General Hospital, Harvard Medical School, 40 Fruit St, WRN 1131, Boston, MA 02114.

REFERENCES

1. Rivera RA, Butt W, Shann F. Predictors of mortality in children with respiratory failure: possible indications for ECMO. *Anaesth Intensive Care.* 1990;18:385-389.
2. Zapol WM, Frikker MJ, Pontoppidan H, et al. The adult respiratory distress syndrome at Massachusetts General Hospital. In: Zapol WM, Lemaire F, eds. *Adult Respiratory Distress Syndrome.* New York, NY: Marcel Dekker Inc; 1991: 367-380.
3. Kolobow T, Moretti MP, Fumagalli R, et al. Severe impairment in lung function induced by high peak airway pressure during mechanical ventilation: an experimental study. *Am Rev Respir Dis.* 1987;135:312-315.
4. Dreyfuss D, Basset G, Soler P, Saumon G. Intermittent positive-pressure hyperventilation with high inflation pressures produces pulmonary microvascular injury in rats. *Am Rev Respir Dis.* 1985;132:880-884.
5. Hill JD, O'Brien TG, Murray JJ, et al. Prolonged extracorporeal oxygenation for acute post-traumatic respiratory failure (shock-lung syndrome): use of the Bramson membrane lung. *N Engl J Med.* 1972;286:629-634.
6. Meyer DM, Jepson ME. Results of extracorporeal membrane oxygenation in children with sepsis: the Extracorporeal Life Support Organization. *Ann Thorac Surg.* 1997;63:756-761.
7. Macha M, Griffith BP, Keenan R, et al. ECMO support for adult patients with acute respiratory failure. *ASAIO J.* 1996;42:M841-M844.
8. Ryan DP, Doody DP. Treatment of acute pulmonary failure with extracorporeal support: 100% survival in a pediatric population. *J Pediatr Surg.* 1992;27:1111-1117.
9. Green TP, Timmons OD, Fackler JC, Moler FW, Thompson AE, Sweeney MF. The impact of extracorporeal membrane oxygenation on survival in pediatric patients with acute respiratory failure: Pediatric Critical Care Study Group. *Crit Care Med.* 1996;24:323-329.
10. Morris AH, Wallace CJ, Menlove KL, et al. Randomized clinical trial of pressure-controlled inverse ratio ventilation and extracorporeal CO_2 removal for adult respiratory distress syndrome. *Am J Respir Care Med.* 1994;149(2 pt 1):295-305.
11. Custer JR, Fackler J. ECLS for children with acute respiratory distress syndrome. In: Zwischenberger JB, Bartlett RH, eds. *ECMO: Extracorporeal Cardiopulmonary Support in Critical Care.* Ann Arbor, Mich: Extracorporeal Life Support Organization; 1995:chap 20.
12. Suchyta MR, Clemmer TP, Orme JF Jr, Morris AH, Elliott CG. Increased survival of ARDS patients with severe hypoxemia (ECMO criteria). *Chest.* 1991;99:951-955.
13. Peek GJ, Sosnowski AW. Extracorporeal membrane oxygenation for pediatric respiratory failure. *Br Med Bull.* 1997;53:745-756.
14. Hickling KG, Henderson SJ, Jackson R. Low mortality associated with low volume pressure limited ventilation with permissive hypercapnia in severe adult respiratory distress syndrome. *Intensive Care Med.* 1990;16:372-377.
15. Bidani A, Tzouanakis AE, Cardenas VJ Jr, Zwischenberger JB. Permissive hypercapnia in acute respiratory failure. *JAMA.* 1994;272:957-962.
16. Zapol WM, Snider MT, Hill JD, et al. Extracorporeal membrane oxygenation in severe acute respiratory failure: a randomized prospective study. *JAMA.* 1979; 242:2193-2196.
17. Bartlett RH, Andrews AF, Toomasian JM, Haiduc NJ, Gazzaniga AB. Extracorporeal membrane oxygenation for newborn respiratory failure: forty-five cases. *Surgery.* 1982;92:425-433.
18. Rosenberg EM, Seguin JH. Selection criteria for use of ECLS in neonates. In: Zwischenberger JB, Bartlett RH, eds. *ECMO: Extracorporeal Cardiopulmonary Support in Critical Care.* Ann Arbor, Mich: Extracorporeal Life Support Organization; 1995.
19. Gattinoni L, Pesenti A, Rossi GP. Treatment of acute respiratory failure with low-frequency positive-pressure ventilation and extracorporeal removal of CO_2. *Lancet.* 1980;2:292-294.
20. Pranikoff T, Hirschl RB, Steimle CN, Anderson HL III, Bartlett RH. Mortality is directly related to the duration of mechanical ventilation before the initiation of extracorporeal life support for severe respiratory failure. *Crit Care Med.* 1997; 25:28-32.
21. Bernard GR, Artigas A, Brigham KL, et al. The American-European Consensus Conference on ARDS: definitions, mechanisms, relevant outcomes, and clinical trial coordination. *Am J Respir Crit Care Med.* 1994;149(pt 1):818-824.
22. Moler FW, Custer JR, Bartlett RH, et al. Extracorporeal life support for severe pediatric respiratory failure: an updated experience, 1991-1993. *J Pediatr.* 1994; 124:875-880.

DISCUSSION

Hardy Hendren, MD, Boston, Mass: The work in each of these ECMO patients, for those of you who have not witnessed it, is absolutely enormous. Yesterday I asked the authors to estimate how many hours they would spend each day at the bedside of 1 of these patients. It is conservatively about 6 hours. A little calculation—6 hours a day for 1 of the 300-hour ECMO-support patients, which is 13 days—indicates that this is roughly the equivalent of doing 20 open heart operations or 10 to 15 Whipple operations, depending on the speed of the operator.

The authors have shown us that a survival of 53% can be achieved in this group of desperately ill patients, for whom the predicted mortality would be 80% otherwise, so this is a significant salvage. They have shown us that multiorgan failure and an immunocompromised state are bad predictors for these patients and that short-term support, that is, less than 13 days, is more apt to result in success than long-term support, that is, more than 300 hours.

I would like to ask the authors 3 questions: First, you've shown that patients younger than 10 years and those in their

30s had a higher likelihood of survival. What's the problem with being in the 10- to 30-year age group?

The second question is, you've shown us that single-organ failure, that is, the lung, and short-term patients do best. Do you have absolute contraindications to the use of ECMO? And how about age? Are about two thirds of the people in this audience beyond the age limit and would you write us off or would you give us a chance with ECMO in the final analysis if it were a single-organ lung failure?

The third question is, when you cross that threshold of 300 hours or 13 days, when and how do you decide to turn off the ECMO?

Pardon Kenney, MD, Boston: Your survival data are obviously impressive. I have a quality-of-life question. How many of your survivors required permanent ventilators, and how many of them actually ended up in a chronic care hospital? How many of these patients have been referred? Are they all based at the Massachusetts General Hospital originally? Can these patients be transported for ECMO, and when would you do that?

Dr Masiakos: To answer Dr Hendren's questions, we find that these diseases cluster by ages, and we suspect that they cluster because of disease predispositions. The group that you speak of, the 10- to 30-year-olds, contains the sickest patients. They are the ones who have fungal sepsis, are immunocompromised after their lung transplants, and are most likely to present with multiorgan failure after trauma. They typically do the worst.

To your second question about the absolute contraindications: The first contraindication is head injury. Children or adults who present with head trauma or intracranial hemorrhage are refused. Irreversible lung damage, as seen by biopsy with indications of pulmonary fibrosis, is also a contraindication. Finally, a patient with an underlying fatal disease like metastatic cancer or end-stage acquired immunodeficiency syndrome would be refused as well.

Age is not an absolute contraindication, and I know you all hate me for saying that, however, it's a patient by patient evaluation and we assume enrollment criteria based on what we find on their lung pathology report.

To your last question, the 300-hour threshold: There's no good way to tell a patient's parents or family members that their life support is going to be withheld or withdrawn. We observe the patients day to day, and if there's no evidence of lung recovery after the second or third week, the patients are offered a lung biopsy. If fibrosis is seen on lung biopsy, we consider that to mean irreversible lung damage, and at that point, we suggest that ECMO be discontinued.

The quality-of-life issues: None of the patients who were survivors after receiving ECMO therapy had poor quality of life, none of them were institutionalized, and none continued to need ventilation therapy for their disease. After they recovered, they would be terminated from ECMO and then subsequently be terminated from ventilator support.

To your question about ECMO referrals, it's imperative to understand that lung damage predisposes these patients to poor outcomes. We suggest that the patients be transferred to an institution where ECMO can be provided if in a short amount of time the patient is deemed not recoverable by the current conventional therapies. To get a patient there promptly results in fewer problems in the transfer than when the patient decompensates later.

PAPER

Outcome of Patients With Melanoma and Histologically Negative Sentinel Lymph Nodes

Michele A. Gadd, MD; A. Benedict Cosimi, MD; Jeanne Yu, BS; Lyn M. Duncan, MD; Lawrence Yu, MB, BS, FRCPA, Dip RC Path; Thomas J. Flotte, MD; Wiley W. Souba, MD, ScD; Mark J. Ott, MD; Lisa S. Wong, BS; Arthur J. Sober, MD; Martin C. Mihm, MD; Frank G. Haluska, MD, PhD; Kenneth K. Tanabe, MD

Hypothesis: Patients with melanoma and histologically negative sentinel lymph nodes identified by lymphatic mapping have a very good prognosis.

Design: Cohort study with follow-up information obtained from medical records and telephone interviews.

Setting and Patients: Of all patients with cutaneous melanoma who underwent intraoperative sentinel lymph node mapping between November 15, 1993, and April 18, 1997, at the Massachusetts General Hospital, Boston, 89 were found to have no evidence of melanoma in their sentinel nodes. Forty-six lesions (51%) were on an extremity and 44 (49%) were of axial location. The median tumor thickness was 1.8 mm (range, 0.36-12.0 mm) and 11 tumors (12%) were ulcerated.

Interventions: Patients underwent intraoperative sentinel lymph node mapping with lymphazurin and radiolabeled sulfur colloid. Sentinel lymph nodes were analyzed by standard hematoxylin-eosin staining. Only 2 patients received adjuvant therapy following wide excision of the primary lesion.

Main Outcome Measures: Site of initial recurrence and time to initial recurrence.

Results: The median follow-up for all patients was 23 months (range, 2-54 months). Eleven patients (12%) developed melanoma recurrences, and 78 (88%) patients remain disease free. Regional lymph nodes were the initial site of recurrence in 7 (8%) of 89 patients, and 7 (7%) of 106 mapped basins. Four patients had recurrence without involvement of regional lymph nodes: 2 with distant metastases and 2 with in transit metastases. The median time to recurrence was 12 months (range, 2-35 months). Sentinel lymph nodes were reanalyzed using serial sections and immunoperoxidase stains in 7 patients with recurrence and metastatic melanoma was identified in 3 (43%).

Conclusions: The risk for melanoma recurrence is relatively low in patients with histologically negative sentinel nodes identified by lymphatic mapping. Longer follow-up will improve our understanding of the prognostic value of this procedure.

Arch Surg. 1999;134:381-387

As with many other malignant neoplasms, melanoma metastasis may develop as a result of either lymphatic or hematogenous dissemination. The most powerful prognostic factor for patients with American Joint Committee on Cancer stage I and II melanoma is the presence or absence of metastatic melanoma in their regional lymph nodes.[1] The hypothesis that some patients may harbor occult regional lymph node metastases prior to the establishment of distant metastases has served as the rationale for performing elective lymph node dissections (ELNDs). However, results of prospective randomized clinical trials designed to evaluate the efficacy of ELND have demonstrated either no survival benefit or survival benefit only to selected subgroups.[2,3] In addition, the development of lymphatic mapping and sentinel lymph node biopsy has provided a less invasive method for determination of whether melanoma has spread to regional lymph nodes.[4]

Several refinements have improved the technical success rate of lymphatic mapping, including the use of radiolabeled sulfur colloid combined with a hand-held gamma detector to guide operative dissection.[5] The predictive value of histopathologic identification of metastatic melanoma within a sentinel lymph node is 100% for determination of whether melanoma has spread to regional lymph nodes. However, the predictive value of the absence of metastatic melanoma within the sentinel lymph node has not been clearly established. In all but 1 published report to date, the accuracy of lymphatic mapping and sentinel lymph node biopsy has

From the Departments of Surgery (Drs Gadd, Cosimi, Souba, Ott, and Tanabe and Mss Yu and Wong), Pathology (Drs Duncan, Yu, Flotte, and Mihm), Dermatology (Dr Sober), and Medicine (Dr Haluska), Massachusetts General Hospital, Harvard Medical School, Boston.

PATIENTS AND METHODS

PATIENTS

We identified 89 consecutive patients who underwent intraoperative lymphatic mapping at the Massachusetts General Hospital (MGH), Boston, for cutaneous melanoma and were found to have no evidence of metastatic melanoma in their sentinel lymph nodes using routine histological techniques. All of the patients were operated on between November 15, 1993, and April 18, 1997. The pathological characteristics of the primary melanoma were reviewed at the MGH for nearly all of the patients in this study. In the few patients whose original primary melanoma tissue was not reviewed at the MGH, ulceration was scored as absent for statistical purposes unless indicated to be present in the referring institution's pathology report. None of the patients had clinical evidence of metastatic melanoma at the time of their lymphatic mapping as assessed by clinical history, physical examination, chest radiograph, and liver function tests. None of these patients underwent a simultaneous ELND.

Nearly all patients were compliant with our follow-up recommendations, which consisted of quarterly history and physical examination, annual chest radiograph, and additional imaging studies for patients with signs or symptoms suggestive of metastatic melanoma. Routine surveillance was recommended every 3 months for the first 2 years, followed by every 6 months for the next 2 years, followed by yearly evaluation. The few patients who were not followed up according to these guidelines were contacted by telephone to determine their disease status.

SENTINEL LYMPH NODE MAPPING TECHNIQUE

One surgeon (K.K.T.) instructed 3 other surgeons (M.A.G., A.B.C., and W.W.S.) in the technique of sentinel lymph node mapping and directly participated in 3 to 5 operations for each. Simultaneous completion ELND was not performed on patients during this period. The patients described in this study represent approximately the first 110 patients who underwent lymphatic mapping for melanoma at the MGH. The number of lymphatic mapping operations performed by each of the surgeons during this period ranged from 15 to 50.

Approximately 3 hours prior to operation, 10.0- to 18.5-MBq technetium Tc 99m sulfur colloid (CIS-US Inc, Bedford, Mass) in a volume of 1 mL was injected into the dermis surrounding the site of the primary melanoma or biopsy scar. The total dose was typically divided into 4 equal parts of 0.25 mL each for injection into 4 sites. For patients with large biopsy scars the total dose was divided into more than 4 parts to permit more injections circumferentially around the scar. Planar gamma images were obtained 5 to 60 minutes following injection to define the location of the sentinel lymph nodes. In the operating room a majority of patients then received an injection of 0.5 to 1.5 mL of 1% lymphazurin dye (Zenith Parenterals, Rosemont, Ill) into the dermis circumferentially around the biopsy scar or melanoma. A handheld gamma detector (Care Wise Medical Products, Morgan Hill, Calif, or Neoprobe Corp, Dublin, Ohio) was used intraoperatively to precisely identify the location of the sentinel lymph nodes. Actual basin counts and lymph node counts varied depending on the gamma probe used and the dose of colloid administered. Basin counts were always at least 1 log order greater than background counts. Sentinel lymph nodes were defined as those that either were stained with lymphazurin dye or concentrated 99mTc sulfur colloid. The lymph node resection bed was scanned carefully to ensure that all radioactive lymph nodes had been removed. Acceptable basin counts after sentinel lymph node excision were defined as less than 10% of the counts of the most radioactive lymph node. In a majority of patients, the entire sentinel lymph node was immediately placed into formalin. However, in a few patients, a portion of the sentinel lymph node was submitted fresh for an initial frozen section analysis. The primary melanoma site was widely excised during the same operation in most patients. The interval between radiolabeled colloid injection and operation typically ranged from 45 minutes to 3 hours.

HISTOLOGICAL ANALYSIS OF SENTINEL LYMPH NODES

Standard analysis of sagittally sectioned paraffin-embedded lymph nodes involved examination of 1 or 2 hematoxylin-eosin–stained sections of the central cut surface of each lymph node. A more detailed analysis of some lymph nodes was subsequently performed on archived tissue as described previously.[10] Briefly, three 4-μm-thick serial tissue sections were obtained from the paraffin-embedded blocks at 3 levels 80 μm apart. One section from each of the 3 levels was stained with hematoxylin-eosin, and the remaining sections were stained with antibodies to S-100, HMB-45, NK1C3, and MART-1.

STATISTICAL ANALYSES

Variables were examined in a univariate analysis using the χ^2 test or Student t test where appropriate. Data from 1 patient in whom 2 separate primary melanomas were mapped during the same operation were analyzed as a single patient for recurrence status; however, the primary tumor characteristics and mapped basins for this patient were each counted individually.

been assessed by simultaneous ELND.[4,6,7] Results of these studies indicate that the false-negative rate of the procedure for detection of metastatic melanoma in regional lymph nodes is approximately 4%, and the predictive value of the absence of metastatic melanoma in the sentinel lymph node is approximately 99%.[4,6] Data from prospective randomized trials designed to evaluate ELND suggest that the false-negative rate as assessed by histopathologic evaluation of lymph nodes may be lower than the false-negative rate as assessed by clinical observation. For example, in WHO (World Health Organization) Melanoma Programme Clinical Trial No. 1, 20% of patients randomized to ELND had metastatic melanoma identified in their regional lymph nodes, whereas 27% of patients randomized to observation subsequently developed regional lymph node metastases.[8,9] This discrepancy in the incidence of regional lymph node metastases as determined by immediate dissection compared with long-term observation suggests that clinical follow-up is necessary to determine the false-negative rate of sentinel

Table 1. Comparison of Clinical and Pathological Characteristics According to Recurrence Status*

Characteristic	Patients With No Recurrence	Patients With Recurrence	All Patients
Sex			
Male	46 (59)	6 (55)	**52** (58)
Female	32 (41)	5 (45)	**37** (42)
Age, y (n = 89)			
Median	51	47	51
Range	22-83	25-73	22-83
Primary tumor site (n = 90)			
Axial	40 (51)	4 (36)	**44** (49)
Extremity	39 (49)	7 (64)	**46** (51)
Tumor thickness, mm (n = 90)			
Mean	2.01	3.82	2.23
Median	1.80	2.85	1.80
Clark level (n = 90)			
II/III	2 (3)	0	**2** (2)
III	9 (11)	1 (9)	**10** (11)
III/IV	6 (8)	1 (9)	**7** (8)
IV	52 (66)	8 (73)	**60** (67)
IV/V	1 (1)	1 (9)	**2** (2)
Unknown	9 (11)	0	**9** (10)
Ulceration (n = 90)			
Present	9 (11)	2 (18)	**11** (12)
Absent	70 (89)	9 (82)	**79** (88)
Mapped lymph node basin (n = 106)			
Head and neck	21 (22)	0	**21** (20)
Axillary	53 (56)	4 (33)	**57** (54)
Inguinal	17 (18)	7 (58)	**24** (23)
Other			
Epitrochlear	2 (2)	0	2 (2)
Chest wall	1 (1)	0	1 (1)
Subscapular	0	1 (8)	1 (1)

**Data are given as number (percentage) unless otherwise indicated.*

lymph node mapping. In addition, long-term follow-up of patients with melanoma who undergo lymphatic mapping will identify those who will have a recurrence in sites other than regional lymph nodes (ie, distant metastases and in transit metastases). In the present study we assessed patterns of failure in a cohort of patients who underwent sentinel lymph node mapping without simultaneous ELND, and were found to have no evidence of melanoma in their sentinel lymph nodes using routine histopathologic analysis.

RESULTS

PATIENT CHARACTERISTICS

No evidence of metastatic melanoma was identified by standard histopathologic evaluation of the sentinel lymph nodes resected from 106 lymph node basins in 89 patients. One patient underwent simultaneous lymphatic mapping of 2 separate primary melanomas, and the sentinel nodes for these 2 lesions were located in separate basins (axillary and inguinal). The clinical and pathological characteristics of the patients are listed in **Table 1**. The median age was 51 years (range, 22-83 years) and 58% of patients were men. The primary melanoma site was on an extremity in 46 (51%) patients and axial location in 44 (49%). The most frequently mapped basin in this cohort of patients was the axilla (54%). Twenty-one patients (20%) underwent mapping of head and neck lymph nodes, and 4 other patients had much less common anatomic locations of their sentinel lymph nodes: epitrochlear, 2; chest wall, 1; and subscapular, 1. The median tumor thickness was 1.80 mm (range, 0.36-12.0 mm) and ulceration was present in 11 lesions (12%).

MELANOMA RECURRENCE

Eleven (12%) of 89 patients subsequently developed a recurrence despite having no evidence of metastatic melanoma with routine histological analysis of their sentinel lymph nodes (**Table 2**). In patients with recurrence, the median time to recurrence was 12 months (range, 2-35 months). The distribution of sex, age, primary melanoma site, and site of mapped lymph node basin was not statistically significantly different between those who developed a recurrence and those who did not (Table 1). Patients whose histologically negative sentinel lymph nodes were harvested from the inguinal lymph node basin accounted for the largest group of patients with subsequent recurrence. Of the 11 patients with subsequent recurrence, 7 (58%) initially underwent lymphatic mapping of the inguinal lymph node basin. The median tumor thickness was greater in patients with recurrence than in those without recurrence (2.85 mm vs 1.80 mm); however, this difference was not statistically significant. No difference was observed in the Clark microstaging level between these 2 groups. Although there was a trend toward a greater frequency of ulceration in the group of patients with recurrence compared with those without recurrence, the number of patients with recurrence was too small to allow a meaningful interpretation of the prognostic significance of this histopathologic feature.

The recurrence rate by site for the 11 patients with recurrence, given as number (percentage) of patients, is shown in the tabulation below.

Site	First Recurrence	Overall Recurrence
Local	0	0
In transit	2(2)	3(3)
Lymph node	7(8)	8(9)
Distant	2(2)	5(6)

Regional lymph node recurrence in a previously mapped basin was the first site of recurrence in 7 patients (8%) with recurrence. Two patients developed distant metastases and 2 other patients developed in transit metastases as their first sites of recurrence. Regional lymph node metastases in a previously mapped basin was the first site of recurrence in 7 (7%) of 106 lymph node basins.

Seven patients developed a single type of recurrence, whereas 4 patients developed more than 1 type of recurrence: 1 patient with in transit metastases subsequently developed regional lymph node metastases and additional in transit metastases, and 3 patients with regional lymph node recurrences subsequently developed distant sites of metastases (Table 2). Accordingly, 8 (9%) of the original 89 patients developed regional lymph node metastases as at least 1 component of their recurrence.

Table 2. Summary of Patients With Recurrences

Patient No./ Sex/Age, y	Primary Site	Procedure Prior to Mapping	Tumor Thickness, mm	Clark Level	Ulceration	Mapped Basin(s)	Time to First Recurrence, mo	Site of First Recurrence
1/M/25	Calf	Wide excision	2.85	IV/V	No	Inguinal	8	In transit
2/F/47	Calf	Biopsy	3.10	IV	No	Inguinal	35	Inguinal nodes
3/F/35	Back	Biopsy	0.86	III/IV	No	Axillary	20	Axillary nodes
4/F/48	Thigh	Biopsy	7.80	IV	Yes	Inguinal	2	Inguinal nodes
5/M/63	Thigh	Biopsy	2.00	IV	No	Inguinal	11	In transit
6/F/72	Upper arm	Biopsy	12.00	IV	No	Inguinal	26	Distant metastases
7/F/35	Chest	Wide excision	1.74	IV	No	Axillary	24	Distant metastases
8/M/73	Shoulder	Biopsy	3.28	IV	Yes	Axillary	1	Axillary nodes
9/M/46	Back	Biopsy	2.10	IV	No	Subscapular	2	Axillary nodes
10/M/30	Ankle	Biopsy	1.65	IV	No	Inguinal	12	Inguinal nodes
11/M/57	Abdominal wall	Biopsy	4.60	IV	No	Axillary and inguinal	4	Inguinal nodes

Of the 5 patients who developed distant metastases as at least 1 component of their recurrence, 3 (60%) had evidence of melanoma in their lymph nodes, and 2 (40%) did not based on routine pathological analysis.

Univariate analyses of the prognostic factors with respect to recurrence revealed that male sex, Clark level greater than III, axial location, presence of ulceration, and mean tumor thickness were not statistically significant ($P>.05$) prognostic factors. The small number of patients with recurrences in this study reduces the statistical power of these analyses.

SURVIVAL

The median follow-up duration for the 89 patients in this study was 23 months (range, 2 54 months), and 78 (88%) of patients remain disease free. The median disease-free survival has not yet been reached. Of the 7 patients whose first recurrence was lymph node metastasis, all underwent regional lymphadenectomy. Four have remained disease free, 2 are alive with disease, and 1 died of disease. Of the 2 patients whose first recurrence was in transit metastasis, 1 underwent surgical resection of the in transit lesions and has remained disease free. The other patient was treated with hyperthermic isolated limb perfusion combined with inguinal lymphadenectomy and subsequently died of complications arising from retroperitoneal metastases.

REEVALUATION OF SENTINEL LYMPH NODES WITH SERIAL SECTIONS AND IMMUNOHISTOCHEMISTRY

The standard pathological assessment of the sentinel nodes in this study consisted of bisection of the lymph node along its long axis and histological examination of 1 or 2 hematoxylin-eosin–stained sections from each cut surface. Careful rereview of the original histological sections did not reveal evidence of metastatic melanoma in any patient in this study. We have also reported a more detailed examination of sentinel lymph nodes, including 78 patients in this study.[10] This examination consisted of deeper sections into the lymph node and immunohistochemical stains with antibodies to S-100, HMB-45, NK1C3, and MART-1. An adequate amount of residual sentinel lymph node tissue was not available for further examination in some patients. Sentinel lymph node reanalysis revealed metastatic melanoma in 9 patients, 6 of whom have not had recurrences to date.

Of the 7 patients who developed regional lymph node metastases as their first site of recurrence, sentinel lymph nodes were reanalyzed in 4, and in 1 (25%) metastatic melanoma was identified in the sentinel node. Of the 2 patients who developed distant metastases as their first site of recurrence, a more detailed analysis of their sentinel lymph nodes revealed metastatic melanoma in 1 but not in the other. Of the 2 patients who developed in transit metastases as their first site of recurrence, metastatic melanoma was identified in 1 of the sentinel lymph nodes, and there was not sufficient additional tissue available for review in the other patient. Overall, of the 11 patients who developed a recurrence, sufficient additional tissue was available for review in 7 patients, and in 3 of them a more detailed pathological assessment of sentinel nodes revealed metastatic melanoma. Therefore, when taking into account the more detailed pathological review of sentinel lymph nodes, regional lymph node metastases in a previously mapped basin was the first site of recurrence in 6 (6%) of 97 lymph node basins harboring histologically negative sentinel lymph nodes. And when analyzed by patient, 86 patients had histologically negative sentinel lymph nodes of whom 6 (7%) subsequently developed regional lymph node metastases in the mapped lymph node basin as their first site of recurrence, and 8 (9%) had overall recurrence. Of the 5 patients who developed distant metastases as at least 1 component of their recurrence, 4 (80%) had evidence of metastastic melanoma in their sentinel lymph nodes using either standard techniques or serial sections with immunohistochemical staining. Only 1 patient presented with distant metastases without evidence of metastatic melanoma in their sentinel node.

COMMENT

In their original description of lymphatic mapping, Morton and colleagues[4,11] used a vital blue dye alone to trace lymphatic channels to the sentinel lymph node. In this landmark study, the authors performed a simultaneous complete lymphadenectomy of the mapped basin to determine the accuracy of the technique. In 38 (95%) of 40 regional node basins containing metastatic melanoma, the sentinel node was found to contain metastatic melanoma using hematoxylin-eosin staining as well as immunohistochemical staining with S-100 and NK1C3. Of 156 basins with histologically negative sentinel lymph nodes, only 2 (1%) had metastatic melanoma in any of the remaining regional lymph nodes, thereby providing a predictive value of a negative result of 99%. In the years following this report, an analysis of published reports on sentinel lymph node mapping for melanoma has revealed interesting trends and concepts. First, the addition of radiolabeled sulfur colloid combined with the intraoperative use of a handheld gamma detector has improved the technical success rate of sentinel lymph node mapping.[5,12-14] In addition, this improvement has presumably reduced the frequency of missed sentinel lymph nodes, especially in patients who have more than a single sentinel lymph node in a basin. Second, most patients are now undergoing sentinel lymph node mapping without simultaneous complete regional lymphadenectomy.[5,7,13,15,16] Third, data have emerged that support the notion that more detailed analyses of sentinel lymph nodes will detect metastatic melanoma more often than routine analyses involving only hematoxylin-eosin staining of 1 or 2 sections.[7,10,17,18]

The false-negative rate of sentinel lymph node mapping may be assessed by simultaneous ELND and comparison of the histological status of the sentinel lymph node with that of the remaining lymph nodes, as was originally described by Morton and colleagues.[4] However, a more clinically relevant assessment of the accuracy of lymphatic mapping requires follow-up of patients who were found to have a histologically negative sentinel lymph node at the time of their lymphatic mapping and did not simultaneously undergo an ELND. The frequency of recurrence in this group of patients provides one measure of the prognostic accuracy of lymphatic mapping. Results from our study are in agreement with those previously published, indicating that the false-negative rate as assessed by clinical follow-up is higher than the false-negative rate as assessed by simultaneous ELND. In our study as well as in the largest follow-up study published to date,[7] approximately 10% of patients with histologically negative sentinel lymph nodes detected by routine techniques have recurrences overall, with only 6% having recurrence in a previously mapped lymph node basin.

There are several possible explanations for false-negative results of lymphatic mapping, and these may be separated into 3 general mechanisms. The first general mechanism that may lead to false-negative results involves the biology of melanoma progression. For example, at the time of lymphatic mapping, metastastic melanoma cells may be within lymphatic channels but have not yet arrived in the regional lymph node basin. Subsequent to resection of a histologically negative sentinel lymph node, these cells may arrive in a regional lymph node and develop into clinically apparent metastases. Another example of melanoma biology that may explain false-negative results involves tumor cells spreading from the sentinel node to "secondary" (nonsentinel) nodes, followed by immune-induced regression of the original focus of metastatic melanoma in the sentinel lymph node. Alternatively, hematogenously circulating melanoma cells may spread to regional lymph nodes after the lymphatic mapping procedure has been performed.

The second general mechanism that may account for false-negative sentinel lymph nodes involves technical aspects of the lymphatic mapping procedure itself. There are several technical errors that may lead to misidentification of sentinel lymph nodes. For example, in patients who undergo lymphatic mapping without intraoperative use of a handheld gamma detector, the surgeon may believe that all of the sentinel lymph nodes have been resected, when in reality, an additional sentinel lymph node remains undetected. The presence of melanoma cells in this missed sentinel lymph node may give rise to a false-negative result. Similarly, the combination of lymphatic mapping using only vital blue dye without any preoperative lymphoscintigraphy may result in failure to identify sentinel lymph nodes residing in alternate lymph node basins or in unusual anatomic locations.[19] Four patients in our series had sentinel lymph nodes located in uncommon anatomic sites. Disruption of the regional lymphatics prior to lymphatic mapping may also lead to misidentification of sentinel lymph nodes. The accuracy of the technique has been demonstrated only in patients in whom the procedure has been performed after a biopsy but prior to a wide excision of the primary melanoma. It is not clear that lymphatic mapping is accurate in patients who have undergone a definitive excision of their melanoma prior to lymphatic mapping. In other words, the lymphatic channels draining the residual scar resulting from a wide excision may not necessarily represent the same lymphatic channels that drained the primary melanoma. Although a radioactive, blue lymph node may be identified and resected in patients who have already undergone a wide excision of their melanoma, this lymph node may not be the primary node that received lymphatic drainage from the melanoma. Two of the patients with false-negative results in this study underwent wide excision of their melanomas prior to lymphatic mapping.

Virtually all investigators are in agreement that the addition of radiolabeled colloid to the technique of lymphatic mapping for melanoma has enhanced the robustness of the technique and shortened the "learning curve."[5,12-14] In general, primary melanomas located on the head and neck region are the most difficult to map because of the close proximity of the primary injection site and sentinel lymph nodes, as well as the technical expertise required to resect sentinel lymph nodes without injury to critical nerves. Conversely, the inguinal lymph node basin tends to serve as the least difficult basin from which to identify and resect sentinel lymph nodes. Interestingly, of the 11 patients in our series with recurrence, 7 had their sentinel lymph nodes resected from the inguinal basin. One possible explanation for this unexpected finding is that after resection of inguinal sentinel lymph nodes, we did not generally resect any additional iliac sentinel lymph nodes.Therefore, it is possible that some patients in our series had iliac sentinel lymph nodes with clinically occult metastases left unresected, thereby giving rise to false-negative results. However, none of the patients in our series developed iliac lymph node recurrences.

A third general mechanism that may give rise to false-negative results of lymphatic mapping involves the failure of routine histopathologic techniques to identify metastatic melanoma in the sentinel lymph node. In some patients, sentinel lymph nodes may contain metastatic melanoma below the limits of resolution for the analytic techniques applied. Although the use of serial sections and immunohistochemical stains clearly enhances the sensitivity of melanoma detection,[7,10,20] these techniques are still limited by the possibility of sampling error, since not all of the lymph node is analyzed. The use of reverse transcription–polymerase chain reaction (RT-PCR) to detect messenger RNA for the tyrosinase gene has been reported to significantly enhance the sensitivity for detection of cells of melanocytic origin. This technique theoretically permits analysis of the entire sentinel lymph node without the limitations of sampling error. However, approximately 10% of patients have benign capsular nevi within their sentinel lymph nodes,[10] thereby giving rise to false-positive results using RT-PCR analysis of the entire node. To help reduce the incidence of false-positive results using RT-PCR, it has been proposed that a portion of the lymph node should still be examined microscopically for capsular nevi. However, setting aside a portion of the lymph node again introduces the possibility of sampling error. Establishing primary cultures of lymph nodes is another sensitive method for detection of metastatic melanoma cells[18]; however, this technique is labor intensive, expensive, and requires facilities that are not available in many hospitals.

The prognostic value of these more sensitive techniques for detection of microscopic melanoma in lymph nodes remains to be established. No long-term follow-up studies have been published of patients whose sentinel lymph nodes were examined by these microstaging techniques. It is possible that in some patients, the microscopic disease detected by these sensitive techniques may have been destroyed by the host immune response if left in situ. It is anticipated that such reports will be forthcoming, given that these microstaging techniques are being used more commonly. Because only a few lymph nodes are typically resected during lymphatic mapping, it has now become more practical to apply these microstaging techniques. One of the specific aims of the Sunbelt Melanoma Trial (Kelly McMasters, MD, PhD, University of Louisville, Louisville, Ky, oral and written communication, 1998) is to define the importance of these molecular techniques for analysis of sentinel lymph nodes.

At the MGH we consider lymphatic mapping for patients with cutaneous melanomas thicker than 1.0 mm and who have not already undergone a wide local excision of the tumor. We will also consider lymphatic mapping for patients with thinner lesions and other adverse prognostic factors including ulceration, axial location, and male sex. Based on the results of this study and others, we recently adopted a standard approach of sentinel lymph node evaluation using serial sections and immunohistochemical stains for S-100 and MART-1, which we believe will reduce the incidence of false-negative results. As indicated above, the false-negative rate may be a function of the rigor with which one examines the sentinel lymph node. However, the false-negative rate is also a function of the duration of clinical follow-up. The median follow-up for this study is only 23 months, and we anticipate that the false-negative rate will continue to rise with longer follow-up. Continued follow-up will also allow us to determine the value of serial sections and immunohistochemistry compared with routine hematoxylin-eosin staining. It is quite interesting that in the entire cohort of patients studied, only a single patient has developed distant metastases in the absence of regional lymph node metastases (excluding the patient in whom metastastic melanoma was identified in the sentinel node retrospectively using microstaging techniques). This supports the notion that melanoma follows an orderly progression of metastases, with disease first appearing in regional lymph nodes, followed by disease appearing in distant sites. However, this temporal relationship does not necessarily imply that regional metastases give rise to distant metastases. The presence of this temporal relationship merely implies that by the time that distant metastases are clinically detectable, melanoma has already spread to regional lymph nodes. These potential mechanisms of disease progression have obvious important ramifications on how complete resection of regional lymph nodes containing metastastic melanoma may or may not influence overall survival.

Presented at the 79th Annual Meeting of the New England Surgical Society, Toronto, Ontario, September 26, 1998.

Reprints: Kenneth K. Tanabe, MD, Division of Surgical Oncology, Cox Building 626, Massachusetts General Hospital, Boston, MA 02114.

REFERENCES

1. Stadelmann WK, Rapaport DP, Soong S-J, et al. Prognostic clinical and pathologic features. In: Balch CM, Houghton AN, Sober AJ, Soong S-J, ed. *Cutaneous Melanoma.* 3rd ed. St Louis, Mo: Quality Medical Publishing Inc; 1998:11-35.
2. Balch CM, Soong S-J, Bartolucci AA, et al. Efficacy of an elective regional lymph node dissection of 1 to 4 mm thick melanomas for patients 60 years of age and younger. *Ann Surg.* 1996;224:255-266.
3. Cascinelli N, Morabito A, Santinami M, MacKie RM, Belli F. Immediate or delayed dissection of regional nodes in patients with melanoma of the trunk: a randomised trial: WHO Melanoma Programme. *Lancet.* 1998;351:793-796.
4. Morton DL, Wen D-R, Wong JH, et al. Technical details of intraoperative lymphatic mapping for early stage melanoma. *Arch Surg.* 1992;127:392-399.
5. Krag DN, Meijer SJ, Weaver DL, et al. Minimal access surgery for staging of malignant melanoma. *Arch Surg.* 1995;130:654-658.
6. Reintgen D, Cruse CW, Wells K, et al. The orderly progression of melanoma nodal metastases. *Ann Surg.* 1994;220:759-767.
7. Gershenwald JE, Colome MI, Lee JE, et al. Patterns of recurrence following a negative sentinel lymph node biopsy in 243 patients with stage I or II melanoma. *J Clin Oncol.* 1998;16:2253-2260.
8. Veronesi U, Adamus J, Bandiera DC, et al. Inefficacy of immediate node dissection in stage I melanoma of the limbs. *N Engl J Med.* 1977; 297:627-630.
9. Veronesi U, Adamus J, Bandiera DC, et al. Delayed regional lymph node dissection in stage I melanoma of the skin of the lower extremities. *Cancer.* 1982;49: 2420-2430.
10. Yu LL, Flotte TJ, Tanabe KK, et al. Detection of microscopic melanoma metastases in sentinel lymph nodes. *Cancer.* In press.
11. Morton DL, Wen D-R, Cochran AJ. Management of early-stage melanoma by intraoperative lymphatic mapping and selective lymphadenectomy. *Surg Oncol Clin North Am.* 1992;1:247-259.
12. Albertini JJ, Cruse CW, Rapaport D, et al. Intraoperative radiolymphoscintigraphy improves sentinel lymph node identification for patients with melanoma. *Ann Surg.* 1996;223:217-224.
13. Alex JC, Krag DN. Gamma-probe-guided localization of lymph nodes. *Surg Oncol.* 1993;2:137-144.
14. Gershenwald JE, Tseng C-H, Thompson W, et al. Improved sentinel lymph node localization in primary melanoma patients with use of radiolabeled colloid. *Surgery.* 1998. In press.

15. Bostick P, Essner R, Sarantou T, et al. Intraoperative lymphatic mapping for early-stage melanoma of the head and neck. *Am J Surg.* 1997;174:536-539.
16. Reintgen D, Rapaport D, Tanabe KK, Ross MI. Lymphatic mapping and sentinel lymphadenectomy. In: Balch CM, Houghton AM, Sober AJ, Soong S-j, eds. *Cutaneous Melanoma.* 3rd ed. St Louis, Mo: Quality Medical Publishing Inc; 1998.
17. Wang X, Heller R, VanVoorhis N, et al. Detection of submicroscopic lymph node metastases with polymerase chain reaction in patients with malignant melanoma. *Ann Surg.* 1994;220:768-774.
18. Heller R, Becker J, Wassalle J, et al. Detection of submicroscopic lymph node metastases in patients with malignant melanoma. *Arch Surg.* 1991;126:1455-1460.
19. Tanabe KK. Lymphatic mapping and epitrochlear lymph node dissection for melanoma. *Surgery.* 1997;121:102-104.
20. Cochran AJ, Wen DR, Herschman JR. Occult melanoma in lymph nodes detected by antiserum to S-100 proteins. *Int J Cancer.* 1984;34:159-163.

DISCUSSION

Dougald MacGillivray, MD, South Portland, Me: Dr Souba and his coauthors have presented the outcome of 89 patients with cutaneous melanoma who had no evidence of metastases to the sentinel lymph nodes. The results of this report support the thesis that lymphatic mapping and sentinel lymph node examination is an accurate method and a logical alternative to elective node dissection for staging the regional lymph node basins in patients with melanoma. At a median follow-up of 23 months, 12% of these patients have had clinical evidence of recurrent disease. Eight patients, or 8.9%, eventually developed a regional nodal metastasis, and 5 patients, or 5.6%, had distant metastases. The rate of recurrent melanoma in this study is similar to that reported by Gershenwald from the M. D. Anderson Cancer Center. In their experience with 243 patients with melanoma who had a negative sentinel lymph node, 11% had recurrent disease over a medial follow-up of 35 months. However, their findings on reevaluation of the sentinel lymph node in those patients who recurred differed from those reported today. In the M. D. Anderson report, 80% of patients who had a regional nodal recurrence as a component of their initial recurrent disease had previously undetected metastases in the sentinel lymph node when it was reevaluated with special techniques, while none of the patients who had in transit or distant metastases as the first sight of recurrence had involvement of the sentinel lymph node on reexamination. In Dr Souba's series, only 1 of 7 patients who had their site of recurrence in the regional nodal basin had occult disease detected on reexamination of the sentinel lymph node, while 4 of 5 patients, or 80%, who developed distant metastases had involvement of the sentinel lymph node. I suspect that some of this difference is due to the number of patients who had an adequate volume of residual tissue available for reexamination. However, of the 11 patients who developed recurrent disease, 8 of those patients, or 73%, had a regional nodal metastasis as a component of their recurrence. Do you think that this was due to a technical problem or failure to identify the sentinel lymph node at the initial procedure, or do you think this was possibly due to secondary involvement of the nodal basin from in transit or systemic disease? Has your experience with this group of patients resulted in a modification of your protocol for sentinel node identification and examination?

It is clear that a more extensive examination of the sentinel lymph node will detect more patients with occult microscopic disease. What is yet to be determined is a clinical significance of lymph node metastases detected by this more intensive scrutiny, particularly metastases detected by immunohistochemistry and molecular techniques.

Have you reexamined the sentinel lymph nodes of those patients who have not recurred to determine the frequency of occult metastatic disease that was not detected on initial examination?

Finally, your recurrence rate of 12% at 2 years of follow-up, while small, is not insignificant, particularly when there is adjuvant treatment that may improve survival in patients with occult metastatic disease. Are you currently investigating or utilizing other prognostic features or techniques such as ulceration, microscopic satellitosis, DNA ploidy, or molecular markers to select high-risk patients with sentinel lymph nodes that are negative who may benefit from adjuvant treatment?

Robert Quinlan, MD, Worcester, Mass: I wonder if this is anything like the breast. Memorial Sloan Kettering has looked at their sentinel node biopsies doing the synchronous dissection in the axilla and have found that, as the primary lesions get larger, up over 1.5 cm to 2 cm, the nonsentinel node is at risk of being positive where the sentinel was negative. And I see that as your melanomas got larger, primarily thicker, you had an increased risk of recurrence. I'm just wondering if you've looked at false-negatives as thickness increased. The numbers are small so you probably haven't looked at it, but I'm wondering if anyone has looked at the question.

Kirby Bland, MD, Providence, RI: I wish you would give us some further information on which of the 2 techniques you think is most sensitive and reproducible in identifying the sentinel node—for instance, is it a lymphazurin dye technique or is it the radio technetium sulfur colloid technique? Have you had methodologic problems in technique as well as administration either of the dye or the radionuclide? Second question, What do you recommend in terms of the type of procedure? Would you do just a superficial node dissection once you identify, by immunohistochemistry, that you have positivity of the node, or should you extend that to a deep dissection and perhaps even if these patients are on protocol do you recommend any type of systemic chemotherapy?

Richard Swanson, MD, Worcester: Do you use rtPCR to analyze the sentinel nodes?

Giles Whalen, MD, Farmington, Conn: The question I have is just a point of technique. Were all of these melanomas in sight when they were injected, or were some of them previously excised and the biopsy site around it injected?

Dr Souba: I would like to thank the discussants for their thoughtful comments. Dr MacGillivray asked about the discrepancy about what M. D. Anderson found and what our group noted in terms of lymph node sections and the presence of melanoma cells. The answer depends, in part, on how hard you look. In the M. D. Anderson study, as many as 200 serial sections were made of the lymph nodes. This explains, at least in part, why they were able to identify melanoma cells more often in their "negative nodes" than we did. There are probably several explanations for false-negatives. One explanation relates to technical issues. There is a learning curve associated with performing lymphatic mapping. Secondly, it is conceivable that the patient has melanoma cells in the different lymphatics which have not reached the sentinel nodes. Under these circumstances, metastatic disease could appear after lymph node resection. The third explanation, as discussed above, relates to the extent to which the nodes are examined. In this light, Dr Swanson asked about reverse transcriptase PCR. This type of molecular biology technique is 1 example of some of the newer efforts that are being employed to examine lymph nodes.

Currently, the guidelines for lymphatic mapping in our group vary somewhat. In general, we map patient [tumors] that are greater than 1 mm in thickness. Those patients who do undergo lymphatic mapping have standard hematoxylin-eosin sections of the lymph node and immunohistochemistry.

Dr MacGillivray asked an interesting question about the significance of nodal micrometastases that are detected only by immunohistochemistry. It is quite possible that many of these patients are cured with surgery alone. However, the significance of micrometastases detected by newer techniques requires further study. As a general rule, patients who have a positive sentinel lymph node undergo a formal lymph node dissection under general anesthesia at a later date.

PAPER

Multimodality Management of Merkel Cell Carcinoma

Mark J. Ott, MD; Kenneth K. Tanabe, MD; Michele A. Gadd, MD; Paul Stark, MS; Barbara L. Smith, MD, PhD; Dianne M. Finkelstein, PhD; Wiley W. Souba, MD, ScD

Hypothesis: Merkel cell carcinoma is a rare dermal neuroendocrine carcinoma whose optimal treatment and prognostic factors are poorly defined. We hypothesize that high-risk patients with Merkel cell carcinoma are best treated with multimodality therapy.

Design: A retrospective review of all patients (N = 33) with Merkel cell carcinoma treated at the Massachusetts General Hospital from January 1, 1980, to August 24, 1997. Median follow-up time was 37 months (range, 6-157 months).

Patients: Adequate data for evaluation were available for 31 patients. Male to female distribution was 14 men and 17 women, with a median patient age of 68 years.

Main Outcome Measure: Stage at presentation; factors associated with recurrence; and the effects of surgery, radiation therapy (XRT), and chemotherapy on recurrence, salvage, and survival rates.

Results: There were 12 extremity, 11 head and neck, and 8 truncal tumors. There were 22 isolated primary tumors, 8 with additional clinically positive lymph nodes, and 1 with distant disease. Therapy was local excision with or without XRT in 19 patients, local resection and lymphadenectomy with or without XRT in 8 patients, and XRT alone in 4 patients with head and neck tumors. Fifteen patients developed recurrences (7 local, 8 nodal, and 10 distant). Median time to recurrence was 8 months (range, 3-48 months). There were 7 tumor-related deaths, 6 of which were associated with truncal lesions ($P<.001$). No locoregional recurrences occurred in patients with margins of resection of 2 cm or greater or adequate XRT. A multivariate analysis selected truncal location ($P = .005$) and nodal disease ($P = .05$) as predictors of mortality. Remission was possible in 5 patients with locoregional and 2 patients with distant recurrences.

Conclusions: Merkel cell carcinoma is an aggressive dermal cancer with frequent nodal metastases; truncal tumors have the worst prognosis. Locoregional recurrence correlates with inadequate margins and lack of XRT, but remission is possible with multimodality therapy.

Arch Surg. 1999;134:388-393

MERKEL CELL carcinoma (MCC), a neuroendocrine carcinoma of the dermis, is an extremely rare and aggressive malignant neoplasm. This tumor has a high propensity for local recurrence (20%-75%), regional nodal metastases (31%-80%), and distant metastases (26%-75%).[1-10] Approximately one third of patients eventually die of their disease.

Toker[11] first described MCC in 1972, and the first published series appeared in 1982.[3] Since that time, slightly over 600 cases have been reported in the literature. Merkel cell carcinoma has a distinctive appearance, presenting clinically as a red to violaceous intradermal nodule. The lesion typically increases rapidly in size over a few weeks to months. Recommended management has usually been surgical excision of the primary lesion, with wide margins (1-3 cm) advocated by most authors.[2,10,12,13] In addition, some have recommended a prophylactic lymphadenectomy due to the propensity for early occult spread to regional nodes.[14,15] More recently, sentinel lymph-node mapping has been used in MCC to detect the presence of regional nodal metastases. This technique allows one to perform selective lymph-node dissection.[16]

Most authors have recommended adjuvant radiation therapy (XRT) for local control, but a survival benefit has not been demonstrated. Meeuwissen et al[17] demonstrated a substantial benefit in both time to recurrence and disease-free survival when XRT was used. While MCC is sensitive to multiple chemotherapy agents (cisplatin, doxorubicin hydrochloride, vindesine sulfate, and fluorouracil), the experience of most authorities is that the response has been short-lived. Owing to the rarity

From the Division of Surgical Oncology, Department of Surgery (Drs Ott, Tanabe, Gadd, Smith, and Souba), and the Department of Biostatistics (Mr Stark and Dr Finkelstein), Massachusetts General Hospital, Harvard Medical School, Boston, Mass.

SUBJECTS AND METHODS

The medical records of 33 patients identified through the cancer data registry with MCC treated at the Massachusetts General Hospital, Boston, from January 1, 1980, to August 24, 1997, were reviewed. Median follow-up was 37 months (range, 6-157 months). Adequate data for evaluation were available for 31 patients (94%). Demographic data were collected and clinical outcomes recorded. Individual physicians were contacted when necessary to complete follow-up data. We determined location and stage at presentation; the incidence of other malignant neoplasms; factors associated with recurrence; and the effects of surgery, XRT, and chemotherapy on recurrence, salvage, and survival rates.

Disease-free survival curves were estimated using the Kaplan-Meier method.[18] Patients who were alive and disease free at the most recent follow-up were treated as censored for this analysis. Factors associated with outcome were compared using a univariate log-rank test Cox regression. An optimal multivariate model was selected using a forward and backward selection procedure. A 2-tailed Fisher exact test was used for analysis of local and regional recurrence.

of this tumor and the lack of a standardized approach to treatment, it has been difficult to adequately evaluate the proper role and regimen for chemotherapy.

The purpose of this study was to analyze our experience with MCC and determine which factors in patient presentation affected outcome and to help clarify the optimal treatment of these patients.

RESULTS

PREDICTORS OF DISEASE-FREE SURVIVAL RATES

The median patient age was 68 years (range, 34-81 years). There were 14 men and 17 women and all patients were white. Thirteen patients (42%) had a total of 17 previously treated or coexisting malignant neoplasms (**Table 1**). The size of the primary lesions varied from 0.5 to 15 cm (median, 2 cm) and did not affect the outcome. Demographic data, tumor location, regional nodal status, and effect of treatment on outcome are presented in **Table 2**. While the incidence of MCC was roughly equal between the sexes, there was a trend for female patients to have a better outcome by univariate analysis ($P = .09$). Twenty-two patients (71%) presented with stage I disease, 8 patients (26%) presented with stage II disease (clinically positive nodes), and only 1 patient (3%) presented with distant disease (stage III) at diagnosis. Primary treatment included local excision with or without XRT in 19 patients, local resection and lymphadenectomy with or without XRT in 8 patients, and XRT alone in 4 patients with head and neck tumors. Fifteen patients (48%) developed recurrences (7 local, 8 nodal, and 10 distant).

Table 1. Other Malignant Neoplasms in Patients With Merkel Cell Carcinoma

Malignant Neoplasms	No. of Occurrences
Squamous cell carcinoma of the skin	3
Breast cancer	3
Endometrial cancer	2
Colon cancer	2
Prostate cancer	2
Chronic lymphocytic leukemia	2
Ovarian clear cell carcinoma	1
Bladder cancer	1
Squamous cell carcinoma of the vocal cord	1

Table 2. Prognostic, Demographic, and Treatment Variables

Characteristics	No. of Patients	No. of Deaths	*P* Univariate	*P* Multivariate
Sex				
Male	14	5	.09	
Female	17	2		
Age, y				
≥55	26	4	.002	
<55	5	3		
Site of tumor				
Extremity	12	0	<.001	.005
Head and neck	11	1		
Trunk	8	6		
Nodal status				
Positive	8	4	.002	.05
Negative	23	3		
Radiotherapy, Gy				
≥45	9	0	.08	
<45	22	7		
Chemotherapy				
Yes	6	3	.02	
No	25	4		
Tumor margin, cm				
≥2	7	2	.69	
<2	24	5		

Univariate, statistically significant predictors of disease-free survival were location of the lesion ($P<.001$), age 55 years or older ($P = .002$), and regional nodal status at the time of diagnosis ($P = .002$). A multivariate survival model selected only truncal location ($P = .005$) and nodal disease ($P = .05$) as statistically significant, independent predictors of survival. With these variables in the model, there were no additional clinical treatments or demographic variables that independently predicted mortality at a significant level. Lesions occurring on the trunk had an extremely poor prognosis (**Figure 1**), with 6 of the 7 deaths occurring in this group and only 2 of the 8 patients with truncal lesions surviving free of disease (at 96 months and 12 months). Both of these patients underwent wide excision of their lesions, with XRT of 45 Gy or more to the tumor bed and regional nodes and adjuvant chemotherapy. Of the 8 patients with clinically positive regional nodes at the time of presentation,

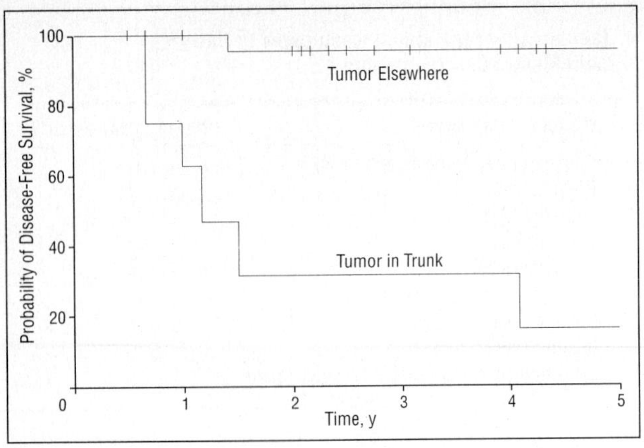

Figure 1. *The effect of tumor location on outcome in patients with Merkel cell carcinoma, using Kaplan-Meier life-table multivariate analysis* (P = .005).

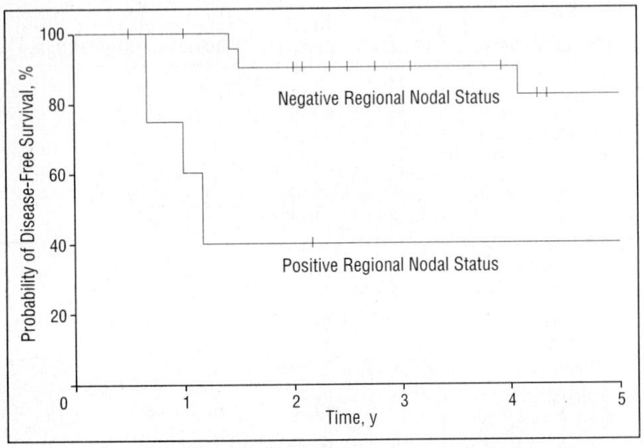

Figure 2. *The effect of regional nodal status on outcome in patients with Merkel cell carcinoma, using Kaplan-Meier life-table multivariate analysis* (P = .05).

only 4 survived (**Figure 2**). Two of these 4 survivors received XRT to the nodal bed, 1 received XRT and a therapeutic lymph-node dissection, and 1 only received a therapeutic lymph-node dissection. Of the 4 patients with positive nodes at the time of diagnosis who did not survive, none received adequate XRT to the nodal bed in the immediate postoperative period. Of the 23 patients who had clinically negative regional nodes at presentation, only 2 subsequently developed nodal disease.

TREATMENT

Radiation therapy of 45 Gy or more to the primary site and/or regional nodes appeared to confer a benefit (*P* = .08), with no treatment failures among the 9 patients who received this dose (**Figure 3**). Within this group, 4 patients had head and neck lesions (4.5 cm on the right cheek, 1.7 cm on the right eyebrow, 1.2 cm on the left upper eyelid [39 Gy], and 3 cm on the left cheek) whose margins were either positive (3 patients) or within 1 mm (1 patient). Due to the limits of resection, XRT was the primary treatment modality in these patients. All of these patients were alive and free of disease at 8, 33, 60, and 92 months, respectively.

Three of 6 patients who received chemotherapy survived, compared with 21 of 25 patients who did not receive chemotherapy. Thus, the administration of chemotherapy was associated with a worse outcome by univariate analysis (*P* = .02). This difference disappeared in multivariate analysis since many of these patients had truncal lesions and positive regional nodes, and that was the main determinant of their outcome. There were in fact 2 patients with distant metastases who were treated with chemotherapy and were free of disease at 33 and 96 months, respectively.

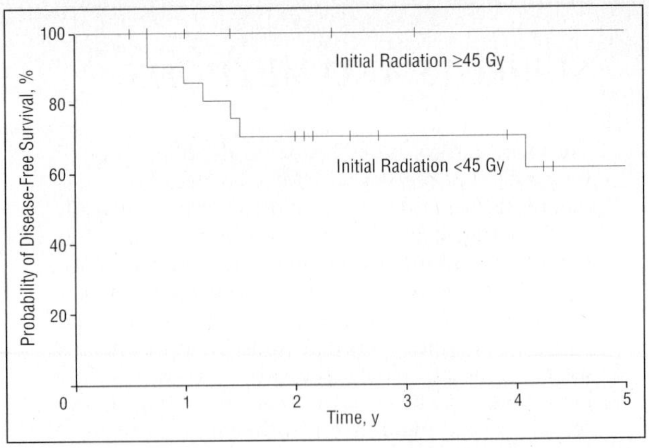

Figure 3. *The effect of perioperative external beam radiation therapy on outcome in patients with Merkel cell carcinoma, using Kaplan-Meier life-table univariate analysis* (P = .08).

Seven patients had margins of resection of 2 cm or larger. None of these patients experienced a local recurrence, compared with 7 local recurrences in 24 patients with margins of resection less than 2 cm (*P* = .16). Two of the 7 patients with wide excisions subsequently died of distant disease. As a result, a margin of resection of 2 cm or larger vs less than 2 cm did not significantly affect the survival rate. Median time to recurrence for the entire series was 8 months (range, 3-48 months).

Recurrence developed locally in 4 patients and in regional nodes only in 1 patient. All 5 of these patients were curable with XRT and/or reexcision (mean disease-free survival, 40 months).

COMMENT

The rarity of Merkel cell carcinoma has contributed to its undertreatment. From both our series of patients and the previously reported combined experience in the literature, it is clear that MCC is an aggressive but also curable lesion. Understaging combined with undertreatment leads to local recurrence and distant failure. Shaw and Rumball[19] point out that, in many respects, MCC is similar to aggressive melanoma. Both skin tumors are of neural tissue origin and found almost exclusively in whites. They both tend to follow a predictable pattern of spread to the regional lymph nodes followed by systemic disease. The occurrence or spread of MCC may reflect a predisposition to developing cancer. Thirteen patients (42%) had previous malignant neoplasms. Four of these patients had experienced 2 prior separate malignant neoplasms. This is a higher multiple cancer rate for this age group than even the expected single cancer rate of 1 in 3 for male and 1 in 4 for female patients. This study represents the first documentation of an increased malignant neoplasm rate among patients with MCC.

WHAT DETERMINES outcome in patients with MCC? In our series, the tumor size had no effect on survival rates, similar to the findings of Victor et al.[14] Six patients with large tumors (4-10 cm) were disease free at 8, 12, 24, 37, 96, and 113 months. By contrast, 3 of the 7 deaths occurred in patients with primary tumors smaller than 2 cm. There was a trend for women to have a better prognosis than men, similar to melanoma.[20] A more favorable prognosis for women with MCC has also been found by other authors.[2,19,21]

Figures 1 and 2 demonstrate that location and nodal status at presentation are correlated with outcome. Again this is similar to melanoma, for which truncal lesions and positive lymph nodes are poor prognostic factors; however, this is the first time truncal location has been shown to carry such a poor prognosis for MCC. Truncal location resulted in mortality in 6 (75%) of 8 patients, compared with no deaths among the 12 patients with extremity lesions and 1 death among the 11 patients with head and neck lesions. The poor outcome of patients with truncal tumors may reflect a wider potential array of lymphatic basins for dissemination relative to extremity and head and neck lesions[16]; it may also be due to earlier systemic spread. Our observation that the 2 truncal lesion survivors received more aggressive therapy than the nonsurvivors suggests that multimodality treatment does make a difference. Both survivors received wide excision and XRT to the tumor bed and regional nodes in excess of 45 Gy, and 1 patient also received chemotherapy. By contrast, of the 6 nonsurvivors, only 1 patient had an optimal wide excision and none received optimal XRT in the perioperative period.

Due to the propensity for early nodal spread and the significant negative impact nodal disease has on outcome, many have felt that prophylactic lymph-node dissection is warranted.[14,15] These authors demonstrate improved locoregional control but no impact on survival. No comment is made about complications of the lymph-node dissection (edema, infection, and pain), so it is not clear at what cost this local benefit was obtained. Our study confirms the findings of the previous studies. Although the 8 patients in our series who underwent lymphadenectomy did not develop nodal recurrences, there was no survival benefit. None of these patients experienced any significant complications from the nodal dissection. At the very least, the information on nodal status may be useful in selecting patients for further adjuvant therapy. In this regard, the report by Messina et al[16] employing the sentinel node technique is promising, with no false negatives, although the follow-up is limited (median, 10.5 months).

Since a truncal location of tumor and node positivity have a significant negative impact on survival, what is the optimal treatment of these high-risk patients as well as all patients with MCC? Almost all authors advocate wide local excision, and we strongly agree with this. This reduces the incidence of local recurrence but does not improve survival. Our findings confirm this and indicate that a 2-cm margin, when possible, is the appropriate width of excision to obtain local control. None of the 7 patients with margins of resection of 2 cm or larger experienced a local recurrence, whereas one third of patients with narrower margins did. In anatomical locations where wide margins cannot technically be obtained, XRT has been useful in local control with long-term survival rates. Our 4 patients with facial lesions treated primarily by XRT suggest that this is a reasonable alternative, although the sample size does not allow a satisfactory statistical analysis.

Radiation therapy is an important component in the treatment of MCC. All 9 patients who received XRT of 45 Gy or greater to the primary tumor bed and to the regional nodal bed were alive and free of disease at the time of this report (Figure 3). This result, in conjunction with the 4 disease-free head and neck primary tumors that were treated primarily with XRT, supports the benefit of XRT for outcome. This is the first time that XRT as the only therapy for MCC has been shown to have a curative role. With a larger sample size, it is likely that the benefit of XRT for survival ($P = .08$) would have achieved statistical significance. While most studies have demonstrated the benefit of XRT for local control, the study by Meeuwissen et al[17] and our study are the only studies also confirming the benefit for survival.

The use of chemotherapy is unproven but advisable for high-risk patients (ie, truncal lesions or nodal disease). Multiple agents have been demonstrated to be active against MCC.[22] Although the administration of chemotherapy was associated with a worse outcome in our series, this clearly reflects a selection bias, as demonstrated by the multivariate analysis. The fact that 2 patients with distant metastatic disease were alive and free of disease at 32 and 96 months may suggest that some lasting benefit is gained from chemotherapy. Given the extremely low incidence of this tumor, it is unlikely that anything more than anecdotal treatment reports will appear in the literature.

When treatments fails with either local recurrence or nodal disease, patient should undergo resection, followed by XRT greater than 45 Gy to the site. At the time of this report, we had 5 such patients, with mean disease-free survival of 40 months. This is in agreement with the 50% to 60% success rate reported by Meland and Jackson.[5]

Our recommendations for the treatment of MCC are based on its aggressive behavior, which requires an aggressive treatment plan. To minimize local recurrence, lesions should, whenever anatomically possible, be widely excised with a 2-cm margin. They should also receive postoperative XRT to the primary site if wide margins have not been obtained or if the primary lesion is located on the trunk. At the time of the resection the status of the draining lymph nodes should be ascertained. Results using the sentinel-node mapping technique suggest that this is as applicable here as it has been shown to be in patients with melanoma. Patients with positive lymph nodes should undergo formal lymph-node dissection, followed by XRT to the nodal bed. Patients who choose not to have a complete lymph-node dissection should probably undergo XRT to the regional nodes, especially if they have a truncal lesion. Patients with truncal lesions or positive nodes are at high risk for distant metastatic disease, and systemic chemotherapy should be seriously considered. When lesions recur, a combined modality approach of reexcision, lymphadenectomy, XRT, and chemotherapy should be used, unless contraindicated. The combination of wide local excision, regional lymphadenectomy, and postoperative XRT has the potential to achieve cure in greater than 90% of patients.

Presented at the 79th Annual Meeting of the New England Surgical Society, Toronto, Ontario, September 26, 1998.

Corresponding author: Mark J. Ott, MD, Division of Surgical Oncology, Department of Surgery, Massachusetts General Hospital, 626 Cox Bldg, 100 Blossom St, Boston, MA 02114 (e-mail: Ott.Mark@MGH.Harvard.Edu).

REFERENCES

1. Cotlar A, Gates J, Gibbs F. Merkel cell carcinoma: combined surgery and radiation therapy. *Am J Surg.* 1986;52:159-164.
2. Hitchcock CL, Bland KI, Laney RG, Daisy F, Harris B, Copeland EM. Neuroendocrine (Merkel cell) carcinoma of the skin: its natural history, diagnosis, and treatment. *Ann Surg.* 1988;207:201-207.
3. Kroll M, Toker C. Trabecular carcinoma of the skin: further clinicopathologic and morphologic study. *Arch Pathol Lab Med.* 1982;106:404-408.
4. Murphy RX Jr, Li JK, Mincer FK, Strauch B. Trabecular (neuroendocrine) carcinoma of the skin: report of 4 cases and review of the literature. *N Y State J Med.* 1990;90:35-38.
5. Meland N, Jackson I. Merkel cell tumor: diagnosis, prognosis, and treatment. *Plast Reconstr Surg.* 1986;77:632-638.
6. Raaf JH, Urmacher C, Knapper WK, Shiu M, Cheng E. Trabecular (Merkel cell) carcinoma of the skin: treatment of primary, recurrent, and metastatic disease. *Cancer.* 1986;57:178-182.
7. Schack RB, Barton RM, Delozier J, Rees R, Lynch J. Is aggressive surgical management justified in the treatment of Merkel cell carcinoma? *Plast Reconstr Surg.* 1994;94:970-974.
8. Sibley RK, Dehner LP, Rosai J. Primary neuroendocrine (Merkel cell?) carcinoma of the skin: a clinicopathologic and ultrastructural study of 43 cases. *Am J Surg Pathol.* 1985;9:95-108.
9. Szadowska A, Wozniak L, Lasota J, Mirecka B, Wolska H. Neuroendocrine (Merkel cell) carcinoma of the skin: a clinico-morphological study of 13 cases. *Histopathology.* 1989;15:483-493.
10. Al-Ghazal SK, Arora DS, Simpson HW, Saxby P. Merkel cell carcinoma of the skin. *Br J Plast Surg.* 1996;49:491-496.
11. Toker C. Trabecular carcinoma of the skin. *Arch Dermatol.* 1972;105:107-110.
12. Queirolo P, Gipponi M, Peressini A, et al. Merkel cell carcinoma of the skin: treatment of primary, recurrent, and metastatic disease: review of clinical cases. *Anticancer Res.* 1997;17:673-678.
13. Marenda SA, Otta RA. Adnexal carcinoma of the skin. *Otolaryngol Clin North Am.* 1993;26:87-116.
14. Victor NS, Morton B, Smith JW. Merkel cell cancer: is prophylactic lymph node dissection indicated? *Am Surg.* 1996;62:879-882.
15. Smith DE, Bielamowicz S, Kagan AR, Anderson PJ, Peddada AV. Cutaneous neuroendocrine (Merkel cell) carcinoma. *Am J Clin Oncol.* 1995;18:199-204.
16. Messina JL, Reintgen DS, Cruse CW, et al. Selective lymphadenectomy in patients with Merkel cell (cutaneous neuroendocrine) carcinoma. *Ann Surg Oncol.* 1997;4:389-395.
17. Meeuwissen JA, Bourne RG, Kearsley JH. The importance of perioperative radiation therapy in the treatment of Merkel cell carcinoma. *Int J Radiat Oncol Biol Phys.* 1995;31:325-331.
18. Kaplan EL, Meier P. Nonparametric estimation from incomplete observations. *J Am Stat Assoc.* 1958;53:457-481.
19. Shaw JH, Rumball E. Merkel cell tumour: clinical behavior and treatment. *Br J Surg.* 1991;78:138-142.
20. Fitzpatrick TB, Milton GW, Balch CM, Shaw HM, McCarthy WH, Sober AJ. Clinical characteristics. In: Balch CM, Houghton AN, Milton GW, Saber AJ, Soong SJ, eds. *Cutaneous Melanoma.* 2nd ed. Philadelphia, Pa: Lippincott-Raven Publishers; 1992:228.
21. Pitale M, Sesions RB, Husain S. An analysis of prognostic factors in cutaneous neuroendocrine carcinoma. *Laryngoscope.* 1992;102:244-249.
22. Krasagakis K, Almond-Roesler B, Zouboulis CC, et al. Merkel cell carcinoma: report of 10 cases with emphasis on clinical course, treatment, and in vitro drug sensitivity. *J Am Acad Dermatol.* 1997;36:727-732.

DISCUSSION

Richard Swanson, MD, Worcester, Mass: I congratulate Dr Ott and his colleagues at the Massachusetts General Hospital for doing an excellent job analyzing data regarding this rare tumor so they they can help us with treatment guidelines. The rarity of this tumor is clear from the fact that only 2 cases per year were seen at the Massachusetts General Hospital over 17 or 18 years. At our own institution, the University of Massachusetts Memorial Health Care Cancer Center, we have seen 5 cases over 7 years. This represents less than 0.1% of all cancer cases seen during this period. Obviously with such a rare tumor it would difficult to conduct a randomized prospective trial to definitively answer questions regarding optimal treatment. Thus, we need to formulate treatment decisions from retrospective analysis such as that presented today.

From your data you've made recommendations about . . . treatment regarding aggressive surgery and radiotherapy. Your suggestions are similar to those found in the literature. From our own small experience, and from my reading of the literature, I'm impressed by the radio-responsiveness of these tumors. This leads me to wonder whether aggressive surgery is necessary if radiotherapy will be used.

Specifically, from your data you recommended . . . excision when possible with postoperative radiotherapy. If all patients receive 45 Gy to the primary, do we need the 2-cm margin? You state that 4 who've had neck cancers were treated primarily with radiotherapy without a wide excision and all are alive without disease. You also stated that 9 patients who had over 45 Gy radiotherapy enjoyed disease-free survival. Other than the 4 head and neck cancer patients, did any of these 9 patients have less than 2-cm margins? Perhaps radiotherapy alone or radiotherapy after a simple excision of the primary without regard to achieving wide margins would be sufficient. I'd appreciate your comments about that point.

You recommended sentinel lymph-node biopsy, or suggest a sentinel lymph-node biopsy would be helpful in determining positive nodes, and then you recommend a formal lymph-node dissection and radiotherapy to the nodal region for positive nodes. I agree that a sentinel-node biopsy is reasonable to identify positive nodes, and I agree that patients with positive nodes should have treatment of those nodes; the question is, what is necessary to treat the sentinel node–positive but clinically negative nodal basin? From your data and the literature I suspect that over 45 Gy in radiotherapy to the nodal region would be sufficient, and dissection would not be necessary. Do you have specific data that argue for the addition of node dissection to radiotherapy in the subset?

In summary, can we treat patients with MCC with excision of the gross tumor without concern about margins followed by sentinel-node biopsy and radiation therapy to the primary and to the node region for positive nodes without formal node dissection?

Peter Deckers, MD, Farmington, Conn: I'd like to speak to just the opposite of what Dr Swanson spoke about. Let me put it this way. I think all of us who have done lymphadenectomies, either in the groin or the axilla, over the years have been impressed with the fact that if you add radiotherapy to well-done axillary dissections or well-done groin dissections, then you don't really gain anything by that from the point of view of survival or local control, but you do significantly increase the morbidity, ie, lymphedema of the arm or lymphedema of the leg. So what I'm asking is can you give me solid evidence that the radiotherapy after an adequate groin dissection or an adequate axillary dissection for clinically positive disease makes a real difference?

Charles Shoemaker, MD, Newport, RI: Just a few observations. One, we reviewed this entity at the New England cancer meeting a couple of years ago, and it's a very rare lesion. I heard the comment, "What does it look like?" Our experience was you took the lesion out, then you found out it was MCC and it was too late to get a picture. Histologically, the lesion starts in the deep layers of the skin, so the top layer of skin may not be involved, so it's just a heaping up of the skin, and looking back at notes, it's sort of pink in color.

The other part of our review supports your last comment—be very aggressive about the recurrences, because some patients are salvageable.

The third comment relates to Dr Deckers' comment. Surgeons from Memorial Sloan-Kettering are very aggressive about doing lymph-node dissection for lesions arising in the head and neck, but do not employ postoperative radiation.

William Cook, MD, North Andover, Mass: It just happens that 2 days ago I had a call from one of our local oncologists, who had an MCC tumor patient they thought was controlled over the past 4 or 5 years and that patient has presented with a solitary nodule in the lung. Dr Ott, would you comment on the nature of your distant metastases as to how often you see, or might expect to see, a solitary pulmonary nodule as an expression of recurrence, or whether I should be thinking about this being a different kind of tumor; obviously, I'll find out. If it turns out to be a recurrence of the MCC tumor, what would you propose besides resection of the lesion as far as additional therapy?

Dougald MacGillivray, MD, Portland, Me: I have 2 questions. One is the method of detection of distant metastases. Have you used octreotide scans in evaluating these patients? We recently had a patient who had an unsuspected distant metastasis detected this way. This patient was on immunosuppression after having a renal transplantation and had very rapid progression of disease. In my review of the literature there have been anecdotal reports of these tumors associated with immunosuppression. Were any of your patients on immunosuppression?

Dr Ott: Thank you very much, Dr Swanson. In terms of the several issues, I'll work back a little bit in reverse order. Several of these patients did have immunosuppressed states. As I said, there was a high incidence of associated malignancies in these patients, and several of them were actually undergoing chemotherapy prior to the development of their MCC. I do think that there probably is some immunosuppression involved with development of this tumor. Certainly, octreotide scans have been reported in the literature as being used clinically to detect metastases. I'm aware of one positive scan similar to yours as well. These do have somatostatin receptors. The octreotide scan is said to be 80% to 85% sensitive in detecting neuroendocrine tumors, and MCC is a neuroendocrine tumor. Only 1 patient in our series had the scan, and it was positive.

In terms of Dr Cook's questions and his patient with the lung metastases, his patient is almost identical to one of the patients in our series. Our patient developed an isolated lung metastasis 26 months after resection of the initial skin lesion. The patient underwent chemotherapy with cisplatin and Adriamycin and is presently at 33 months disease free. The patient did not have resection of that isolated lesion as part of the patient's treatment.

Merkel cell cancer, when it's looked at by a pathologist, looks exactly like small cell carcinoma lung. In fact, when a skin lesion is detected, it's very important to make sure that the patient does not have a primary somewhere else and that the skin lesion is not a metastasis. Neuroendocrine tumors of the gut and small cell of the lung can metastasize to the skin, so it is important to exclude these other tumors.

In terms of the metastatic pattern, we've had metastases to the lung. We've had them to the bone. We've had them to other areas of the skin, to the liver, to the small bowel, to the kidney, to the brain, and to nodes. So in a sense it behaves very similar to an aggressive melanoma, and it can basically show up anywhere.

Dr Shoemaker's comments about the lesion's appearance on the skin: Yes, it's an intradermal lesion. The Merkel cell receptor is located at the base of the hair follicle, and it's believed to arise in that area, and it does cause a heaping up of the skin with sort of a reddish/purple discoloration. The vast majority of times, the lesion is excised, believing that it's a benign intradermal process. When it ultimately comes back as MCC, it is usually a surprise. So you're right; it's very uncommon to have a great photograph of an MCC until it's in the pathology lab.

In terms of the whole question of surgery and radiation therapy, this is an extremely radiosensitive tumor. In the 4 cases of the head and neck lesions, 2 of those cases had clinically positive neck nodes, and all of those cases received radiation to the primary as well as to the neck on that side. All 4 patients had regression of the primary or nodal disease. All 4 patients are now alive at 8, 33, 60, and 92 months out and are free of disease. I think there is certainly room for treating these patients with radiation as the primary form of therapy. There was 1 patient who had a positive single lymph-node biopsy in the groin and then received subsequent radiation to that area without surgical resection and is among the patients who are disease free 3 to 4 years out from their initial treatment. Certainly this is a radiosensitive tumor, but due to the small numbers, it is difficult to test whether surgery vs radiotherapy is better or whether they should be combined.

As to my own opinion of using both surgery and radiation therapy, yes, there is a higher incidence of lymphedema and morbidity from that combined approach. And, yes, there are patients in our series who had just lymphadenectomy without radiation therapy and are free of disease at 3 to 4 years. I can think of 2 in our series of survivors who did not have radiation. Having reviewed the data, my point is that more of these patients could have been cured. Due to the rarity of this disease, we're never going to know how little we can get away with. We are therefore stuck with erring on the side of being more aggressive and combining therapies. That was the basis of this entire paper. That applies particularly to the nodal disease. To Dr Swanson's question about whether it is adequate just to simply excise the primary and give radiation therapy to control the primary, I think the answer to that is probably yes. All of us here are surgeons, and we would feel much more comfortable doing a wide excision of 2 cm which will also cure the primary. Certainly curative surgery is preferable to surgery and radiation when possible in treating the primary tumor. It is nice to have a tumor which gives one both options.

Mechanism of Adrenal Insufficiency Following Trauma and Severe Hemorrhage

Role of Hepatic 11β-Hydroxysteroid Dehydrogenase

Ping Wang, MD; Zheng F. Ba; Doraid Jarrar, MD; William G. Cioffi, MD; Kirby I. Bland, MD; Irshad H. Chaudry, PhD

Background: Although adrenal insufficiency may not occur with moderate hypotension, it does occur with severe hemorrhage. Since hepatocellular function is depressed following severe hemorrhage, it remains unknown whether the liver plays any role in regulating adrenal function after trauma and hemorrhagic shock.

Hypothesis: Hepatic 11β-hydroxysteroid dehydrogenase (11β-HSD), a microsomal enzyme responsible for the degradation of bioactive corticosterone, plays a major role in the development of adrenal insufficiency following trauma and severe hemorrhage.

Design, Interventions, and Main Outcome Measures: Male rats underwent laparotomy to induce trauma before hemorrhage. They were then bled to and maintained at a blood pressure of 40 mm Hg until 40% of the maximal bleed-out volume was returned in the form of Ringer lactate. The rats were then resuscitated with 4 times the volume of maximal bleed-out with Ringer lactate during a 60-minute period. Plasma levels of corticosterone and corticotropin were measured at various intervals. In additional groups, corticotropin-induced corticosterone release, adrenal contents of corticosterone and cyclic adenosine monophosphate (cAMP), hepatic 11β-HSD activity, and plasma levels of corticosterone-binding globulin were determined at 1.5 hours after resuscitation. Moreover, a model of moderate hypotension (blood pressure, 80 mm Hg) was used to determine whether adrenal function is depressed under such conditions.

Results: At the time of maximal bleed-out, plasma corticosterone and corticotropin levels increased by 245% ($P<.001$) and 293% ($P<.001$), respectively. Despite corticotropin levels being similar to those of the animals undergoing sham operation after resuscitation, corticosterone levels in hemorrhaged animals remained elevated up to 4 hours after resuscitation (by 158%-207%; $P<.001$). In addition, corticotropin-induced corticosterone release decreased by 78% at 1.5 hours after resuscitation ($P=.009$). In contrast, moderate hypotension did not reduce corticotropin-induced corticosterone release. Adrenal corticosterone content and cAMP levels (ie, the second messenger of corticotropin action) decreased by 55% ($P<.001$) and 25% ($P=.03$), respectively. Hepatic 11β-HSD activity decreased significantly at 1.5 hours after resuscitation ($P<.001$).

Conclusions: Sustained increase in plasma corticosterone levels following hemorrhage and resuscitation may be, in part, due to the decreased hepatic 11β-HSD activity. The high level of corticosterone negatively regulates corticotropin release, further reducing adrenal responsiveness to corticotropin stimulation. Thus, the liver appears to play an important role in regulating adrenal function following trauma and severe hemorrhage.

Arch Surg. 1999;134:394-401

From the Center for Surgical Research and Department of Surgery, Brown University School of Medicine and Rhode Island Hospital, Providence.

DESPITE MAJOR advances in the management of trauma, a large number of trauma patients subsequently die of the ensuing sepsis, septic shock, and multiple organ failure.[1-3] Although early and rapid fluid resuscitation remains the cornerstone of the treatment of trauma victims, studies have indicated that hepatocellular dysfunction (ie, the depressed clearance of indocyanine green), which occurs early after hemorrhage, persists despite crystalloid resuscitation.[4,5] In addition, circulating levels of liver enzymes (alanine aminotransferase and aspartate aminotransferase) increase significantly following trauma and hemorrhagic shock,[6] indicating hepatocyte damage under such conditions. Although adrenal insufficiency occurs frequently during sepsis and septic shock,[7-9] and although administration of hydrocortisone in patients with sepsis has been reported to reverse the altered hemodynamics during late septic shock,[10] it is a common notion that adrenal insufficiency occurs rarely after trauma and surgery.[11,12] However, recent studies by Barquist and Kirton[13] have indicated that although the overall inci-

MATERIALS AND METHODS

ANIMAL MODEL OF TRAUMA AND SEVERE HEMORRHAGE

We used a nonheparinized model of trauma-hemorrhage and resuscitation in the rat, as described previously,[5] with minor modifications. Briefly, male Sprague-Dawley rats (Charles River Laboratory, Wilmington, Mass) weighing 275 to 325 g were not fed for 16 hours before the experiment but were allowed water ad libitum. The animals were anesthetized using methoxyflurane inhalation; they underwent a 5-cm ventral midline laparotomy to induce tissue trauma before the onset of hemorrhage. The abdominal incision was then closed in layers. Both femoral arteries were cannulated using polyethylene-50 tubing for bleeding or monitoring of mean arterial pressure. All incisions were then closed and bathed with 1% lidocaine hydrochloride to provide analgesia throughout the experiment. The animals were then bled to a mean arterial pressure of 40 mm Hg (ie, severe hypotension) within 10 minutes. The blood pressure of 40 mm Hg was maintained by removing more blood until the animal was no longer able to maintain its blood pressure at that level (ie, maximal bleed-out). At that point, the blood pressure was further maintained by returning fluid in the form of Ringer lactate solution (RL) intravenously until 40% of the shed blood volume was returned in that form. Following this, the animals were resuscitated with RL at 4 times the volume of maximal bleed-out during a period of 60 minutes. Animals undergoing sham operation (hereafter referred to as sham animals) underwent the same surgical procedure but were not bled or resuscitated. The time required for maximal bleed-out was approximately 45 minutes, the volume of maximal bleed-out was approximately 60% of the calculated circulating blood volume,[17] and the total hemorrhage time was approximately 90 minutes. Blood samples were collected at various time points for measurement of plasma corticosterone and adrenocorticotropic hormone (corticotropin) levels. In additional groups of animals, adrenal glands were harvested at 1.5 hours after the completion of hemorrhage and resuscitation for determination of tissue corticosterone and corticotropin levels. Moreover, corticotropin-induced release of corticosterone was assessed at 1.5 hours after resuscitation in separate groups of animals. There were 6 to 8 rats in each group at each time, and the rats were killed using an overdose of intravenous pentobarbital sodium at the end of each experiment. The experiments described herein were performed in adherence to the National Institutes of Health guidelines for the use of experimental animals. This project was approved by the Institutional Animal Care and Use Committee of Rhode Island Hospital, Providence.

EXPERIMENTAL MODEL OF MODERATE HYPOTENSION

To determine whether adrenal insufficiency occurs only following severe hemorrhagic shock, a model of moderate hypotension was also used in additional groups of animals. Briefly, male Sprague-Dawley rats (275-325 g) were not fed overnight before the experiment but were allowed water ad libitum. The rats were anesthetized using methoxyflurane inhalation before the induction of trauma (ie, 5-cm midline laparotomy). Following cannulation of various blood vessels, the rats were bled to and maintained at a mean arterial pressure of 80 mm Hg for 90 minutes (moderate hypotension). The animals were then resuscitated using RL at 4 times the volume of the withdrawn blood (5.46 ± 0.45 mL/rat; approximately 30% of the calculated blood volume) during a 60-minute period. Blood samples were taken at various times for measuring corticosterone and corticotropin levels. At 1.5 hours after resuscitation, corticotropin-induced corticosterone release was determined in additional groups of animals. There were 5 to 8 rats in each group at each time.

DETERMINATION OF CORTICOSTERONE AND CORTICOTROPIN LEVELS

Blood samples for corticosterone and corticotropin assays were collected at 2 to 4 PM, when plasma levels were similar to the 24-hour average.[15] Plasma levels of corticosterone and corticosterone contents in the adrenal tissues were determined using a commercially available double-antibody radioimmunoassay kit specifically for rat corticosterone (Immuchem; ICN Biomedicals Inc, Costa Mesa, Calif). Plasma samples (10 μL each) were assayed in duplicates. The cross-reactivity of the radioimmunoassay for rat corticosterone was 100%. For other steroids, the cross-reactivity was as follows: desoxycorticosterone, 0.34%; testosterone, 0.10%; cortisol, 0.05%; aldosterone, 0.03%; progesterone, 0.03%; and all other tested steroids, less than 0.01%. Plasma levels of corticotropin were measured using a specific radioimmunoassay kit from Peninsula Labs

Continued on next page

dence of adrenal insufficiency was less than 1% in surgical intensive care units, 11% of the patients older than 55 years and with intensive care unit stays of 14 days or longer were found to have adrenal insufficiency. It is also reported that postoperative adrenal insufficiency is more common in patients than currently recognized.[14] Thus, investigation of the mechanism responsible for adrenal insufficiency following trauma and hemorrhage is important for improved management of severe trauma.

The enzyme 11β-hydroxysteroid dehydrogenase (11β-HSD) is expressed extensively in the liver[15] and catalyzes the conversion of 11β-hydroxysteroids—cortisol in humans and corticosterone (the main glucocorticoid in rodents) in the rat—into their inactive forms, cortisone and 11-dehydrocorticosterone, respectively.[16] Although previous studies have demonstrated that hepatocellular dysfunction occurs early after the onset of hemorrhage and persists even after fluid resuscitation,[4] it remains unknown whether the depressed hepatocellular function is associated with a decrease in 11β-HSD activity. Our aim, therefore, was to determine whether hepatic 11β-HSD activity is reduced following hemorrhage and resuscitation and, if so, whether the decreased 11β-HSD activities are associated with adrenal insufficiency under such conditions.

(Belmont, Calif). Briefly, a 1.5-mL blood sample was collected into a polypropylene tube containing ethylenediaminetetraacetic acid (1 mg/mL) and aprotinin (500 KIU/mL) at various times during and after hemorrhage, and plasma was separated. The extraction of corticotropin was performed using columns packed with C18 sorbent. The corticotropin was eluted with 60% acetonitrile and 1% trifluoroacetic acid. Eluates were evaporated to dryness using a centrifugal concentrator. Rat corticotropin assay has less than 0.1% cross-reactivity with other tested peptides.

CORTICOTROPIN-STIMULATED RELEASE OF CORTICOSTERONE

At 1.5 hours after the completion of hemorrhage and resuscitation or a corresponding time in the sham animals, 100 μg of porcine corticotropin (1-39; 90 IU/mg; Sigma-Aldrich Corporation, St Louis, Mo) in 0.2-mL isotonic sodium chloride solution vehicles was injected intravenously.[18] Blood samples were taken before and 30 minutes after corticotropin administration for corticosterone assays, as described. Studies have indicated that the plasma concentrations of corticosterone increased rapidly following corticotropin administration, reaching a peak at 15 to 30 minutes and returning to basal levels by 90 minutes.[19] Our preliminary experiments indicated that plasma corticosterone levels reached a peak 30 minutes after intravenous injection of porcine corticotropin in sham animals (data not shown).

MEASUREMENT OF CYCLIC ADENOSINE MONOPHOSPHATE LEVELS

To determine the levels of cyclic adenosine monophosphate (cAMP) in the adrenal tissue, both adrenal glands were homogenized at 4°C with isotonic sodium chloride solution (1 mL of homogenate). The cAMP levels were determined radioimmunologically according to the manufacturer's instructions (a nonacetylated-procedure, cAMP radioimmunoassay kit; Du Pont/NEN, Boston, Mass), as described previously.[20]

DETERMINATION OF HEPATIC 11β-HSD ACTIVITY

Hepatic 11β-HSD activity was determined by assessing the rate of conversion of cortisol to cortisone.[21] Briefly, approximately 0.2 g of hepatic tissue was homogenized in 4 mL of ice-cold sodium phosphate buffer (10 mmol/L; pH, 7.0) containing 0.25-mol/L sucrose. Each assay tube contains approximately 150 000 counts per minute tritiated cortisol (Du Pont/NEN), 1.0 μmol/L nonradioactive cortisol, and 250-μmol/L β-nicotinamide adenine dinucleotide phosphate. Sodium phosphate buffer (0.1 mol/L) was added to bring the volume up to 0.4 mL. After 10-minute incubation at 37°C, 100 μL hepatic homogenate containing 1.0 mg of protein was added. After further incubation for 30 minutes, the reaction was arrested by rapidly transferring the tubes onto ice. The steroids were then extracted with 4 mL ethyl acetate containing a 40-μg mixture of nonradioactive cortisol and cortisone as carrier steroids. The extracts were dried, and the residues were resuspended in 100 μL of methanol. A fraction of the resuspension was spotted on a thin layer chromatography plate, which was developed in chloroform-methanol (volume-volume ratio, 9:1). The bands containing the labeled cortisol and cortisone were identified by UV light of the cold carriers, cut out into scintillation vials, and counted. The conversion rate of cortisol to cortisone was calculated from the specific activity of the labeled cortisol and the radioactivity of cortisone, and the results are expressed as the amount of cortisone (picomoles) formed per milligram of protein in 30 minutes.

DETERMINATION OF CORTICOSTERONE-BINDING GLOBULIN AND PLASMA PROTEIN LEVELS

Plasma levels of corticosterone-binding globulin (CBG) were assayed by using a saturation analysis.[22] Briefly, endogenous steroids were removed from the samples by dilution (1:100) in a slurry of dextran-coated charcoal (DCC). After the centrifugation to remove DCC, aliquots (100 μL) of the supernatant were incubated with 10-nmol/L tritiated cortisol (Du Pont/NEN) in the presence or absence of 2-μmol/L unlabeled cortisol. Separation of CBG-bound steroid was achieved by incubation for 10 minutes at 0°C with 600 μL of DCC, followed by centrifugation. The supernatants were subjected to liquid scintillation counting. Plasma levels of protein were measured according to the method of Lowry et al.[23]

STATISTICAL ANALYSIS

One-way analysis of variance and Tukey test or Student *t* test were used, and the differences were considered significant at $P \leq .05$. Results are presented as mean ± SEM.

RESULTS

ALTERATIONS IN PLASMA LEVELS OF CORTICOSTERONE AND CORTICOTROPIN

As shown in **Figure 1**, plasma levels of corticosterone increased by 245% ($P < .001$) at the time of maximal bleed-out. The significantly increased levels of corticosterone persisted after fluid resuscitation, ie, 158% to 207% at 0 to 4 hours after the completion of fluid resuscitation ($P < .001$) (Figure 1). Similar to the changes in plasma corticosterone levels, corticotropin levels increased by 293% ($P < .001$) at the time of maximal bleed-out (**Figure 2**). However, circulating levels of corticotropin decreased by 52% to 58% ($P < .001$) at 0 to 4 hours after the completion of fluid resuscitation, compared with the levels at the time of maximal bleed-out (Figure 2). In addition, these levels were not significantly different from the values in sham animals (Figure 2).

CORTICOTROPIN-INDUCED CORTICOSTERONE RELEASE AND ADRENAL CONTENTS OF CORTICOSTERONE AND cAMP

At 30 minutes after the intravenous administration of porcine corticotropin, plasma levels of corticosterone increased by 101% in sham animals (from 4.31 ± 0.70 to 8.68 ± 0.98 ng/mg protein; $P = .005$) (**Figure 3**). At 1.5

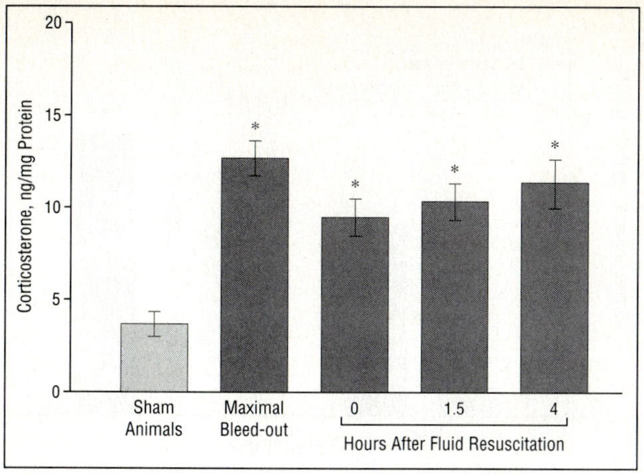

Figure 1. *Alterations in plasma levels of corticosterone in animals undergoing sham operation (sham animals), at the time of the maximal bleed-out, and 0, 1.5, and 4 hours after the completion of fluid resuscitation. Data are presented as mean ± SEM and compared using 1-way analysis of variance and Tukey test. Asterisk indicates* P<*.05 vs sham animals.*

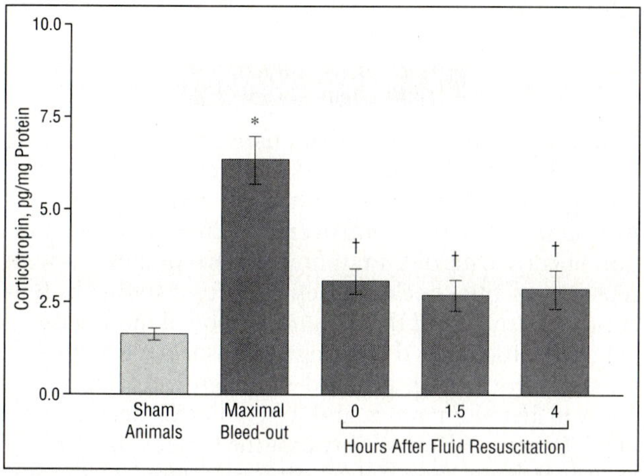

Figure 2. *Alterations in plasma levels of adrenocorticotropic hormone (corticotropin) in animals undergoing sham operation (sham animals), at the time of the maximal bleed-out, and 0, 1.5, and 4 hours after the completion of fluid resuscitation. Data are presented as mean ± SEM and compared using 1-way analysis of variance and Tukey test. Asterisk indicates* P<*.05 vs sham animals; dagger,* P<*.05 vs time of maximal bleed-out.*

hours after hemorrhage and resuscitation, however, corticotropin-induced release of corticosterone only increased by 8% (from 12.36 ± 0.96 to 13.34 ± 0.59 ng/mg protein; $P = .41$) (Figure 3). Thus, corticotropin-induced net increase of corticosterone levels was reduced by 78% from 4.37 ± 0.73 to 0.98 ± 0.75 ng/mg protein ($P = .009$). In addition, adrenal corticosterone levels decreased by 55% at 1.5 hours after hemorrhage and resuscitation ($P < .001$) (**Figure 4**, top). Similarly, the basal cAMP levels in the adrenal tissue decreased significantly following hemorrhage and resuscitation (Figure 4, bottom).

ALTERATIONS IN HEPATIC 11β-HSD ACTIVITY

As shown in **Figure 5**, hepatic 11β-HSD activity was 81.3 ± 2.6 pmol/mg protein in 30 minutes in sham animals. At 1.5 hours after the completion of hemorrhage and resuscitation, however, hepatic 11β-HSD levels decreased by 31% ($P < .001$) (Figure 5).

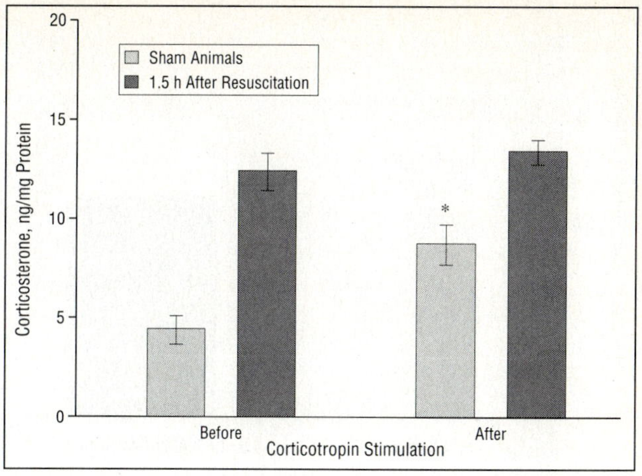

Figure 3. *Alterations in corticotropin-stimulated increase in plasma corticosterone levels in animals undergoing sham operation (sham animals) and at 1.5 hours after the completion of hemorrhage and resuscitation. Data are presented as mean ± SEM and compared using 1-way analysis of variance and Tukey test. Asterisk indicates* P<*.05 vs the respective corticosterone level before corticotropin administration.*

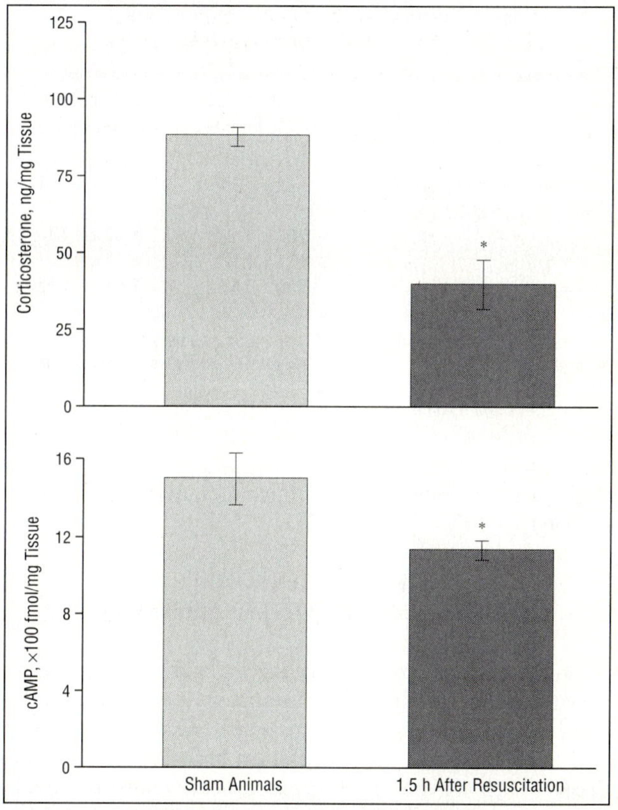

Figure 4. *Alterations in adrenal corticosterone contents (top) and adrenal cyclic adenosine monophosphate (cAMP) levels (bottom) in animals undergoing sham operation (sham animals) and at 1.5 hours after the completion of hemorrhage and resuscitation. Data are presented as mean ± SEM and compared using unpaired Student* t *test. Asterisk indicates* P<*.05 vs sham animals.*

ALTERATIONS IN PLASMA CGB LEVELS

The plasma levels of CGB were found to be 30.25 ± 2.76 pmol/mL in sham animals. Although plasma CBG levels increased to 45.50 ± 6.74 pmol/mL at 1.5 hours after the completion of hemorrhage and resuscitation, such an in-

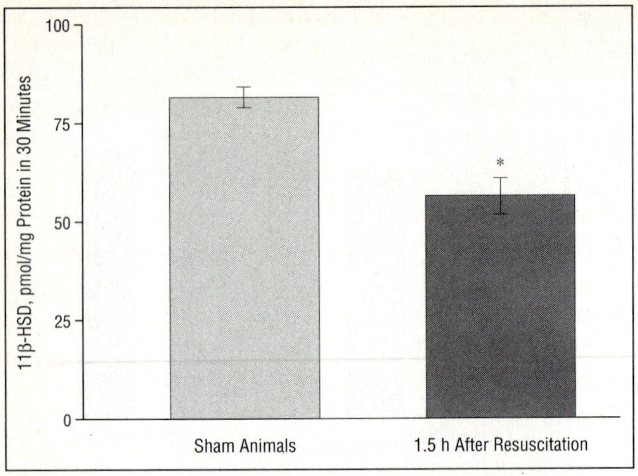

Figure 5. *Alterations in hepatic 11β-hydroxysteroid dehydrogenase (11β-HSD) activity in animals undergoing sham operation (sham animals) and at 1.5 hours after the completion of hemorrhage and resuscitation. Data are presented as mean ± SEM and compared using unpaired Student* t *test. Asterisk indicates* P<*.05 vs sham animals.*

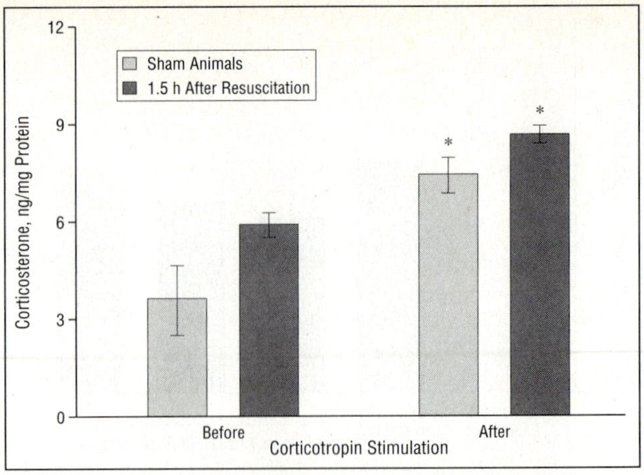

Figure 6. *Alterations in corticotropin-stimulated increase in plasma corticosterone levels in animals undergoing sham operation (sham animals) and at 1.5 hours after the completion of hemorrhage and resuscitation in a model of moderate hypotension. Data are presented as mean ± SEM and compared using 1-way analysis of variance and Tukey test. Asterisk indicates* P<*.05 vs the respective corticosterone level before corticotropin administration.*

Alterations in Plasma Levels of Corticosterone and Corticotropin During and After Moderate Hypotension*

	Corticosterone, ng/mg Protein	Corticotropin, pg/mg Protein
After sham operation	3.57 ± 1.11	1.54 ± 0.16
During 45-min hemorrhage	8.22 ± 0.30†	2.39 ± 0.13†
After resuscitation, h		
0	6.63 ± 0.39†	1.67 ± 0.13
1.5	6.25 ± 0.52†	1.58 ± 0.12
4	5.81 ± 0.47	2.44 ± 0.24†

**Data are presented as mean ± SEM and compared using 1-way analyses of variance and Tukey test. Moderate hypotension indicates mean arterial pressure of 80 mm Hg for 90 minutes.*

†P<.05 vs sham values.

crease was not statistically significant (6 animals per group; *P* = .06).

ADRENAL RESPONSES AFTER MODERATE HYPOTENSION

Similar to the severe hemorrhage, plasma levels of corticosterone in moderate hypotension increased significantly during the hemorrhage period and persisted at 0 and 1.5 hours after the completion of fluid resuscitation (**Table**). However, the increased corticosterone levels were not statistically different from those of the sham animals at 4 hours after resuscitation (Table). Plasma levels of corticotropin were also significantly elevated during hemorrhage and at 4 hours after resuscitation (Table). Despite the similarity in the responses of corticosterone and corticotropin after moderate hypotension vs after severe hemorrhage, corticotropin induced a significant increase in corticosterone release in sham (*P* = .014) and hemorrhaged animals (*P*<.001) (**Figure 6**). The corticotropin-induced net increase of corticosterone levels was 3.81 ± 0.98 ng/mg protein in sham animals and 2.76 ± 0.32 ng/mg protein in hemorrhaged animals (reduced by 28%) (*P* = .34).

COMMENT

A number of studies have demonstrated that circulating levels of corticosterone increase following trauma, hemorrhage, and other adverse circulatory conditions.[12,13,24-30] Although it remains controversial whether administration of corticosteroids in trauma victims or patients with sepsis and septic shock is beneficial, recent studies by Bollaert et al[10] indicated that administration of modest doses of hydrocortisone in the setting of pressor-dependent septic shock for 4 days resulted in a significant improvement in hemodynamics and a beneficial effect on survival. Despite the possibility that the beneficial effects of hydrocortisone may not be directly related to the improvement in adrenocortical insufficiency,[10] it has been demonstrated that the incidence of adrenal insufficiency increases in critically ill patients at the surgical intensive care unit.[13] Furthermore, adrenal insufficiency appears to occur during the progression of multiple organ failure in trauma victims. Although adrenal insufficiency occurs after various adverse circulatory conditions such as septic shock and severe trauma or major surgery,[31] and although it has been clearly demonstrated that hepatocellular dysfunction and hepatic failure occur under such conditions,[1,4] it remains unknown whether there is any correlation between adrenal insufficiency and hepatocellular dysfunction following trauma-hemorrhage and resuscitation. Our aim, therefore, was to determine whether the hepatocellular dysfunction observed following hemorrhagic shock plays any role in the development of adrenal insufficiency.

Our results indicate that at the time of maximal bleedout, plasma levels of corticosterone and corticotropin increased significantly. However, despite the fact that corticotropin levels decreased to levels similar to those of sham animals after resuscitation, plasma corticosterone levels remained significantly elevated up to 4 hours after resuscitation. The lack of the sustained high levels of corticotropin may be due to the negative feedback of the high levels of plasma corticosterone. Hepatic 11β-HSD is responsible for the degradation of circulating corticosterone in the rat. Thus, the reduced 11β-HSD activity may play a partial role in producing the sustained levels of plasma corticosterone after resuscitation. Since our results demonstrate that hepatic 11β-HSD activity was decreased significantly after hemorrhage and resuscitation, the reduction of hepatic 11β-HSD activity may be responsible for the increased levels of plasma corticosterone. The increased corticosterone levels, therefore, decreased the levels of corticotropin after resuscitation compared with the levels at the time of maximal bleed-out, through a negative feedback mechanism. Moreover, adrenal insufficiency occurred at 1.5 hours after fluid resuscitation in hemorrhaged animals, as evidenced by the decrease of corticotropin-induced corticosterone release by 78%. In addition, adrenal corticosterone content and cAMP levels (ie, the second messenger of the corticotropin action) decreased by 55% and 25%, respectively. These results, taken together, suggest that the sustained increase in plasma corticosterone levels following resuscitation may be due to the decreased hepatic 11β-HSD activity. The high level of corticosterone negatively regulates corticotropin release,[32,33] further reducing adrenal responsiveness to corticotropin stimulation. Thus, the liver appears to play an important role in regulating adrenal function following trauma and severe hemorrhagic shock.

Under normal conditions, corticotropin is secreted by the anterior pituitary gland following the stimulation of corticotropin-releasing hormone, a peptide secreted from the hypothalamus. Corticotropin then stimulates the secretion of glucocorticoid hormones, which by a negative feedback mechanism regulate release of corticotropin-releasing hormone and corticotropin.[34] The short-term effect of corticotropin on the release of corticosterone from the adrenal cortex is due to the rapid mobilization of cholesterol by binding to the membrane receptors, activating adenylate cyclase, and elevating intracellular cAMP levels. As a result, cholesterol is liberated and penetrates into the P-450 system of the inner mitochondrial membrane, thus providing more substrate for steroidogenesis within minutes.[15] In the long term (hours), corticotropin regulates the activity of the adrenal steroid hydroxylase system by elevating intracellular cAMP levels.[15] However, the corticotropin-induced corticosterone release test, which we used, appears to assess the short-term effects of corticotropin on the adrenal cortex.

Our results indicate that the basal level of adrenal cAMP decreased significantly after severe hemorrhage and fluid resuscitation. Although it remains unknown whether corticotropin-stimulated cAMP accumulation is also reduced under such conditions, our findings that corticotropin-stimulated release of corticosteroid and basal cAMP levels in adrenal tissue decreased significantly suggest that corticotropin-stimulated cAMP accumulation may have decreased. Further studies are needed to determine whether corticotropin-stimulated cAMP accumulation indeed decreases after trauma and hemorrhagic shock and, if so, whether this is due to down-regulation of corticotropin receptors, decrease of levels of adenylate cyclase and/or G proteins in the adrenal tissues, or reduction in adrenal adenosine triphosphate levels. It could be argued that the elevated levels of plasma corticosterone following severe hemorrhage may not reflect adrenal insufficiency, since a maximal corticosterone response may have been achieved without the stimulation of exogenous corticotropin. Although our study cannot rule out this possibility, other studies have clearly indicated that adrenal insufficiency occurs in combination with the elevated levels of circulating corticosterone.[7,31] In our study, the adrenal insufficiency observed after severe hemorrhage is characterized by not only the reduced corticotropin-stimulated release of corticosterone, but also the decreased adrenal contents of its second messenger, cAMP, and reduced adrenal levels of corticosterone. In addition, the occurrence of adrenal insufficiency suggests that the adrenal glands may not meet the demands for further increasing corticosterone release when a second hit (eg, sepsis) develops following trauma and hemorrhagic shock. In contrast to severe hemorrhage, adrenal insufficiency did not occur following moderate hypotension, despite significantly increased plasma levels of corticosterone under those conditions. Since 11β-HSD is responsible for degradation of circulating corticosterone, and since its activity in the hepatic tissue is reduced following trauma-hemorrhage and resuscitation, it is most likely that the reduced hepatic 11β-HSD activity is, in part, responsible for producing the elevated levels of plasma corticosterone under such conditions. In this regard, we propose that the reduced hepatic 11β-HSD activity plays an important role in maintaining the sustained high level of plasma corticosterone. The increased levels of corticosterone thus negatively regulate corticotropin-releasing hormone release from the hypothalamus and corticotropin release from the anterior pituitary gland, thereby reducing the circulating levels of corticotropin. The combination of the decreased levels of plasma corticotropin, adrenal corticosterone, and cAMP contents reduces adrenal function (ie, adrenal corticotropin responsiveness) following trauma and hemorrhagic shock. Thus, the reduced hepatic 11β-HSD activity, as the result of hepatocellular dysfunction following trauma and hemorrhagic shock, appears to have an important impact on adrenal function. Also, β-glycyrrhetinic acid is a potent inhibitor of 11β-HSD activity.[15] To further confirm the role of 11β-HSD in producing adrenal insufficiency following severe hemorrhage, β-glycyrrhetinic acid should be administered to healthy animals to determine whether the inhibition of 11β-HSD results in an elevated level of corticosterone and reduced corticotropin-induced corticosterone release.

More than 75% of the circulating corticosterone is bound to CBG under normal conditions.[15] Although it is unknown whether the ratio between bound and unbound corticosterone changes following adverse circulatory conditions in which plasma levels of corticosterone increase markedly, studies have indicated that plasma levels of CBG decrease significantly during sepsis and septic shock, but do not decrease in patients without sepsis.[34] In line with that study, we did not find plasma levels of CBG to be reduced following trauma-hemorrhage and fluid resuscitation. In contrast, the plasma CBG level was approximately 50% higher than that in sham ani-

Statement of Clinical Relevance

Despite advances in the understanding of the mechanisms responsible for cell and organ dysfunction and failure following trauma and hemorrhagic shock, a large number of trauma victims subsequently die of sepsis, septic shock, and ensuing multiple organ failure. Although adrenal insufficiency may not occur with mild trauma and moderate hypotension, it does occur following severe trauma, hemorrhagic shock, and/or major surgery. Since hepatocellular function is depressed early after hemorrhage and persists after fluid resuscitation, it is important to determine whether the depressed hepatocellular function under such conditions plays any role in the development of adrenal insufficiency. In this regard, our results indicate that the sustained increase in plasma corticosterone levels following resuscitation may be partially due to the decreased hepatic 11β-HSD activity observed under such conditions. The high level of corticosterone negatively regulates corticotropin release, further reducing adrenal responsiveness to corticotropin stimulation. Thus, the liver appears to play an important role in regulating adrenal function following trauma and severe hemorrhage. In view of this, we propose that maintenance of hepatocellular function (thereby preventing the reduction in hepatic 11β-HSD activity) may reverse the negative feedback mechanism and thereby improve adrenal corticotropin responsiveness.

mals, although such an increase was not statistically significant. It is possible that the elevated plasma CBG levels represent a compensatory mechanism that attempts to reduce the unbound corticosterone levels in the circulation. Because the measured plasma levels of corticosterone represent both bound and unbound portions of corticosterone, it remains unknown whether the increased CBG levels alter the ratio of bound and free corticosterone following trauma and hemorrhagic shock.

Our results suggest that the sustained increase in plasma corticosterone levels following resuscitation may be, in part, due to the decreased hepatic 11β-HSD activity. The high level of corticosterone negatively regulates corticotropin release, further reducing adrenal responsiveness to corticotropin stimulation. Thus, the liver appears to play an important role in regulating adrenal function following trauma and severe hemorrhagic shock.

This investigation was supported by grant RO1 GM 39519 (Dr Chaudry) and Independent Scientist Award KO2 AI 01461 (Dr Wang), National Institutes of Health, Bethesda, Md.

Presented at the 79th Annual Meeting of the New England Surgical Society, Toronto, Ontario, September 27, 1998.

Reprints: Ping Wang, MD, Center for Surgical Research, Rhode Island Hospital, Middle House II, 593 Eddy St, Providence, RI 02903 (e-mail: pwang@lifespan.org).

REFERENCES

1. Baue AE, Durham R, Faist E. Systemic inflammatory response syndrome (SIRS), multiple organ dysfunction syndrome (MODS), multiple organ failure (MOF): are we winning the battle? *Shock.* 1998;10:79-89.
2. Deitch EA. Multiple organ failure: pathophysiology and potential future therapy. *Ann Surg.* 1992;216:117-134.
3. Hechtman HB, Shepro D. Lung metabolism and systemic organ function. *Circ Shock.* 1982;9:457-467.
4. Wang P, Hauptman JG, Chaudry IH. Hepatocellular dysfunction occurs early after hemorrhage and persists despite fluid resuscitation. *J Surg Res.* 1990;48:464-470.
5. Wang P, Singh G, Rana MW, Ba ZF, Chaudry IH. Preheparinization improves organ function after hemorrhage and resuscitation. *Am J Physiol.* 1990;259:R645-R650.
6. Wang P, Ba ZF, Zhou M, Tait SM, Chaudry IH. Pentoxifylline restores cardiac output and tissue perfusion following trauma-hemorrhage and decreases susceptibility to sepsis. *Surgery.* 1993;114:352-359.
7. Aygen B, Inan M, Doganay M, Kelestimur F. Adrenal functions in patients with sepsis. *Exp Clin Endocrinol Diabetes.* 1997;105:182-186.
8. Carlson DE. Adrenocorticotropin correlates strongly with endotoxemia after intravenous but not after intraperitoneal inoculations of *E coli. Shock.* 1997;7:65-69.
9. Briegel J, Schelling G, Haller M, Mraz W, Forst H, Peter K. A comparison of the adrenocortical response during septic shock and after complete recovery. *Intensive Care Med.* 1996;22:894-899.
10. Bollaert PE, Charpentier C, Levy B, Debouverie M, Audibert G, Larcan A. Reversal of late septic shock with supraphysiologic doses of hydrocortisone. *Crit Care Med.* 1998;26:645-650.
11. Claussen MS, Landercasper J, Cogbill TH. Acute adrenal insufficiency presenting as shock after trauma and surgery: three cases and review of the literature. *J Trauma.* 1992;32:94-100.
12. Murphy JF, Purdue GF, Hunt JL. Acute adrenal insufficiency in the patient with burns. *J Burn Care Rehabil.* 1993;14:155-157.
13. Barquist E, Kirton O. Adrenal insufficiency in the surgical intensive care unit patient. *J Trauma.* 1997;42:27-31.
14. Merry WH, Caplan RH, Wickus GG, et al. Postoperative acute adrenal failure caused by transient corticotropin deficiency. *Surgery.* 1994;116:1095-1100.
15. Hierholzer K, Buhler H. Metabolism of cortical steroid hormones and their general mode of action. In: Greger R, Windhorst U, eds. *Comprehensive Human Physiology.* Vol 1. New York, NY: Springer-Verlag NY Inc; 1996:403-429.
16. Mujaso F, Neri G, Tortorella C, Mazzocchi G, Nussdorfer GG. Intra-adrenal 11 β-hydroxysteroid dehydrogenase plays a role in the regulation of corticosteroid secretion: an in vitro study in the rat. *Life Sci.* 1996;59:1401-1406.
17. Wang P, Ba ZF, Lu M-C, Ayala A, Harkema JM, Chaudry IH. Measurement of circulating blood volume in vivo after trauma-hemorrhage and hemodilution. *Am J Physiol.* 1994;266:R368-R374.
18. Putnam CD, Brann DW, Mahesh VB. Acute activation of the adrenocorticotropic-adrenal axis: effect on gonadotropin and prolactin secretion in the female rat. *Endocrinology.* 1991;128:2558-2566.
19. Cavallaro S, Korneyev A, Guidotti A, Costa E. Diazepam-binding inhibitor (DBI)–processing products, acting at the mitochondrial DBI receptor, mediate adrenocorticotropic hormone-induced steroidogenesis in rat adrenal gland. *Proc Natl Acad Sci U S A.* 1992;89:10598-10602.
20. Wang P, Tait SM, Ba ZF, Chaudry IH. ATP-$MgCl_2$ administration normalizes macrophage cyclic AMP and β-adrenergic receptors after hemorrhage and resuscitation. *Am J Physiol.* 1994;267:G52-G58.
21. Yang K, Berdusco ETM, Challis JRG. Opposite effects of glucocorticoid on hepatic 11 β-hydroxysteroid dehydrogenase mRNA and activity in fetal and adult sheep. *J Endocrinol.* 1994;143:121-126.
22. Hammond GL, Lähteenmäki PLA. A versatile method for the determination of serum cortisol binding globulin and sex hormone binding globulin binding capacities. *Clin Chim Acta.* 1983;132:101-110.
23. Lowry OH, Rosebrough NJ, Farr AL, Randall RJ. Protein measurement with the Folin phenol reagents. *J Biol Chem.* 1951;193:265-275.
24. Carlson DE, Babus JK, Nguyuza N, Melhem-Stancofski H, Eastridge BJ. Role of endotoxin in the response to experimentally induced bacteremia in chronically prepared rats. *Am J Physiol.* 1997;272:R1562-R1570.
25. Wichmann MW, Zellweger R, DeMaso CM, Ayala A, Chaudry IH. Melatonin administration attenuates depressed immune functions after trauma-hemorrhage. *J Surg Res.* 1996;63:256-262.
26. Hauger RL, Thrivikraman KV, Plotsky PM. Age-related alterations of hypothalmic-pituitary-adrenal axis function in male Fischer 344 rats. *Endocrinology.* 1994;134:1528-1536.
27. Sharma AC, Bosmann HB, Motew SJ, Hales KH, Hales DB, Ferguson JL. Steroid hormone alterations following induction of chronic intraperitoneal sepsis in male rats. *Shock.* 1996;6:150-154.
28. Webster JB, Bell KR. Primary adrenal insufficiency following traumatic brain injury: a case report and review of the literature. *Arch Phys Med Rehabil.* 1997;78:314-318.
29. Darlington DN, Barraclough CA, Gann DS. Hypotensive hemorrhage elevates corticotropin-releasing hormone messenger ribonucleic acid (mRNA) but not vasopressin mRNA in the rat hypothalamus. *Endocrinology.* 1992;130:1281-1288.
30. Komaki G, Gottschall PE, Somogyvari-Vigh A, Tatsuno I, Yatohgo T, Arimura A. Rapid increase in plasma IL-6 after hemorrhage, and posthemorrhage reduction of the IL-6 response to LPS, in conscious rats: interrelation with plasma corticosterone. *Neuroimmunomodulation.* 1994;1:127-134.
31. Lilly MP, Gann DS. The hypothalamic-pituitary-adrenal-immune axis: a critical assessment. *Arch Surg.* 1992;127:1463-1474.
32. Rivier C, Vale W. Diminished responsiveness of the hypothalmic-pituitary-adrenal axis of the rat during exposure to prolonged stress: a pituitary-mediated mechanism. *Endocrinology.* 1987;121:1320-1328.

33. Lilly MP. Effect of surgery on the pituitary-adrenal response to repeated hemorrhage. *Am J Physiol.* 1994;266:R1976-R1984.
34. Perrot D, Bonneton A, Dechaud H, Motin J, Pugeat M. Hypercortisolism in septic shock is not suppressible by dexamethasone infusion. *Crit Care Med.* 1993; 21:396-401.

DISCUSSION

Herbert Hechtman, MD, Boston, Mass: The authors have revisited the question of adrenal insufficiency following trauma and hemorrhage. The data are intriguing but fall a little short of supporting a definitive conclusion. The main issue is the need to prove causality with regard to the approximately 30% decline of the hepatic dehydrogenase as a mechanism of the 3- to 4-fold rise in corticosterone. These percentage changes do not appear to be in synchrony. What would be the effect of partial or complete hepatectomy therapy, removing all or part of liver dehydrogenase activity, on adrenal function? Is the significance of corticosterone a negative regulator in the setting of trauma and hemorrhage? In sham animals, would an infusion of corticosterone, sufficient to raise circulating levels 3 to 4 times normal, not lead to a reduction of corticotropin below normal values? In contrast, corticotropin levels in your severe hemorrhage animals remain elevated to 2 times baseline.

The fascinating question is why the elevated corticosterone levels following trauma and hemorrhage lead to adrenal unresponsiveness to corticotropin in only 1½ hours. Have you shown the same phenomena by a corticosterone infusion to mimic levels seen following trauma?

Finally, you might reconsider the confusing description of these data as adrenal insufficiency, since there are high levels of adrenal hormone.

Armour Forse, MD, Boston: This is indeed an interesting paper, but a few questions are important to make it clear what degree of shock you are dealing with in this model. The model you used, particularly the severe shock, has a mortality of 50% or 60%. Could you provide us with some information about the cardiovascular parameters in this animal model? I am particularly concerned that the models not only reflect shock but also severe anemia, as the animals were resuscitated with RL. Could you give us some indication of what the hematocrit was in these animals?

Are you hypothesizing that one cause for the results was changes in hepatic function? Could you give us more information about the liver? Did you measure liver function parameters? Do you have any liver histology? Finally, did you perform any histology on the adrenal gland? This would be important in interpreting your results.

Dr Wang: In his opening remarks, Dr Hechtman questioned whether there is a cause-and-effect relationship between the decreased hepatic 11β-HSD activity and adrenal insufficiency following trauma and hemorrhagic shock. I would like to point out that the primary aim of this study was not to examine the cause-and-effect relationship, but to determine whether hepatic 11β-HSD activity is reduced following hemorrhagic shock, and, if so, whether the decreased hepatic 11β-HSD is associated with adrenal insufficiency. Our data have clearly indicated that hepatic 11β-HSD activity decreases significantly following trauma-hemorrhage and fluid resuscitation, which is associated with adrenal insufficiency. Additional studies are, however, needed to determine whether inhibition of hepatic 11β-HSD by its inhibitors, such as β-glycyrrhetinic acid, in normal animals, produces adrenal insufficiency.

Dr Hechtman suggested that we should examine the effects of partial or complete hepatectomy (ie, partial or complete removal of hepatic 11β-HSD) on adrenal function. Although studies utilizing models of partial or complete hepatectomy may provide some mechanistic insights into the role of hepatic 11β-HSD in producing adrenal insufficiency, the inhibition of 11β-HSD activity by β-glycyrrhetinic acid may be a better approach, since hepatectomy in itself will significantly affect systemic metabolisms and host defense mechanisms.

Another question of Dr Hechtman's was whether or not administration of corticosterone in normal animals reduces plasma corticotropin below normal values. Although it has been well documented that the synthesis and release of corticotropin are negatively regulated by circulating levels of corticosterone, it remains unknown whether plasma corticotropin decreases below the basal level when plasma corticosterone increases 3 to 4 times higher than the basal level. The fact that plasma corticotropin decreased significantly after fluid resuscitation as compared to the levels at the time of maximal bleedout would suggest that the sustained high levels of plasma corticosterone negatively regulate corticotropin synthesis/release following hemorrhage and resuscitation.

Dr Hechtman also raised the issue that adrenal unresponsiveness to corticotropin stimulation occurs as early as 1.5 hours after the completion of hemorrhage and resuscitation. Since hemorrhage time was approximately 90 minutes, and the time required for fluid resuscitation was 60 minutes, 1.5 hours after resuscitation represents approximately 4 hours from the onset of hemorrhage. With regard to the reduced adrenal responsiveness to corticotropin after hemorrhage, we propose this is probably due to a combination of the decrease in corticotropin receptor number and/or affinity, uncoupling between corticotropin receptor and adenylate cyclase, decrease in intracellular levels of cAMP, and reduction in the adrenal corticosterone levels. However, it remains to be determined whether administration of corticosterone in normal animals can mimic the reduced adrenal responsiveness to corticotropin which is observed following trauma and hemorrhage.

With regard to Dr Hechtman's last question, adrenal insufficiency is defined as a condition in which corticotropin-induced release of corticosterone is significantly reduced. In this study, although plasma levels of corticosterone remained significantly elevated, corticotropin-induced corticosterone release decreased by 78% at 1.5 hours after the completion of hemorrhage and resuscitation. Thus, the occurrence of adrenal insufficiency suggests that the adrenal glands will not meet the demands for further increasing corticosterone release when a second hit (eg, sepsis) develops following trauma and hemorrhagic shock.

Dr Forse's question dealt with cardiovascular and hepatic responses following trauma-hemorrhage and resuscitation. We have indeed performed various studies to determine alterations in cardiovascular and hepatocellular functions in the hemorrhage model used in this study. Our results indicate that cardiac performance, cardiac output, and organ blood flow decrease significantly after hemorrhage, despite crystalloid resuscitation. In addition, hepatocellular function, as determined by indocyanine green clearance, decreases during hemorrhage and persists following resuscitation. Our preliminary results also indicate that oxygen delivery decreases significantly following hemorrhage and resuscitation. The systemic hematocrit decreases by more than 50% following fluid resuscitation in the hemorrhaged animals. Thus, tissue hypoxia may occur in this model of hemorrhage. Although liver histology shows focal necrosis and neutrophil infiltration, we have not examined adrenal histology after trauma-hemorrhage and resuscitation.

PAPER

Interval or Permanent Nonoperative Management of Acute Type A Aortic Dissection

Frank G. Scholl, MD; Michael A. Coady, MD, MPH; Ryan Davies; John A. Rizzo, PhD; Graeme L. Hammond, MD; Gary S. Kopf, MD; John A. Elefteriades, MD

Hypothesis: Selected patients with acute type A (ascending) aortic dissection who are treated with delayed operation or nonoperative therapy may have better early and short-term outcomes than was previously expected.

Design and Setting: Retrospective cohort at a university hospital.

Subjects: Data on 75 patients with acute or chronic type A aortic dissection treated at one institution from January 1, 1985, to November 30, 1997, were analyzed. Of these 75 patients, 34 (21 male and 13 female, with a mean age of 65.5 years) did not undergo initial operative treatment, and 15 (10 male and 5 female, with a mean age of 72.6 years) never underwent surgery. For the 19 patients who underwent delayed surgery, the mean period between aortic dissection and intervention was 11.4 ± 4.83 days. The follow-up period ranged from 0.27 to 149 months, with a mean of 20.2 months.

Main Outcome Measures: Vascular complications, hospital mortality, and early survival.

Results: Reasons for interval delay in surgical treatment included initial misdiagnosis or delay in diagnosis (13 [68%] of 19), need to address significant comorbidity (4 [21%] of 19), and initial refusal of operative intervention (2 [11%] of 19). For the 15 patients treated entirely by medical therapy, reasons for electing nonoperative management included extensive comorbidity (5 [33%] of 15), refusal of surgical intervention (6 [40%] of 15), and misdiagnosis or long delay in diagnosis (4 [27%] of 15). Of the 34 patients, 15 (44%) presented with moderate or severe aortic insufficiency, 5 (14%) had evidence of pericardial effusion, 6 (21%) had evidence of concomitant coronary ischemia on electrocardiogram, and 8 (24%) had extension of the dissection into the descending aorta. Four patients (11.8%) died while in the hospital. Of the 34 patients, 30 (88%) who underwent either delayed or no surgery received aggressive medical treatment (β-adrenergic blocking agents and afterload-reducing agents) and were discharged from the hospital. All patients who were operative candidates in the interval treatment group survived to reach definitive operation. There was no statistically significant difference in short-term survival between the group of patients undergoing delayed surgery or medical treatment only and the group of 41 patients undergoing early operation ($P = .42$).

Conclusions: Immediate surgical therapy is still recommended for acceptable operative candidates with acute type A aortic dissection who seek immediate treatment. However, this study permits the following 2 conclusions: (1) patients with type A aortic dissection who are referred or whose conditions are diagnosed several days after presentation have survived the early dangerous period and can safely undergo surgery semielectively (rather than emergently); and (2) selected patients who are not considered operative candidates and who survive the initial type A aortic dissection without complication may be treated with aggressive medical therapy and achieve acceptable early and short-term outcomes, which is better than previously expected.

Arch Surg. 1999;134:402-406

From the Department of Surgery, Section of Cardiothoracic Surgery (Drs Scholl, Coady, Hammond, Kopf, and Elefteriades and Mr Davies) and the Department of Epidemiology and Public Health (Dr Rizzo), Yale University School of Medicine, New Haven, Conn.

EARLY EXPERIENCE[1,2] indicated an extremely high immediate mortality from acute ascending (type A) aortic dissection. Accordingly, acute type A aortic dissection is generally considered a surgical emergency. The results of surgical treatment have shown significant improvement during recent years,[3-5] and, now, patients with acute type A aortic dissection usually undergo urgent surgical repair.

Because of the urgent surgical treatment, the natural history of acute type A aortic dissection treated with nonsurgical therapy in the current era is not well known. Current medical management with aggressive anti-impulse therapy and blood pressure control may influence significantly the early morbidity and mortality of type A aortic dissection treated with nonoperative therapy. The patient who survives an initial episode of aortic dissection may be at lower risk of death than previously thought if aggressive medical treatment is begun.

We examined the outcome of patients at our institution with acute type A aortic dissection who, because of a variety of rea-

PATIENTS AND METHODS

A computerized database is maintained as part of ongoing studies at the Yale Center for Thoracic Aortic Disease, New Haven, Conn.[6] This database currently includes 1962 imaging studies in 598 patients with diseases of the thoracic aorta. From this database, 75 patients with acute and chronic type A aortic dissection treated from January 1, 1985, to November 30, 1997, were identified. Forty-one patients were treated by immediate surgical intervention. Of these patients, 34 (21 male and 13 female) were treated with early medical therapy without initial operative treatment. Of these patients, 15 (10 male and 5 female) never underwent surgical intervention, while 19 patients (11 male and 8 female) underwent interval operation more than 48 hours after the aortic dissection. The time and date of onset of the acute aortic dissection were assumed to be coincident with the onset of pain.

The medical regimen for anti-impulse therapy included intravenous β-adrenergic blocking agents (or calcium antagonists when β-adrenergic blocking agents were contraindicated) as well as afterload-reducing agents. The regimen was administered until the patient had a target heart rate less than 60 beats/min and systolic blood pressure less than 100 mm Hg, unless oliguria or evidence of organ ischemia occurred. Oral medications were used after 48 hours of treatment.

Follow-up was obtained via telephone conversations with patients, physicians, or family members and through office and hospital chart review and was available in 99% (74 of 75) of patients. The overall mean follow-up was 20.2 months, with a range of 0.27 to 149 months.

sons, did not undergo standard early operative treatment and had delayed surgical intervention or nonoperative treatment of the aortic dissection. The purpose of this study is to determine the clinical outcome of this group of patients and to form clinical correlates regarding appropriate management.

RESULTS

Patients treated nonoperatively were older as a group than those treated with either delayed operative treatment or with initial surgery. Demographic data are shown in **Table 1**. The reasons for electing either nonoperative treatment or delayed surgical treatment are listed in **Table 2**. Major reasons for nonoperative treatment included delay in diagnosis, usually at an outside institution, patient's or family's refusal of surgery, and significant comorbidity. The 34 patients treated without initial operation sought treatment a mean of 4.2 days (range, 2-20) after the initial aortic dissection. In the patients who underwent interval operation, the mean time from aortic dissection to surgical intervention was 11.4 ± 4.83 days.

Of the 34 patients, 15 (44%) had moderate or severe aortic insufficiency, 5 (14%) had evidence of pericardial effusion, 6 (21%) had evidence of concomitant coronary ischemia on an electrocardiogram, and 8 (24%) had extension of the dissection into the descending aorta.

Table 1. Patient Demographics*

Characteristic	Initial Surgical Treatment	Initial Nonoperative Treatment: Interval Operative Treatment	Initial Nonoperative Treatment: Medical Treatment Only
Patients (M/F)	41 (28/13)	19 (11/8)	15 (10/5)
Age, mean ± SD, y	59.49 ± 15.84	58.33 ± 22.40	72.64 ± 15.49†
Interval from aortic dissection until surgical intervention, mean ± SD	<24 h	11.4 ± 4.8 d	. . .

**Ellipses indicate not applicable.*
†*Significant difference in age (P = .01).*

Table 2. Reasons for Nonoperative or Delayed Operative Management*

Reason	No. (%) of Patients: Interval Operative Treatment (n = 19)	No. (%) of Patients: Medical Treatment (n = 15)
Extensive comorbidity	4 (21)	5 (33)
ARF/encephalopathy	. . .	1 (7)
Severe COPD	2 (11)	3 (20)
CHF	2 (11)	1 (7)
Refusal of operation	2 (11)	6 (40)
Initial misdiagnosis or delay in diagnosis	13 (68)	4 (27)

**ARF indicates acute renal failure; COPD, chronic obstructive pulmonary disease; CHF, congestive heart failure, which was historical and not a consequence of aortic dissection; and ellipses, not applicable.*

An outcome flow diagram for the study is presented in **Figure 1**. The hospital mortality rate for the patients treated with delayed surgical intervention was 5.2% (1/19). The cause of death was disseminated intravascular coagulation and massive hemorrhage at the time of operation. All patients who were operative candidates in the interval treatment group survived to reach definitive operation. For patients undergoing medical therapy exclusively, the hospital mortality rate was 20% (3 /15). The causes of death were extension of the aortic dissection with cardiac tamponade in 2 patients and acute renal failure and ongoing cardiac ischemia in 1 patient. For the patients undergoing immediate surgical treatment, the hospital mortality rate was 19.5% (8/41). These mortality rates are not statistically different ($P = .84$; $\chi^2 = 0.33$). The short-term survival rate (**Figure 2**) after hospital discharge as determined by the log-rank test did not show a significant difference between the 41 patients treated with initial operative intervention and the 34 patients treated with either interval operation or medical treatment alone. The 1- and 2-year actuarial survival rates for the patients treated with initial operation are 82%. Actuarial survival is 74% at 1 and 2 years for those treated

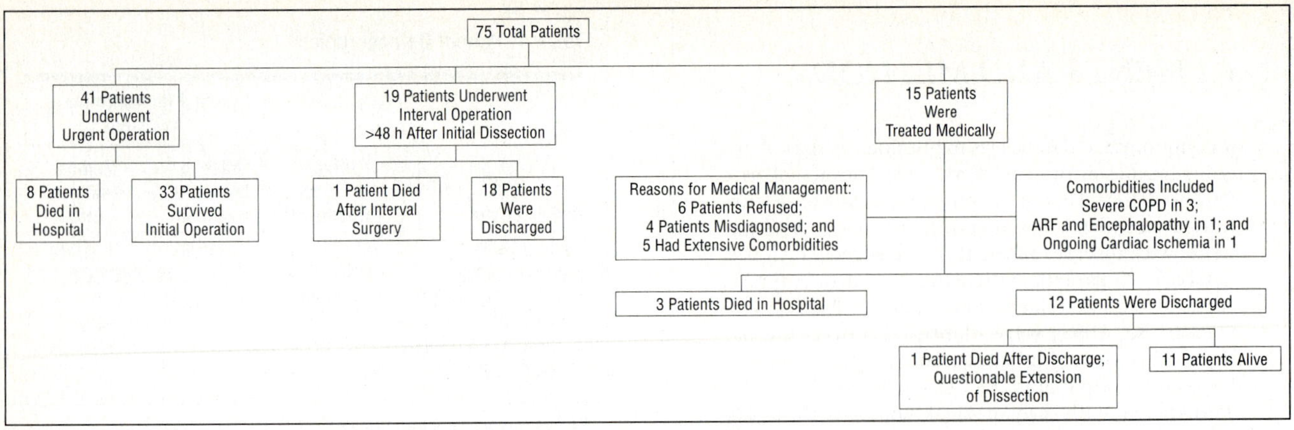

Figure 1. *Outcome of all patients treated for acute type A aortic dissection. COPD indicates chronic obstructive pulmonary disease; ARF, acute renal failure.*

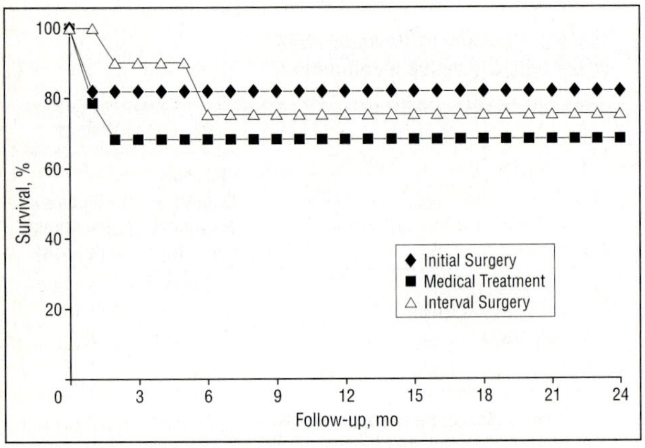

Figure 2. *Kaplan-Meier actuarial survival curve from date of initial presentation and treatment. Comparision made using log-rank test (*P *= .44).*

without initial operation ($P = .42$). Only 1 medically treated patient died following discharge from the hospital during the follow-up period; the cause of death was a suspected extension of the aortic dissection.

COMMENT

Most patients with type A aortic dissection are brought to the operating room for urgent surgical correction. This course of treatment is the standard policy at our institution. We continue to recommend such immediate surgical intervention for suitable operative candidates presenting early following type A aortic dissection. This report focuses on those patients presenting later in the course of acute type A aortic dissection and those patients who, for other reasons, are not suitable operative candidates.

The well-known complications of acute type A aortic dissection, for example, intrapericardial rupture, acute aortic valve insufficiency, coronary ischemia, and branch vessel occlusion, are often lethal without prompt surgical intervention. This report is not intended to refute in any way the conventional wisdom that acute type A aortic dissection represents a surgical emergency.[7,8] This retrospective review is intended to provide a snapshot of 2 distinct groups of patients: those who seek medical attention or whose conditions are diagnosed several days after the onset of acute type A aortic dissection and those who are not appropriate for surgical correction secondary to advanced age, debility, or comorbidity. Scant information is available in the literature regarding these specific subgroups of patients with type A aortic dissection.

The subgroup profile of patients in this report should not be interpreted to reflect general patterns of this disease, because there is likely a selection bias inherent in the referral pattern of a tertiary referral center serving a broad geographic area. Specifically, the patients presented in this report are those who have survived long enough to have their conditions diagnosed and be referred and transported. Thus, the relative size of the group of patients who did not undergo initial operation may be exaggerated by this selection bias.

The decision about the timing of surgery when a patient with acute type A aortic dissection is referred 2 days into the disease course is difficult. Usually, the decision revolves around whether the patient should be taken to the operating room at night or undergo operation semielectively the next day when a full complement of staff can assist in the challenging procedure. This report suggests that after 48 hours the aortic dissection may have passed the most critical phase and can be aggressively managed with anti-impulse therapy and operated on semielectively. The absence of mortality prior to operation in the subgroup of patients undergoing interval operation supports this reasoning. The low operative mortality in this subgroup (5.2%) likely represents both self-selection of a more stable group of patients and the benefits of a semielective optimal operative environment.

Because most patients with acute type A aortic dissection undergo urgent surgical management, few current data are available regarding the group of patients treated solely with medical therapy. The group of medically treated patients in this report is different from patients with chronic type A aortic dissection who present months or years after the acute event. These patients' conditions were all diagnosed during the acute phase of the aortic dissection shortly after the initial event. The data in this series show that the outlook for these patients, at least in the short term, may be better than previously expected both during hospitalization and after discharge from the hospital. This conclusion is consistent with data from Masuda and colleagues,[9] who reported that survival of medically treated patients with acute type A aortic dissection who survived the first week did not differ from the survival of patients with medically treated type B (descending) aortic dissection. Again, these patients may have passed the critical phase of the aortic dissection and proved their ability to survive the initial dangerous period. Since the acutely lethal consequences of type A aortic dissection, such as rupture with tamponade, acute aortic insufficiency, and coronary ischemia, are usually early events, it is not unreasonable to conclude that the natural history after the first week may resemble that of type B aortic dissection.

This is a retrospective review of a highly selected group of patients and is subject to the errors inherent in such a design. The groupings were made based on retrospective chart review and not in advance or during the course of treatment. Additionally, although the number of patients in this report may be adequate considering the highly selected subgroups of interval and permanent medical management, these results and suggestions must be viewed as preliminary. It is the intent of this article to add some insight into the relative void of information on this complex topic.

CONCLUSIONS

Acute type A aortic dissection is an indication for urgent operation and we advocate prompt surgical treatment for patients with acute type A aortic dissection. However, the results of the current study suggest the following: (1) patients with type A aortic dissection who present for treatment several days after initial aortic dissection have survived the initial dangerous period and can safely undergo surgery semielectively rather than emergently; and (2) those patients who are not operative candidates due to age, overwhelming comorbidity, or refusal may be treated with anti-impulse therapy and achieve reasonable early and short-term outcomes, which is better than previously expected.

Presented at the 79th Annual Meeting of the New England Surgical Society, Toronto, Ontario, September 27, 1998.

Reprints: John A. Elefteriades, MD, Section of Cardiothoracic Surgery, Yale University School of Medicine, 333 Cedar St, New Haven, CT 06510.

REFERENCES

1. Shennan T. *Dissecting Aneurysms.* London, England: Medical Research Council; 1934. Special Report Series No. 193.
2. Hirst AJ, Johns VJ Jr, Kime SW Jr. Dissecting aneurysms of the aorta: a review of 505 cases. *Medicine (Baltimore).* 1958;37:217-279.
3. Svensson LG, Crawford ES, Hess KR, et al. Dissection of the aorta and dissecting aortic aneurysms: improving early and long-term surgical results. *Circulation.* 1990;82(suppl 5):IV24-IV38.
4. Miller DC, Mitchell RS, Oyer PE, Stinson EB, Jamieson SW, Shumway NE. Independent determinants of operative mortality for patients with aortic dissections. *Circulation.* 1984;70(3, pt 2):I153-I164.
5. Kouchoukos NT, Wareing TH, Murphy SF, Perrillo JB. Sixteen-year experience with aortic root replacement: results of 172 operations. *Ann Surg.* 1991;214:308-318.
6. Coady M, Rizzo J, Hammond G, et al. What is the appropriate size criterion for resection of thoracic aortic aneurysm? *J Thorac Cardivasc Surg.* 1997;113:476-491.
7. Ergin M, Griepp R. Dissections of the aorta. In: Baue AE, Geha AS, Hammond GL, Laks H, Nawnheim KS, eds. *Glenn's Thoracic and Cardiovascular Surgery.* East Norwalk, Conn: Appleton & Lange; 1996.
8. Stone C, Borst H. Dissecting aortic aneurysm. In: Edmunds LJ, ed. *Cardiac Surgery.* New York, NY: McGraw-Hill Book Co; 1997.
9. Masuda Y, Yamada Z, Morooka N, Watanabe S, Inagaki Y. Prognosis of patients with medically treated aortic dissections. *Circulation.* 1991;84(suppl 5):III7-III13.

DISCUSSION

Alan Hilgenberg, MD, Boston, Mass: Patients with aortic dissections are divided into acute and chronic types, depending upon the timing of their presentation. Patients with acute aortic dissection are traditionally defined as those presenting within 2 weeks of the onset of symptoms; the logic of this definition is derived from the fact that most of the mortality associated with acute aortic dissection involving the ascending aorta occurs within the first 2 weeks. In untreated patients, the mortality rate is about 70%, with death most commonly due to intrapericardial aortic rupture. The typical patient experiences acute pain, presents to an emergency room, the diagnosis is confirmed by transesophageal echocardiography, and an emergency operation is usually done to replace the ascending aorta, generally without preoperative angiography. The authors of this paper are to be commended for focusing attention on a group of patients who still fit into the definition of acute aortic dissection but who have survived the initial few days of their disease without benefit of diagnosis or treatment. Thus, there has been some biologic selection so that they probably are not representative of the entire population of patients with acute aortic dissection. In this study, the hospital mortality and 2-year survival rates were not statistically different for 3 groups of patients: those treated with emergency surgery, delayed surgery, or medical treatment. The 3 deaths in the medically treated patients were due to predictable causes: aortic rupture, extension of dissection, and renal failure.

Our experience at the Massachusetts General Hospital is somewhat different, with hospital mortality lower for surgically treated patients then for a small group of medically treated patients. During a recent 3-year period, 1995 to 1997, we treated 45 patients with acute type A dissections. Forty of them had emergency surgery, usually within 1 hour of diagnosis, and there were 3 deaths, a 7.5% mortality rate. Five had medical treatment with 2 hospital deaths, a 40% mortality rate.

I have a few questions. What is the advantage to the patient or to the surgeon in delaying operation more than just a few hours or perhaps 1 day after diagnosis in those patients who are to undergo delayed surgery?

Were the operative procedures in the delayed patients different from those in the immediate surgery group? For example, was one group more likely to need aortic valve replacement or composite aortic root replacement, as opposed to just simply an ascending aortic graft? Was bleeding less in the delayed patients, perhaps because the aortic tissue was more substantial? And finally, based on this retrospective study, do you plan to make any changes in your future management strategy of these patients who present several days after the onset of symptoms?

Once again I commend the authors for bringing this rather unusual and very interesting and important material to our attention.

Arun Singh, MD, Providence, RI: All acute dissection does not need to be operated on, if the patients present in stable condition. Our experience is similar; we had 32 patients with acute dissection, operated on in the last 3 years with a mortality of 8%. Five patients had delayed presentation. Three of them were followed up for 2 years and are still alive and doing well. Two of the patients subsequently operated on have survived and done well.

This series goes back to 1985 to 1995, so what was the long-term follow-up of the medically treated patients, because your data show survival up to only 2 years?

Dr Scholl: I'd like to thank Dr Hilgenberg and Dr Singh for their excellent comments.

With regards to your initial question, Dr Hilgenberg, the advantages to the patients in delaying the operation, we find that once some of these patients are admitted to the hospital, the dissection occurred some time ago and they have been hemodynamically stable without evidence of end-organ ischemia. If we then treat them with aggressive medical therapy, the operation can be safely delayed until such time as they can be operated on in a semielective fashion, with a fresh operative team and all available resources on hand to assist in their care. Also, this allows time for more accurate and sometimes multiple diagnostic studies of these complex patients.

However, the fact is, as you mentioned in your comments, that these patients have biologically self-selected themselves by the simple fact that they are hemodynamically stable and have withstood the initial dissection without significant end-organ injury. We also have no way of knowing how many of these patients died before arriving at the hospital

Regarding your question as to the types of operations required, the acutely operated-on patients tended to require more valve replacements due to the fact that some of them were brought to the operating room with significant aortic insufficiency or very proximal dissection with tamponade.

As far as the future management of patients with ascending aortic dissections, we continue to advocate prompt surgical treatment for all patients who present with acute type A dissection. We feel that the patients with acute type A dissections who present at a later time and who are hemodynamically stable without signs of end-organ damage can be safely managed with aggressive anti-impulse therapy and semielective operation as the operating room schedule permits. We will continue to follow this group of patients, as well as the group treated with medical therapy alone, and critically evaluate their long-term outcomes.

In response to Dr Singh's comments, the majority of the medically treated patients were treated more recently, thus follow-up on this group is relatively short; in addition we have a few patients lost to follow-up. Thus, we don't yet have a good idea of the long-term prognosis of these medically treated patients as the number of patients who are out at the longer follow-up intervals is quite small. We will be looking at these patients closely over the next few years to see if they succumb to complications of their dissection.

PAPER

Cavernous Hemangioma of the Liver

Anatomic Resection vs Enucleation

Roberto Gedaly, MD; James J. Pomposelli, MD, PhD; Elizabeth A. Pomfret, MD, PhD; W. David Lewis, MD; Roger L. Jenkins, MD

Hypothesis: Patient outcome and the development of major intra-abdominal postoperative complications following removal of cavernous hemangiomas of the liver are affected by methods of resection.

Design: Case-control study.

Setting: Hepatobiliary surgery and liver transplantation unit in a tertiary care referral medical center.

Patients: Between December 1, 1987, and December 1, 1997, 28 patients underwent the surgical removal of cavernous hemangioma either by hepatic resection or enucleation. Indications for the operation were pain, enlarging tumors, uncertain diagnosis, or rupture.

Main Outcome Measures: The technique of tumor removal, hospital course, and the development of intra-abdominal complications. Independent factors influencing the development of complications were ascertained by multivariate analysis.

Results: Twenty-four female and 4 male patients (age, 47.5 ± 12.4 [mean ± SD] years) underwent either enucleation (n = 23) or liver resection (n = 5). Lesions ranged from 2 to 16 cm in their postresection diameter. No surgical (30-day) mortality was observed. Four major intra-abdominal complications were found: 1 episode of intraoperative bleeding requiring abdominal packing and 3 intra-abdominal fluid collections requiring percutaneous drainage. Enucleation was the only independent factor found by univariate and multivariate analyses to be associated with a reduction in the number of intra-abdominal complications ($P = .04$).

Conclusions: Cavernous hemangiomas of the liver can be removed safely by either hepatic resection or enucleation. Enucleation is associated with fewer intra-abdominal complications and should be the technique of choice when tumor location and technical factors favor enucleation.

Arch Surg. 1999;134:407-411

CAVERNOUS hemangiomas represent the most common benign tumor of the liver.[1,2] These lesions consist of large vascular spaces lined by a monolayer of endothelial cells. Because most of these tumors are asymptomatic, the diagnosis is most commonly made by ultrasonography, computed tomographic (CT) scan, or during laparotomy for other intra-abdominal disease.[3] Occasionally, patients present with abdominal pain, early satiety, or a sensation of an abdominal mass. Rarely, a patient may present with consumptive coagulopathy (Kasabach-Merritt syndrome) resulting from sequestration and the destruction of platelets related to giant hemangiomas.[4,5]

For most patients, the natural history of cavernous hemangiomas in the liver remains uneventful, and surgical intervention can be avoided. The observation of asymptomatic lesions with routine follow-up with CT scan or ultrasonography is often sufficient.[2] Indications for the surgical removal of hemangioma may include the development of pain, especially in patients with rupture, rapidly enlarging lesions, profound thrombocytopenia, or an uncertain diagnosis of a liver mass.[6-8] In this study, we evaluated the outcome of patients who underwent the surgical removal of cavernous hemangioma and assessed factors affecting major complications postoperatively.

RESULTS

In 17 patients (61%), the tumor was located in the right lobe and, in 9 patients (32%), in the left lobe. Bilobar location was found in 2 patients (7%). Indications for surgical resection were pain alone in 16 patients (57%), pain and tumor growth in 3 patients (11%), uncertain diagnosis in 7 patients (25%), and rupture in 2 patients (7%).

The surgical removal of the tumors was by enucleation in 23 patients and anatomic liver resection in 5 patients. In the

From the Division of Hepatobiliary Surgery and Liver Transplantation, Department of Surgery, Beth Israel Deaconess Medical Center, Harvard Medical School, Boston, Mass.

PATIENTS AND METHODS

PATIENTS

Between December 1, 1987, and December 1, 1997, 28 patients (24 women and 4 men) underwent surgical removal of a hepatic cavernous hemangioma in the Hepatobiliary Surgery and Liver Transplantation Unit at the Beth Israel Deaconess Medical Center, Boston, Mass. Patients underwent surgical removal by either anatomic resection (n = 5) or enucleation (n = 23). Patient medical records were reviewed for demographics, characteristics of the tumor (location and size), indication for the operation, the technique of removal (resection or enucleation), operative variables (operation time, amount of blood loss, transfusion requirement, and inflow occlusion time), hospital length of stay, and postoperative complications. Indications for the operation included pain, rapidly enlarging mass, uncertain diagnosis, and hemorrhage. No patient in the current series presented with coagulopathy associated with Kasabach-Merritt syndrome.

Methods for diagnosis included ultrasonography, CT scan, magnetic resonance imaging (MRI) scan, or combinations of more than 1 technique. Scanning using erythrocytes labeled with technetium Tc 99m was done in 4 patients to assist with the preoperative pathological diagnosis. Our current diagnostic preference is ultrasonography and dynamic CT scanning, followed by MRI, if necessary.

For patients who underwent anatomic resection, the following definitions are used for consistency[9]: *right hepatic lobectomy* includes the resection of Couinaud segments[10] 5, 6, 7, and 8, whereas *left hepatic lobectomy* refers to the resection of segments 2, 3, and 4. *Extended left hepatic lobectomy* refers to the resection of segments 2, 3, and 4 and portions of segments 5 and 8, whereas *extended right hepatic lobectomy* refers to the resection of segments 5, 6, 7, and 8 and portions of segment 4. *Left lateral segmentectomy* is limited to the resection of segments 2 and 3.[9] *Enucleation* refers to the creation of a plane between the normal liver parenchyma and the hemangioma without the removal of any normal hepatic parenchyma. *Major intra-abdominal complications* were defined as intra-abdominal infection, hemorrhage requiring reoperation and packing, and major bile leakage.

OPERATIVE TECHNIQUE

Enucleation

A right subcostal incision is used, with extension to the left side as needed. After the abdominal cavity is explored, the liver is fully mobilized by dividing the suspensory ligaments. Intraoperative ultrasonography is frequently used to assist with the identification of the lesion and its relations to intraparenchymal venous structures. Following the initial assessment of the location of the lesion, a 2.5-cm Penrose drain is placed around the hepatoduodenal ligament to provide inflow occlusion as indicated (Pringle maneuver). The capsule of the liver is coagulated with cautery to demarcate the extent of the resection and to initiate the development of a plane between the tumor and the hepatic parenchyma. The tumor is progressively separated from the parenchyma with a finger or a blunt instrument. Small bridging vessels are divided with the cautery, and the relatively few larger vessels are controlled with silk ligatures. After the hemangioma is removed, the residual cavity is manually compressed for several minutes to facilitate hemostasis. Residual bleeding points are controlled with suture ligatures, electrocautery, or argon-beam coagulation. For large defects, omentum can be placed in the bed of the cavity. A closed suction drain is placed to monitor for bile leaks and bleeding.

Hepatic Resection

Anatomic resection is performed using standard resection techniques. We prefer complete mobilization of the liver and the routine use of intraoperative ultrasonography to identify portal and hepatic venous structures. This is especially useful during right hepatic lobe resections, when large inferior right hepatic veins can be easily identified.

Once the extent of resection is decided, dissection of the porta hepatis is carried out. Generally, the portal vein and hepatic artery on the affected side are divided before bile duct division. This minimizes the risk of injury to the bile duct on the contralateral side. After the inflow vessels are divided, we generally prefer to control the hepatic veins at their level of entry into the inferior vena cava before hepatic parenchyma division. This reduces blood loss considerably and may obviate the need for total inflow occlusion (Pringle maneuver).

After the hepatic parenchyma is removed, manual compression of the cut surface is used to facilitate hemostasis. Residual bleeding sites are controlled with simple sutures, electrocautery, or argon-beam coagulation. We do not use large transhepatic compression sutures to avoid ischemic injury to the remaining segments.

STATISTICAL ANALYSIS

Results are expressed as mean ± SD. Continuous variables were compared by the Student t test. Univariate analysis was performed using the Fisher exact test for dichotomized variables. Multivariate analysis using logistic regression was performed to identify independent factors affecting abdominal complications. Differences were considered significant at $P<.05$ in all cases.

group undergoing anatomic resection, 2 patients had right hepatic lobectomies, 1 patient had extended right hepatic lobectomy, 1 patient had extended left hepatic lobectomy, and 1 patient had left lateral segmentectomy. The lesions ranged from 2 to 16 cm as measured after resection. Given the propensity for these vascular lesions to empty of blood during resection, the diameter of the lesions before resection was always much greater, with the largest lesion having a radiologically measured diameter of 45 cm.

Vascular inflow occlusion (Pringle maneuver) was used in 11 (48%) of 23 patients in the group having enucleation, for a mean of 14.7 minutes (range, 0-50 minutes), and in 3 (60%) of 5 patients in the group having resection, for a mean of 19.2 minutes (range, 0-45 minutes). Transfusion requirement, operative time, and length

Table 1. Tumor Characteristics and Indications for Surgery Between the Group Undergoing Enucleation (n = 23) and the Group Undergoing Anatomic Resection (n = 5)*

Variable	Enucleation	Resection
Age, mean ± SD, y	47.6 ± 13.4†	47.2 ± 7.2†
Tumor size, mean ± SD, cm	6.0 ± 3.7†	8.6 ± 5.4†
Location		
Right lobe	14 (61)	3 (60)
Left lobe	8 (35)	1 (20)
Bilateral extension	1 (4)	1 (20)
Indications		
Pain	13 (56)	3 (60)
Uncertain diagnosis	6 (26)	1 (20)
Rapid growth	3 (13)	0
Rupture	1 (4)	1 (20)

**Data are given as number (percentage) of patients except as noted.*
†Values are not statistically different by Student t *test.*

Table 2. Operative and Hospital Course in the Group Undergoing Enucleation (n = 23) and the Group Undergoing Anatomic Resection (n = 5)*

Course	Enucleation	Resection
Blood loss, mL	922.7 ± 1032.5†	2080.0 ± 1138.9†
Blood transfusion, U	1.2 ± 3.6	2.6 ± 2.8
Operative time, h	3.4 ± 1.2	4.3 ± 1.5
Time of vascular control, min	14.1 ± 17.8	19.2 ± 19.5
Hospital stay, d	8.2 ± 3.9	9.4 ± 2.2

**Data are given as mean ± SD.*
†Blood loss statistically significant by Student t *test,* P *= .04.*

of hospital stay are summarized in the following tabulation. Packed red blood cells (PRBC) were administered to 10 patients, and 3 patients received only autologous blood.

Course	Mean ± SD (Range)
PRBC transfused, U	1.29 ± 2.88 (0-14)
Autologous blood, U	1.46 ± 3.47 (0-17)
Operative time, h	3.58 ± 1.31 (1.6-6.8)
Hospital stay, d	8.39 ± 3.65 (5-21)

As shown in **Table 1**, demographics, characteristics of the tumor, and indications for surgical resection were similar in the group of patients undergoing enucleation compared with those undergoing anatomic resection. Perioperative variables like amount of blood loss, transfusions, operative time, time of vascular inflow occlusion, and hospital stay between these 2 groups demonstrated that blood loss was significantly greater in the group undergoing anatomic resection than in the group undergoing enucleation ($P = .04$). **Table 2** demonstrates the tendency of a longer operative time, greater blood product usage, and prolonged vascular inflow occlusion and hospital stays in the group of patients treated with anatomic resection, without showing statistical significance.

Four major intra-abdominal complications were encountered. These included 1 case of persistent intraoperative bleeding that required packing and reoperation 24 hours later for pack removal; 2 patients in whom infected intra-abdominal fluid collections developed that were treated by percutaneous drainage under CT guidance, and 1 patient with a biloma in whom a bronchobiliary fistula eventually developed, requiring reoperation. There was no operative (30-day) mortality. Other significant complications included 1 nonfatal case of pulmonary embolus, 3 cases of atelectasis, 1 of urinary tract infection, 1 of postoperative ileus, 1 of antibiotic reaction resulting in anaphylaxis, and 1 of wound infection.

Table 3. Univariate Analysis of Variables Predicting Major Complications After Surgical Removal of Hepatic Hemangiomas

Parameter*	*P*
Operative time, h	
≥3.6 / <3.6	.12
Blood loss, mL	
≥1565 / <1565	.06
Resection vs enucleation	.01†
Vascular control time, min‡	
>15 / ≤15	.30
Transfusions	
Yes / No	.32
Vascular control used	
Yes / No	.20

**The mean value was used as the threshold value for operative time, blood loss, and time of vascular control.*
†Type of surgical resection significant by Fisher exact test, $P<.05$.
‡Vascular control time refers to minutes with inflow occlusion (Pringle maneuver).

UNIVARIATE AND MULTIVARIATE ANALYSIS

Univariate analysis revealed that enucleation of hemangiomas was associated with significantly fewer intra-abdominal complications compared with anatomic resection (**Table 3**). Enucleation was the only independent risk factor found by multivariate analysis to be associated with fewer intra-abdominal complications ($P = .04$). Although there was a strong trend for blood loss of greater than 1500 mL to be associated with a higher complication rate, this did not reach statistical significance ($P = .06$).

COMMENT

Hepatic hemangiomas are common tumors and have an incidence of 0.4% to 7.0% in the general population.[11,12] For most persons, these tumors remain asymptomatic and are discovered incidentally during a surgical procedure or imaging studies for unrelated problems. When symptomatic, abdominal pain, early satiety, and distention are most common.[1] Rarely, platelet sequestration with thrombocytopenia or spontaneous rupture with intraperitoneal or intrahepatic hemorrhage can occur and can be life-threatening.[2] In this study, 2 patients (7%) presented with severe pain and intrahepatic hemorrhage due to rupture.

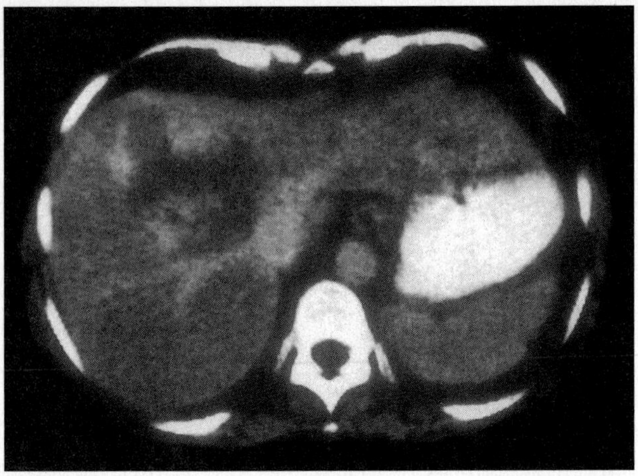

A computed tomographic scan showing a nodular peripheral enhancement with hypodense center after the administration of contrast medium, typically seen in hepatic hemangiomas.

The strategic approach to diagnose these lesions varies among institutions, with ultrasonography, CT scan, erythrocyte scanning, and MRI scanning used alone or in combination.[13-17] Rarely is arteriography necessary to ascertain the diagnosis or resectability. The precise diagnostic criteria for cavernous hemangiomas of the liver vary with each diagnostic procedure. For lesions found on ultrasonography, small hemangiomas are described as hyperechoic homogeneous masses.[14] Large or massive hemangiomas have heterogeneous areas interspersed within the hyperechoic mass on ultrasonography.[18] With contrast-enhanced CT scans, a peripheral nodular pattern of enhancement with a hypodense center is often seen[19] (**Figure**). Scintigraphic studies using red blood cells tagged with technetium Tc 99m show delayed filling from the periphery of the lesion, whereas a hyperintense signal is seen during T_2-weighted MRI scanning.[14,20]

The diagnostic algorithm used in our institution has been to focus on ultrasonography to assess initial tumor characteristics, followed by dynamic CT scanning to better identify anatomic relationships. We generally restrict the use of MRI to adjunctive use if the diagnosis is in doubt or if a more complete delineation of the tumor's relationship to hepatic venous structures is desired. Scanning with technetium-labeled erythrocytes has been used less extensively in recent years because improved CT and MRI scanning techniques have evolved. Core biopsy and fine-needle aspiration are reportedly safe but may be associated with pain or bleeding, and we do not recommend them for diagnosis.[21-23]

Because most patients with cavernous hepatic hemangiomas remain asymptomatic, the decision to remove these lesions surgically has been a point of controversy in previous reports.[6,24] In this series, only hemangiomas causing severe abdominal pain or those with an indeterminate diagnosis or hemorrhage were removed. In these patients, the benefit of palliating pain, excluding the diagnosis of a possible malignant tumor, or controlling life-threatening hemorrhage, justifies the risk of surgery. In an asymptomatic patient with a secure diagnosis of a cavernous hemangioma, surgical resection cannot be justified.

Once the decision to remove a symptomatic hemangioma has been made, an important surgical management issue relates to the technique of removal. Both anatomic resection and enucleation can be effective in removing the lesion. In this study, enucleation was found to be associated with fewer complications postoperatively compared with anatomic resection. Occasionally, the tumor location precludes safe enucleation, and anatomic resection can be performed more expeditiously. Given the potential for life-threatening intraoperative and postoperative complications, the surgical treatment of hepatic cavernous hemangiomas should be performed by surgeons comfortable with their removal using a variety of techniques, which will ensure a low rate of morbidity and mortality.

Presented at the 79th Annual Meeting of the New England Surgical Society, Toronto, Ontario, September 27, 1998.

Corresponding author: Roger L. Jenkins, MD, Division of Hepatobiliary Surgery and Liver Transplantation, Beth Israel Deaconess Medical Center, 110 Francis St, Suite 8C, Boston, MA 02215.

REFERENCES

1. Belli L, De Carlis L, Beati C, Rondinara G, Sansalone V, Brambilla G. Surgical treatment of symptomatic giant hemangiomas of the liver. *Surg Gynecol Obstet.* 1992;174:474-478.
2. Weimann A, Ringe B, Klempnauer J, et al. Benign liver tumors: differential diagnosis and indications for surgery. *World J Surg.* 1997;21:983-991.
3. Iqbal N, Saleem A. Hepatic hemangioma: a review. *Tex Med.* 1997;93:48-50.
4. Larsen EC, Zinkham WH, Eggleston JC, Zitelli BJ. Kasabach-Merritt syndrome: therapeutic considerations. *Pediatrics.* 1987;79:971-980.
5. Mewes T, Moldenhauer H, Pfeifer J, Papenberg J. The Kasabach-Merritt syndrome: severe bleeding disorder caused by celiac arteriography: reversal by heparin treatment. *Am J Gastroenterol.* 1989;84:965-971.
6. Moreno Egea A, Del Pozo Rodriguez M, Vicente Cantero M, Abellan Atenza J. Indications for surgery in the treatment of hepatic hemangioma. *Hepatogastroenterology.* 1996;43:422-426.
7. Andersson R, Bengmark S. Surgical treatment of cavernous hemangioma of the liver. *Acta Chir Scand.* 1988;154:577-579.
8. Kuo PC, Lewis WD, Jenkins RL. Treatment of giant hemangiomas of the liver by enucleation. *J Am Coll Surg.* 1994;178:49-53.
9. Strasberg SM. Terminology of liver anatomy and liver resections: coming to grips with hepatic Babel [published erratum appears in *J Am Coll Surg.* 1997;185:309]. *J Am Coll Surg.* 1997;184:413-434.
10. Couinad C. Lobes et seqments hepatiques: note sur l'architecture anatomique et chirurgicale du foie. *Press Med.* 1954;63:709.
11. Schwartz SI, Husser WC. Cavernous hemangioma of the liver: a single institution report of 16 resections. *Ann Surg.* 1987;205:456-465.
12. Jenkins RL, Johnson LB, Lewis WD. Surgical approach to benign liver tumors. *Semin Liver Dis.* 1994;14:178-189.
13. Ferrucci JT. Liver tumor imaging: current concepts. *AJR Am J Roentgenol.* 1990;155:473-484.
14. Egglin TK, Rummeny E, Stark DD, Wittenberg J, Saini S, Ferrucci JT. Hepatic tumors: quantitative tissue characterization with MR imaging. *Radiology.* 1990;176:107-110.
15. Gaa J, Saini S, Ferrucci JT. Perfusion characteristics of hepatic cavernous hemangioma using intravenous CT angiography (IVCTA). *Eur J Radiol.* 1991;12:228-233.
16. Samad SA, Maimunah A, Zulfiqar A, Zaharah M. Ultrasound (US) and computed tomographic (CT) appearances of large (giant) hepatic cavernous hemangiomas. *Med J Malaysia.* 1995;50:82-86.
17. Sirisriro R, Kim EE, Podoloff DA. Radioimmunoscintigraphy in the differential diagnosis of hepatic mass lesion. *Eur J Nucl Med.* 1995;22:385-388.
18. Lise M, Feltrin G, Da Pian PP, et al. Giant cavernous hemangiomas: diagnosis and surgical strategies. *World J Surg.* 1992;16:516-520.
19. Leslie DF, Johnson CD, Johnson CM, Ilstrup DM, Harmsen WS. Distinction between cavernous hemangiomas of the liver and hepatic metastases on CT: value of contrast enhancement patterns. *AJR Am J Roentgenol.* 1995;164:625-629.

20. Moinuddin M, Allison JR, Montgomery JH, Rockett JF, McMurray JM. Scintigraphic diagnosis of hepatic hemangioma: its role in the management of hepatic mass lesions. *AJR Am J Roentgenol.* 1985;145:223-228.
21. Tung GA, Cronan JJ. Percutaneous needle biopsy of hepatic cavernous hemangioma. *J Clin Gastroenterol.* 1993;16:117-122.
22. Taavitsainen M, Airaksinen T, Kreula J, Paivansalo M. Fine-needle aspiration biopsy of liver hemangioma. *Acta Radiol.* 1990;31:69-71.
23. Cronan JJ, Esparza AR, Dorfman GS, Ridlen MS, Paolella LP. Cavernous hemangioma of the liver: role of percutaneous biopsy. *Radiology.* 1988;166:135-138.
24. Farges O, Daradkeh S, Bismuth H. Cavernous hemangiomas of the liver: are there any indications for resection? *World J Surg.* 1995;19:19-24.

DISCUSSION

Giles Whalen, MD, Farmington, Conn: Dr Gedaly and colleagues focused their gaze on this rather uncommon problem. It is the most common benign liver tumor, but it is an uncommon clinical problem, as indicated by only 28 patients during a 10-year period. It is even more uncommonly operated on. The reason is that these are often large tumors. They are bloody, may be awkwardly situated, and, perhaps most important, their natural history is not as worrisome as used to be thought. It is clear that these generally do not go on to rupture, which was previously a fear. Interestingly, you have 2 patients in this series who did appear to have rupture. Because the usual precipitating event, at least in most of the literature, has been a biopsy, or mucking around with it in some way, I would be interested in knowing whether or not those patients who had presented with a rupture, in fact, had had a previous biopsy, or were they being watched? As is expected, the most common indication for operating on 1 of these tumors is pain. I would like to hear how much pain did the patients need to be in to have an operation? Some of the pain is perhaps due to thrombosis of the vessels. The natural history of the tumor in patients with pain is not entirely clear, and it can be a difficult call. You performed these operations with your expected success and excellence, a 14% major abdominal morbidity rate and no mortality. These are large operations with large incisions, and you have demonstrated how well the technique of enucleation works. The rest of my questions go directly to your central claim: Why do you think enucleation is a better technique for these operations? Even though there is a nice univariate and multivariate analysis, I feel a bit statistically challenged. Five of the operations are resections, and there are only 4 complications. I wonder whether the operations that were resections were performed for an emergency rupture, in which case one might expect to find a higher morbidity.

The other question is, if it is such a wonderful technique, are there times when you would not use it? Are there particular circumstances when you feel that it is not indicated? If you have embarked on it and have encountered some technical difficulties, do you have any tricks that you would like to impart as to how to get out of trouble while enucleating the tumor?

Mark Callery, MD, Worcester, Mass: Dr Whalen makes some important points in this mysterious lesion. My question pivots on your patient selection. How much pain do they have to have for you to operate on them? And what are your results from relieving the pain? How do you know which patients are probably going to have a good result?

Robert Beazley, MD, Boston, Mass: I have grown up with the fear that hemangiomas may rupture, but I have never heard of one or seen one that has ruptured. These are the first 2 cases I have heard reported. Would you give us some background on the cause of the rupture, whether they were iatrogenic, steering wheel, or what?

My other question is more of a philosophical one. I think enucleation is a major advance in the management of these tumors because it is so much better than a resectional approach, so much easier and less bloody. I question whether you might know if anyone has started to do these laparoscopically?

Richard Swanson, MD, Worcester: One question on the indications. You talked about pain. Do you use size alone as an indication, or a change in size? Was that 45-cm tumor operated on purely because of the size?

Dougald MacGillivray, MD, South Portland, Me: If uncertainty in the diagnosis was the reason for operation, did you approach these lesions with plans for enucleation, or were those the patients who had resection?

Dr Gedaly: I had 2 questions concerning rupture as the cause of the surgical intervention. We have 2 patients in our series with this rare and unusual complication, representing 7% of our patients. I have found only 29 other cases of spontaneous rupture of these tumors that have been reported in the literature. Most cases of hemorrhage from hemangiomas are iatrogenic, associated with biopsies or trauma, as described in previous studies.

Another important issue is, how much pain do patients have to have to need surgery and is there any way to anticipate good results in these patients? Let me answer the second part of the question first. It is essential that the surgeon rule out other important causes of pain in the right upper quadrant, even in those patients with giant tumors that obviously seem to be the source of their symptoms. This should be performed to have a certain amount of confidence that the hemangioma is the cause of pain and to subsequently optimize the results. Some authors have described the pain as severe or incapacitating to justify surgery. Yes, we think that enucleation is an excellent operation for benign tumors, not just because it was associated with a low rate of intra-abdominal complications compared with anatomic resection in both univariate and multivariate analyses in this series. We have demonstrated that this procedure can be performed with a low major morbidity rate and no mortality, with excellent results in terms of the resolution of the symptoms.

As I said in the conclusions, both anatomic resection and enucleation can be effective in removing these tumors, and enucleation should be considered the technique of choice. In some patients, however, the location of the tumor and technical aspects preclude safe enucleation. A good example may be total lobar replacement by the hemangioma or nearly total replacement of 1 lobe in a patient with a suggestion of a malignant neoplasm in which the only way to get adequate margins is to perform a right or left hepatic lobectomy. In these circumstances, anatomic resection is a reasonable alternative, but each case should be evaluated individually.

Changing to the next question regarding laparoscopic resection of hepatic hemangiomas, I have found only a few reports of laparoscopic removal of these tumors in studies regarding laparoscopic resection of hepatic tumors. The last question was in respect to the size as an indication of surgery. Size itself is not an indication. Rapid growth may increase the suspicion that you are dealing with a hepatic cancer. In this case, uncertainty of diagnosis is the real indication for surgical exploration. I want to be clear in this particular point: indications for surgery are severe abdominal pain, uncertain diagnosis, rupture, and profound thrombocytopenia and coagulopathy associated with Kasabach-Merritt syndrome.

Dr Jenkins: The important thing is to make sure that you take your time doing this. You cannot push with your fingers very much, but it really is extraordinarily easy to develop this plane and skeletonize everything so that when you look down at the end of it with a large tumor, you have a view of the vena cava, hepatic veins, and biliary radicals. Obviously, if you get into a difficult situation, you might have to do a major hepatic resection, but this is much easier. I get calls every year from surgeons who have cut across a hemangioma at the base of it as they were doing a liver resection. They call me from the operating room and say, "What shall we do now? The patient's bleeding to death." Enucleation is a much safer way to do this.

PAPER

Perioperative Strokes After 1001 Consecutive Carotid Endarterectomy Procedures Without an Electroencephalogram

Incidence, Mechanism, and Recovery

Allen D. Hamdan, MD; Frank B. Pomposelli, Jr, MD; Gary W. Gibbons, MD; David R. Campbell, MD; Frank W. LoGerfo, MD

Hypothesis: That alternative methods of cerebral protection, especially routine shunting of all patients undergoing general anesthesia or shunting on the basis of neurologic assessment with the patient awake under cervical plexus block, result in outcomes of carotid endarterectomy comparable with those reported using electroencephalographic monitoring.

Design: Retrospective review of cases from a vascular registry established in 1990.

Setting: Tertiary care center.

Patients: Consecutive sample of 1001 patients who underwent carotid endarterectomy.

Interventions: Carotid endarterectomy procedures were performed without electroencephalographic monitoring, using general anesthesia with routine shunting or using regional anesthesia.

Main Outcome Measures: Overall stroke and mortality rates and cause and consequence of the postoperative strokes.

Results: There were 14 nonfatal strokes (1.4%) and 2 deaths (0.2%), for a combined stroke and death rate of 1.6%. Nine (64%) of the 14 strokes appeared to result from a technical error during the endarterectomy. Mild deficits were noted after 7 strokes (50%), with the remainder resulting in deficits that required inpatient rehabilitation. Twelve patients with strokes (86%) eventually returned home without need for assistance.

Conclusions: Most postoperative strokes in this series were due to technical errors. Overall, even in patients with strokes initially requiring inpatient rehabilitation, there was good recovery of function. Low stroke and mortality rates can be achieved in carotid endarterectomy without the use of electroencephalographic monitoring.

Arch Surg. 1999;134:412-415

WITH THE results of 2 major, randomized prospective trials reporting the expected benefits of carotid endarterectomy (CEA) vs medical management for symptomatic and asymptomatic carotid stenosis,[1,2] the number of patients undergoing this procedure has increased. For the benefits of surgery to be realized, however, the operation must be performed with a low complication rate in regard to stroke and mortality.[3] Since it is likely that in some instances placement of an indwelling shunt will prevent the development of postoperative stroke, the method of cerebral protection or cerebral monitoring is a topic of interest. Cerebral monitoring in general is conducted with an electroencephalogram (EEG) or use of regional anesthesia in an awake patient.[4,5] Carotid artery stump pressures also have been used to determine the need for shunt placement based on predetermined thresholds.[6] The rationale for monitoring is to identify a subgroup of patients most likely to benefit from shunt placement. Some patients will demonstrate significant cerebral hypoperfusion, as measured by EEG changes, on carotid clamping. The presumption is that in the absence of a shunt, a small number of these patients will have a postoperative neurologic deficit. Electroencephalographic monitoring, however, requires additional equipment and expertise and generates a cost. Another method, which abrogates the need for cerebral monitoring, is the use of general anesthesia with routine shunting. At our institution, we have used regional anesthesia with shunting based on a neurologic change during the procedure, but we now perform CEA with general anesthesia and routine shunting almost exclusively. We reviewed 1001 consecutive CEAs performed during a 7-

From the Department of Vascular Surgery, Beth Israel Deaconess Medical Center, West Campus, Harvard Medical School, Boston, Mass.

PATIENTS, MATERIALS, AND METHODS

A computerized vascular registry was established in January 1990. Data from all patients who have undergone vascular procedures at the West Campus of the Beth Israel Deaconess Medical Center (formerly The New England Deaconess Hospital), Boston, Mass, were prospectively entered. We reviewed all consecutive patients who underwent CEA from January 1, 1990, through August 31, 1997. Patients who underwent combined procedures (coronary artery bypass grafting), aortic arch procedures, or operations for recurrent carotid stenosis were not included in this review. The 1001 CEAs were performed during these 7 years by 4 of the 5 of us (F.B.P., G.W.G., D.R.C., and F.W.L.) at our hospital. Patients who underwent bilateral CEAs during the study interval had their risk factors and results entered separately at the time of each operation. Most patients underwent general anesthesia with routine shunting. Proper function of the shunt was confirmed using a hand-held continuous-wave doppler. Some CEAs were performed under regional anesthesia with shunting on the basis of continuous neurologic assessment. A patch closure was used at the discretion of the individual surgeons based on the diameter of the internal carotid artery. Recently, all arteries are patched, most commonly with collagen-impregnated Dacron fabric. Typically, postoperative patients recovered overnight in the postanesthesia care unit or the vascular intensive care unit (a specialized vascular ward for stable, unintubated patients) and then were discharged to home or transferred to the floor.

Patient demographics and preoperative risk factors were also evaluated, including history of coronary artery disease or congestive heart failure and presence of diabetes mellitus. Data were obtained by registry review and additional review of hospital records in certain cases. Indications for CEA were classified as asymptomatic, symptomatic (which included transient ischemic attacks [TIAs] and amaurosis fugax), or completed stroke. We characterized patients who presented with unclear or nonlateralizing symptoms as asymptomatic.

Categorization of the extent of disability due to a postoperative stroke was as follows: mild indicates deficit limited to 1 extremity, requiring no inpatient rehabilitation or in-home assistance; moderate, deficits requiring inpatient rehabilitation for motor skills or speech; or severe, profound deficits requiring skilled nursing facilities, including ventilatory and nutrition support. Other complications tracked include congestive heart failure, myocardial infarction, arrhythmia, hyperperfusion syndrome, and severe cranial nerve injuries (requiring rehabilitation). The number of minor cranial nerve injuries was not present in the current database. The average length of hospital stay (LOS) includes all postoperative days, including those incurred during a second consecutive procedure after a CEA such as a peripheral bypass.

year period without the use of EEG. In addition, an attempt was made to characterize the cause of perioperative stroke as well as the resultant deficits.

RESULTS

PATIENTS

Mean age of patients was 70.5 years (range, 39-94). Other overall characteristics of the 1001 patients with regard to preoperative risk factors are listed in the following tabulation:

Characteristics	% of Patients
Male	61
Female	39
Diabetes	38
Hypertension	70
Congestive heart failure	10
Previous coronary artery bypass graft	22
Overt coronary artery disease	46
Indications for CEA	
Asymptomatic	42.6
Symptomatic	49
Completed stroke	8.4

LENGTH OF HOSPITAL STAY

For the whole group, the average LOS was 3.1 days (range, 0-62 days). Six hundred seventy-seven (67.7%) of the patients were discharged by postoperative day 2.

COMPLICATIONS AND MORBIDITY

Complications are given in the following tabulation:

Complication	No. (%) of Patients
Nonfatal strokes	14 (1.4)
Death	2 (0.2)
TIA	4 (0.4)
Myocardial infarction	5 (0.5)
Congestive heart failure	8 (0.8)
Arrhythmia	8 (0.8)
Hyperperfusion syndrome	3 (0.3)
Severe cranial nerve injury	1 (0.1)

Overall, 14 strokes and 4 TIAs totaled 18 neurologic complications (1.8%).

Transient Ischemic Attacks

Two of the 4 patients with TIAs presented with symptomatic stenosis, 2 were asymptomatic, and all underwent CEA with an indwelling shunt. On reexploration, an intimal dissection was noted in 2 patients, no abnormality in one patient, and only an occluded external carotid artery in the other.

Strokes

Eleven (79%) of the 14 patients who suffered a postoperative stroke presented with a symptomatic stenosis, yielding stroke rates for asymptomatic and symptomatic patients of 0.7% and 1.9%, respectively. General endotracheal anesthesia with shunting was used in 11 patients (79%), with regional anesthesia used in the remainder. None of the strokes in the regional group was preceded by intraoperative clinical changes, and therefore the patients did not undergo shunting.

In those patients who underwent reexploration for ipsilateral postoperative neurologic deficits, several causes of the strokes were noted. In 5 patients, there was internal carotid artery thrombosis or the presence of fresh clot without an intimal flap. In 2 patients, a distal intimal flap with clot was apparent. In 1 patient, a distal kink with obstruction of flow was found, and, in another, the stroke resulted from an embolus or hypoperfusion, since no operative defect was identified, and since the patient did not undergo shunting.

The other 5 patients did not undergo reexploration, but some information was available. Heparin-induced thrombocytopenia and complete thrombosis of the internal carotid artery developed in 1 patient after a subsequent peripheral bypass graft 14 days after CEA. There was 1 intracerebral bleed noted on postoperative day 8. Emboli or hypoperfusion was presumed to be the cause of strokes in the other 3 patients, since all had patent internal carotid arteries radiologically. Thus, of the 14 postoperative strokes, 9 (64.3%) were likely due to technical errors during the endarterectomy and closure, since these patients had intimal flaps or presence of clot.

The initial manifestations of the strokes were as follows: 7 mild deficits (50%) that did not require any inpatient rehabilitation but prolonged the LOS to 6.3 days; 2 moderate deficits (14%) that required an LOS of 14 days and a subsequent period of inpatient rehabilitation; and 5 severe deficits (36%) that required intensive rehabilitation and, in 2 patients (14%), tracheostomy and gastrostomy tube placement. Their average LOS was 12.2 days before transfer to a skilled nursing facility. In the mild deficit category, all 7 patients showed continued recovery of motor or speech deficits, with 2 patients eventually having no recognizable deficit. In 1 patient, however, occlusion of his carotid repair developed, and he died of multiple-system organ failure as a complication of sepsis and renal failure 4 months after surgery. In the moderate deficit group, 1 patient showed some recovery of motor and speech loss and, although she eventually went home, she was still significantly debilitated. The other patient experienced a full recovery. In the severe deficit group, 1 patient suffered a subsequent ipsilateral TIA and, despite occlusion of the operative repair, the paresis improved and she did not require inpatient rehabilitation. Two patients were able to return home in less than 1 month and recovered most function except the ability to write in 1 patient and some speech disability in the other. Of the 2 patients who required tracheostomy and gastrostomy, 1 patient now lives at home with assistance from a health aide, whereas the other died at the rehabilitation center 2 months after surgery.

Death

There were 2 deaths within 30 days after surgery. One patient with severe renal insufficiency died in the recovery room from a suture line bleed, resulting in a respiratory arrest. The other patient died 8 days after surgery from complications of a myocardial infarction.

TYPE OF ANESTHESIA OR SHUNT

Eleven patients (79%) underwent general anesthesia; the remainder underwent regional anesthesia. Stroke rates for both groups were 1.5% and 1.2%, respectively. Six (43%) of 14 patients underwent patching.

COMMENT

Our report presents data on 1001 CEAs performed without using EEG as a cerebral monitoring technique. Most of the operations were performed under general anesthesia with routine shunting, but some were performed under regional anesthesia. The stroke rate was 1.4%; the combined stroke and death rate, 1.6%. These results were very similar to those of the Asymptomatic Carotid Atherosclerosis Study,[1] in which all patients were asymptomatic, and to those of the Cleveland Clinic report on 1924 CEAs,[7] in which most were performed with routine shunting. The stroke rates reported in these series, including ours, represent clinically apparent strokes, since it is not standard practice to obtain preoperative and postoperative computed tomographic or magnetic resonance imaging scans in all patients. In 1 study, this practice increased the infarct rate from 2% to 12%.[8] The significance of asymptomatic strokes is not exactly clear, but when comparing results between series, one must realize that the so-called silent stroke rate may vary considerably.

Results of series in which selective shunting was used based on EEG changes reveal combined stroke and mortality rates ranging from 1.4% to 2.7%.[4,9] However, it is clear in these series and others that EEG is not 100% sensitive for predicting postoperative strokes.[10] Also, EEG changes do not always occur immediately on clamping, but can happen several minutes later, which can cause technical problems if it occurs during the actual endarterectomy. In addition, it is clear from series exclusively using regional anesthesia that some patients will not show signs of cerebral ischemia during CEA but still suffer a perioperative stroke.[11] Accordingly, these patients would not undergo shunting during the procedure. This occurred in 3 patients who suffered postoperative strokes after CEA performed under regional anesthesia in our study. The causes of the strokes in the regional group, however, were similar to those noted in the routine shunting group.

Overall, the data suggest that although only a small number of patients will benefit from shunting, there is no preoperative clinical factor or intraoperative technique, including close observation under regional anesthesia, that reliably identifies those patients. Based on this, our current practice is to use general endotracheal anesthesia with routine shunting in most cases. Since it is also evident that series using different techniques have similarly low morbidity rates, we do not believe that routine shunting is the only acceptable method. However, since all patients receiving general anesthesia undergo shunting, we concentrate on widely exposing the distal internal carotid artery to avoid the potentially dangerous situation of having to urgently insert a shunt in an environment with inadequate distal exposure. Some of the technical errors were possibly contributed to by the shunt itself, but the rate is extremely low.

Another observation that can be made from these data is that, as noted by Riles et al,[12] a number of the strokes were due to a technical error with the endarterectomy or the distal end point. Thus, the already low stroke rates may be even lower.

In conclusion, performing CEA without EEG monitoring is a safe and reliable method. The results are likely due in part to the fact that CEAs were performed at a tertiary care center with a high volume of carotid procedures and reflect a multidisciplinary approach, including experienced nurses and anesthesiologists. However, technical errors still account for a large proportion of postoperative strokes after CEA, emphasizing the need for technical precision. Accordingly, more attention should be directed toward performing a precise endarterectomy and less to the method of cerebral monitoring. When strokes do occur, most patients can be expected to make a reasonable recovery and return to a level of function where they can live at home.

Presented at the 79th Annual Meeting of the New England Surgical Society, Toronto, Ontario, September 27, 1998.

Reprints: Frank B. Pomposelli, Jr, MD, Harvard Medical School, Department of Vascular Surgery, Beth Israel Deaconess Medical Center, West Campus, 110 Francis St, Suite 5B, Boston MA, 02215 (e-mail: fpomposelli@bidmc.harvard.edu).

REFERENCES

1. Executive Committee for the Asymptomatic Carotid Atherosclerosis Study. Endarterectomy for asymptomatic carotid artery stenosis. *JAMA*. 1995;273:1421-1428.
2. North American Symptomatic Carotid Endarterectomy Trial Collaborators. Beneficial effect of carotid endarterectomy in symptomatic patients with high-grade stenosis. *N Engl J Med*. 1991;325:445-453.
3. Moore WS, Barnett HJM, Beebe HG, et al. Guidelines for carotid endarterectomy. *Stroke*. 1995;26:188-201.
4. Whittemore AD, Kaufman JL, Kohler TR, Mannick JA. Routine electroencephalographic (EEG) monitoring during carotid endarterectomy. *Ann Surg*. 1982;197:707-713.
5. Benjamin ME, Silva MB Jr, Watt C, et al. Awake patient monitoring to determine the need for shunting during carotid endarterectomy. *Surgery*. 1993;114:673-681.
6. Harada RN, Comerota AJ, Good GM, et al. Stump pressure, electroencephalographic changes and the contralateral carotid artery. *Am J Surg*. 1995;170:148-153.
7. Hertzer NR, O'Hara PJ, Mascha EJ, et al. Early outcome assessment for 2228 consecutive carotid endarterectomy procedures. *J Vasc Surg*. 1997;26:1-10.
8. Berguer R, Sieggreen MY, Lazo M, Hodakowski BA. The silent brain infarct in carotid surgery. *J Vasc Surg*. 1986;3:442-447.
9. Green RM, Messick WJ, Ricotta JJ, et al. Benefits, shortcomings and costs of EEG monitoring. *Ann Surg*. 1985;201:785-792.
10. McCarthy WJ, Park AE, Koushanpour E, et al. Carotid endarterectomy. *Ann Surg*. 1996;224:297-307.
11. Lawrence PF, Alves JC, Jicha DJ, et al. Incidence, timing, and causes of cerebral ischemia during carotid endarterectomy with regional anesthesia. *J Vasc Surg*. 1998;27:329-337.
12. Riles TS, Imparato AM, Jacobowitz GR, et al. The cause of perioperative stroke after carotid endarterectomy. *J Vasc Surg*. 1994;19:206-216.

DISCUSSION

Jack Huse, MD, Meriden, Conn: The North American Symptomatic Carotid Endarterectomy Trial (NASCET) and the Asymptomatic Carotid Atherosclerosis Study (ACAS) have verified what surgeons have intuitively believed for decades, namely, that properly selected patients with high-grade carotid stenosis, regardless of symptoms, have a longer stroke-free survival with operative vs nonoperative therapy. This concept is valid only when surgical management results in a stroke and combined stroke and death rate of 1% to 3%. The maintenance of optimal cerebral profusion is generally regarded as the critical factor for the successful carotid endarterectomy outcomes. How to best monitor this optimal cerebral profusion has been the topic of countless articles in the surgical literature. Moore and Hall, in 1969, proposed the use of internal carotid artery stump pressure as an index of collateral cerebral circulation during carotid clamping. Since that time, other authors have championed transcranial doppler ultrasonography (TCD) to monitor blood flow in the basal cerebral arteries. Pertinent to this morning's paper, the EEG has been shown to be an exquisitely sensitive measure of cerebral blood flow. Despite its sensitivity, the value of an EEG interoperatively to reduce CEA complication rates is rightfully being called into question.

Dr Hamdan and his colleagues from the Beth Israel Deaconess Medical Center have provided a meticulous analysis of over 1000 cases of CEAs safely performed without the use of intraoperative EEG monitoring. Unfortunately, the sensitivity of an EEG to predict a postoperative stroke is not 100%. In fact, there are a number of papers documenting minimal or no evidence of intraoperative EEG changes in patients who have demonstrated significant neurologic deficits postoperatively. Conversely, there are papers documenting patients with substantial intraoperative EEG changes who did not develop any postoperative neurologic deficits. When faced with this mind-boggling dilemma (before having had the opportunity to read Dr Hamdan's paper), I did what all good scientists do, I asked my colleagues in Connecticut what they were doing referable to EEG monitoring. I'm pleased to report, at least on this issue, Massachusetts and Connecticut agree. The routine use of EEG monitoring in the operating room is not currently utilized in Hartford, New Haven, New Britain, or, I suspect, in other hospitals within the state that I failed to contact.

Cost-effectiveness is certainly important to all of this in this day and age, but patient safety and excellence of outcomes has always been our goal. It is therefore important we document the efficacy of CEA, without the added expense of intraoperative EEG monitoring. I believe this paper has successfully defended that position.

I have several questions for the authors. When you reviewed the technical errors that contributed to the incidence of postoperative neurologic deficits, did you discover any features which might be helpful in reducing future technical problems? And secondly, do you have any experience with the use of high-dose thiopental anesthesia as a method of cerebral protection during CEA?

Padiath Aslam, MD, Augusta, Me: I'd like to know if the same uniform technique was used with a classical longitudinal incision, or eversion endarterectomy had been done in later cases, as it is becoming popular? And also, whether any intraoperative arteriogram or intraoperative duplex scanning has been employed to see the adequacy of the endarterectomy?

Dr Hamdan: As for the technical errors that we identified, the most common one was a problem with the distal end point. One thing that we have discovered, especially when you are using a patch, is to extend the initial arteriotomy beyond the distal end point so that when you are sewing in the patch, or starting your primary closure, you are not closing directly over the area of concern. Other than that, I don't have other tips on avoiding technical errors except for being as precise with the endarterectomy and closure as possible.

As far as use of thiopental anesthesia, I apologize, but I'm not really familiar with that technique, and we don't have any experience with that at our institution.

To answer the second group of questions, this is a standard endarterectomy with a longitudinal arteriotomy. We don't perform eversion endarterectomies, although that has been shown to be a very successful technique.

We do not routinely evaluate the adequacy of our repair and closure with intraoperative duplex scan or arteriography. We do use a handheld continuous wave doppler at the end of the procedure. When there is a concern about the repair, we will perform an intraoperative arteriogram. However, this has been the case in only a small percentage of our patients.

PAPER

Distal Splenorenal Shunt

Role, Indications, and Utility in the Era of Liver Transplantation

Roger L. Jenkins, MD; Roberto Gedaly, MD; James J. Pomposelli, MD, PhD; Elizabeth A. Pomfret, MD, PhD; Fredric Gordon, MD; W. David Lewis, MD

Hypothesis: The distal splenorenal shunt (DSRS) continues to play an important role in the management of recurrent variceal bleeding with minimal negative impact on subsequent orthotopic liver transplantation (OLT).

Design: Case-control study.

Setting: Hepatobiliary surgery and liver transplantation unit in a tertiary referral medical center.

Patients: From August 1, 1985, through October 31, 1997, a single team of surgeons performed 81 DSRS procedures for recurrent variceal hemorrhage. Eleven patients undergoing OLT subsequent to DSRS were compared with a group of 274 patients undergoing OLT without any previous shunt during the same period.

Main Outcome Measures: Operative time, use of blood products, length of hospital stay, perioperative complications, and survival rates.

Results: Operative (30-day) mortality for DSRS was 6% (n = 5). From follow-up information available for 74 patients, the 1- and 5-year survival rates were 86.4% (n = 64) and 74.3% (n = 55), respectively. Recurrent variceal bleeding and hepatic encephalopathy occurred in 5 (6.8%) and 11 patients (14.9%), respectively, after DSRS. In 9 patients, DSRS was used as salvage for failed transjugular intrahepatic portosystemic shunt.

Conclusions: Distal splenorenal shunt is a safe, durable, and effective treatment for controlling recurrent variceal hemorrhage in patients with acceptable operative risk and good liver function. It does not compromise future liver transplantation and can considerably delay the time until transplantation is required. Given the early occlusion rate and need for constant surveillance, transjugular intrahepatic portosystemic shunting should be reserved for patients with Child C classification cirrhosis with chronic hemorrhage or intractable ascites or as an emergency procedure for patients with uncontrollable bleeding using endoscopic therapy.

Arch Surg. 1999;134:416-420

From the Division of Hepatobiliary and Transplantation Surgery, Department of Surgery, Beth Israel Deaconess Medical Center, Harvard Medical School, Boston, Mass.

TREATMENT OPTIONS for the patient with variceal bleeding and portal hypertension have changed dramatically during the past decade. Historically, medical therapy, balloon tamponade, and emergency portal decompression procedures were the mainstay of treatment for the patient with refractory variceal bleeding but were associated with significant morbidity and mortality.[1-4] Refinements in endoscopic sclerotherapy and pharmacological intervention led to an increasing number of patients successfully treated without the need for emergency surgical shunt procedures.[5,6]

More recently, the development of transjugular intrahepatic portosystemic shunting (TIPS) has added substantially to the armamentarium of therapeutic options for patients with complications of chronic liver disease. Transjugular intrahepatic portosystemic shunting has demonstrated efficacy as an emergency modality for the patient with refractory variceal bleeding, or as the primary therapy for the patient in whom operative risk is considered poor. The use of TIPS is limited, however, by the need for constant surveillance, frequent revisions, and a high rate of early thrombosis.[7,8]

See Invited Critique at end of article

For the patient with relative preservation of hepatic function and minimal ascites, selective portosystemic shunting still should be considered for the management of variceal bleeding when pharmacological therapy and sclerotherapy have failed.[9,10] Although orthotopic liver transplantation (OLT) remains the definitive treatment for the patient with liver failure, many patients with portal hypertension and esophageal bleeding may not require OLT for many years.[11]

PATIENTS AND METHODS

From August 1, 1985, through October 31, 1997, DSRS was performed in 81 patients in the liver transplantation unit at the Beth Israel Deaconess Medical Center, Boston, Mass. Patient medical records were reviewed for demographics, cause of the liver disease, Child classification, indication for shunting, intraoperative blood loss, transfusion requirement, perioperative surgical complications, length of hospitalization, postoperative encephalopathy, and rebleeding rates. A group of 11 patients undergoing OLT subsequent to DSRS (DSRS was performed at the study center in 6 patients and at referring hospitals in 5) was compared with a group of 274 patients who underwent OLT only during the same interval. Thirty-day operative mortality and long-term survival rates were evaluated.

The primary indication for DSRS was recurrent variceal bleeding. In 9 patients, however, DSRS was used for salvage after TIPS and subsequent development of acute occlusion and rebleeding (**Figure 1**).

Seven of 81 patients were unavailable for follow-up and were excluded from statistical analysis. Of the 74 patients in whom complete data were available, Child classification was A in 57 (77%) and B in 17 (23%) at the time of surgery. Endoscopy showed esophageal varices alone in 52 patients (70%) and esophageal and gastric varices in 22 (30%). Primary sclerotherapy was performed in all patients to control initial bleeding episodes. In cases of medical failure with recurrent hemorrhage refractory to sclerotherapy, TIPS or DSRS was considered. Distal splenorenal shunting was performed only in patients with Child A or B classification. Patients were selected for transplantation based on the development of end-stage liver failure in accordance to guidelines promulgated by the United Network for Organ Sharing.[14]

Unless otherwise indicated, all data are presented as mean ± SEM. Continuous data were compared using Student t test. Thirty-day survival data were compared using χ^2 test. Statistical significance was set at $P<.05$ in all cases. Survival data were calculated using the Kaplan-Meier product-limit method.

Each year the number of patients waiting for liver transplants increases, yet the number of available organs from suitable donors remains relatively unchanged.[12] This places a premium on the development of strategies for treating patients with portal hypertension to delay the need for transplantation. The goal should be to maintain the functional reserve of the remaining liver while minimizing recurrent bleeding without compromising the ability to perform a remedial transplantation. The distal splenorenal shunt (DSRS) procedure developed by Warren et al[13] in 1967 fulfills these criteria.

In this study, we review a single center's experience in performing DSRS during a 12-year period in a single institution with an active liver transplantation program. We explore the utility of DSRS in the management of recurrent variceal bleeding, outcome analysis, and impact on subsequent OLT.

RESULTS

Fifty-two men (64%) and 29 women (36%) had a mean age of 56.9 ± 1.2 years (range, 35-88 years) at the time of surgery. The primary causes of portal hypertension and variceal bleeding are summarized in the following tabulation:

Cause	No. (%) of Patients
Alcohol	34 (42)
Cryptogenic liver disease	15 (18)
Hepatitis C	11 (14)
Primary sclerosing cholangitis	8 (10)
Primary bilary cirrhosis	4 (5)
Hepatitis B	3 (4)
Autoimmune hepatitis	3 (4)
Portal vein thrombosis	1 (1)
Budd-Chiari syndrome	1 (1)
Hemochromatosis	1 (1)
Total	**81 (100)**

Hepatitis C disease assumed increasing importance in later years and undoubtedly contributed to cirrhosis in patients with cryptogenic or alcoholic liver disease before serologic markers became routinely available.

Hospital course is summarized in the following tabulation:

Factor	Mean ± SEM (Range)
Operative time, h	5.68 ± 0.12 (2.75-8.00)
Estimated blood loss, mL	1209 ± 176 (100-5000)
Packed red blood cells, U	2.1 ± 0.3 (0-15)
Length of hospital stay, d	16.1 ± 1.8 (4-71)

Perioperative and long-term complications are summarized in **Table 1**. Most complications developed during the perioperative phase and required observation or short-term treatment. Operative 30-day mortality was 6% (n = 5). Child classification in 3 of these patients was A; in 2, B. Causes of death included adult respiratory distress syndrome and multiple organ failure (n = 2), coagulopathy and uncontrolled bleeding (n = 2), and cardiac arrhythmia (n = 1). Of particular note is the finding that thrombosis of the portal vein developed within the first week of surgery in 5 patients, contributing to delay in resolution of postoperative ascites in all. Three of these 5 patients have subsequently required OLT. One of these patients required an iliac vein graft to reconstruct the portal vein, whereas the other 2 underwent thrombectomy and standard anastomosis.

Long-term complications included recurrent variceal bleeding and hepatic encephalopathy, which occurred in 6.8% (n = 5) and 14.9% (n = 11) of patients, respectively. These data reflect occurrences throughout a mean survival time of 6.5 years. **Figure 2** shows the Kaplan-Meier survival curve for all patients who underwent successful DSRS. The 1- and 5-year survival rates were 86.4% (n = 64) and 74.3% (n = 55), respectively.

During the study, 11 patients underwent OLT a median of 5.1 years following DSRS (range, 0.4-10.1 years). We compared these patients with 274 patients who underwent OLT during the same period without any preexisting shunt. The relative impact of previous DSRS on operative outcome of OLT is shown in **Table 2**. There was no significant statistical impact on duration of sur-

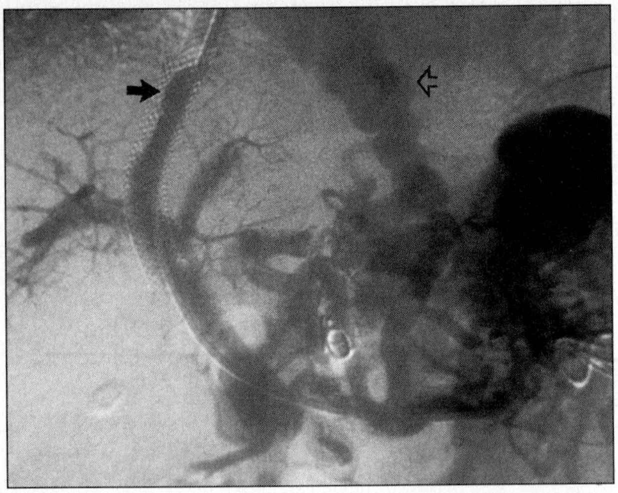

Figure 1. *Angiographic study in patient presenting with third variceal bleed following transjugular intrahepatic portosystemic shunting. Large varices remain despite placement of multiple coils (open arrow). Laminated thrombus is visible within lumen of stent. Distal splenorenal shunting was performed subsequently (solid arrow).*

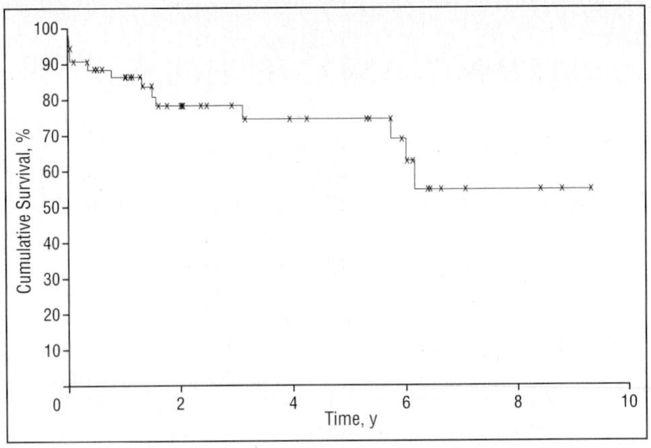

Figure 2. *Survival curve after distal splenorenal shunting. Patients were observed for a mean of 6.5 years and censored according to Kaplan-Meier methods. The 1- and 5-year survival rates were 86.0% and 74.2%, respectively.*

Table 1. Early and Late Postoperative Complications*

Complications	No. of Patients
Perioperative	
Abdominal	
Portal vein thrombosis	5
Pancreatitis	2
Ascites requiring readmission	2
Retroperitoneal bleeding	1†
Variceal bleeding	1†
Pancreatic pseudocyst	1
Adynamic ileus	1
Cardiopulmonary	
ARDS and MOF	2†
Nonfatal arrhythmia	1
Fatal arrhythmia	1†
Aspiration	1
Pneumonia	1
Wound infection	2
Renal	
Urinary tract infection	2
Renal	1
Late complications	
Hepatic encephalopathy	11
Recurrent variceal bleeding	4

**ARDS indicates adult respiratory distress syndrome; MOF, multiple organ failure. Thirty-four of 81 patients had at least 1 complication, for a perioperative morbidity rate of 42%. Perioperative complications are defined as those within 30 days of surgery. Late complications are those after 30 postoperative days and represent occurrences throughout a mean follow-up of 6.5 years. One patient had recurrent variceal bleeding after surgery and died. Encephalopathy developed in 15 of 74 patients.*

†Indicates patients who died (perioperative mortality, 6%).

Table 2. Liver Transplant Outcome After DSRS vs No Previous Shunt*

	Mean ± SD			
Group†	Operative Time, h	PRBC, U	FFP, U	30-Day Mortality, %
DSRS	7.4 ± 2.5	12.0 ± 8.6	14.1 ± 10.7	0
No-shunt	6.5 ± 2.0	17.4 ± 15.6	18.9 ± 15.9	12

**Mortality was not significant using χ^2 analysis. Operative variables were not significant by Student t test. No-shunt group represents 274 patients undergoing liver transplantation during the same period. DSRS indicates distal splenorenal shunt; PRBC, packed red blood cells; and FFP, fresh frozen plasma.*

†Described in the "Results" section.

gery, use of blood products, or 30-day operative mortality. The DSRS was ligated after hepatic revascularization in 5 patients, and was left intact in the remaining 6.

COMMENT

Management of portal hypertension and variceal bleeding is complicated by the variable degree of hepatic synthetic disruption by a diverse group of chronic liver diseases and the number of treatment options available. For the patient with recurrent variceal hemorrhage but adequate hepatic function, controversy exists as to the best method of prophylaxis against future bleeding.[1,15,16] In patients with unsuccessful pharmacological and endoscopic control of variceal bleeding, TIPS has evolved recently as a relatively convenient treatment modality, and in many institutions its use is not restricted to patients with poor hepatic reserve. Emerging data suggest the frequent need for TIPS revision for stenosis or thrombosis within the first 1 to 2 years (20%-50%) and the potential for life-threatening complications.[7,17-22] These observations should temper enthusiasm for the use of TIPS in good-risk patients who have the potential for long-term survival once portal hypertension is controlled. Properly used, TIPS should play its pivotal role in the treatment of patients with recurrent variceal hemorrhage who are not candidates for transplantation, in bleeding patients desperately awaiting liver replacement, and in selected patients with intractable ascites.[23]

Whereas liver transplantation offers the best long-term solution to portal hypertension, end-stage liver failure may not develop for many years in many patients after their first bleeding episode. Therefore, any treatment option to control variceal hemorrhage should reduce the incidence of bleeding, maintain hepatic reserve, and remain durable for years.

There are several advantages to a selective DSRS over other selective and nonselective shunts in controlling variceal bleeding. First, selective decompression of gastroesophageal varices via the splenic circulation maintains prograde portal flow into the liver while effectively decompressing esophageal and gastric varices.[24] Maintenance of portal flow may better preserve the delivery of hepatotrophic factors that, in turn, are responsible for preservation of hepatic architecture and function.[25] Second, DSRS avoids extensive hepatic hilar mobilization, which might significantly complicate any future transplantation effort. Some caution in the use of DSRS is suggested by the low incidence of postoperative portal vein thrombosis, which occurred in 5 of our patients. Although recanalization of the portal vein may occur during several months, complete or partial thrombosis of the portal vein adds complexity to a subsequent liver transplantation.[26,27]

Our study confirms that DSRS can be performed in select patients with low operative mortality and a 6.8% rate of rebleeding during a mean follow-up of 6.5 years. Encephalopathy, which occurs frequently after nonselective shunts such as portocaval shunts and TIPS, occurred in only 14.9% of our patients during follow-up and was readily managed by dietary restriction and lactulose.[28,29] In patients with DSRS undergoing later transplantation, adhesions may increase the technical difficulties of recipient hepatectomy, but operative times, use of blood products, and survival rates are equivalent to those of the population undergoing liver transplantation as the primary treatment.

Our present algorithm for the management of variceal hemorrhage uses most of the available treatment options, with an emphasis on the immediate identification of patients who are anticipated to need urgent or late transplantation. Octreotide infusion and endoscopic sclerotherapy or banding is used initially in all patients presenting with variceal bleeding. Patients with Child A classification and in whom endoscopic variceal control fails are offered DSRS surgery in anticipation that they will not need transplantation for a prolonged period. Attempts are made to optimize patients with Child B classification who may then also be candidates for DSRS. Patients with Child C classification who are poor candidates for transplantation and patients actively waiting on the transplant list with uncontrollable bleeding are offered TIPS. Surgical portocaval shunts are restricted to rare patients in whom TIPS or DSRS fails or patients with salvageable Budd-Chiari syndrome.[30]

Given the long waiting times on many transplant lists, evaluation for potential liver transplantation should be instituted early in the patient's clinical course. Patients with chronic liver failure who are referred near the end of their disease process often will not survive the waiting period before a donor organ becomes available.

Distal splenorenal shunting continues to be a safe and effective procedure for controlling recurrent variceal hemorrhage and should be the treatment of choice for patients with acceptable operative risk and good liver function. It also serves as an excellent salvage procedure for patients with favorable Child classification in whom injudiciously placed TIPS fail. Furthermore, DSRS is a durable bridge to transplantation, with a greater than 5-year interval between surgical decompression and OLT in our series.

Presented at the 79th Annual Meeting of the New England Surgical Society, Toronto, Ontario, September 25, 1998.

Corresponding author: Roger L. Jenkins, MD, Division of Hepatobiliary and Transplantation Surgery, Beth Israel Deaconess Medical Center, 110 Francis St, Suite 8C, Boston, MA 02215 (e-mail: rjenkins@caregroup.harvard.edu).

REFERENCES

1. Henderson JM. Portal hypertension and shunt surgery. *Adv Surg.* 1993;26:233-257.
2. Orloff MJ, Orloff MS, Orloff SL, Rambotti M, Girard B. Three decades of experience with emergency portacaval shunt for acutely bleeding esophageal varices in 400 unselected patients with cirrhosis of the liver. *J Am Coll Surg.* 1995;180:257-272.
3. Spina GP, Henderson JM, Rikkers LF, et al. Distal spleno-renal shunt versus endoscopic sclerotherapy in the prevention of variceal rebleeding: a meta-analysis of 4 randomized clinical trials. *J Hepatol.* 1992;16:338-345.
4. Rikkers LF, Jin G. Emergency shunt: role in the present management of variceal bleeding. *Arch Surg.* 1995;130:472-477.
5. Besson I, Ingrand P, Person B, et al. Sclerotherapy with or without octreotide for acute variceal bleeding. *N Engl J Med.* 1995;333:555-560.
6. Conn HO, Lebrec D, Terblanche J. The treatment of oesophageal varices: a debate and a discussion. *J Intern Med.* 1997;241:103-108.
7. Rossle M, Siegerstetter V, Huber M, Ochs A. The first decade of the transjugular intrahepatic portosystemic shunt (TIPS): state of the art. *Liver.* 1998;18:73-89.
8. Rosemurgy AS II, Bloomston M, Zervos EE, et al. Transjugular intrahepatic portosystemic shunt versus H-graft portacaval shunt in the management of bleeding varices: a cost-benefit analysis. *Surgery.* 1997;122:794-800.
9. Abouljoud MS, Levy MF, Rees CR, et al. A comparison of treatment with transjugular intrahepatic portosystemic shunt or distal splenorenal shunt in the management of variceal bleeding prior to liver transplantation. *Transplantation.* 1995;59:226-229.
10. Mercado MA, Morales-Linares JC, Granados-Garcia J, et al. Distal splenorenal shunt versus 10-mm low-diameter mesocaval shunt for variceal hemorrhage. *Am J Surg.* 1996;171:591-595.
11. Hermann RE, Henderson JM, Vogt DP, Mayes JT, Geisinger MA, Agnor C. Fifty years of surgery for portal hypertension at the Cleveland Clinic Foundation: lessons and prospects. *Ann Surg.* 1995;221:459-468.
12. Harper AM, Rosendale JD. The UNOS OPTN waiting list and donor registry: 1988-1996. In: Cecka JM, Terasaki P, eds. *Clinical Transplants.* Los Angeles, Calif: UCLA Tissue Typing Laboratory; 1996:69-90.
13. Warren WD, Zeppa R, Fomon JJ. Selective trans-splenic decompression of gastroesophageal varices by distal splenorenal shunt. *Ann Surg.* 1967;166:437-455.
14. Blumstein JF. Government's role in organ transplantation policy. *J Health Polit Policy Law.* 1989;14:5-39.
15. Rees CJ, Hudson M, Record CO. Therapeutic modalities in portal hypertension. *Eur J Gastroenterol Hepatol.* 1997;9:9-11.
16. Navarro VJ, Garcia-Tsao G. Variceal hemorrhage. *Crit Care Clin.* 1995;11:391-414.
17. Kerlan RK Jr, LaBerge JM, Gordon RL, Ring EJ. Transjugular intrahepatic portosystemic shunts: current status. *AJR Am J Roentgenol.* 1995;164:1059-1066.
18. Sanyal AJ, Freedman AM, Luketic VA, et al. The natural history of portal hypertension after transjugular intrahepatic portosystemic shunts. *Gastroenterology.* 1997;112:889-898.
19. Sanyal AI, Freedman AM, Luketic VA, et al. Transjugular intrahepatic portosystemic shunts compared with endoscopic sclerotherapy for the prevention of recurrent variceal hemorrhage: a randomized controlled trial. *Ann Intern Med.* 1997;126:849-857.
20. Cosenza CA, Hoffman AL, Friedman ML, et al. Transjugular intrahepatic portosystemic shunt: efficacy for the treatment of portal hypertension and impact on liver transplantation. *Am Surg.* 1996;62:835-839.
21. LaBerge JM, Somberg KA, Lake JR, et al. Two-year outcome following transjugular intrahepatic portosystemic shunt for variceal bleeding: results in 90 patients. *Gastroenterology.* 1995;108:1143-1151.

22. Foshager MC, Ferral H, Nazarian GK, Castaneda-Zuniga WR, Letourneau JG. Duplex sonography after transjugular intrahepatic portosystemic shunts (TIPS): normal hemodynamic findings and efficacy in predicting shunt patency and stenosis. *AJR Am J Roentgenol.* 1995;165:1-7.
23. Bataller R, Arroyo V, Gines P. Management of ascites in cirrhosis. *J Gastroenterol Hepatol.* 1997;12:723-733.
24. Rikkers LF, Jin G, Langnas AN, Shaw BW Jr. Shunt surgery during the era of liver transplantation. *Ann Surg.* 1997;226:51-57.
25. Starzl TE, Porter KA, Kashiwagi N. Portal hepatotrophic factors, diabetes mellitus and acute liver atrophy, hypertrophy and regeneration. *Surg Gynecol Obstet.* 1975;141:843-858.
26. Lerut JP, Mazza D, van Leeuw V, et al. Adult liver transplantation and abnormalities of splanchnic veins: experience in 53 patients. *Transpl Int.* 1997;10:125-132.
27. Langnas AN, Marujo WC, Stratta RJ, et al. A selective approach to preexisting portal vein thrombosis in patients undergoing liver transplantation. *Am J Surg.* 1992;163:132-136.
28. Pomier-Layrargues G. TIPS and hepatic encephalopathy. *Semin Liver Dis.* 1996;16:315-320.
29. Riggio O, Merlli M, Pedretti G, et al. Hepatic encephalopathy after transjugular intrahepatic portosystemic shunt: incidence and risk factors. *Dig Dis Sci.* 1996;41:578-584.
30. Hemming AW, Langer B, Greig P, et al. Treatment of Budd-Chiari syndrome with portosystemic shunt or liver transplantation. *Am J Surg.* 1996;171:176-180.

Invited Critique

The article by Jenkins et al reports a single center's experience with distal splenorenal shunt (DSRS) over a 12-year period. It helps to define the effect of shunt surgery in the overall scheme of management of patients with portal hypertension, variceal bleeding, and liver disease. The authors define which patients have been selected for shunts, what outcomes have been achieved, and where DSRS fits in the scheme of endoscopic therapy, transjugular intrahepatic portosystemic shunt (TIPS), and transplantations.

Child class A and B patients with recurrent variceal bleeding were candidates for DSRS, and as reported in other surgical series, the authors achieved a low operative mortality rate (6.2%) and good long-term survival rates, 86% at 1 year and 74% at 5 years. The rebleeding rate was 6.8%, the encephalopathy rate was 14.9%, and the transplantation rate was 13.6%, with a median follow-up time of approximately 5 years, indicating what can be achieved in a highly selected group of patients.

Eleven of their 81 patients underwent orthotopic liver transplantation (OLT), and the data presented support the current literature indicating that patients with DSRS who undergo OLT are at no disadvantage. Operative time, blood loss, and early mortality are not significantly different from those in the transplantation population as a whole. The fact that only 13.6% of their DSRS population needed OLT over 5 years indicates that this operation did not accelerate this group's need for OLT.

An interesting aside is the number of patients who required surgical rescue for TIPS thrombosis. Nine of the 81 DSRS patients fell into this category, but unfortunately, we do not have the the total number of TIPS procedures performed during this time. The lesson learned is that DSRS can be successfully achieved when TIPS has failed, and failed TIPS does not necessarily lead to a need for OLT.

Where does this leave us in the use of DSRS? This group has documented that a "Hepatobiliary Surgery and Transplant Unit"—as they define themselves—can and should have this surgical option available as part of their repertoire. As Jenkins et al point out, it is important that the full breadth of options be available to patients, and liver transplant surgeons should provide this expertise for appropriately selected patients.

J. Michael Henderson, MD
Cleveland, Ohio

Reticuloendothelial System Activity and Organ Failure in Patients With Multiple Injuries

Hans-Christoph Pape, MD; Dierk Remmers, MD; Martin Grotz, MD; Jörg Kotzerke, MD; Sabine von Glinski, MD; Martijn van Griensven, PhD; Michael Dahlweid, MD; Susanne Sznidar, MD; Harald Tscherne, MD

Hypothesis: Reticuloendothelial system function is altered in patients with multiple trauma and organ failure.

Design: Prospective cohort study.

Setting: Surgical intensive care unit at a level I trauma center.

Patients: Patients with multiple blunt trauma and injury severity scores greater than 20, with no referrals.

Interventions: Every second day reticuloendothelial system (RES) clearance capacity and liver blood flow were determined by administering labeled human albumin. Liver function was measured by enzymatic decay of indocyanine green, and levels of plasma tumor necrosis factor α were evaluated.

Results: In nonsurviving patients with blunt trauma, RES function was altered and was associated with organ dysfunction and infectious complications. Of 61 patients, 42 survived and 19 did not. Sixteen patients (84%) died of multiple organ failure. Significantly elevated RES activity (colloid clearance rate) was present between day 5 and day 13 after trauma in nonsurvivors (0.86 ± 0.16 [mean ± SD] on day 7, $P = .003$) compared with survivors (0.48 ± 0.08 on day 7) and 20 healthy volunteers (0.47 ± 0.06); RES activity then decreased to subnormal levels in nonsurvivors. Tumor necrosis factor α plasma levels were elevated early after injury only in nonsurvivors (on day 1: nonsurvivors, 1.2 ± 0.4 ng/mL [mean ± SD]; survivors, 0.5 ± 0.2 ng/mL; $P = .02$). Indocyanine green half-life values increased late after trauma, indicating late organ failure (on day 19: nonsurvivors, 111 ± 29 minutes [mean ± SD]; survivors, 12 ± 4 minutes; $P < .001$).

Conclusions: Early after trauma, nonsurviving patients demonstrated increased proinflammatory cytokine levels, followed by a state of pathological hyperactivation of the reticuloendothelial system prior to death. These results indicate that the stationary host defense system is involved in the mechanisms causing organ failure after severe trauma.

Arch Surg. 1999;134:421-427

From the Department of Trauma Surgery, Hannover Medical School, Hannover, Germany (Drs Pape, Remmers, Grotz, Griensven, Dahlweid, Sznidar, and Tscherne); Department of Nuclear Medicine, Ulm University, Ulm Germany (Dr Kotzerke); and the San Francisco Orthopaedic Residency Program, San Francisco, Calif (Dr von Glinski). *The authors have no commercial, proprietary, or financial interest in the products or companies described in this article.*

THE PATHOGENESIS of multiple organ failure (MOF) has been attributed to disturbances of the intestinal barrier and the systemic immunologic response.[1] These mechanisms suggest that a loss of intestinal barrier function associated with increased intestinal permeability allows systemic invasion of intestinal pathogens.[2-5] In turn, intestinal permeability damage, which has been demonstrated after trauma and burns, may pave the way for further translocation of intestinal bacteria and bacterial endotoxin.[1,2,6] In combination with other stimuli, endotoxin is able to cause MOF in sheep.[7] Some authors have attributed the development of organ failure to overwhelming invasion of bacteria and endotoxins, exceeding the capacity of bacterial clearance of the reticuloendothelial system (RES).[8]

Other authors have doubted the clinical significance of these findings, since clinical studies have failed to prove a relationship between intestinal bacteria and later organ failure or death.[9,10] Moreover, bacterial translocation to mesenteric lymph nodes and to the portal system was documented in human organ donors, suggesting that bacterial translocation may occur despite an anatomically intact gastrointestinal tract.[11]

Irrespective of the controversial discussion about the clinical significance of the "gut-liver axis," the changes in function of the RES in response to trauma and hemorrhagic shock have been well described.[12-14] Altered RES function has also been reported following low-grade intravascular coagulation or ischemia reperfusion damage.[15,16] In these studies, the stimulus caused impairment of

MATERIALS AND METHODS

The study was performed according to the international guidelines of the declaration of Helsinki. Informed consent was obtained from each patient's closest relative prior to the start of the study. Patients with multiple injuries were prospectively studied based on the following inclusion criteria: an injury severity score of more than 20; an initial Glasgow Coma Scale score greater than 8; primary admission and intensive care at our institution; no death due to hemorrhagic shock; a survival rate greater than 14 days after trauma; no liver or bowel disease or abdominal surgery; and no hepatic or colorectal malignant neoplasms or alcoholism.

DEFINITIONS

Adult respiratory distress syndrome and sepsis were defined according to scoring systems.[18,19] Severity of injury was categorized by the injury severity score (ISS)[20] and the Glasgow Coma Scale score.[21] Multiple organ failure was defined according to the criteria described by Knaus and Wagner.[22] Changes of organ function during the course of intensive care were also documented according to a multiple organ dysfunction score.[23]

All measurements were done every second day during intensive care therapy, starting on the day of injury. The study period encompassed the intensive care unit stay. In our institution, early intubation and prophylactic ventilation are routinely performed. Using standard laboratory tests, total serum bilirubin level, total protein level, and serum-platelet counts were determined, along with ventilatory parameters and gas analyses.

The patients were separated into 2 groups: survivors and nonsurvivors.

RES CLEARANCE

Determination of the uptake of radioactively labeled albumin into the liver allows for quantification of the phagocytic function of the hepatic RES in vivo.[24-27]

A fresh preparation of 100 MBq (2.7 mCi) of technetium Tc 99m bound to human albumin was obtained to measure RES clearance capacity and was administered as an intravenous bolus into the central venous catheter. For serial measurements at comparable body areas, after verification of both liver lobes by ultrasound, portable Geiger-Müller counters were placed on each lobe, at the center of the aorta, on the heart, and across the right lung. The additional Geiger-Müller counters were used to account for natural ^{99m}Tc decay or any influence caused by variations of circulation. All data were sampled in a portable bedside computer system (Engypan Forschunyszcntrum, Karlsruhe, Germany), and the rate of radioactive emission was constantly recorded during 18 minutes in 15-second increments. These data were corrected for the time-dependent decay of ^{99m}Tc. Time-activity curves were generated for the entire liver. A monoexponential fit was performed to calculate the uptake of colloid into the liver. If the tracer is extracted entirely by the liver and perfusion does not change during measurement, the uptake time unit is dependent only on the colloid clearance rate (K_2): $K_2 = Ln\ 2/t_{½}$, where $t_{½}$ is given as 1/minutes. The invasion constant of RES activity was calculated (normal range, 0.42±0.06, determined by measurement of 20 healthy controls).

LIVER PERFUSION

For quantification of the arterial and venous fractions of total hepatic blood flow a liver perfusion value (K_1) was

clearance functions and subsequent downregulation of RES capacity.[12-16] Other studies have revealed that RES function, based on measurements in isolated Kupffer cells, responds to endotoxemia and tumor necrosis factor α (TNF-α) stimulation by an increase in oxygen radical production.[17] These results suggest that changes in RES clearance capacity may not depend on alterations of the intestinal barrier.

Human data on the RES and its possible role in MOF are sparse. Therefore, our prospective clinical study compares the function of the RES in patients with multiple trauma who develop late organ failure and death with the function of the RES in patients who demonstrate an uneventful clinical course.

RESULTS

Between October 15, 1994, and April 15, 1997, consecutive patients who met the inclusion criteria were investigated. Of 68 patients, 4 died before 14 days after trauma and 3 died of hemorrhagic shock and were excluded. Sixty-one patients with multiple trauma were studied, with 42 survivors (29 men, 13 women) and 19 nonsurvivors (11 men, 8 women). Demographic data revealed no statistically significant difference in the severity of injury, the degree of head injury on the scene, and the duration of intubation and intensive care therapy. The amount of intravascular fluid received during rescue was significantly higher in nonsurvivors (**Table 1**).

Adult respiratory distress syndrome occurred in 6 survivors and 3 nonsurvivors. Renal failure requiring hemofiltration was found only in association with late organ failure. Hemofiltration was performed in 7 survivors and 3 nonsurvivors. There was a significantly higher rate of pulmonary infections among nonsurvivors. The other data associated with infectious complications revealed no differences between groups (Table 1). **Table 2** demonstrates the course of the MOF score in patients who did and who did not survive.

Serum bilirubin levels were normal early after trauma and remained normal in survivors. Among nonsurvivors, a statistically significant increase followed until the end of the third week after trauma ($P<.003$ compared with survivors, $P<.001$ compared with baseline). The liver perfusion values demonstrated no statistically significant difference between patient groups during the entire study period (**Table 3**). The independent measure of intestinal blood flow by Doppler ultrasound revealed large SDs despite the fact that a mean of 3 measurements was calculated. Therefore, these data were not used and are not shown.

All coagulation values were significantly altered early after trauma in both groups of patients. Nonsurvivors calculated. Three points on the time-activity curve were investigated: the beginning of arterial liver perfusion, the beginning of portal venous perfusion, and the beginning of recirculation effects at the end of the first portal passage.

As an independent measure of perfusion, Doppler ultrasound examination of the hepatic vein was also performed (Sonoline AC, No. U3-040.201.01.01, Siemens Corp, Erlangen, Germany), using a 5-MHz device. Three sequential measurements were made and the mean of these measurements was calculated.

PROINFLAMMATORY CYTOKINE

Tumor necrosis factor α levels were determined using an enzyme-linked immunosorbent assay technique (polyclonal rabbit anti–human TNF-α coating, Polysan-TNF BPS 30; Biochrom KG, Berlin, Germany). Also, recombinant TNF-α (standard, 10 μg per vial [Bissendorf KG, Hannover, Germany]) and monoclonal mouse Fab anti–human TNF-α peroxidase 20 (No. 1198688; Boehringer Mannheim GmbH, Mannheim, Germany) was used.

INDOCYANINE GREEN TEST

Indocyanine green (ICG), an anionic water-soluble dye, was freshly dissolved prior to each measurement. Following initial blood sampling, the sterile preparation of ICG was injected intravenously at 0.5 mg/kg body weight (ICG Pulsion; Pulsion Medicine Systems KG, Munich, Germany) .At 5, 10, 15, and 20 minutes, 5 mL of blood was withdrawn from the antecubital vein and the serum concentrationwas determined enzymatically at 800 nm (Beckmann DU-6 photometer; Beckmann GmbH, Hövelhof, Germany). Calibration was performed using control blood. The plasma disappearance rate was calculated by linear regression analysis of the plasma concentrations at 5, 10, and 15 minutes.

COAGULATION STUDIES

Platelet-poor plasma was prepared from 4.5 mL of blood mixed with 0.5 mL of 0.1-mol/L sodium citrate in a siliconized glass tube and centrifuged at 2600 rpm for 20 minutes.

Antithrombin III was measured by means of the Coamatic LR Antithrombin test kit (Cromogenix AB, Mölndal, Sweden) using the CobasFara chemistry analyzer (Hoffmann–La Roche Ltd, Basel, Switzerland). This test is based on the blocking effect of the activity of factor Xa by the antithrombin-heparin complex. Samples from patients with multiple trauma were compared with samples from 20 healthy controls.

The activity of protein C was measured using the Berichrom kit (Behring Diagnostics, Frankfurt, Germany). A sodium citrate solution was carefully mixed at a 1:9 ratio with venous blood. Subsequently, the mixture was centrifuged at 3000g for 10 minutes. Plasma samples were stored at −20°C; at this temperature the sample is stable for at least 1 month.

The measurement of D-dimer cross-linked fibrin degradation products was performed using a D-dimer enzyme-linked immunosorbent assay kit (American Diagnostica Inc, Greenwich, Conn).[28]

STATISTICS

Paired and unpaired *t* tests were performed. Probabilities less than .05 were considered significant. Values are expressed as mean±SEM.

Table 1. Demographic and Infection Rate Data for Study Participants*

	Nonsurvivors	Survivors
No. of patients	19	42
Age, y	39.2 ± 4.5	36.7 ± 4.9
Injury severity score	32.8 ± 6.1	27.8 ± 6.9
Glasgow Coma Scale score	12.3 ± 3.8	11.4 ± 5.3
Prehospital rescue time, min	64 ± 48	59 ± 43
Prehospital intravenous fluids, mL†	4620 ± 440	1770 ± 890
Infections during intensive care unit stay, No. (%)		
Pneumonia‡	11 (58)	8 (19)
Sepsis	2 (11)	3 (7)
Wound infection	5 (26)	7 (17)

*Values are expressed as mean ± SEM unless otherwise indicated.
†P=.03.
‡P=.04.

Table 2. Clinical Course of Patients With Multiple Trauma as Determined by Multiple Organ Dysfunction Score*†

	Multiple Organ Dysfunction Score	
Day	Nonsurvivors	Survivors
1	4.9 ± 4.1	4.3 ± 3.9
3	5.2 ± 3.0	4.9 ± 3.8
5	6.4 ± 3.8	6.5 ± 3.8
7	8.8 ± 6.3	8.2 ± 2.6
9	12.5 ± 7.9	7.3 ± 7.0
14	19.7 ± 8.9	5.9 ± 5.4
21	22.2 ± 8.6	5.5 ± 5.2

*Values are expressed as mean ± SEM.
†Marshall et al.[23]

demonstrated lower protein C values and higher levels of D-dimer cross-linked fibrin degradation products at days 1 and 3 than survivors (**Table 4**).

Figure 1 demonstrates changes in RES function. Early after trauma, data were normal. Among nonsurvivors, an increase developed within the first week after injury (day 7, 0.86±0.1; *P*=.003) compared with survivors (day 7, 0.48±0.08) and controls (0.47±0.06). During the third week, values among nonsurvivors decreased to subnormal levels.

The central venous levels of plasma TNF-α were significantly higher among nonsurvivors than among survivors until day 5 after injury (day 1: nonsurvivors,1.2±0.4 ng/mL; survivors, 0.5±0.2 ng/mL; *P*=.02). Following the first week, no difference was found between nonsurvivors and survivors (**Figure 2**).

Table 3. Liver Excretory Function Based on Serum Bilirubin Levels*

	Bilirubin, µmol/L (mg/dL)		Liver Perfusion Constant†	
Day	Nonsurvivors	Survivors	Nonsurvivors	Survivors
1	22.3 ± 11 (1.3 ± 0.6)	21 ± 6 (1.2 ± 0.4)	1.8 ± 0.1	1.8 ± 0.2
3	32.8 ± 30 (1.9 ± 1.8)	21 ± 8 (1.2 ± 0.5)	1.9 ± 0.3	1.7 ± 0.3
5	53.4 ± 38 (3.1 ± 2.2)	24 ± 10 (1.4 ± 0.6)	2.1 ± 0.4	1.8 ± 0.3
7	80.3 ± 68 (4.7 ± 4.0)	38 ± 12 (2.2 ± 0.7)	2.0 ± 0.1	1.9 ± 0.4
9	112.0 ± 59 (6.5 ± 3.5)	29 ± 7 (1.7 ± 0.4)‡	1.8 ± 0.2	1.9 ± 0.3
14	187.0 ± 67 (10.9 ± 3.9)	34 ± 16 (2.0 ± 0.9)§	2.1 ± 0.2	2.0 ± 0.3
21	245.0 ± 89 (14.3 ± 5.2)	26 ± 12 (1.5 ± 0.7)‖	1.8 ± 0.1	1.9 ± 0.2

**Values are expressed as mean ± SEM.*
†*Calculated from the uptake of technetium Tc 99m decay.*
‡P = .04.
§P = .007.
‖P = .003.

Table 4. Parameters Indicative of Coagulatory Changes*

	Antithrombin III, %†		Protein C, mg/L		D-Dimer, ng/mL	
Day	Nonsurvivors	Survivors	Nonsurvivors	Survivors	Nonsurvivors	Survivors
1	50 ± 21	61 ± 26	0.2 ± 0.1	1.3 ± 0.2‡	2520 ± 530	870 ± 490§
3	78 ± 30	83 ± 28	0.6 ± 0.2	1.7 ± 0.3‖	1800 ± 780	450 ± 240‡
7	85 ± 28	91 ± 22	2.2 ± 1.1¶	2.9 ± 0.4¶	460 ± 210¶	520 ± 300
14	107 ± 37¶	130 ± 26¶	3.7 ± 1.2¶	4.0 ± 1.1¶	230 ± 50¶	210 ± 70¶
21	95 ± 29¶	126 ± 22¶	3.8 ± 1.1¶	4.9 ± 1.2¶	80 ± 30¶	60 ± 30¶

**Values are expressed as mean ± SEM.*
†*Percent of normal activity.*
‡P = .03.
§P = .02.
‖P = .04.
¶*Significant change from day 1 (P<.05).*

Indocyanine green values were normal in both groups early after trauma. No significant changes from baseline occurred in survivors during the entire course of intensive care. Nonsurvivors showed a significant increase compared with baseline and with survivors (**Figure 3**).

COMMENT

Death from MOF continues to represent an unsolved problem in critically ill patients, affecting 15% of patients admitted to intensive care units in the United States and Europe.[22] In the present study, we attempted to investigate whether there is a difference in RES clearance capacity between patients who demonstrate an uneventful clinical course and patients who die late after severe trauma, generally from MOF.

To our knowledge, the only clinical study measuring RES function after blunt trauma involved patients with liver injuries.[29] One severe problem with this study was the inability to perform RES measurements in the intensive care unit. Since a bedside system was not available, all patients had to be transferred to the department of nuclear medicine. This influenced the selection criteria; patients could only be investigated if their cardiorespiratory status was stable enough for transport. Moreover, patient transport immediately prior to investigation may have influenced the results obtained.

These difficulties were avoided in the present study. The method we used to evaluate RES function is reliable[24-27] and has been used in previous experimental investigations.[30] In a previous study undertaken at our hospital, this method was able to assess the alterations of RES function in liver transplant recipients.[31] In our study, normal levels in the control group were reproducible and showed a mean RES function of 0.42±0.06. Nevertheless, the presence of multiple sources of hemorrhage, as in patients with multiple trauma, may influence the results obtained. Our study considered the effects of hemorrhagic shock.

We assumed that both liver perfusion (K_1) and RES function (K_2) values are influenced by splanchnic perfusion.[24,29,30] In contrast, other authors have argued that only the accumulation of tracer is influenced by the liver's sinusoidal blood flow, whereas the elimination of tracer from the liver is much less altered in cases of decreased blood flow. It was unlikely that the effects of slowed splanchnic perfusion played a major role, because the time-activity curve was calculated over 15 minutes.[26] Moreover, clinical studies have found no correlation between hepatic blood flow and the removal constant of radioactive tracer.[25]

Nevertheless, we tried to account for the possible effects of impaired liver blood flow and performed an ICG test parallel to the measurements of RES function in all

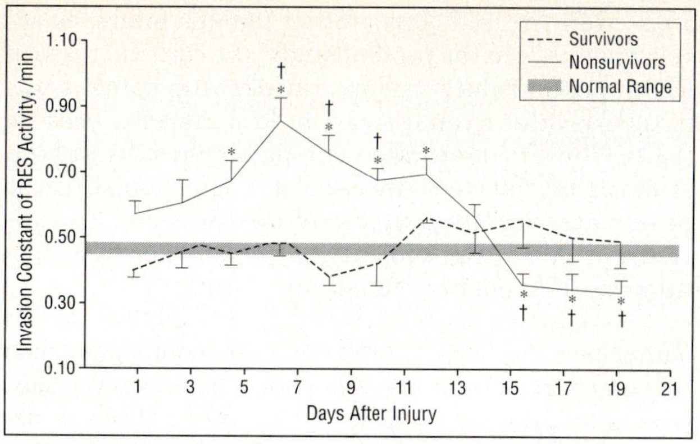

Figure 1. *Changes of the reticuloendothelial system (RES) clearance capacity, based on the hepatic uptake of 100 MBq (2.7 mCi) of technetium Tc 99m bound to human albumin (invasion constant). Normal levels in a group of healthy volunteers were 0.42±0.06. Asterisk indicates significant (P<.05) differences between groups; dagger, significant differences from baseline (day 1 after trauma).*

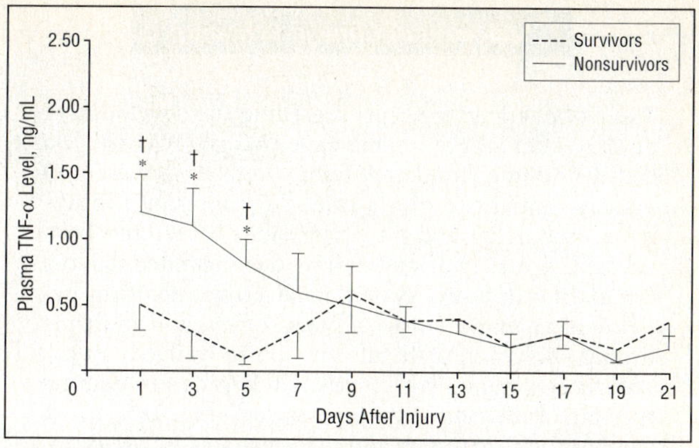

Figure 2. *Posttraumatic course of the central venous plasma concentration of the proinflammatory cytokine tumor necrosis factor α (TNF-α) in surviving and nonsurviving patients with severe blunt trauma. Asterisk indicates significant (P<.05) differences between groups; dagger, significant differences from baseline (day 1 after trauma).*

patients. The ICG test is a well-established method for evaluation of liver blood flow.[32,33] Splanchnic perfusion can be quantified because ICG is removed from the blood solely by the liver and is excreted without biotransformation and uptake occurs through a flow-limited mechanism.[34,35] The results of RES function measurements were deemed reliable only if the ICG test result was normal. In view of these prerequisites, we feel that it is justified to draw conclusions concerning RES function from the data obtained.

We measured several parameters indicative of posttraumatic coagulatory changes to account for impaired microvascular blood flow secondary to disseminated intravascular coagulation.

Antithrombin III is well known to decrease after trauma and hemorrhage.[36] Protein C levels were also measured because protein C has a similar function to antithrombin III but is more sensitive because it has a shorter half-life (half-life of antithrombin III, 2.5 days; half-life of protein C, 4-6 hours).[37] Moreover, the measurement of D-dimer cross-linked fibrin degradation products is a sensitive indicator of hypercoagulability in trauma patients.[38] All data were corrected for hematocrit to exclude effects due to dilution secondary to therapy for shock. Observed decreases of the activity of various substrates are in fact due to their consumption during an increased coagulatory response. Our results demonstrate alterations of the coagulatory response early after injury that we attributed to hemorrhagic shock. All 3 parameters were abnormal early after trauma and normalized thereafter. Among nonsurviving trauma patients, the early state of hypercoagulability was worse at days 1 and 3. At time points when RES function was different between groups, the coagulatory response was comparable. Therefore, according to the coagulation studies, it is unlikely that the disseminated intravascular coagulation influenced the hepatic microvascular perfusion following the first 3 days after injury.

Our principal result is a biphasic response in RES activity in among nonsurviving patients. During the first week after injury, the RES function in nonsurvivors was significantly increased in comparison with survivors and with the control group. Later during the clinical course,

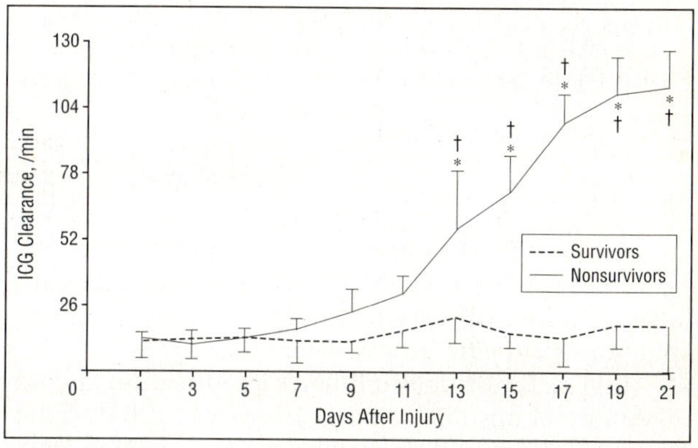

Figure 3. *Changes of liver function indicated by the enzymatic clearance of indocyanine green (ICG). Nonsurvivors developed a profound disturbance of the capacity to metabolize ICG late after injury. Asterisk indicates significant (P<.05) differences between groups; dagger, significant differences from baseline (day 1 after trauma).*

nonsurvivors demonstrated a decrease in RES function to subnormal levels. Also, a higher incidence of pulmonary infections was found in among nonsurvivors. In 9 of the 11 nonsurviving patients with pneumonia, the onset of infection occurred between day 3 and day 10, suggesting that an impaired immune defense was present despite RES hyperactivation during this period. No changes of ICG levels occurred in either group during the first week after trauma. We conclude that during this period liver perfusion was not impaired, and that changes in RES function results were due to increased RES activity. The late decrease in RES function values may be related to cardiocirculatory changes or impairment of liver function, because serum bilirubin concentrations and ICG levels showed pathologic values following the second week after injury. The finding of increased RES function is in accordance with a previous animal study from our laboratory.[30] Moreover, increased RES phagocytic capacity has also been observed in patients with peritonitis.[39]

In contrast, other authors have reported a decreased phagocyte response following a variety of stimuli. Kaplan and Saba[12,40] described transient RES dysfunction after intravascular coagulation, which was ex-

Statement of Clinical Relevance

The pathogenetic concepts regarding the development of MOF after severe trauma have changed over the last decades. While circulatory failure and sepsis were previously thought to play a role, the importance of immune dysfunction and gut barrier failure has recently been stressed. A variety of studies have demonstrated that the circulating immune system is severely altered in patients after major surgery, burn injury, and multiple trauma; however, little information is available on the stationary system. The current study provides data on the role of the stationary immune system (RES) in severely injured patients and demonstrates hyperactivation of the RES, especially in those patients who later die as a result of MOF. This may be viewed as the body's response to external pathogens. Whether this reaction is the result of a disturbance of the gut barrier function or whether other stimuli are important cannot be determined from our data. Whatever the exact cause may be, our study demonstrates that the hyperactive state of the RES does not prevent the patient with severe injuries from developing late organ failure.

plained by decreased hepatic Kupffer cell clearance. It was argued that the stationary system can sufficiently explain these changes, since previous in vivo studies also have indicated depressed Kupffer cell function in response to traumatic hemorrhagic shock.[12,14]

Several factors may influence RES function, including failure of opsonic activity, phagocytic cell dysfunction, and failure of the test substance to be delivered to the hepatic sinusoid area, where it would be cleared by Kupffer cells. The latter may be caused by sinusoidal blood flow secondary to splanchnic malperfusion, sinusoidal congestion, or disseminated coagulation.[15] The studies describing suppression of RES function as a uniform reaction to a variety of insults[12,14,40] have to be considered in view of these principles. Splanchnic vasoconstriction is known to occur despite normal systemic blood pressure. Impaired hepatic perfusion should be considered to have influenced RES function in these studies; however, the effect of splanchnic perfusion cannot be determined since no data were available in these investigations.[12,14,40]

Trauma and hemorrhagic shock have been demonstrated to cause aggregation of polymorphonuclear leukocytes to liver endothelial cells, which may cause impairment of microvascular blood flow.[41] Moreover, in a study investigating intravascular coagulation, impaired sinusoidal blood flow is likely to occur and influence the degree of impairment of RES function.[15]

In our investigation, the opsonizing activity in the stationary defense system is not measurable, since liver biopsy is not acceptable in these patients for ethical reasons. In contrast, data on opsonizing activity are available for the circulating defense system (polymorphonuclear leukocytes [PMNLs]). In PMNLs isolated from central venous blood, the opsonizing capacity was not different on the day of injury regardless of whether organ failure developed.[42] Further clinical studies showed a state of increased activation of PMNLs following severe trauma.[43] In the present study, the early increase in RES function values among nonsurviving patients was most likely due to an increase in RES capacity, because the ICG test demonstrated comparable results in both groups. Disseminated intravascular coagulation as a cause of impaired intrahepatic blood flow was also considered, but did not play a role at time points when RES function was different between groups (Table 4).

As a further cause of changed RES function, the accumulation of activated PMNLs on liver endothelium must be considered. Hemorrhagic shock has been demonstrated to induce significant adhesion of PMNLs to hepatic endothelial cells.[41] The associated impaired microvascular perfusion is known to develop prior to histologic evidence of hepatocellular injury.[44] In our patients, liver perfusion was adequate during the course of intensive care; however, this may not have been the case during the resuscitation period. The amount of intravenous fluid administration during rescue was significantly higher among nonsurviving patients. Sufficient volume replacement obviously was performed, since there was no difference between groups in admission blood pressures, which adequately reflected the severity of hemorrhagic shock (data not shown).[45] The assumption that initial hemorrhagic shock was different between groups is supported by the fact that there was a higher degree of activation of the inflammatory response (TNF-α) in nonsurvivors. These results are consistent with previous reports.[46] Production of TNF-α is known to be inducible by endotoxin.[47] It has been suggested that lipopolysaccharide activates gut-associated macrophages on translocation and causes further activation of Kupffer cells, which consequently produce more TNF-α.[46] This effect would explain the clinical course of RES data in the present study. Moreover, a similar response has been confirmed in previous studies of blunt trauma in both patients and animals subjects.[29,30]

Whether gut barrier failure leading to the passage of viable enteric bacteria and endotoxin is responsible for the altered RES function seen in our study cannot be determined on the basis of our results, because endotoxin levels and bacterial translocation were not determined. The activation of the RES measured in nonsurvivors, most of whom died of MOF, may constitute indirect evidence for the necessity to clear bacteria and endotoxins. As postulated above, the late decrease in hepatic function is likely to have influenced RES function, but a disturbance in the clearance capacity may have been present independent of perfusion.

No clinical study has proven that changes in the intestinal barrier cause MOF.[9,10] Among other host defense mechanisms, a pathologic increase in the systemic posttraumatic inflammatory response has been documented[48] that might involve the RES. Whether direct stimulation of RES function occurs or whether invading PMNLs following shock might affect RES function, as previously discussed,[41] remains speculative.

Our results demonstrate that a sustained increase in the clearance capacity of the reticuloendothelial system occurred in patients who died after severe trauma, predominantly from late MOF. Despite this increased RES capacity, a higher pulmonary infection rate was found in nonsurvivors, suggesting impaired defense mechanisms. Reticuloendothelial system function does not depend on liver perfusion. Further studies may clarify whether these findings are a result of failure of the gut-liver axis or whether hyperactivation of the RES is part of a generalized hyperinflammatory reaction.

Corresponding author: Hans-Christoph Pape, MD, Department of Trauma Surgery, Hannover Medical School, Carl Neubergstrasse 1, 30625 Hannover, Germany.

REFERENCES

1. Meakins JL, Marshall JC. The gastrointestinal tract: the motor of multiple organ failure. *Arch Surg.* 1986;121:197-201.
2. Ziegler TR, Smith RJ, O'Dwyer ST, Demling RH, Wilmore DW. Increased intestinal permeability associated with infection in burn patients. *Arch Surg.* 1988; 123:1313-1319.
3. LeVoyer T, Cioffi WG Jr, Pratt L, et al. Alterations in intestinal permeability after thermal injury. *Arch Surg.* 1992;127:26-30.
4. Pape HC, Remmers D, Kleemann W, Goris RJA, Tscherne H. Post-traumatic multiple organ failure: a report on clinical and autopsy findings. *Shock.* 1994;2:228-234.
5. Pape HC, Dwenger A, Regel G, et al. Increased intestinal permeability after multiple trauma. *Br J Surg.* 1994;87:850-852.
6. Deitch EA, Winterton J, Li MA, Berg A. The gut as a portal entry for bacteria. *Ann Surg.* 1987;205:681-685.
7. Pape HC, Grotz M, Remmers D, et al. Multiple organ failure (MOF) after severe trauma: a sheep model. *Intensive Care Med.* 1998;24:590-598.
8. Lanser ME. Reticuloendothelial system failure. In: Deitch EA, ed. *Multiple Organ Failure: Pathophysiology and Basic Concepts of Therapy.* New York, NY: Thieme-Stratton Inc; 1990:72-86.
9. Moore FA, Moore EE, Pogetti R. Gut bacterial translocation via the portal vein: a clinical perspective with major torso trauma. *J Trauma.* 1991;31:629-638.
10. Brathwaite CE, Ross SE, Nagele R, Mure AJ, O'Malley KF, Garcia-Perez FA. Bacterial translocation occurs in humans after traumatic injury: evidence using immunofluorescence. *J Trauma.* 1993;34:586-590.
11. van Goor H, Rosman C, Grond J, Kooi K, Wubbels GH, Bleichrodt RP. Translocation of bacteria and endotoxin in organ donors. *Arch Surg.* 1994;129:1063-1066.
12. Kaplan JE, Saba TM. Humoral deficiency and reticuloendothelial depression after traumatic shock. *Am J Physiol.* 1976;230:7-14.
13. Pape HC, Remmers D, Grotz M, et al. Levels of antibodies to endotoxin and cytokine release inpatients with severe trauma: does posttraumatic dysergy contribute to organ failure. *J Trauma.* In press.
14. Loegering DJ. Humoral factor depletion and reticuloendothelial depression during hemorrhagic shock. *Am J Physiol.* 1977;232:H283-H287.
15. Kaplan JE, Saba TM. Low grade intravascular coagulation and reticuloendothelial function. *Am J Physiol.* 1978;234:H323-H329.
16. Thompson PN, Cho E, Blumenstock FA, Shah DM, Saba TM. Liver and spleen phagocytic depression after peripheral ischemia and reperfusion. *Am J Surg.* 1992; 164:248-253.
17. Bautista AP, Schuler A, Spolarics Z, Spitzer J. Tumor necrosis factor-α stimulates superoxide anion generation by perfused rat liver and Kupffer cells. *Am J Physiol.* 1991;261:G891-G895.
18. Murray JF, Matthay MA, Luce JM, Flick MR. An expanded definition of the adult respiratory distress syndrome. *Am Rev Respir Dis.* 1988;138:720-723.
19. Stevens LE. Gauging the severity of surgical sepsis. *Arch Surg.* 1983;118:1190-1192.
20. Baker SP, O'Neill B, Haddon W, Long WB. The injury severity score: a method for describing patients with multiple injuries and evaluating emergency care. *J Trauma.* 1974;14:187-196.
21. Teasdale G, Jennett B. Assessment of coma and impaired consciousness: a practical scale. *Lancet.* 1974;2:81-84.
22. Knaus WA, Wagner DP. Multiple systems organ failure: epidemiology and prognosis. *Crit Care Clin.* 1989;5:221-232.
23. Marshall JC, Cook DJ, Christou NV, Bernard GR, Sprung CL, Sibbald WJ. Multiple organ dysfunction score: a reliable descriptor of a complex clinical outcome. *Crit Care Med.* 1995;23:1638-1652.
24. Gratz FK, Schober O, Schwarzrock R. Nuklearmedizinische Untersuchungen in der Transplantationschirurgie. *ROFO Fortschr Geb Rontgenstr Nuklearmed.* 1987; 10:47-59.
25. Bolognesi M, Merkel C, Gatra A. The use of human albumin millimicrospheres tagged with 99m TC in the evaluation of the removal capacity of the reticuloendothelial system. *Eur J Nucl Med.* 1987;13:254-257.
26. Reske SN, Vysna K, Feinendegen LE. In vivo assessment of phagocytic properties of Kupffer cells. *J Nucl Med.* 1981;22:405-410.
27. Scheffel U, Rhodes BA, Natarajan TK, Wagner HN Jr. Albumin microspheres for study of the reticuloendothelial system. *J Nucl Med.* 1987;13:498-503.
28. Whitaker AN, Elms MJ, Masci PP. Measurement of cross linked fibrin derivatives in plasma: an immunoassay using monoclonal antibodies. *J Clin Pathol.* 1984;37:882-886.
29. Regel G, Gratz KF, Pohlemann T, Sturm JA, Tscherne H. Changes in RES capacity associated with liver dysfunction in multiple trauma. In: Sturm JA, ed. *ARDS: An Aspect of Multiple Organ Failure.* New York, NY: Springer-Verlag NY Inc; 1991: 156-168.
30. Regel G, Nerlich ML, Dwenger A, Tscherne H. Phagocytic function of PMNL and the RES in endotoxemia. *J Surg Res.* 1987;42:74-78.
31. Kuse ER, Kemnitz J, Kotzerke J, et al. Fat emulsions in parenteral nutrition after liver transplantation: the recovery of the allografts RES function and histological observations. *Clin Nutr.* 1990;9:331-336.
32. Leevy CM, Smith F, Longueville J, Paumgartner G, Howard MM. Indocyanine green clearance as a test for hepatic function: evaluation by dichromatic ear densitometry. *JAMA.* 1967;200:236-240.
33. Moody FG, Rikkers LF, Aldrete JS. Estimation of the functional reserve from the liver. *Ann Surg.* 1974;180:592-598.
34. Paumgartner G, Probst P, Kraines R, et al. Kinetics of indocyanine green removal from the blood. *Ann N Y Acad Sci.* 1970;170:134-147.
35. Kawamoto S, Inohue M, Tashiro S. Inhibition of ischemia and reflow induced liver injury by an SOD derivative that circulates bound to albumin. *Arch Biochem Biophys.* 1990;277:160-165.
36. Miller RS, Weatherford DA, Stein D, Crane M, Stein M. Antithrombin III and trauma patients: factors that determine low levels. *J Trauma.* 1994;37:442-445.
37. Barhels M, Poliwoda H. Die Verbrauchskoagulopathie. In: Barthels M, ed. *Gerinnungs-analysen.* Stuttgart, Germany: Georg Thieme Verlag; 1993:57-72.
38. Enderson BL, Chen JP, Robinson R, Maull KI. Fibrinolysis in multisystem trauma patients. *J Trauma.* 1991;31:1240-1246.
39. Schildt B, Gertz I, Wide L. Differentiated RES function in some critical surgical conditions. *Acta Chem Scand.* 1974;140:611-617.
40. Saba TM. Reticuloendothelial host defense following surgery and traumatic shock. *Circ Shock.* 1975:2:91-108.
41. Marzi I, Takei Y, Knee J, et al. Assessment of reperfusion injury by intravital fluorescence microscopy following liver transplantation in the rat. *Transplant Proc.* 1990;22:2004-2005.
42. Seidel J, Mirkhani J, Behrmann M, Stangel M. Functional changes in PMNL function following severe polytrauma. In: Sturm JA, ed. *ARDS: An Aspect of Multiple Organ Failure.* New York, NY: Springer-Verlag NY Inc; 1991:156-168.
43. Dwenger A, Schweitzer G, Regel G. Bronchoalveolar lavage fluid and plasma proteins, chemiluminescence response and protein contents of polymorphonuclear leukocytes from blood and lavage fluid in traumatized patients. *J Clin Chem Clin Biochem.* 1986;24:73-88.
44. Asher EF, Rowe RL, Garrison RN, Fry DE. Experimental bacteremia and hepatic nutrient blood flow. *Circ Shock.* 1986;20:43-49.
45. Hall RC, Hodge RL. Changes in catecholamine and angiotensin levels in the cat and dog during hemorrhage. *Am J Physiol.* 1971;221:1305-1309.
46. Chaudry IH, Ayala A, Ertel W, Stephan RN. Hemorrhage and resuscitation: immunological aspects. *Am J Physiol.* 1990;259:663-678.
47. Bottoms GD, Gimarc S, Pfeifer C. Plasma concentrations of endotoxin following jugular or portal injections of endotoxin and following gastrointestinal ischemia due to hemorrhage. *Circ Shock.* 1991;33:1-6.
48. Roumen RMH, Hendriks T, Wevers RA, Goris RJA. Intestinal permeability after severe trauma and hemorrhagic shock is increased without relation to septic complications. *Arch Surg.* 1993;128:453-457.

ORIGINAL ARTICLE

Perioperative Immunonutrition in Patients Undergoing Cancer Surgery

Results of a Randomized Double-blind Phase 3 Trial

Marco Braga, MD; Luca Gianotti, MD, ScD; Giovanni Radaelli, PhD; Andrea Vignali, MD; Gilberto Mari, MD; Oreste Gentilini, MD; Valerio Di Carlo, MD

Hypothesis: Perioperative administration of a supplemented enteral formula may reduce the rate of postoperative infections.

Design: Prospective, randomized, double-blind clinical trial.

Setting: Department of surgery at a university hospital.

Patients: Two hundred six patients with neoplasm of colorectum, stomach, or pancreas.

Intervention: Patients were randomized to drink 1 L/d of either a control enteral formula (n = 104) or the same formula enriched with arginine, RNA, and ω3 fatty acids (n = 102) for 7 consecutive days before surgery. The 2 diets were isoenergetic and isonitrogenous. Jejunal infusion with the same formulas was started 6 hours after operation and continued until postoperative day 7.

Main Outcome Measures: Rate of postoperative infectious complications and length of hospital stay.

Results: Both groups were comparable for age, sex, weight loss, Karnofsky scale score, nutritional status, hemoglobin level, duration of surgery, blood loss, and rate of homologous transfusion. Intent-to-treat analysis showed a 14% (14/102) infectious complication rate in the supplemented group vs 30% (31/104) in the control group ($P = .009$). In the eligible population, the postoperative infection rate was 11% (9/85) in the supplemented group vs 24% (21/86) in the control group ($P = .02$). The mean ± SD length of postoperative stay was 11.1 ± 4.4 days in the supplemented group and 12.9 ± 4.6 in the control group ($P = .01$).

Conclusion: Perioperative administration of a supplemented enteral formula significantly reduced postoperative infections and length of stay in patients undergoing surgery for cancer.

Arch Surg. 1999;134:428-433

DESPITE SEVERAL reports[1-7] that the early postoperative administration of enteral diets enriched with arginine, ω3 fatty acids, and nucleotides resulted in improved host defense mechanisms, the effectiveness of postoperative immunonutrition in terms of clinical benefit is a matter of debate.[1,7-18] This is probably because the amount of substrates delivered in the first days after operation may not be sufficient to stimulate a prompt burst of the immune response. In fact, in patients fed supplemented formulas, the up-regulation of the immune system becomes evident only some days after operation, while the impairment of the host defense mechanisms occurs immediately after major surgery.[2-5]

In a recent phase 2 trial, Braga et al[19] reported that when the provision of immunonutrients was anticipated before surgery the early postoperative immune impairment was effectively controlled, the postoperative inflammatory response was modulated, and gut microperfusion and oxygen metabolism were up-regulated. However, data supporting translation of these biologic benefits to clinical advantages are warranted. Thus, a phase 3 trial was designed to evaluate whether the perioperative administration of immunonutrition could reduce postoperative infections after major surgery for cancer. Both well-nourished and malnourished patients were included in the study because the immunoenhancing diet was not given perioperatively to simply provide energy and proteins but mainly to counteract the postoperative immune and metabolic alterations that also occur in well-nourished patients.[1,3,5,19]

From the Department of Surgery, Scientific Institute San Raffaele Hospital (Drs Braga, Gianotti, Vignali, Mari, Gentilini, and Di Carlo), and Department of Informative Systems, University of Milan (Dr Radaelli), Milan, Italy.

RESULTS

Six patients (4 in the supplemented group and 2 in the control group) who did not

PATIENTS AND METHODS

This was a prospective, randomized, double-blind clinical trial. Enrolled in the study were 206 consecutive patients of both sexes, aged between 18 and 75 years, with neoplasm of colorectum, stomach, or pancreas and who were candidates for elective curative surgery. Exclusion criteria were alterations of the pulmonary, cardiovascular, renal, or hepatic function; history of recent immunosuppressive therapy (including preoperative radiochemotherapy) or immunological diseases; ongoing infection; emergency operation; and preoperative evidence of widespread metastatic disease, as previously described.[11] Patients were required to sign a written informed consent after the details of the protocol were fully explained. The protocol was approved by the Ethical Committee of the San Raffaele Institute, Milan, Italy.

By means of sealed envelopes, patients were randomized to drink 1 L/d for 7 consecutive days of either a supplemented liquid diet (Impact; Novartis Nutrition, Bern, Switzerland) or a control isonitrogenous, isoenergetic liquid diet. In addition to the 2 liquid diets, the patients of both groups were advised to consume standard food as desired. One liter of Impact contains the following: 12.5 g of arginine, 3.3 g of ω3 fatty acids, and 1.2 g of RNA. The kilojoule-to-milliliter ratio is 1:1. The preoperative treatment was carried out as outpatient therapy. Hospital admission was scheduled 2 days before surgery. The preoperative diets were provided by the manufacturer in powder form, to be mixed with water before drinking. The envelopes containing the 2 different powders were coded with 2 different letters. To ensure the double-blind nature of the study, the 2 formulas were prepared to obtain a liquid suspension with the same taste and appearance. The control diet was specially formulated to meet those characteristics and it was not commercially available.

The fish oil was encapsulated in microcaplets to avoid its smell or taste in the experimental diet.

Palliative surgery for intraoperative evidence of metastatic disease or unresectable primary tumor, and the lack of preoperative feeding were considered protocol violations.

Eight days before surgery (day −8), the following baseline measures were determined in all patients: plasma levels of albumin, retinol-binding protein, prealbumin, transferrin, cholinesterase activity, hemoglobin, and C-reactive protein. Serum levels of interleukin 6 (IL-6) were measured in the first 60 patients by a commercially available enzyme-linked immunoabsorbent assay (Genzyme Diagnostics, Cambridge, England). Patients with weight loss of 10% or more of usual body weight were considered as malnourished.[20] Performance status was assessed in all patients according to the Karnofsky scale. Baseline measures were reassessed 1 day before surgery (−1) and 1 (+1) and 8 (+8) days after surgery.

Intestinal washout with an iso-osmotic solution (3 L) was carried out the day before operation in patients undergoing colorectal surgery. The evening before and the morning of operation, patients were also treated with enema. These patients received antibiotic prophylaxis with a single intravenous dose (2 g) of cefotetan disodium 30

Continued on next page

complete preoperative intake of the liquid diets and 14 patients (10 in the supplemented group and 4 in the control group) with intraoperative evidence of metastatic disease or unresectable primary tumor were excluded from the study for protocol violation. To avoid possible biases linked to surgical technical problems, 15 patients (5 in the supplemented group and 10 in the control group) who had clinical or radiological anastomotic leak were excluded from the analysis of postoperative infections.

Table 1 lists the baseline (day −8) and surgical characteristics of the remaining 171 eligible patients (85 in the supplemented group and 86 in the control group). Both groups were comparable as to age, sex, performance status (Karnofsky scale), weight, rate of malnutrition, hemoglobin level, cancer site, surgical parameters, and blood transfusions.

One hundred thirty-nine patients (81.3%) did not report any adverse effects related to enteral feeding. Abdominal distension occurred in 11 patients (6.4%), abdominal cramping in 10 (5.8%), diarrhea in 4 (2.3%), inadvertent removal of the nasojejunal feeding tube in 4 (2.3%), and emesis in 3 (1.7%). Temporary discontinuation or lowering of the infusion rate usually allowed symptoms to regress, so that the daily volume of 1500 mL was reached after 4.5 ± 0.7 days and 4.7 ± 0.5 days in the control and supplemented groups, respectively ($P = .63$). Seven patients (3 in the supplemented group and 4 in the control group) failed to reach the volume of 1500 mL/d for emesis (n = 3), diarrhea (n = 1), persisting abdominal cramps (n = 1), or displacement of the nasojejunal tube (n = 2). In these patients, enteral nutrition was interrupted permanently. **Table 2** describes the distribution of the adverse effects in the 2 groups. The daily mean postoperative volume infused was 1038 ± 352 mL in the control group vs 1060 ± 309 mL in the supplemented group ($P = .58$).

The intent-to-treat analysis of postoperative infections and the results of the eligible patients are shown in **Table 3**. The intent-to-treat analysis included the 6 patients who did not complete the preoperative diet regimen, the 14 patients who underwent palliative surgery, and the 15 patients with anastomotic leak. In the eligible population (171 patients), 31 infections occurred in a total of 30 patients (17.5%). There was a significantly lower number of patients who developed postoperative infections in the supplemented group (9/85; 11%) than in the control group (21/86; 24%) ($P = .02$; $\chi^2 = 4.801$). The mean duration of antibiotic therapy needed to treat postoperative infections was 6.7 ± 1.7 days in the supplemented group vs 9.0 ± 2.5 days in the control group ($P = .001$). The mean length of postoperative stay was significantly shorter in the patients receiving the supplemented formula than in the control group (11.1 ± 4.4 days vs 12.9 ± 4.6 days, respectively; $P = .01$). The post hoc analysis of postoperative infections in both well-nourished and malnourished patients showed that the administration of the supplemented diets significantly reduced the rate of postoperative infections regardless of the baseline nutritional status (**Figure**).

Table 4 shows the distribution of postoperative noninfectious complications. No significant difference was minutes before surgery. Patients undergoing gastric or pancreatic surgery were treated with intestinal washout (1 L) the day before operation and antibiotic prophylaxis with a single intravenous dose (2 g) of cefazolin sodium 30 minutes before surgery. A second dose of antibiotic was given if the duration of the surgical procedures was longer than 4 hours.

Just before suturing the abdominal wall, an enteral feeding tube (2.6-mm outer diameter) (Kangaroo; Sherwood Medical, Tullamore, Ireland) was inserted through the nose and advanced by the surgeon to reach the jejunum in patients undergoing gastric or colorectal surgery. In the patients undergoing gastric surgery (all with Roux-en-Y reconstruction), the tip of the feeding tube was placed approximately 10 cm above the jejunoileal anastomosis. In all patients undergoing pancreaticoduodenectomy, a feeding jejunostomy was performed. Operative blood loss, duration of surgery, and the amount of homologous blood transfused were recorded in all patients. The decision to give homologous blood transfusion was based on the perioperative hemoglobin level (<80 g/L) or the clinical condition of the patient.[21]

Postoperative enteral feeding with either a supplemented or control diet was started 6 hours after surgery with an infusion rate of 10 mL/h, which was progressively increased up to a volume of 1500 mL/d on postoperative day 3. Intravenous fluids and electrolytes were administered according to clinical requirement as integration of enteral diets. Oral food intake was allowed on postoperative day 7. None of the patients received parenteral nutrition before or after surgery.

Side effects from enteral feeding, such as abdominal cramping, bloating, diarrhea (defined as more than 3 liquid stools per day), and emesis, were recorded. If any side effect appeared, jejunal infusion was reduced or discontinued for 4 hours and then resumed at a lower infusion rate.

The following postoperative infectious complications were recorded by the surgical staff who were not involved in the study: abdominal abscess, peritonitis, surgical wound infection, urinary tract infection, pneumonia, bacteremia, and sepsis, as defined by the American College of Chest Physicians/Society of Critical Care Medicine Consensus Conference[22]; and overinfection of pancreatic fistula. Patients were followed up for infectious complications for 30 days after hospital discharge by serial in-hospital visits. Noninfectious complications were also recorded.

It was assumed that postoperative infections would occur in approximately 25% of the patients if not treated.[11] A reduction of 50% in the incidence rate would be considered to indicate the efficacy of treatment. Detecting a difference of this magnitude admitting a type I error level of 0.05 and a power of 0.90 required the presence of 70 patients in each group.[23] The Student *t* test and the Mann-Whitney *U* test were used to compare continuous variables, and the χ^2 test and Fisher exact test were used to compare discrete variables. Values of $P<.05$ were considered to indicate statistical significance (2-tailed test). The SPSS 7.5 package for Windows (SPSS Inc, Chicago, Ill) was used for statistical analysis. Data are given as mean ± SD.

observed between the 2 groups. Reoperation was necessary in 3 patients (2%) (1 in the supplemented group for gastrointestinal tract bleeding and 2 in the control group—1 for fascial dehiscence and 1 for hemoperitoneum).

Postoperative mortality was 0.6% (1 patient in the control group died of septic shock secondary to pneumonia).

Table 5 reports the variations of nutritional values, C-reactive protein, and IL-6. The IL-6 and C-reactive protein plasma levels sharply rose on day +1 in both groups but rose to a lesser extent in the supplemented group. On day +8, the IL-6 concentration returned to similar preoperative values in the supplemented group and remained elevated in the control group. None of the nutritional values were affected by the preoperative feeding. Surgical trauma caused a decline in all measures, although preoperative transferrin values were not significantly different compared with preoperative values. Eight days after operation the concentration of both prealbumin and retinol-binding protein were significantly higher in the supplemented group than in the control group.

COMMENT

In the last years, standard enteral preparations have been modified by adding immunonutrients, such as arginine, glutamine, ω3 fatty acids, nucleotides, and others. These substrates have been shown to up-regulate host immune response, to control inflammatory response, and to modulate nitrogen balance and protein synthesis after injury.[1-8,24-28] All of these substrates, tested separately or in different combinations, improved septic morbidity and mortality in animal models.[26,29-32]

In different phase 2 clinical trials, the effect of dietary supplementation with arginine, ω3 fatty acids, and nucleotides on host immune response after injury or surgery has been evaluated. The administration of this supplemented formula allowed a more rapid recovery of the postsurgical immune depression than a standard diet. However, the superiority of the supplemented diet appeared only from the fourth postoperative day. Conversely, in the first days after surgery the impairment of phagocytosis ability, the alteration of cytokine profiles, the reduction of immunoglobulin levels, the number of activated T and B cells, and the lymphocyte mitogenesis were similar in patients fed supplemented diets and those given standard diets.[1-7]

Twelve prospective randomized studies have investigated the effects of immunonutrition on outcome either after major operation for cancer (6 trials)[1,7,11-14] or after severe injury (4 trials of intensive care unit [ICU] patients and 2 trials of burn patients).[8,9,15-18] Gottschlich et al[9] (burn patients) and Moore et al[15] and Kudsk et al[16] (ICU patients) reported a significant reduction of septic complications in immunonourished patients. In a large multicenter trial of ICU patients, Bower and colleagues[8] found that the patients fed the supplemented diet had a substantial reduction of length of stay and significant reduction of frequency of acquired infections if the patients had septic complications on admission to the study; however, there was no difference between treated and control groups in the intent-to-treat analysis. Conversely, no beneficial effects by immunonutrition were reported by Mendez et al[18] (ICU patients) and by Saffle et al[17] (burn patients). In cancer patients undergoing elective surgery, Daly et al reported, in 2 different studies,[1,7] a significant reduction of postoperative infections in patients who were given immunonutrition early after surgery. A multicenter study from Germany[14] showed a slight reduction of overall postoperative complication rate in the immunonutrition group (22% vs 31% in the control group). When the authors grouped complications occurring before or after postoperative day 5, the immunonutrition group had a significantly less incidence of late postoperative complications, whereas no difference was found in the early postoperative complication rate. These results seem consistent with the hypothesis that some days of feeding are necessary to improve the host defense and subsequently to reduce infections. Heslin et al,[13] who studied 195 patients undergoing elective cancer surgery, did not find a significant difference in postoperative infectious and noninfectious complications by comparing groups treated with either an early postoperative immunoenhancing diet or simple crystalloid fluid replacement. However, in the immunonutrition group the average postoperative energy intake was 60% of the nutritional goal and only 30% was given with the immunoenhancing diet. In our experience[11,12] the early postoperative administration of enteral immunonutrition compared with a control enteral diet significantly reduced both severity of infections and postoperative stay, while the reduction of postoperative infection rate was not significant.

The differences in results among these trials might be attributed to the different populations studied and to several other variables, but a constant that associates all these studies is that the amount of immunoenhancing substrates given in the first days following operation is quite limited and therefore it may be not sufficient to allow a prompt burst of the immune system and an effective bacterial clearance shortly after surgery.[1-7] As any other substance with supposed pharmacological action, immunonutrients should reach suitable tissue and plasma concentration to be active. For this reason we believed that a key point could have been to anticipate the provision of immunonutrients before surgery to obtain adequate levels at the time of surgical stress when the need for stimulation of the immune system is maximal.

Experimental studies demonstrated that the efficacy of immunonutrients was superior when they were given both before and after injury than solely in the postinjury period.[26,29-33] In our recent randomized, double-blind trial[19] the preoperative supplementation with an enteral diet enriched with arginine, ω3 fatty acids, and RNA prevented the early postoperative decline of both the

Table 1. Baseline and Surgical Characteristics of the 2 Groups*

	Supplemented Group (n = 85)	Control Group (n = 86)
Age, y	60.9 ± 11.9	60.8 ± 9.7
Male:female	50:35	56:30
Karnofsky scale, %	76 ± 12	78 ± 11
Weight, kg	65.8 ± 10.9	67.6 ± 11.2
Malnourished patients, No.	22	18
Hemoglobin, g/L	125 ± 19	129 ± 17
Cancer site, No. of patients		
Stomach	28	28
Colon	27	21
Rectum	20	25
Pancreas	10	12
Time of surgery, min	234 ± 66	215 ± 82
Operative blood loss, mL	541 ± 410	605 ± 467
Transfused patients, No.	20	20
Blood transfused, U	2.3 ± 1.0	2.8 ± 1.2

Data are given as mean ± SD unless otherwise specified.

Table 2. Adverse Effects of Postoperative Enteral Feeding

	Supplemented Group (n = 85)	Control Group (n = 86)
Abdominal cramping	4	6
Abdominal distention	5	6
Diarrhea	2	2
Emesis	1	2
Inadvertent removal of feeding tube	2	2
Overall	**14** (16%)	**18** (21%)

*P = .58 control group vs supplemented group.

Table 3. Distribution of Postoperative Infections

	Intent-to-Treat Patients		Eligible Patients	
	Supplemented Group (n = 102)	Control Group (n = 104)	Supplemented Group (n = 85)	Control Group (n = 86)
Wound infection	4	6	3	6
Pneumonia	4	10	4	9
Urinary tract infection	3	3	2	3
Sepsis	2	5	0	2
Intra-abdominal abscess	2	4	0	2
Peritonitis	3	6	0	0
Overall infections	**18**	**34**	**9**	**22**
With any complications	14 (14%)	31 (30%)*	9 (11%)	21 (24%)†

*P = .009 (χ^2 = 6.908) control group vs supplemented group (intent to treat).
†P = .02 (χ^2 = 4.801) control group vs supplemented group (eligible).

phagocytosis ability and the respiratory burst of polymorphonuclear cells, significantly increased the nitric oxide plasma concentration and the CD4/CD8 ratio immediately after operation, reduced the synthesis of postoperative C-reactive protein, and improved both intestinal microperfusion, as directly measured by intraoperative laser Doppler flowmetry technique, and postoperative gut mucosal oxygen metabolism as measured by jejunal tonometry. In a similarly designed study, Wachtler et al[34] reported that preoperative immunonutrition improved postoperative generation of leukotriene B_5 from peripheral neutrophils and reduced the leukotriene B_4–leukotriene B_5 ratio.

The reduced production of IL-6 and C-reactive protein early after operation and the increased synthesis of prealbumin and retinol-binding protein in the supplemented group suggest a switch from the synthesis of acute-phase proteins to constitutive visceral proteins, probably as an effect of ω3 fatty acids on eicosanoid balance.[35]

We speculate that the reduction of postoperative infections, which has been found in the supplemented group, is the translation of the immunologic and metabolic advantages reported in patients receiving perioperative supplementation with immunonutrition.[19] The provision of immunoenhancing substrates before surgery appears to play a key role in reducing postoperative infections by a substantial activation of the immune response. Our data also suggest that perioperative immunonutrition is efficacious regardless of the baseline nutritional status of the patients. In fact, preoperative administration of immunoenhancing diets reduced postoperative infections also in well-nourished patients in whom a severe postoperative impairment of the host defense mechanisms has been reported.[1,3-5,19]

In conclusion, the perioperative administration of the supplemented diet improved the synthesis of constitutive visceral proteins and significantly reduced the rate of postoperative infections and the length of stay in patients undergoing surgery for cancer.

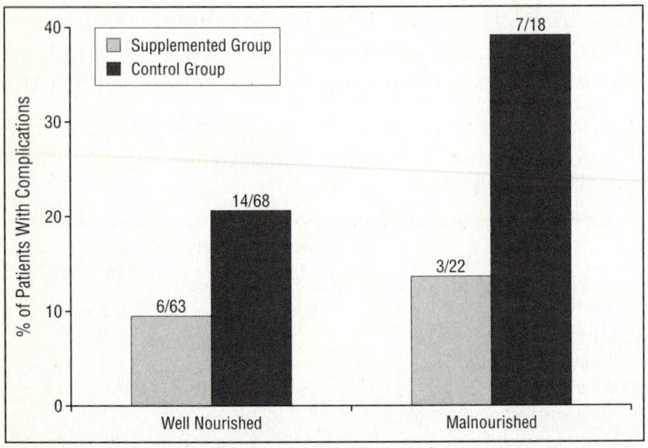

Distribution of postoperative infections according to preoperative nutritional status. P = .05, well-nourished supplemented patients vs well-nourished controls and malnourished supplemented patients vs malnourished controls.

Table 4. Postoperative Noninfectious Complications in Eligible Patients

	Supplemented Group (n = 85)	Control Group (n = 86)
Fascial dehiscence	0	1
Sterile pancreatic fistula	2	1
Hemoperitoneum	0	1
Heart failure	2	2
Gastrointestinal tract bleeding	1	1
Ileus	1	2
Pleural effusion/atelectasis	1	0
Delayed gastric emptying	2	1
Patients with any complications	7 (8%)	8 (9%)*

*P = .98 control group vs supplemented group.

The diets were generously provided by Novartis Nutrition, Bern, Switzerland.

Presented at the 18th Annual Meeting of the Surgical Infection Society, New York, NY, April 30, 1998.

Table 5. Variations of Nutritional and Inflammatory Values

		Days (Before or After Surgery), mean ± SD			
	Group	−8	−1	+1	+8
Albumin, g/L	Supplemented	39.3 ± 4.2	39.4 ± 4.0	34.6 ± 5.0*	37.3 ± 3.6
	Control	39.1 ± 4.6	39.3 ± 4.4	35.1 ± 4.3*	36.7 ± 3.8
Cholinesterase activity, U/L	Supplemented	7.85 ± 1.74	7.74 ± 1.62	5.84 ± 1.41*	6.15 ± 1.08
	Control	7.88 ± 2.17	7.61 ± 2.04	5.76 ± 1.66*	5.94 ± 1.57
Transferrin, g/L	Supplemented	2400 ± 480	2510 ± 360	2110 ± 580	2230 ± 480
	Control	2500 ± 500	2550 ± 470	1980 ± 470	2180 ± 520
Prealbumin, g/L	Supplemented	0.24 ± 0.06	0.25 ± 0.04	0.18 ± 0.05*	0.23 ± 0.04‡
	Control	0.23 ± 0.05	0.24 ± 0.04	0.17 ± 0.06*	0.18 ± 0.04*†
Retinol-binding protein, mg/mL	Supplemented	45.2 ± 12.5	46.3 ± 13.8	31.5 ± 12.7*	37.8 ± 11.7‡
	Control	44.4 ± 13.7	45.9 ± 15.7	32.1 ± 13.4*	32.9 ± 10.4*†
Interleukin, pg/mL	Supplemented	32 ± 9	46 ± 12	89 ± 41*	46 ± 15‡
	Control	30 ± 11	41 ± 10	151 ± 62*†	97 ± 39*†
C-reactive protein, mg/L	Supplemented	5.2 ± 2.4	5.9 ± 1.8	68 ± 25*	49 ± 19*
	Control	4.9 ± 2.2	5.4 ± 2.0	118 ± 57*†	72 ± 30*†

*P<.05 vs days −8 and −1.
†P<.05 vs supplemented group.
‡P<.05 vs day +1.

Reprints: Marco Braga, MD, Department of Surgery, Scientific Institute San Raffaele Hospital, Via Olgettina 60, 20132 Milan, Italy (e-mail: braga.marco@hsr.it).

REFERENCES

1. Daly JM, Lieberman MD, Goldfine J, et al. Enteral nutrition with supplemental arginine, RNA, and ω 3 fatty acids in patients after operation: immunologic, metabolic and clinical outcome. *Surgery.* 1992;112:56-67.
2. Vignali A, Braga M, Gianotti L, Cestari A, Profili M, Di Carlo V. Impact of an enriched enteral formula on immune function and nutritional status in cancer patients following surgery. *Riv Ital Nutr Parenter Enter.* 1995;13:25-31.
3. Braga M, Vignali A, Gianotti L, Cestari A, Profili M, Di Carlo V. Immune and nutritional effects of early enteral nutrition after major abdominal operations. *Eur J Surg.* 1996;162:105-112.
4. Kemen M, Senkal M, Homann HH, et al. Early postoperative enteral nutrition with arginine, ω-3 fatty acids and ribonucleic acid-supplemented diet versus placebo in cancer patients: an immunologic evaluation of Impact®. *Crit Care Med.* 1995; 23:652-659.
5. Senkal M, Kemen M, Homann HH, et al. Modulation of postoperative immune response by enteral nutrition with a diet enriched with arginine, RNA, and ω-3 fatty acids in patients with upper gastrointestinal cancer. *Eur J Surg.* 1995;161:115-122.
6. Cerra FB, Lehmann S, Konstantinides N, et al. Improvement in immune function in ICU patients by enteral nutrition supplemented with arginine, RNA, and menhaden oil is independent of nitrogen balance. *Nutrition.* 1991;7:193-199.
7. Daly JM, Weintraub FN, Shou J, Rosato EF, Lucia M. Enteral nutrition during multimodality therapy in upper gastrointestinal cancer patients. *Ann Surg.* 1995; 221:327-338.
8. Bower RH, Cerra FB, Bershadsky B, et al. Early enteral administration of a formula (Impact®) supplemented with arginine, nucleotides, and fish oil in intensive care unit patients: results of a multicenter, prospective, randomized, clinical trial. *Crit Care Med.* 1995;23:436-449.
9. Gottschlich MM, Jenkins M, Warden GD, et al. Differential effects of three dietary regimens on selected outcome variables in burn patients. *JPEN J Parenter Enteral Nutr.* 1990;14:225-236.
10. Braga M, Vignali A, Gianotti L, Cestari A, Profili M, Di Carlo V. Benefits of early postoperative enteral feeding in cancer patients. *Infusionther Transfusionmed.* 1995;22:280-284.
11. Gianotti L, Braga M, Vignali A, et al. Effect of route of delivery and formulation of postoperative nutritional support in patients undergoing major operations for malignant neoplasm. *Arch Surg.* 1997;132:1222-1230.
12. Braga M, Gianotti L, Vignali A, Cestari A, Bisagni P, Di Carlo V. Artificial nutrition after major abdominal surgery: impact of route of administration and composition of the diet. *Crit Care Med.* 1998;26:24-30.
13. Heslin MJ, Latkany L, Leung D, et al. A prospective randomized trial of early enteral feeding after resection of upper gastrointestinal malignancy. *Ann Surg.* 1997; 226:567-580.
14. Senkal M, Mumme A, Eickhoff U, et al. Early postoperative immunonutrition: clinical outcome and cost-comparison analysis in surgical patients. *Crit Care Med.* 1997;25:1489-1496.
15. Moore FA, Moore EE, Kudsk KA, et al. Clinical benefits of an immune-enhancing diet for early postinjury enteral feeding. *J Trauma.* 1994;37:607-615.
16. Kudsk KA, Minard G, Croce MA, et al. A randomized trial of isonitrogenous enteral diets after severe trauma. *Ann Surg.* 1996;224:531-543.
17. Saffle JR, Wiebke G, Jennings K, Morris E, Barton RG. Randomized trial of immunoenhancing enteral nutrition in burn patients. *J Trauma.* 1997;42:793-802.
18. Mendez C, Jurkovich GJ, Garcia I, et al. Effects of immuno-enhancing diet in critically injured patients. *J Trauma.* 1997;42:933-941.
19. Braga M, Gianotti L, Cestari A, et al. Gut function, immune and inflammatory responses in patients perioperatively fed with supplemented formulas. *Arch Surg.* 1996;131:1257-1265.
20. Gianotti L, Braga M, Radaelli G, et al. Lack of improvement of prognostic performance of weight loss when combined with other nutritional parameters. *Nutrition.* 1995;11:12-16.
21. Braga M, Gianotti L, Vignali A, et al. Evaluation of recombinant human erythropoietin to facilitate autologous blood donation before surgery in anaemic patient with cancer of the gastrointestinal tract. *Br J Surg.* 1995;82:1637-1640.
22. American College of Chest Physicians/Society of Critical Care Medicine Consensus Conference. Definition for sepsis and organ failure and guidelines for the use of innovative therapies in sepsis. *Crit Care Med.* 1992;20:864-873.
23. Armitage P, Berry G. *Statistical Methods in Medical Research.* 2nd ed. London, England: Blackwell Scientific Publications; 1987.
24. Moncada S, Higgs A. The L-arginine-nitric oxide pathway. *N Engl J Med.* 1993; 329:2002-2012.
25. Kenler AS, Swails WS, Driscoll DF, et al. Early feeding in postsurgical cancer patients: fish oil structured lipid-based polymeric formula versus a standard polymeric formula. *Ann Surg.* 1996;223:316-333.
26. Gianotti L, Alexander JW, Pyles T, Fukushima R. Arginine-supplemented diets improve survival in gut-derived sepsis and peritonitis by modulating bacterial clearance: the role of nitric oxide. *Ann Surg.* 1993;217:644-654.
27. Hall JC, Heel K, McCauley R. Glutamine. *Br J Surg.* 1996;83:305-312.
28. Kinsella JE, Lokesh B, Broughton S, Whelan J. Dietary polyunsaturated fatty acids and eicosanoids: potential effect on the modulation of inflammatory and immune cells: an overview. *Nutrition.* 1990;6:24-44.
29. Gennari R, Alexander JW, Eaves-Pyles T. Effect of different combinations of dietary additives on bacterial translocation and survival in gut-derived sepis. *JPEN J Parenter Enteral Nutr.* 1995;19:319-325.
30. Braga M, Gianotti L, Costantini E, et al. Impact of enteral nutrition on intestinal bacterial translocation and mortality in burned mice. *Clin Nutr.* 1994;13:256-261.
31. Gianotti L, Alexander JW, Pyles T, et al. Dietary fatty acids modulate host bactericidal response, microbial translocation and outcome following blood transfusion and thermal injury. *Clin Nutr.* 1996;15:291-296.
32. Gianotti L, Alexander JW, Gennari R, et al. Effect of oral glutamine on gut barrier function following thermal injury and immunosuppression. *JPEN J Parenter Enteral Nutr.* 1995;19:69-74.
33. Gianotti L, Braga M, Vaiani R, Profili M, Socci C, Di Carlo V. Effect of composition of enteral solutions and timing of administration on outcome and bacterial translocation. *Riv Ital Nutr Parenter Enter.* 1996;14:191-195.
34. Wachtler P, Axel R, König W, Bauer H, Kemen M, Köller M. Influence of a preoperative enteral supplementation on functional activities of peripheral leukocytes from patients with major surgery. *Clin Nutr.* 1995;14:275-282.
35. Wigmore SJ, Fearon KCH, Ross JA. Modulation of human hepatocyte acute phase protein production by ω-3 and ω-6 polyunsaturated fatty acids. *Ann Surg.* 1997; 225:103-111.

Clinical Implications of Hemoglobin as a Nitric Oxide Carrier

Nirmal K. Veeramachaneni, BS; Alden H. Harken, MD; Charles B. Cairns, MD

Hemoglobin is perhaps the most intensively studied of the biologically important molecules. Much is known of its structure, its function, and its regulation. In addition to well-characterized processes of oxygen, carbon dioxide, and carbon monoxide transport, new data suggest a key role of hemoglobin as a carrier of nitric oxide. In this review, we describe the basis of this interaction, as well as its clinical relevance to such problems as acute respiratory distress syndrome, percutaneous transluminal coronary angioplasty, and transplant allograft survival.

Arch Surg. 1999;134:434-437

Hemoglobin is essential to life. Recent observations relating hemoglobin-bound nitric oxide (NO) to vascular dynamics and oxygen delivery have emphasized the central role of this multipurpose carrier molecule in health and disease. The purposes of this review are (1) to examine the essential features of hemoglobin function, (2) to delineate the novel relationship between hemoglobin and NO, and (3) to focus on these NO-hemoglobin functions as they relate to pathological states encountered in surgical practice.

STRUCTURE AND FUNCTION OF HEMOGLOBIN

Adult hemoglobin is a tetramer of 2 α and 2 β subunits. Each subunit of the hemoglobin tetramer contains a pocket in which the iron-containing ring (heme) is suspended. The central iron (Fe^{2+}) is covalently attached to nitrogen groups in the heme, and pulled slightly above the ring by a histidine of the hemoglobin subunit. Without the Fe^{2+} in heme, the protein portion of hemoglobin could not bind or transport oxygen. Similarly, the heme portion alone, without the globin protein, would rapidly react with oxygen to form water and ferric heme (methemoglobin, Fe^{3+}).

From the School of Medicine (Mr Veeramachaneni), Department of Surgery (Dr Harken), and Division of Emergency Medicine and Colorado Emergency Medicine Research Center (Dr Cairns), University of Colorado Health Sciences Center, Denver.

The complementary nature of the heme moiety to globin protein interaction is illustrated by carbon monoxide (CO) poisoning. The potentially paralyzing effect of CO on cellular electron transport is prevented by virtue of the structure of the globin molecule. Free heme binds CO with an affinity 25 000 times that of oxygen. Steric hindrance by the globin protein reduces the essentially irreversible CO-heme interaction to a hemoglobin affinity for CO of only 200 times that of oxygen.[1] In this fashion, hemoglobin protects cells from lethal CO exposure while permitting CO release from hemoglobin in the lung, albeit slowly.

All of the available hemoglobin sites for oxygen binding are saturated in the lungs. When a single oxygen molecule binds the hemoglobin tetramer, the oxygen affinity of the hemoglobin increases, making it more likely that second, third, and fourth oxygen molecules will also bind. Conversely, in the peripheral tissue, where oxygen tension is lower, the release of 1 oxygen molecule enhances the release of the other oxygen molecules. Cooperative, noncovalent interactions between the globin subunits result in this familiar sigmoidal relationship of hemoglobin oxygen saturation and oxygen pressure. Oxygen binding pulls the iron, normally suspended above the porphyrin ring, into the heme plane. This motion of the iron and the attached histidine triggers a conformational change in the entire hemoglobin tetramer that increases its affinity for oxygen.

The affinity for oxygen is also influenced by the microenvironment of tissues. As respiring cells produce carbon dioxide, carbamate is formed at the N terminus of the hemoglobin molecule. When the N terminus is no longer positively charged and salt bridges form between the α and β subunits, oxyhemoglobin affinity decreases. This is the basis of the Bohr effect that facilitates hemoglobin uptake of oxygen in the lungs and release of oxygen in the tissues.

LIFE AND DEATH OF NO

Nitric oxide is generated from multiple endogenous and exogenous sources and has diverse physiologic functions.[2,3] Vascular endothelial cell–derived NO acts directly on adjacent vascular smooth muscle via a cyclic guanosine monophosphate mechanism to cause vasorelaxation, with an increase in regional blood flow and oxygen delivery.[4] Macrophages use NO in the destruction of phagocytosed material, while the central nervous system uses NO as a neurotransmitter. Platelet aggregation and activation is known to be inhibited by NO, while bronchoconstriction is attenuated.[2] Other cell types, including hepatocytes, and myocardial cells, are known to possess different forms of NO-producing enzymes.[2,3] The differential regulation of these enzyme systems by various cytokines and other cell signals is crucial to the biological effect of NO.[3] While NO plays a role in physiologically appropriate diastolic relaxation, NO also mediates the aberrant myocardial depression during the inflammatory response.[5-7] In the liver, NO plays a protective role during oxidative stress, during inflammatory injury, and is able to inhibit cytokine-induced apoptosis.[8,9] Nitroglycerin, nitroprusside, and amyl nitrite serve as clinically accessible exogenous NO donors available to the surgeon.

Nitric oxide reacts with a number of biologically important molecules. When NO combines with free oxygen, nitrite species are formed.[10] Covalent interaction with thiol groups leads to formation of S-nitrosylated proteins, thus both modulating their function, and creating a reservoir of NO.[11] Superoxide oxygen radicals interact with NO to form cytotoxic peroxynitrite ($ONOO^-$).[2] When NO combines directly with the heme of oxyhemoglobin, ferrous iron (Fe^{2+}) is reduced to form ferric methemoglobin ($Hb[Fe^{3+}]$). Conversely, NO combines with the heme site of deoxyhemoglobin to form $Hb[Fe^{2+}]NO$.[12] This scavenging of NO by hemoglobin results in vasoconstriction[13] (**Figure 1**).

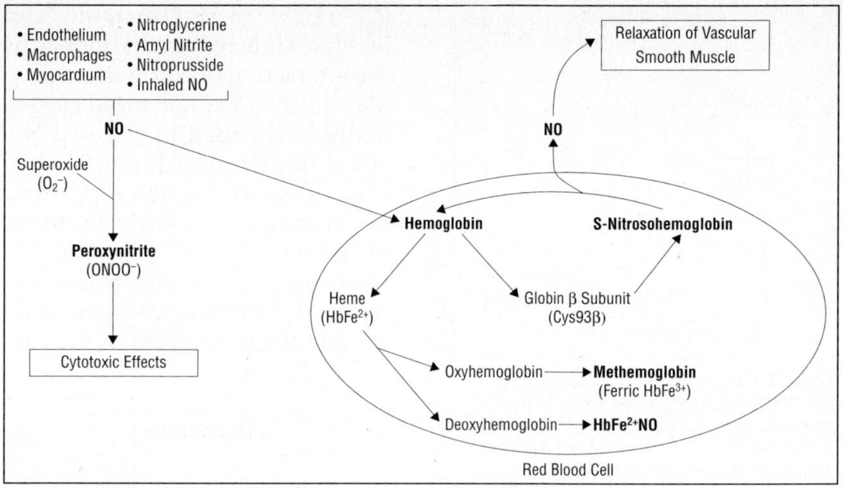

Figure 1. *Nitric oxide (NO) is derived from exogenous and endogenous sources. While S-nitrosohemoglobin increases blood flow by delivery of NO to vascular smooth muscle, the heme portion of hemoglobin scavenges NO, resulting in vasoconstriction. Free radicals react with NO, forming cytotoxic peroxynitrite.*

HEMOGLOBIN IS AN NO DONOR

By comparing the structure of hemoglobin across many species, a surprisingly limited number of amino acid sequences are constant. The most phylogenetically constant amino acids (and, by inference, the most crucial to function) include those surrounding the heme pocket, as well as a cysteine at position 93 on the surface of the β subunit (cys93β).[14] This cysteine, a thiol, is capable of binding NO and forming S-nitrosohemoglobin (SNO-Hb). While heme rapidly scavenges local endothelial cell–generated NO, inducing vasoconstriction when hemoglobin is perfused through isolated aortic segments, SNO-Hb exhibits vasodilatory properties when perfused through the same in vitro system.[14] Furthermore, the deletion of cys93β of the perfused hemoglobin results in vasoconstriction. Jia et al[14] and Stamler et al[15] have proposed that the role for this highly conserved cysteine is to bind NO in the lungs, and to deliver NO to peripheral tissues as a fundamental mechanism of blood flow and blood pressure control.

In a physiologically predictable fashion, the deoxygenated form of SNO-Hb is more apt to release NO and cause vasodilation than the oxygenated form.[14] When SNO-Hb is infused into animals breathing room air, they exhibit an increase in cerebral blood flow. In contrast, there is no alteration in cerebral blood flow with infusion of SNO-Hb in animals under hyperoxic conditions.[15] Furthermore, endogenous SNO-Hb is detected in the arterial blood alone, while $Hb[Fe^{2+}]NO$ is present in venous blood in animals breathing room air; SNO-Hb predominates in both sides of the circulation under hyperoxic conditions. These data imply formation of SNO-Hb in the lung, by a yet unidentified mechanism, with subsequent release of NO from cys93β in the tissue arterioles to cause vasodilation, counteracting the decreased blood flow from NO scavenging by heme. This process occurs only when peripheral oxygen tension is low, such as with breathing room air, ensuring a balance between oxygen delivery and demand[15] (**Figure 2**).

Nitric oxide released from hemoglobin does not simply diffuse out of red blood cells and into vascular smooth muscle to promote vasodilatation. Plasma NO is bound to al-

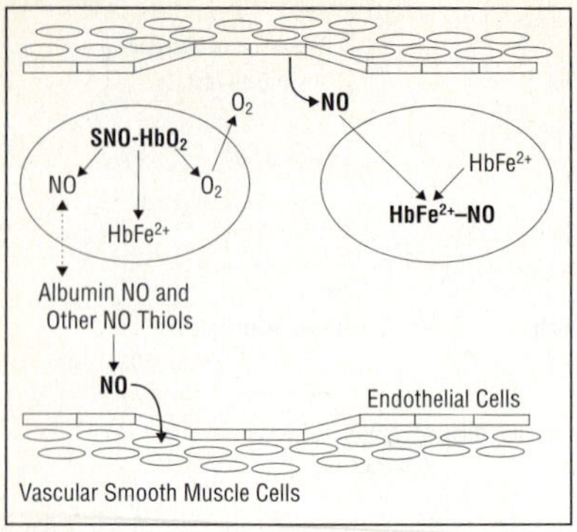

Figure 2. *Oxygenated S-nitrosohemoglobin (SNO-HbO_2) is formed in the lungs. In the peripheral vasculature, both nitric oxide (NO) and oxygen (O_2) are released. Nitric oxide delivery causes vasodilation and counteracts scavenging of NO by hemoglobin ($HbFe^{2+}$-NO) to ensure oxygen delivery matches oxygen demand.*

bumin and other cysteine containing low molecular weight proteins (thiols). Data suggest NO is sequentially transferred from hemoglobin to plasma protein thiols, and to vascular smooth muscle cells.[16-19] The specific mechanism of the NO transfer remains to be elucidated.

CLINICAL IMPLICATIONS OF SNO-Hb

Acute Respiratory Distress Syndrome

Inhaled NO is an attractive potential treatment for patients with acute respiratory distress syndrome (ARDS). Nitric oxide should not only direct pulmonary blood flow toward ventilated alveoli, enhancing oxygen uptake in the lung, but also vasodilate peripherally, via SNO-Hb, promoting systemic oxygen delivery. Indeed, NO is purported to lower pulmonary hypertension, a central feature of ARDS.[20,21] Improvement in peripheral tissue oxygen delivery, as well as enhanced mitochondrial utilization of oxygen in the periphery, has been reported with inhaled NO therapy in patients with ARDS.[22] Surprisingly, recent randomized clinical trials on the use of inhaled NO in patients with ARDS conclude no effect on mortality or duration of mechanical ventilation.[23-25] Furthermore, any positive effect on the lung's ability to oxygenate blood appears transient, lasting hours to days.[23,26] This therapeutic failure is consistent with the generation of the unstable, and highly toxic peroxynitrite, formed by the interaction of NO and superoxide radicals.[2] The enhanced oxygen delivery afforded by inhaled NO could impair mitochondrial electron transport through these toxic by-products.[22] Ultimately, the therapeutic potential of exogenous NO will depend on striking a balance between NO-enhanced oxygen delivery and the production of destructive NO radicals.

Angioplasty

Percutaneous transluminal coronary angioplasty for the treatment of coronary artery disease is limited by the high incidence of restenosis. Restenosis is the result of endothelial cell injury, release of cytokines, and resultant proliferation and migration of smooth muscle cells underlying the damaged endothelium.[27,28] Interestingly, this post–percutaneous transluminal coronary angioplasty vascular remodeling does not lead to clinically relevant blockage in all patients.[27]

Nitric oxide may modulate this process of intimal hyperplasia and restenosis. Addition of an NO donor reduces the degree of intimal thickening, and enhances the regeneration of the endothelial cells, reforming the surface of the injured blood vessel.[29] Similar attenuation of restenosis has been reported following administration of an NO-albumin conjugate, and with gene transfection of the NO-generating enzyme, NO synthase, into endothelial cells.[30-32] Furthermore, prolonged inhalation of NO has been shown to attenuate intimal proliferation after angioplasty in the rat.[33] This latter beneficial effect of augmenting NO delivery to the injured blood vessel may be mediated by SNO-Hb. However, the specific role of SNO-Hb in modulating vessel injury remains undefined.

Cardiac Transplantation

A diffuse coronary arterial intimal hyperplasia affects 40% of transplanted hearts and is the dominant limitation to donor organ survival. Endothelial injury appears to be the inciting event of posttransplantation neointimal hyperplasia. Studies of human heart recipients 1 to 3 years after cardiac transplantation reveal defects in endothelium dependent, NO-mediated vasodilation.[34] Theories invoking reaction to major histocompatibility complex antigens on the endothelial cells of the donor organ, unanswered variable expression of adhesion molecules on the endothelium, or bystander damage to the endothelium from reaction to donor white blood cells have been proposed to explain this diffuse allograft vasculopathy. Surprisingly, work in inbred animals indicates that the transplant vasculopathy progresses even if the donor organ is protected from the recipient immune system by donor organ replacement back into the donor strain.[35] Conversely, vasculopathy is prevented if the allograft is transplanted back into the donor strain within 4 days (but not later) of the original transplant. This time dependence suggests that early injury to the endothelium of the transplanted organ is responsible for the diffuse vasculopathy. Indeed, cardiac endothelial dysfunction (decreased NO activity) at 2 weeks after human heart transplantation predicts the development of cardiac vasculopathy at 1 year.[36]

Thus, decreased NO activity is not only a marker for endothelial dysfunction, but it may play a role in the pathogenesis of allograft vasculopathy. Inhibition of NO synthase in animals exacerbates renal, cardiac, and aortic allograft rejection, while transfection of NO synthase suppresses vasculopathy.[37-39] Thus, an NO delivery system used early in the posttransplantation period is a promising strategy to attenuate allograft vasculopathy.

Hemoglobin-Based Blood Substitutes

The development of stroma-free hemoglobin (SFH) as a blood substitute has been limited by the prominent side effect of systemic hypertension. Stroma-free hemoglobin becomes an unregulated scavenger of NO in the vasculature. Although this hypertension may be mediated partially by α_2-adrenergic receptors, the hypertensive effects of SFH involve an interaction at the heme site of artificial hemoglobin with NO.[13,40,41]

Intraluminal scavenging of NO alone may be insufficient to bring about all of the hypertensive effects of SFH.[13] Gould et al[42] postulate that extravasation of SFH across the endothelial cell barrier with binding of NO at its vascular smooth muscle target is the cause of hypertensive effects. Thus, polymerized forms of SFH that prevent extravasation should promote normotensive oxygen delivery. A preliminary clinical trial supports this hypothesis.[42]

Sickle Cell Anemia

In addition to vascular dynamics, NO may influence the oxygen affinity of some altered forms of hemoglobin. It is clear that improving the oxygen affinity of sickle cell hemoglobin will prevent the characteristic polymerizing disfigurement of deoxygenated sickle cell hemoglobin molecules, with resultant sickle cell crisis.[43] Head and colleagues[44] have reported that inhaled NO in doses up to 80 ppm for 5 minutes enhances the oxygen affinity of sickle cell hemoglobin, but predictably, does not influence the oxygen-hemoglobin relationship of normal adult hemoglobin. The clinical administration of NO could both prevent and treat sickle-cell crisis.

This work was supported by a Center for Excellence Award from the Emergency Medicine Foundation, Dallas, Tex; and grant 6M-4922 and a Student Research Grant from the National Institutes of Health, Bethesda, Md.

Corresponding author: Charles B. Cairns, MD, B-211, University of Colorado Health Sciences Center, 4200 E Ninth Ave, Denver, CO 80262 (e-mail: Charles.Cairns@UCHSC.edu).

REFERENCES

1. Derewenda Z, Dodson G, Emsley P, et al. Stereochemistry of carbon monoxide binding to normal human adult and Cowtown haemoglobins. *J Mol Biol.* 1990;211:515-519.
2. Singh S, Evans TW. Nitric oxide, the biological mediator of the decade: fact or fiction? *Eur Respir J.* 1997;10:699-707.
3. Geller DA, Billiar RT. Molecular biology of nitric oxide synthases. *Cancer Metastasis Rev.* 1998; 17:7-23.
4. Palmer RM, Ferrige AG, Moncada S. Nitric oxide release accounts for the biological activity of endothelium-derived relaxing factor. *Nature.* 1987; 327:524-526.
5. Meldrum DR. Tumor necrosis factor in the heart. *Am J Physiol.* 1998;274(3 pt 2):R577-R595.
6. Balligand JL, Cannon PJ. Nitric oxide synthases and cardiac muscle: autocrine and paracrine influences. *Arterioscler Thromb Vasc Biol.* 1997; 17:1846-1858.
7. Ikeda U, Shimada K. Nitric oxide and cardiac failure. *Clin Cardiol.* 1997;20:837-841.
8. Farghali H, Hynie S, Vohnikova Z, Masek K. Possible dual role of nitric oxide in oxidative stress injury: a study in perfused hepatocytes. *Int J Immunopharmacol.* 1997;19:599-605.
9. Kim YM, Talanian RV, Billiar TR. Nitric oxide inhibits apoptosis by preventing increases in caspase-3-like activity via two distinct mechanisms. *J Biol Chem.* 1997;272:31138-31148.
10. Kon K, Maeda N, Shiga T. Effect of nitric oxide on the oxygen transport of human erythrocytes. *J Toxicol Environ Health.* 1977;2:1109-1113.
11. Stamler JS. Redox signaling: nitrosylation and related target interactions of nitric oxide. *Cell.* 1994; 78:931-936.
12. Chiodi H, Mohler JG. Effects of exposure of blood hemoglobin to nitric oxide. *Environ Res.* 1985; 37:355-363.
13. Gould SA, Moss GS. Clinical development of human polymerized hemoglobin as a blood substitute. *World J Surg.* 1996;20:1200-1207.
14. Jia L, Bonaventura C, Bonaventura J, Stamler JS. S-nitrosohaemoglobin: a dynamic activity of blood involved in vascular control. *Nature.* 1996;380:221-226.
15. Stamler JS, Jia L, Eu JP, et al. Bloodflow regulation by S-nitrosohemoglobin in the physiological oxygen gradient. *Science.* 1997;276:2034-2037.
16. Scharfstein JS, Keaney JF, Slivka A, et al. In vivo transfer of nitric oxide between a plasma-bound reservoir and low molecular weight thiols. *J Clin Invest.* 1994;94:1432-1439.
17. Stamler JS, Simon DI, Osborne JA, et al. S-nitrosylation of proteins with nitric oxide: synthesis and characterization of biologically active compounds. *Proc Natl Acad Sci U S A.* 1992;89:444-448.
18. Stamler JS, Jaraki O, Osborne J, et al. Nitric oxide circulates in mammalian plasma primarily as an S-nitroso adduct of serum albumin. *Proc Natl Acad Sci U S A.* 1992;89:7674-7677.
19. Minamiyama Y, Takemura S, Inoue M. Albumin is an important vascular tonus regulator as a reservoir of nitric oxide. *Biochem Biophy Res Commun.* 1996;225:112-115.
20. Rossaint R, Falke KJ, Lopez F, Slama K, Pison U, Zapol WM. Inhaled nitric oxide for the adult respiratory distress syndrome. *N Engl J Med.* 1993; 328:399-405.
21. McIntyre RC, Moore FA, Moore EE, Piedalue F, Haenel JS, Fullerton DA. Inhaled nitric oxide variably improves oxygenation and pulmonary hypertension in patients with acute respiratory distress syndrome. *J Trauma.* 1995;39:418-425.
22. Cairns CB, Veeramachaneni N, Walther JM, McIntyre R, Harken AH. Inhaled nitric oxide improves peripheral tissue oxygenation in patients with the acute respiratory distress syndrome [abstract]. *Ann Emerg Med.* 1997;30:374.
23. Dellinger RP, Zimmerman JL, Taylor RW, et al. Effects of inhaled nitric oxide in patients with acute respiratory distress syndrome: results of a randomized phase II trial. *Crit Care Med.* 1998;26:15-23.
24. Groupe d'Etude sur le NO inhale au cours de l'ARDS. Inhaled NO in ARDS: presentation of a double blind randomized multicentric study [abstract]. *Am J Respir Crit Care Med.* 1996;153:A590.
25. Lundin S, Mang H, Smithies M, Stenqvist O, Frostell C. Inhalation of nitric oxide in acute lung injury: preliminary results of a European multicenter study. *Intensive Care Med.* 1997;23 (suppl 1):S2.
26. Michael JR, Barton RG, Saffle JR, et al. Inhaled nitric oxide versus conventional therapy: effect on oxygenation in ARDS. *Am J Respir Crit Care Med.* 1998;157:1372-1380.
27. Liu MW, Roubin GS, King SB. Restenosis after coronary angioplasty: potential biological determinants and role of intimal hyperplasia. *Circulation.* 1989;79:1374-1387.
28. Casscells W. Migration of smooth muscle and endothelial cells: critical events in restenosis. *Circulation.* 1992;86:723-729.
29. Guo JP, Milhoan KA, Tuan RS, Lefer AM. Beneficial effect of SPM-5185, a cysteine-containing nitric oxide donor, in rat carotid artery intimal injury. *Circulation Res.* 1994;75:77-84.
30. Marks DS, Vita JA, Folts JD, Keaney JF, Welch GN, Loscalzo J. Inhibition of neointimal proliferation in rabbits after vascular injury by a single treatment with a protein adduct of nitric oxide. *J Clin Invest.* 1995;96:2630-2638.
31. Von Der Leyen HE, Gibbons GH, Morishita R, et al. Gene therapy inhibiting neointimal vascular lesion: in vivo transfer of endothelial cell nitric oxide synthase gene. *Proc Natl Acad Sci U S A.* 1995; 92:1137-1141.
32. Shears LL, Kibbe MR, Murdock AD, et al. Efficient inhibition of intimal hyperplasia by adenovirus-mediated inducible nitric oxide synthase gene transfer to rats and pigs in vivo. *J Am Coll Surg.* 1998;187:295-306.
33. Lee JS, Adrie C, Jacob HJ, Roberts JD Jr, Zapol WM, Bloch KD. Chronic inhalation of nitric oxide inhibits neointimal formation after balloon-induced arterial injury. *Circ Res.* 1996;78:337-342.
34. Treasure CB, Vita JA, Ganz P, et al. Loss of the coronary microvascular response to acetylcholine in cardiac transplant patients. *Circulation.* 1992;86:1156-1164.
35. Izutani H, Miyagawa S, Shirakura R, et al. Evidence that graft coronary arteriosclerosis begins in the early phase after transplantation and progresses without chronic immunoreaction. *Transplantation.* 1995;60:1073-1079.
36. Davis SF, Yeung AC, Meredith IT, et al. Early endothelial dysfunction predicts the development of transplant coronary artery disease at 1 year posttransplant. *Circulation.* 1996;93:457-462.
37. Stojanovic T, Grone HJ, Gieseler RK, et al. Enhanced renal allograft rejection by inhibitors of nitric oxide synthase: a nonimmunologic influence on alloreactivity. *Lab Invest.* 1996;74:496-512.
38. Paul LC, Myllarniemi M, Muzaffar S, Benediktsson H. Nitric oxide synthase inhibition is associated with decreased survival of cardiac allografts in the rat. *Transplantation.* 1996;62:1193-1195.
39. Shears LL, Kawaharada N, Tzeng E, et al. Inducible nitric oxide synthase suppresses the development of allograft arteriosclerosis. *J Clin Invest.* 1997;100:2035-2042.
40. Sharma AC, Gulati A. Yohimbine modulates diaspirin crosslinked hemoglobin-induced systemic hemodynamics and regional circulatory effects. *Crit Care Med.* 1995;23:874-884.
41. Ketcham EM, Cairns CB. Hemoglobin-based oxygen carriers: development and clinical potential. *Ann Emerg Med.* 1999;33:326-337.
42. Gould SA, Moore EE, Hoyt DB, et al. The first randomized trial of human polymerized hemoglobin as a blood substitute in acute trauma and emergent surgery. *J Am Coll Surg.* 1998;187:113-120.
43. Sunshine HR, Hofrichter J, Eaton WA. Requirements for therapeutic inhibition of sickle haemoglobin gelation. *Nature.* 1978;275:238-240.
44. Head CA, Brugnara C, Martinez-Ruiz R, et al. Low concentrations of nitric oxide increase oxygen affinity of sickle erythrocytes in vitro and in vivo. *J Clin Invest.* 1997;100:1193-1198.

Surgery in Argentina

Enrique M. Beveraggi, MD

This article will provide a brief background on Argentina and then summarize the country's medical and surgical history, undergraduate and postgraduate training programs, residency programs, surgical associations, research, and the *Argentinean Journal of Surgery (Revista Argentina de Cirugía)*. Surgery in Argentina is at the same level as that of most developed countries although transplantation, traumatology, and laparoscopic surgery have been emphasized.

Arch Surg. 1999;134:438-444

Surgery is an essential discipline in the field of medicine in which solutions are difficult to find since they depend primarily on the socioeconomic, cultural, educational, and environmental conditions that interact with one another. Therefore, I find it necessary to provide a general background of Argentina before discussing the central topic of this article.

Argentina is located in the southernmost part of South America, has a surface of 3 000 000 km^2, and 36 million inhabitants (**Figure 1**). The population distribution is irregular, with over half of the country's inhabitants concentrated in the city of Buenos Aires and the surrounding suburbs. Only about 20% of the population resides in rural areas. Argentina is a young country with a very small Native American population; most of its inhabitants are of European descent, mainly Italian and Spanish, but a substantial number are of other ethnic origin.

Argentina has a federal republican representative form of government. The official language is Spanish and most Argentineans are Catholic, although they are free to worship as they please. The country allocates 7% of its gross domestic product to health care, which amounts to $650 per capita per year. Despite the fact that this is the highest amount allocated for health care services in Latin America, 35% of the population does not have medical insurance (**Figure 2**).

From the Hospital Italiano de Buenos Aires, Servicio de Cirugía, Gascón 450, Buenos Aires, Argentina.

HISTORICAL BACKGROUND

Native American medicine did have not a substantial influence on modern medicine in Argentina, as it was not as developed as it was in other Latin American countries such as Mexico or Peru. During the colonial times, Spanish and Portuguese physicians introduced medical knowledge acquired in Europe. Simultaneously, Argentineans practiced self-medication, preparing their own medicines and caring for patients in their homes. They also consulted traditional healers.

As in most countries, surgery was practiced in the most primitive form by these traditional healers and others responsible for the health of the community. Before the country's emancipation from Spain, there were reports of occasional surgical procedures, performed mainly by missionary Jesuit priests of European origin, in the 17th and 18th centuries. Most of these priests and the first surgeons were Spanish and some were Portuguese. Later, some British surgeons came in slave ships and settled in Argentina. Toward the end of the 18th century, the Buenos Aires Board of Physicians, which was in charge of regulating and monitoring medical practice, was created.

The wars leading to the country's independence and consolidation created the need for military surgeons, the best known being Cosme Argerich (1756-1820).

The first medical school, established in 1821, was modeled after Spanish, British, and French university cur-

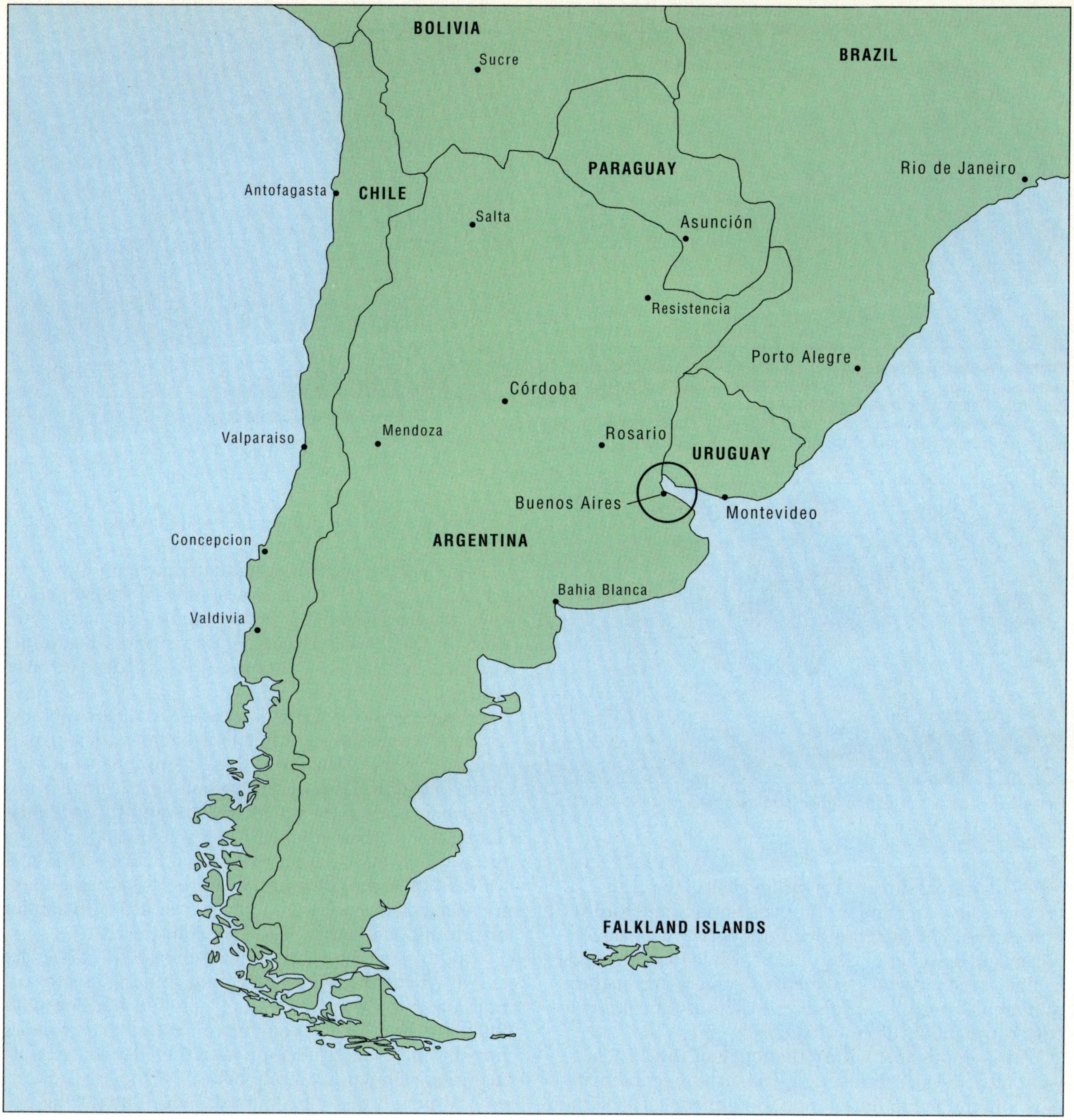

Figure 1. *Argentina. More than half of the country's population is concentrated within the encircled area.*

ricula, ie, the academic bases of the medical profession in Argentina were universal, a characteristic that still prevails. The Academia Argentina de Medicina was founded in 1822. The first official surgery courses were taught by the Spanish surgeon Agustín Fabre (1749-1820) at the turn of the 19th century. In 1829, Juan José Montes de Oca (1806-1875) started teaching surgery and performing autopsies. One of his disciples, Ignacio Pirovano (1844-1895), came to be known as the father of Argentinean surgery. He started a trend of Argentinean graduates visiting Europe (mainly Paris, London, and Vienna).

Beginning in 1890, great progress ensued, led by Pirovano's disciples Enrique Bazterrica, Andrés Llobet, Alejandro and Máximo Castro, Marcelino Herrera Vegas, and Alejandro Posadas. The latter was an exceptional surgeon who died at age 31 years, leaving behind many followers and original techniques.

After World War I, French medicine had a marked influence on local practice. Between World War I and World War II, the main influences were from France, Germany, Austria, Italy, England, and the United States; the latter became the primary influence in 1945.

In the second decade in the 20th century, Argentinean physicians made important and original contributions to the medical field. Three of them were awarded the Nobel prize: Bernardo A. Houssay (1947), in medicine and physiology; Luis Federico Leloir (1969), in chemistry; and Cesar Milstein (1984), in medicine.

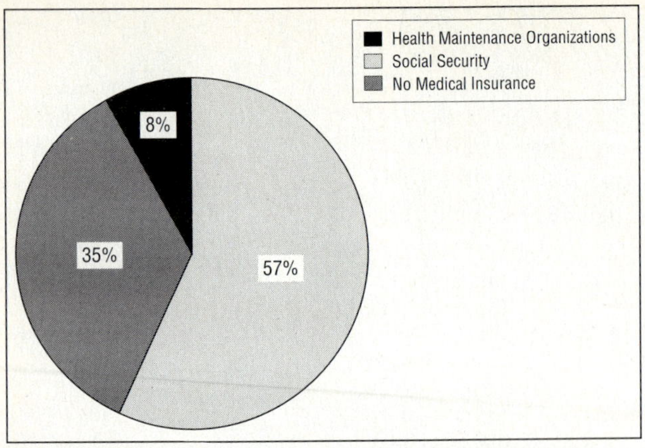

Figure 2. *Pie graph of the percentage of the Argentinean population who are uninsured and must receive care at public hospitals, receive social security benefits (including those in the pensioners' social security system), or belong to health maintenance organizations. Total health expenditure in Argentina, 7% gross domestic product ($21.9 billion in US dollars).*

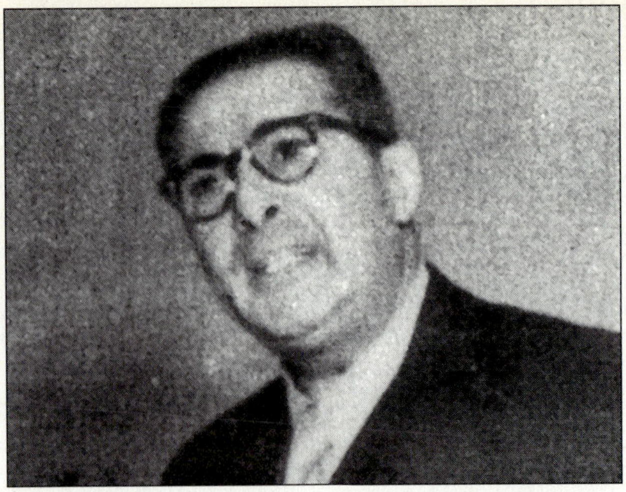

Figure 4. *Pablo Mirizzi, MD, who introduced the first intraoperative cholangiography in 1931.*

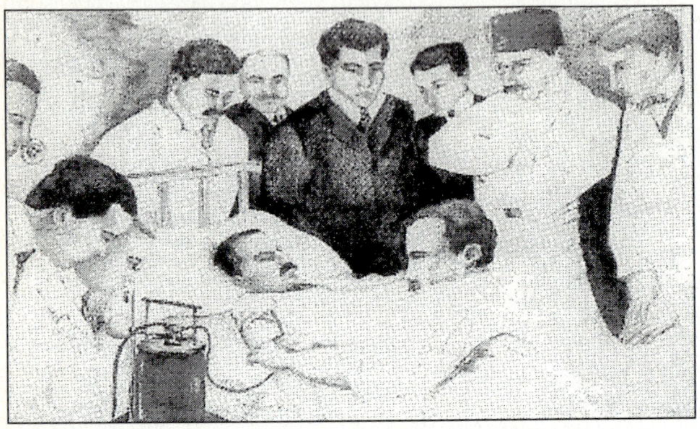

Figure 3. *First citrated blood transfusion, performed in Argentina in 1914.*

Three great surgeons of the first half of the 20th century were José Arce and the brothers Enrique and Ricardo Finochietto. The elder brother, Enrique, was a great technician and designer of instruments, while Ricardo was a brilliant teacher who systematized surgery and had innumerable disciples who spread their art and knowledge throughout the country.

It is impossible within the range of this article to name all of the most brilliant Argentinean surgeons, many of whom trained in Europe and the United States. Some of the best, however, are mentioned below.

In 1914, Luis Agote performed the first transfusion with citrate to prevent coagulation (**Figure 3**). In 1931, Pablo Mirizzi performed the first intraoperative cholangiography, a procedure that was adopted worldwide (**Figure 4**). In 1932, Julio Diez described the technique of lumbar sympathectomy for peripheral vascular disease.

MEDICAL SCHOOLS AND UNDERGRADUATE SURGICAL TRAINING

In 1613, the Jesuits established the first university in Córdoba, a city located in the center of the country. At present, Argentina has 36 state and 40 private universities. There are 8 medical schools that are part of state universities and 11 private medical schools, 9 created since 1990.

In general, the undergraduate curriculum for the training of general physicians requires 6 years of study and, at some schools, a 1-year internship with rotations in the 4 basic departments (internal medicine, surgery, pediatrics, and tocogynecology) is also required.

Some schools, particularly those in the private sector, have admission requirements such as tests or prerequisite courses. However, these requirements are not uniform and the issue of how to standardize them is under debate both in the university community and in the public forum. This problem is also being addressed by the National Association of Medical Schools (AFACIMERA), an organization formed by the deans of the country's medical schools, who have close ties with similar organizations in other American countries.

Both general surgery and the surgical specialties are taught during the last 3 years of the undergraduate curriculum (clinical cycle) in university hospitals or in affiliated institutions. Neither the contents of these courses nor the methods used for evaluating student performance are similar in all schools.

Although there is a high dropout rate during undergraduate studies (approximately 40%), an average of 4000 new physicians graduate every year. The diploma granted by the universities is the physician's medical license, ie, it is the only requirement to practice. Provincial or local authorities usually require other credentials, such as completion of residency or additional courses to authorize the practice.

A surplus of new physicians graduate each year, and there are already more than 100 000 active physicians in Argentina, ie, 1 physician for every 360 inhabitants. Their geographical distribution is grossly distorted, as most physicians are concentrated in urban areas. In some major cities, the ratio of physicians to inhabitants is alarming. This constitutes a challenge for physicians seeking postgraduate education, since at present there are only about 1500 positions, both in public and private institutions, for the training of residents in the various specialties and subspecialties.

POSTGRADUATE TRAINING

In the first half of the 20th century, postgraduate training was conducted by medical schools in cooperation with public hospitals. The quality and number of these programs increased during the last 30 years with the participation of all the public medical schools and some private ones together with most of the national, municipal, private, and community hospitals.

Augusto Moreno started the first residency in surgery in 1951, but it was only in 1958 that surgical residences were officially introduced under the leadership of thoracic surgeon Mario Brea at the Teaching Hospital of the University of Buenos Aires. Together with Andrés Santas, they represented a strong modernizing force in medical education in Argentina. Since then, numerous residency programs in different specialties were established throughout the country. In 1967, the Residency Subcommittee of the Argentinean Medical Association (Asociación Medica de Argentina) and the National Council for Medical Residencies (Consejo Nacional de Residencias Médicas) were founded to supervise the establishment of new programs and to control the approval and evaluation of medical procedures.

In 1989, the Argentinean Association of Surgery (Asociación Argentina de Cirugía [AAC]) created the Residency Committee, which included representatives from several surgical disciplines, to assess and categorize residency programs. Of 105 programs in general surgery, 69 have been registered since 1989.

Admission to a residency program is based on the grade point average obtained during undergraduate studies, a multiple-choice examination of general medical knowledge, and a personal interview. There are residency programs in gynecology (which is becoming increasingly independent of the residency of general surgery), urology, orthopedics, traumatology, otorrhinolaryngology, and plastic, thoracic, cardiovascular, and pediatric (closely associated with the residence in pediatrics) surgery. To be admitted to these residency programs, physicians must have completed at least a partial residence in general surgery.

The different programs, which include a final year as chief resident, take from 4 to 5 years to complete. At the completion of the programs, the residents are not granted certification as specialists, since that is done by the corresponding surgical association.

In 1997, the Association for the Certification and Assessment of Postgraduate Medical Training in Argentina (ACAP), which encompasses all medical disciplines, was created. This strengthens the current trend toward increased involvement of scientific societies in medicine, which, with the proper legal support, will have a more active role in postgraduate training during the next century.

ARGENTINEAN ASSOCIATION OF SURGERY (ASOCIACIÓN ARGENTINA DE CIRUGÍA)

The AAC, which was founded in 1930, has 3566 members; 2314 of them are full members and 1232 are associate members. The number of surgeons in Argentina has reached about 6000. To become a full AAC member, each applicant must have a minimum of 5 years of surgical training, submit a list of operations performed during the previous year, and pass a theoretical and practical examination. Moreover, the applicant must have the support of 6 full AAC members. A program for the recertification of surgeons was started in 1990, and 1496 members have been recertified as of 1997.

One of the main objectives of the AAC has been the organization of the Argentinean annual meeting of surgery, the main surgical meeting in the country. At the meeting, 2 official presentations on the state of the art of important surgical problems are discussed. Roundtables, lectures, colloquiums, postgraduate courses, television forums, and other activities are organized with the cooperation of sister scientific societies depending on the topics being discussed. More than 3000 surgeons from Argentina and neighboring countries attend the meeting, and surgeons from abroad with worldwide recognition are invited to participate every year. Major topics of recent meetings have been continuous education, residencies, recertification, bioethics, and the organization of surgical departments, as well as other issues that contribute to the improvement of the professional standing of surgeons, individually and as a group.

In the last few decades, the AAC has become actively involved in issues related to surgical practice as indicated, eg, by the central topic of the 1999 meeting: the role of the AAC in surgical practice. Recently, the AAC has entered a stage of active professionalization with the

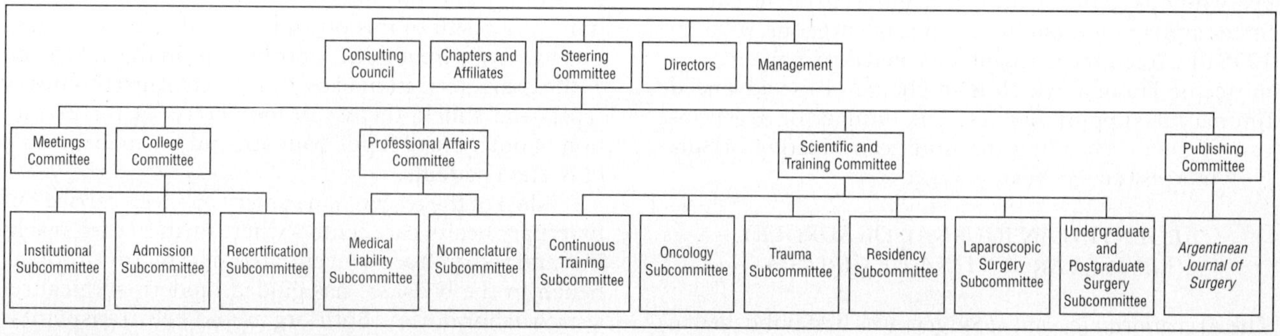

Figure 5. *Structure of the Argentinean Association of Surgery.*

appointment of a surgeon as permanent director and the development of a complex organizational structure (**Figure 5**). The influence of the American College of Surgeons (ACS) was evident after 1970.

ARGENTINEAN ACADEMY OF SURGERY (ACADEMIA ARGENTINA DE CIRUGÍA)

The Argentinean Academy of Surgery is the highest academic institution in surgery in Argentina. It was founded on September 30th, 1911, to promote the study and development of surgery. Initially called the Surgical Society of Buenos Aires (Sociedad de Cirugía de Buenos Aires), it was renamed the Argentinean Academy of Surgery in 1942. Regular meetings are held every Wednesday from 7 to 8:30 PM, and sessions run from the first Wednesday in April to the last Wednesday in November. During these meetings, appointed members read their papers or those submitted by nonmembers for discussion. Most of the papers are published in the *Argentinean Journal of Surgery*. The Academy is consists of 70 principal academics, 40 associates, 40 national correspondents, 40 foreign correspondents, and an unlimited number of emeritus and honorary academics. The vacancies are filled based on qualification and depending on availability in each category. The Academy awards prizes and fellowships on the basis of the regulations established in its rules of proceedings.

ARGENTINEAN CHAPTER OF THE AMERICAN COLLEGE OF SURGEONS

In October 1954, a group of Argentinean surgeons, the Fellows of the ACS, developed the Argentinean chapter of the ACS, with Juan Martín Allende as the first governor and Rodolfo E. Pasman as the first chairman. At present, the Argentinean chapter consists of 171 fellows and is the largest in Latin America after the Mexican chapter. There are also 178 associate members. The Argentinean chapter has always worked closely with the AAC in an attempt to inspire it with the basic ACS objectives and to encourage Argentinean surgeons to become fellows. The Argentinean chapter has more recently organized special sessions during the annual meeting of surgery on topics essential for the improvement of surgery.

Also, it is worth highlighting the following events: the National Meeting on Medical Residencies (1963), the First Joint Meeting of South American Chapters (1966), the Fourth Latin American Meeting of ACS Fellows (1992), and the International Chapter Course carried out every June as of 1993 with special guests from the United States and a numerous attendance of surgeons. Also, in 1995 the Argentinean Chapter created the Chapter Committee of Trauma, which is in charge of the advanced trauma life support courses. The number of Argentinean surgeons attending the American Meeting of Surgery increases every year.

ARGENTINEAN JOURNAL OF SURGERY (REVISTA ARGENTINA DE CIRUGÍA)

The *Argentinean Journal of Surgery* was first published in 1960 and is now the official journal of the AAC, which also publishes the documents by the Argentinean Academy of Surgery. This journal is published in 2 annual volumes of 4 issues, 3800 copies each. Also, there is a special edition that includes the presentations from the Argentinean Annual Meeting of Surgery . The journal is distributed to the associated members and all medical school libraries in Latin America and around the world. Although it is written in Spanish, all of its articles also include an abstract and key words translated into English.

The *Argentinean Journal of Surgery* is listed in the Latin American *Index Medicus*, and since 1991 has adopted the guidelines of the International Committee of Biomedical Editors. The Editor-in-Chief is the only Argentinean member of the Council of Biology Editors and will belong to its membership council until 2001. The journal has been included in a special CD-ROM package, along with other Argentinean journals such as *Anestesiología*, *Cardiología*, and *Medicina de Buenos Aires*, of which the 1995 volumes are comprised.

RESEARCH IN SURGERY

The incorporation of surgery and the development of related research at academic medical centers has followed essentially the same pattern as in other countries. Until about 1950, general surgery was considered a technical practice and, although Argentinean surgeons made significant contributions to the field, they were restricted to the description of new surgical procedures or to reports by specialized surgeons.

In the 1960s, surgery became a separate specialty at universities and, as did surgeons in the rest of the world, Argentinean surgeons started to play a key role in research, particularly in the field of critical care. With the first intensive care units, surgeons became actively involved in the interdisciplinary analysis of problems such as shock, infections, multisystem dysfunction, nutrition, and others, when the units devoted to experimental surgery were instrumental in the development of cardiovascular surgery and the emerging field of organ transplantation.

Since 1966, a Forum on Surgical Research, conceived and chaired by Andrés Santas until his death, is organized every year at the Argentinean Meeting of Surgery.

The interaction between surgical and other academic departments was strengthened in the 1980s when surgeons and basic scientists from areas such as molecular biology and physiology started a fruitful cooperation. As a result of this ongoing shared interest, Argentina has made important contributions in the field, such as the characterization of oxygen reactive metabolites in sepsis and shock, the use of tonometry for the prediction of outcome of septic patients, and the management of burned patients.

Most of the research in surgery has been carried out in tertiary health care centers where medical care, teaching, and research are concentrated. The motto "from the bench to the bedside" has guided modern surgical research laboratories. Both organ and cell transplantations are routinely performed, the physiopathology of criti-

Rate of Organ and Tissue Donation*		
	Donors per Million Inhabitants	
Year	Organs and Tissue	Solid Organs
1995	11.70	. . .
1996	12.33	. . .
1997	13.31	6.08

*Ellipses indicate not applicable.

cal patients is investigated, and tools derived from molecular biology are increasingly used for both diagnostic procedures and the development of techniques aimed at experimental gene transfer.

LAPAROSCOPIC SURGERY

In the past few years, laparoscopic surgery has represented a phenomenon that has affected the bases of traditional surgery and, therefore, the professional associations of surgeons.

The AAC immediately understood that laparoscopic surgery as well as endoscopic and mini-invasive surgery are variants of traditional surgery and should be handled by the general surgeon in the simplest cases (eg, cholecistectomy and appendectomy), and by the specialist in the most complex cases. Laparoscopic surgery is, therefore, not regarded as a new surgical discipline, but as a new surgical technique.

Under this view, the AAC has carried out and sponsored basic and advanced training courses in laparoscopic surgery. Certificates are granted after a committee evaluates the applicants' skills, completion of required courses, and experience as a surgeon and assistant in laparoscopic surgery. The committee also monitors the laparoscopic surgery programs that are part of the residency, as approved by the AAC. Monitoring and certification of the laparoscopic practice is the role of the laparoscopic subcommittee, which is encompassed by the steering committee of the AAC. This subcommittee has organized 2 national consensus conferences, the first in 1996 on "Training and Certification in Surgery," and the second in 1997 on "Laparoscopic Treatment of Gastroesophageal Reflux Disease." This system is unlike that in most other countries, where specific associations have been created to regulate laparoscopic surgery.

TRANSPLANTATION

The first kidney transplantation in Argentina was performed in 1955. Toward the end of the 1980s and at the beginning of the 1990s, the first liver, heart, and lung transplantations were performed, and more recently pancreatic and renopancreatic transplantations have been performed. By 1980 and particularly as of 1990, the National Institute for the Coordination of Ablations and Transplantations (INCUCAI), within purview of the Ministry of Public Health, has been doing an excellent job educating society members in the area of organs donation. Nevertheless, the rate of organ and tissue donations in Argentina is growing at a low pace (**Table**).

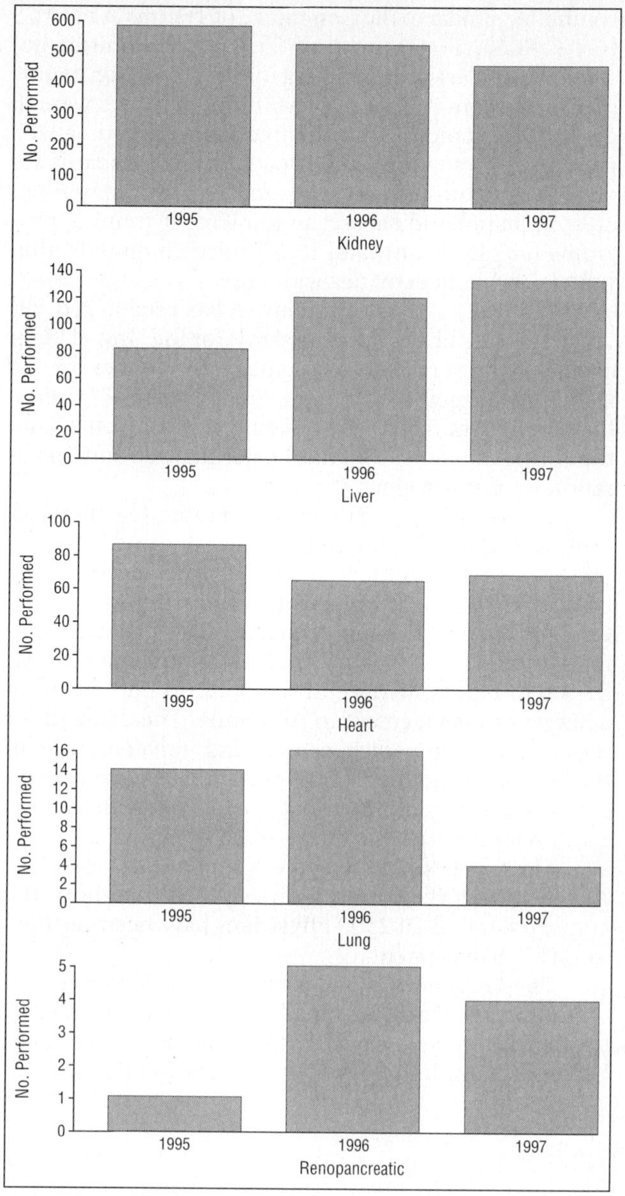

Figure 6. *Solid organ transplantations between 1995 and 1997.*

Figure 6 shows the number of solid organ transplantations carried out in 1995, 1996, and 1997. Kidney and heart transplantations are performed at various centers throughout the country. On the other hand, liver, lung, and pancreas transplantations are only performed in a few academic centers in Buenos Aires. Live related-donor transplantations have been performed in Argentina since 1992. Transplantation outcomes are generally comparable to world standards.

TRAUMA

Statistics show that trauma is the most common cause of death during the 3 first decades of life, and the third most common cause of death at any age worldwide. This is an issue of serious concern in Argentina, and Argentinean surgeons have always taken the lead in the management of trauma. In 1982, a group of surgeons from the AAC, led by Miguel Angel Gomez, organized a trauma committee similar to the Committee of Trauma at the ACS (COT-ACS). Thus, the AAC Trauma Committee became the first academic and organic approach for trauma management in Argentina. The initial purposes were to divulge the standards for the treatment of traumatized patients; to set, adapt, and broadcast the standards for the categorization of patients and medical centers; to create a national database; to implement training programs for physicians; and to organize communication centers and joint activities with other associations.

The AAC Trauma Committee has established, divulged, and published the standards for the "Initial Management of Traumatized Patients," "Guidelines for the Definite Management of Traumatized Patients," "Guidelines for Air Transportation of Traumatized Patients," and the "Principles for the Medical Coordination and Preparation for Catastrophes."

In 1989, the AAC Trauma Committee, together with professionals belonging to the Argentinean Chapter of the ACS, organized the first course of advanced trauma life support trainers, and, through a joint effort with the Chapter Trauma Committee, started a professional training program for the management of the traumatized patient that represented a turning point in the history of emergency management in Argentina. The demand for these courses in medical centers and universities in all the provinces and the most important cities in the country has made Argentina one of the countries with the fastest developing trauma committees.

There are 40 ATLS trainers, and an average of 20 ATLS courses are conducted per year throughout the country. More than 2500 physicians have been certified in ATLS management.

The 3 Argentinean and the 2 Pan-American meetings on trauma that have been held and the meeting planned for the current year show that trauma management has become a multidisciplinary activity. The fact that specialists are interested in various disciplines encourages and fosters the creation of trauma committees in different professional associations. The acceptance by governmental organizations of the standards established by scientific associations has opened the door for trauma committees to influence national law in the areas of prevention, training, and certification. The close cooperation that has always existed between the AAC Trauma Committee and the COT-ACS is an example worth imitating.

PEDIATRIC TRAUMA PROGRAM

The Pediatric Trauma program was launched in 1989 within the framework of the Argentinean Association of Child Surgery (Asociación Argentina de Cirugía Infantil), the Argentinean Society of Pediatrics (Sociedad Argentina de Pediatría), and the AAC. Among its achievements are the Registry of Pediatric Trauma, the Advanced Courses of Initial Management of Traumatized Patients (24 courses conducted to date), the 2 advanced trauma life support trainers' courses, the Interassociation Project of Trauma (a project that targets small communities), and the "Official Guidelines for the Initial Management of the Traumatized Pediatric Patient". The Pediatric Trauma program has extended to other centers in Argentina, bordering countries, and Spain and has become a referential model at national and international levels.

I thank the AAC, its Residency, Publishing, Trauma, and Laparoscopic Committees and Subcommittees, the Academia Argentina de Cirugía, the Argentinean Chapter of the ASC, the National Institute for the Coordination of Ablations and Transplantations, and all of the professionals who have cooperated for the preparation of the manuscript.

Corresponding author: Enrique M. Beveraggi, MD, Hospital Italiano de Buenos Aires, Servicio de Cirugía, Gascón 450, Buenos Aires, CP 1181 Argentina.

The Value of Physician Assistants to Surgical Education in Teaching Hospitals

SEVERAL MONTHS ago, a commentary appeared in this journal[1] estimating the dollar replacement value of surgical residents to community teaching hospitals, and comparing the cost of supporting junior faculty with the cost of replacing surgical residents with physician assistants. Some readers may have misinterpreted the commentary as being anti–physician assistant. In fact, the opposite is true. The author is a strong proponent of increasing the physician assistant participation in patient care in teaching hospitals, and creating mechanisms for the simultaneous training of physician assistants alongside surgical residents.

Eighty-three percent of American health care is at community, nonteaching hospitals, yet the graduate medical education of most specialists is structured as if all program graduates will become professors at the nearest medical school. Particularly in surgery, it is common to find high-quality, sophisticated care at community hospitals, which may have decided to "showcase" or emphasize a particular program as part of their overall competitive position or community mission. In these institutions, a combination of assistant surgeons, "house surgeons," physician assistants, nurse-clinicians, nurse-clinician specialists, and surgical assistants are essential to the function of the team. While training, credentialing, and privileging of surgeons is a major emphasis of most hospitals' medical staff office, it is surprising how unregulated and haphazard the training, credentialing, and privileging of these assistants is. These individuals may perform reasonably invasive procedures with some element of risk independently, without a surgeon in immediate attendance.

Patients in all hospitals have a right to expect that anyone who lays a hand on them has been properly trained to do any procedures involving risk. And hospitals need to reassure both the community as a whole and the patient who has had an adverse experience that bad outcomes are part of the unavoidable risk of all procedures, and are not related to the inexperience or poor supervision of the practitioner. These goals can be met through a simple adaptation of the hospital's credentialing and privileging process to include physician assistants. There are immediate problems encountered, however, in any attempts to credential and privilege individuals in a totally different department (nursing) to perform procedures normally performed by physicians. We would advocate that all surgical assistants be credentialed and privileged through the relevant department of surgery. Furthermore, we would advocate the hospital staffs consider creating "allied health" or "dependent practitioner" status, as voluntary members of their surgical staff may have physician assistants who should be brought into the clinical community of the hospital. Some surgical departments have even decided to make physician assistants voting members of the department and participants in all department decision making, but the specifics of membership, credentialing, and privileging need to be worked out at both the medical staff and departmental level.

But it is in the specific area of surgical physician assistant residencies that the greatest clinical and educational good may be accomplished. Many physicians have no idea of the rigors and standards of physician assistant education. The state of Florida recently performed an interesting experiment in allowing nonlicensed international medical graduates to take the physician assistant qualifying examination, necessary for licensure and practice in that state. Inasmuch as taking the examination was voluntary, one would expect that only motivated and well-prepared individuals would take it. Unfortunately, the passage rate was only 3.6%,[2] which raises profound problems for those who claim that house surgeons are equivalent or superior to properly trained physician assistants. Certainly, in terms of the fund of medical knowledge and practice testable by examination, this does not seem to be the case.

The principal need for physician assistant residencies seems to be in specialty and subspecialty education. In data presented at the 1998 Clinical Congress of the American College of Surgeons, of 2500 physician assistant respondents to a questionaire from the American Academy of Physician Assistants, 35% were practicing in orthopedics, 23% in cardiac surgery, 17% in general surgery, 7% in neurosurgery, and the remaining 18% throughout other surgical disciplines. The training of many of these individuals was "on the job," usually by the physician signatory of their license. While there are currently 10 surgical physician assistant residencies in the country, there will be an increased need for trained physician assistants in the future, and the educational needs will increase apace.

In most teaching hospitals, the service needs of the surgical service have traditionally been provided by residents. But as the service needs of hepatic transplantation programs and cardiac surgical programs have diverged from the fundamental goals of educating the next generation of general surgeons, a haphazard pattern of providing service has emerged. The residency review committee for surgery and the Association of Program Directors in Surgery are in the process of ensuring that the focus of general surgical residency remains on learning general surgery rather than addressing the service needs of the hospital. They are also addressing the excess of preliminary surgical residency positions beyond the needs of the surgical subspecialties or the opportunities for candidates to finish in a categorical slot. This has created a significant group of competent individuals with good scores on the in-training examination and good recommendations from their program director with no place to go. The fact that so many of these individuals are international medical graduates raises concerns about fairness and exploitation that have risen to the level of Immigration and Naturalization Services and the Educational Council on Foreign Medical Graduates.

The logical alternative to excessive preliminary residents is physician assistants, yet we have argued in the previous commentary that this can be expensive. The expense can be significantly offset by billing and collecting on behalf of the physician assistant, who can now collect 13.6% of the surgeon's fees for Medicare and Medicaid patients. To do this, the physician assistant must not be claimed in the Medicare cost report filed by the hospital, or "double-dipping" will have occurred. But if a group or surgical practice plan employs the individual, this is not a problem. In most states, while Medicare reimburses the teaching hospital for surgical residents, it is the expectation that a resident of sufficient training and skill will be available to help. If this is not the case, a bill can be submitted on behalf of an appropriately trained assistant surgeon or physician assistant. In some states, a letter must be signed by the chief of surgery every time this occurs, but in others retrospective review of hospital records in any audit may suffice. In our experience, these collections for clinical services may underwrite the entire cost of the physician assistant's salary and benefits.

The real crux of the matter is training physician assistant residents alongside surgical residents. In many hospitals, the exact cases that are judged by residents to be of marginal educational value are the very cases on which surgical physician assistants will earn their living. Examples include vascular access for hemodialysis, routine coronary artery bypass surgery, and arthroscopy. Vascular access cases are illustrative of the problem. In many ways, dialysis patients are the "outpatient critically ill"—they have complex illnesses, multiple problems, and multiple procedures, but may be employed and vigorous members of society. Most access procedures are relatively minor technical undertakings, but these are the patient's lifeline and should not be underestimated in their overall importance. With patients now commonly living with dialysis for 20 years or more, repeated loss of vascular conduit due to imprecise technical skills or clinical decisions can reach life-threatening (or life-shortening) proportions.

Safe performance of vascular access surgery requires communication with the dialysis unit and nephrologist, coordination with the anesthesiologist, and communication with both patient and dialysis unit postoperatively. For the tiny number of patients who will encounter a surgical or (more likely) medical problem in the course of their procedure, a capsulized summary of their medical history and current medical issues on their medical record is essential. There are specific procedures to be learned, such as the Allen test, a careful vascular history, and interpretation of noninvasive vascular evaluations. All of these skills can be formalized, documented, and reviewed to prove that the physician assistant is often considerably more knowledgeable in his or her specific area of responsibility than the average postgraduate year 1 or 2 surgical resident usually assigned to the case. It will often be the case that a trained physician assistant will be the person to whom residents look for advice on quality standards and problem solving. It is also obvious that the implementation of "best clinical practices" is a natural complement to this process, and should achieve significant economies of utilization and scale.

But how to get to that point? Most physician assistants have only completed 6- to 8-week surgical rotations during their training, similar to medical school rotations. We would argue that a 1-year course of training for surgical physician assistants should exist alongside surgical residencies. In rotations involving 4 to 6 months of general surgery, 1 to 2 months of critical care, 1 to 2 months of emergency department evaluation of surgical problems, and 2 to 4 months of electives, together with clinic and office experience, programs such as Norwalk Hospital, Norwalk, Conn, and Martin Luther King Medical Center, Los Angeles, Calif, have turned out mature, experienced professionals. Norwalk Hospital created a program as an alternative to a physician surgical residency, but future programs should consider training physician assistants and residents in a "blended" manner. There are several reasons for this. If 83% of health care is provided at the community hospital level, the sooner surgical residents begin to think of physician assistants as colleagues and integrated members of the surgical team, the better. Educational needs in surgery require case conferences, didactics, bedside teaching, quality assurance, and review. These all preexist in resident teaching programs, under the guidance and standards of the Accreditation Council on Graduate Medical Education and its residency review committees. In the same way that the residency review committee for surgery insists that the training of surgical fellows not interfere with the training of general surgery residents, the educational goals and oversite of physician assistant surgical residencies in surgical teaching hospitals should be similarly monitored for intrinsic volume, quality, standards, and beneficial effect on the surgery resident's program. The very cases the residents feel overburdened with in terms of service-to-education value may be the exact type of service or subspecialty cases in which the physician assistants will earn their living. If there is a really large volume of surgical educational opportunity in a specific area uncovered by residents, it may be appropriate to create a second year of physician assistant fellowship in such focused areas as orthopedic surgery, cardiac surgery, vascular surgery, trauma surgery, critical care, or pediatric surgery. As hospital networks increasingly mature, fellowship-trained physician assistants may become an important link in the evaluation, safe transfer, and coordination of tertiary care between community hospital and teaching hospital.

The imperative to downsize postgraduate medical education is on us, and preemptive strategies to deal with the service workload at teaching hospitals are essential. We believe that an increased formal reliance on physician assistants, with an associated increase in postgraduate medical education for physican assistants, will be an important and cost-effective tool in this process, and will have the net effect of improving the overall quality of surgical education and surgical care at teaching hospitals, community teaching hospitals, and community hospitals.

Marvin A. McMillen, MD
Paul West, PA-C
Chicago, Ill

Corresponding author: Marvin McMillen, MD, Department of Surgery, Montefiore Medical Center, 111 E 210th St, Bronx, NY 10467-2490.

REFERENCES

1. McMillen MA. The value of surgical residencies to community teaching hospitals. *Arch Surg.* 1998; 133:1039-1040.
2. Teaching IMGs to practice as PAs. *Clinician News.* 1998;1:1.

Comprehensive Vascular Exposures

by Ronald J. Stoney, MD, and David J. Effeney, MBBS, FRACS, 208 pp, with 248 illus, $110, ISBN 0-397-51342-9, Philadelphia, Pa, Lippincott-Raven Publishers, 1998.

Few would argue with the proposition that safe, appropriate, and adequate exposure remains a cornerstone to successful outcome in vascular surgery. This well-written and appropriately illustrated volume focuses exclusively on the anatomical and technical details relating to the regional exposure of blood vessels required for most procedures in the repertoire of the vascular surgeon. Within less than 200 pages, 10 chapters cover approaches on a regional basis and are supported by more than 200 illustrations, a highlight of this book. These illustrations, the work of Eileen Natuzzi, MD, a vascular trainee, consist of large, beautifully executed, and anatomically correct color drawings and line drawings that emphasize important points in the text. Additional illustrations include intraoperative and cadaveric dissection photographs. In almost all cases, the illustrations are conveniently juxtaposed with the relevant text.

Each of the 7 chapters relating to regional exposures is formatted in a similar way, covering relevant and often detailed surgical anatomy, positioning of the patient, details of incisions, dissection, and the use of appropriate retractors. Each section concludes with a note on methods of normal closure. Chapter 2, "Practical Application of the Principles," describes in detail the surgical approach to exposure of the femoral vessels in the groin (the point where most trainees cut their vascular teeth) and stresses vascular surgical principles, including methods of scissors and forceps dissection, planes of dissection, the handling of tributary veins and lymphatics, and the use of diathermy, suture, vascular slings and clamps, and appropriate retraction. There is a section on techniques used in the reoperative groin and the lateral-sartorius border approach to the profunda femoris and superficial femoral artery. This chapter is appropriately placed. By describing principles of dissection common to all approaches, it largely avoids repetition in subsequent chapters.

Other chapters explore (1) neck surgery, including the approach to carotid bifurcation and the common carotid artery, with a note on the authors' preferred method of exposure of the distal internal carotid artery; (2) temporomandibular subluxation or dislocation; (3) surgery of the base of the neck, including exposure of the subclavian artery, brachial plexus, and first rib; (4) mediastinum surgery, including median sternotomy, ascending aorta, brachiocephalic artery, and neck extensions; and (5) thoracic surgery, including the left transthoracic approach to the left subclavian artery and descending aorta. The chapter on the abdomen is, in my opinion, the best in this book. It shows approaches to the infrarenal, juxta, and suprarenal aorta, thoracoabdominal exposure, and medial visceral rotation, together with approaches to the inferior vena cava and major tributaries of the portal system.

The chapters on the upper and lower extremities are good. In the latter chapter, there is considerable overlap with chapter 2. The approach to the crural vessels is particularly well described.

The last chapter briefly describes aortofemoral, femorofemoral, and axillofemoral tunnels. It also has a brief description of thoracoretroperitoneal routes and the authors' preferred route for deep and anatomical infrainguinal bypass.

I did have a few minor quibbles with the book. I suspect that the authors, in describing their own preferred basic approaches, avoided a description of the pros and cons of alternative or less commonly used approaches, which would have added to the size and cost of this publication. A bibliography for other approaches, such as the transaxillary approach to the first rib and its structures, vertebral artery approaches, skull-base approach to the internal carotid artery, and obturator bypass, among others, would have enhanced the value of this book. Reading descriptive anatomy without accompanying illustrations was irksome. Rereading these sections with an accompanying anatomy atlas greatly assisted comprehension and is recommended. The color photographs of cadaveric dissections, in my view, do not add to the text and vary in tonal quality.

This book is well written and the illustrations are notable. By limiting its scope to vascular exposures, it neatly fills a niche. This would be on my prescribed short list as a basic book for residents rotating through a vascular unit and for vascular fellows. I also suspect that many established vascular surgeons will purchase and use this book.

Edward J. Immelman, FCSSA, FRCSE
Cape Town, South Africa

Safe Answers for the American Board of Surgery Certifying Exam

4th ed, by Sarmad Aji, MD, 263 pp, $74.95, 1998. [Available only by mail order: PO Box #1920, Clintwood, VA 24228.]

Although not a surgical text in the traditional sense, this practical reference will serve many readers' needs. This work has recently been published in a much improved and updated fourth edition and represents a commendable effort on the part of Sarmad Aji, MD.

This reference is designed to review the commonly asked questions on the American Board of Surgery Certifying Examination. The author states that he interviewed countless numbers of examinees and board examiners and gathered together their experiences with questions commonly asked on the examination. Dr Aji has sought to present these topics in a logical, consistent, and thoughtful style that he hopes will allow the reader to answer the rare question not covered in the chapters. This edition, in contrast to previous versions, is improved by its complete table of contents and its correct use of English. The previous editions suffered from rampant typographical and grammatical errors, although the surgical management strategies presented were sound. This book is not written in a strict question and answer format, but does often offer an example of a generic patient (whom you might even think that you recognize) to lead off the discussion about the workup of each particular topic, such as a 35-year-old woman with a breast mass.

This tool is not limited to those preparing for their first certifying examination. Chief residents in general surgery will find the information in this text invaluable during morning reports and morbidity and mortality conferences, allowing them to present at least one reasonable way to address nearly every surgical predicament. Those taking the recertifying examination as well as those just out into practice will also enjoy this source for its clarity and ability to refresh and quickly present the workups (ie, ordering the correct studies) for common surgical problems encountered during a busy clinic day.

The author has assumed a certain baseline knowledge of surgical disease that is appropriate for the intended audience. This text therefore limits its focus to the diagnosis and therapy of common and not-so-common surgical diseases, appropriately leaving in-depth historical and pathophysiologic discussions for more comprehensive texts. I would prefer that this book be offered in a more portable bound format, but it is very easy to reduce its size to 8.5×11 in using a photocopier.

This text is well written and can form an excellent supplement for self-preparation for the board examination. It is enjoyable to use and gives readers the feeling that they are taking a look inside the mind of an experienced clinical general surgeon.

Brian S. Cain, MD
Oakland, Calif

An Update of Tumor Metastasis to the Breast Data

We read with interest the article on carcinoid tumor metastatic to the breast by Rubio et al[1] published in the October 1998 issue of the ARCHIVES. For the benefit of the readers, we would like to update the data on tumor metastasis to the breast.

Using the MEDLINE database and other reports,[2] we have reviewed 24 articles presenting data from 1855 to 1998. We found a total of 431 cases of tumor metastasis to the breast. The primary sites for metastasis were malignant melanoma (87 cases), lung (78 cases), ovary (50 cases), prostate (39 cases), kidney (24 cases), stomach (15 cases), ileum (13 cases), thyroid (12 cases), cervix (12 cases), and other (101 cases). On the basis of this review, we found an unusually high number of malignant melanoma metastases to the breast.

Suraj Alva, MD
Neetha Shetty-Alva, MD
Providence, RI

1. Rubio IT, Korourian S, Brown H, Cowan C, Klimberg VS. Carcinoid tumor metastatic to the breast. *Arch Surg.* 1998;133:1117-1119.
2. Shetty MR, Ahmed MI, Khan FR. Metastatic tumors to the breast: a review: 1855 AD to 1993 AD. In: *Proceedings of the XVI UICC International Cancer Congress, New Delhi, India.* Bologna, Italy: Monduzzi Editore. 1994:1577-1581. International Proceedings Series.

From Tennis Courts to Transplants

PROFESSOR JANNIE LOUW and Hamilton Naki were my guides and greatest helpers throughout my postgraduate surgical career. "Hami" Naki was born on June 26, 1926, in the district of Kentani in what was then Transkei. He was 1 of the 3 children of Mduna and Ainei. He attended school near his home and completed standard 6 (junior high school) at age 14 years. He worked with his parents for a few years and then came to Cape Town, South Africa, at age 18 years to seek employment. His first job was to help in the garden of the University of Cape Town, and his specific task was to roll the grass tennis courts.

While doing this one day, he was summoned by Robert Goetz, MD, who was the first and only J. S. Marais traveling fellow and who had left Europe to take a position in the new surgical laboratory. There were limited funds and almost no experts to consult, but Goetz was a remarkable innovator and inventor with ideas and abilities ahead of his time. Young Hamilton helped him in any way possible and absorbed his ability to make something out of nothing. These were exciting years. Most of the research was done with dogs, which he learned to anesthetize, and he is one of the few surgical researchers who helped operate on a giraffe (to dissect the jugular venous valves to determine why giraffes do not faint when bending to drink).

When Goetz left, Hamilton became both the surgical and the anaesthetic research assistant. For several years, work in the laboratory was sporadic, as different young surgeons with minimal funds and few ideas came and went. Then came

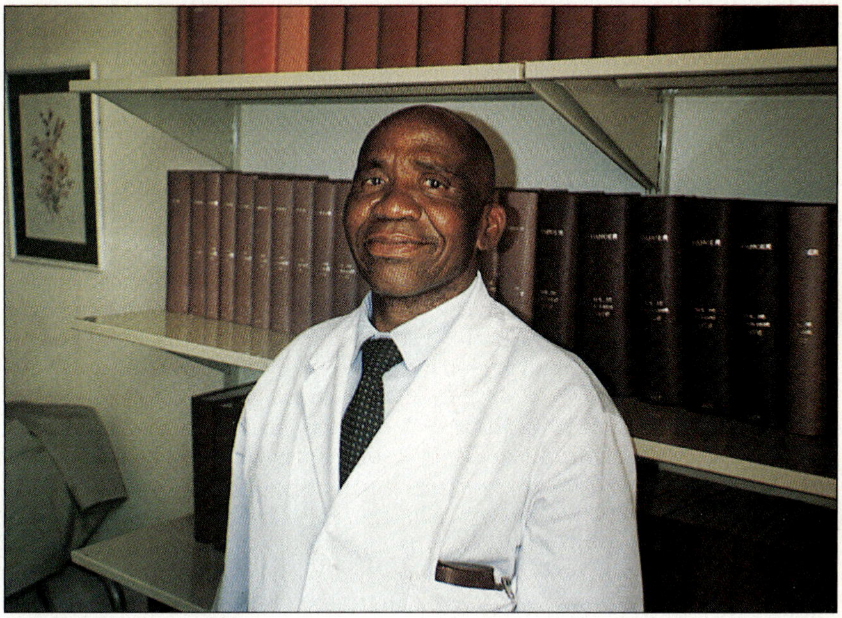

Hamilton Naki

Hamilton's second break. A young cardiac surgeon, Christiaan Barnard, MD, began to introduce to South Africa the new techniques of open heart surgery and cardiopulmonary bypass surgery, which he had learned in the United States. His anesthetist was Hamilton, his surgical assistant Victor Fick, and his pump technician Prescott Madlingozi, ably assisted by "Boots" Clifford Snyders and John Roussouw. In those days, finger pumps circulated blood through heat exchangers warmed or cooled by great steel tanks of water of the required temperature. The techniques were perfected and then introduced clinically to establish cardiac surgery on a firm footing. Ten to 15 years later, these techniques and Barnard's skill and guts gave South Africa, the University of Cape Town, and the J. S. Marais laboratory international attention when the first heart transplantation was performed there in 1967. One of the people closest to Barnard in many of the photographs was Hamilton, now relieved of his anesthetic duties and appointed principal surgical assistant of the laboratory because of his remarkable skill and dexterity.

The next few years brought visitors from around the world to the laboratory and the walls rang with tongues from countries that the assistants had never heard of. In 1968, the cardiac surgical research team moved to sparkling new headquarters in the Heart Disease and Organ Transplantation building funded by the Anglo American Corporation, Johannesburg, Gauteng. Hamilton was involved in the evolution of the heterotopic "piggyback" heart transplantation technique, but because of a personality clash between himself and an ill-mannered young researcher, he moved back to the J. S. Marais laboratory. Their loss was our inestimable gain—the liver transplantation technique learned by John Terblanche, MD, in Bristol, England, needed to be developed in Cape Town and Hamilton applied his attention to this area. Despite his limited conventional education, he had an amazing ability to learn anatomical names and recognize anomalies. His skills ranged from assisting to operating and he frequently prepared the donor animal (sometimes single-handedly) while another team worked on the recipient. He helped to train and guide Gerald de Vos, Edward Henry, Nolan Hendricks, Thomson Magxala, and Johannes Williams as a highly competent team of assistants.

He must have been principal surgical assistant at as many liver transplantation operations as most operating nurses and his sterile techniques and care of instruments rivaled many. He was also probably unique in once assisting with a delicate hepatic arterial anastomosis while gently rocking my baby's cradle.

When he retired in 1991, there was some question about the duration of his pension contributions. This was not helped by the fact that complete records were not kept when he started working; indeed, the buildings that housed the financial department were not even in existence.

Hamilton arrived at work at 6 AM come rain, shine, or strike and no matter how far he had to travel he almost never missed a day. In latter days when strikes disrupted the public transportation system, he left so early in the morning that the blockades had not yet been erected.

He was always immaculately dressed in a suit, tie, and hat and his shoes sparkled, which often put to shame young researchers dressed in tattered jeans and scuffed sneakers. When not operating, he would read his Bible at work, and was a senior and respected member of his church community. He was known as one of the longest-serving members of the university community and was beloved by all. He tried to influence the vagrants who slept in the cemetery behind the medical school, sometimes with success, and could often be seen in long discussions with them on the benches along the road.

Since his retirement, he has commuted between Cape Town in Langa, where his house is in the special single quarters, and Kentani, where some of his family lives. In Kentani, he has helped the community in many ways, such as in the construction of a school and in the provision of a mobile clinic for the thousands of people for whom the previous closest medical care was 70 km away on foot.

He is truly a remarkable man whose great influence and patient teaching skills will never be forgotten by any of the visiting or local surgical researchers, consultants, or registrars.

When asked by a news reporter how he had managed to learn all the surgical skills that he had without formal training, he smiled and said quietly, "I stole with my eyes."

Rosemary Hickman, MD
Cape Town, South Africa

Medical Education in Early 19th Century America

AFTER 1800, in an attempt to upgrade the level of formal medical education in America, medical colleges were being founded wherever there seemed to be large enough populations to financially support them. By 1810, 7 medical schools (University of Pennsylvania [1765]; King's College, now Columbia [1767]; Harvard [1782]; Dartmouth [1797]; College of Physicians and Surgeons of New York City [1807]; University of Maryland [1807]; and the short-lived institution at Brown University [1807]) were providing course work. The total number of medical students in attendance was approximately 650, 406 of whom were at the University of Pennsylvania.

Following the War of 1812, the growth of new facilities continued unabated, especially in sparsely settled areas of the country. This demand for institutions in the frontier led to the establishment of the College of Physicians and Surgeons of the Western District at Fairfield, Herkimer County, New York (1813); the Medical Department of Transylvania University, Lexington, Ky (1818); Castleton Medical College Castleton, Vt (1818); and the Medical College of Ohio, Cincinnati (1819). By 1845, almost 40 medical schools were in existence, scattered from Maine down to Georgia, out to Louisiana and Missouri, and up to Illinois. Although many of these medical "colleges" were associated with academic institutions of higher standards than medical education itself could claim, the connection was largely nominal. Quite simply, a group of local practitioners who wished to start a medical school would approach a "name" academic institution and seek permission to grant degrees under its charter, or would obtain a license from the state as an independent educational institution authorized to award the medical degree.

More often than not, these "proprietary" schools consisted of a single large room suitable for lectures, a small library containing books on loan from a local faculty member, and an adjoining, underequipped space for anatomical or chemical demonstrations. Clinical instruction was strictly by lecture and rote learning from textbooks. The standard curriculum consisted of 7 courses (anatomy, physiology, and pathology; materia medica, therapeutics, and pharmacy; chemistry; medical jurisprudence; theory and practice of medicine; principles and practice of surgery; and obstetrics and the diseases of women and children). There was no consideration of scientific research or other nonpractical matters.

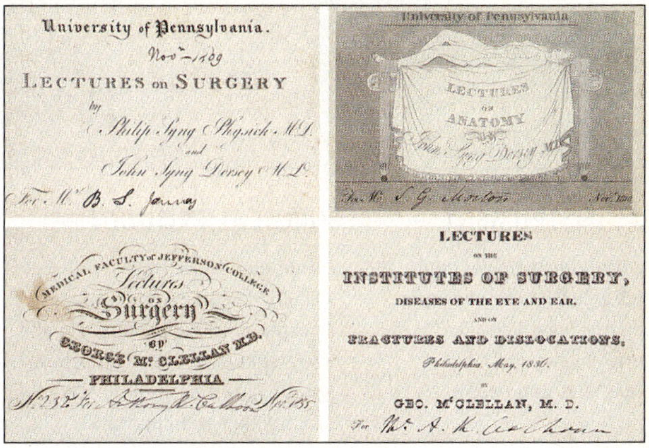

Early 19th century medical students were admitted to clinical lecture series by showing individually purchased attendance cards. Some of the cards were quite ornate; others were ordinary in appearance (Courtesy of Historical Collections, College of Physicians of Philadelphia, Pa).

Such modern-day necessities as the ever-present classroom laboratory were unheard of, nor did the concept of bedside clinical instruction even exist. Instead, students endured 6 to 8 hours daily of a humdrum existence. The entire student body would be assembled in the large amphitheater to sit and listen to one lecturer after another, with this routine lasting from mid October to the beginning of March. Following a second year of this monotonous existence, with the second term identical in course content to the first, the student became eligible to receive his medical degree. Other specific requirements varied from one school to another, but usually entailed the writing of a "thesis" on some subject connected with the science of medicine. Any semblance of hands-on clinical instruction could only be obtained by the student becoming a private pupil or apprentice to a local practitioner and observing their interaction with patients.

Ira M. Rutkow, MD, MPH, DrPH

PRODUCTS & SERVICES

The information given here is supplied by the companies cited. Publication of these notices does not imply endorsement or warranty by the American Medical Association, publishers of the *Archives of Surgery*.

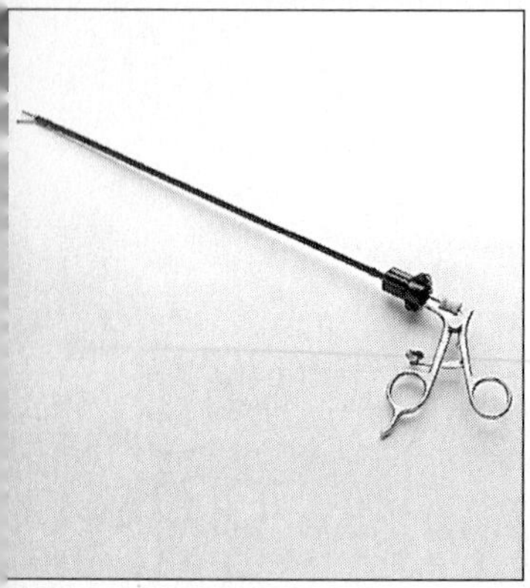

SURGICAL INSTRUMENT —

Aslan Medical Technologies has introduced a locking scissors-grip handle for the new VersaLap™ line of instruments used in laparoscopic and endoscopic surgery.

The stainless-steel handle is an alternative to the company's new Sensor™ handles, which offer a radical (and comfortable) straight-line design.

Unlike disposable instruments, it can be sterilized in an autoclave and re-used for a net reduction in instrument costs and medical waste. A non-locking insulated model is also available for electrocautery use.

Aslan Medical Technologies manufactures a growing line of custom instruments for minimally invasive surgery.

For information write
ASLAN MEDICAL TECHNOLOGIES
4110 South 9th Street
Kalamazoo, MI 49009

Call toll free
800-551-4561

Fax
616-372-9639

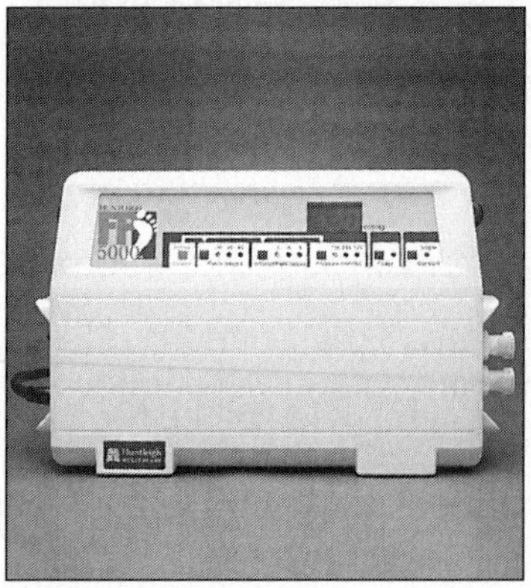

SURGICAL PRODUCT —

Huntleigh Healthcare introduces its FP5000™ Pump System in-service poster as an educational aid and reference guide for the hospital staff. Providing step-by-step instruction and application procedures, this tool aids the hospital staff in properly utilizing the FP5000 Pump System for the prevention of deep vein thrombosis (DVT).

The FP5000 Pump System, provides external intermittent pneumatic compression of the foot. It is the ideal prophylactic modality when use of standard calf or thigh length garments is inappropriate.

The pump is equipped with state-of-the-art microprocessor technology featuring smart alarms, readout of true therapy pressures and the ability to operate the pump in single leg mode when only one garment is needed. A range of pressure, inflation and cycle time options can be easily programmed.

Huntleigh Healthcare is a wholly-owned subsidiary of Huntleigh Technology, plc, a prominent manufacturer of a variety of healthcare products used in homes, hospitals and extended care facilities.

For information write
HUNTLEIGH HEALTHCARE
Attn: Steve Clavelle
227 Route 33 East
Manalapan, NJ 07726-8362

Call toll free
800-223-1218 x170

Fax
732-446-1938

Web site
www.huntleigh-healthcare.com

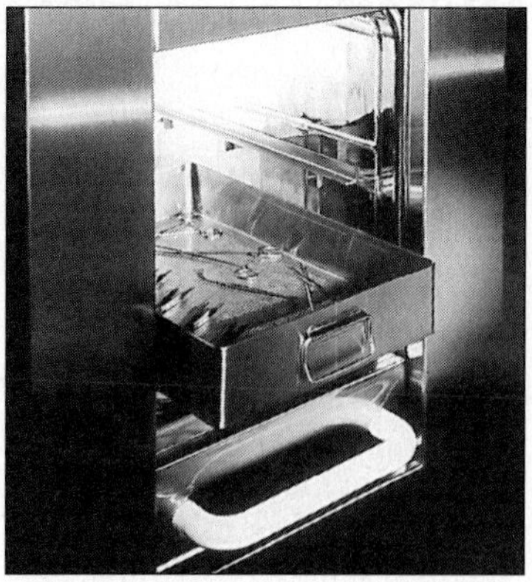

STERILIZATION PRODUCT —

Primus Sterilizer Company, Inc. announces their new "Stat-Cycle"™ flash sterilization cycle, for their small and medium sized sterilizers.

Primus sterilizers, already known for their uncomplicated design and reliable service, now offer flash sterilization cycles that can be minutes faster than with older style inefficient cylindrical chambers. When the need arises to flash-sterilize instruments or apparatus "stat," Primus' "Stat-Cycle"™ uses their volume-efficient rectangular chamber, to reduce start-to-finish cycle times. A single push-button initiates the Stat-Cycle™, which has been preset to preferred time and temperature parameters.

The volume efficient chamber also provides operational economies. The Primus sterilizer consumes less steam per cycle, and when used with the integral electric steam boilers, electricity consumption is also reduced.

The Primus sterilizer with Stat-Cycle™ includes a polished type 316L stainless steel chamber with a Pri-Mirror™ mirror-reflective surface.

For information write
PRIMUS STERILIZER COMPANY, INC
Attn: Connie Mansfield
117 South 25th Street
Omaha, NE 68131

Phone
402-344-4200

Fax
402-344-4242

E-mail
primussales@nfinity.com

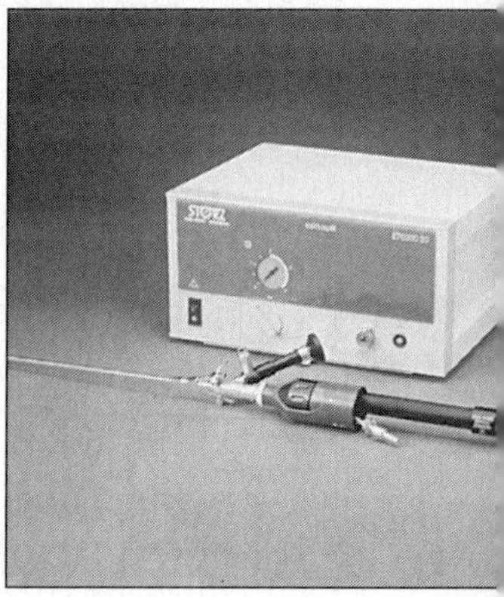

SURGICAL INSTRUMENT —

Karl Storz Endoscopy-America, Inc introduces the Calcusplit™ Pneumatic Lithotriptor for effective intracorporeal stone management. Driven by compressed air, the Calcusplit™'s pneumatic energy source disintegrates even the hardest stones quickly and effectively without heat, thus preventing possible tissue damage.

Calcusplit™ utilizes a variety of reusable probes available in solid or hollow styles starting at an 0.8 mm diameter. The probes are compatible with existing ureteroscopes and percutaneous nephroscopes and are completely autoclavable to withstand the rigors of day-to-day sterilization procedures.

Calcusplit™'s simple design is easy to use, clean and sterilize, and it can operate either from the hospital's existing compressed air supply or E-cylinder. The Calcusplit™ also comes with an exclusive adapter to provide ergonomic, one-handed operation with ureteroscopes.

For information write
KS ENDOSCOPY-AMERICA, INC
600 Corporate Pointe
Culver City, CA 90230-7600

Call toll free
800-421-0837

Web site
www.karlstorz.com

Classified Advertising

Academic/Faculty
Cardiovascular/Thoracic Surgery
CME Corner
Chiefs/Department Heads/ Directors
Courses/Symposia/Seminars
Facial Plastic Surgery
Graduate Training/ Residencies/Fellowships
Locum Tenens Wanted
Multiple Specialties/Group Practice
Neurosurgery
Notices
Othopedic Surgery
Pediatric Surgery
Plastic Surgery
Practices For Sale
Surgical Specialities
Thoracic Surgery
Vascular Surgery

Sales Information

1999 CLASSIFIED ADVERTISING RATES

Regular	1x 1.65/wd	*3x 1.55/wd
Bold	1x 1.85/wd	*3x 1.75/wd

*In order to receive the 3-time frequency price, the request must be made upon initial placement. The minimum charge is 20 words. A word consists of one or more letters surrounded by space on each side. For information on display advertising and our network buys contact an account representative.

POLICY

Orders for classified advertising must be submitted in writing. Although the American Medical Association believes the classified advertisements in these pages to be from reputable sources, the Association does not investigate the offers made and assumes no liability concerning them. Acceptance of advertising is restricted to professional opportunities, practices for sale, and medical office space available. The Association reserves the right to decline, withdraw, or edit advertisements at its discretion. Every care is taken to avoid mistakes but responsibility cannot be accepted by the Association for clerical or printer's errors.

REPLY BOX SERVICE

Confidential box numbers are available for an additional $25 per issue, plus the words: Box ________, c/o SUR. When responding to a box number, please send to Archives of Surgery, Box ________, c/o SUR, 515 N State St, Chicago, IL 60610.

CANCELLATIONS/CHANGES

Cancellations/changes must be received in writing at least 25 days prior to the date of the issue. In order to expedite, please fax to 312-464-5909 to the attention of your account representative.

GENERAL INFORMATION

To contact a Classified Advertising account representative, call 312-464-2475/2490/2491/4485 or 800-AMA-2260. Or fax your insertion order to 312-464-5909. Mail your materials to AMA Classified Advertising, 12th Floor, 515 N State St, Chicago, IL 60610.

ACADEMIC/FACULTY

SPARTANBURG REGIONAL HEALTHCARE SYSTEM. SURGICAL EDUCATION. SOUTH CAROLINA - GENERAL SURGERY RESIDENCY PROGRAM: An exceptional opportunity for a board-certified Surgeon with an emphasis in general surgery and critical care medicine to join the Surgical Education Faculty at Spartanburg Regional Medical Center. The physician will be responsible for teaching general surgery residents as well as conducting a limited private practice. Affiliated with the Medical University of South Carolina and the University of South Carolina. Exceptional call coverage arrangement. A previous academic appointment will be a plus. Trauma experience is necessary, as Spartanburg Regional Medical Center is one of four Level I Trauma facilities in the state of South Carolina. Outstanding salary based upon background and experience, as well as an excellent comprehensive benefits package including relocation expenses, CME and professional liability insurance. Research opportunities are also available. For confidential consideration please contact Cathy K. Benson, CMSR, Spartanburg Regional Medical Center, 800-890-0138 or Fax your CV: 864-560-7472. Cbenson@srhs.com EOE.

SURGICAL CRITICAL CARE/TRAUMA. ASSISTANT/ASSOCIATE PROFESSOR: The Department of Surgery at Robert C. Byrd Health Sciences Center of WVU/Charleston Division/Charleston Area Medical Center, is seeking a general surgeon with interest in surgical critical care and trauma. Fellowship training with eligibility or added certification qualifications in Surgical Critical Care required. Charleston Area Medical Center is a State, Level I trauma center with helicopter and ACGME accredited General Surgery Residency. Opportunities for clinical research, resident and student education, and general surgery practice are available. Application Deadline: Position will remain open until filled. Send curriculum vitae to James P. Boland, MD, Professor and Chairman, Department of Surgery, 3110 MacCorkle Ave, SE, Charleston, WV 25304. Phone: 304-347-1233, Fax: 304-347-1343. E-mail: james .boland@camcare.com

ANNOUNCEMENT

Call for Crossword Puzzle Creators

We are looking for persons interested in creating ophthalmic-oriented crossword puzzles for the *Archives of Ophthalmology*. If you are interested in generating crossword puzzles on an ongoing basis, please contact the editorial office at *Archives of Ophthalmology*, 2870 University Ave, Suite 102, Madison, WI 53705; telephone: (608) 262-7769; fax: (608) 265-5896; e-mail: archives@eyesee.ophth.wisc.edu

HEMATOLOGY & ONCOLOGY

SPARTANBURG REGIONAL HEALTHCARE SYSTEM. SURGICAL EDUCATION. SURGICAL ONCOLOGIST: South Carolina - General Surgery Residency Program: An exceptional opportunity for a board-certified Surgical Oncologist to join the Surgical Education Faculty at Spartanburg Regional Medical Center. The physician will be responsible for teaching general surgery residents as well as conducting a limited private practice. Affiliated with the Medical University of South Carolina and the University of South Carolina. Exceptional call coverage arrangement. A previous academic appointment will be a plus. Trauma experience is necessary, as Spartanburg Regional Medical Center is one of four Level I Trauma facilities in the state of South Carolina. The system offers a range of specialized healthcare services that is unrivaled in its five-county service region, featuring world-class specialty centers, including the Regional Cancer Center, a 100,000+ square foot state-of-the-art facility scheduled to open in June of 1999. Outstanding salary based upon background and experience, as well as an excellent comprehensive benefits package including relocation expenses, CME and professional liability insurance. Research opportunities are also available. For confidential consideration please contact Cathy K. Benson, CMSR, Spartanburg Regional Medical Center, 800-890-0138 or Fax your CV: 864-560-7472. Cbenson@srhs.com EOE.

LEGAL SERVICES

LOCUM TENENS WANTED

LOCUM TENENS OPPORTUNITIES: are available throughout the US for Physicians of all specialties. Please Fax CV to Staff Exchange @ 770-751-6695 or call: 888-842-4049.

PRACTICES FOR SALE

SENIOR SOLO: General Surgeon in Atlanta area wishes to sell practice totally. FAX inquires to 770-739-2803.

SURGERY: GENERAL

FOX RIVER VALLEY, WI: Town of 14,000 (draw 50,000) thirty minutes from Green Bay. Join another surgeon in 14-physician group, proven caseload. Endoscopy, laparoscopy required, C-sections preferred, vascular a plus. For consideration, call Kari Donovan, 800-765-3055, ID#6378AR, Fax: 314-726-3009, e-mail: kdonovan@cejka.com Visit our website: www.cejka.com

GENERAL SURGERY, ACADEMIC POSITION: Immediate opening for a General Surgeon at Scott & White Clinic and Texas A&M University Health Science Center at the assistant-associate professor level. Scott & White is the largest multispecialty clinic in the Southwest with over 500 physicians and boasts over a century of patient care. Our not-for-profit HMO, which currently contributes about 30% of our business, has over 165,000 members and has been ranked as one of the best in the nation. Interested candidates should have an academic background and a strong interest in teaching residents and medical students. The operative case load is 500+ per year and includes general and advanced laparoscopic surgery. No vascular, thoracic or endoscopic experience is required. Call is 1/6. Please respond with curriculum vitae and three letters of reference to Mike Nichols, Director of Physician Recruitment, Scott & White Clinic, 2401 S 31st St, Temple, TX 76508, or Fax: 254-724-4974. For more information about Scott & White, please visit our web site at http://www.sw.org Scott & White is an equal opportunity employer. Women & minority candidates are encouraged to apply. No J-1 opportunities available.

GENERAL SURGERY, PORTLAND, ORGEON: Northwest Permanente, PC, a physician-managed multispecialty group serving the members of Kaiser Permanente in the Northwest Division, has two excellent opportunities for BC/BE general and/or vascular surgeons. Our new associate will practice with the 21 general surgeons at Kaiser Permanente's affiliated hospitals in the Portland/Vancouver metropolitan area. The Northwest Division has a total of 24 general surgeons providing quality care to over 435,000 plan members in Oregon and Washington. Ours is a collegial and professionally stimulating practice in one of the most successful managed care programs in the country. In addition to a lifestyle inherent to the beautiful Pacific Northwest, we offer a predictable work schedule, and a competitive salary and benefit package which includes professional liability coverage, a comprehensive pension program, sabbatical leave and more. For additional information please forward CV to A. S. Weiland, MD, Regional Medical Director, NORTHWEST PERMANENTE, PC, 500 NE Multnomah, Ste 100, Portland, OR 97231-2099. EOE.

GENERAL SURGICAL GROUP seeking Board Certified surgeon with Trauma and ICU experience. Please send Curriculum Vitae to Flint Surgical Specialists, PC, 5210 Lapeer Rd, Burton, MI 48509.

HOSPITAL IN BEAUTIFUL SOUTHERN COLORADO COMMUNITY OF 4,000: near the foothills of the Rockies is adding a General Surgeon to their staff of 6 primary care physicians. Coverage w/another surgeon from a nearby community is available. Competitive salary & benefits, commensurate w/experience. Call Tony Stajduhar w/Summit Medical Consultants at 800-598-6610 for information.

LOGAN, UTAH: One BE/BC general surgeon needed for an outstanding practice opportunity. Employment position in a multi-specialty clinic within Intermountain Health Care's Physician Division. Practice in an area where many people visit to ski, fish, hike, camp and enjoy the beauty of the area. A low crime rate and family oriented culture makes this an ideal place in which to live. A negotiable salary and generous benefits package are offered with moving costs negotiable. For more information, send/Fax a CV to IHC Physician Services, Attn: Wilf Rudert, 36 S State St, 20th Fl, Salt LakeCity, UT 84111. 800-888-3134 #1. Fax: 801-442-2999. E-mail:comdixon@ihc.com Internet: http://www.ihc.com/phys_recruit

OPPORTUNITY IN NORTHEASTERN OKLAHOMA LAKE COUNTRY: Strong 70 bed JCAHO accredited not-for-profit hospital has an opportunity for 1 general surgeon. General surgery service area of 60,000+. 12 BC physicians on staff including an anesthesiologist. 40 minutes from Tulsa. Negotiable financial arrangements. Call Stan Schuermann at INTEGRIS Baptist Medical Center at 800-332-8663.

ANNOUNCEMENT

Volunteer Services Needed

CommunityHealth, a free primary care clinic serving uninsured and medically underserved patients, is seeking family practitioners and specialists to volunteer services at their north side Chicago location.

For information, contact Anna Hoeskstra, Volunteer Coordinator; telephone (773) 395-4840.

OPPORTUNITY FOR SEASONED, progressive, BC/BE general surgeon to immediately join busy, well established, private surgical practice. Located in Northern Michigan on the Great Lakes. Spectacular four season recreation, safe, caring, family oriented community. Supportive and friendly hospital and professional staff with over forty referring physicians and excellent ER, ICU, and diagnostic imaging support. Efficient, state-of-the-art office suite in new medical office building connected to hospital. Competitive salary with full benefits. Send cover letter and curriculum vitae to T. M. Burandt, DO & Associates, PC, 810 South Main Street, Suite#1, Cheboygan, MI 49721, Facsimile: 616-627-7758, E-mail: tburandt@cdimed.com

PIEDMONT NORTH CAROLINA: General Surgeon. Ideal candidate should have a strong vascular interest. You would be co-located with a solo general surgeon who has built a tremendous practice since moving here from residency nearly three years ago. This position will offer a guaranteed salary for the first year and a partnership tract. Candidates should have completed medical school at a LCME-accredited program and residency at a ACGME-accredited program. Safe, family-oriented community enjoys excellent school system, low crime, 97%+ employment, and many recreational activities in the beautiful rolling hills of NC. Mail CV to Randy Mitchell, Randolph Hospital, 364 White Oak St, Asheboro, NC 27203. Or Fax: 336-626-7664. Or call: 336-633-7777. E-mail: rlm@atomic.net Visit our website at www.randolphhospital.org

THREE PHYSICIAN GENERAL/VASCULAR PRACTICE: seeking surgeon with expert skills in breast and laparoscopic surgery. Board certified or Board eligible. Fax resume to 908-722-8676.

SURGERY: ORTHOPEDIC

OPPORTUNITY IN NORTHEASTERN OKLAHOMA LAKE COUNTRY: Strong not-for-profit hospital has an opportunity for 1 orthopedic surgeon. Orthopedic surgery service area of 60,000+. 70 bed JCAHO accredited hospital with 12 BC physicians on staff including an anesthesiologist. 40 minutes from Tulsa. Negotiable financial arrangements. Call Stan Schuermann at INTEGRIS Baptist Medical Center at 800-332-8663.

SURGERY: SURGICAL SPECIALTIES

TWO-SURGEON PRACTICE, located in central New York, seeks general surgeon with laparoscopic, vascular, and/or thoracic capabilities. Recent fellowship training desirable. Based in the scenic and cosmopolitan home of Cornell University. The practice serves two progressive medical centers. Excellent lifestyle opportunities abound in housing, education, and recreation. Reply to Box 323, c/o JAMA, 515 N State St, 12th Fl, Chicago, IL 60610.

SURGERY: THORACIC

LONG ISLAND - THORACIC SURGEON: BC/BE Thoracic Surgeon to join a busy 7 surgeon group practicing thoracic/vascular/general surgery 45 minutes from Manhattan. Send CV to Long Island Thoracic Surgeon, Ste 26, 375 E Main St, Bay Shore, NY 11706.

SURGERY: VASCULAR

DERRY, NH: Seeking BC/BE Vascular/General Surgeon for single specialty practice. Competitive compensation and benefits package. Call 1:3. Less than one hour from Boston. Contact: Cheryl DeVita at 800-678-7858; Fax: 314-726-0026; E-mail: cdevita@cejka.com ID#6486SURG. Visit our website at www.cejka.com

ANNOUNCEMENT

Notice to Authors of Reports From Clinical Trials

The Journal of the American Medical Association (JAMA) and the *Archives of Ophthalmology* function as an editorial consortium. With one submission and one set of reviews, your clinical trial manuscript will be considered for publication in both *JAMA* and the *Archives of Ophthalmology*.

Submit your paper to the journal of your choice according to the appropriate Instructions for Authors and the following guidelines will apply: 1. If your manuscript is accepted by *JAMA*, it will be considered for an editorial or commentary in *JAMA*. Your abstract will also be published in the *Archives of Ophthalmology* with a commentary or editorial. 2. If your manuscript is accepted by the *Archives of Ophthalmology*, it will be considered for an editorial or commentary in the *Archives of Ophthalmology*. Your abstract will also be considered for publication in *JAMA* and may be accompanied by a commentary or editorial in *JAMA*.

SPARTANBURG REGIONAL HEALTHCARE SYSTEM: SURGICAL EDUCATION. VASCULAR SURGEON: South Carolina - General Surgery Residency Program: An Exceptional opportunity for a board-certified Vascular Surgeon to join the Surgical Education Faculty at Spartanburg Regional Medical Center. The physician will be responsible for teaching general surgery residents as well as conducting a limited private practice. Affiliated with the Medical University of South Carolina and the University of South Carolina. Exceptional call coverage arrangement. A previous academic appointment will be a plus. Trauma experience is necessary, as Spartanburg Regional Medical Center is one of four Level I Trauma facilities in the state of South Carolina. The system offers a range of specialized healthcare services that is unrivaled in its five-county service region, featuring world-class specialty centers, including the Regional Heart Center. Outstanding salary based upon background and experience, as well as an excellent comprehensive benefits package including relocation expenses, CME and professional liability insurance. Research opportunities are also available. For confidential consideration please contact Cathy K. Benson, CMSR, Spartanburg Regional Medical Center, 800-890-0138 or Fax your CV: 864-560-7472. Cbenson@srhs.com EOE.

VASCULAR SURGEON: Beautiful Central Florida. Easy access to Orlando and Tampa. Moss-draped oak trees line hundred year old streets in our beautiful city. Practice vascular surgery and some general surgery as the third surgeon in a busy practice. Affiliate with two hospitals with more than 550 beds in the community. Call Robert Estes at 800-321-2460. FAX CV to 407-253-9055.

ANNOUNCEMENT

Call for Abstracts: Public Health Dentistry

The American Association of Public Health Dentistry (AAPHD) is inviting submissions of programmatic and scientific papers on a broad range of topics at its 62nd annual session. Topics include science-based and evidence-based approaches to health promotion, disease prevention and management, utilization of care, delivery systems, cost benefit and cost-effectiveness of programs, surveillance and epidemiology, health policies, knowledge, attitudes, and practices of the public and the profession, and education of health personnel, the public, and policy makers. The meeting will be held October 6 through 8, 1999, in Honolulu, Hawaii. The theme is Improving Public Health Through Global Partnerships.

The deadline is May 1, 1999. For a copy of the abstract form or further information, contact the AAPHD National Office, 3760 SW Lyle Ct, Portland, OR 97221, telephone: (503) 242-0712; fax: (503) 242-0721; e-mail: natoff@aol.com.

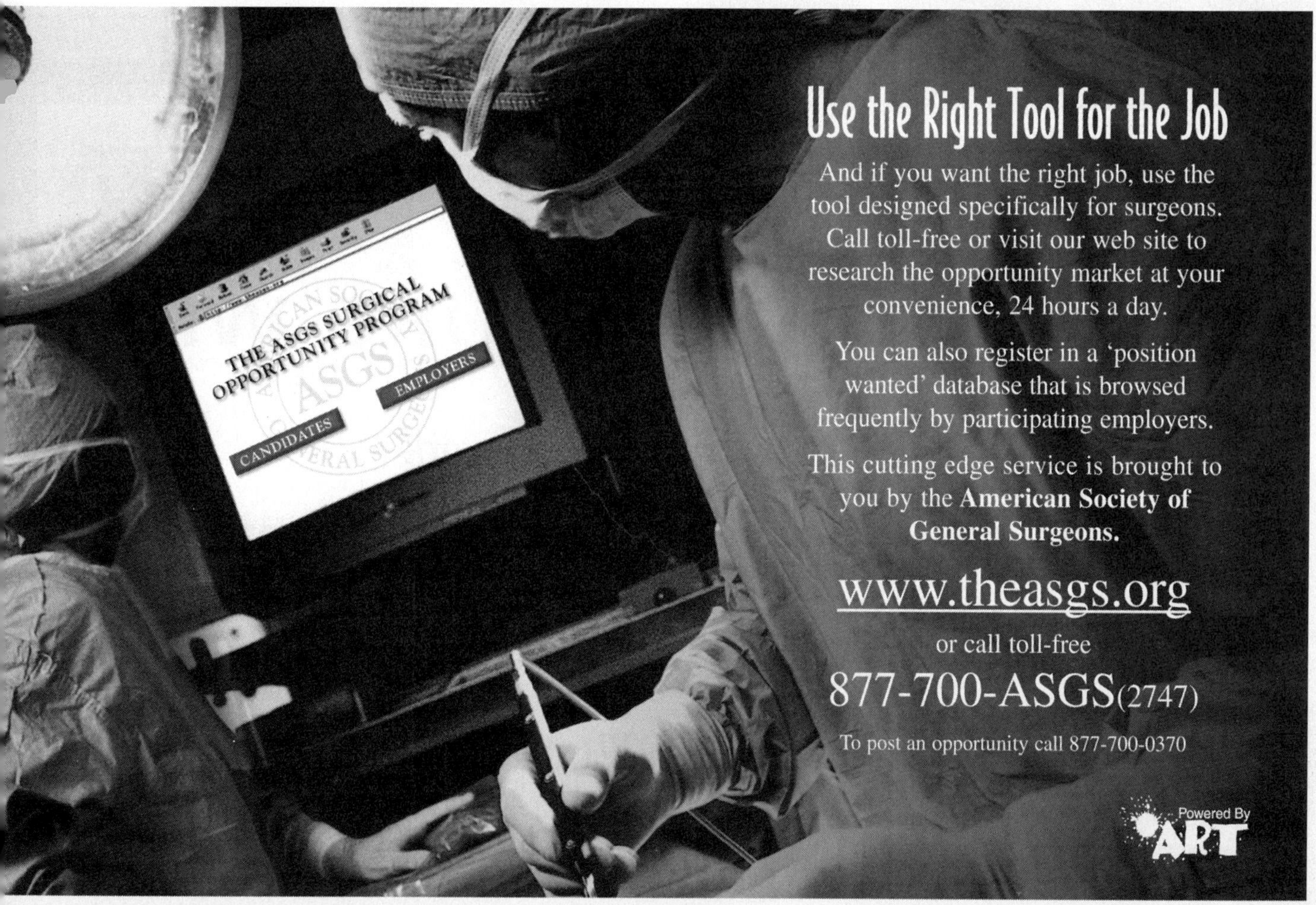

Index of Advertisers

CLASSIFIED ADVERTISING 455-460
http://www.ama-assn.org

ETHICON INC
Suture Assist 347

GLAXO WELLCOME
Panorex 349
Zofran .... Cover 2-345

PFIZER, US PHARMACEUTICAL GROUP
http://www.pfizer.com
Trovan .... Cover 4

While every precaution is taken to ensure accuracy, we cannot guarantee against the possibility of an occasional change or omission in the preparation of this index.

Document Delivery Information

Copies of individual articles are available from the following:

UnCover
Tel: 800-787-7979
303-758-3030
Fax: 303-758-5946
URL: http://uncweb.carl.org
e-mail: uncover@carl.org

Institute for Scientific Information (ISI)
Tel: 800-336-4474
215-386-0100
Fax: 215-386-6362
URL: http://www.isinet.com

TROVAN®
(trovafloxacin)

KC286D98

Pfizer U.S. Pharmaceuticals

ARCHIVES OF SURGERY

MAY 1999

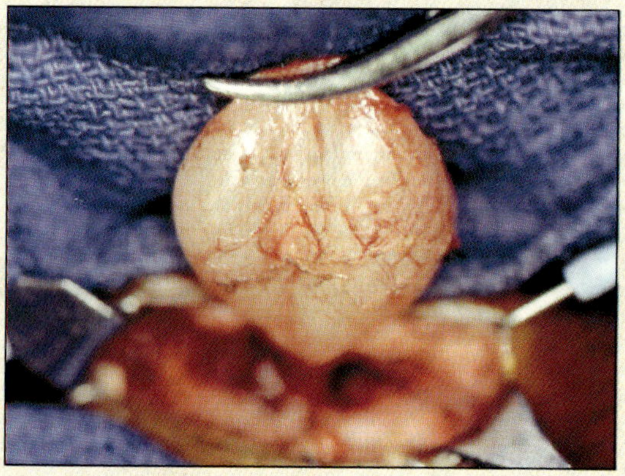

Thyroglossal duct cyst.

VANADATE AND THE ABSENCE OF MYOFIBROBLASTS IN WOUND CONTRACTION

WHOLE-BODY PET IMAGING WITH [18F]FLUORODEOXYGLUCOSE IN MANAGEMENT OF RECURRENT COLORECTAL CANCER

TUMOR OF THE AMPULLA OF VATER: EXPERIENCE WITH LOCAL OR RADICAL RESECTION IN 171 CONSECUTIVELY TREATED PATIENTS

TOLERANCE OF THE LIVER TO INTERMITTENT PRINGLE MANEUVER IN HEPATECTOMY FOR LIVER TUMORS

REASONS WHY TRAUMA SURGEONS FAIL TO SCREEN FOR ALCOHOL PROBLEMS

SURGERY IN BELGIUM

COMPLETE TABLE OF CONTENTS INSIDE

American Medical Association

Physicians dedicated to the health of America

www.ama-assn.org/surgery

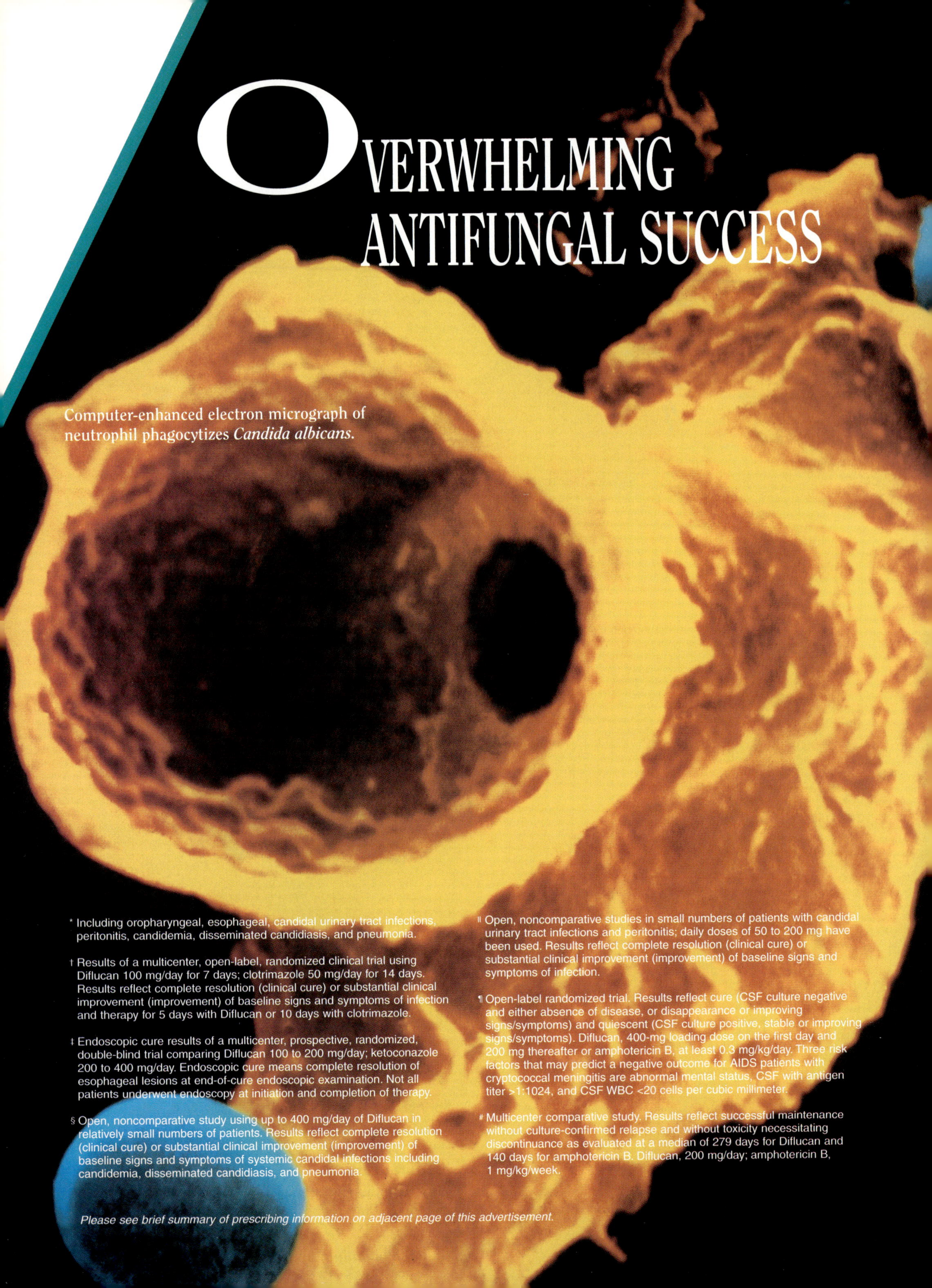

OVERWHELMING ANTIFUNGAL SUCCESS

Computer-enhanced electron micrograph of neutrophil phagocytizes *Candida albicans.*

* Including oropharyngeal, esophageal, candidal urinary tract infections, peritonitis, candidemia, disseminated candidiasis, and pneumonia.

† Results of a multicenter, open-label, randomized clinical trial using Diflucan 100 mg/day for 7 days; clotrimazole 50 mg/day for 14 days. Results reflect complete resolution (clinical cure) or substantial clinical improvement (improvement) of baseline signs and symptoms of infection and therapy for 5 days with Diflucan or 10 days with clotrimazole.

‡ Endoscopic cure results of a multicenter, prospective, randomized, double-blind trial comparing Diflucan 100 to 200 mg/day; ketoconazole 200 to 400 mg/day. Endoscopic cure means complete resolution of esophageal lesions at end-of-cure endoscopic examination. Not all patients underwent endoscopy at initiation and completion of therapy.

§ Open, noncomparative study using up to 400 mg/day of Diflucan in relatively small numbers of patients. Results reflect complete resolution (clinical cure) or substantial clinical improvement (improvement) of baseline signs and symptoms of systemic candidal infections including candidemia, disseminated candidiasis, and pneumonia.

‖ Open, noncomparative studies in small numbers of patients with candidal urinary tract infections and peritonitis; daily doses of 50 to 200 mg have been used. Results reflect complete resolution (clinical cure) or substantial clinical improvement (improvement) of baseline signs and symptoms of infection.

¶ Open-label randomized trial. Results reflect cure (CSF culture negative and either absence of disease, or disappearance or improving signs/symptoms) and quiescent (CSF culture positive, stable or improving signs/symptoms). Diflucan, 400-mg loading dose on the first day and 200 mg thereafter or amphotericin B, at least 0.3 mg/kg/day. Three risk factors that may predict a negative outcome for AIDS patients with cryptococcal meningitis are abnormal mental status, CSF with antigen titer >1:1024, and CSF WBC <20 cells per cubic millimeter.

\# Multicenter comparative study. Results reflect successful maintenance without culture-confirmed relapse and without toxicity necessitating discontinuance as evaluated at a median of 279 days for Diflucan and 140 days for amphotericin B. Diflucan, 200 mg/day; amphotericin B, 1 mg/kg/week.

Please see brief summary of prescribing information on adjacent page of this advertisement.

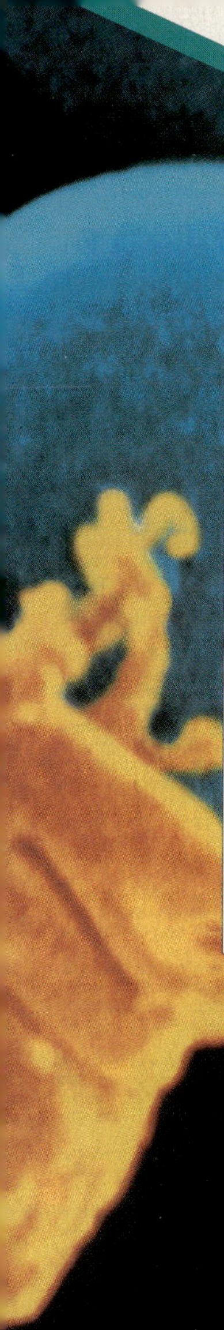

Excellent clinical success in a wide range of candidal infections* and cryptococcal meningitis

MUCOSAL CANDIDIASIS	OROPHARYNGEAL[1†] *P*<.001		ESOPHAGEAL[2‡] (endoscopic cures) *P*<.001	
	DIFLUCAN (212/221) Cured 81% Improved 15%	96%	DIFLUCAN (58/64)	96%
	clotrimazole (79/91) Cured 65% Improved 14%	79%	ketoconazole (34/65)	52%
SYSTEMIC CANDIDAL INFECTIONS	CANDIDEMIA[1§]		DISSEMINATED[3§]	
	DIFLUCAN (29/32) Cured 69% Improved 22%	91%	DIFLUCAN (22/31) Cured 52% Improved 19%	71%
OTHER CANDIDAL INFECTIONS	URINARY TRACT[1‖]		PERITONITIS[1‖]	
	DIFLUCAN (30/38) Cured 53% Improved 26%	79%	DIFLUCAN (32/35) Cured 66% Improved 25%	91%
CRYPTOCOCCAL MENINGITIS	ACUTE THERAPY[4¶] *P*=NS		MAINTENANCE TO PREVENT RELAPSE[1,5#] *P*<.001	
	DIFLUCAN (78/131) Cured 34% Quiescent 26%	60%	DIFLUCAN (103/111)	93%
	amphotericin B Cured 40% Quiescent 27% (212/221)	67%	amphotericin B (52/78)	67%

Extensive penetration to key tissues, organs, and fluids

Distribution throughout the body approximates that of total body water after oral or IV dosing.[1] Oral bioavailability of Diflucan is >90% and unaffected by agents that increase gastric pH.[1]

Excellent clinical safety

In more than 4,000 patients who received multiple-dose Diflucan, the most common adverse events were nausea (3.7%), headache (1.9%), skin rash (1.8%), vomiting (1.7%), abdominal pain (1.7%), and diarrhea (1.5%).

Diflucan has been associated with rare cases of serious hepatic toxicity, including fatalities primarily in patients with serious underlying medical conditions. Patients who develop abnormal liver function tests should be monitored for the development of more severe hepatic injury. Patients have rarely developed exfoliative skin disorders during treatment with Diflucan. Coadministration of terfenadine is contraindicated in patients receiving Diflucan at multiple daily doses of 400 mg or higher. Coadministration of cisapride is contraindicated in patients receiving Diflucan.

ONCE-A-DAY

Diflucan® (fluconazole) ORAL / IV

100/200 mg Tablets, 10/40 mg/mL Oral Suspension, 200/400 mg IV Injection

Overwhelming antifungal success

References: **1.** Data available on request from Roerig. **2.** Laine L, Dretler RH, Conteas CN, et al. Fluconazole compared with ketoconazole for the treatment of *Candida* esophagitis in AIDS: a randomized trial. *Ann Intern Med.* 1992;117:655-660. **3.** Stevens DA. Fungal infections in AIDS patients. *Br J Clin Pract.* 1990;44(suppl 71):11-22. **4.** Saag MS, Powderly WG, Cloud GA, et al. Comparison of amphotericin B with fluconazole in the treatment of acute AIDS-associated cryptococcal meningitis. *N Engl J Med.* 1992;326:83-89. **5.** Powderly WG, Saag MS, Cloud GA, et al. A controlled trial of fluconazole or amphotericin B to prevent relapse of cryptococcal meningitis in patients with the acquired immunodeficiency syndrome. *N Engl J Med.* 1992;326:793-798.

Diflucan® (fluconazole)

100/150/200 mg Tablets, 10/40 mg/mL Oral Suspension, 200/400 mg IV Injection

BRIEF SUMMARY

Once-daily dosing for a wide range of patients

Indication	Loading dose	Daily therapy
Oropharyngeal candidiasis	**200 mg**	100 mg
Esophageal candidiasis	**200 mg**	100 mg*
Candidal UTI and peritonitis	†	50 to 200 mg‡
Systemic candidal Infections†	†	up to 400 mg
Cryptococcal meningitis (acute)§	**400 mg**	200 mg*
Cryptococcal meningitis (maintenance to prevent relapse)		200 mg
Bone marrow transplant prophylaxis‖		400 mg

*Doses up to 400 mg/day may be used, based on medical judgment of the patient's response to therapy.

†In general, a loading dose of twice the daily dose is recommended on the first day of therapy to result in plasma concentrations close to steady-state by the second day of therapy.

‡Including candidemia, disseminated candidiasis, and pneumonia.

§Three risk factors that may predict a negative outcome for AIDS patients with cryptococcal meningitis are abnormal mental status, CSF with antigen titer >1:1024, and CSF WBC <20 cells per cubic millimeter.

‖Therapy should be continued for 7 days after neutrophil count rises above 1000 cells/mm³. Patients who are anticipated to have severe granulocytopenia (<500 neutrophils/mm³) should start Diflucan prophylaxis several days before the anticipated onset of neutropenia and continue for 7 days after the neutrophil count rises above 1000 cells per cubic millimeter.

Pediatric patient dose conversion

Pediatric patients	Adults
3 mg/kg	100 mg
6 mg/kg	200 mg
12 mg/kg‖	400 mg

‖Some older children may have clearances similar to that of adults. Absolute doses exceeding 600 mg/day are not recommended.

INDICATIONS AND USAGE

DIFLUCAN (fluconazole) is indicated for the treatment of:

1. Vaginal candidiasis (vaginal yeast infections due to *Candida*).
2. Oropharyngeal and esophageal candidiasis. In open noncomparative studies of relatively small numbers of patients, DIFLUCAN was also effective for the treatment of *Candida* urinary tract infections, peritonitis, and systemic *Candida* infections including candidemia, disseminated candidiasis, and pneumonia.
3. Cryptococcal meningitis. Before prescribing DIFLUCAN for AIDS patients with cryptococcal meningitis, please see CLINICAL STUDIES section (in full prescribing information). Studies comparing DIFLUCAN to amphotericin B in non-HIV infected patients have not been conducted.

Prophylaxis. DIFLUCAN is also indicated to decrease the incidence of candidiasis in patients undergoing bone marrow transplantation who receive cytotoxic chemotherapy and/or radiation therapy.

Specimens for fungal culture and other relevant laboratory studies (serology, histopathology) should be obtained prior to therapy to isolate and identify causative organisms. Therapy may be instituted before the results of the cultures and other laboratory studies are known; however, once these results become available, anti-infective therapy should be adjusted accordingly.

CONTRAINDICATIONS

DIFLUCAN is contraindicated in patients who have shown hypersensitivity to fluconazole or to any of its excipients. There is no information regarding cross-hypersensitivity between fluconazole and other azole antifungal agents. Caution should be used in prescribing DIFLUCAN to patients with hypersensitivity to other azoles. Coadministration of terfenadine is contraindicated in patients receiving DIFLUCAN at multiple doses of 400 mg or higher based upon results of a multiple dose interaction study. Coadministration of cisapride is contraindicated in patients receiving DIFLUCAN. (See PRECAUTIONS below.)

WARNINGS

(1) Hepatic injury: DIFLUCAN has been associated with rare cases of serious hepatic toxicity, including fatalities primarily in patients with serious underlying medical conditions. In cases of DIFLUCAN-associated hepatotoxicity, no obvious relationship to total daily dose, duration of therapy, sex or age of the patient has been observed. DIFLUCAN hepatotoxicity has usually, but not always, been reversible on discontinuation of therapy. Patients who develop abnormal liver function tests during DIFLUCAN therapy should be monitored for the development of more severe hepatic injury. DIFLUCAN should be discontinued if clinical signs and symptoms consistent with liver disease develop that may be attributable to DIFLUCAN.

(2) Anaphylaxis: In rare cases, anaphylaxis has been reported.

(3) Dermatologic: Patients have rarely developed exfoliative skin disorders during treatment with DIFLUCAN. In patients with serious underlying diseases (predominantly AIDS and malignancy) these have rarely resulted in a fatal outcome. Patients who develop rashes during treatment with DIFLUCAN should be monitored closely and the drug discontinued if lesions progress.

PRECAUTIONS

General: Single Dose. The convenience and efficacy of the single dose oral tablet of fluconazole regimen for the treatment of vaginal yeast infections should be weighed against the acceptability of a higher incidence of drug related adverse events with DIFLUCAN (26%) versus intravaginal agents (16%) in U.S. comparative clinical studies. (See ADVERSE REACTIONS.)

Drug Interactions: Clinically or potentially significant drug interactions between DIFLUCAN and the following agents/classes have been observed. These are described in greater detail below: Oral hypoglycemics, coumarin-type anticoagulants, phenytoin, cyclosporine, rifampin, theophylline, terfenadine, cisapride, astemizole, rifabutin, tacrolimus.

Oral hypoglycemics: Clinically significant hypoglycemia may be precipitated by the use of DIFLUCAN with oral hypoglycemic agents; one fatality has been reported from hypoglycemia in association with combined DIFLUCAN and glyburide use. DIFLUCAN reduces the metabolism of tolbutamide, glyburide, and glipizide and increases the plasma concentration of these agents. When DIFLUCAN is used concomitantly with these or other sulfonylurea oral hypoglycemic agents, blood glucose concentrations should be carefully monitored and the dose of the sulfonylurea should be adjusted as necessary.

Coumarin-type anticoagulants: Prothrombin time may be increased in patients receiving concomitant DIFLUCAN and coumarin-type anticoagulants. Careful monitoring of prothrombin time in patients receiving DIFLUCAN and coumarin-type anticoagulants is recommended.

Phenytoin: DIFLUCAN increases the plasma concentrations of phenytoin. Careful monitoring of phenytoin concentrations in patients receiving DIFLUCAN and phenytoin is recommended.

Cyclosporine: DIFLUCAN may significantly increase cyclosporine levels in renal transplant patients with or without renal impairment. Careful monitoring of cyclosporine concentrations and serum creatinine is recommended in patients receiving DIFLUCAN and cyclosporine.

Rifampin: Rifampin enhances the metabolism of concurrently administered DIFLUCAN. Depending on clinical circumstances, consideration should be given to increasing the dose of DIFLUCAN when it is administered with rifampin.

Theophylline: DIFLUCAN increases the serum concentrations of theophylline. Careful monitoring of serum theophylline concentrations in patients receiving DIFLUCAN and theophylline is recommended.

Terfenadine: Because of the occurrence of serious cardiac dysrhythmias secondary to prolongation of the QTc interval in patients receiving azole antifungals in conjunction with terfenadine, interaction studies have been performed. One study at a 200-mg daily dose of fluconazole failed to demonstrate a prolongation of QTc interval. Another study at a 400-mg and 800-mg daily dose of fluconazole demonstrated that DIFLUCAN taken in doses of 400 mg per day or greater significantly increases plasma levels of terfenadine when taken concomitantly. The combined use of fluconazole at doses of 400 mg or greater with terfenadine is contraindicated. (See CONTRAINDICATIONS.) The coadministration of fluconazole at doses lower than 400 mg/day with terfenadine should be carefully monitored.

Cisapride: There have been reports of cardiac events, including torsade de pointes in patients to whom fluconazole and cisapride were coadministered. The combined use of fluconazole and cisapride is contraindicated. (See CONTRAINDICATIONS.)

Astemizole: The use of fluconazole in patients concurrently taking astemizole or other drugs metabolized by the cytochrome P450 system may be associated with elevations in serum levels of these drugs. In the absence of definitive information, caution should be used when coadministering fluconazole. Patients should be carefully monitored.

Rifabutin: There have been reports of uveitis in patients to whom fluconazole and rifabutin were coadministered. Patients receiving rifabutin and fluconazole concomitantly should be carefully monitored.

Tacrolimus: There have been reports of nephrotoxicity in patients to whom fluconazole and tacrolimus were coadministered. Patients receiving tacrolimus and fluconazole concomitantly should be carefully monitored.

Fluconazole tablets coadministered with ethinyl estradiol-and levonorgestrel-containing oral contraceptives produced an overall mean increase in ethinyl estradiol and levonorgestrel levels; however, in some patients there were decreases up to 47% and 33% of ethinyl estradiol and levonorgestrel levels. The data presently available indicate that the decreases in some individual ethinyl estradiol and levonorgestrel AUC values with fluconazole treatment are likely the result of random variation. While there is evidence that fluconazole can inhibit the metabolism of ethinyl estradiol and levonorgestrel, there is no evidence that fluconazole is a net inducer of ethinyl estradiol or levonorgestrel metabolism. The clinical significance of these effects is presently unknown.

Physicians should be aware that interaction studies with medications other than those listed in the CLINICAL PHARMACOLOGY section (in full prescribing information) have not been conducted, but such interactions may occur.

Carcinogenesis, Mutagenesis and Impairment of Fertility: Fluconazole showed no evidence of carcinogenic potential in mice and rats treated orally for 24 months at doses of 2.5, 5 or 10 mg/kg/day (approximately 2-7x the recommended human dose). Male rats treated with 5 and 10 mg/kg/day had an increased incidence of hepatocellular adenomas.

Fluconazole, with or without metabolic activation, was negative in tests for mutagenicity in 4 strains of *S. typhimurium*, and in the mouse lymphoma L5178Y system. Cytogenetic studies *in vivo* (murine bone marrow cells, following oral administration of fluconazole) and *in vitro* (human lymphocytes exposed to fluconazole at 1000 µg/mL) showed no evidence of chromosomal mutations.

Fluconazole did not affect the fertility of male or female rats treated orally with daily doses of 5, 10 or 20 mg/kg or with parenteral doses of 5, 25 or 75 mg/kg, although the onset of parturition was slightly delayed at 20 mg/kg PO. In an intravenous perinatal study in rats at 5, 20 and 40 mg/kg, dystocia and prolongation of parturition were observed in a few dams at 20 mg/kg (approximately 5-15x the recommended human dose) and 40 mg/kg, but not at 5 mg/kg. The disturbances in parturition were reflected by a slight increase in the number of still-born pups and decrease of neonatal survival at these dose levels. The effects on parturition in rats are consistent with the species specific estrogen-lowering property produced by high doses of fluconazole. Such a hormone change has not been observed in women treated with fluconazole.

Pregnancy: Teratogenic Effects. Pregnancy Category C: Fluconazole was administered orally to pregnant rabbits during organogenesis in two studies, at 5, 10 and 20 mg/kg, and at 5, 25, and 75 mg/kg respectively. Maternal weight gain was impaired at all dose levels, and abortions occurred at 75 mg/kg (approximately 20-60x the recommended human dose); no adverse fetal effects were detected. In several studies in which pregnant rats were treated orally with fluconazole during organogenesis, maternal weight gain was impaired and placental weights were increased at 25 mg/kg. There were no fetal effects at 5 or 10 mg/kg; increases in fetal anatomical variants (supernumerary ribs, renal pelvis dilation) and delays in ossification were observed at 25 and 50 mg/kg and higher doses. At doses ranging from 80 mg/kg (approximately 20-60x the recommended human dose) to 320 mg/kg embryolethality in rats was increased and fetal abnormalities included wavy ribs, cleft palate and abnormal cranio-facial ossification. These effects are consistent with the inhibition of estrogen synthesis in rats and may be a result of known effects of lowered estrogen on pregnancy, organogenesis and parturition.

There are no adequate and well controlled studies in pregnant women. There have been reports of multiple congenital abnormalities in infants whose mothers were being treated for 3 or more months with high dose (400-800 mg/day) fluconazole therapy for coccidioidomycosis (an unindicated use). The relationship between fluconazole use and these events is unclear. DIFLUCAN® (fluconazole) should be used in pregnancy only if the potential benefit justifies the possible risk to the fetus.

Nursing Mothers: Fluconazole is secreted in human milk at concentrations similar to plasma. Therefore, the use of DIFLUCAN in nursing mothers is not recommended.

Pediatric Use: An open-label, randomized, controlled trial has shown DIFLUCAN to be effective in the treatment of oropharyngeal candidiasis in children 6 months to 13 years of age.

The use of DIFLUCAN in children with cryptococcal meningitis, *Candida* esophagitis, or systemic *Candida* infections is supported by the efficacy shown for these indications in adults and by the results from several small noncomparative pediatric clinical studies. In addition, pharmacokinetic studies in children have established a dose proportionality between children and adults. (See DOSING.)

In a noncomparative study of children with serious systemic fungal infections, most of which were candidemia, the effectiveness of DIFLUCAN was similar to that reported for the treatment of candidemia in adults. Of 17 subjects with culture-confirmed candidemia, 11 of 14 (79%) with baseline symptoms (3 were asymptomatic) had a clinical cure; 13/15 (87%) of evaluable patients had a mycologic cure at the end of treatment but two of these patients relapsed at 10 and 18 days, respectively, following cessation of therapy.

The efficacy of DIFLUCAN for the suppression of cryptococcal meningitis was successful in 4 of 5 children treated in a compassionate-use study of fluconazole for the treatment of life-threatening or serious mycosis. There is no information regarding the efficacy of fluconazole for primary treatment of cryptococcal meningitis in children.

The safety profile of DIFLUCAN in children has been studied in 577 children ages 1 day to 17 years who received doses ranging from 1 to 15 mg/kg/day for 1 to 1,616 days. (See ADVERSE REACTIONS.)

Efficacy of DIFLUCAN has not been established in infants less than 6 months of age. A small number of patients (29) ranging in age from 1 day to 6 months have been treated safely with DIFLUCAN.

ADVERSE REACTIONS

In Patients Receiving a Single Dose for Vaginal Candidiasis: During comparative clinical studies conducted in the United States, 448 patients with vaginal candidiasis were treated with DIFLUCAN, 150 mg single dose. The overall incidence of side effects possibly related to DIFLUCAN was 26%. In 422 patients receiving active comparative agents, the incidence was 16%. The most common treatment-related adverse events reported in the patients who received 150 mg single dose fluconazole for vaginitis were headache (13%), nausea (7%), and abdominal pain (6%). Other side effects reported with an incidence equal to or greater than 1% included diarrhea (3%), dyspepsia (1%), dizziness (1%), and taste perversion (1%). Most of the reported side effects were mild to moderate in severity. Rarely, angioedema and anaphylactic reaction have been reported in marketing experience.

In patients receiving multiple doses for other infections: Sixteen percent of over 4000 patients treated with DIFLUCAN in clinical trials of 7 days or more experienced adverse events. Treatment was discontinued in 1.5% of patients due to adverse clinical events and in 1.3% of patients due to laboratory test abnormalities.

Clinical adverse events were reported more frequently in HIV infected patients (21%) than in non-HIV infected patients (13%); however, the patterns in HIV infected and non-HIV infected patients were similar. The proportions of patients discontinuing therapy due to clinical adverse events were similar in the two groups (1.5%).

The following treatment-related clinical adverse events occurred at an incidence of 1% or greater in 4048 patients receiving DIFLUCAN for 7 or more days in clinical trials: nausea 3.7%, headache 1.9%, skin rash 1.8%, vomiting 1.7%, abdominal pain 1.7%, and diarrhea, 1.5%.

The following adverse events have occurred under conditions where a causal association is probable: *Hepatobiliary:* In combined clinical trials and marketing experience, there have been rare cases of serious hepatic reactions during treatment with DIFLUCAN. (See WARNINGS.) The spectrum of these hepatic reactions has ranged from mild transient elevations in transaminases to clinical hepatitis, cholestasis and fulminant hepatic failure, including fatalities. Instances of fatal hepatic reactions were noted to occur primarily in patients with serious underlying medical conditions (predominantly AIDS or malignancy) and often while taking multiple concomitant medications. Transient hepatic reactions, including hepatitis and jaundice have occurred among patients with no other identifiable risk factors. In each of these cases, liver function returned to baseline on discontinuation of DIFLUCAN.

In two comparative trials evaluating the efficacy of DIFLUCAN for the suppression of relapse of cryptococcal meningitis, a statistically significant increase was observed in median AST (SGOT) levels from a baseline value of 30 IU/L to 41 IU/L in one trial and 34 IU/L to 66 IU/L in the other. The overall rate of serum transaminase elevations of more than 8 times the upper limit of normal was approximately 1% in fluconazole-treated patients in clinical trials. These elevations occurred in patients with severe underlying disease, predominantly AIDS or malignancies, most of whom were receiving multiple concomitant medications, including many known to be hepatotoxic. The incidence of abnormally elevated serum transaminases was greater in patients taking DIFLUCAN concomitantly with one or more of the following medications: rifampin, phenytoin, isoniazid, valproic acid, or oral sulfonylurea hypoglycemic agents.

Immunologic: In rare cases, anaphylaxis has been reported.

The following adverse events have occurred under conditions where a causal association is uncertain: *Central Nervous System:* seizures. *Dermatologic:* Exfoliative skin disorders including Stevens-Johnson Syndrome and toxic epidermal necrolysis (see WARNINGS), alopecia. *Hematopoietic and Lymphatic:* leukopenia, including neutropenia and agranulocytosis, thrombocytopenia. *Metabolic:* hypercholesterolemia, hypertriglyceridemia, hypokalemia.

Adverse Reactions in Children: In Phase II/III clinical trials conducted in the United States and in Europe, 577 pediatric patients, ages 1 day to 17 years were treated with DIFLUCAN at doses of up to 15 mg/kg/day for up to 1,616 days. Thirteen percent of children experienced treatment-related adverse events. The most commonly reported events were vomiting (5%), abdominal pain (3%), nausea (2%), and diarrhea (2%). Treatment was discontinued in 2.3% of patients due to adverse clinical events and in 1.4% of patients due to laboratory test abnormalities. The majority of treatment-related laboratory abnormalities were elevations of transaminases or alkaline phosphatase.

Percentage of Patients With Treatment-Related Side Effects

	Fluconazole (N=577)	Comparative Agents (N=451)
With any side effect	13.0	9.3
Vomiting	5.4	5.1
Abdominal pain	2.8	1.6
Nausea	2.3	1.6
Diarrhea	2.1	2.2

Pfizer U.S. Pharmaceuticals

Ad Code: FC152A99

Rev. October 1998
PI Code: FX055A98

ARCHIVES OF SURGERY

The ARCHIVES OF SURGERY is a member of the consortium of AMA journals listed below. The complete text of all AMA journals is available online from Dialog Information Services and Information Access Company.

The Journal of the American Medical Association (JAMA)
Archives of Dermatology
Archives of Facial Plastic Surgery
Archives of Family Medicine
Archives of General Psychiatry
Archives of Internal Medicine
Archives of Neurology
Archives of Ophthalmology
Archives of Otolaryngology–Head & Neck Surgery
Archives of Pathology & Laboratory Medicine
Archives of Pediatrics & Adolescent Medicine
Archives of Surgery

The ARCHIVES OF SURGERY (ISSN 0004-0010) is published monthly by the American Medical Association, 515 N State St, Chicago, IL 60610, and is an official publication of the Association. The ARCHIVES OF SURGERY reaches more than 19 000 readers in over 69 countries each month. Periodicals postage paid at Chicago, IL, and at additional mailing offices. GST registration number 12622 5556 RT. Canada Post International Publications Mail (Canadian Distribution) Sales Agreement No. 319309. Printed in the USA.

Official Publication of the New England Surgical Society, Pacific Coast Surgical Association, Surgical Infection Society, Western Surgical Association.

SUBSCRIPTION RATES—The personal subscription rates for the ARCHIVES OF SURGERY are $145 for 1 year (12 issues) in the United States and US possessions; $195 in the Americas; £125 outside the Americas. The institution rates for 1 year are $245 in the US; $345 in the Americas; £195 outside the Americas. Special rates for residents and medical students are available. Address all subscription communications to: Subscriber Services Center, American Medical Association, PO Box 10946, Chicago, IL 60610-0946. Phone: (800) 262-2350. Fax: (312) 464-5831. E-mail: ama-subs@ama-assn.org. For mailing addresses outside the United States and US possessions, see International Subscription Information.

CHANGE OF ADDRESS—POSTMASTER, send all address changes to ARCHIVES OF SURGERY, c/o Subscriber Services, American Medical Association, 515 N State St, Chicago, IL 60610. Please notify us of address change at least 6 weeks in advance to ensure uninterrupted service. Include both old and new addresses, a recent mailing label, and new ZIP code. For mailing addresses outside the United States and US possessions, see International Subscription Information.

SUBSCRIBER SERVICES—For information about subscribing to any of the AMA publications, change of address, missing issues, or purchasing back issues, please contact Subscriber Services Center, American Medical Association, PO Box 10946, Chicago, IL 60610-0946, or call (800) 262-2350 or (312) 670-SUBS (670-7827) between 8:30 AM and 4:30 PM CST. Fax: (312) 464-5831. E-mail: ama-subs@ama-assn.org. For mailing addresses outside the United States and US possessions, see International Subscription Information.

INTERNATIONAL SUBSCRIPTION INFORMATION—Subscriptions outside the United States and US possessions are served according to geographic region. Please address correspondence to the following 2 offices based on delivery address: (1) For delivery in North America, Central America, and South America, contact Subscriber Services, AMA, PO Box 10946, Chicago, IL 60610-0946. Phone: (312) 670-7827. Fax: (312) 464-5831. E-mail: ama-subs@ama-assn.org. (2) For delivery outside the Americas contact JAMA & Archives Journals, Reader Services Centre, PO Box 299, London WC1H 9TD, England. Phone: +44 (0)171-383-6270. Fax: +44 (0)171-383-6402. E-mail: jama-archives@dial.pipex.com.

REPRINTS—Authors place their reprint order at the time the edited typescript is reviewed and should allow 4 to 6 weeks for delivery following publication. Requests for individual reprints should be sent directly to the author at the address shown in the article.

For bulk reprint orders for distribution by commercial organizations, please contact Wanda Bartolotta, 500 Fifth Ave, #2210, New York, NY 10110. Phone: (212) 354-0050. Fax: (212) 354-1169. E-mail: wanda_bartolotta@ama-assn.org. For reprint orders in limited quantities for distribution by educational organizations and for author reprints, please contact Reprint Coordinator, 515 N State St, Chicago, IL 60610. Phone: (312) 464-4594. Fax: (312) 464-4849.

PERMISSIONS—Contact Rhonda Bailey, Permissions Assistant, 515 N State St, Chicago, IL 60610. Phone: (312) 464-2513.

ADVERTISING PRINCIPLES—Each advertisement in this issue has been reviewed and complies with the principles governing advertising in AMA scientific publications. A copy of these principles is available on request. The appearance of advertising in AMA publications is not an AMA guarantee or endorsement of the product or the claims made for the product by the manufacturer.

WORLD WIDE WEB ADDRESS—http://www.ama-assn.org.
SURGERY HOME PAGE—http://www.ama-assn.org/surgery.

ARCHIVES OF SURGERY

www.ama-assn.org/surgery

VOL 134 NO. 5, MAY 1999

MISSION STATEMENT

To promote the art and science of surgery by publishing relevant peer-reviewed clinical and basic science information to assist the surgeon in optimizing patient care. The *Archives of Surgery* will also serve as a forum for the discussion of issues that involve ethics, teaching, surgical history, and socioeconomic concerns.

*Approved by the Editorial Board, *Archives of Surgery*, July 19, 1996.

PAPERS

Laparoscopic Colectomy: Indications for Conversion to Laparotomy 471
Sonal Pandya, MD; John J. Murray, MD; John A. Coller, MD; Lawrence C. Rusin, MD

Handoscopic Surgery: A Prospective Multicenter Trial of a Minimally Invasive Technique for Complex Abdominal Surgery 477
Southern Surgeons' Club Study Group

Invited Critique 486
Manuel Trías Folch; Eduardo Mª Targarona

Surgical Management of Phyllodes Tumors 487
Abeel A. Mangi, MD; Barbara L. Smith, MD, PhD; Michele A. Gadd, MD; Kenneth K. Tanabe, MD; Mark J. Ott, MD; Wiley W. Souba, MD, ScD

ORIGINAL ARTICLES

Vanadate and the Absence of Myofibroblasts in Wound Contraction 494
H. Paul Ehrlich, PhD; Kerry A. Keefer, MS; Roland L. Myers, MS; Anthony Passaniti, PhD

American Medical Association
Physicians dedicated to the health of America

All articles published, including editorials, letters, and book reviews, represent the opinions of the authors and do not reflect the policy of the American Medical Association, the Editorial Board, or the institution with which the author is affiliated, unless this is clearly specified.

Whole-Body PET Imaging With [18F]Fluorodeoxyglucose in Management of Recurrent Colorectal Cancer 503
Peter E. Valk, MB, BS; Elma Abella-Columna, MD; Michael K. Haseman, MD; Thomas R. Pounds, MD; Ruth D. Tesar; Richard W. Myers, MD; Hani B. Greiss, MD; Glenn A. Hofer, MD

Invited Critique 511
Steven D. Wexner, MD

Senna vs Polyethylene Glycol for Mechanical Preparation the Evening Before Elective Colonic or Rectal Resection: A Multicenter Controlled Trial 514
Alain Valverde, MD; Jean-Marie Hay, MD; Abe Fingerhut, MD; Marie-Jeanne Boudet, MD; Roberta Petroni, MD; Xavier Pouliquen, MD; Simon Msika, MD; Yves Flamant, MD; for the French Association for Surgical Research

Acceleration of Wound Healing With Topically Applied Deoxyribonucleosides 520
E. Alexandria Chen, MD; Lily Zhao, MD; Michael Bamat, PhD; Reid von Borstel, PhD; Thomas Mustoe, MD

Tumor of the Ampulla of Vater: Experience With Local or Radical Resection in 171 Consecutively Treated Patients 526
Hans G. Beger, MD; Frank Treitschke, MD; Frank Gansauge, MD; Nobuhiko Harada, MD; Naoki Hiki, MD; Torsten Mattfeldt, MD

Tolerance of the Liver to Intermittent Pringle Maneuver in Hepatectomy for Liver Tumors 533
Kwan Man, MB, PhD; Sheung-Tat Fan, MS, MD, FRCS(Glasg & Edin); Irene O. L. Ng, MD, FRCPath; Chung-Mau Lo, MBBS, MS, FRCS(Edin), FRACS; Chi-Leung Liu, MBBS, FRCS(Edin); Wan-Ching Yu, MB; John Wong, PhD, FRACS, FRCS(Edin)

Major Surgery Suppresses Maximal Production of Helper T-Cell Type 1 Cytokines Without Potentiating the Release of Helper T-Cell Type 2 Cytokines 540
Ramon Berguer, MD; Capt Normita Bravo, MS, USAF; Mark Bowyer, MD; Craig Egan, MD; Tom Knolmayer, MD; David Ferrick, PhD

ARCHIVES OF SURGERY

ARCHIVES OF SURGERY

Peritoneal Expansion by Artificially Produced Ascites During Perfusion Chemotherapy 545
Dimitris Tsiftsis, MD, PhD; Eelco de Bree, MD; John Romanos, MD; Anastasios Petrou, MD; Elias Sanidas, MD; John Askoxylakis, MD; Konstantinos Zervos, MD; Dimitris Michaloudis, MD

Invited Critique 550
John S. Spratt, MD

Staging Investigations in Patients With Breast Cancer: The Role of Bone Scans and Liver Imaging 551
Rajiv Samant, MD; Pradip Ganguly, MD

Invited Critique 554
Philip Z. Israel, MD

Improved Continuity of Care in a Community Teaching Hospital Model 555
Vijay Mittal, MD; Whitney David, MD; Shun Young, MD; Alasdair McKendrick, MD; Thomas Gentile, Jr, MSA; Robert Casalou, MPH

Laparoscopic Reoperation for Failed Antireflux Procedures 559
Myriam J. Curet, MD, FACS; Robert K. Josloff, MD; Othmar Schoeb, MD; Karl A. Zucker, MD

Reasons Why Trauma Surgeons Fail to Screen for Alcohol Problems 564
Per E. Danielsson, MD; Frederick P. Rivara, MD, MPH; Larry M. Gentilello, MD; Ronald V. Maier, MD

SPECIAL ARTICLE

Surgery in Belgium 569
Pierre Mendes da Costa, MD; Roger Detry, MD; Jacques Gruwez, MD; Luc Harper, MD; Patrick Rutten, MD

CORRESPONDENCE AND BRIEF COMMUNICATIONS

The Value of Physician Assistants in the Modern Surgical Setting 575
Stephan C. Crane, PhD, MPH

In Reply 575
Marvin A. McMillen, MD

Somatostatin Receptor Scintigraphy and Endoscopic Ultrasonography for Occult Carcinoid Tumor 575
Carmine Volpe, MD; Ralph J. Doerr, MD

SURGICAL REMINISCENCES

Cattell and Surgical Technique 577
John W. Braasch, MD

MOMENTS IN SURGICAL HISTORY

Crawford Williamson Long 578
Ira M. Rutkow, MD, MPH, DrPH

DEPARTMENTS

Surgical Anatomy 519

Products & Services 579

Classified Advertising 580

Index to Advertisers 584

Instructions for Authors—
See January 1999 issue, page 107, or visit the Web site at http://www.ama-assn.org/surgery.

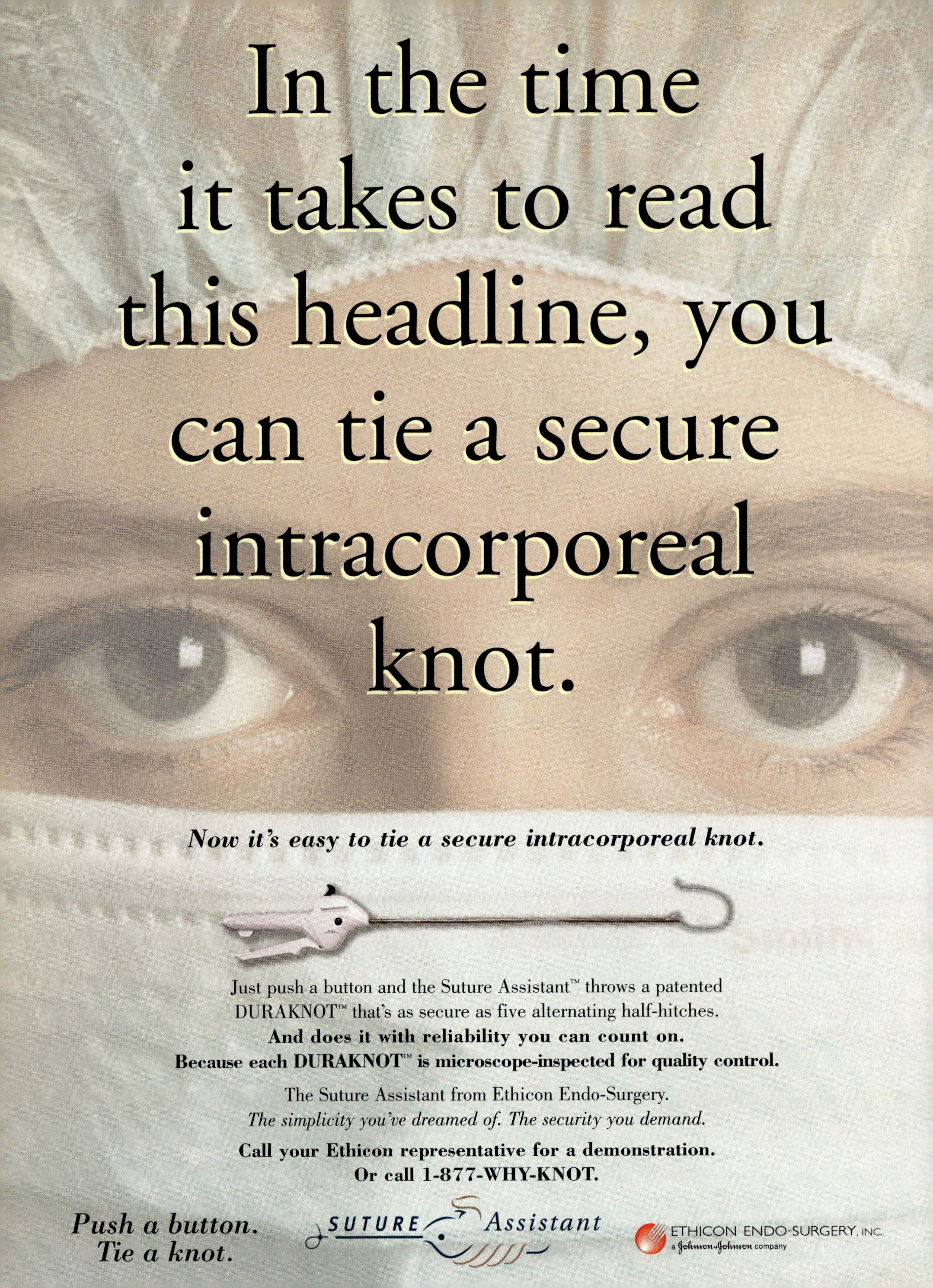
In the time it takes to read this headline, you can tie a secure intracorporeal knot.
Now it's easy to tie a secure intracorporeal knot.
Just push a button and the Suture Assistant™ throws a patented DURAKNOT™ that's as secure as five alternating half-hitches.
And does it with reliability you can count on.
Because each DURAKNOT™ is microscope-inspected for quality control.
The Suture Assistant from Ethicon Endo-Surgery.
The simplicity you've dreamed of. The security you demand.
Call your Ethicon representative for a demonstration.
Or call 1-877-WHY-KNOT.
Push a button.
Tie a knot.
SUTURE Assistant
ETHICON ENDO-SURGERY, INC.
a Johnson & Johnson company

PAPER

Laparoscopic Colectomy

Indications for Conversion to Laparotomy

Sonal Pandya, MD; John J. Murray, MD; John A. Coller, MD; Lawrence C. Rusin, MD

Hypothesis: Although experience with laparoscopic colectomy continues to accumulate, criteria for patient selection for the procedure have yet to be developed. We propose that review of indications for conversion to laparotomy during laparoscopic colectomy should define some of the current technical limitations of the procedure. This information may facilitate development of selection criteria for laparoscopic colon and rectal surgery.

Design: Single-institution retrospective medical records review.

Setting: Tertiary referral center.

Patients: Two hundred patients who underwent laparoscopic colon surgery, in 47 (23.5%) of whom the procedure was converted to laparotomy.

Interventions: A registry of 200 patients who have undergone laparoscopic colon surgery was analyzed. Medical records of 47 patients whose procedure was converted were reviewed to assess indications for conversion and identify factors contributing to the need for conversion.

Results: Between July 1, 1991, and September 30, 1998, 200 laparoscopic colon procedures were performed: 78 ascending colectomies, 74 descending or sigmoid colectomies, 14 diverting stomas, and 34 "other procedures." The 200 patients were divided into 4 cohorts of 50 consecutive patients to analyze changes with time. The conversion rate was statistically greater in the first quarter (18 patients [36.0%]) than in subsequent quarters (16.0%; $P < .05$). The rate of conversion to laparotomy for segmental resection of the ascending and descending colon (31/153 [20.3%]) has been equivalent and less than the conversion rate for other procedures (16/33 [48.5%]; $P < .05$). The distribution of patients by operative indication has been fairly constant. The indication for operation has not influenced the need for conversion. The indications for conversion were technical problems in 15 patients (hypercarbia, unclear anatomy, and stapler misfire), laparoscopic complications in 9 patients (bleeding, cystotomy, and enterotomy), and problems that exceeded the limits of laparoscopic dissection in 23 patients (phlegmon, adhesions, obesity, and adjacent organ involvement by cancer).

Conclusions: Our conversion rate has decreased during our experience, and currently the need for conversion to laparotomy is most frequently caused by situations such as excessive tumor bulk, adhesions, and diverticular phlegmon that exceed the technical limitations of laparoscopic dissection. Colorectal reanastomosis following a Hartmann resection and procedures involving resection of the distal rectum are unlikely to be successfully completed. Although obesity accentuates the technical limitations of laparoscopic dissection, it is an infrequent cause for conversion to laparotomy.

Arch Surg. 1999;134:471-475

From the Departments of General Surgery (Dr Pandya) and Colon and Rectal Surgery (Drs Murray, Coller, and Rusin), Lahey Clinic, Burlington, Mass.

THERAPEUTIC laparoscopy has substantially altered the treatment of many gastrointestinal disorders. Colectomy is arguably the most challenging procedure to be attempted laparoscopically on a large scale. Although experience with laparoscopic colectomy is expanding rapidly, several issues must be clarified.

The evaluation of results of laparoscopic colectomy has primarily focused on demonstrating that the operative goals are technically achievable and that the purported advantages of decreased hospital stays and shorter postoperative disability can be realized. As experience with laparoscopic colectomy accumulates, there is increasing pressure to demonstrate that the procedure is cost-effective. To maximize the therapeutic and economic benefits, criteria for disease and patient selection must be defined.

There are 2 prerequisites for establishing selection criteria for any therapeutic procedure. The technical limitations of the procedure must be defined, and the results of the procedure must be critically analyzed in a representative cohort of patients. Given the evolving nature of laparoscopic technology, the relatively limited experience with laparoscopic colectomy to date, and the unresolved controversy regarding the safety of laparoscopic surgery in patients with malignant disease, it has not been possible to establish criteria for patient selection.

PATIENTS AND METHODS

Between July 1, 1991, and September 30, 1998, 200 patients underwent laparoscopic colon procedures at the Lahey Clinic, Burlington, Mass. A registry of all laparoscopic operations is maintained prospectively. Registry data include the indication for surgery, the presence of comorbid conditions, the type of procedure, perioperative morbidity, the need for conversion to a laparotomy, and details relating to postoperative convalescence. For the purpose of this review, our primary outcome measure has been conversion to a laparotomy. To identify changes in our results with time, the experience has been analyzed in 4 cohorts of 50 consecutive patients. The medical records of all patients whose procedure was converted to a laparotomy have been analyzed to identify the indication for conversion and to assess patient or disease characteristics influencing conversion. In some patients, multiple factors contributed to the need for conversion, but the operating surgeon usually identified the primary problem precipitating the need for a laparotomy.

A precise definition of laparoscopic colectomy has not been clearly established. We have proposed a fairly narrow definition of the procedure.

With our approach, the segment of colon to be resected is mobilized, and the mesentery is divided intracorporeally. The specimen is extracted through a 5.0- to 7.5-cm muscle-splitting incision in the right or left flank. For ascending colectomy, an extracorporeal stapled anastomosis is performed through the flank incision. For resections of the distal colon or rectum, the proximal end of the divided colon is delivered through the flank incision. The anvil of the circular anastomotic stapler is inserted in the colon and secured with a purse-string suture. After the flank incision is closed, an anastomosis is performed intracorporeally. Any variation from this description of the technique has been labeled a conversion.

Data have been analyzed for statistical significance ($P<.05$) using a 2-tailed Student t test.

Although the conversion to laparotomy may represent sound and appropriate surgical judgment, it has been used as an indication of failure in performing laparoscopic surgery. Experience has shown that the timing of conversion influences morbidity and operative costs, both of which are increased in patients with prolonged laparoscopic dissection before conversion.[1] The recognition of patient, disease, or procedural characteristics that influence the need for converting to a laparotomy may help to define criteria for patient selection and identify indications for early conversion to a laparotomy so that the therapeutic benefits and cost-effectiveness of the procedure can be maximized.

We have reviewed our experience with laparoscopic colectomy, with particular attention to those patients who required conversion to a laparotomy. We have attempted to identify patient or disease characteristics influencing the need for conversion and to evaluate changes in the frequency of conversion and in the indications for conversion during our experience.

RESULTS

Of 200 laparoscopic colon procedures performed at the Lahey Clinic, conversion to a laparotomy was required in 47 patients (23.5%). Although the procedure of 18 (36.0%) of our first 50 patients was converted, the rate of conversion for our subsequent 150 patients has averaged 19.3% (29 patients) (8/50-11/50 [16.0%-22.0%]), which represents a statistically significant improvement ($P=.02$).

Table 1 lists the laparoscopic procedures comprising our experience. In 33 patients, the procedures are designated as "other." These include several procedures that are performed infrequently, often for a variety of indications. We have grouped these other procedures into 3 categories: those requiring mobilization and resection of the entire colon (total abdominal colectomy with ileostomy or ileorectal anastomosis, total proctocolectomy with ileostomy, and total proctocolectomy with ileal pouch–anal anastomosis); procedures that involve resection of the middle or distal rectum (low anterior resection and abdominoperineal resection), and procedures involving colorectal anastomosis following a Hartmann resection. Aside from a slight decrease in the number of other procedures performed during the last 2 quarters, the distribution of patients per quarter has been fairly stable. No patient undergoing a laparoscopic-assisted ileostomy or colostomy has required conversion to a laparotomy.

The rate of conversion for segmental resection of the ascending and descending colon has been equivalent (20.3% [31/153 patients]) and significantly less than the 48.5% conversion ratio (16/33 patients) for other procedures ($P<.05$). There has been a statistically significant difference in the conversion ratio for other procedures during the first half of our experience (63.6% [14/22 patients]) compared with results from the second half (18.2% [2/11 patients]; $P<.01$). This difference may reflect the decrease in the number of low anterior resections and abdominoperineal resections performed during the second half of our experience. The conversion rates for procedures involving resection of the distal rectum and those involving colorectal anastomosis following a Hartmann resection have remained relatively stable. The need for conversion for procedures involving total colectomy with or without proctectomy and for colectomy with an ileal pouch–anal anastomosis has decreased. Five of these procedures performed during the first quarter of our experience required conversion. By contrast, 7 subsequent procedures performed during the second half of the study have been completed successfully.

Table 2 lists the indications for operation. Except for a slight decrease in the number of procedures performed for cancer and for inflammatory bowel disease, the distribution of patients by operative indication has been fairly constant. Overall, resection for neoplastic disease (polyps and cancer) has accounted for about half of our experience. Inflammatory disorders (inflammatory bowel disease and diverticulitis) have been the indication for operation in a third of patients, and the treatment of functional problems has accounted for the remaining patients. The indication for operation has not influenced the rate of conversion, except for those procedures performed for cancer. In the first quarter, 7 (53.8%) of 13 patients having resection for cancer required conversion to a laparotomy, whereas

Table 1. Conversion of Laparoscopic Procedures (n = 47) to a Laparotomy

	Patient Cohort Quarter*				
Procedure Site	**1**	**2**	**3**	**4**	**Total, No. (%)**
Ascending colon	5/22	2/17	4/20	3/19	**14/78** (17.9)
Descending or sigmoid colon	4/15	3/22	4/19	6/19	**17/75** (22.6)
Stoma	0	0/2	0/7	0/5	**0/14** (0)
Other†	9/13	5/9	0/4	2/7	**16/33** (48.5)‡
Total, No. (%)	**18/50** (36.0)§	**10/50** (20.0)	**8/50** (16.0)	**11/50** (22.0)	**47/200** (23.5)

*Data are given as the number of patients whose procedure was converted to laparotomy/the number of patients in that quarter having the procedure.
†Low anterior resection or abdominoperineal resection (7 of 15 patients); total abdominal colectomy, total proctocolectomy, or ileal pouch–anal anastomosis (5 of 12 patients); and Hartmann reanastomosis (4 of 6 patients).
‡$P<.05$.
§$P = .02$.

only 3 (10.3%) of 29 patients in the subsequent 3 quarters of our experience have required a conversion. This difference is statistically significant ($P <.05$).

Table 3 lists the reasons for converting to a laparotomy. As previously mentioned, several factors contributed to the need for conversion in some patients. A review of the operative report, however, usually identified the primary problem precipitating the decision to convert. The indications for conversion have been grouped in 3 categories. Of 47 patients, 15 (31.9%) had their procedure converted for technical problems. In 6 patients, the procedure was converted to a laparotomy because of the development of an uncorrectable respiratory acidosis. Pneumoperitoneum decreases the functional residual capacity of the lung.[2-5] The decrease in the functional residual capacity combined with carbon dioxide absorption can produce substantial respiratory acidosis in patients with limited pulmonary reserve. Through less reliance on Trendelenburg positioning and improved operative management of these patients by anesthesiologists, there have been no conversions for respiratory acidosis in the latter half of our experience.

Other technical problems requiring conversion included equipment malfunction, inability to expose and identify the ureter, and 1 instance of incorrect location of a colonic neoplasm. This error was identified after the segment of colon had been mobilized but before it was transected. Five patients listed in the category of "too ambitious" included 2 who had proctocolectomies with an ileal pouch–anal anastomosis and 3 with total abdominal colectomies, previously described. Although these operations were proceeding uneventfully at the time of conversion, the projected time required to complete the procedure was judged to be excessive, precipitating a decision to convert to a laparotomy. All 5 of these patients were from the first quarter of our experience, and this result most likely reflects the consequence of limited experience. There have been no subsequent conversions for this reason. Seven similar procedures have been completed successfully.

Nine patients (19.1%) required conversion to a laparotomy to manage intraoperative complications. Most frequently, this was due to persistent bleeding from a mesenteric or retroperitoneal vessel that could not be adequately managed with laparoscopic techniques. Three patients required conversion for an unintentional enterotomy or cystotomy.

In 23 (48.9%) of the 47 patients, the decision to proceed with a laparotomy was precipitated by findings that were thought to exceed the technical limits of laparoscopic dissection. Five patients undergoing sigmoid colectomy for complications of diverticulitis required conversion because of a large paracolic phlegmon. Despite the fact that 105 patients (52.5%) in our series of 200 had previously undergone a laparotomy, only 5 patients required conversion to laparotomy because of extensive intra-abdominal adhesions. Four of these 5 patients had extensive, dense adhesions obliterating the pelvic cavity following a Hartmann resection for pelvic sepsis.

In 3 patients, conversion to a laparotomy was required because operative exposure and laparoscopic

Table 2. Influence of Operative Indication on Converting to a Laparotomy*

	Patient Cohort Quarter				
Indication	**1**	**2**	**3**	**4**	**Total, No. (%)**
Polyp	2/14	2/13	4/14	2/16	**10/57** (17.5)
Cancer	7/13	2/12	0/10	1/7	**10/42** (23.8)
Diverticulitis	1/7	2/15	3/14	5/14	**11/50** (22.0)
Inflammatory bowel disease	3/6	1/4	0/2	1/3	**5/15** (33.3)
Other†	5/10	3/6	1/10	2/10	**11/36** (30.6)

*Data are given as the number of patients whose procedure was converted to laparotomy/the number of patients in that quarter having a procedure for the operative indication.
†Incontinence, colonic inertia, rectal prolapse, sigmoid volvulus, and lower gastrointestinal tract bleeding.

Table 3. Indications for Converting to a Laparotomy (n = 47)

Indication	No. of Patients (%)	Description (No. of Patients)
Technical problems	15 (31.9)	Hypercarbia (6) Unclear anatomy (2) Stapler misfire (2) "Too ambitious" (5)
Operative complications	9 (19.1)	Bleeding (6) Cystotomy (1) Enterotomy (2)
Technical limitations	23 (48.9)	Phlegmon (5) Adhesions (5) Obesity, unfavorable body habitus (3) Inadequate cancer operation (10)

Table 4. Indications for Conversion to a Laparotomy (n = 47) by Quarter*

Indication	Patient Cohort Quarter 1	2	3	4	Total
Technical problems	9 (50)	3 (30)	1 (13)	2 (18)	**15** (32)
Complications	2 (11)	3 (30)	2 (25)	2 (18)	**9** (19)
Technical limitations	7 (39)	4 (40)	5 (62)	7 (64)	**23** (49)
Total Conversions	**18 (100)**	**10 (100)**	**8 (100)**	**11 (100)**	**47 (100)**

*Data are given as number (percentage) of patients.

dissection were compromised by the patient's obesity. Obesity increases the technical difficulty of laparoscopic and open surgery. Attempts to quantify the effects of an unfavorable body habitus on laparoscopic surgery and identify an objective measure that could be applied to patient selection have been unsuccessful. We have evaluated the effects of the body mass index (BMI; defined as the patient's weight in kilograms divided by height in meters squared) on the need for conversion to a laparotomy. Obesity is defined as a BMI of more than 29. The 3 patients in our series whose procedure was converted because of obesity had BMIs of 35, 27, and 26. Whereas all of these indexes are above normal (reference range, 19-24), only 1 patient meets the definition of obesity. The BMI correlated with the need for conversion, however. Of 95 patients, 14 (14.7%) with a BMI of less than 28 required conversion, whereas of 58 patients, 16 (27.6%) with a BMI of less than 29 had their operation converted to an open procedure. This difference is statistically significant ($P<.05$). Furthermore, 25 (53.2%) patients who required conversion had a BMI of less than 29, reflecting the fact that obesity accentuates the technical limitations of laparoscopic dissection.

Ten patients required conversion because of concerns about the ability to complete an adequate cancer resection. This was due to extensive adhesions that compromised exposure, adjacent organ involvement by the tumor, or the presence of a bulky tumor that interfered with exposure and mobilization of the colon and adjacent mesentery.

Although the analysis of data regarding changes in the indications for conversion during our experience is hampered by the small number of cases in individual categories, several interesting observations can be made. As our experience has increased, technical problems have become a less frequent indication for conversion, and factors identified as technical limitations of the method have accounted for an increasing proportion of converted operations. Of 15 patients requiring conversion because of technical problems, 9 were from our initial group of 50 patients (**Table 4**). Technical problems accounted for 9 (50%) of the 18 conversions in the first quarter compared with 2 (18%) of the 11 conversions in the last quarter. On the other hand, technical limitations accounted for 7 (39%) of the 13 conversions in the first quarter and 7 (64%) of the 11 converted cases in the latter half of our experience. As we have progressed along the learning curve of our experience, these technical limitations have become the primary factor influencing the need for conversion to a laparotomy.

COMMENT

The precise role of laparoscopic surgery in the treatment of diseases of the colon and rectum has yet to be defined. Several features of colon surgery make it amenable to laparoscopic techniques. Colectomy is a commonly performed procedure, providing surgeons the opportunity to develop and maintain their technical skills for laparoscopic resection. The colon is relatively accessible to laparoscopic manipulation compared with other intra-abdominal organs. Most important, the development of laparoscopic stapling instruments permits the application of techniques for intestinal anastomosis similar to those used for standard intestinal resections.

Although a reasonable volume of experience with laparoscopic colectomy has been recorded, criteria for patient selection for the procedure have yet to be defined. In part, this reflects uncertainty regarding the role of laparoscopic surgery in the treatment of malignant neoplasms. In an initial attempt to develop selection criteria for laparoscopic colectomy, we have sought to identify factors that influence the successful completion of laparoscopic procedures. The number of patients is small, and several variables may have influenced results, but we have made several interesting observations.

Although the learning curve for laparoscopic colectomy has not been defined precisely, it appears to be long and relatively flat. Estimates have ranged from 10 to 50 patients or more.[6,7] Looking at our experience, 50 patients seem to be an appropriate estimate, given the change in frequency of conversion between our first quarter and subsequent quarters.

Based on our results, no segment or extent of the colon is beyond the scope of laparoscopic resection. Our conversion ratio for ascending and descending colectomy is equivalent. The high conversion rate in our initial experience with total abdominal colectomy was probably a reflection of the learning curve. Laparoscopic dissection is often tedious, and the time required to complete these procedures can be excessive. As we have gained greater experience, the limitations encountered in performing total abdominal colectomy have been overcome. We no longer consider this procedure too ambitious. On the other hand, procedures that involve resection of the distal rectum challenge the current limitations of laparoscopic technology. Although other authors have reported success with laparoscopic abdominoperineal resection, this has not been our experience.[8] Despite improved exposure in the pelvis with laparoscopy, we have encountered a high rate (40% [4/10]) of conversion to a laparotomy. This may reflect patient selection. Most of the patients having proctectomies have had inflammatory bowel disease. An inflammatory reaction in the adjacent mesentery with the obliteration of normal dissection planes has been the most frequent indication for conversion. Difficulty mobilizing and transecting the distal mesorectum has been the usual cause for converting low anterior resections. Constraints imposed by a narrow pelvis and a lack of compact articulating stapling instruments make this dissection difficult, especially when treating malignant disease. For these reasons, the technical requirements for low anterior resection probably exceed the limits of current laparoscopic technology. At our institution, Hartmann procedures are usually reserved for patients with advanced pelvic sepsis from complicated diverticulitis. Patients presenting with distal obstruction are usually treated with intraoperative colonic lavage and single-stage resection. This treatment strategy may have influenced our results with laparoscopic colorectal anastomosis following a Hartmann procedure. Based on our experience, the extensive adhesive reaction that may accompany a Hartmann procedure presents a substantial technical challenge. We no longer recommend a laparoscopic attempt at colorectal reanastomosis following a Hartmann resection. If laparoscopy is undertaken, we recommend early conversion to a laparotomy if extensive adhesions are encountered.

The indication for operation does not appear to influence the need for conversion. In our experience, the whole spectrum of colorectal diseases has been treated by laparoscopic resection. As mentioned previously, the role of laparoscopy in the treatment of potentially curable malignant lesions remains controversial. Several investigators[8,9] have confirmed that the length of colon and the extent of mesentery resected laparoscopically can be equivalent to that removed during a standard laparotomy. Whether proximal ligation of the vascular pedicle can be accomplished as successfully with laparoscopy is as yet unproved. Reports of port site and incisional metastases following laparoscopic resection of abdominal malignant neoplasms have raised additional concerns about the safety of the laparoscopic treatment of colorectal carcinoma.[10-13] Although more careful analysis of available data suggests that the risk of abdominal wall metastases is not significantly greater with laparoscopic surgery, this has not been established conclusively.[14] The multi-institutional prospective randomized trial[15,16] currently under way may resolve several of these questions.

We maintain a prospective institutional audit of all patients undergoing laparoscopic resection of colon carcinomas. Mean follow-up exceeds 48 months. There have been no cancer deaths in our series except for patients presenting with incurable disease. There have been no port site or incisional metastases in our series. Coincident with reports regarding port site metastases following laparoscopic colon resections for cancer, the number of laparoscopic resections performed for cancer during the latter half of our experience has decreased. The likelihood of conversion has not been influenced by the pathological stage of malignant disease, but the need for conversion is increased when treating bulky tumors that are difficult to mobilize or too large to remove through a small flank incision. When the tumor invades the retroperitoneum or involves adjacent organs, the technical limits of laparoscopic dissection are compromised, and conversion to a laparotomy is indicated.

A review of the change in indications for conversion during our experience suggests that technical problems that reflect the initial learning curve have now become a less frequent indication for conversion, whereas those factors reflecting the technical limitations of the method—large phlegmon, dense adhesions, bulky tumor, and adjacent organ involvement—account for an increasingly greater proportion of conversions to a laparotomy. If these findings are identified preoperatively, then a laparotomy should be the initial procedure. When these abnormalities are encountered during laparoscopic surgery, early conversion to a laparotomy is recommended.

Obesity has been identified as a relative contraindication to laparoscopic surgery. We have found obesity to be an infrequent indication for conversion, but our results suggest that obesity, as defined by a BMI of greater than 29, accentuates the technical limitations of laparoscopic colectomy.

CONCLUSIONS

As experience with laparoscopic colectomy accumulates, it is increasingly apparent that the procedure is a technically feasible option for treating a wide array of colorectal disorders. Although controversy regarding the treatment of cancer remains unresolved, there are few strict contraindications to the application of laparoscopic technology for the treatment of disorders of the large intestine. Experience with laparoscopic colectomy has been similar to that of other laparoscopic procedures. Evolving technology has made it possible to accomplish goals that were previously unattainable. We expect that current technical limitations of the procedure will be overcome as the methods continue to develop. It is likely that a laparoscopic approach may become the preferred method for treating a variety of colorectal disorders.

Presented at the 79th Annual Meeting of the New England Surgical Society, Toronto, Ontario, September 26, 1998.

Corresponding author: John J. Murray, MD, Department of Colorectal Surgery, Lahey Clinic, 41 Mall Rd, Burlington, MA 01805 (e-mail: John.murray@lahey.org).

REFERENCES

1. Slim K, Pezet D, Riff Y, Clark E, Chipponi J. High morbidity rate after converted laparoscopic colorectal surgery. *Br J Surg.* 1995;82:1406-1408.
2. Fitzgerald SD, Andrus CH, Baudendistel LJ, Dahms TE, Kaminski DL. Hypercarbia during carbon dioxide pneumoperitoneum. *Am J Surg.* 1992;163:186-190.
3. Wahba RWM, Mamazza J. Ventilatory requirements during laparoscopic cholecystectomy. *Can J Anaesth.* 1993;40:206-210.
4. Putensen-Himmer G, Putensen C, Lammer H, Lingnau W, Aigner F, Benzer H. Comparison of postoperative respiratory function after laparoscopy or open laparotomy for cholecystectomy. *Anesthesiology.* 1992;77:675-680.
5. Kent RB III. Subcutaneous emphysema and hypercarbia following laparoscopic cholecystectomy. *Arch Surg.* 1991;126:1154-1156.
6. Simons AJ, Anthone GJ, Ortega AE, et al. Laparoscopic-assisted colectomy learning curve. *Dis Colon Rectum.* 1995;38:600-603.
7. Senagore AJ, Luchtefeld MA, MacKeigan JM. What is the learning curve for laparoscopic colectomy? *Am Surg.* 1995;61:681-685.
8. Lord SA, Larach SW, Ferrara A, Williamson PR, Lago CP, Lube MW. Laparoscopic resections for colorectal carcinoma: a three year experience. *Dis Colon Rectum.* 1996;39:148-154.
9. Milsom JW, Bohm B, Decanini C, Fazio VW. Laparoscopic oncologic proctosigmoidectomy with low colorectal anastomosis in a cadaver model. *Surg Endosc.* 1994;8:1117-1123.
10. Nduka CC, Monson JRT, Menzies-Gow N, Darzi A. Abdominal wall metastases following laparoscopy. *Br J Surg.* 1994;81:648-652.
11. Wexner SD, Cohen SM. Port site metastases after laparoscopic colorectal surgery for cure of malignancy. *Br J Surg.* 1995;82:295-298.
12. Cirocco WC, Schwartzman A, Golub RW. Abdominal wall recurrence after laparoscopic colectomy for colon cancer. *Surgery.* 1994;116:842-846.
13. Jones DB, Guo LW, Reinhard MK, et al. Impact of pneumoperitoneum on trocar site implantation of colon cancer in hamster model. *Dis Colon Rectum.* 1995;38:1182-1188.
14. Reilly WT, Nelson H, Schroeder G, Wieand HS, Bolton J, O'Connell MJ. Wound recurrence following conventional treatment of colorectal cancer: a rare but perhaps underestimated problem. *Dis Colon Rectum.* 1996;39:200-207.
15. Stocchi L, Nelson H. Laparoscopic colectomy for colon cancer: trial update. *J Surg Oncol.* 1998;68:255-267.
16. Nelson H, Weeks JC, Wieand HS. Proposed phase III trial comparing laparoscopic-assisted colectomy versus open colectomy for colon cancer. *J Natl Cancer Inst Monogr.* 1995;No. 19:51-56.

Handoscopic Surgery

A Prospective Multicenter Trial of a Minimally Invasive Technique for Complex Abdominal Surgery

Southern Surgeons' Club Study Group

Hypothesis: We hypothesized that hand-assisted laparoscopic surgery (a new technique that involves a surgeon's hand passing through a pneumoperitoneum-protecting sleeve device and assisting in laparoscopic surgery) is feasable and outcomes are comparable to purely laparoscopic procedures in selected cases.

Design: A prospective, multicenter, nonrandomized, noncontrolled study was conducted with the participation of expert laparoscopic surgeons.

Setting: Academic and community medical centers in 16 states.

Patients: Any patient 18 years or older requiring abdominal surgery and determined to be suitable for laparoscopic surgery.

Main Outcome Measures: Incision size, duration of the procedure, conversion rate to an open technique, detection of subtle disease, return of bowel function, length of hospital stay, complication rate, and subjective evaluation.

Results: The device was used in 58 patients for 24 different procedures, most commonly during colectomy (n = 21) and splenectomy (n = 7). Twenty-two percent of cases required conversion to open technique because of failure to maintain pneumoperitoneum or failure to complete the anticipated operation by this method. Average incision size was 7.6 cm. Mean duration of all procedures was 223 minutes (range, 110-415 minutes) and for nonconverted procedures was 178 minutes (range, 65-540 minutes). Preoperatively undetectable, subtle disease was palpated in 14 patients (24%). Mean length of hospital stay for all patients was 7.9 days and for the nonconverted group was 6.7 days. Twenty-four percent of patients developed complications, most commonly either wound complications (n = 4) or prolonged ileus (n = 3). In 58% of cases, surgeons thought that the technique shortened surgery, and 88% of surgeons found the technique "helpful" in all the completed procedures.

Conclusions: This technique seems to be a useful tool in the management of cases that either are too complex or take too long to be managed with purely minimally invasive techniques. To further define the potential benefits of this technique in selected procedures, prospective randomized trials are needed.

Arch Surg. 1999;134:477-485

MINIMALLY INVASIVE surgery has revolutionized general surgery during the past 10 years. Laparoscopic cholecystectomy is currently the operation of choice for symptomatic gallstone disease, and the laparoscopic approach has also been used in the management of appendicitis, hernias, gastroesophageal reflux, and numerous other disease processes.[1-5] In fact, laparoscopic surgery is increasingly being used as an alternative to conventional open surgery because of several advantages over conventional open procedures: less trauma and pain, reduced hospitalization, and quicker recovery.

However, for more advanced surgical procedures, the acceptance of the minimally invasive approach has been slower than expected. This slow acceptance reflects a number of factors. First, performing major organ resections requires exceptional technical skills in laparoscopic tissue handling and manipulation. Given the limited number of training programs currently available for advanced laparoscopic surgery, only a select group of surgeons will acquire the necessary expertise in the foreseeable future. Second, current laparoscopic instrumentation is often inadequate for proper visualization and complex manipulation of intra-abdomi-

See Invited Critique at end of article

A complete list of the members of the Southern Surgeons' Club Study Group is given at the end of this article.

PATIENTS, MATERIALS, AND METHODS

A national, collaborative, single-arm study was organized through the Southern Surgeons' Club Study Group, with industry supplying the sleeve device and initial training. Surgeons were trained at either Duke University Medical Center, Durham, NC, or the Advanced Laparoscopy Training Center in Marietta, Ga. The study was conducted at academic and community medical centers and was approved by the institutional review boards of the participating institutions. The 27 surgeons involved in the study practiced in the following states: California (n = 4), Colorado (n = 2), Florida (n = 1), Georgia (n = 2), Kansas (n = 1), Massachusetts (n = 2), Mississippi (n = 1), Missouri (n = 1), Nebraska (n = 2), North Carolina (n = 2), Ohio (n = 2), Pennsylvania (n = 1), Texas (n = 2), Virginia (n = 1), Washington (n = 2), and Wisconsin (n = 1). All the surgeons had reasonable experience in advanced laparoscopic procedures.

In total, 63 patients requiring abdominal surgery were found to be suitable for laparoscopic surgery in conjunction with the Dexterity Pneumo Sleeve system and were enrolled in the study. General inclusion criteria included (1) being 18 years or older and (2) undergoing any abdominal surgery. General exclusion criteria included (1) being younger than 18 years, (2) participating in another study with any investigational device within the past 30 days, and (3) having a contraindication for treatment with the Dexterity Pneumo Sleeve and protector retractor (eg, a dermatologic condition because of the adhesive component). Patients who fulfilled the above inclusion and exclusion criteria signed an informed consent form. The surgeons tested the device under conditions in which they faced difficulties in completing procedures in a purely laparoscopic approach or, given the complexity of the cases and the need for tactile feedback, decided to start with the hand-assisted technique.

The sterile and disposable trial device had 6 components: the Dexterity Pneumo Sleeve, a protector retractor, absorbent roll, incision template, gown sleeve cover, and sterile lubricant (**Figure**). The incision template is a disk of paper or a similar material that is used to mark the incision site and the location for the sleeve application. The protector retractor has an open-ended cylinder with a flexible ring at each end. One ring is inserted through the incision into the peritoneal cavity and the other remains outside the incision. The retractor lines the wound and holds the incision open and protects it against wound contamination.

The Dexterity Pneumo Sleeve device is approximately 86.36 cm long and 24.13 cm wide and is made of a biocompatible, sealable, polyolifin-type material. The distal (patient) side of the sleeve has a fenestration and an adhesive flange for attaching to the patient's abdomen. A valve located in the sleeve's lumen is constructed to close as carbon dioxide escapes from the peritoneum through the fenestration. The proximal (surgeon) end of the sleeve has a cuff (constructed of a Velcro strap or molded plastic) that is designed to secure the sleeve to the surgeon's arm to prevent leakage of carbon dioxide. The absorbent roll is 10.16 cm long and 0.95 cm in diameter. It is tucked under the top (outside) ring of the protector retractor to prevent fluids from contacting the skin in the area on which the adhesive will be placed.

The gown sleeve cover is a sterile, disposable device that can only be used in conjunction with surgery gowns that are gas permeable. It is placed over the surgeon's arm to prevent leakage of insufflation gas through the gown material. The sterile lubricant is used to facilitate insertion of the surgeon's hand through the protector retractor. It is best applied to the retractor with a standard gauze bandage before the Dexterity Pneumo Sleeve is attached to the patient.

Surgeons chose to use the sleeve device either to improve the efficiency of a currently accepted laparoscopic procedure or to perform a more complex procedure not usually done with minimally invasive techniques. Use of the trial device was discontinued during surgery when any of the following occurred: (1) inability to perform the surgery, (2) intolerable adverse effects, or (3) inadequate functioning of the device. Discontinuation of use of this device did not indicate withdrawal from the trial.

The effectiveness of the treatment was assessed with regard to the evaluation of multiple end points, which included length of incision, number and size of trocars, duration of the operation, tissue removal and size, conversions to an open procedure, product evaluation, surgeon glove size, insufflation pressure, complications, infection, bowel function, and length of hospital stay.[1]

Statistical analysis was performed using the Student *t* test assuming unequal variances as appropriate, with $P<.05$ representing significance.

nal organs, and the inappropriate use of these instruments may jeopardize patients' safety. Third, many surgeons, other physicians, and third-party payers argue that increased surgery time and surgical costs associated with complex laparoscopic procedures may negate the benefits of minimal access surgery,[6] despite the documentation that operating time can effectively be reduced with training and expertise.[7] Finally, the lack of tactile feedback, which is an essential means by which surgeons identify structures and maintain safe dissection, prevents many surgeons from performing advanced minimally invasive procedures. The oncologic safety of laparoscopic procedures has become an additional source of debate.[8]

The previous observations led to the development of a device that allows insertion of a hand into the abdominal cavity while maintaining pneumoperitoneum, enabling the surgeon to perform the operation according to the principles of open surgery while retaining many of the advantages of a laparoscopic procedure. The Dexterity Pneumo Sleeve and protector retractor (Pilling Weck Corp, Raleigh, NC) functions similar to a trocar cannula. The device provides access to the abdominal cavity while maintaining pneumoperitoneum. Unlike the trocar cannula, the device allows the surgeon's hand to pass through a relatively small abdominal incision. Once in the abdominal cavity, the surgeon's hand provides haptic feedback, which assists in the performance of the procedure. Use of this technique may provide major advantages during laparoscopic surgery.

Initial reports about this technique were favorable,[9-11] and to further evaluate the usefulness of the Dexterity Pneumo Sleeve system and the efficacy of hand-assisted laparoscopic surgery we initiated a prospective, multicenter, noncontrolled clinical trial. In this study we report our experience based on 24 different types of hand-assisted laparoscopic procedures performed in 58 patients.

RESULTS

GENERAL RESULTS

A total of 62 patients were enrolled in the study, but the device was not used in 4 patients. The most common reason for not using hand-assisted surgery was because the surgeon thought that the procedure could be adequately done with a purely laparoscopic approach. Overall, 24 distinct procedures were performed in 58 patients (**Table 1**). The average age of patients was 57 years (range, 32-84 years), and their mean weight was 79 kg (range, 45-172 kg).

The most common procedure performed using the Dexterity Pneumo Sleeve device was colectomy (n = 24), either as a single procedure (n = 19) or in combination with another operation (n = 5). Splenectomy was carried out in 7 patients, and Nissen fundoplication and gastric bypass were each performed 3 times. In 3 patients, laparoscopic cholecystectomy was undertaken first, followed by a hand-assisted procedure (1 common bile duct exploration, 1 ileal resection, and 1 partial gastrectomy). In addition, 2 Whipple procedures and various other complex operations were performed using the hand-assisted laparoscopic technique. A summary of cases with general patient data and mean operation times is shown in Table 1.

HAND-ASSISTED TECHNIQUE–RELATED RESULTS

Average incision size to introduce a hand was 7.6 cm (range, 7.0-9.5 cm), which corresponded well with the average glove size of 7.4 cm. The exact positioning of the hand-assisted device depended on various factors, such as the surgeon's dexterity, comfort, and target area. The incision was placed in the midline in 19 patients, on the right side in 12 patients, on the left side in 17 patients, and in either the horizontal or vertical suprapubic position in 8 patients. In general, 2 to 3 additional laparoscopic trocars were introduced based on the situation and the surgeon's preference. Average insufflation pressure was 13.3 mm Hg (range, 8.3-15.0 mm Hg). The major function of the assisting hand included tissue manipulation (100%) and abdominal exploration (84%). Previously undetected disease was identified in 14 patients (24% of all patients). Of 25 patients diagnosed as having cancer, 5 (20%) were found to have previously undetected disease (**Table 2**).

Participating surgeons were asked to quantify the relevance of the presence of their hand in the abdomen while performing laparoscopic surgery. On a scale from 1 to 5 (5 being the best), for the purpose of abdominal exploration the overall satisfaction rate was 4.36. The assisting hand's utility in retraction and blunt dissection were equally rated as 4.60. The role of the hand-assisted laparoscopic technique in the control of hemorrhage was

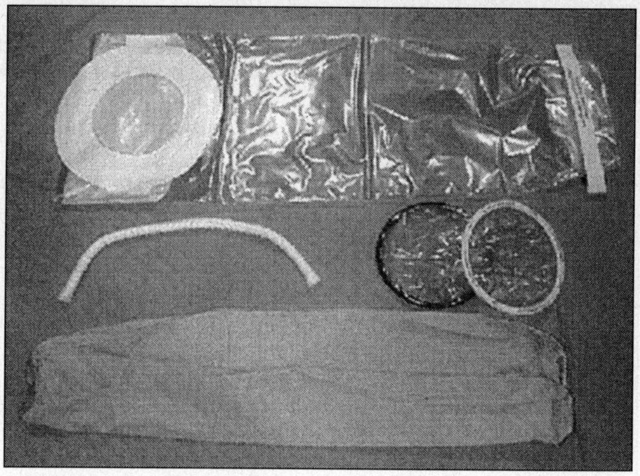

The Dexterity Pneumo Sleeve system.

rated as 4.05. In 33 cases the operating surgeon had the impression that use of the hand-assisted technique considerably shortened operation time, by an average of 70 minutes.

Overall, 13 operations (22%) had to convert to an open procedure for various reasons, which are listed in **Table 3**. In 4 of these operations there was an initial plan to convert to an open procedure because certain parts of the procedures were easily performed through the limited incision of the Dexterity Pneumo Sleeve device. Four cases were converted because of leakage of pneumoperitoneum through the device. Other cases that required conversion to an open procedure included 2 liver resections for hemangioma, a paraesophageal hernia repair, a gastric bypass procedure for morbid obesity, and a total abdominal colectomy for pseudocolonic obstruction.

DEVICE-RELATED RESULTS

Tissue removal through the protector retractor was carried out in 37 cases (64%) (**Table 4**). In 8 cases, 11 additional Dexterity Pneumo Sleeve devices were needed to complete the procedure. Reasons for device replacement included gas leakage (n = 6), problems with applying the device (n = 3), enlargement of the incision (n = 1), and the device being accidentally dropped on the floor (n = 1).

Inadequate sealing and gas leakage was the most commonly encountered device-related problem during the trial. Adhesive leakage was noted in 14 cases (24%), sleeve leakage in 10 cases (17%), and cuff leakage in 4 cases (7%). Although the mean weight of patients was higher in those in whom leakage problems were recorded (83.3 vs 75.7 kg), the difference was not statistically significant ($P = .28$). Overall impression of participating surgeons with the device was rated 4.5.

POSTOPERATIVE RESULTS

Skin complications (blistering and rash) at the site of the adhesive were recorded in 2 patients. At the site of the Dexterity Pneumo Sleeve, there was 1 wound infection (a vertical banded gastroplasty performed for morbid obesity in a diabetic patient), and a seroma was noted in

Table 1. Procedures Performed Using the Hand-Assisted Technique*

Diagnosis	Procedure	Length of Surgery, min	Patient Characteristics: Age, y	Race	Sex	Weight, kg
Recurrent colon cancer	Colon resection (splenic flexure)	115	58	W	F	69.9
Rectal carcinoma	Very low anterior resection	240	69	W	F	65.3
Redundant sigmoid colon	Sigmoid colon resection	120	43	W	F	65.8
Sigmoid polyp (3 cm)	Low anterior resection	141	77	W	F	83.9
Midtransverse colon tumor	Transverse colectomy	150	78	W	M	61.2
Right colon cancer with liver metastases	Right hemicolectomy, liver biopsy	N/A	49	W	F	54.4
Pseudocolonic obstruction	Total abdominal colectomy with ileoanal anastomosis	N/A	41	W	M	79.8
Familial polyposis	Ileoanal pull-through	NA	17	W	F	50.8
Metastatic colon cancer	Exploration, liver biopsy, right hemicolectomy	110	69	W	M	69.4
Colon cancer	Exploration, omentectomy, left hemicolectomy	180	80	W	F	45.4
Sigmoid villous adenoma with adenocarcinoma	Sigmoid colectomy	205	77	W	M	67.1
Hartmann pouch after colon cancer	Closure of colostomy, intraoperative ultrasound	240	66	W	M	81.6
Squamous cell carcinoma of vulva	Abdominal perineal resection	N/A	38	W	F	100.7
Cecal volvulus	Laparoscopic right hemicolectomy	95	82	W	F	47.6
Diverticulitis, colovaginal fistula	Sigmoid colectomy and repair of fistula	157	68	W	F	58.1
Diverticulitis, enterovesical fistula	Sigmoid colectomy, repair of bladder fistula	220	79	W	F	55.8
Diverticulitis, colovesical fistula	Sigmoid colectomy, bladder repair	130	60	W	M	72.6
Perforated sigmoid diverticulitis	Hartmann sigmoid colectomy	190	74	W	F	58.1
Perforated sigmoid diverticulitis	Hartmann sigmoid colectomy	155	44	W	M	145.2
Diverticulitis, chronic and acute	Sigmoid colectomy	130	65	W	F	73.5
Diverticulitis	Sigmoid colectomy, liver biopsy	94	48	W	M	112.5
Diverticulitis	Sigmoid colectomy	100	38	W	M	106.6
Diverticulitis	Sigmoid colectomy	168	41	W	F	76.2
Crohn colitis	Total abdominal colectomy	180	38	W	F	73.9
Crohn disease with enteroenteral fistula	Ileocolectomy with repair of ileocolic fistula	135	32	W	F	65.3
Crohn colitis, Crohn ileitis	Subtotal abdominal colectomy with ileosigmoid anastomosis	180	55	W	F	85.7
Splenic abscesses with periabscess fibrosis	Splenectomy	247	61	W	F	46.7
Idiopathic hemolytic anemia	Splenectomy	N/A	41	W	F	119.8
Hereditary spherocytosis	Splenectomy	160	42	W	M	88.0
Hypersplenism	Splenectomy	145	69	W	M	48.5
Thrombocytopenia, splenomegaly, lymphoma	Splenectomy	148	56	W	M	79.8
Lymphoma	Splenectomy	170	70	W	M	81.6
Hodgkin disease, thrombocytopenia	Splenectomy	154	53	W	F	N/A
GERD	Nissen fundoplication	65	69	W	F	73.5
GERD	Nissen fundoplication	170	45	W	F	66.2
GERD, cholelithiasis	Laparoscopic cholecystectomy, then hand-assisted Nissen fundoplication	185	38	W	F	98.0
Cholecystolithiasis	Laparoscopic cholecystectomy, then hand-assisted resection of ileum	155	72	W	F	73.5
Cholecystolithiasis, gastric leiomyoma	Laparoscopic cholecystectomy, then hand-assisted partial gastrectomy	140	79	W	M	66.7
Gallbladder mass	CBD exploration, stone extraction, cholecystectomy	136	75	B	F	45.8
Biliary obstruction	Exploration, liver biopsy, choledochojejunostomy	N/A	65	W	F	70.3
Liver hemangioma	Liver resection (converted to open)	N/A	41	W	F	59.0
Liver hemangioma	Laparoscopy, liver resection	N/A	64	W	F	79.4
Periampullary tumor	Whipple procedure	540	71	W	M	68.9
Pancreatic cancer	Whipple procedure	350	64	W	F	80.7
Pancreatic cancer	Exploration to determine resectability	130	57	W	M	86.2
Gastric lymphoma	Subtotal gastrectomy	360	66	W	F	118.8
Incisional hernia associated with morbid obesity	Gastric bypass and ventral hernia repair	390	44	W	M	172.4
Morbid obesity	Gastric bypass	N/A	32	W	F	107.1
Severe obesity	Gastric bypass	N/A	44	W	F	117.0
Metastatic tumor of the small bowel	Small-bowel resection	160	43	W	M	63.5
Severe obesity, diabetes, HTN, depression	Vertical banded gastroplasty	120	57	W	F	149.7
Esophageal cancer	Laparoscopic transhiatal esophagectomy	320	67	W	M	69.4
Paraesophageal hernia	Repair of paraesophageal hernia	N/A	50	W	M	79.4
Pseudoarthrosis L4-5	Anterior spinal fusion (L4-5)	N/A	36	W	M	N/A
Failed laminectomy syndrome	Anterior discectomy/fusion	N/A	32	W	M	74.8
Partial small-bowel obstruction	Adhesiolysis	N/A	67	W	F	66.2
Small-bowel obstruction	Exploratory laparoscopy, adhesiolysis	110	84	W	M	60.3
Retroperitoneal adenopathy	Exploration, biopsy	48	80	W	M	74.8

**W* indicates white; B, black; F, female; M, male; N/A, not available; GERD, gastroesophageal reflux disease; CBD, common bile duct; and HTN, hypertension.*

another patient after a sigmoid resection for diverticulitis. Infection at the skin staple site was noted in a patient who underwent gastric bypass procedure for morbid obesity. The postoperative complications are listed in **Table 5**.

The average number of postoperative days before return to a regular diet and the average hospital stay for uncomplicated cases of left colectomy, splenectomy, and Nissen fundoplication (which were the most commonly performed procedures in the series) are listed in **Table 6**.

COMMENT

The evolution of laparoscopic surgery experienced its peak during the early 1990s with the rapid acceptance of laparoscopic cholecystectomy.[12] This change in surgical practice was followed shortly by other procedures, such as inguinal and abdominal hernia repair, appendectomy, colon resection, and Nissen fundoplication. The transition to more complex laparoscopic operations has apparently slowed down, which mainly reflects the technical difficulties and the safety concerns associated with these advanced procedures.

The recent introduction of the Dexterity Pneumo Sleeve device allows one to insert a hand (usually the nondominant hand) into the abdominal cavity during a laparoscopic procedure without the subsequent loss of pneumoperitoneum. Although the technique is appealing, immediate concerns were raised regarding the efficacy and the minimal invasiveness of the resulting operation. This national, prospective, multicenter, noncontrolled clinical trial was initiated by the Southern Surgeons' Club Study Group to identify potential applications, advantages, and disadvantages for the hand-assisted laparoscopic technique.

Colorectal cases constituted almost half of the entire series of 58 patients (26 cases). Despite the considerable caseload, laparoscopic colorectal surgery has not gained popularity among most colorectal surgeons. This only partly reflects the lack of technical expertise in advanced laparoscopic procedures. Controversial results regarding oncologic safety, including port site recurrence, and excessive operating time and associated costs have discouraged many to approach colorectal malignancies with the minimal access technique.[13] The hand-assisted laparoscopic technique may provide a solution to some of these concerns.[14]

In our series, the average operating time for hand-assisted laparoscopic sigmoid colectomies (149 minutes) and the average length of hospital stay (6.4 days) were similar to those of most published laparoscopic colectomy series.[7,15] Although this is only an initial experience with the technique, these results suggest that the purely laparoscopic and the hand-assisted techniques do not significantly differ in terms of minimal invasiveness for colon resections. These findings give credence to the belief that insertion of a hand will make the surgeon more efficient because initial experience with the hand-assisted technique resulted in operating times that have been achieved only after considerable experience in the laparoscopic series. This reflects a steeper learning curve for hand-assisted laparoscopic surgery for colon resections.[16] The fact that almost half of the total series were colorectal cases (and only 2 of them required conversion to open surgery) indicates that colorectal surgery may be the subspecialty that could benefit most from the hand-assisted technique.

Table 2. Previously Undetected Disease Identified During Hand-Assisted Laparoscopic Surgery

Preoperative Diagnosis	Procedure	Previously Undetected Disease Found
Gallbladder mass	CBD* exploration, stone extraction, cholecystectomy	Choledocholithiasis, cholelithiasis
Biliary obstruction	Exploration, liver biopsy, choledochojejunostomy	Liver cyst, cystic neoplasm of the pancreas
Liver hemangioma	Liver resection (converted to open)	Size of hemangioma
Liver hemangioma	Laparoscopy, liver resection	Liver cyst
Diverticulitis	Sigmoid colectomy	Degree of inflammation
Sigmoid polyp (3 cm)	Low anterior resection	Benign hepatic cysts
Retroperitoneal adenopathy	Exploration, biopsy	Yes, not specified
Failed laminectomy syndrome	Anterior discectomy/fusion	Yes, not specified
Esophageal cancer	Transhiatal esophagectomy	Splenic nodule
Perforated sigmoid diverticulitis	Hartmann sigmoid colectomy	Metastatic implant on bowel
Small-bowel obstruction	Lysis of adhesions	Multiple adhesions
Metastatic colon cancer	Right hemicolectomy, liver biopsy	Tumor was in hepatic flexure and not in cecum as thought
Pancreatic cancer	Exploration	Celiac plexus found to be encased in tumor
Colon cancer	Left hemicolectomy, omentectomy	Yes, metastatic tumor

**CBD indicates common bile duct.*

Because a limited laparotomy is required to remove the resected specimen, it seems logical to make the small incision at the beginning of the procedure. This may address concerns regarding operating time, related costs, and oncologic safety. Inserting a hand makes tissue manipulation (exploration, blunt dissection, and retraction) considerably easier and, therefore, increases the surgeon's confidence. Should a hemorrhagic complication occur, a bleeding vessel can more easily be controlled and blood loss minimized, providing the surgeon with valuable time to plan a strategy for problem resolution—even conversion, if necessary. After the colon has been fully mobilized, an extracorporal anastomosis can be performed through the small incision.

Port site recurrence has been a major argument against laparoscopic surgery for malignant lesions. Results of a recent prospective randomized trial,[17] however, demonstrate that wound recurrence in open surgery and port site recurrence in laparoscopic surgery have an equal probability. Although in vitro evidence is con-

Table 3. Reasons for Conversions to Open Procedures

Diagnosis	Procedure	Reason for Conversion to an Open Procedure
Biliary obstruction	Exploration, liver biopsy, choledochojejunostomy	Leakage of Pneumo Sleeve valve
Squamous cell carcinoma of vulva	Abdominal perineal resection	Difficulty with getting adequate adhesion of device and visualization
Severe obesity	Laparoscopic gastric bypass	Failure to maintain pneumoperitoneum
Idiopathic hemolytic anemia	Splenectomy	Inability to maintain pneumoperitoneum, obesity, pancreas too close to spleen
Paraesophageal hernia	Repair of paraesophageal hernia	Unable to reduce spleen from chest
Liver hamangioma	Liver resection (converted to open)	Size of hemangioma
Liver hemangioma	Laparoscopy, liver resection	To ensure patient safety
Morbid obesity	Laparoscopic gastric bypass	Difficulty in positioning stapler across proximal stomach
Pseudocolonic obstruction	Total abdominal colectomy with ileoanal anastomosis	Time-consuming dissection to get to colon
Familial polyposis	Ileoanal pull-through	It was a planned conversion for pelvic dissection; there was no need to enlarge incision
Partial small-bowel obstruction	Adhesiolysis	Small-bowel resection was performed conveniently through Dexterity incision
Failed laminectomy syndrome	Anterior discectomy/fusion	Vena caval retraction/mobilization performed through Dexterity incision
Right colon cancer with liver metastases	Right hemicolectomy and liver biopsy	Planned extracorporeal anastomosis

Table 4. Tissue Removed Through the Protector-Retractor Device During Surgery*

Procedure	Tissue
Colorectal cases	
Sigmoid colectomy, low anterior resection, Hartmann procedure	Sigmoid colon (13 cases)
Exploration, omentectomy, low anterior resection	Sigmoid colon, omentum
Colon resection (splenic flexure)	Left colon
Right hemicolectomy	Right colon (3 cases)
Right hemicolectomy and liver biopsy	Right colon, liver tissue
Subtotal abdominal colectomy with ileosigmoid anastomosis	Entire colon and terminal ileum
Ileoanal pull-through	Colon and rectum
Splenectomy	Spleen (6 cases)
Other advanced minimally invasive procedures	
Whipple procedure	Head of pancreas, duodenum (2 cases)
Laparoscopic transhiatal esophagectomy	Esophagus
Subtotal gastrectomy	Stomach
Small-bowel resection	Small bowel
Laparoscopic cholecystectomy, then hand-assisted Nissen fundoplication	Gallbladder
Laparoscopic cholecystectomy, then hand-assisted partial gastrectomy	Gallbladder, stomach
CBD exploration, stone extraction, cholecystectomy	Gallbaldder, CBD stones
Laparoscopic cholecystectomy, then hand-assisted resection of ileum	Ileum

**CBD indicates common bile duct.*

troversial, it is increasingly accepted that it is more likely to be inadequate surgical technique and wound protection that account for tumor recurrence at the port site or in the abdominal incision.[18,19] In general, we believe that resected specimens should only be removed in a specimen bag (or through a protected port) and that direct contact between the abdominal wall and the resected tissue should be avoided. Specimen removal through the protector retractor was performed in 36 cases (Table 4). The protector retractor portion of the Dexterity Pneumo Sleeve system provides excellent wound protection throughout the procedure by covering the entire surface of the incision. If a specimen containing neoplastic tumor cells is being removed through the protected wound, the likelihood of tumor seeding in the incision should be minimal. Our study does not contain long-term follow-up information, and, therefore, this issue needs to be addressed by long-term randomized prospective trials in the future.

One of the major arguments against the use of laparoscopy in the management of malignant disease is the lack of tactile sensation, which has been an essential tool of the surgeon in the detection of covert metastases in open operations. The lack of the opportunity to blindly explore abdominal contents and to identify accidental findings not otherwise seen with the laparoscope has discouraged many surgeons from the routine application of the minimally invasive technique in their practice.

A major advantage of the hand-assisted technique over the purely laparoscopic approach is the ability to identify previously undetected disease only recognizable by palpation (Table 2). In our series, previously undetected and unsuspected lesions were identified in 14 cases, half of which had oncologic relevance. Metastatic implants, tumor extension, or even incidental findings can effectively be localized by palpation. These findings confirm the potential utility of the hand-assisted technique in the minimal access management of malignant tumors.

Seven splenectomies were performed during the trial. The average operating time was 171 minutes, although almost all the operations were performed on enlarged spleens, which typically are associated with longer operating times. One surgeon would not have attempted the laparoscopic approach without the Pneumo Sleeve device, and another case would have been converted to open surgery because of technical difficulties related to the enlarged spleen. One of the challenges of laparoscopic splenectomy is the successful retraction of the spleen. Cur-

Table 5. Postoperative Complications

Diagnosis	Procedure	Complications
Wound complications		
Diverticulitis, chronic and acute	Sigmoid colectomy	Seroma at Pneumo Sleeve site
Severe obesity, diabetes, hypertension, depression	Vertical banded gastroplasty	Wound infection at Pneumo Sleeve site
Squamous cell carcinoma of vulva	Abdominal perineal resection	2-cm wound separation
Morbid obesity	Gastric bypass	Staple site infection
Ileus		
Carcinoma of the rectum	Very low anterior resection	Ileus
Right colon cancer with liver metastases	Right hemicolectomy and liver biopsy	Ileus
Small-bowel obstruction	Exploration, adhesiolysis	Ileus, partial small-bowel obstruction
Abdominal complications		
Metastatic tumor of the small bowel	Small-bowel resection	Pelvic seroma
Crohn colitis	Total abdominal colectomy	Anastomotic leak
Pancreatic cancer	Whipple procedure	Pancreatic leak
Other complications		
Splenic abscesses with periabscess fibrosis	Splenectomy	Anemia, hyponatremia
Liver hemangioma	Liver resection (converted to open)	Bleeding, inferior vena cava thrombus, pulmonary complications
Incisional hermia associated with morbid obesity	Gastric bypass and hernia repair	Postoperative pneumonia, respiratory insufficiency
Esophageal cancer	Transhiatal esophagectomy	Pneumothorax

rent laparoscopic retractors often do not safely deal with large spleens. Having a hand inside the abdomen is the best potential retractor, and the ability to identify major vessels by palpation is helpful in avoiding serious bleeding complications. The spleen was successfully removed through the protector retractor either whole or morcellated, depending on its size. Only 1 (14%) of 7 cases had to be converted in the series. Average hospital stay after the procedure was 3.8 days, which is slightly longer than what has been reported by most series of laparoscopic splenectomies.[20] Recent series[21,22] report mean operating times of 190 to 265 minutes, with conversion rates ranging between 25% and 50% for enlarged spleens. Given the fact that the hand-assisted laparoscopic cases in our series consisted almost exclusively of enlarged spleens, which would be difficult, if not impossible to remove purely laparoscopically, the results seem superior to those of laparoscopic splenectomy. Preoperative embolization before laparoscopic splenectomy recommended by some authors is not necessary if the hand-assisted approach is used.[21] Overall, the hand-assisted technique proved to be a useful tool in minimal access splenectomy, seemingly making the procedure safer and shorter, especially in cases of splenomegaly.

Three Nissen fundoplications were performed successfully using the technique. The operating times and hospital stays were slightly longer than those of laparoscopic Nissen fundoplication.[23] Two surgeons found that the hand-assisted technique was difficult and experienced setup problems (hands were too close to camera). It seems now that the skills necessary to perform laparoscopic Nissen fundoplication can be easily developed, and because recent studies confirm the excellent long-term results with the purely laparoscopic approach, the hand-assisted technique will not be needed in the management of gastroesophageal reflux disease.[5,23,24]

The technique was successfully used for other advanced procedures such as liver resections, Whipple procedures, gastric bypass, partial gastrectomy, and others (Table 1). Overall impression about the technique was favorable, but based on this limited experience it is still too early to form a definitive statement about the utility of hand-assisted laparoscopy in the management of these cases. Sporadic reports confirm our findings that the assisting hand proved to be useful in the precise localization of tumors, adhesiolysis, organ retraction and manipulation, and hemorrhage control.[11,25-27] Although, our series did not include hand-assisted laparoscopic nephrectomies, some reports have been published with favorable experiences.[28] More experience is required to explore the pitfalls and benefits, but the initial results are encouraging.

Table 6. Average Hospital Stays for the Most Commonly Performed Uncomplicated Procedures

Hand-Assisted Laparoscopic Procedure	Postoperative Days Before Regular Diet Initiated, Mean	Hospital Stay, Mean, d
Colectomy (19 cases)	3.5	6.4
Splenectomy (6 cases)	3.2	3.8
Nissen fundoplication (3 cases)	3.7	3.3

Thirteen operations were converted to an open technique for various reasons; however, 4 of these were planned conversions, either to perform extracorporal anastomosis or to do a part of the procedure in an open fashion. One of the key elements of successful minimal access surgery is flexibility and quick adaptation of existing possibilities. This may include rearranging instruments using the existing ports, placing new ports, or, in the case of hand-assisted laparoscopic surgery, using the incision for the Dexterity Pneumo Sleeve device to perform open surgery. This flexibility is perceived as a major advantage of hand-assisted laparoscopic surgery.

Five cases required conversion when the surgeons could not safely complete the procedures. In 4 cases conversion was needed because the device did not function properly and pneumoperitoneum could not be maintained. In fact, air leakage was the most commonly encountered problem during the entire trial. Leakage was noted at the adhesive, at the cuff, or at the sleeve in 28 cases, forcing replacement of the device 6 times. In addition, problems with applying the device and eventual replacement were noted in 3 cases. These difficulties may be a result of insufficient experience, but it was the major determinant of surgeon satisfaction and overall success. Device leakage was unrelated to patient weight. It is our belief that difficulties with leakage and application of the device will need to be addressed in subsequent generations of the product, otherwise these annoying and distracting events may eventually discourage surgeons from using the device.

Fourteen postoperative complications were noted in the entire series, and most occurred after complex abdominal surgery. Only 2 minor wound infections occurred at the site of the incision: 1 seroma and 1 wound infection after a sigmoid colectomy and a vertical banded gastroplasty, respectively.

CONCLUSIONS

These data support the concept that hand-assisted laparoscopic surgery is a useful adjunct in the armamentarium of the general surgeon. Based on our limited initial experience, we recommend possible use of the hand-assisted technique in the following situations: (1) any major solid or hollow organ resection that will require a limited incision for specimen removal; (2) complex laparoscopic procedures that currently have extensive operating time, higher costs, and higher conversion rates than open procedures; (3) as a replacement to conversion to open surgery in cases in which temporary tactile feedback of manual assistance is required; and (4) major abdominal procedures considered too difficult for laparoscopic surgery. In this study, there was an apparent benefit for selected cases of splenectomy when there is splenomegaly, for colorectal resections, and other isolated complex cases with this approach. To further define the potential benefits of this technique in the management of oncologic problems, prospective randomized trials are needed. The availability of this device may encourage some surgeons who have not developed enough advanced laparoscopic expertise to pursue minimally invasive procedures. However, at this time we recommend use of hand-assisted laparoscopy only for experts in laparoscopic surgery and for procedures that either are too complex or take too long to be managed with purely laparoscopic surgery.

This study was partially sponsored by a grant from the Pilling Weck Corp, Raleigh, NC.

Presented at the 79th Annual Meeting of the New England Surgical Society, Toronto, Ontario, September 25, 1998.

The members of the Southern Surgeons' Club Study Group are as follows: William C. Meyers, MD, David P. Foley, MD, Andras Sandor, MD, Demetrius E. M. Litwin, MD, Mark P. Callery, MD, and Steven M. Yood, MD, University of Massachusetts Medical School, Worcester; Michel Gagner, MD (formerly with the Cleveland Clinic Foundation), Antonio Garcia, MD, Jeffrey W. Milson, MD, and Tekeshi Naitoh, MD, Mt Sinai Medical Center, New York, NY; Clark D. Gerhart, MD, private practice, Hazleton, Pa; Barry Feig, MD, Alice Madary, RN, and Paul Mansfield, MD, University of Texas M. D. Anderson Cancer Center, Houston; Eugene Foley, MD, Anna Miller, RN, and Bruce Schirmer, MD, University of Virginia Health Science Center, Charlottesville; Robert Fitzgibbons, Jr, MD, Anthony Lowham, MD, and Muhammed Ashraf Memon, MD, Creighton University School of Medicine, Omaha, Neb; Joseph Wasselle, MD, Holmes Regional Medical Center, Melbourne, Fla; Gene Branum, MD, Atlanta VA Hospital, Decatur, Ga; William P. Chalfant III, MD, Cabarrus Memorial Hospital, Concord, NC; Daniel T. Dempsey, MD, Temple University Hospital, Philadelphia, Pa; Quan-Yung Duh, MD, VA Medical Center, San Francisco, Calif; Michael Holzman, MD, Vanderbilt University Medical School, Nashville, Tenn; Santiago Horgon, MD, Carlos A. Pellegrini, MD, and Mika Sinanan, MD, University of Washington, Seattle; John D. Hunter, MD, Emory Clinic, Atlanta, Ga; Namir Katkhouda, MD, and Hesham Soliman, MD, University of California Healthcare Consultation Center, Los Angeles; Amy Andersen, MS, David Mahvi, MD, and Stephen Nakada, MD, University of Wisconsin Hospital, Madison; Robert McIntyre, MD, and Greg Steigman, MD, University of Colorado Health Center, Denver; Joseph Petelin, MD, Shawnee Mission Medical Center, Shawnee Mission, Kan; Anthony Petro, MD, and Carl R. Voyles, MD, Mississippi Baptist Medical Center, Jackson; Nathaniel Soper, MD, Washington University, St Louis, Mo; Mary Stanley, MD, Medical Center of Central Massachusetts; Joyce Stevens, MS; Lawrence W. Way, MD, University of California at San Francisco Medical School; Carol Eliadi, RN, University of Massachusetts Medical School, Worcester; Mary Ann Iannacchione, RN, Duke University Medical Center, Durham, NC; William B. Saye, MD, Advanced Laparoscopic Training Center, Marietta, Ga.

Corresponding author: William C. Meyers, MD, Department of Surgery, University of Massachusetts Medical Center, 55 Lake Ave N, Worcester, MA 01655.

REFERENCES

1. A prospective analysis of 1518 laparoscopic cholecystectomies: the Southern Surgeons' Club [published erratum appears in *N Engl J Med.* 1991;325:1517-1518] [see comments]. *N Engl J Med.* 1991;324:1073-1078.
2. Litwin DE, Girotti MJ, Poulin EC, Mamazza J, Nagy AG. Laparoscopic cholecystectomy: trans-Canada experience with 2201 cases. *Can J Surg.* 1992;35:291-296.
3. Johnson AB, Peetz ME. Laparoscopic appendectomy is an acceptable alternative for the treatment of perforated appendicitis. *Surg Endosc.* 1998;12:940-943.
4. Wellwood J, Sculpher MJ, Stoker D, et al. Randomised controlled trial of laparoscopic versus open mesh repair for inguinal hernia: outcome and cost. *BMJ.* 1998;317:103-110.
5. McKernan JB, Champion JK. Minimally invasive antireflux surgery. *Am J Surg.* 1998;175:271-276.
6. Philipson BM, Bokey EL, Moore JW, Chapuis PH, Bagge E. Cost of open versus laparoscopically assisted right hemicolectomy for cancer. *World J Surg.* 1997; 21:214-217.
7. Fielding GA, Lumley J, Nathanson L, Hewitt P, Rhodes M, Stitz R. Laparoscopic colectomy. *Surg Endosc.* 1997;11:745-749.
8. Luck A, Hensman C, Hewett P. Laparoscopic colectomy for cancer: a review. *Aust N Z J Surg.* 1998;68:318-327.
9. Bemelman WA, Ringers J, Meijer DW, de Wit CW, Bannenberg JJ. Laparoscopic-assisted colectomy with the Dexterity Pneumo Sleeve. *Dis Colon Rectum.* 1996; 39(suppl 10):S59-S61.
10. Kusminsky RE, Boland JP, Tiley EH, Deluca JA. Hand-assisted laparoscopic splenectomy. *Surg Laparosc Endosc.* 1995;5:463-467.

11. O'Reilly MJ, Saye WB, Mullins SG, Pinto SE, Falkner PT. Technique of hand-assisted laparoscopic surgery. *J Laparoendosc Surg.* 1996;6:239-244.
12. Nagy AG, Poulin EC, Girotti MJ, Litwin DE, Mamazza J. History of laparoscopic surgery. *Can J Surg.* 1992;35:271-274.
13. Wexner SD, Cohen SM. Port site metastases after laparoscopic colorectal surgery for cure of malignancy [see comments]. *Br J Surg.* 1995;82:295-298.
14. Boulez J, Espalieu P, Fontaumard E, Meeus P. Laparoscopic colorectal surgery: analysis of 113 cases. *Hepatogastroenterology.* 1997;44:40-44.
15. Stevenson AR, Stitz RW, Lumley JW, Fielding GA. Laparoscopically assisted anterior resection for diverticular disease: follow-up of 100 consecutive patients. *Ann Surg.* 1998;227:335-342.
16. Mooney MJ, Elliott PL, Galapon DB, James LK, Lilac LJ, O'Reilly MJ. Hand-assisted laparoscopic sigmoidectomy for diverticulitis. *Dis Colon Rectum.* 1998; 41:630-635.
17. Lacy AM, Delgado S, Garcia-Valdecasas JC, et al. Port site metastases and recurrence after laparoscopic colectomy. *Surg Endosc.* 1998;12:1039-1042.
18. Lee SW, Southall J, Allendorf J, Bessler M, Whelan RL. Traumatic handling of the tumor independent of pneumoperitoneum increases port site implantation rate of colon cancer in a murine model. *Surg Endosc.* 1998;12:828-834.
19. Gellman L, Salky B, Edye M. Laparoscopic assisted colectomy. *Surg Endosc.* 1996; 10:1041-1044.
20. Szold A, Sagi B, Merhav H, Klausner JM. Optimizing laparoscopic splenectomy: technical details and experience in 59 patients. *Surg Endosc.* 1998;12:1078-1081.
21. Poulin EC, Mamazza J. Laparoscopic splenectomy: lessons from the learning curve [see comments]. *Can J Surg.* 1998;41:28-36.
22. Targarona EM, Espert JJ, Balague C, Piulachs J, Artigas V, Trias M. Splenomegaly should not be considered a contraindication for laparoscopic splenectomy. *Ann Surg.* 1998;228:35-39.
23. Peters JH, DeMeester TR, Crookes P, et al. The treatment of gastroesophageal reflux disease with laparoscopic Nissen fundoplication: prospective evaluation of 100 patients with "typical" symptoms. *Ann Surg.* 1998;228:40-50.
24. Leggett PL, Churchman-Winn R, Ahn C. Resolving gastroesophageal reflux with laparoscopic fundoplication: findings in 138 cases. *Surg Endosc.* 1998;12:142-147.
25. Naitoh T, Gagner M. Laparoscopically assisted gastric surgery using Dexterity Pneumo Sleeve. *Surg Endosc.* 1997;11:830-833.
26. Watson DI, Game PA. Hand-assisted laparoscopic vertical banded gastroplasty: initial report. *Surg Endosc.* 1997;11:1218-1220.
27. Memon MA, Fitzgibbons RJ Jr. Hand-assisted laparoscopic surgery (HALS): a useful technique for complex laparoscopic abdominal procedures. *J Laparoendosc Adv Surg Tech A.* 1998;8:143-150.
28. Wolf JS Jr, Moon TD, Nakada SY. Hand assisted laparoscopic nephrectomy: comparison to standard laparoscopic nephrectomy. *J Urol.* 1998;160:22-27.

DISCUSSION

Dougald Macgillivray, MD, South Portland, Me: What we have seen today is the experience of the Southern Surgeons' Club in a multicenter feasibility trial of a device that allows for the surgeon to use his or her hand during complex laparoscopic procedures. These results indicate that this device can be used successfully in a variety of complex laparoscopic operations. The operative times reported for the most part are compatible with what one would expect had the procedures been done using an open approach.

This is remarkable for a new technical device that was being used by many different surgeons on relatively few cases. The device seems to be safe in that the reported complications were mostly minor or ones that you would expect to be related to the procedure itself rather than to the utilization of the device. One could question the judgment of using a new technical device that is still unproven in some of these challenging operations, but, as was pointed out, this was a feasibility trial.

I agree with Dr Foley that if an incision is required to remove a specimen or to perform anastomosis that it is sensible to make the incision early and to use it for the difficult portion of the dissection. This device allows for the utilization of a needed incision while maintaining pneumoperitoneum. It allows for the protection of the wound, which appears to be important in reducing tumor implantation. The ability to use tactile sensation during the larapascopic procedure is a major potential advantage of this device. However, I think they slightly overemphasize their ability to detect lesions in the manuscript.

Twenty-seven surgeons participated in this study, but the device was only used in 58 patients.

What factors limited the acceptance for utilization of this technique? A conversion rate of 22% is high for a motivated group of highly skilled laparoscopic surgeons. A technical failure of the device seemed to be a reason for many of these conversions. Has the device recently been modified or improved?

In a group of patients who had a colon resection a regular diet was started on postoperative day 3.5, but the average hospital stay was 6.4 days. What accounted for the delay in discharge of this group of patients?

One could argue that some of these procedures could have been accomplished using a purely laparoscopic approach or by extending the incision 2 or 3 cm by an entirely open approach. Do you think that by reducing an abdominal incision by a few centimeters the operative morbidity will be reduced enough to justify the use of this device? And do you plan on conducting a randomized trial to more rigorously test the potential benefits of this device?

Dr Foley and his associates have presented an interesting and innovative technique and they have challenged us to consider expanding the field of minimally invasive surgery to more complex operations.

Dr Foley: To answer your questions in regard to the number of surgeons who participated and why only 58 patients underwent the procedure, the device was supplied by industry and there was a limit on the number of devices supplied. We are currently working with Smith & Nephew Inc at the University of Massachusetts Medical Center to improve the device and minimize gas leakage. The new device has an additional bubble that lies in the abdominal cavity up against the abdominal wall and when insufflated prevents leakage of gas during the procedure.

As far as the delay in discharge, it's unclear exactly why these patients actually started their diet on average postoperative day 3.5 and they went home on postoperative day 6. There were a wide variety of surgeons in the study, and we couldn't really delineate the reason for delay in discharge.

As far as the justification for the use of the device, we don't know if the operative morbidity will be less than that with laparotomy. This is the question we hope to answer in future studies. With full laparotomy it is unclear exactly why patients develop postoperative ileus or complications from a larger incision. Is it due to desiccation, or increased abdominal retraction, etc? By actually reducing the incision size and maintaining adequate exposure via laparoscopy, we are able to perform these procedures, and these data suggest that potentially it would be of benefit. Also, we have an ongoing, randomized trial at the University of Massachusetts Medical Center, randomizing patients either to laparascopic colectomy or to hand-assisted laparascopic colectomy, so we should have some data from that in the near future.

Walter Goldfarb, MD, Portland, Me: This is the first prospective 1-armed study reported!

Charles Shoemaker, MD, Newport, RI: One of the problems with this new explosive technology is how to get it out into the community. Having been there and seen the pressure both from patients and industry, perhaps this concept of handscopic surgery is the way to go. Trying to introduce this pure laparascopic surgery into the community is very difficult. Your hospital has not given you credentials for a new procedure, and it is difficult to bring down an expert from Brown [University] each time a new procedure is introduced. This is a nice intermediate way to get the traditional surgeon, who's comfortable feeling the tissue, to gradually move in the direction of laparascopic surgery. It's a concept that we really must pay attention to.

Blake Cady, MD, Providence, RI: I can't resist. I can foresee the next technical advance in modern surgery, the introduction of both hands into the abdominal cavity! My question is, how soon do you think that new advance will occur?

Dr Foley: We actually have 2 single-arm studies in progress trying to answer that question.

Invited Critique

The Southern Surgical Club has recruited many patients to assess the clinical utility of hand-assisted laparoscopic surgery. This device permits the surgeon to recover the tactile feeling, maintaining the advantages of laparoscopy. The cases chosen include a variety of procedures performed and levels of complexity, which complicate analysis, as reflected by the high conversion rate (22%). Some indications are difficult to accept (eg, hiatal hernia) when results with the standard laparoscopic approach are satisfactory. The best message comes from the analysis of 2 accepted indications: colectomy and splenectomy. The results after colectomy are promising, especially when they include more difficult situations (eg, diverticulitis and intestinal fistula). The authors do not state the characteristics of spleens approached with the hand port, but 4 of 7 were benign, and they could be morcellated. The accessory incision in splenic surgery should be considered only for cases of massive spleen or for retrieval of the intact organ, and it is in this selected group of patients that use of the hand port may be beneficial. Probably the most important data of this work is the surgeon's subjective feeling that this device facilitated the procedure in 88% of cases, with a score higher than 4 on a scale from 0 to 5.

A shortcoming is that conversion in 4 of 13 cases was caused by malfunction of the device; in 8 cases, an additional 11 devices were required, increasing the already expensive cost of laparoscopic surgery.

Hand-assisted laparoscopic surgery opens a new area of interest in minimally invasive surgery. The next step is randomized comparison with standard open or laparoscopic procedures to investigate the clinical place of this hybrid type of surgery, and to know whether it is an initial tool for the trainee laparoscopic surgeon or a last resort for the experienced laparoscopic surgeon.

A final comment about the title: "Handoscopic or Laparohand?" The scope does not end with the hand; a simple "hand-assisted laparoscopic surgery" might be more appropriate.

Manuel Trías Folch
Eduardo Mª Targarona
Service of Surgery
Hospital of Sant Pau
Sant Antoni M. Claret 167
08025 Barcelona
Spain

PAPER

Surgical Management of Phyllodes Tumors

Abeel A. Mangi, MD; Barbara L. Smith, MD, PhD; Michele A. Gadd, MD; Kenneth K. Tanabe, MD; Mark J. Ott, MD; Wiley W. Souba, MD, ScD

Hypothesis: Although phyllodes tumors have minimal metastatic potential, we hypothesized that they have a proclivity for local recurrence and should be excised with a wide margin. We reviewed the clinical and radiological appearance of phyllodes tumors and analyzed the role of surgical treatment in their management.

Design: Medical records, imaging studies, pathology reports, and interventions were reviewed.

Setting: A large tertiary care teaching hospital.

Patients: Between 1980 and 1997, 40 patients with phyllodes tumors were identified through the tumor registry at the Massachusetts General Hospital, Boston.

Main Outcome Measures: Surgical resection margins, rates of local recurrence, incidence of distant metastases, and survival.

Results: All 40 patients were female, with a mean age of 41 years. Each patient had a palpable mass or a mammographic finding that was indistinguishable from a fibroadenoma on examination. Tumor size ranged from 5 mm to 28 cm. Local recurrence correlated with excision margins ($P<.05$), but not with tumor grade or size. Local recurrence occurred in 5 patients, each of whom had positive margins or margins less than 1 cm after excision. After reexcision with a 1-cm margin, these individuals remained free of recurrence. One patient developed metastatic disease after total mastectomy and died after chemotherapy.

Conclusions: Phyllodes tumors mimic fibroadenomas and are often excised with close margins. Primary excision or reexcision with a 1-cm margin is recommended. Mastectomy is indicated for patients with large lesions. Lymph node metastases are unusual and occur secondary to necrotic tumor. Chemotherapy is based on guidelines for the treatment of sarcomas, not breast adenocarcinoma.

Arch Surg. 1999;134:487-473

THE PHYLLODES tumor, a lesion limited to mammary tissue, was first described by Muller in 1838. It is a rare condition, with an incidence of 1 in 100 000, and its cause remains unclear. It is a disease almost exclusively of women and occurs most often in the third and fourth decades of life, although there are reports of occurrences in adolescents. Epidemiological data suggest that the incidence of phyllodes tumors may be higher in whites in general and in Latina whites and East Asians in particular.[1,2]

Most patients have a smooth, round, firm, well-defined, motile, painless mass on examination. These lesions do not have any pathognomonic mammographic or ultrasonographic features. They are difficult, if not impossible, to distinguish from fibroadenoma on physical examination or by radiological studies except when quite large. In addition, the biological behavior of phyllodes tumors cannot be assessed on the basis of their radiological appearance.[3-5] There are case reports of accumulation of technetium 99 in primary[6] and metastatic[7] phyllodes tumors. Whether imaging modalities that use radiolabeled substances have a role in the treatment of these patients remains to be determined.

Palpable axillary lymph nodes are encountered in 20% of patients with phyllodes tumors, but histological evidence of malignancy is encountered in less than 5% of axillary lymph node dissections for clinically positive nodes. The remainder of the findings are caused by necrosis of the primary tumor. The stromal component of the phyllodes tumor is monoclonal and neoplastic.[8] Structural[9] and cytogenetic[10] studies of constituent

From the Division of Surgical Oncology, Department of Surgery, Massachusetts General Hospital, Harvard Medical School, Boston.

PATIENTS AND METHODS

All patients diagnosed and treated for phyllodes tumors at the Massachusetts General Hospital, Boston, from January 1, 1980, through December 31, 1997, were identified by means of the institution's tumor registry. Forty cases were identified and their medical records were examined. Data were analyzed retrospectively with review of breast imaging studies, pathology slides, and therapeutic interventions. Tumor grade was categorized as low, intermediate, or high on the basis of 5 criteria: stromal cellularity, stromal atypia, microscopic appearance of the margin of tumor (infiltrating, effacing, or bulging), mitoses per 10 high-power fields, and macroscopic size of the tumor. The main outcomes measured were local and distant recurrence rates and survival. A MEDLINE study search on the world literature on phyllodes tumors from 1966 to 1998 was also performed. The Fisher exact test was used for statistical analysis. A *P* value less than .05 was considered to be statistically significant.

cells have demonstrated similarities between fibroadenomas and phyllodes tumors, and there is evidence that certain fibroadenomas have the ability to progress into phyllodes tumors.[11] Fine-needle aspiration is usually nondiagnostic, primarily because of the difficulty in obtaining adequate numbers of stromal cells for cytogenic analysis.[12] This usually does not alter treatment plans, as most patients eventually undergo excisional biopsy or mastectomy.

The optimal treatment of patients with phyllodes tumors remains unclear. The purpose of this study is to examine the relationship between patient characteristics, surgical resection margins, tumor size and grade, rates of local recurrence, incidence of distant metastases, and survival in patients with a definitive diagnosis of phyllodes tumor.

RESULTS

DEMOGRAPHICS

All 40 patients in our series were female. The average age was 41.3 years (age range, 17-74 years). Thirty of the 40 patients were premenopausal. Thirty-five of the patients were non-Hispanic white, 2 were East Asian, 1 was African American, 1 was Middle Eastern, and 1 was Hispanic. Average age at menarche was 13.2 years (range, 10-16 years). Gravidity and parity were documented in 15 cases. The average number of pregnancies was 2.7 (range, 0-7), and the average number of deliveries was 1.9 (range, 0-6).

MEDICAL HISTORY

Twelve patients reported a personal history of having had at least 1 breast mass excised in the past. Seven patients had a previous fibroadenoma. Each of these patients had an average of 3.7 fibroadenomas excised (range, 1-13; median, 3; mode, 1). These had been excised an average of 11.1 years before the patient was found to have a phyllodes tumor (range, 5-26 years). The remaining 5 patients gave a history of pathologically documented fibrocystic disease. Biopsies had been performed 1 to 12 years before the patient was found to have a phyllodes tumor. No patient gave a history of previous breast malignant neoplasm. Eleven of these patients went on to develop low-grade phyllodes tumors. Only 1 went on to develop an intermediate-grade tumor. Three patients had a history of a malignant neoplasm of nonbreast origin. One had had a right-upper-extremity melanoma, 1 a prolactinoma, and 1 an acoustic neuroma. All of these patients went on to develop low-grade phyllodes tumors.

Eight patients reported a family history of breast cancer. Only 1 of these patients went on to develop an intermediate-grade phyllodes tumor. The other 7 developed low-grade tumors. One of the 8 patients reported a family history of gynecologic malignant neoplasms. Two individuals reported a family history of colon carcinoma; one of these patients went on to develop an intermediate-grade phyllodes tumor, and the other developed a low-grade lesion.

Five patients had used or were using oral contraceptives; 3 patients had been or were taking postmenopausal hormone replacement therapy at the time of diagnosis. One of the patients using oral contraceptives developed an intermediate-grade phyllodes tumor. The other 7 patients developed low-grade tumors.

INITIAL COMPLAINT AND PHYSICAL FINDINGS

Thirty-seven patients were initially examined because of a palpable breast mass, and 7 of these patients had pain at the site of the mass. Three were asymptomatic but had a mass detected on routine mammographic screening. The length of time between detection of the mass and diagnosis was reported in 10 cases (median, 14 weeks; mode, 12 weeks).

Of the 34 patients with low-grade tumors, 17 had a left-sided and 14 a right-sided lesion. The site in 3 patients was unknown. In the group with left-sided lesions, 13 (76%) were in the upper outer quadrant, and in the group with right-sided lesions, 9 (64%) were in the upper outer quadrant. The entire breast was occupied by the mass in 1 patient with an intermediate-grade lesion and in 1 patient with a high-grade lesion.

Of the patients with low-grade tumors (n = 34), 10 had masses that measured 0 to 2 cm, 18 had masses greater than 2 to 5 cm, and 3 had masses greater than 5 cm (**Table 1**). In 3 of these 34 patients, size was not accurately reported. Of the patients with intermediate-grade tumors (n = 3), 2 had masses greater than 2 to 5 cm, and 1 had a mass greater than 5 cm. Of the patients with high-grade tumors (n = 3), 2 had masses greater than 2 to 5 cm and 1 had a mass greater than 5 cm.

RADIOLOGICAL FINDINGS

Mammograms were performed in 15 patients with low-grade phyllodes tumors, in 1 patient with an intermediate-grade tumor, and in 1 patient with a high-grade tumor. The tumors were described as round or lobulated and solid, with sharp, well-defined borders and occasional "popcornlike" calcifications. No differences were noted between the low-, intermediate-, and high-grade tumors. Ultrasonography was performed in 4 patients with low-grade tumors and in 1 patient with an intermediate-grade tumor. Well-defined anechoic masses were noted in all 5 studies. No differences were noted between the low- and intermediate-grade tumors.

CYTOLOGICAL EXAMINATION

Fine-needle aspiration was performed in 3 patients with low-grade phyllodes tumors confirmed by excisional biopsy. One cytological finding was negative, 1 was consistent with a fibroadenoma, and the third disclosed atypical stromal cells. The results did not alter the course of treatment for the patients, all of whom went on to have complete open excision. Fine-needle aspiration was performed in 2 patients with high-grade tumors. In one it showed atypical spindle and epithelioid stromal cells and sheets of hyperplastic epithelium; in the other it was negative for malignant cells.

SURGICAL TECHNIQUE, EXTENT OF RESECTION MARGIN, RECURRENCE, AND SURVIVAL

Thirty-four patients with low-grade tumors were identified. After surgical resection, 4 developed local recurrences and 1 patient developed a systemic recurrence. There were 3 deaths in this group. Only 1 was attributable to the patient's phyllodes tumor.

The initial therapy in 16 of the 34 patients was simple excision (**Table 2**). Eleven patients remained free of disease at an average of 32 months (range, 12-73 months). Four local recurrences, as well as the single distant recurrence, were seen in this group; all of these patients had narrow resection margins (**Table 3**). These patients remained free of disease an average of 57 months (range, 24-84 months) after treatment of their recurrence.

Eleven patients with low-grade tumors were treated with excision followed by immediate wide local excision. These patients were all free of disease at an average of 54 months (range, 26-73 months). Five of the 34 patients with low-grade tumors were treated by simple excision followed by immediate total mastectomy. All of these patients were free of disease at a mean follow-up of 48 months (range, 26-132 months). Two patients with low-grade tumors were treated with immediate total mastectomy. They both remained free of disease at an average of 35 months (range, 34-36 months) of follow-up. There was 1 death in this group secondary to metastatic breast adenocarcinoma that developed in the contralateral breast.

Three patients with intermediate-grade phyllodes tumors were identified (Table 2). One patient had a simple

Table 1. Distribution of Tumors Based on Size and Grade*

	No. of Tumors by Tumor Size, cm		
Tumor Grade	**0-2**	**>2-5**	**>5**
Low†	10	18	3
Intermediate	0	2	1
High	0	2	1

**Criteria used for grading: stromal cellularity, stromal atypia, tumor edge characteristics, mitoses per 10 high-power fields, and macroscopic size.*
†Size in 3 tumors was not specified.

Table 2. Outcome Based on Surgical Procedure

	Outcome, No.				
Tumor Grade	**No Evidence of Disease**	**Local Recurrence**	**Metastasis**	**Death**	**Total**
Simple excision					
Low	11	4	1	2*	**16**
Intermediate	1	0	0	0	**1**
High	0	1	0	0	**1**
Simple excision followed by immediate wide local excision					
Low	11	0	0	0	**11**
Intermediate	1	0	0	0	**1**
High	1	0	0	0	**1**
Simple excision followed by immediate total mastectomy					
Low	5	0	0	0	**5**
Intermediate	1	0	0	0	**1**
High	0	0	0	0	**0**
Total mastectomy					
Low	2	0	0	1	**3**
Intermediate	0	0	0	0	**0**
High	1	0	0	0	**1**

**One of these patients had a local recurrence and died of squamous cell carcinoma of the mandible. The other developed systemic recurrence and died of complications related to phyllodes tumor.*

Table 3. Characteristics of Patients With Local Recurrence and Metastatic Disease*

Tumor Grade	Size, cm	Initial Treatment	Margins, mm	Disease-Free Interval, mo	Treatment of Recurrence	Outcome
			Recurrent Disease			
Low	4	Simple excision	3	44	WLE	NED, DOD
Low	4	Simple excision	<1	2	WLE	Recurred 5 y, WLE, now NED
Low	2	Simple excision	<1	22	TM	NED, 6 y
Low	2	Simple excision	<1	60	TM	NED, 24 mo
High	2	Simple excision	+	76	WLE, XRT	NED, 84 mo
			Metastatic Disease			
Low	2	Simple excision	<1	36	TM, XRT	DOD

**WLE indicates wide local excision; NED, no evidence of disease; DUD, died of unrelated disease; TM, total mastectomy; plus sign, microscopically positive margin for tumor; XRT, radiotherapy; and DOD, died of disease.*

Table 4. Predictors of Local Recurrence, Metastatic Disease, and Death*

	Correlation With		
Patient Characteristics	Recurrence	Metastases	Death
History of fibroadenoma	NS	NS	NS
History of fibrocystic disease	NS	NS	NS
Physical findings	NS	NS	NS
Low grade tumor	NS	NS	NS
Tumor grade	NS	NS	NS
Tumor size	NS	NS	NS
Presence of tumor at excision margin	$P<.05$	NS	NS
Excision margin <1 cm	$P<.05$	NS	NS

**NS indicates* $P>.05$.

excision of the mass, 1 patient had simple excision followed by wide local excision, and 1 patient had an incisional biopsy followed by modified radical mastectomy and intermediate reconstruction. There was no evidence of disease at a mean follow-up of 57 months (range, 29-75 months).

Three patients with high-grade phyllodes tumors were identified. Two patients were disease-free and 1 developed a local recurrence. One patient had simple excision followed by wide local excision, and 1 had a total mastectomy; they remained disease-free at a median follow-up of 45 months. The third patient had a lumpectomy initially. She developed a local recurrence treated by wide local excision after being free of disease for 76 months. She also received 7000 cGy of external beam radiation therapy to the chest wall and was free of recurrent disease at 84 months (Table 3).

We were unable to demonstrate a statistically significant correlation between age, race, pain, or size of the mass; family history of breast cancer, a personal history of breast disease, a history of oral contraceptive use, or postmenopausal hormone replacement therapy; and local recurrence, metastatic disease, or death (**Table 4**).

CHEMOTHERAPY AND RADIATION THERAPY IN THE MANAGEMENT OF PHYLLODES TUMORS

Only 1 patient received systemic therapy that was administered after the diagnosis of metastatic disease (Table 3). The treatment regimen included prophylactic whole-brain irradiation, and chemotherapy consisting of mesna, doxorubicin hydrochloride, and ifosfamide. The patient died of disease 2 months after the diagnosis of metastatic disease. One patient with a high-grade tumor received chest wall radiation for a local recurrence that could not be completely extirpated surgically. The patient remained free of disease 84 months after recurrence.

COMMENT

Phyllodes tumors are mesenchymal tumors of the breast that exhibit a range of clinical and pathological presentations. When viewed as part of a broad spectrum, low-grade phyllodes tumors might be conceptualized as being further along a continuum than a hypercellular fibroadenoma, while high-grade phyllodes can be thought of as connective-tissue tumors that are less aggressive than most sarcomas. Despite this gradation, as arbitrary as it might be, the influence of patient age, histopathological features, DNA content, and resection margins on local recurrence in patients undergoing surgical excision for phyllodes tumors is controversial. Unlike some previous studies[13-16] but similar to others,[17-20] we were unable to demonstrate a correlation between pathological grade of phyllodes tumor and clinical behavior. The inability to demonstrate a relationship, which makes it difficult to make specific treatment recommendations based on grade, may result from an insufficient number of patients with high-grade phyllodes tumors and differences in histological grading between pathologists.

A mean systemic recurrence rate of 13.6% (range, 3.2%-25%) for phyllodes tumors has been reported in the international literature. In our study, the recurrence rate was 15%; all of these recurrences were in patients with resection margins around the primary tumor that were less than 1 cm. This is not to say that a patient with an 8-mm margin is destined to have a recurrence; however, it is apparent from our data that patients who did have recurrences had narrow margins and those with margins of 1 cm (or greater) did not have local recurrences. While the exact margin was not specified in all of the patients in this latter group, margins greater than 1 cm do not appear to be necessary when a phyllodes tumor is resected, irrespective of size or grade.

Metastatic disease can involve the lungs,[13] thigh,[21] pleura, sacrum,[22] axial skeleton, pancreas,[23] central nervous system,[24] and mandible.[25] Statistically significant correlations between tumor grade[26,27]—specifically, stro-

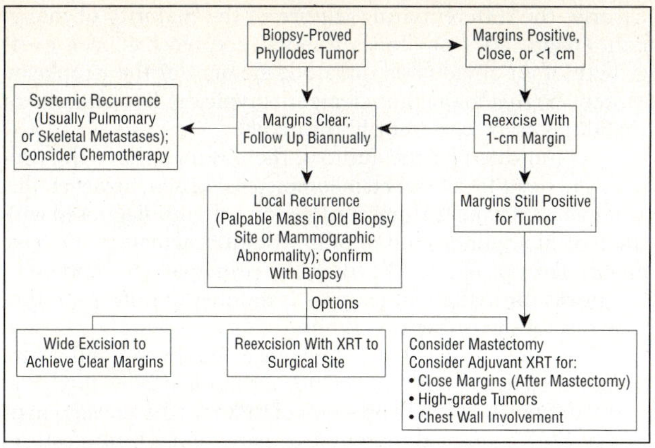

Proposed treatment of patients with a diagnosis of phyllodes tumor. XRT indicates radiotherapy.

mal overgrowth,[28-30] high mitotic rate, cytological atypia,[25] and metastatic disease—have been demonstrated in the literature. The designation *stromal overgrowth*, a microscopic term indicating that the stroma has replaced the glandular elements of the breast, is thought to be an important determinant of metastatic potential.

Salvage therapy may be useful in the setting of recurrent phyllodes tumors. We treated 1 patient with residual tumor on the chest wall who received external beam radiation and was disease-free at 12 years. There are sporadic reports in the literature of responses to radiation therapy for chest wall recurrences.[31] Chemotherapy has not been proved to be of benefit in this disease and does not appear to have any adjuvant role. Doxorubicin[32] has been used with some success in the setting of uncontrolled systemic dissemination. The use of chemotherapy in the treatment of patients with metastatic phyllodes tumors is based on guidelines for the treatment of sarcomas, not breast cancer. Hormonal therapy has not been described in this setting, but the literature reports approximately 20% to 40% of phyllodes tumors as being estrogen receptor positive and 100% as being progesterone receptor positive.[33,34] This may make antiprogestational agents particularly useful in setting of phyllodes tumors. In view of the rarity of this tumor, it would be difficult to conduct a clinical trial that addresses the potential role of hormonal therapy.

In our study, the behavior of low-grade tumors was similar to that previously reported with the exception of a subgroup that behaved aggressively, resulting in 6 episodes of local recurrence in 4 patients and 1 death from metastatic disease. Patients with these aggressive low-grade tumors demonstrated a greater likelihood of experiencing notable pain at the site of the mass or of having a history of hormonal therapy or oral contraceptive use. None of these associations reached statistical significance. There may also be a tendency to undertreat these lesions, as they continued to recur despite repeated wide local excisions. On completion mastectomy, however, patients remained free of disease at long-term follow-up.

In summary, the diagnosis of phyllodes tumor should be considered in all patients with a history of a firm, rounded, well-circumscribed, solid (noncystic) lesion in the breast. Simple excisional biopsy should be performed if aspiration fails to return cyst fluid or if ultrasound demonstrates a solid lesion. Because phyllodes tumors mimic fibroadenomas, they are often enucleated or excised with a close margin. If a 1-cm margin has not been obtained after examination of the permanent section, the patient should undergo reexcision to obtain wider margins. Otherwise, a recurrence rate of 15% to 20% can be expected. If the mass of breast tissue is such that simple excision cannot be accomplished without gross cosmetic deformity, or if the tumor burden is too large, a simple mastectomy may be performed. If mastectomy does not yield a 1-cm margin, or if chest wall invasion is noted, postoperative radiation therapy with a boost to the surgical bed should at least be considered (**Figure**). Axillary lymph node dissection is to be reserved for clinically palpable nodes only.

This approach should be adequate for all age groups and for all grades of tumor. Patients with a diagnosis of phyllodes tumors should be followed up closely with physical examinations and mammograms. If there is a concern of local recurrence, simple excisional biopsy with the aim of 1-cm margins is the surgical goal. If this is not possible without residual cosmetic deformities or because of the tumor burden, completion mastectomy should be performed. A "watch and wait" policy may be adopted after a first recurrence. After a second recurrence, total mastectomy must be considered for definitive local control. Breast reconstruction may be performed at the time of mastectomy.

Presented at the 79th Annual Meeting of the New England Surgical Society, Toronto, Ontario, September 26, 1998.

Corresponding author: Wiley W. Souba, MD, ScD, Division of Surgical Oncology, Massachusetts General Hospital, Cox 626, 100 Blossom St, Boston, MA 02114.

REFERENCES

1. Bernstein L, Deapen D, Ross RK. The descriptive epidemiology of malignant cystosarcoma phyllodes tumors of the breast. *Cancer.* 1993;71:3020-3024.
2. Chua CL. Cystosarcoma phyllodes: Asian variations. *Aust N Z J Surg.* 1988;58:301-305.
3. Liberman L, Bonnaccio E, Hamele-Bena D, Abramson AF, Cohen MA, Dershaw DD. Benign and malignant phyllodes tumors: mammographic and sonographic findings. *Radiology.* 1996;198:121-124.
4. Buchberger W, Strasser K, Heim K, Muller E, Schroksnadel H. Phyllodes tumor: findings on mammography, sonography, and aspiration cytology in 10 cases. *AJR Am J Roentgenol.* 1991;157:715-719.
5. Page JE, Williams JE. The radiological features of phyllodes tumor with clinicpathologic correlation. *Clin Radiol.* 1991;44:8-12.
6. Lerman SH, Morris D, Johnston GS. Tc99m diphosphonate uptake in primary malignant cystosarcoma phyllodes. *Clin Nucl Med.* 1982;7:425.
7. Ohta H, Komibuchi T, Adachi R, et al. ^{99m}Tc-HMDP accumulation in a phyllodes tumor of the breast, a case report. *Ann Nucl Med.* 1993;7:51-52.
8. Noguchi S, Motomura K, Inaji H, Imaoka S, Koyama H. Clonal analysis of fibroadenoma and phyllodes tumor of the breast. *Cancer Res.* 1993;53:4071-4074.
9. Silverman JS, Tameness A. Mammary fibroadenoma and some phyllodes tumor stroma are composed of CD34+ fibroblasts and factor XIIIa+ dendrophages. *Histopathology.* 1996;29:411-419.
10. Dietrich CU, Pandis N, Bardi G, et al. Karyotypic changes in phyllodes tumors of the breast. *Cancer Genet Cytogenet.* 1994;78:200-206.
11. Noguchi S, Yokouchi H, Aihara T, et al. Progression of fibroadenoma to phyllodes tumor demonstrated by clonal analysis. *Cancer.* 1995;76:1779-1785.
12. Shimizu K. Cytologic evaluation of phyllodes tumors as compared to fibroadenomas of breast. *Acta Cytol.* 1994;38:891-897.
13. Reinfuss M, Mitus J, Smolak K, Stelmach A. Malignant phyllodes tumors of breast:

a clinical and pathologic analysis of 55 cases. *Eur J Cancer.* 1993;29(suppl A): 1252-1256.
14. Terrier P, Terrier-Lacombe MJ, Mouriesse H, Friedman S, Spielmann M, Contesso G. Primary breast sarcoma: a review of 33 cases with immunohistochemistry and prognostic factors. *Breast Cancer Res Treat.* 1989;13:39-48.
15. Cohn-Cedermark G, Rutqvist LE, Rosendahl I, Silfversward C. Prognostic factors in cystosarcoma phyllodes: a clinicopathologic study of 77 patients. *Cancer.* 1991;68:2017-2022.
16. el-Naggar AK, Ro JY, McLemore D, Garnsy L. DNA content and proliferative activity of cystosarcoma phyllodes of the breast: potential prognostic significance. *Am J Clin Pathol.* 1990;93:480-485.
17. Layfield LJ, Hart J, Neuwirth H, Bohman R, Trumbull WE, Giuliano AE. Relation between DNA ploidy and the clinical behavior of phyllodes tumors. *Cancer.* 1989; 64:1486-1489.
18. Chu JS, Chang KJ, Lee WJ, Hsu HC. Clinicopathologic study of phyllodes tumors of the breast. *J Formos Med Assoc.* 1995;94:238-242.
19. Modena S, Prati G, Mainente M, et al. Phyllodes tumors of the breast: problems of differential diagnosis and therapeutic approach from an analysis of 17 cases. *Eur J Surg Oncol.* 1993;19:70-73.
20. Ciatto S. Phyllodes tumor of the breast: a multicenter series of 59 cases. *Eur J Surg Oncol.* 1992;18:545-549.
21. Buchanan EB. Cystosarcoma phyllodes and its surgical management. *Ann Surg.* 1995;61:350-355.
22. Rainville E. Metastatic cystosarcoma phyllodes: a case report. *Acta Cytol.* 1993; 37:555-558.
23. Wolfson P, Rybak BJ, Kim U. Cystosarcoma phyllodes metastatic to the pancreas. *Am J Gastroenterol.* 1978;70:184-187.
24. Rhodes RH, Frankel KA, Davis RL, Tatter D. Metastatic cystosarcoma phyllodes: a report of 2 cases presenting with neurological symptoms. *Cancer.* 1978;41: 1179-1187.
25. Abemayor E, Nast CC, Kessler DJ. Cystosarcoma phyllodes metastatic to the mandible. *J Surg Oncol.* 1988;39:235-240.
26. McGregor GI. Sarcoma and cystosarcoma phyllodes tumors of the breast: a retrospective review of 58 cases. *Am J Surg.* 1994;167:477-480.
27. Rowell MD, Perry RR, Hsiu JG, Barranco SC. Phyllodes tumors. *Am J Surg.* 1993; 165:376-379.
28. Hawkins RE. The clinical and histologic criteria that predict metastases from cystosarcoma phyllodes. *Cancer.* 1992;69:141-147.
29. Grimes MM. Cystosarcoma phyllodes tumor of the breast: histologic features, flow cytometric analysis and correlations. *Mod Pathol.* 1992;5:232-239.
30. Ward RM, Evans HL. Cystosarcoma phyllodes: a clinicopathological study of 26 cases. *Cancer.* 1986;58:2282-2289.
31. Stockade AD, Leader M. Phyllodes tumor of the breast: response to radiotherapy. *Clin Radiol.* 1987;38:287.
32. Orsini JM, Perloff M, Rybak B. Cystosarcoma phyllodes: a case presentation. *Med Pediatr Oncol.* 1981;9:449-453.
33. Rao BR, Meyer JS, Fry CG. Most cystosarcoma phyllodes and fibroadenomas have progesterone receptors but lack estrogen receptor: stromal localization of progesterone receptor. *Cancer.* 1981;47:2016-2021.
34. Brentani MM, Nagai MA, Oshima CT, Pacheco MM, Goes JC, Lemos LB. Steroid receptors in cystosarcoma phyllodes. *Cancer Detect Prev.* 1982;5:211-219.

DISCUSSION

Kirby I. Bland, MD, Providence, RI: When the term *phyllodes tumor* was first coined by Muller in 1838, the term meant only a "fleshy" tumor. The general use of the term to mean a tumor with predicted malignant behavior did not arise until several decades later. Pathologists now regard the term *cystosarcoma* as an example of outmoded 19th-century descriptive medical terminology—*phyllodes tumor* is now the preferred designation.

The histological appearance of this neoplasm seems to be identical to that of the large fibroadenoma unless specific characteristics are sought. Fechner suggested that phyllodes tumors exhibit stroma of great cellularity and cell activity, while fibroadenomas show 3 or 4 mitoses per high-power field. Page et al also adhere to this definition and suggest that the factor defining a phyllodes tumor is the close application of a particularly cellular connective tissue element to the basement membrane of the epithelial elements. Authorities suggest that size of the tumor should have no part in differentiating between these mixed tumors of the breast. Clearly, the differentiating feature of the majority of malignant (metastatic) phyllodes tumors reported has been overgrowth of an obvious sarcomatous element of the neoplasm. Moreover, this malignant element is typically liposarcoma or rhabdomyosarcoma—not fibrosarcoma.

As indicated by the authors, these tumors have the proclivity to recur locally when incompletely excised; however, distant metastases are uncommon. Hence, patients diagnosed with the typical phyllodes tumor of low or intermediate grade have an excellent prognosis. Further, the principal determinant of prognosis for malignant features is number of mitoses, rather than size of the presenting tumor.

The predictors of local recurrence, metastasis, and death, as indicated by the authors, include 2 pathological features that correlate statistically: (1) presence of tumor at the excision margin and (2) a surgical margin less than 1 cm. Of interest, recurrence, metastasis, and death are unrelated to grade or size of the presenting tumor. My first question: The authors observed that mitoses/HPF or grade does not correlate with recurrence, metastases, or death. Is this suggestive of a β error due to the small (total) number of cases in the subsets? Do these limited parameters allow such differentiation of statistical outcomes?

Clearly, the size of the neoplasm may determine whether compromised or generous surgical tumor margins are attained. The presence of a large tumor in a small or medium-size breast may afford only minimal surgical margins, and therefore may require total mastectomy. Do you recommend immediate reconstruction following total mastectomy? Further, are there individuals in whom you recommend low-level (level I and I-II) axillary dissections in clinically negative axillae? Are there circumstances (high grade, size of tumor) in which you would recommend sampling or resection of low or multiple levels of nonpalpable nodal disease? Do grade and nodal palpability enter into this decision process?

The margins of resection that you recommend (1-2 cm) are those that surgeons typically strive to achieve for DCIS and for invasive lobular/ductal carcinoma. Do you consider adding adjuvant radiation therapy when tumors closely approximate the chest wall or when attainable margins are less than 1 cm? Please give us more details of your experience and recommendations for radiotherapy in the treatment of these high-grade tumors.

Blake Cady, MD, Providence: I would like to question the author on the diagnosis of low-grade small-sized lesions in patients who had multiple previous fibroadenomas and how their pathologists reliably distinguish this lesion from fibroadenomas. I wonder if these were prospective data in any case, or were these retrospective analyses of obviously large numbers of fibroadenomas? I would question whether the presence of a local recurrence, which can also be seen in a fibroadenoma if it's not taken out with reasonable margins, is the definition of the term *sarcoma.*

Robert Quinlan, MD, Worcester, Mass: Do all the surgeons of the Society believe fibroadenomas should be removed in young people, if it's a classic presentation in a young woman? (Show of hands.) Is there anyone who would disagree with the routine removal of a classic fibroadenoma? Dr Deckers, I would be impressed with whether you would suggest we remove all small clinical fibroadenomas in young women, based on the fact that we might miss an early cystosarcoma. I should also alert the membership, there is a randomized study going on from Dartmouth . . . numbers of cystosarcoma are very minimal in New England, and Dr Barth of Dartmouth is looking for as many patients as possible. Dr Barth is doing a study on routine use of radiation therapy after excision for these "sarcomas."

Dr Mangi: To refer to Dr Bland's first question, that of the small number of our study, we feel that is limited by the rare occurrence of this tumor. This study was one of the largest single institutional studies that we reported, and certainly one of the limitations of it is that the numbers of intermediate-grade and high-grade tumors are relatively low, and that certainly does impact on the data that we've presented.

Regarding the issue of immediate reconstruction, it's difficult to comment definitively on this given the limited number of cases. There are reports of immediate reconstruction after resection of phyllodes tumor, and it would seem to be more feasible in the setting of low-grade tumors once it has been definitively shown that clear margins have been achieved. That certainly would be an option due to the fact this disease is seen in younger women predominately.

Regarding the issue of axillary dissections, palpable lymphadenopathy is encountered in less than 20% of patients, and less than 5% of those patients actually have metastatic disease in their lymph nodes, so we would not recommend axillary dissection in the setting of nonpalpable lymph nodes.

Regarding the issue of planned radiation vs chemotherapy, again we're limited by the rarity of this tumor. The situations in which we would recommend it would be (1) a high-grade tumor, (2) the presence of tumor at the chest wall where adequate resection margins cannot be attained, and (3) in a patient adamantly opposed to mastectomy, who would undergo lumpectomy with radiation therapy.

Regarding Dr Cady's question of distinguishing between fibroadenoma and phyllodes tumor, certainly that is an issue of much contention, and 7 of our patients had had multiple excisions of what were called fibroadenomas and may have actually been phyllodes tumors. We did not go back and actually review that data, but our pathologists used the standard criteria, especially mitotic activity, invasion, and stomach overgrowth in attempting to differentiate between fibroadenoma and phyllodes tumors in our resected specimens.

Finally, addressing the question proposed by Dr Quinlan, whether or not we would advocate removal of small fibroadenomas in young women, certainly this tumor is seen most commonly in women in their third and fourth decades of life, and interestingly enough, the patients with the most clinically aggressive tumors actually have low-grade tumors, so there may be an argument to be made for actually excising fibroadenomas in young women for the purpose of establishing diagnosis and making sure that a low-grade tumor is not missed.

IN OTHER AMA JOURNALS

JAMA

Analysis of Missed Cases of Abusive Head Trauma

Carole Jenny, MD, MBA; Lt Col Kent P. Hymel, MD, USAF, MC; Alene Ritzen, MD, JD; Steven E. Reinert, MS; Thomas C. Hay, DO

Context: Abusive head trauma (AHT) is a dangerous form of child abuse that can be difficult to diagnose in young children.
Objectives: To determine how frequently AHT was previously missed by physicians in a group of abused children with head injuries and to determine factors associated with the unrecognized diagnosis.
Design: Retrospective chart review of cases of head trauma presenting between January 1, 1990, and December 31, 1995.
Setting: Academic children's hospital.
Patients: One hundred seventy-three children younger than 3 years with head injuries caused by abuse.
Main Outcome Measures: Characteristics of head-injured children in whom diagnosis of AHT was unrecognized and the consequences of the missed diagnoses.
Results: Fifty-four (31.2%) of 173 abused children with head injuries had been seen by physicians after AHT and the diagnosis was not recognized. The mean time to correct diagnosis among these children was 7 days (range, 0-189 days). Abusive head trauma was more likely to be unrecognized in very young white children from intact families and in children without respiratory compromise or seizures. In 7 of the children with unrecognized AHT, misinterpretation of radiological studies contributed to the delay in diagnosis. Fifteen children (27.8%) were reinjured after the missed diagnosis. Twenty-two (40.7%) experienced medical complications related to the missed diagnosis. Four of 5 deaths in the group with unrecognized AHT might have been prevented by earlier recognition of abuse.
Conclusion: Although diagnosing head trauma can be difficult in the absence of a history, it is important to consider inflicted head trauma in infants and young children presenting with nonspecific clinical signs. *(1999;281:621-626)* www.jama.com

Corresponding author and reprints: Carole Jenny, MD, MBA, Hasbro Children's Hospital, MOC-140, 593 Eddy St, Providence, RI 02903 (e-mail: cjenny@lifespan.org).

ORIGINAL ARTICLE

Vanadate and the Absence of Myofibroblasts in Wound Contraction

H. Paul Ehrlich, PhD; Kerry A. Keefer, MS; Roland L. Myers, MS; Anthony Passaniti, PhD

Hypothesis: Fibroblasts, not myofibroblasts, are responsible for wound contraction. Only myofibroblasts express a smooth muscle actin for which vanadate blocks its expression. Wound contraction in vanadate-treated rats will proceed normally in the absence of myofibroblasts.

Design: Laboratory study using rats.

Methods: Wound healing in rats receiving vanadate parenterally, an inhibitor of tyrosine phosphate phosphatases, was investigated. For 21 days, treated rats received drinking water containing vanadate, 0.2 mg/mL, in isotonic sodium chloride solution, and the control rats received isotonic sodium chloride solution alone. On day 7, 4 square, full-excision wounds were made dorsally and measured, then 2 polyvinyl alcohol sponges were placed ventrally in subcutaneous pockets.

Results: After 2 weeks, the wound area in the rats receiving vanadate measured 7.1 ± 1.8 U (mean ± SD), and the wound area in the control rats measured 7.2 ± 2.2 U. The control rats' granulation tissue (GT) had myofibroblasts, or α-smooth muscle (α-SM) actin-positive fibroblasts, whereas the vanadate-treated group's fibroblasts were devoid of α-SM actin. By Western blot analysis, GT homogenates in the vanadate-treated group contained less α-SM actin. By electron microscopy, control rats' GT showed classic myofibroblast populations, and the collagen fiber bundles were randomly organized. In contrast, the wounds in the vanadate-treated group showed unencumbered fibroblast populations and neatly ordered, parallel collagen fiber bundles. By polarized light microscopy, the GT of the vanadate-treated group displayed orderly collagen fiber bundles.

Conclusions: The differentiation of fibroblasts into myofibroblasts requires the dephosphorylation of selected tyrosine phosphate residues. In the absence of myofibroblasts, the rate of rat wound contraction is normal, and collagen fiber bundles have a more orderly arrangement. Myofibroblasts are not required for wound contraction.

Arch Surg. 1999;134:494-501

THE WOUND healing process advances by an overlapping sequence of events referred to as "lag," "proliferative," and "remodeling" phases of repair. The lag phase is characterized by inflammation, which checks infection and initiates the proliferative phase of repair. The proliferative phase is characterized by the migration and division of fibroblasts and the synthesis and deposition of a new, vascularized connective tissue matrix. The remodeling phase of repair involves the organization of that new connective tissue matrix into a scar. The connective tissue organization in scar differs from dermis; a parallel arrangement of scar collagen fiber bundles replaces the basket-weave collagen fiber bundles of dermis. With few exceptions, dermal loss is replaced with scar and not dermal regeneration. The amount of scar deposited in full excisional wounds in rats is limited because of wound contraction, in which normal skin is pulled into the defect. Skin is pulled into the wound site by forces generated through the continued reorganization of the newly deposited collagen fibers in granulation tissue (GT),[1] rather than through cell contraction. The requirement of a specialized fibroblast, the myofibroblast, that has been proposed to generate those processes is the subject of this report.

Cell "crawling" is required for the migration of fibroblasts into the wound site during the early proliferative phase of repair. Cell crawling involves polymerized actin organized into a filamentous network at the cell's leading edge. Actin-binding proteins play important roles in the polymerization of actin into highly branched networks seen in the leading edge of ambulatory fibroblasts.[2] In sedentary fibroblasts, actin filaments are organized into cytoplasmic microfilaments that aggregate into thick stress fibers. These actin bundles in stress fibers demonstrate minimal branching and terminate at focal adhesion plaques near the plasma mem-

From the Division of Plastic Surgery, Departments of Surgery (Dr Ehrlich and Mr Keefer) and Neurosciences and Anatomy (Mr Myers), Milton S. Hershey Medical Center, Pennsylvania State University College of Medicine, Hershey; and the Laboratory of Biological Chemistry, National Institute on Aging, Baltimore, Md (Dr Passaniti).

MATERIALS AND METHODS

Adult male Sprague-Dawley rats (weight, 375-400 g) were purchased (Charles River Labs, Wilmington, Mass). The rats were weighed and then placed in pairs in cages. The treatment group rats (n = 8) were given sodium orthovanadate (Sigma-Aldrich Corp, St Louis, Mo), 0.2 mg/mL, in sodium chloride, 150 mmol/L, in their drinking water for 1 week before wounding and for 2 weeks after wounding, when the experiment was terminated. Control rats (n = 7) received sodium chloride, 150 mmol/L, in their drinking water during the same period. The salted water was necessary to make the vanadate palatable. Unlike other animals, rats tolerate the long-term ingestion of sodium chloride solution in place of water.

Rats were placed under anesthesia with an intraperitoneal injection of pentobarbital sodium (Nembutal), 50 mg/kg of body weight, and their backs and abdomens were shaved. On the back of each rat, 4 full-thickness excision wound squares of 15 × 15 mm were made with scissors. The wound edges were tattooed and photographed with a ruler in place. An incision was made on the abdominal surface, and subcutaneous pockets were made on each side of the midline. A PVA sponge (Unipoint Laboratories, High Point, NC) was cut into disks of 3 mm thick and 12 mm in diameter. Sponge disks were boiled in distilled water, blotted with sterile gauze, and each weighed to the nearest milligram. These were placed into the subcutaneous pockets, and the entry wound was sutured closed. The rats were returned to their cages after complete recovery from anesthesia and remained on their drinking water regimen.

Two weeks later, the rats were killed with an overdose of pentobarbital and then weighed. The healing wounds were rephotographed with a ruler in place, and the healed wound sites and PVA sponges were harvested. The sponges and wounds were bisected. Half were processed for biochemical analysis, and the other half were processed for histological evaluation. Tissues to undergo biochemical analysis were homogenized in lysis buffer (0.1% sodium dodecyl sulfate; Tris hydrochloride, 10 mmol/L; at pH 6.8), boiled, cleared by centrifugation, and stored frozen (−80°C) until analyzed. The wound and sponge halves used for histological analysis were divided into pieces for paraffin and frozen sections. Only specimens from open wound tissue were processed for transmission electron microscopy (TEM; Phillips 400 Electron Microscope; Philips Technologies, Cheshire, Conn). The paraffin sections were fixed in 10% formaldehyde, embedded, sectioned, and stained with hematoxylin-eosinor Sirius redor fast green, as previously described.[6] Specimens for frozen sectioning were placed in cassettes, submerged in tissue cryo-embedding liquid (Fisher Scientific, Springfield, NJ), frozen in liquid nitrogen, and stored at −80°C. Frozen sections were cut 4 to 6 μm thick with a cryostat, fixed in buffered 4% paraformaldehyde, permeabilized with 0.1% Triton X-100 detergent (Sigma-Aldrich Corp), and immunostained with monoclonal antibody directed to α-SM actin and β-actin (Sigma-Aldrich Corp). The α-SM actin–antibody complex was identified by a fluorescein-conjugated second antibody (sheep antimouse $F[ab]_2$; Jackson ImmunoResearch Labs, Inc, West Grove, Pa) directed to mouse IgG, and filamentous actin was demonstrated by rhodamine-phalloidin staining (Molecular Probes, Inc, Eugene, Ore). The wound tissue specimens for TEM were cut into 1-mm cubes and fixed for 2 hours in Karnovsky fixative, then postfixed in 1% osmium tetroxide or 1.5% potassium ferrocyanide, dehydrated in ethanols, stained with 1% aqueous uranium acetate, embedded in Spurrs resin (Polysciences, Inc, Warrington, Pa), sectioned, and examined by TEM.

To measure wound areas, photographic slides taken immediately following wounding and 2 weeks later were projected. Their sizes were equalized by the included ruler, so all images were at the same magnification. The images were then traced on plain white paper. The tracings were cut out and weighed to the nearest 0.1 g. The mean ± SD weight from the wound tracings was calculated.

For Western blot analysis (immunoblotting), the protein concentrations were determined for the cleared homogenates using the Bradford method.[7] Equal amounts of protein were run by sodium dodecyl sulfate–polyacrylamide gel electrophoresis with a Tris hydrochloride–glycine buffer on a mini-Protean II cell system (Bio Rad Labs, Hercules, Calif) following instructions from the supplier. Protein transfer was made to a PVDF membrane (Millipore Corp, Bedford, Mass). The membrane underwent sequential stainings with primary antibodies directed to α-SM actin and β-actin. The membrane was treated with 5% dried milk to block nonspecific protein-binding sites before incubating with primary antibody. After being incubated with primary antibody, the membrane was rinsed and then incubated with an antimouse IgG peroxidase-conjugated secondary antibody. The membrane was finally washed before developing with an electrochemiluminescence system (Amersham Life Sciences, Arlington Heights, Ill) following the manufacturer's instructions.

brane of a cell. These focal adhesion plaques contain several proteins that are involved in cell signaling.[3] Tyrosine phosphorylation and dephosphorylation of proteins in focal adhesions act as switches in the transfer of information between the cell and its extracellular matrix.[4] Tension is maintained on a substratum by cells through the formation of cytoplasmic stress fibers.[5]

The formation of α-smooth muscle (α-SM) actin–containing stress fibers in myofibroblasts may require the dephosphorylation of selected tyrosine phosphate residues. Vanadate is a potent inhibitor of phosphatase that dephosphorylates tyrosine phosphate residues. We examined the possibility of altering wound contraction and the character of GT deposited in polyvinyl alcohol (PVA) sponge implants in rats ingesting vanadate. For 1 week, rats in the experimental group received vanadate in their drinking water, and the control group received isotonic sodium chloride solution in their drinking water before open wounds were made and PVA sponges were implanted. Two weeks later, the rats were killed, the wound sizes were recorded, and tissue specimens were biochemically and histologically analyzed. The following questions are addressed: Does an inhibitor of tyrosine phosphate turnover block myofibroblast formation? Are myofibroblasts critical for wound contraction? Are there differences between myofibroblasts and fibroblasts in organizing collagen fiber bundles within GT?

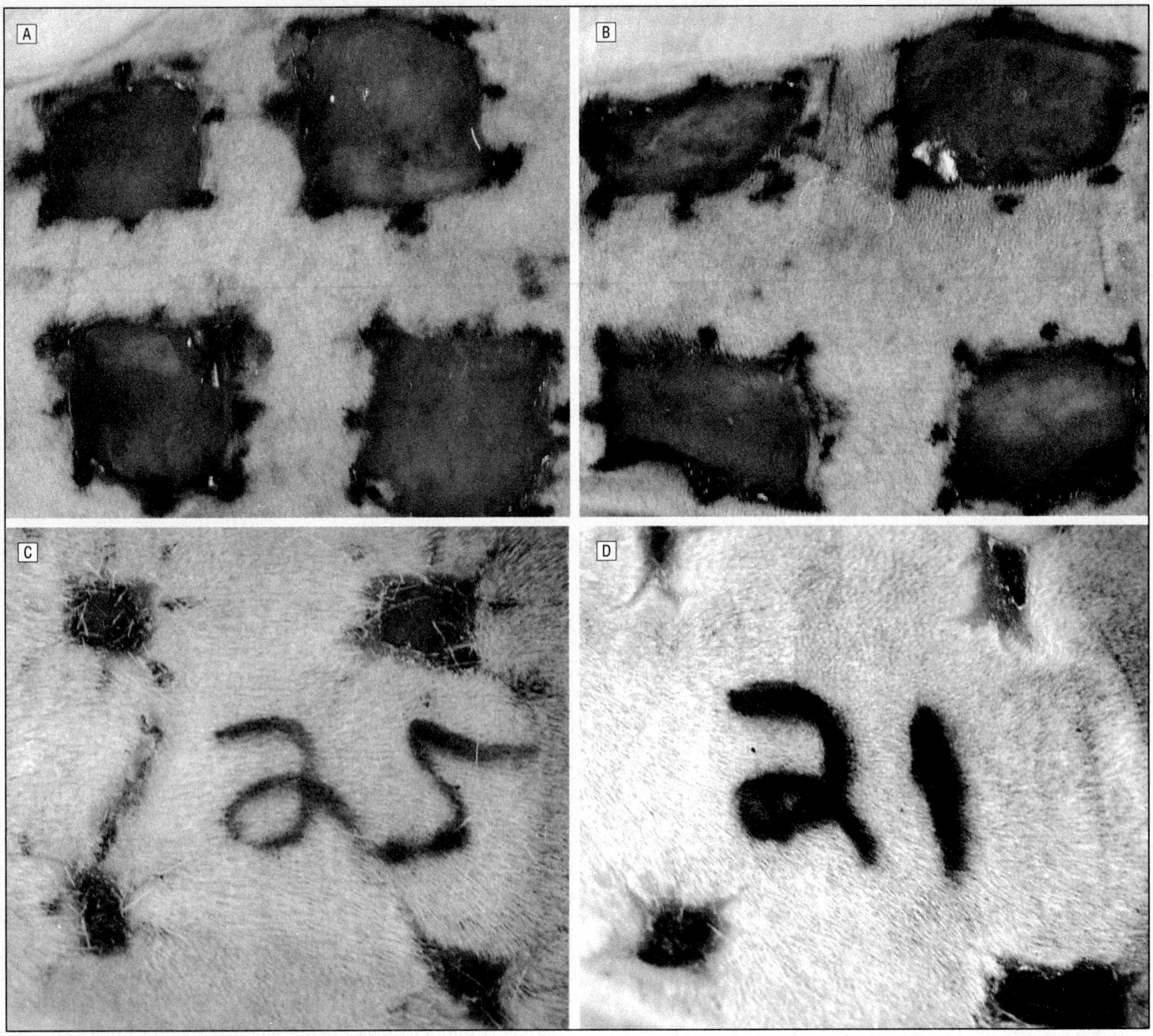

Figure 1. *Wounds immediately after wounding in (A) a control rat and (B) a vanadate-treated rat. Those same wounds 2 weeks later from control rats maintained on sodium chloride solution (C) and from the vanadate-treated rat (D).*

RESULTS

Rats ingesting sodium chloride solution or sodium chloride solution containing vanadate, 0.2 mg/mL, for 3 weeks had similar weight gains. During the 2 weeks after wounding, the group given sodium chloride solution alone (control group) gained 21 ± 5 g (n = 7), and the vanadate-treated group gained 15 ± 3 g (n = 8) (all data are expressed as mean ± SD). The difference between the 2 groups' weight gain was not significant ($P>.05$; Student *t* test).

The full-excision open wounds healed mostly by wound contraction. **Figure 1** shows representative wounds made on the backs of rats from the 2 experimental groups immediately and 2 weeks after wounding. Wounds from both groups contracted about 75% during the 2 weeks. The noncontracted wound area was determined by weighing tracings, and 1 area unit equaled 1 g. The initial wound size averaged 27.6 U for both groups, and at 2 weeks, the control wounds contracted to 7.2 ± 2.2 U (n = 12), whereas the wound size of the vanadate-treated group was 7.1 ± 1.8 U (n = 12). Administering vanadate parenterally did not alter wound contraction. In both treated and control groups, open wounds closed by wound contraction.

The weights of PVA sponges at the time of implantation and harvesting at 2 weeks were recorded as a measure of GT deposited. The GT weight of sponges from the control group was 63 ± 36 mg and from the vanadate-treated group, 77 ± 40 mg. The amount of GT deposited in the PVA sponge implants was similar between groups; ie, there was no significant difference ($P>.05$; Student *t* test). The ingestion of vanadate did not alter the amount of GT deposited in PVA sponge implants.

Vanadate treatment, however, altered the structure of cells and the organization of collagen fibers bundles in GT. In normal dermis, fibroblasts do not exhibit cytoplasmic stress fibers, but in GT they do. Rhodamine-phalloidin–stained stress fibers within fibroblasts and smooth muscle cells of blood vessel from a 2-week-old

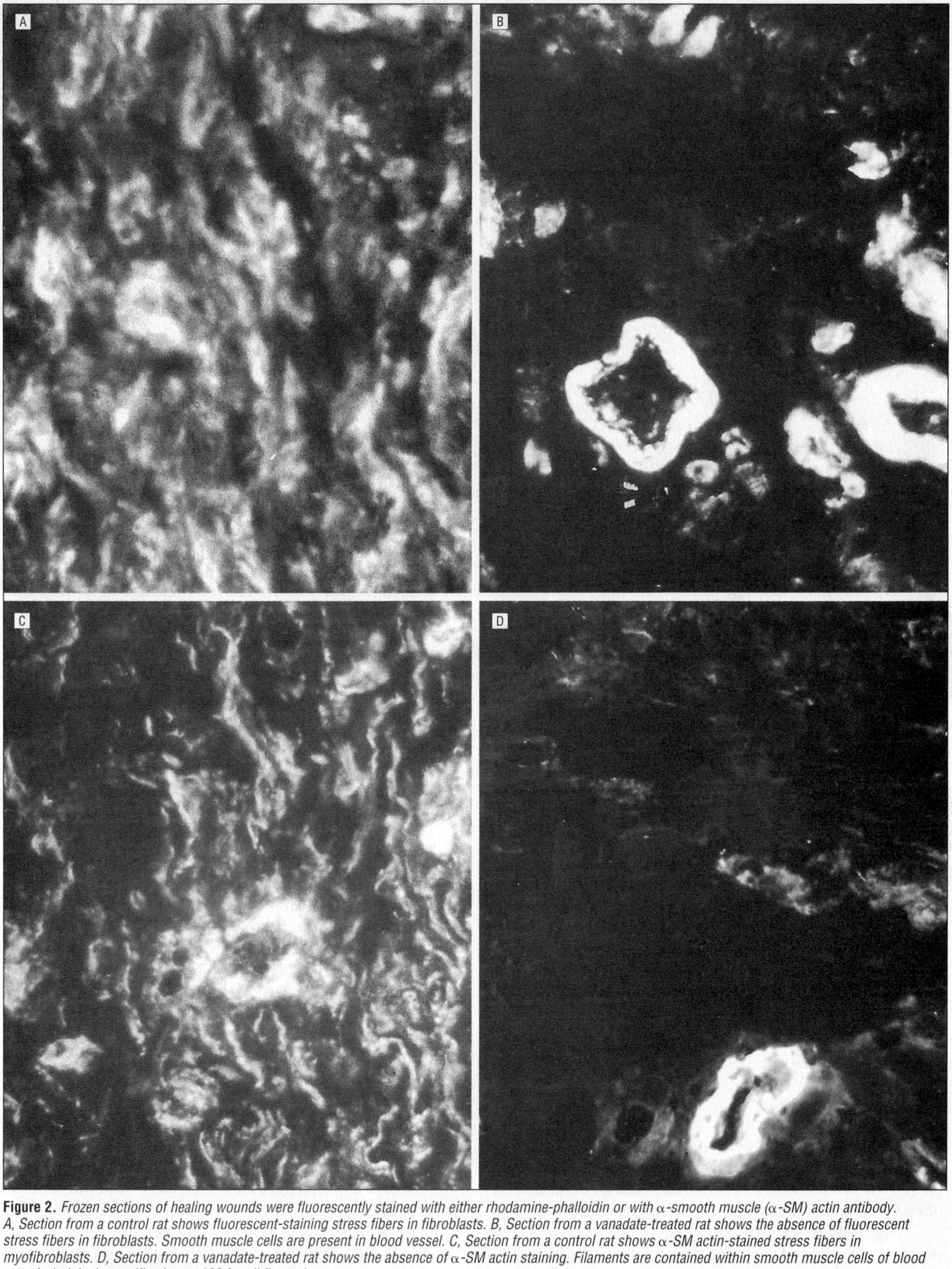

Figure 2. *Frozen sections of healing wounds were fluorescently stained with either rhodamine-phalloidin or with α-smooth muscle (α-SM) actin antibody. A, Section from a control rat shows fluorescent-staining stress fibers in fibroblasts. B, Section from a vanadate-treated rat shows the absence of fluorescent stress fibers in fibroblasts. Smooth muscle cells are present in blood vessel. C, Section from a control rat shows α-SM actin-stained stress fibers in myofibroblasts. D, Section from a vanadate-treated rat shows the absence of α-SM actin staining. Filaments are contained within smooth muscle cells of blood vessels (original magnification, ×100 for all figures).*

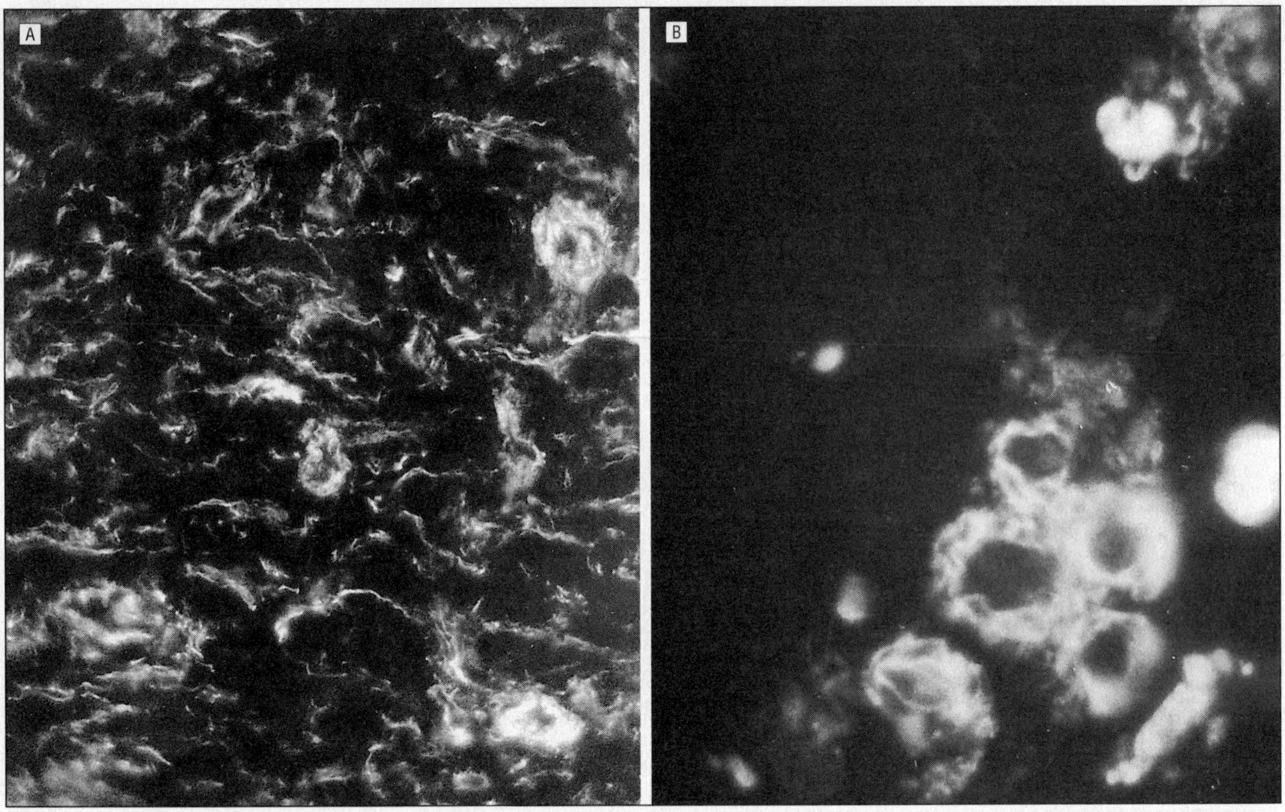

Figure 3. *Frozen sections of 2-week-old polyvinyl alcohol sponge implants were processed for α-smooth muscle (α-SM) actin immunostaining. A, Section from a control rat demonstrates myofibroblast populations with cytoplasmic α-SM actin filaments running parallel to one another. B, Section from a vanadate-treated rat shows the α-SM actin staining limited to smooth muscle cells contained in blood vessels (original magnification ×360).*

healing open-wound GT are shown in **Figure 2**. In contracting wounds from control rats, prominently stained stress fibers in the myofibroblasts and in the smooth muscle cells of vessel walls were evident (Figure 2, A). In contrast, the GT of open wounds from vanadate-treated rats (Figure 2, B) was devoid of stained stress fibers within fibroblasts. Vanadate blocked the development of stress fibers forming in fibroblasts but had no effect on stress fibers within smooth muscle cells of blood vessels. Although the degree of wound contraction was identical in the open wounds of treated and control rats, a major structural difference was that vanadate ingestion prevented the appearance of stress fibers in the fibroblasts of the GT of contracting wounds.

Myofibroblasts have been characterized in GT and hypertrophic scar by their prominent cytoplasmic stress fibers, which contain α-SM actin.[8] Myofibroblasts were readily identified in control rat GT by stress fibers showing α-SM actin (Figure 2, C). On the other hand, in the fibroblast populations of GT from vanadate-treated rats, α-SM actin stress fibers were absent (Figure 2, D). The absence of α-SM actin–staining fibroblasts was not due to flawed immunostaining because the smooth muscle cells of the vessel wall did contain that antigen (Figure 2, D).

Granulation tissue from 2-week-old PVA sponge implants was examined to confirm the open wound findings. The PVA implants from control rats contained a high density of myofibroblasts (**Figure 3**, A). In contrast, GT from PVA sponge harvested from the vanadate-treated rats contained fibroblasts devoid of α-SM actin (Figure 3, B). Like the GT of open wounds, the smooth muscle cells in the vessel wall showed α-SM actin, demonstrating an internal control for immunostaining. In all slides examined from vanadate-treated rats, the GT of both open wounds and PVA sponge implants was devoid of myofibroblasts, but all blood vessel smooth muscle cells contained α-SM actin.

Western blot analysis was used to determine the expression of 3 different cytoskeletal proteins in PVA sponge homogenates: the focal adhesion plaque protein vinculin; α-SM actin; and the microfilament protein β-actin. Twenty micrograms of protein from GT homogenate, from either control or vanadate-treated rats, was analyzed and compared. As shown in **Figure 4**, A, the ingestion of vanadate specifically reduced the levels of α-SM actin compared with those in controls, due to the absence of myofibroblasts. Vanadate did not affect the levels of vinculin, indicating no alteration in its expression in focal adhesion plaques (Figure 4, B). By the expression of equivalent densities of β-actin bands (Figure 4, C), equal quantities of cell microfilaments were applied to the polyacrylamide gels. It appears that the expression of α-SM actin is specifically reduced in GT from vanadate-treated rats.

Biopsy specimens of 2-week-old contracting wounds were examined by TEM. Granulation tissue of contracting wounds from control rats showed typical myofibroblast cell populations. Characteristic, numerous cell-cell associations and indentations of the cells' nuclei were seen (**Figure 5**, A). These myofibroblasts showed aggregated microfilaments contained in stress fibers in an area immediately below the plasma membrane of the cell,

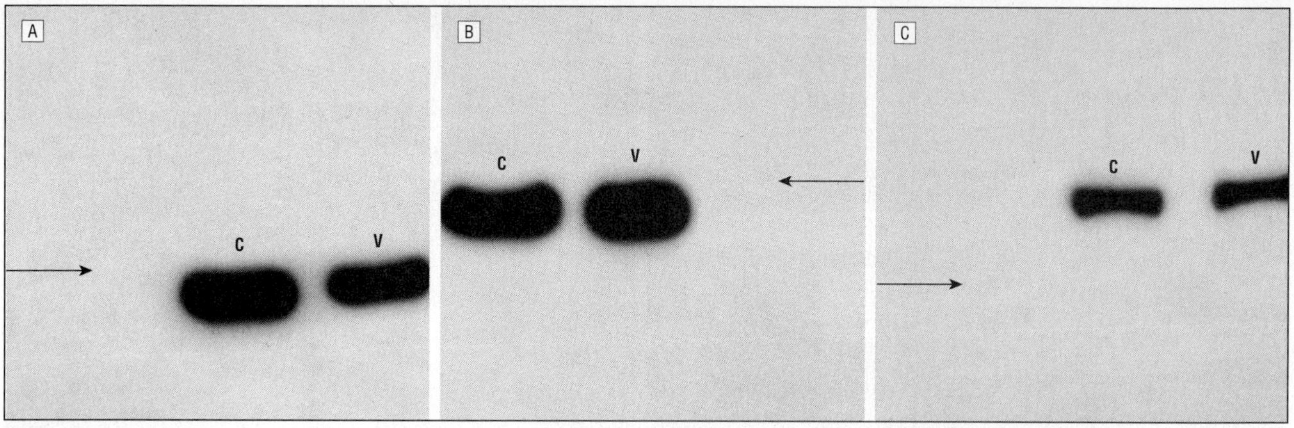

Figure 4. *Western blot analysis of α-smooth muscle (α-SM) from granulation tissue. Tissue homogenates of protein, 20 μg, from vanadate-treated or control rats underwent immunoblot analysis. A, Following vanadate treatment, levels of α-SM actin are reduced in lane V (vanadate) compared with those in lane C (control). B, The densities of β-actin bands in lanes C and V of tissue homogenates were equivalent. C, The levels of vinculin, a focal adhesion protein, were equivalent between the 2 treatment groups. The arrows in all 3 indicate the location of the 66 000 molecular weight marker.*

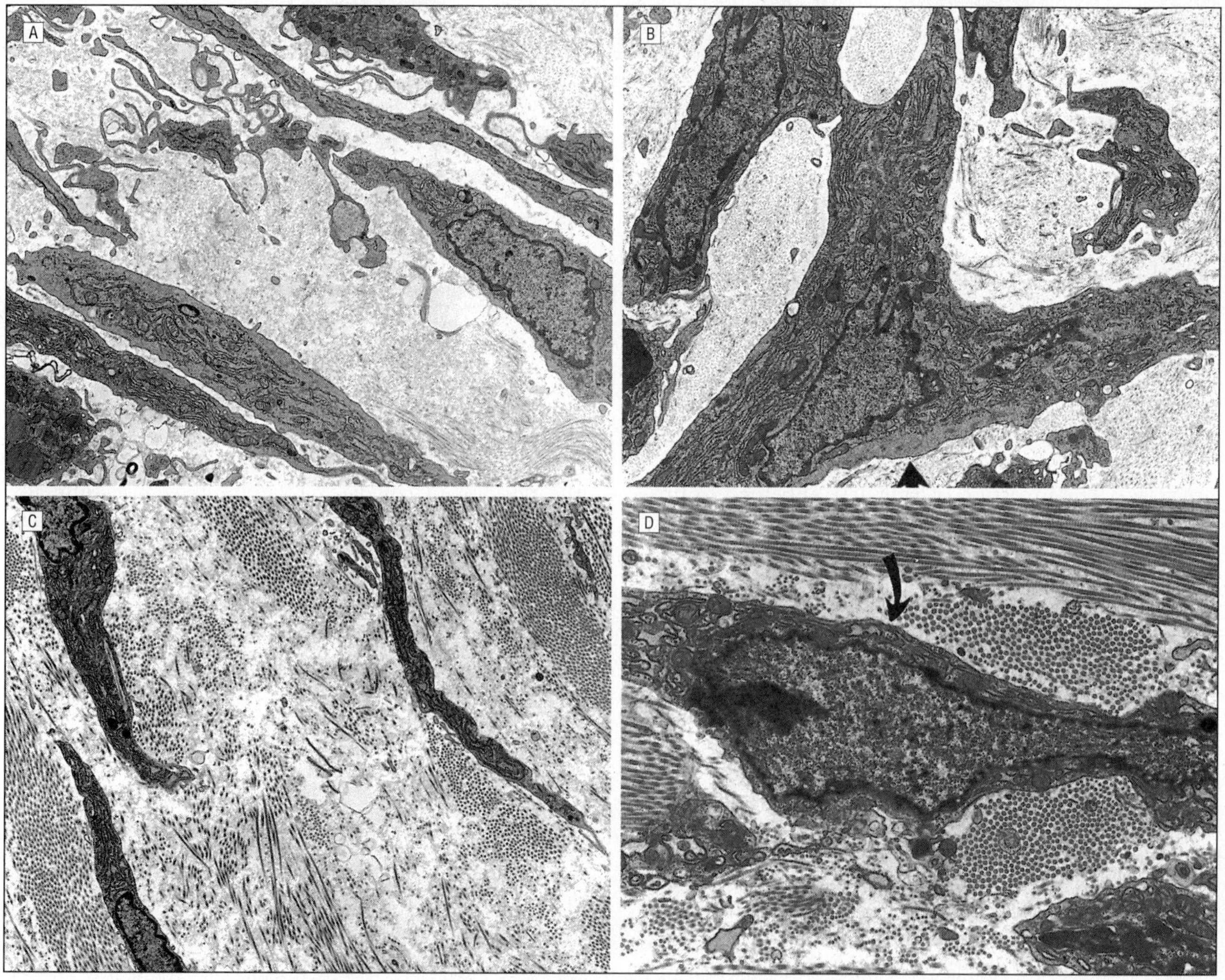

Figure 5. *Transmission electron microphotographs of granulation tissue from 2-week-old contracting open wounds from a control rat (A, original magnification ×4600, and B, original magnification ×6000). Cells are attached to one another, the collagen fiber bundles are arranged randomly, and there is an area just beneath the plasma membrane of the cell that is devoid of subcellular organelles. Sections from a vanadate-treated rat are shown (C, original magnification ×4600, and D, original magnification ×7700). Cells do not touch one another, the collagen fiber bundles are arranged in a parallel manner, and just beneath the plasma membrane of the cell are numerous subcellular organelles (arrow).*

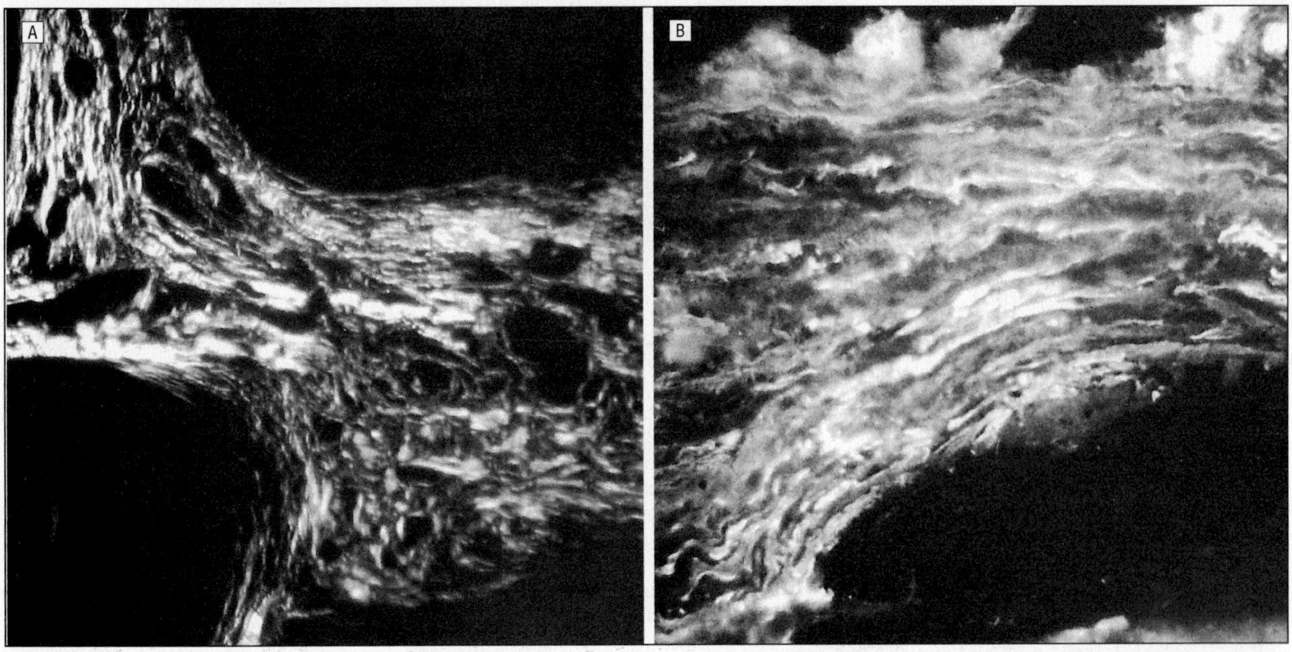

Figure 6. *Formalin-fixed sections from 2-week-old polyvinyl alcohol sponge implants were stained with Sirius red and viewed with polarized light optics (original magnification, ×50). A, The birefringence pattern is shown from a control rat. B, The birefringence pattern from a vanadate-treated rat is more intense because of thicker, more parallel collagen fiber bundle packing.*

which was devoid of other subcellular organelles (Figure 5, B). In addition, the extracellular compartment contained collagen fiber bundles that were randomly arranged. In contrast, the GT from vanadate-treated rats contained cell populations displaying minimal cell-cell associations and the absence of cytoplasmic stress fibers, and the area just beneath the plasma membrane of the cell contained subcellular organelles (Figure 5, C). The arrangement of collagen fiber bundles was striking because they were organized in a parallel manner (Figure 5, D). The ingestion of vanadate appeared to promote the arrangement of collagen fibers in distinctively ordered parallel bundles.

By light microscopy, hematoxylin-eosin–stained sections of healing open wounds showed no obvious differences in the cell types, cell density, or orientation of blood vessels within the GT between the 2 treatment groups (not shown). The PVA sponge implants from both treatment groups showed similar levels of GT ingrowth, density of cell populations, number of blood vessels, and character of connective tissue. By Sirius red–polarized light microscopy, however, differences in the packing and organization of collagen fiber bundles were apparent between treatment groups. The collagen fiber bundles of GT from a control rat's PVA sponge implants showed modest intensity of greenish yellow birefringence, and the collagen fiber bundles were finely organized (**Figure 6**, A). The implants harvested from vanadate-treated rats demonstrated greater greenish yellow birefringent intensity, and the collagen fiber bundles were organized in an orderly parallel manner (Figure 6, B). The greater birefringence in the vanadate-treated rats compared with the control rats was the more ordered arrangement of the collagen fiber bundles. These differences in birefringence paralleled the TEM findings, in which more ordered collagen fiber bundles were evident in the vanadate-treated group.

COMMENT

The ingestion of vanadate in drinking water for 3 weeks apparently was not toxic to adult rats because no differences in weight gain were noted. Despite ingesting sodium chloride solution in place of water for 3 weeks, both groups of rats gained weight at equivalent rates. Likewise, the ingestion of vanadate neither inhibited nor stimulated the closure of open wounds or the amount of GT deposited in PVA sponge implants. At the microscopic level, however, the long-term ingestion of vanadate altered both the structure of cells and the organization of collagen fiber bundles in GT. Parenteral vanadate inhibits the conversion of fibroblasts to myofibroblasts, which have been proposed to be responsible for wound contraction.[9] The findings presented here support the hypothesis that myofibroblasts are not required for wound contraction.

Vanadate added in vitro to cultured fibroblasts prevents the appearance of cytoplasmic stress fibers and large focal adhesion plaques.[10] Human fibroblasts in monolayer culture normally show prominent stress fibers, but the inclusion of vanadate prevents their appearance. Vanadate inhibits phosphatases that remove phosphate groups from selected phosphorylated tyrosine residues in proteins. Vanadate also down-regulates p125 focal adhesion kinase, which is associated with the retarded appearance of both stress fibers and focal adhesions.[11] This implies that the removal of selected tyrosine phosphate groups is involved with the appearance of stress fibers and the expression of α-SM actin within fibroblasts of GT.

The in vivo ingestion of vanadate does not prevent stress fibers from developing in the smooth muscle cells of new blood vessels. This implies that the development of stress fibers in fibroblasts requires signals different from those required for these structures to appear in smooth muscle cells. With vanadate ingestion, α-SM actin expression occurred in smooth muscle cells of new vessels but not in fibroblasts developing into myofibroblasts. Although ingested vanadate does not alter smooth muscle cell structure, it reportedly[12] enhances the proliferation and the contractility of vascular smooth muscle cells. Others report[4,13,14] that the phosphorylation of the tyrosine residues in focal adhesion proteins can be related to cell shape, microfilament organization, and cell locomotion. Transmission electron microscopic studies reveal that vanadate affects the organization of microfilaments in treated ovarian granulosa cells that show fragmented actin filaments.[15]

More important, the persistence of selected tyrosine phosphate residues in fibroblasts of GT promotes the better organization of collagen fiber bundles. Evidence supports a relationship between the phosphorylation of tyrosine residues and cell function in wound healing. The binding of cells to extracellular matrix is associated with increased phosphorylation of focal adhesion–associated tyrosine kinase.[16] Mouse fibroblasts receiving high concentrations of platelet-derived growth factor display alterations in the levels of tyrosine phosphate residues in focal adhesion proteins, show the absence of cytoplasmic stress fibers, and demonstrate better attachment to their surrounding matrix.[17]

It has been proposed that cell "tractional forces" describe the mechanical force[18] that organizes collagen fiber bundles required for the evolution of scar integrity, the contraction of open wounds, and the advancement of scar contractures.[1,19,20] The organization and orientation of collagen fibrils into scar matrix occur through forces generated by resident cells. Fine microfilaments are present in fibroblasts, generating the tractional forces involved in the translocation of collagen fibrils, whereas fibroblasts with stress fibers are poor at translocating collagen fibrils.[19] Parenteral vanadate prevents fibroblasts from developing into myofibroblasts, while promoting the more orderly organization of collagen fiber bundles.

By both TEM and polarized light optics, collagen fiber bundles were more organized in the wound specimens of the vanadate-treated group. Vanadate therapy does not change the cell density of GT, as revealed by hematoxylin-eosin–staining patterns. The maturation of fibroblasts in rat GT and the development of stress fibers apparently occur through the dephosphorylation of selected tyrosine phosphate residues. Hence, a change occurs in the interaction of cells and collagen fiber bundles when these tyrosine residues lose phosphate. Vanadate preserves selected tyrosine phosphate groups and prolongs the interaction of cells with collagen fiber bundles, producing a more orderly connective tissue matrix.

The closure of open wounds in tight-skin mice by wound contraction was shown to proceed in the absence of myofibroblasts.[21] It was concluded from that study that myofibroblasts do not actively participate in wound contraction. The hypothesis for wound contraction is that collagen is reorganized by the cytoskeletal contractile unit of the fibroblast, where fine microfilaments attached to small focal adhesion structures linked to $\alpha_{2\beta1}$ integrin, the collagen receptor, translocates collagen fiber bundles. The mechanism for the reorganization of collagen fibers into thicker fiber bundles is the translocation of collagen fibrils over the cell surface. When collagen fibers reach a point where there is sufficient resistance to the further translocation of collagen fiber bundles, the collagen is released from its attachment to $\alpha_{2\beta1}$ integrins, which causes the intracellular clustering of focal adhesions into large plaques, the aggregation of microfilaments into stress fibers, and the expression of α-SM actin.[22]

We acknowledge the technical assistance of Gretchen M. Allison and the helpful suggestions of Robert L. Trelstad, MD.

Reprints: H. Paul Ehrlich, PhD, Department of Surgery, Mail Code H113, Hershey Medical Center, 500 University Dr, Hershey, PA 17033-0850 (e-mail: pehrlich @psu.edu).

REFERENCES

1. Ehrlich HP. Granulation tissue maturation and wound contraction. *J Surg Pathol.* 1997;2:243-249.
2. Stossel TP. On the crawling of animal cells. *Science.* 1993;260:1086-1094.
3. Sefton BM, Hunter T, Ball EH, Singer SJ. Vinculin: a cytoskeletal target of the transforming protein of Rous sarcoma virus. *Cell.* 1981;24:165-174.
4. Romer LH, McLean N, Turner CE, Burridge K. Tyrosine kinase activity, cytoskeletal organization, and motility in human vascular endothelial cells. *Mol Biol Cell.* 1994;5:349-361.
5. Fukui Y, Lynch TJ, Brzeska H, Korn ED. Myosin I is located at the leading edges of locomoting *Dictyostelium amoebae. Nature.* 1989;341:328-331.
6. Ehrlich HP, Desmouliere A, Diegelmann RF, et al. Morphological and immunochemical differences between keloids and hypertrophic scar. *Am J Pathol.* 1994; 145:105-113.
7. Bradford H. A rapid and sensitive method for the quantitation of μg quantities of proteins, using the principle of protein-dye binding. *Anal Biochem.* 1976;72:248-254.
8. Darby I, Skalli O, Gabbiani G. α-Smooth muscle actin is transiently expressed by myofibroblasts during experimental wound healing. *Lab Invest.* 1990;63:21-29.
9. Majno G, Gabbiani G, Hirschel BJ, Ryan GB, Statkov PR. Contraction of granulation tissue in vitro: similarity to smooth muscle. *Science.* 1971;173:548-550.
10. Maher PA, Pasquale EB, Wang JYJ, Singer SJ. Phosphotyrosine-containing proteins are concentrated in focal adhesions and intercellular junctions in normal cells. *Proc Natl Acad Sci U S A.* 1985;82:6576-6580.
11. Retta SF, Barry ST, Critchley DR, Defilippi P, Silengo L, Tarone G. Focal adhesion and stress fiber formation is regulated by tyrosine phosphatase activity. *Exp Cell Res.* 1996;229:307-317.
12. Jin N, Siddiqui RA, English D, Rhoades RA. Communication between tyrosine kinase pathway and myosin light chain kinase pathway in smooth muscle. *Am J Physiol.* 1996;271(pt 2):H1348-H1355.
13. DeClue JE, Martin GS. Phosphorylation of talin at tyrosine in Rous sarcoma virus–transformed cells. *Mol Cell Biol.* 1987;7:371-378.
14. Enomoto T, Okamoto T, Sato JD. Vascular endothelial growth factor induces the disorganization of actin stress fibers accompanied by protein tyrosine phosphorylation and morphological change in Balb/C3T3 cells. *Biochem Biophys Res Commun.* 1994;202:1716-1723.
15. Aharoni D, Dantes A, Amsterdam A. Cross-talk between adenylate cyclase activation and tyrosine phosphorylation leads to modulation of the actin cytoskeleton and to acute progesterone secretion in ovarian granulosa cells. *Endocrinology.* 1993;133:1426-1436.
16. Kornberg L, Earp HS, Parsons JT, Schaller M, Juliano RL. Cell adhesion or integrin clustering increases phosphorylation of a focal adhesion-associated tyrosine kinase. *J Biol Chem.* 1992;267:23439-23442.
17. Rankin S, Rozengurt E. Platelet-derived growth factor modulation of focal adhesion kinase ($p125^{FAK}$) and paxillin tyrosine phosphorylation in Swiss 3T3 cells: bell-shaped dose response and cross-talk with bombesin. *J Biol Chem.* 1994; 269:704-710.
18. Harris AK, Wild P, Stopak D. Silicone rubber substrata: a new wrinkle in the study of cell locomotion. *Science.* 1980;208:177-179.
19. Ehrlich HP, Rajaratnam JBM. Cell locomotion forces versus cell contraction forces for collagen lattice contraction: an in vitro model of wound contraction. *Tissue Cell.* 1990;22:407-417.
20. Yamato M, Adachi E, Yamamoto K, Hayashi T. Condensation of collagen fibrils to the direct vicinity of fibroblasts as a cause of gel contraction. *J Biochem (Tokyo).* 1995;117:940-946.
21. Hembry RM, Bernanke DH, Hayashi K, Trelstad RL, Ehrlich HP. Morphologic examination of mesenchymal cells in healing wounds of normal and tight skin mice. *Am J Pathol.* 1986;125:81-89.
22. Ehrlich HP, Cremona O, Gabbiani G. The expression of $\alpha_{2\beta1}$ integrin and α smooth muscle actin in fibroblasts grown on collagen. *Cell Biochem Funct.* 1998;16:129-137.

ORIGINAL ARTICLE

Whole-Body PET Imaging With [^{18}F]Fluorodeoxyglucose in Management of Recurrent Colorectal Cancer

Peter E. Valk, MB, BS; Elma Abella-Columna, MD; Michael K. Haseman, MD; Thomas R. Pounds, MD; Ruth D. Tesar; Richard W. Myers, MD; Hani B. Greiss, MD; Glenn A. Hofer, MD

Hypothesis: Metabolic imaging by positron emission tomography (PET) using [^{18}F]fluorodeoxyglucose will be more accurate than anatomic imaging by computed tomography (CT) for detection of recurrent colorectal cancer. More accurate staging of recurrent tumor by PET will lead to more appropriate management decisions.

Design: Prospective blinded study comparing PET with CT, using histologic diagnosis, serial CT imaging, and clinical follow-up as criterion standards, with a fully blinded, retrospective reinterpretation of PET studies. Changes in diagnosis resulting from PET findings were correlated with subsequent treatment and surgical findings. Potential cost savings resulting from use of PET for preoperative staging were calculated.

Setting: Private practice in an outpatient tertiary referral center.

Patients: A group of 155 consecutive patients with imaging for diagnosis or staging of recurrent colorectal cancer. Twenty-one patient (14%) were excluded due to lack of a criterion standard. Computed tomographic scans were available for comparison for 115 patients.

Results: Positron emission tomographic scan sensitivity and specificity were 93% and 98%, respectively, compared with 69% and 96% for CT. Ninety-five percent confidence intervals for the differences between the modalities were 16% to 32% for sensitivity and 1% to 5% for specificity. The sensitivity of both modalities varied with anatomic site of recurrence. Positron emission tomographic scans were true positive in 12 (67%) of 18 patients with elevated serum carcinoembryonic antigen levels and negative CT findings. In 23 (29%) of 78 preoperative studies in which CT showed a single site of recurrence, PET showed tumor at additional sites. At surgery, nonresectable, PET-negative tumor was found in 7 (17%) of 42 patients who had PET evidence of localized recurrence only. Potential savings resulting from demonstration of nonresectable tumor by PET were calculated at $3003 per preoperative study.

Conclusions: Positron emission tomography was more sensitive and specific than CT for detection of recurrent colorectal cancer. Preoperative detection of nonresectable tumor by PET may avoid unnecessary surgery, and thereby reduce the cost of patient treatment.

Arch Surg. 1999;134:503-511

From the Northern California PET Imaging Center (Drs Valk, Abella-Columna, Haseman, Pounds, Myers, Greiss, and Hofer and Ms Tesar); the Radiological Associates of Sacramento (Drs Valk, Haseman, Pounds, Myers, Greiss, and Hofer); and Sutter Cancer Center (Drs Greiss and Hofer), Sacramento, Calif.

Peter E. Valk, MD, and Ruth D. Tesar are stockholders of PETNet Pharmaceutical Services LLC, Norcross, Ga.

POSITRON EMISSION tomography (PET) with [^{18}F]fluorodeoxyglucose (FDG) has potential for demonstrating tumor metabolic activity before structural changes can be detected by computed tomographic (CT) imaging. Previous evaluations of FDG PET for diagnosis and staging of recurrent colorectal cancer have demonstrated higher sensitivity and specificity than CT.[1-5] We now

See Invited Critique at end of article

report a prospective evaluation of the accuracy of PET in 134 studies that were performed in patients with known or suspected recurrent colorectal cancer, together with assessment of the impact of PET findings on patient treatment and treatment cost.

RESULTS

PREVALENCE OF TUMOR RECURRENCE AND IMAGE ABNORMALITIES

One hundred fifteen patients underwent both PET and CT. The PET study was performed after CT in most patients, and the interval between PET and CT ranged from 0 to 56 days, with a median interval of 22 days. Validation procedures established a diagnosis of recurrent tumor at 157 sites in 101 patients and no tumor in 14 patients. Validated recurrence was found at 149 of 171 sites that were abnormal by

MATERIALS AND METHODS

PATIENT POPULATION

All 155 PET studies that were performed at the Northern California PET Imaging Center between October 27, 1992, and May 16, 1996, for evaluation of known or suspected recurrent colorectal cancer were included in the study. No independent diagnosis was available for 21 studies (14%), and these were excluded from analysis. Study subjects included 66 men and 68 women with a median age of 67 years (range, 31-93 years). Seventy-one primary tumors had been located in the ascending, transverse, or descending colon and 63 in the sigmoid colon or rectum. Median time of presentation after resection of the primary tumor was 22 months (range, 1 month to 8 years). Informed consent was obtained from all participating subjects.

An independent final diagnosis was obtained for 134 studies (86%) that were performed in 127 patients. One hundred twenty-one patients were studied once, 5 patients were studied twice, and 1 patient was studied 3 times. Excluded patients consisted of 6 patients who had less than 1 year of follow-up after studies with negative findings, 6 who were lost to follow-up, 5 who died without validation of sites of tumor involvement, and 4 who were treated by radiation or chemotherapy without further validation of findings. Computed tomography findings were available for comparison with PET findings in 115 patients.

INDICATIONS FOR PET IMAGING

Preoperative Staging

Seventy-eight studies were performed for preoperative assessment in patients who were under consideration for resection of recurrent tumor. In 76 cases, the patient had a localized CT abnormality at a single site that was considered to be potentially resectable.

Serum Carcinoembryonic Antigen Elevation

Thirty-two patients were being evaluated because of elevated serum carcinoembryonic antigen (CEA) levels. In 18 patients, prior CT findings had been negative. Fourteen patients had not been examined by CT.

Other Indications

Twenty-four studies were performed for other indications. Nine patients were undergoing restaging after surgery, 6 patients were thought to have nonresectable disease on the basis of multiple CT abnormalities, and 5 patients were being evaluated prior to radiation therapy. Four patients were studied because of symptoms or abnormal physical findings.

PET IMAGING

Imaging was performed with an ECAT EXACT 921 PET system (CTI Inc, Knoxville, Tenn). This system has an axial field of view of 16.2 cm, with intrinsic transverse resolution of 6.0 mm and axial resolution of 5.5 mm full width at half maximum. Direct and cross-plane data obtained from 24 detector rings were used to reconstruct 47 image sections, separated by 3.4 mm center to center. When images were reconstructed using a Hann filter with 0.4 cutoff, image resolution was approximately 10 mm full width at half maximum. Data acquisition, image reconstruction, and image display were performed using standard system software. Patients fasted for at least 4 hours prior to intravenous injection of FDG, 5.29 MBq/kg (0.14 mCi/kg), for an average dose of 0.37 MBq (10 mCi). Non–attenuation-corrected whole-body imaging at 4 minutes per bed position was commenced 30 minutes after injection. At the conclusion of whole-body imaging, 1 to 3 static 10- to 20-minute emission acquisitions were performed in regions of high suspicion. Transmission data were acquired for 10 to 20 minutes, depending on the activity of transmission sources. In the first 42 patients, transmission imaging was performed prior to tracer injection. In subsequent patients, transmission acquisition was performed at the end of the emission studies.

CT IMAGING

Computed tomographic imaging of the abdomen and pelvis had been performed prior to the PET study in 115 cases, usually at 1 of 7 different hospital radiology departments or outpatient imaging centers in the Sacramento region. The scanners in use at these sites were all GE 8900 or GE HiLight Advantage systems (GE Medical Systems, Milwaukee, Wis) during the first 18 months of the study. Subsequently, GE HiSpeed Advantage helical systems were used at 3 sites. The 1-cm contiguous-image sections were obtained in 2 to 4 seconds with the earlier scanners, and 7-mm sections were obtained in 1 second with the high-speed systems. Studies were performed after intravenous injection of 100 to 200 mL of contrast material. Standard scanning parameters were used.

PET IMAGE INTERPRETATION

All PET images were interpreted at the time of the study by 1 or 2 of us (P.E.V., E.A.C., T.R.P., M.K.H., or R.W.M.) who had access to clinical data. Images were viewed in axial, coronal, and sagittal planes using an interactive video display system. Since most PET studies were performed for further evaluation of CT findings, PET images were read in conjunction with CT images whenever possible.

PET, CT, or both and at 8 sites that were normal by both modalities.

A final diagnosis of no recurrence was established at 22 sites of image abnormality. Seventeen of these were abnormal by CT only, 3 were abnormal by PET only, and 2 were abnormal by both modalities. Five patients without recurrence who had normal PET and CT scans remained clinically disease free for more than 1 year after imaging.

DIAGNOSTIC ACCURACY OF PET AND CT

Sensitivity and Specificity

Sensitivity and specificity of PET and CT on a patient-by-patient basis are shown in **Table 1**. **Table 2** and **Table 3** show sensitivity and specificity of PET and CT by site of recurrence, as well as the difference between the 2 mo-

Standardized uptake values (SUVs) and target-to-background ratios (T-B ratios) were determined for lesions that were more than 1 cm in diameter. The SUV is a semiquantitative measure of uptake that is obtained by dividing maximum activity detected in the lesion (microcuries per milliliter) by injected dose corrected for body weight (microcuries per gram). Standardized uptake values were not calculated for smaller lesions because the recovery coefficient decreases rapidly with size below 1 cm. To obtain measurements that were not affected by small lesion size, only lesions that were clearly more than 1 cm in diameter in the PET images were included. Standardized uptake values and T-B ratios were also determined for 19 sites with false-positive CT findings.

To obtain tumor activity values for calculation of SUVs and T-B ratios, circular regions of interest 1 cm in diameter were placed over the region of increased uptake, centered on the point of highest visible activity, and the maximum pixel activity within the region was determined. To obtain background activity values for calculation of ratios, the region of interest was placed just outside the area of visible tumor uptake.

All images were reread at the conclusion of the study by 2 of 3 investigators (E.A.C., P.E.V., and M.K.H.) reading independently, without knowledge of patient identity, clinical data, CT findings, histologic data, or the results of the initial reading. Readings were subsequently compared and consensus was reached by discussion. At rereading, images were read by comparison of lesion activity to adjacent normal activity and were graded as positive or negative for tumor. Involvement of an organ or an anatomic region (eg, pelvis) was considered a single site of disease, regardless of the number of individual lesions. Each lung was considered as a separate site.

CT IMAGE INTERPRETATION

Since CT imaging had been performed at many different imaging facilities, CT scans were reinterpreted by 2 experienced readers (G.A.H. and H.B.G.), to ensure uniformity of interpretation. Computed tomographic images were read as positive or negative for each of the same anatomic regions as the PET scans. Readers were blinded to clinical, histologic, and PET data.

VALIDATION OF IMAGING FINDINGS

A final diagnosis was established at 171 sites that were positive for tumor by PET and/or CT. A further 8 tumor sites that were negative by PET and CT were confirmed surgically. The diagnosis was established histologically at 103 sites (57%), surgically at 93 sites, and by needle biopsy at 10 sites. Abnormal imaging findings at 45 sites (25%) were validated by demonstration of progression (38 sites) or no progression (7 sites) at a second CT imaging. In 7 patients with advanced disease, who died during the course of the study, clinical evidence of tumor progression was accepted as positive evidence at 20 sites of imaging abnormality (11%). Clinical evidence of absence of disease for 1 year or more after the PET study was accepted as negative evidence at 13 sites of imaging abnormality (7%) and in 5 patients who had normal PET and CT findings.

DATA ANALYSIS

For comparison of the accuracy of PET and CT, only the 115 studies in which patients had been imaged by both modalities were considered. All 134 studies were considered in evaluation of the effect of PET findings on patient treatment.

Means and SDs of SUVs and T-B ratios of lesions that were clearly greater than 1 cm in diameter were calculated. Mean SUVs and T-B ratios were also calculated for 19 sites with false-positive findings by CT. Analysis of variance was used to determine whether significant differences existed between mean SUVs and T-B ratios of tumor foci at different anatomic sites and between the false-positive CT sites and true sites of tumor.[6] Where differences were detected, post hoc tests were used to identify sites of difference.[6]

Sensitivity and specificity of PET and CT for the detection of tumor were calculated patient by patient and site by site. The differences in sensitivity and specificity between the 2 modalities were calculated. Ninety-five percent confidence intervals (CIs) were calculated according to the method described by Berry,[7] to evaluate the precision of the difference values and to determine statistical significance.[8] Sensitivity was also determined separately for sites where the final diagnosis had been established by histologic examination only.

IMPACT OF PET FINDINGS ON SURGICAL TREATMENT AND MANAGEMENT COST

The effect of PET findings on surgical treatment was determined by review of pre- and post-PET clinical records and discussion of those records with surgeons. Positron emission tomographic findings were correlated with subsequent surgical treatment and surgical findings. To determine the effect of the PET findings on the cost of patient treatment, it was assumed that recurrence at more than 1 site would be regarded as nonresectable. The cost of the surgical procedures that would be avoided was compared with the cost of PET imaging. These costs were determined from Medicare reimbursement rates for hospitalization, professional services (surgery and anesthesia), and pathologic examination of surgical specimens.[9-11] Since there was no Medicare reimbursement for oncologic PET during the time of the study, PET costs were based on average reimbursement for whole-body PET examination at our center during the study period.

dalities and 95% CI for the difference. One hundred four sites were true positive by both PET and CT. Forty-two (88%) of 48 sites that were false negative by CT were true positive by PET and 5 (45%) of 11 sites that were false negative by PET were true positive by CT. Ninety-five percent CIs for the differences between PET and CT (Table 2) showed that PET was more sensitive than CT at the .05 confidence level at all anatomic locations except the lungs and the liver. The 95% CI for lesions in the liver was close to statistical significance at −1% to 22%. A difference is significant at the .05 level if the 95% CI does not include 0.[8] When only tumor sites that had been validated histologically were considered, sensitivity was 91% (90/99) for PET and 66% (65/99) for CT.

Positron emission tomographic scans were false negative at 11 sites, 6 of which were also negative by

Table 1. Sensitivity and Specificity of Positron Emission Tomographic and Computed Tomographic Scans by Patients

	Positron Emission Tomographic Scan, No. (%)	Computed Tomographic Scan, No. (%)	Difference (95% CI*), %
Sensitivity	96/101 (95)	79/101 (78)	17 (7 to 25)
Specificity	11/14 (79)	7/14 (50)	29 (−11 to 69)

*CI indicates confidence interval.

Table 2. Sensitivity of Positron Emission Tomographic and Computed Tomographic Scans by Sites of Tumor Recurrence

Site	Positron Emission Tomographic Scan, No. (%)	Computed Tomographic Scan, No. (%)	Difference (95% CI*), %
Liver	54/57 (95)	48/57 (84)	11 (−1 to 22)
Pelvis	30/31 (97)	21/31 (68)	29 (9 to 49)
Abdomen	22/28 (79)	13/28 (46)	33 (11 to 54)
Retroperitoneum	12/12 (100)	7/12 (58)	42 (10 to 74)
Lungs	16/17 (94)	16/17 (94)	0 (−19 to 19)
Other†	12/12 (100)	4/12 (33)	67 (36 to 98)
Total	**146/157** (93)	**109/157** (69)	24 (16 to 32)

*CI indicates confidence interval.
†Other sites include hila and mediastinum (n = 4), bone (n = 4), abdominal wall (n = 2), and adrenal glands (n = 2).

CT. Hepatic metastases were missed in 3 patients. Computed tomography findings were negative in 1 patient and positive in the other 2. There were false-negative PET findings at 6 sites in the abdomen. In one instance, a largely necrotic 4-cm lesion was diagnosed by CT but not by PET. The other 5 patients had diffuse peritoneal spread or small nodules of less than 1 cm that were negative by CT as well. One patient had a metastatic lung nodule of less than 1 cm that was negative by PET and positive by CT, and another had a 3-cm, PET-negative pelvic tumor mass that was positive by CT. Five of the 11 patients who had false-negative PET findings proved to have disease at a single site only. The other 6 false-negative findings occurred in patients who had other, PET-positive lesions.

There were false negative CT findings at 48 sites, 6 of which were also negative by PET. In 4 of 9 instances in which hepatic CT images were false negative for tumor, the images showed no abnormalities. In 5 cases, the CT images showed benign changes, including heterogeneous fatty infiltration in 2 patients, postoperative changes in 2 patients, and multiple small hepatic cysts in 1 patient; coexisting tumors were not diagnosed. In 8 of the 9 patients with false-negative CT results in the liver, the PET study was true positive. The largest number of false-negative CT findings occurred in the abdomen, pelvis, and retroperitoneum, where 30 (42%)of 71 disease sites were not detected. Twenty-one of these sites (70%) were positive by PET.

Positron emission tomography was more specific than CT at all sites except the retroperitoneum, but the differences were smaller than the differences in sensitivity, ranging from 1% to 6%. Only in the lungs was the difference statistically significant (Table 3). The difference was also significant when all sites were considered together. There were 5 false-positive PET results, including 3 in patients who proved to be free of tumor recurrence at all sites. Three of these false-positive foci were found in the pelvis. The positive predictive value of PET findings was 97% (146/151) on a site-by-site basis and 97% (96/99) on a patient-by-patient basis. The negative predictive value was 69% (11/16) patient by patient.

Table 3. Specificity of Positron Emission Tomographic and Computed Tomographic Scans by Sites of Tumor Recurrence

Site	Positron Emission Tomographic Scan, No. (%)	Computed Tomographic Scan, No. (%)	Difference (95% CI*), %
Liver	58/58 (100)	55/58 (95)	5 (−1 to 12)
Pelvis	81/84 (96)	76/84 (90)	6 (−2 to 13)
Abdomen	87/87 (100)	85/87 (98)	2 (−2 to 6)
Retroperitoneum	103/103 (100)	103/103 (100)	0 (0 to 0)
Lungs	97/98 (99)	94/98 (96)	3 (1 to 5)
Other	103/104 (99)	101/104 (98)	1 (−1 to 1)
Total	**529/534** (99)	**514/534** (96)	3 (1 to 5)

*CI indicates confidence interval.

There were 19 false-positive CT findings, including 7 in patients who proved to have no tumor recurrence at any site. Eight occurred in the pelvis, 4 in the lungs, 2 in the abdomen, and 3 in the liver. Two patients had benign, enlarged adrenal glands. One false-positive finding in the pelvis was also false positive by PET; all others were negative by PET. The positive predictive value of CT findings was 85% (109/128) on a site-by-site basis and 93% (79/85) on a patient-by-patient basis. The negative predictive value was 24% (7/29) patient by patient.

Blinded Reinterpretation of PET Images

Blinded reinterpretation resulted in change in diagnosis in 9 (7%) of 134 studies at 9 (5%) of 178 sites of imaging abnormality.

In 5 patients who had been initially diagnosed as having recurrences at 2 or more sites, an additional site of tumor was noted at rereading. An independent diagnosis could not be established at these sites at the time of reinterpretation; however, all 5 patients were already known to have nonresectable tumors, so that the changes in interpretation would not have affected treatment decisions. In 3 patients who had no abnormality at the initial reading, solitary foci of abnormal activity were noted at rereading. In 1 of these patients, an initially false-negative site in the liver was correctly reinterpreted as positive, and this change could have affected treatment. The other 2 findings proved to be false positive on the basis of more than 1 year of disease-free follow-up. In 1 patient, an initial false-positive finding in the pelvis was correctly reinterpreted as representing bowel uptake.

Table 4. Standardized Uptake Values and Target-to-Background Ratios by Sites of Tumor Recurrence

Site	No. of Lesions	Standardized Uptake Value, Mean ± SD (Range)	Target-to-Background Ratio, Mean ± SD (Range)
Liver	79	6.05 ± 1.89 (3.3-12.7)	2.68 ± 0.67 (1.5-4.7)
Abdomen	39	6.35 ± 2.40 (2.4-11.1)	4.43 ± 1.70 (1.6-9.3)
Pelvis	32	6.51 ± 3.45 (2.4-19.6)	5.28 ± 2.46 (2.5-10.6)
Lung	13	5.48 ± 3.10 (1.7-11.3)	6.02 ± 3.18 (2.8-15.5)
All sites	163	6.17 ± 2.48 (1.7-19.6)	3.87 ± 2.08 (1.5-15.5)

SUVs and T-B Ratios of Tumor Sites

Standardized uptake values and T-B ratios are shown by site of recurrence in **Table 4**. Only sites where there was a total of more than 10 lesions more than 1 cm in diameter were included. The mean ± SD SUV for all tumor sites was 6.17 ± 2.48, and the mean ± SD T-B ratio was 3.87 ± 2.08. The mean ± SD SUV at 19 sites of false-positive CT findings was 1.97 ± 0.81, and the mean ± SD T-B ratio was 1.26 ± 0.60. Analysis of variance of SUVs by tumor location showed no statistically significant differences between mean SUVs at different anatomic sites. Analysis of variance and post hoc tests showed that SUVs and T-B ratios of false-positive CT sites were significantly lower than SUVs and T-B ratios of tumor at any location ($P<.001$). Target-to-background ratios of liver lesions were lower than T-B ratios of tumor at all other sites ($P<.001$), as would be expected from the relatively higher uptake in normal liver compared with most other normal tissues.

There was overlap between the mean SUV of identifiable bowel, which was 2.91 ± 1.44 (range, 1.11-5.30), and the mean SUV of abdominal tumor, which was 6.35 ± 2.40 (range, 2.43-11.19). In these cases, diagnostic confusion was avoided by clear visual differences in the distribution of activity, which followed a characteristic linear pattern in the case of bowel and was focal in the case of tumor. There were 3 cases in which a false-positive diagnosis could have resulted from unrecognized focal bowel uptake.

IMPACT OF PET FINDINGS ON PATIENT TREATMENT

Preoperative Assessment of Tumor Recurrence

Seventy-eight patients were referred specifically for preoperative evaluation prior to attempted curative resection of recurrent tumor at a single site. In 76 patients, tumor recurrence had been demonstrated by CT. The PET findings in these patients are summarized in **Table 5**. In 47 of these patients (60%), PET imaging also showed a single, localized site of recurrence. In 23 patients (29%), PET demonstrated other, unsuspected sites of recurrence, and in 2 patients with hepatic metastases (3%), PET demonstrated extensive, bilobar disease, where only localized tumor had been detected by CT. Six patients (8%) had no evidence of tumor on PET. **Figure 1** shows CT and PET images obtained in a patient with CT evidence of hepatic metastasis only, while PET correctly demonstrated retroperitoneal metastasis as well.

Table 5. Results of Preoperative Positron Emission Tomographic Scan Evaluation in 78 Patients

Site	Positron Emission Tomographic Scan Results, No.			
	Single Site of Recurrence	Recurrence at Other Sites	No Recurrence	Total, No.
Liver	24*	12†	2‡	**38**
Pelvis	11	4	3‡	**18**
Abdomen	4	3	1	**8**
Retroperitoneum	2	2	0	**4**
Lung	7	2	0	**9**
Abdominal wall	1	0	0	**1**
Total (%)	**49*** (63)	**23†** (29)	**6§** (8)	**78**

**Two patients (3%) with focal recurrence in one lobe by computed tomographic scan had extensive bilobar recurrence by positron emission tomographic scan.*

†One pulmonary abnormality proved to be a false-positive positron emission tomographic scan result.

‡One proved to be a false-negative positron emission tomographic scan.

§Two proved to be false-negative positron emission tomographic scans.

Surgery was undertaken in 42 (89%) of 47 patients with evidence of localized recurrence at a single site. At surgery, it was found that PET had underestimated the extent of tumor recurrence in 11 (26%) of 42 patients, and 7 of these patients (17%) proved to have nonresectable tumor. Two patients with known liver metastases also had diffuse peritoneal tumor and 1 had multiple small liver lesions that had not been detected by PET. Three patients with focal pelvic recurrence and 1 with focal abdominal recurrence on PET also had undetected diffuse tumor that could not be resected.

One patient each with hepatic, pelvic, abdominal, and pulmonary recurrence had more focal lesions than PET had demonstrated, which were then resected. Resection for cure was undertaken in 35 (83%) of 42 patients, representing 45% of the original group of 78 patients referred for preoperative assessment.

Thirteen of the 23 patients with PET evidence of tumor at multiple sites were subsequently evaluated at surgery, with confirmation of PET findings in 12 (92%) of 13 cases. One patient who had liver and lung abnormalities by PET and CT was found to have a resectable hepatic recurrence and a benign granulomatous lung lesion. In the other 10 patients, PET findings were confirmed by imaging and clinical follow-up. No CT-negative PET abnormalities proved to be false positive.

There were 6 patients with hepatic, pelvic, or abdominal CT abnormalities in whom PET showed no tumor. Subsequent surgery demonstrated a 3-cm pelvic tumor mass in one of these patients and a 3.5-cm hepatic metastasis in another. On PET imaging, the hepatic metastasis had shown lower FDG uptake than normal liver. Of the other 4 patients, 2 had no evidence of tumor at surgery, and all remained clinically tumor free at 14 to 32 months after PET.

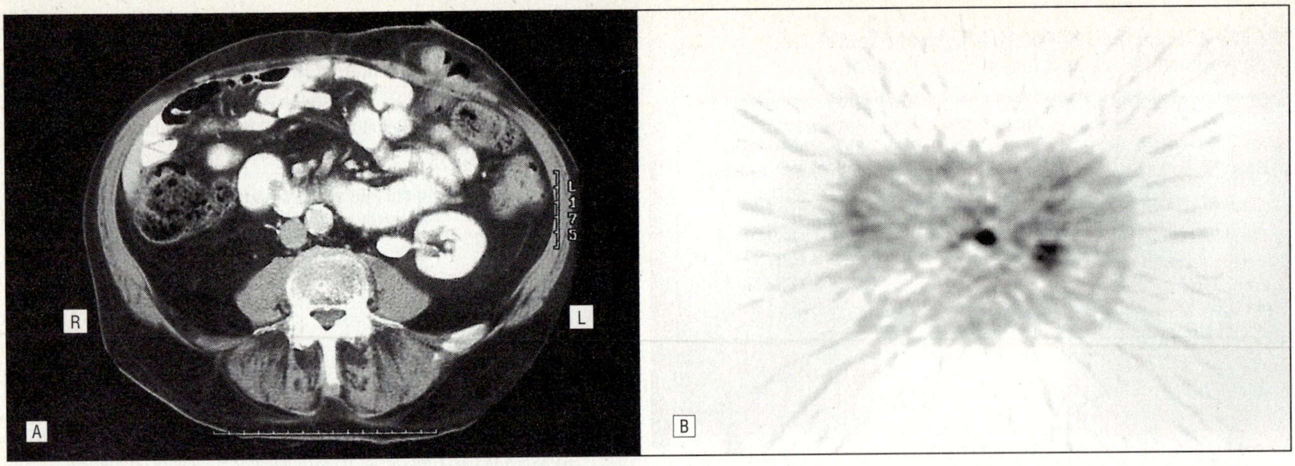

Figure 1. *A, A computed tomographic scan shows no evidence of retroperitoneal tumor in a patient who had computed tomographic scan evidence of a solitary hepatic metastasis and was undergoing preoperative evaluation. B, A corresponding positron emission tomographic image section shows a retroperitoneal tumor focus. Retroperitoneal foci were also seen in 3 other positron emission tomographic image sections. Surgery was not performed, and a second computed tomographic image 14 weeks later demonstrated interim enlargement of retroperitoneal lymph nodes.*

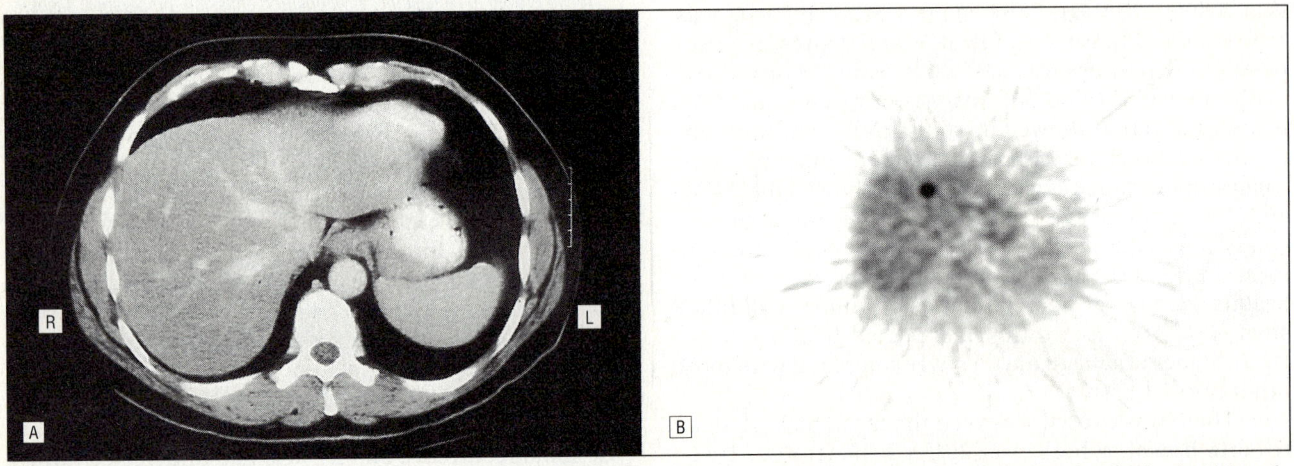

Figure 2. *A, A computed tomographic scan of the liver shows no abnormality in a patient with an elevated serum carcinoembryonic antigen level and a history of colon carcinoma. B, A corresponding positron emission tomographic image section demonstrates a hepatic tumor focus. Hepatic tumor foci were also seen in 2 other positron emission tomographic image sections. A second computed tomographic image 13 weeks later confirmed hepatic recurrence at these locations.*

Elevated Serum CEA Level

Thirty-two patients underwent PET imaging for investigation of serum CEA elevation. Eighteen had negative CT findings, and 14 did not undergo CT. Positron emission tomography findings were positive in 12 (67%) of 18 and 7 (50%) of 14 patients, respectively, and negative in the other 13. Thirteen patients had recurrence at 1 anatomic site only, but in 2 of these patients, tumor was extensive and not amenable to resection. Six patients had recurrences at multiple sites. **Figure 2** shows true-positive PET findings, with false-negative CT findings in the liver of a patient with an elevated serum CEA level.

Nine patients with PET evidence of localized recurrence at a single site underwent surgery, and resection with curative intent was performed in 7 cases. One patient was found to have diffuse, nonresectable abdominal tumor as well as a PET-positive focal lesion, and 1 pelvic PET abnormality proved to be false positive. Three patients with PET evidence of tumor at multiple sites also underwent surgical evaluation, with confirmation of PET findings in each case. Follow-up for 1 year or more showed no recurrence in 11 of 13 patients with negative PET results. The other 2 patients subsequently underwent surgery 33 and 58 days after the PET scans and were both found to have extensive abdominal tumor recurrence that had not been demonstrated by PET.

In the patients who were studied because of elevated serum CEA levels, PET sensitivity was 90% (18/20) and specificity was 92% (11/12) patient by patient. The positive predictive value was 95% (18/19) and the negative predictive value was 85% (11/13).

Impact of Preoperative PET Imaging on Cost of Surgical Treatment

In a management algorithm in which recurrence at more than 1 site is treated as nonresectable, the PET findings in the 78 preoperative patients would translate into avoidance of surgery for nonresectable tumor in 25 patients (32%). Surgery would be avoided in 14 patients with hepatic, 4 with pelvic, 3 with abdominal, 2 with

Table 6. Net Savings Resulting From Use of Positron Emission Tomographic Scans for Preoperative Staging

	Cost/Savings, $
Savings from avoided surgery	374 596
Total cost of positron emission tomographic studies	140 400
Net savings from avoided surgery	234 196
Net savings per patient	3003

retroperitoneal, and 2 with pulmonary lesions. On the basis of published surgical findings,[12] it was assumed that half of the patients with hepatic recurrence and unsuspected tumor at a second site would be found to have nonresectable tumors at surgery, so that the avoided procedure would be laparotomy only, without hepatic resection.

The total Medicare costs of surgical procedures at these sites amounted to $20 668 for hepatic resection, $15 508 for pulmonary resection, and $12 916 for pelvic or abdominal resection. Average reimbursement for whole-body PET examination at our center during the period of the study was $1800. The savings that resulted from elimination of surgical procedures amounted to $374 596 (**Table 6**). The per-patient savings were $3003 after subtraction of PET costs. If the 4 cases in which CT was false positive and PET was true negative are included in determining the procedures that were avoided, net savings would be $3764 per patient.

COMMENT

Positron emission tomography was significantly more sensitive than CT for detection of recurrent tumor, with a difference of 24% (95% CI, 16% to 32%). Positron emission tomography was also more specific than CT, with a smaller difference of 3% (95% CI, 1% to 5%). The largest difference between the 2 modalities was found in the abdomen and pelvis, where more than one third of sites that were true positive by PET were false negative by CT. Computed tomography also had 10 false-positive findings in the abdomen and pelvis, compared with 3 by PET. In the liver, the difference between the modalities was smaller, at 11% (95% CI, –1% to 22%), and in some cases resulted from difficulty in differentiating benign from malignant abnormalities by CT. In the lungs, both modalities failed to detect 1 metastatic lesion, but CT had more false-positive findings.

Although PET is more sensitive than CT, PET sensitivity is also limited by minimum detectable lesion size. Detectability of tumor by PET depends on 2 factors: tumor size and uptake of FDG. In our study, PET failed to detect 7 lesions that were less than 1 cm in diameter and 4 lesions that were larger. One of these larger lesions had only a narrow rim of viable tumor around a necrotic center while the other 3 were solid and showed low tracer uptake. Also, in 5 patients with PET-positive abdominal or pelvic recurrence, PET underestimated the extent of tumor. Each of these patients had diffuse peritoneal or pelvic spread that was missed by PET and by CT.

Physiologic tracer accumulation in normal structures, particularly the intestine and urinary tract, is another possible source of error in interpretation of PET images. In 3 of our patients, false-positive findings in the pelvis may have represented focal bowel activity, and in 1 of these cases, the pelvic activity was correctly read as intestinal uptake at reinterpretation; however, in most cases, bowel activity was identifiable by its characteristic linear pattern. Artifacts resulting from high bladder activity can interfere with interpretation of non–attenuation-corrected pelvic images, but we did not find this to be a problem when attenuation correction was used. Ureteric activity also did not interfere with interpretation.

Our findings regarding the accuracy of PET and CT are similar to those obtained by other investigators. Schiepers et al[2] compared PET findings with those obtained by conventional imaging, which included CT and ultrasound imaging of the liver, CT of the pelvis, and chest radiography. Reported sensitivities of PET and conventional imaging were 94% and 85%, respectively, for liver metastasis, and 93% and 60% for pelvic recurrence. Also, PET demonstrated unsuspected tumor at other sites in 10 (13%) of 76 patients.

Delbeke et al[5] found in 61 patients that PET was more accurate than CT for detection of liver metastases (92% vs 78%) and extrahepatic metastases (92% vs 71%). Altogether, PET detected unsuspected metastases in 17 (28%) of 61 studies. Similarly, Lai et al[4] demonstrated unsuspected extrahepatic tumor in 11 (32%) of 34 patients with known hepatic metastases.

An unbiased determination of the accuracy of PET and CT cannot be obtained from studies of this type, in which many patients are selected for PET imaging because of positive CT findings. This case-selection bias results in overrepresentation of positive CT findings, both true and false, with consequent overestimation of CT sensitivity and underestimation of specificity. However, study of a biased population of this type is appropriate when the purpose is to determine the impact of adding a new modality to the patient treatment algorithm and does demonstrate which test is more accurate in the relevant clinical context.

A more difficult issue in quantifying sensitivity and specificity in disseminated malignant disease arises from problems in verification of imaging findings.[13] Often there are no means of detecting tumor sites that are nonsymptomatic and that are not detected by either imaging modality, so that the findings of the more sensitive technique essentially provide their own criterion standard. This results in high values for sensitivity, such as the values that were reported for CT when it was first introduced[14] and the values that we are finding for PET at the present time. Specificity may also be overestimated, since it is not possible to verify all abnormalities in a patient with a disseminated tumor.

It is desirable to use histologic diagnosis as the only reference test in measuring the performance of a diagnostic modality, but this can lead to another type of verification bias in the study population.[15] When patients have clinical and imaging evidence of extensive recurrence, it is usual for only one lesion, and sometimes no lesions, to be verified pathologically. If sites of pathologically nonverified lesions are excluded from the study, positive PET and CT findings at the corresponding anatomic sites will be underrepresented, thereby reducing the measured sensitivity of both modalities in these regions. To reduce this bias, we included results at sites where a reference diagnosis was obtained by clinical and imaging follow-up, as suggested by Begg and McNeill.[15]

These forms of bias affected the evaluations of both imaging modalities equally, without biasing the comparison of PET and CT results. There were other possible sources of bias that could have favored PET over CT, including the interval between CT and PET imaging, unequal skills in test performance, variations in CT technology, and bias in test interpretation.

AS A RESULT of the interval between the CT and PET examinations, the tumor was an average of 24 days more advanced by the time of the PET study. This imaging sequence favored PET but accurately reflected the results that could be expected when PET is used for preoperative evaluation of patients with known CT abnormalities. Some degree of inequality in PET and CT performance was also likely, since the study was conducted in a PET imaging center, and the investigators had no control over the performance of the CT examinations. The PET operators were involved in the evaluation of a new imaging technology, while the CT examinations were performed as routine procedures at multiple clinical sites.[15,16]

The findings did not reflect the maximum CT performance that was technologically possible, since only some of the examinations were performed with helical CT scanners. Indeed, when Vitola et al[3] compared PET and helical CT in 24 patients with hepatic recurrence, they found a smaller difference in sensitivity of hepatic tumor detection (90% vs 86%) than we did; however, the increase in CT sensitivity was accompanied by a decrease in specificity to 58%, indicating that there was increased detection of benign as well as malignant lesions. Positron emission tomography also detected unsuspected extrahepatic tumor in 17% of their patients. Thus, it seems that existing technologic improvements in CT could narrow the gap between the modalities but would not be likely to eliminate it.

Availability of CT images at the time of initial PET interpretation was a potential source of interpretation bias. In the preoperative patients, this was an essential part of the algorithm that was under study, according to which PET was used for further evaluation of CT abnormalities. Only negative CT images were available in the patients who were being studied for elevated CEA levels. This study was initially undertaken as a prospective field study of PET imaging rather than a fully controlled comparison of the 2 modalities. Field studies that observe conventional clinical practices are more likely to be directly generalizable than studies in a controlled environment.[15] A controlled comparison of PET and CT was achieved by the retrospective, fully blinded reinterpretation of images.

In our evaluation of the impact of PET on management decisions, preoperative PET imaging correctly demonstrated unsuspected tumor at other sites in 29% of patients and more extensive nonresectable tumor at the same site in 3%. In a treatment algorithm according to which recurrence at more than 1 site is treated as nonresectable, this would translate into avoidance of nonindicated surgery by demonstration of nonresectable tumor in 32% of patients. At Medicare reimbursement rates, the cost of avoided surgery would exceed the cost of PET studies, resulting in net savings of $3003 per patient.

Similar findings were obtained in 3 previous studies that evaluated the effect of PET findings on management decisions. Beets et al[17] found that PET findings affected treatment in 15 (43%) of 35 patients with liver or pelvic recurrence and demonstrated unsuspected, nonresectable tumor in 6 (25%) of 24 preoperative patients. In staging suspected liver metastasis only, Vitola et al[3] found that PET altered surgical plans in 6 (25%) of 24 patients, avoiding surgery in 3 patients (13%). In the study by Lai et al,[4] PET avoided inappropriate hepatic resection in 11 (32%) of 34 patients.

In published reports of surgical findings, approximately 40% to 50% of patients who were thought to have resectable hepatic metastases and 30% to 40% of patients with limited local recurrences by CT were found to have nonresectable tumor at surgery.[12,18] In our study, PET reduced the proportion of patients with nonresectable tumor at surgery to 17%. Whether PET will also reduce the rate of rerecurrence by reducing the rate of undetected residual tumor after surgery remains to be determined.

In the past, serum CEA monitoring of patients with colorectal cancer has been regarded as controversial[19]; however, practice guidelines determined by the American Society of Clinical Oncology now recommend that CEA levels be monitored postoperatively if resection of liver metastasis would be clinically indicated.[20] Similarly, the National Comprehensive Cancer Network recommends monitoring serum CEA levels to evaluate patients who have an elevated serum CEA level preoperatively and whose level has decreased after surgery.[21]

When serum CEA is used for patient monitoring, positive results should be further assessed by the most accurate imaging modality available, and our findings suggest that this modality should be PET. Positron emission tomography findings were true positive in 67% of patients with elevated serum CEA levels and negative CT findings. A whole-body PET study is more expensive to perform than a CT study, but PET may reduce the overall cost of patient treatment by reducing the cost of repeated imaging after false-negative results, as well as the cost of unnecessary surgery.

All findings published to date have shown that PET imaging with FDG is more accurate than CT for diagnosis and staging of recurrent colorectal cancer. This and other studies have demonstrated the effectiveness of PET for determining resectability of recurrent tumor, and our results suggest that PET will also be more effective for initial diagnosis of recurrence.

This work was supported in part by a grant from the Sutter Institute of Medical Research, Sacramento, Calif (Dr Valk).

Corresponding author: Peter E. Valk, Northern California PET Imaging Center, 3195 Folsom Blvd, Sacramento, CA 95816.

REFERENCES

1. Strauss LG, Clorius JH, Schlag P, et al. Recurrence of colorectal tumors: PET evaluation. *Radiology.* 1989;170:329-332.
2. Schiepers C, Penninckx F, De Vadder N, et al. Contribution of PET in the diagnosis of recurrent colorectal cancer: comparison with conventional imaging. *Eur J Surg Oncol.* 1995;21:517-522.
3. Vitola JV, Delbeke D, Sandler MP, et al. Positron emission tomography to stage suspected metastatic colorectal carcinoma to the liver. *Am J Surg.* 1996;171: 21-26.
4. Lai DTM, Fulham M, Stephen MS, et al. The role of whole-body positron emission tomography with [18F]fluorodeoxyglucose in identifying operable colorectal cancer metastases to the liver. *Arch Surg.* 1996;131:703-707.
5. Delbeke D, Vitola JV, Sandler MP, et al. Staging recurrent metastatic colorectal carcinoma with PET. *J Nucl Med.* 1997;38:1196-1201.
6. Keppel G. *Design and Analysis: A Researcher's Handbook.* Englewood Cliffs, NJ: Prentice-Hall International Inc; 1982.
7. Berry CC. A tutorial on confidence intervals for proportions in diagnostic radiology. *AJR Am J Roentgenol.* 1990;154:477-480.
8. Metz CE. Quantification of failure to demonstrate statistical significance: the usefulness of confidence intervals. *Invest Radiol.* 1993;28:59-63.
9. Johnson C, Bowers CR, Swann KL, Kukucka RM, eds. *St Anthony's DRG Guidebook.* Reston, Va: St Anthony's Publishing Inc; 1997.
10. *International Classification of Diseases, Ninth Revision, Clinical Modification.* Washington, DC: Public Health Service, US Dept of Health and Human Services; 1988.
11. *Medicare Participating Provider Program: California Physician Fee Schedule (Area 4).* Washington, DC: Public Health Service, US Dept of Health and Human Services; 1997.
12. Steele GJ, Bleday R, Mayer RJ, Lindblad A, Petrelli N, Weaver D. A prospective evaluation of hepatic resection for colorectal carcinoma metastases to the liver: Gastrointestinal Tumor Study Group Protocol 6584. *J Clin Oncol.* 1991; 9:1105-1112.
13. Valk PE. Sense and sensitivity: issues in technology assessment [editorial]. *J Nucl Med.* 1996;37.
14. Moss AA, Thoeni RF, Schnyder P, Margulis AR. Value of computed tomography in the detection and staging of recurrent rectal carcinomas. *J Comput Assist Tomogr.* 1981;5:870-874.
15. Begg CB, McNeill BJ. Assessment of radiologic tests: control of bias and other design considerations. *Radiology.* 1988;167:565-569.
16. Gelfand DW, Ott DJ. Methodologic considerations in comparing imaging methods. *AJR Am J Roentgenol.* 1985;144:1117-1121.
17. Beets G, Penninckx F, Schiepers C, et al. Clinical value of whole-body positron emission tomography with [18F]fluorodeoxyglucose in recurrent colorectal cancer. *Br J Surg.* 1994;81:1666-1670.
18. Steele G Jr. Standard postoperative monitoring of patients after primary resection of colon and rectum cancer. *Cancer.* 1993;71(suppl 12):S4225-S4235.
19. Moertel CG, Fleming TR, Macdonald JS, Haller DG, Laurie JA, Tangen C. An evaluation of the carcinoembryonic antigen (CEA) test for monitoring patients with resected colon cancer. *JAMA.* 1993;270:943-947.
20. American Society of Clinical Oncology. Clinical practice guidelines for the use of tumor markers in breast and colon cancer. *J Clin Oncol.* 1996;14:2843-2877.
21. Engstrom P. Comprehensive cancer network colorectal cancer practice guidelines. *Oncology.* 1996;10(suppl):140-178.

Invited Critique

Valk et al are certainly to be congratulated for their fervent enthusiasm for this new privately held technology. The skeptic might assume that since these private physicians are based in a PET imaging center, they would bias a study by design to favor PET scan; however, it is important to put aside all such potentially cynical prejudices in favor of academic interpretation of a large number of patients carefully assessed by a variety of means and numerous statistical tests. It is particularly important to do so in light of the scope of this problem. Colorectal cancer is the second most common noncutaneous malignant neoplasm, anticipated to affect approximately 165 000 people this year.[1] It can also be anticipated that more than 40% of patients, despite seemingly curative resections, will experience a recurrence of their disease.[2-4] The most common sites of recurrence are the pelvis, liver, and lungs. Over the past several decades, numerous new technologies have been introduced in an attempt to better identify and therefore more appropriately treat patients with recurrences in each of these areas. The primary tool for both preoperative and postoperative evaluation of patients with rectal carcinoma is rectal ultrasonography.[5-7] The potential problem with rectal ultrasound is that whether the focal length is 5.0, 7.0, 7.5, or 10.0 MHz, the best clarity is in the layers of the rectal wall as opposed to within the pelvis itself. Local recurrences tend to occur not at the suture line or anastomosis but actually in the pelvis.[8] Therefore, any intraluminal evidence of tumor tends to show the tip of the iceberg rather than the major nidus of tumor.

The most common extrapelvic and potentially resectable tumor site is the liver. Finlay and McArdle[9] and others[10,11] have demonstrated very high rates of sensitivity and specificity of ultrasonography for liver metastasis. More recently, intrahepatic ultrasonography by either laparotomy or laparoscopy[12,13] has enabled avoidance of unnecessary hepatic resection in many patients. Even with multiple bilobar lesions, a 5-year survival rate of 35% can be anticipated, provided that a curative liver resection can be accomplished.[8] In addition to CT scan and extracorporeal and intraoperative hepatic ultrasonography, other modalities exist to evaluate the presence of any liver lesions. These tests include liver-spleen scan and, recently, radioimmunoguided surgery.[14,15] The main use of the latter technology is for detection of unresectable deposits, such as retroperitoneal tumor spread and periportal tumor involvement, both of which would preclude attempted curative hepatic resection. Lung metastasis can also be treated for cure, with an anticipated survival rate only slightly worse than that after resection of liver metastases.[16,17] The optimal test for detection of these pulmonary metastases is regarded by some thoracic surgeons as helical CT scan.[18]

Continued on next page

These authors have elected to compare their privately held technological investment with a single modality: CT scan. There are multiple problems with this type of study design, some of which have been mentioned by the authors, and others of which have been overlooked. I would like to address these problems on an individual basis. First, the study has been designed to include as the criterion standard positives not only histopathologically proven tumor but also clinical evidence of tumor progression (11%), clinical evidence of absence of disease for 1 year or more after the PET study was accepted as negative evidence (7%), and demonstration of progression (38 sites) or no progression (7 sites) at a second imaging. Although a final diagnosis was established in 171 sites, in 78 of those sites, no histopathologic confirmation was ever obtained. Thus, the denominator of the study is skewed in favor of the interpretive design of the study. Therefore, the authors should have eliminated from their denominator all of the patients in whom histopathologic confirmation was not obtained. Had they done so, I imagine that their sensitivity rate for the remaining 93 patients would have approximated that of CT scan.

Second, the follow-up of patients in whom "clinical evidence of absence of disease for 1 year or more" was accepted was suspect. For example, slow tumor growth could have well accounted for a patient who had a 1-cm recurrence 8 years after surgery and still had a 1-cm recurrence 9 years after surgery. Had that patient been evaluated at 10 years, the tumor might have continued to slowly enlarge; 1 year is an inappropriately short interval. As a much more important issue, the length of follow-up after attempted curative surgery for recurrent disease was not even mentioned. This factor is crucial to ascertain the true accuracy of the PET scan. For example, a patient may have undergone an attempted curative pelvic exenteration for isolated pelvic disease and remained disease-free for 6 months, after which hepatic recurrence may have been noted. Therefore, the length of follow-up should have been supplied along with rigorous postresectional imaging studies to confirm the authors' conclusions. Was re-recurrence defined as only clinically evident or was it vigorously sought?

Third, the authors have made an assumption in their definitions that if more than a single site was involved by tumor, that patient was "unresectable." As a surgeon, I would certainly challenge this assumption. Two of many possible examples include bilateral 1-cm peripheral pulmonary metastases 5 years after initial resection and a true anastomotic recurrence with a single perianastomotic tumor focus 2 years after the initial operation. The authors should have been more specific in their discussion of the positive sites and should have included all potentially resectable patients, as jointly judged by a surgeon and radiologist and not as judged in isolation by a radiologist.

Fourth, although the authors have accepted some culpability for the mean 22-day delay between CT scan and PET scan, I feel that this problem is minor relative to other flaws in the study design. I do not think that within 3 weeks, any major tumor growth would occur, and if such growth indeed were so rapid, it would most likely render the patient incurable. Once again, the problem is that the parameters seem to have been set forth exclusively by radiologists, without consultation from a surgical oncologist, colorectal surgeon, or general surgeon.

Fifth, in a similar light, the authors have assumed in their cost analysis that surgery would be performed based on a positive PET scan result without surgeons having performed other tests. Perhaps the surgeons in Sacramento are so enamored and convinced of this technology that they would not require additional studies, such as CT portography, radioimmunoguided surgery, diagnostic laparoscopy, or other modalities; however, most surgeons would indeed be loath to operate based on a single positive study result. Accordingly, the cost of those additional confirmatory investigations should have been factored into their cost analysis.

Sixth, one of the most major problems was the inequivalence in performance of the CT scan. It is well accepted in surgery that the more one performs a procedure, the better the results will be. Heald et al[19,20] have quite convincingly and repeatedly demonstrated local recurrence rates after curative resection of rectal carcinoma well below 5%. By adoption of these meticulous surgical techniques and high-volume procedure performance, others have been able to reproduce these laudable results.[21-24] Merely by standardization and repeated performance of the same operation, all of these investigators have been able to demonstrate markedly lower recurrence rates than even the most widely touted North American intergroup study.[25] Thus, following an identical method, the authors, who clearly have significant expertise and a vested financial interest in this technology, have compared their obviously carefully selected equipment, their standardized technique, and their impressive interpretative skills with a myriad hybrid of scans performed at an unknown number of institutions by countless radiologists and technicians. Obvious differences may exist in terms of thickness of the "cuts"; use or lack of use of intravenous, oral, or rectal contrast; and performance of additional cuts to investigate any questionable areas, contingent on the level of interest and expertise of the radiologist. In point of fact, the radiologist is often guided by a sometimes inadequate amount of clinical information supplied by the surgeon and/or oncologist. In every instance, these investigators had available to them not only their own machine and technicians using a standardized approach, but also the previously performed CT scans in every instance. Although they state that this study design is appropriate, they also admit the potential source of interpretation bias. Clearly, a more accurate study would be designed to include randomization of patients to undergo 1 of the 2 studies first, followed by the other. In both instances, the scan would be performed by "experts" using the best and newest possible machines with the highest resolution using standardized techniques and blinded to the results of the other study.

In terms of the results, the authors tout the 93% sensitivity of PET scanning against the 69% sensitivity of CT scan. They gloss over the fact that the specificity rates of the 2 studies (98% and 96%, respectively) were virtually identical. Once again, because of flaws in the study design, the sensitivity of PET scanning for the liver, pelvis, abdomen, and retroperitoneum might not have been better compared with other modalities, such as magnetic resonance imaging,[26] transanal rectal ultrasound,[27] radioimmunoguided surgery,[15] or CT portography.[28] Much in the way that the Krook et al[25] study had an unacceptably high rate of local recurrence in the surgery alone group, the CT specificity rate shown in Table 1 was among the worst I have seen, undoubtedly due to the problems I have previously cited.

Additional problems with the results include the fact that in 11 (26%) of 42 patients, resection for cure was undertaken but found to be impossible. That cost should clearly be factored out of their cost/savings equation. The 69% negative pre-

Continued on next page

dictive value should also be discussed as clearly less than ideal. Furthermore, in 30% of PET scan–negative patients, tumor was apparently found in the pelvis, abdomen, or retroperitoneum. This group also needs to be subtracted out of the cost/savings equation. Last, in 5 of 11 sites that were deemed negative by PET scan, the tumors were judged to be true positive by CT scan. This portion of the discussion was again not highlighted within the cost/savings equation. A greater problem is that the cost analysis is really based on Medicare reimbursement and therefore is related exclusively to local charges and in no direct way to cost. A discussion of relative value units or a distillation of indirect and direct costs would be much more meaningful in the current context of health care economics than the new reporting of Medicare reimbursement rates. Medicare reimbursement is of course exclusively related to charges but not to cost. Therefore, although throughout this article the authors used the word *cost*, they are in fact presenting discounted charges.

Based on this analysis, PET scan may well have a role in selected patients with suspected recurrence after attempted curative surgery for colorectal carcinoma. A prerequisite might be the availability of radiologists with the level of expertise of the authors. Regardless, I do not feel that PET scan should be widely adopted without more convincing evidence of true cost savings, or before comparison with many of the other modalities. The authors have elected to use their expertise against a single, poorly controlled modality rather than against any or all of the other tools that are currently available and in widespread use for the identical purpose of detection of recurrent disease. To their credit, they admit to this problem in the "Comment" section, where they mention the study of Vitola et al,[28] in which PET scan was compared with helical CT scan, and the sensitivity rates were 90% vs 86%, respectively. Hopefully, more appropriately designed prospective randomized trials will better define the role of this promising new technology.

Steven D. Wexner, MD
Fort Lauderdale, Fla

1. Landis SH, Murray T, Bolden S, Wingo PA. Cancer statistics, 1998. *CA Cancer J Clin.* 1998;48:6-29.
2. Galandiuk S, Wieand HS, Moertel CG. Patterns of recurrence after curative resection of carcinoma of the colon and rectum. *Surg Gynecol Obstet.* 1992;174:27-32.
3. Marsh PJ, James RD, Schofield PF. Definition of local recurrence after surgery for rectal cancer. *Br J Surg.* 1995;82:465-468.
4. Obrand DI, Gordon PH. Incidence and patterns of recurrence following curative resection for colorectal carcinoma. *Dis Colon Rectum.* 1997;40:15-24.
5. Beynon J. An evaluation of the role of rectal endosonography in rectal cancer. *Ann R Coll Surg Engl.* 1989;71:131-139.
6. Saitoh N, Okui K, Sarashina H, Suzuki M, Arai T, Nunomura M. Evaluation of echographic diagnosis of rectal cancer using intrarectal ultrasonic examination. *Dis Colon Rectum.* 1986;29:234-242.
7. Hildebrandt U, Fiefel G, Schwartz HP, Scherr O. Endorectal ultrasound: instrumentation and clinical aspects. *Int J Colorectal Dis.* 1986;1:203-207.
8. Chandler PJ, Orkin BA. Rectal carcinoma: operative treatment. In: Beck DE, Wexner SD, eds. *Fundamentals of Anorectal Surgery*. New York, NY: McGraw-Hill Book Co; 1992:301-367.
9. Finlay IG, McArdle CS. The role of occult hepatic metastases in staging colorectal carcinoma. *Scand J Gastroenterol Suppl.* 1988;149:150-154.
10. Goel AK, Seenu V, Bal S, Shukla NK. Hepatic metastases from colorectal cancer: an overview of surgical management. *Trop Gastroenterol.* 1994;15:121-129.
11. Takeuchi N, Ramirez JM, Mortensen NJ, Cobb R, Whittlestone T. Intraoperative ultrasonography in the diagnosis of hepatic metastases during surgery for colorectal cancer. *Int J Colorectal Dis.* 1996;11:92-95.
12. Foley EF, Kolecki RV, Schirmer BD. The accuracy of laparoscopic ultrasound in the detection of colorectal cancer liver metastases. *Am J Surg.* 1998;176:262-264.
13. Lo CM, Lai EC, Liu CL, Fan ST, Wong J. Laparoscopy and laparoscopic ultrasonography avoid exploratory laparotomy in patients with hepatocellular carcinoma. *Ann Surg.* 1998;227:527-532.
14. Martin EW Jr, Mojzisik CM, Hinkle GH Jr, et al. Radioimmunoguided surgery using monoclonal antibody. *Am J Surg.* 1988;156:386-392.
15. Nieroda CA, Mojzisik C, Hinkle G, Thurston MO, Martin EW Jr. Radioimmunoguided surgery (RIGS) in recurrent colorectal cancer. *Cancer Detect Prev.* 1991;15:225-229.
16. Attiyeh FF, Wanebo HJ, Stearns MW. Hepatic resection for metastasis from colorectal cancer. *Dis Colon Rectum.* 1978;21:160-162
17. Brister SJ, de Varennes B, Gordon PH, Sheiner NM, Pym J. Contemporary operative mangement of pulmonary metastases of colorectal origin. *Dis Colon Rectum.* 1988;31:786-792.
18. Mori K, Sasagawa M, Moriyama N. Detection of nodular lesions in the lung using helical computed tomography: comparison of fast couch speed technique with conventional computed tomography. *Jpn J Clin Oncol.* 1994;24:252-257.
19. Heald RJ, Moran BJ, Ryall RD, Sexton R, MacFarlane JK. Rectal cancer: the Basingstoke experience of total mesorectal excision, 1978-1997. *Arch Surg.* 1998;133:894-899.
20. Heald RJ, Husband EM, Ryall RD. The mesorectum in rectal cancer surgery: the clue to pelvic recurrence? *Br J Surg.* 1982;69:613-616.
21. Enker WE, Havenga K, Polyak T, Thaler H, Cranor M. Abdominoperineal resection via total mesorectal excision and autonomic nerve preservation for low rectal cancer. *World J Surg.* 1997;21:715-720.
22. Arbman G, Nilsson E, Hallbook O, Sjodahl R. Local recurrence following total mesorectal excision for rectal cancer. *Br J Surg.* 1996;83:375-379.
23. Leo E, Belli F, Andreola S, et al. Total rectal resection, mesorectum excision, and coloendoanal anastomosis: a therapeutic option for the treatment of low rectal cancer. *Ann Surg Oncol.* 1996;3:336-343.
24. Bernstein MA, Amarnath B, Weiss EG, Nogueras JJ, Wexner SD. Total mesorectal excision without adjuvant therapy for local control of rectal cancer: a North American experience. *Tech Coloproctology*. 1998;2:11-15.
25. Krook JE, Moertel CG, Gunderson LL, et al. Effective surgical adjuvant therapy for high-risk rectal carcinoma. *N Engl J Med.* 1991;324:709-715.
26. Soyer P, Levesque M, Caudron C, Elias D, Zeitoun G, Roche A. MRI of liver metastases from colorectal cancer vs CT during arterial portography. *J Comput Assist Tomogr.* 1993;17:67-74.
27. Nogueras JJ. Endorectal ultrasonography: technique, image, interpretation, and expanding indications in 1995. *Semin Colon Rectal Surg.* 1995;6:70-77.
28. Vitola JV, Delbeke D, Sandler MP, et al. Positron emission tomography to stage suspected metastatic colorectal carcinoma to the liver. *Am J Surg.* 1996;171:21-26.

Senna vs Polyethylene Glycol for Mechanical Preparation the Evening Before Elective Colonic or Rectal Resection

A Multicenter Controlled Trial

Alain Valverde, MD; Jean-Marie Hay, MD; Abe Fingerhut, MD; Marie-Jeanne Boudet, MD; Roberta Petroni, MD; Xavier Pouliquen, MD; Simon Msika, MD; Yves Flamant, MD; for the French Association for Surgical Research

Hypothesis: Senna is more efficient than polyethylene glycol as mechanical preparation before elective colorectal surgery.

Design: Prospective, randomized, single-blind study.

Setting: Multicenter study (18 centers).

Patients: Five hundred twenty-three consecutive patients with colonic or rectal carcinoma or sigmoid diverticular disease, undergoing elective colonic or rectal resection followed by immediate anastomosis.

Intervention: Two hundred sixty-two patients were randomly allotted to receive senna (1 package diluted in a glass of water) and 261 to receive polyethylene glycol (2 packages diluted in 2-3 L of water), administered the evening before surgery. All patients received 5% povidone iodine antiseptic enemas (2 L) the evening and the morning before surgery. Ceftriaxone sodium and metronidazole were given intravenously at anesthetic induction.

Main Outcome Measures: Degree of colonic and rectal cleanliness.

Results: Colonic cleanliness was better ($P = .006$), fecal matter in the colonic lumen was less fluid ($P = .001$), and the risk for moderate or large intraoperative fecal soiling was lower ($P = .11$) with senna. Overall, clinical tolerance did not differ significantly between groups, but 20 patients receiving polyethylene glycol (vs 16 with senna) had to interrupt their preparation, and 15 patients (vs 8 with senna) complained of abdominal distension. Senna, however, was better tolerated ($P = .03$) in the presence of stenosis. There was no statistically significant difference found in the number of patients with postoperative infective complications (14.7% vs 17.7%) or anastomotic leakage (5.3% vs 5.7%) with senna and polyethylene glycol, respectively.

Conclusion: Mechanical preparation before colonic or rectal resection with senna is better and easier than with polyethylene glycol and should be proposed in patients undergoing colonic or rectal resection, especially patients with stenosis.

Arch Surg. 1999;134:514-519

Several controlled studies have shown beyond any doubt that abdominal infective complications after colonic and rectal surgery were decreased by systemic antibiotic prophylaxis.[1] Antiseptic enemas such as povidone iodine also have been shown to be bacteriologically[2] and clinically[3,4] efficient. Mechanical preparation plays a role as well, ensuring adequate colonic and rectal cleanliness.[5,6] Although it has never been shown that endoluminal cleanliness decreased the rate of postoperative complications,[7-12] most authors agree that mechanical cleansing is preferable before performing colonic resection,[7] and it is used by 30% to 51% of North American colorectal surgeons.[13-15] Several mechanical cleansing preparations are available, and these can be divided into volume-induced agents, such as mannitol or polyethylene glycol, and secretory and stimulant agents (laxatives), such as sodium phosphate or senna, sometimes used in association with various types of enemas (tap water, saline solution, or povidone iodine).[3,4,16] Polyethylene glycol is used by many endoscopists because the fluid contents can easily be aspirated.[17] Controlled studies in elective colorectal surgery have shown that cleanliness was better with polyethylene glycol than with water enema alone[17] and better with senna compared with mannitol.[16] However, to our knowledge, there are no prospective, controlled studies comparing polyethylene glycol with senna, particularly the evening before surgery. We therefore

From the Departments of Surgery, Hôpital Louis Mourier, Colombes (Drs Valverde, Hay, Boudet, Msika, and Flamant), Centre Hospitalier Intercommunal, Poissy (Dr Fingerhut), Hôpital Tenon, Paris (Dr Petroni), and Hôpital Victor Dupouy, Argenteuil (Dr Pouliquen), France. A complete listing of participants from the French Association for Surgical Research appears on page 516.

PATIENTS, MATERIALS, AND METHODS

PATIENTS AND DISEASE

From February 1, 1992, to October 1, 1996 (56 months), 548 consecutive patients (279 men and 269 women; mean age, 64 ± 12 years; age range, 32-93 years) were eligible for this prospective trial. Although all 18 centers (2 university hospitals, 14 teaching hospitals, and 2 private clinics) participating in this study did not start at the same time, they all finished on October 1, 1996, which explains that a median of 27 patients (range, 11-82) were entered per center and that a median of 19 (range, 11-46) patients were entered per year and per center. Twenty-five surgeons performed or supervised all operations.

All patients undergoing elective surgery for carcinoma of the colon or the proximal or middle rectum or for sigmoid diverticular disease were eligible for this study. All patients underwent resection, with palliative or curative intent in the case of carcinoma, followed by immediate anastomosis.

Ileocolonic, colocolonic, colorectal or ileorectal, or coloanal anastomoses were performed, sometimes protected by a diverting stoma, and sometimes covered by omentoplasty. The degree of stenosis was quantified by the surgeon clinically, after opening the resected intestinal specimen, as narrowing of the lumen of less than one third, one third to two thirds, and more than two thirds of normal caliber, and endoscopically as narrowing of the lumen precluding the passage of an adult-size colonoscope. The degree of stenosis was not a reason for noninclusion, any more than the presence of organ (heart, pulmonary, kidney, hepatic, or other) compromise. Patients with specific or ulcerative colitis, benign tumor, or familial polyposis without carcinoma; patients who did not undergo resection or immediate anastomosis (eg, the Hartmann procedure or abdominoperineal resection); and patients who underwent emergency resection (for obstruction or peritonitis), reversal of the Hartmann procedure, or simple closure of colostomy were not considered for the study.

TECHNIQUE OF PREPARATION

Patients received senna solution (X Prep Sarget) (one 120-mg package of flavored powder diluted in a glass of water or 2 packages for obese patients) or polyethylene glycol (ColoPeg Nicholas SA) (two 59-g packages of flavored powder diluted in 2-3 L of water) on the evening before surgery. All patients received 2 L of 5% povidone iodine enema on the evening before and on the morning before (at least 2 hours) surgery.[4] Single-dose ceftriaxone sodium (1 g) and metronidazole (1 g), diluted in 125 mg saline solution infused for 15 minutes, were administered to all patients intravenously at anesthetic induction.[4] Patients with previously recognized allergy to 1 of these or related drugs were not included.

OUTCOME MEASURES

The main outcome measure was the degree of colonic and rectal cleanliness as judged by the operating surgeon in the upstream and downstream intestinal segments and defined according to Hollender et al[18] as follows: 0 indicates no fecal matter; plus sign, small amounts of fecal matter, not bothersome to the surgeon; and 2 plus signs, fecal matter bothersome to the surgeon. A 0 and/or a plus sign in the upstream and/or downstream segments were considered to be satisfactory cleanliness. The quantity and consistency of fecal matter were assessed in the proximal and distal segments through the opening made in the intestine for manual anastomosis, to introduce the mechanical stapling devices for side-to-end or end-to-end anastomoses, or after confection of the purse string in circular mechanical anastomoses. In the double-stapling technique, the endoluminal contents were assessed when the anvil was inserted through the anus. The surgeon was unaware of the type of colonic preparation administered. Secondary outcome measures included (1) consistency of fecal matter defined as solid, soft, or fluid; (2) the rate and magnitude of intraoperative fecal soiling, defined as nil, minimal, moderate, or large; (3) tolerance of the preparation as attested by the absence of abdominal pain, distension, malaise, vomiting, need to discontinue the preparation, or other complications; and (4) the rate of abdominal infective complications (including wound abscess or disruption, local deep abscess or generalized peritonitis, blood-borne infection, clinical or radiological anastomotic leakage [all patients received a routine diatrizoate sodium enema between days 8 and 10]), repeated operations, or death occurring during the hospital stay or the 30 days following hospital discharge.[19] All patients who died in the hospital underwent an autopsy.

RANDOM ALLOTMENT

Patients were divided into 2 strata, ie, those with carcinoma and those with sigmoid diverticular disease. At the latest on the evening before surgery, patients were randomly allotted to their colonic preparation by unfolding the previously stapled upper corner of a questionnaire in preference to the envelope method,[20] under which "senna" or "polyethylene glycol," determined by random number tables, was hidden. Random assignment was balanced every 6 patients by center and by stratum.

NUMBER OF PATIENTS

Based on the 14% difference between the previous 66% rate for colonic cleanliness after senna preparation[16] and the previous mean 80% rate after polyethylene glycol preparation,[21,22] the number of patients required was calculated to be 226 per group, ie, 452 patients in all, with an α and β risk equal to .05, in a 2-tailed test.[23]

STATISTICAL METHODS

Preoperative and postoperative patient demographics and secondary outcome measures were compared within both groups using the χ^2 test for categorical values and the Student t test for continuous variables. This study was approved by the ethical committee of the coordinating center. The center effect was analyzed.

Participants From the French Association for Surgical Research

Eaubonne: Patrice Baillet, MD. *Aulnay-sous-Bois:* André Elhadad, MD, Didier Brassier, MD, Elias Habib, MD. *Thonon les Bains:* Christian Dilin, MD. *Poissy:* Abe Fingerhut, MD, FRCS. *Dinan:* Jacques Francin, MD. *Romorantin:* Henri Hennet, MD. *Créteil:* Michel Julien, MD, Pierre-Louis Fagniez, MD, Nelly Rotman, MD, Marie-Jeanne Boudet, MD. *Chatellerault:* Marc Kalfon, MD. *Corbeil:* Gérard Kohlmann, MD. *Pau:* Yves Laborde, MD. *Paris:* Hughes Levard, MD. *Meulan:* Simon Msika, MD. *Besançon:* Edouard Pelissier, MD. *Senlis:* Patrick Peyramaure, MD. *Vernon:* Claude Rey, MD. *Nice:* Jean-Louis Sicard, MD. *Montmorency:* Yves Soulier, MD. *Colombes:* Jean-Marie Hay, MD, Yves Flamant, MD, Guy Zeitoun, MD.

Table 1. Patient Demographics*

	Group	
	Senna (n = 262)	Polyethylene Glycol (n = 261)
Sex ratio, M:F	134:128	132:129
Age, y		
Mean ± 1 SD	68 ± 13	68 ± 12
Range	32-82	33-93
Disease		
Carcinoma	202	199
Diverticular disease	60	62
Factors affecting healing		
Obesity >15% theoretical weight	85	76
Weight loss >15% usual weight	78	88
Corticosteroid, chemotherapy, or radiation therapy	17	10
Risk factors		
Cirrhosis	12	7
Carcinomatosis	5	5
Ascites	1	1
Respiratory failure	24	18
Heart disorders	27	27
Site of anastomosis		
Ileocolic	53	62
Colocolic	34	31
Proximal colorectal	123	114
Distal colorectal	45	44
Ileorectal	7	10

Unless otherwise indicated, data are given as number of patients.

Table 2. Degree of Cleanliness of Intestinal Segments*

	Group, No. (%) of Patients	
	Senna (n = 262)	Polyethylene Glycol (n = 261)
Quantity of matter upstream†		
0	131 (50.0)	106 (40.6)
+	107 (40.8)	99 (37.9)
++	23 (8.8)	52 (19.9)
Unknown‡	1 (0.4)	4 (1.5)
Quantity of matter downstream		
0	117 (44.6)	115 (44.1)
+	114 (43.5)	112 (42.9)
++	25 (9.5)	29 (11.1)
Unknown	6 (2.3)	5 (1.9)
Upstream/downstream cleanliness§		
0/0, 0/+, +/0	182 (69.5)	150 (57.5)
+/+, +/++, ++/+, ++/++	73 (27.9)	101 (38.7)
Unknown‡	7 (2.7)	10 (3.8)

Indicates quantity of fecal matter according to Hollender et al,[18] ie, 0 indicates no fecal matter; plus sign, small amounts of fecal matter, not bothersome to the surgeon; and double plus sign, fecal matter bothersome to the surgeon. Percentages have been rounded and may not sum 100.

†$P = .04$.

‡*Because of clamp.*

§$P = .006$.

undertook this prospective, randomized multicenter study to compare both types of mechanical colonic preparations as regards colonic cleanliness in elective colonic or rectal resection.

RESULTS

Twenty-five patients were withdrawn from the study after random allotment (12 in the senna group and 13 in the polyethylene glycol group) because of benign tumor (n = 7), absence of resection or anastomosis (n = 11), or a random allotment error (n = 7). Five hundred twenty-three patients remained for final analysis.

Both groups of patients were comparable as regards sex, age, disease, factors affecting healing, and risk factors (**Table 1**).

Senna was significantly more efficient in providing intestinal cleanliness in the upstream ($P = .04$) and in both intestinal segments taken together ($P = .006$) (**Table 2**). Conversely, the difference in the downstream segment was not statistically significant (Table 2).

Senna significantly decreased the rate of fluid matter in the upstream and downstream ($P = .001$) or both intestinal segments ($P = .001$), whereas there was no statistically significant difference found in the rate of fecal soiling between groups (**Table 3**). When spillage did occur, however, soiling was more often nil or minimal with senna than moderate or large ($P = .11$) (Table 3).

Overall clinical tolerance was similar between groups, but fewer patients receiving senna had to discontinue their preparation or complained of abdominal distension (16 and 8 vs 20 and 15 with polyethylene glycol, respectively) (**Table 4**). Neither difference, however, was statistically significant.

Stenosis was found in 59.7% of our patients. Comparing the patients with or without stenosis (**Table 5**), stenosis was significantly associated with less cleanliness ($P = .001$), smaller soiling ($P = .001$), and poorer tolerance ($P = .06$) compared with patients without stenosis. The results in favor of senna were similar, irrespective of the presence or absence of stenosis (Tables 2 and 3). Compared with polyethylene glycol, however, senna was tolerated significantly better ($P = .03$) in the presence of stenosis.

There was no significant difference found between senna compared with polyethylene glycol as regards the rate of each postoperative infective complication, anastomotic leakages, repeated operations, or deaths, as well as the rate of patients with at least 1 infective complication (**Table 6**).

No center effect was found concerning patient demographics or results.

COMMENT

Senna preparation was significantly associated with more effective intestinal cleanliness (Table 2), and, when fecal matter persisted, it was less fluid (Table 3), decreasing the risk for moderate or large soiling when intraoperative spillage occurred (Table 3). The tolerance and the rate of postoperative complications did not differ significantly between groups (Tables 4 and 6). However, senna was better tolerated in case of stenosis.

The 69.5% satisfactory cleanliness rate that we found for senna (Table 2) was comparable with results (66%) of a previous study.[16]

The cleanliness provided using polyethylene glycol has been reported to be subjectively good, very good, or excellent in 72%,[22] 90%,[21] and 100%[24] of patients, rates that were higher than those found in our study. Our 57.8% upstream-downstream cleanliness rate with polyethylene glycol, however, was close to the 61% (33/54) cleanliness rate found by Wolters et al.[12] Possible explanations for these

Table 3. Fecal Matter Consistency

	Group, No. (%) of Patients	
	Senna (n = 262)	Polyethylene Glycol (n = 261)
Upstream fecal matter		
None	131 (50.0)	96 (36.8)
Solid	11 (4.2)	4 (1.5)
Soft	47 (17.9)	32 (12.3)
Fluid*	72 (27.5)	125 (47.9)
Unknown†	1 (0.4)	4 (1.5)
Downstream fecal matter*		
None	117 (44.6)	105 (40.2)
Solid	6 (2.3)	2 (0.8)
Soft	42 (16.0)	18 (6.9)
Fluid	91 (34.7)	121 (46.4)
Unknown†	6 (2.3)	15 (5.7)
Fluid in both segments, irrespective of the quantity of fecal matter*	67 (25.6)	105 (40.2)
Intraoperative soiling*		
Nil	212 (80.9)	216 (82.8)
Minimal	27 (10.3)	11 (4.2)
Moderate to large	23 (8.8)	34 (13.0)

*$P = .001$.
†*Because of clamp.*

Table 4. Tolerance

	Group, No. (%) of Patients	
	Senna (n = 262)	Polyethylene Glycol (n = 261)
Complete tolerance	206 (78.6)	207 (79.3)
Discomfort*	55 (21.0)	55 (21.1)
Vomiting	12 (4.6)	7 (2.7)
Abdominal pain	35 (13.4)	30 (11.5)
Distension	8 (3.0)	15 (5.7)
Malaise	23 (8.8)	15 (5.7)
Miscellaneous	6 (2.3)	7 (2.7)
Need to discontinue colonic preparation	16 (6.1)	20 (7.7)
Stenosis		
No stenosis	106 (40.4)	105 (40.2)
Stenosis, diameter	156 (59.5)	156 (59.8)
Less than one third of normal	42 (26.9)	33 (21.2)
One third to two thirds of normal	61 (39.1)	57 (36.5)
More than two thirds of normal	53 (34.0)	66 (42.3)
Colonoscopy		
Not performed	51 (19.5)	50 (19.2)
Performed	211 (80.5)	211 (80.8)
Stenosis impossible to pass through	70 (26.7)	75 (28.7)

**Some patients had more than 1 symptom.*

Table 5. Cleanliness, Fecal Matter Consistency, Intraoperative Soiling, and Discomfort According to Presence of Stenosis

	Patient Groups					
	Stenosis (n = 312)			No Stenosis (n = 211)		
	Senna, No. (n = 156)	Polyethylene Glycol, No. (n = 156)	Total No. (%)	Senna, No. (n = 106)	Polyethylene Glycol, No. (n = 105)	Total No. (%)
Cleanliness of 0/0, 0/+, or +/0	99*	73*	**172** (55.1)†	83‡	77†	**160** (75.8)†
Fluid in both segments	40§	62§	**102** (32.7)	27‖	43‖	**70** (33.2)
Moderate to large soiling	7	17	**24** (7.7)‖	16	17	**33** (15.6)‖
Discomfort	29§	45§	**74** (23.7)¶	26¶	10¶	**36** (17.1)¶

*$P < .003$.
†$P < .001$.
‡$P < .40$.
§$P = .03$.
‖$P = .004$.
¶$P = .06$.

Table 6. Postoperative Course

	Group, No. (%) of Patients	
	Senna (n = 262)	Polyethylene Glycol (n = 261)
Complications		
Wound abscess	4 (1.5)	16 (6.1)
Wound disruption	7 (2.7)	5 (1.9)
Deep abscess	6 (2.3)	5 (1.9)
Generalized peritonitis	4 (1.5)	5 (1.9)
Blood-borne infection	7 (2.7)	13 (5.0)
Anastomotic leakage	14 (5.3)	15 (5.7)
Clinical	7 (2.7)	6 (2.3)
Radiological alone	7 (2.7)	9 (3.4)
Patients with ≥1 complication	38 (14.5)	46 (17.6)
Repeated operation	22 (8.4)	13 (5.0)
Deaths		
Overall	6 (2.3)	8 (3.1)
With leakage	0	1 (0.4)

discrepancies include use of the semiquantitative grading system of Hollender et al[18] in our study (Table 3), less subjective than that used by others,[12,22,24] and the high rate of stenosis (59.5%) (Table 4) observed in our series, which significantly ($P = .001$) limited intestinal cleanliness (55.1% [172/312] in patients with stenosis vs 75.8% in patients without stenosis) (Table 5). Only 1 study[25] on polyethylene glycol reported a cleanliness rate of 58% with stenosis vs 68% without stenosis, especially in the left compared with the right colon, where feces are more fluid. In other reports,[21,22,24] the rate and degree of stenosis were not evaluated. Moreover, stenosis is probably seen more often in the surgical population than in the overall colonoscopic population.[21,22] The quantity of fluid retained in the upstream segment after preparation was directly proportional to the amount of cleansing fluid administered,[12] and, notably in the case of stenosis, explained why upstream fluid endoluminal contents after 1 glass of senna were significantly ($P = .001$) (Table 2) less than after 2 to 3 L of polyethylene glycol. Conversely, cleanliness in the downstream segment, similar in both groups, was undoubtedly due to the amounts (2 L) and efficacy of associated enemas. The 100% cleanliness rate observed by Beck et al[24] was obtained with polyethylene glycol administered until clean effluent was evacuated, followed by a bisacodyl capsule in a small group of 30 patients without significant stenosis. In the same study,[24] senna was administered 48 hours before surgery, whereas it has been shown that the maximal action of senna takes place 6 to 12 hours after administration.[26] Sodium phosphate also is more efficient when administered twice, with the latter dose given the morning before surgery.[27]

A further advantage of senna is that when the residual fecal contents of the colon are less fluid (Tables 3 and 5), the risk for spillage into the operative field is lower,[7] potentially reducing the threat of anastomotic leakage.[11] This is why, in agreement with several authors,[5,7,28] we believe that endoluminal fluid contents should be avoided in surgery. This contrasts with the expectations of colonoscopists who, conversely, easily can aspirate fluid contents as opposed to solid or soft contents.[17]

As in other types of mechanical preparations, clinical tolerance depends on the agent itself, as well as on the quantity of fluid administered and the use of associated preparations (enemas) or medications (metoclopramide hydrochloride).[24] In our series, tolerance of polyethylene glycol was comparable with that reported in the literature for traditional 3-day preparations, including enemas,[17] mannitol preparations,[18,29,30] and polyethylene glycol when used alone.[21,22,24] Our overall rate of patient discomfort (21.0%) (Table 4) was very close to those found in the literature, ie, 20.7%,[14] 24%,[22] and 25%.[24] Our rate of vomiting was the same as that found by Solla and Rothenberger[14] (2.7%), but lower than those found by others, ie, 6%,[21] 10%,[24] and 11%.[22] In contrast, Wolters et al[12] reported no vomiting. The nausea rate in their series, however, was high, 33% of 54 patients, but the quantity of fluid administered was often abundant (1.3-7 L) until clean fluid was evacuated. In conclusion, satisfactory tolerance of polyethylene glycol seems to depend on the relatively moderate quantity of the fluid ingested in our study (2-3 L).

In the literature, senna tolerance has been judged to be excellent because there were no major complaints recorded.[3,4] Our study shows that clinical tolerance of senna and polyethylene glycol was similar (Table 4). However, in other randomized studies,[31,32] sodium phosphate has been shown to be significantly better tolerated than polyethylene glycol for colonoscopy preparation. In our study, it is difficult to ascertain and to evaluate the tolerance of senna or polyethylene glycol alone, because the few, minor discomforts observed may in fact be observed or enhanced due to associated povidone iodine enemas.[3,4] Enemas were used not only for their mechanical action,[13-15] but also for their local antiseptic properties.[2-4] In our series, senna was tolerated better than polyethylene glycol, especially in the presence of stenosis (Table 5), which confirms that the quantity of fluid ingested plays a role in tolerance. Last, when studying tolerance, one must take into account the number of patients for whom it is necessary to discontinue the preparation. This occurred in 6.9% of patients in our series (Table 4), with no significant difference between senna and polyethylene glycol, comparing favorably with the 0% to 25% of cases in the survey conducted by Beck and Fazio,[13] but the exact number of patients receiving laxatives or polyethylene glycol (43% of the overall population) was not known. On the other hand, 27% of patients receiving polyethylene glycol for colonoscopy[33] and 63% of patients undergoing resection[34] had to discontinue their colonic preparation, but this was with 4 L of fluids.

We did not study the cost-effectiveness of both preparations. Compared with oral sodium phosphate,[32] senna is easy to administer and relatively less expensive and may be used as an outpatient bowel preparation,[21,35] thus reducing costs and preoperative hospital stay.

In our study, there was no significant difference found between groups of patients as concerns the rate of postoperative infective complications (Table 6). To the best of our knowledge, no clinical study to date has shown that mechanical preparation alone, excepting povidone enemas,[3,4] can reduce postoperative abdominal infective complications. Oral mechanical preparation in itself did not decrease the bacterial load or their type.[10,11]

Cleanliness of the intestines and the consistency of residual fecal matter are important factors to consider, especially in laparoscopic colonic resection, because of the difficulty in ensuring adequate clamping of the colonic segments in this technique.

As with 90 mL of sodium phosphate,[34] senna can be considered the standard for elective colonic or rectal resection. Further progress can be expected when senna vs sodium phosphate, various combinations of oral and systemic antibiotics, and other antiseptic enemas (povidone vs hypochlorite)[36] are compared.

Reprints: Jean-Marie Hay, MD, Associations de Recherche en Chirurgie, 8 Avenue des Peupliers 92270 Bois-Colombes, France.

REFERENCES

1. Baum ML, Anish DS, Chalmers TC, Sacks HS, Smith H, Fagerstrom RM. A survey of clinical trials on antibiotic prophylaxis in colon surgery: evidence against further use of no-treatment controls. *N Engl J Med.* 1981;305:795-799.
2. Hay JM, Boussougant Y, Roverselli D, et al. Povidone-iodine enema as a preoperative bowel preparation for colorectal surgery: a bacteriologic study. *Dis Colon Rectum.* 1989;32:9-13.
3. French Association for Surgical Research, Rodary M, Fingerhut A, Hay JM. Povidone-iodine enema and one-day antibiotic prophylaxis: a continuous search for the ideal bowel preparation for elective colonic surgery: a multicenter controlled trial. *Coloproctology.* 1991;13:5-12.
4. Fingerhut A, Hay JM, the French Association for Surgical Research. Single-dose ceftriaxone, ornidazole, and povidone-iodine enema in elective left colectomy: a randomized multicenter controlled trial. *Arch Surg.* 1993;128:228-232.
5. Irvin TT, Goligher JC. Aetiology of disruption of intestinal anastomoses. *Br J Surg.* 1973;60:461-464.
6. Hares MM, Alexander-Williams J. The effect of bowel preparation on colonic surgery. *World J Surg.* 1982;6:175-181.
7. Irving AD, Scrimgeour D. Mechanical bowel preparation for colonic resection and anastomosis. *Br J Surg.* 1987;74:580-581.
8. Duthie GS, Foster ME, Price-Thomas JM, Leaper DJ. Bowel preparation or not for elective colorectal surgery. *J R Coll Surg Edinb.* 1990;35:169-171.
9. Mansvelt B, Arrigo E, Passelecq E, Gavelli A, Harb J, Huguet C. Préparation intestinale a minima avant colectomie pour cancer: expérience de 189 cas. *Ann Chir.* 1992;46:592-595.
10. Burke P, Mealy K, Gillien P, Joyce W, Traynor O, Hyland J. Requirements for bowel preparation in colorectal surgery. *Br J Surg.* 1994;81:907-910.
11. Santos JCM, Batista J, Sirimarco MT, Guimaraes AS, Levy CF. Prospective randomized trial of mechanical bowel preparation in patients undergoing elective colorectal surgery. *Br J Surg.* 1994;81:1673-1676.
12. Wolters U, Keller HW, Sorgatz S, Raab A, Pichlmaier H. Prospective randomized study of preoperative bowel cleansing for patients undergoing colorectal surgery. *Br J Surg.* 1994;81:598-600.
13. Beck DE, Fazio VW. Current preoperative bowel cleansing methods: results of a survey. *Dis Colon Rectum.* 1990;33:12-20.
14. Solla JA, Rothenberger DA. Preoperative bowel preparation: a survey of colon and rectal surgery. *Dis Colon Rectum.* 1990;33:154-159.
15. Nichols RL, Smith JN, Garcia RY, Waterman RS, Holmes JW. Current practices of preoperative bowel preparation among North American colorectal surgeons. *Clin Infect Dis.* 1997;24:609-619.
16. French Association for Surgical Research, Rodary M, Fingerhut A, Hay JM. Mechanical and antibiotic preparation of the bowel for elective colorectal surgery: three-day versus one-day preparation: a multicenter controlled trial. *Coloproctology.* 1988;10:271-276.
17. Fleites RA, Marshall JB, Eckhauser ML, Mansour EG, Imbembo AL, McCullough AJ. The efficacy of polyethylene glycol electrolyte lavage solution versus traditional mechanical bowel preparation for elective colonic surgery: a randomized, prospective, blinded clinical trial. *Surgery.* 1985;98:708-716.
18. Hollender LF, Calderoli H, Philippides J, Jamart J. Advantages of whole gut irrigation in colorectal surgery. *Curr Probl Surg.* 1980;37:227-233.
19. Evans MC, Pollock AV. Trials on trial: a review of trials of antibiotic prophylaxis. *Arch Surg.* 1984;119:109-113.
20. Cancer Research Campaign Working Party. Trials and tribulations: thoughts on the organization of multicentre clinical studies. *BMJ.* 1980;281:918-920.
21. Lirzin P, Salas H, Dahlab MR. Préparation colique par Fortrans prise unique ou deux prises fractionnées. *Acta Endosc.* 1989;5:373-376.
22. Di Palma JA, Marshall JB. Comparison of a new sulfate-free polyethylene glycol electrolyte lavage solution versus a standard solution for colonoscopy cleansing. *Gastrointest Endosc.* 1990;3:285-289.
23. Schwartz D, Flamant R, Lellouch J. *Clinical Trials.* Orlando, Fla: Academic Press Inc; 1980.
24. Beck DE, Harford FJ, Di Palma JA. Comparison of cleansing methods in preparation for colonic surgery. *Dis Colon Rectum.* 1985;7:491-495.
25. Sakanoue Y, Kusuniki M, Shosi Y, Yamamura T, Utsynomiya J. The efficacy of whole gut irrigation with polyethylene glycol electrolyte solution in elective colorectal surgery for cancer. *Acta Chir Scand.* 1990;156:463-466.
26. Frexinos J, Staumont G, Fioramonti J, Bueno L. Effects of sennosides on colonic myoelectrical activity in man. *Dig Dis Sci.* 1989;34:214-219.
27. Frommer D. Cleansing ability and tolerance of three bowel preparations for colonoscopy. *Dis Colon Rectum.* 1995;40:101-104.
28. Dorudi S, Wilson NM, Heddle RM. Primary restorative colectomy in malignant left-sided large bowel obstruction. *Ann R Coll Surg Engl.* 1990;72:393-395.
29. French Association for Surgical Research, Rodary M, Hay JM, Fingerhut A, Oberlin P. Conventional mechanical preparation versus whole-gut irrigation for elective colonic resections: a multicentric prospective controlled trial. *Coloproctology.* 1986;2:87-93.
30. Crapp AR, Tillotson P, Powis SJA, Cooke WT, Alexander WJ. Preparation of the bowel by whole-gut irrigation. *Lancet.* 1975;20:1239-1240.
31. Henderson JM, Barnet JL, Turgeon DK, et al. Single-day, divided dose oral sodium phosphate laxative versus intestinal lavage as preparation for colonoscopy: efficacy and patient tolerance. *Gastrointest Endosc.* 1995;42:238-243.
32. Golub RW, Kerner BA, Wise WE Jr, et al. Colonoscopic bowel preparations: which one? a blinded, prospective, randomized trial. *Dis Colon Rectum.* 1995;38:594-599.
33. Saunders BP, Masaki T, Fukumot M, Halligan S, Williams CB. The quest for a more acceptable bowel preparation: comparison of a polyethylene glycol–electrolyte solution and a mannitol–Micolax mixture for colonoscopy. *Postgrad Med J.* 1995;71:476-479.
34. Oliveira L, Wexner SD, Daniel N, et al. Mechanical bowel preparation for elective colorectal surgery: a prospective randomized surgeon blinded trial comparing sodium phosphate and polyethylene glycol based oral lavage solutions. *Dis Colon Rectum.* 1997;40:585-591.
35. Frazee RC, Roberts J, Symmonds R, Snyder S, Hendriche J, Smith R. Prospective, randomized trial of inpatients vs outpatients bowel preparation for elective colorectal surgery. *Dis Colon Rectum.* 1992;35:223-226.
36. Scammel BE, Phillips RP, Brown R, Burdon DW, Keighley MRB. Influence of rectal washout on bacterial counts in the rectal stump. *Br J Surg.* 1985;72:548-550.

Surgical Anatomy

The boundaries of the **gastrinoma triangle** are:
(1) third portion of the duodenum,
(2) porta hepatis, and
(3) neck of the pancreas.

ORIGINAL ARTICLE

Acceleration of Wound Healing With Topically Applied Deoxyribonucleosides

E. Alexandria Chen, MD; Lily Zhao, MD; Michael Bamat, PhD; Reid von Borstel, PhD; Thomas Mustoe, MD

Hypothesis: We hypothesized that a topical mixture of purified deoxyribonucleosides would accelerate wound healing in an open wound model.

Design: Full-thickness 6-mm wounds were made on the ears of young adult rabbits. In some experiments, 2 of the 3 arteries in each ear were divided to induce wound ischemia.

Interventions: An equiweight mixture containing all 4 of the major deoxyribonucleosides (deoxyadenosine, deoxycytidine, deoxyguanosine, and thymidine), designated PN105, or other subgroups of deoxyribonucleosides, or vehicle (saline) was applied to wounds on 1 ear every 2 days, with the other ear serving as a control.

Main Outcome Measures: Wound tissue was processed for histological examination 7 days after the initial wounding. Granulation tissue formation and epithelialization were measured in histological cross sections of wounds.

Results: Treatment of wounds with PN105 resulted in a 191% increase in total new granulation tissue ($P<.05$) and a higher incidence of complete wound reepithelialization (67% vs 37%; $P<.05$) when compared with controls, and a similar increase under ischemic conditions on day 7. Wound ischemia markedly impairs healing; PN105 treatment resulted in a 242% increase in the amount of new granulation tissue formed by day 7 in ischemic wounds, relative to the appropriate controls ($P<.05$). All 4 of the major deoxyribonucleosides were required for optimum activity; mixtures with 3 or 2 were less active or inactive.

Conclusions: Topically applied deoxyribonucleosides reproducibly accelerate wound healing in normal and ischemic wounds, and to a magnitude equivalent to that of recombinant growth factors such as platelet-derived growth factor, previously studied in this model. In view of their safety, availability, and efficacy, deoxyribonucleosides hold considerable promise for improving healing of chronic wounds.

Arch Surg. 1999;134:520-525

From the Division of Plastic Surgery, Northwestern Medical School, Chicago, Ill (Drs Chen, Zhao, and Mustoe); and Pro-Neuron Inc, Gaithersburg, Md (Drs Bamat and von Borstel). Drs Bamat and von Borstel are employees of Pro-Neuron Inc. Pro-Neuron Inc owns the rights to and supplied the PN105 wound healing agent for the studies reported in this article.

WOUND exudate adhering to surgical dressings provided the material in which DNA was first reported by Miescher in 1871.[1] Dumont[2] proposed that extracellular DNA in wound exudate might contribute to the initiation of fibroplasia in wounds, and provided evidence that topically applied DNA (isolated either from rabbit peritoneal inflammatory exudate or from calf thymus) stimulated the formation of granulation tissue in full-thickness excision wounds in rabbits. Independently, Marshak and Walker[3] and Nicolau and Badaniou[4] also reported that topical DNA preparations accelerated the development of granulation tissue in full-thickness wounds in rats.

It is implausible that exogenous DNA, especially from a different species, could affect wound healing via uptake into cells followed by gene expression. It is more likely that DNA or its degradation products affect wound healing either indirectly by eliciting production and release of growth factors (analogous to induction of interferons in mammalian cells by exogenous double-stranded RNA) or by entering into cellular metabolism and thereby affecting cell proliferation.[5,6] We report herein that particular mixtures of purified deoxyribonucleosides significantly accelerate both granulation and epithelialization in the rabbit ear dermal ulcer model of wound healing. An equiweight mixture of the 4 major deoxyribonucleosides (deoxyadenosine, deoxycytidine, deoxyguanosine, and thymidine), designated PN105, was found to be effective in both ischemic healing-impaired ulcers and in nonischemic dermal ulcers. In contrast to the activity of deoxyribonucleosides, mixtures of ribonucleosides were relatively ineffective. The mechanism through which exogenous deoxyribo-

MATERIALS AND METHODS

The rabbit ear dermal ulcer model developed by Ahn and Mustoe[7] and Mustoe and colleagues[8] was used for evaluation of wound healing activity of test compounds. This quantitative wound healing model has been validated and extensively used for testing the relative and absolute activities of a variety of putative wound healing factors.[9-14] Young adult female New Zealand white rabbits (Hazelton-Dutchland, Inc, Denver, Pa), weighing 2.7 to 3.4 kg were acclimated and housed under standard conditions, per experimental protocol approved by the Northwestern University Animal Care and Use Committee (Chicago, Ill).

Surgery was performed under sterile conditions after rabbits were anesthetized with ketamine hydrochloride, 60 mg/kg (Sigma-Aldrich Corp, St Louis, Mo) and xylazine hydrochloride, 5 mg/kg (Sigma-Aldrich Corp). Three or 4 full-thickness (to bare cartilage) excisional wounds were made on the interior surface of each ear with a 6-mm tissue punch. Immediately after surgery (day 0), and at days 2 and 4, mixtures of nucleosides (each nucleoside at 10 mg/mL) in physiological saline (Pro-Neuron Inc, Gaithersburg, Md) or vehicle (sterile saline) were applied to wounds in a volume of 10 μL. Wounds were then covered with an occlusive dressing (Tegaderm; 3M Corp, Minneapolis, Minn). In some experiments, persistent ischemia was produced in rabbit ears before creation of the circular excision wounds by dividing the central and rostral arteries and dermal circulation.[1] On day 7 after wounding, the animals were killed and the wounds were fixed in 10% formalin. Histological cross sections of wounds, stained with hematoxylin-eosin, were used for quantitative evaluation of wound healing by an observer blinded to treatment. Values for total new granulation tissue and new wound epithelium at 7 days were derived from measurements of (1) depth or height of new granulation tissue (P), (2) lateral distance from the wound margin covered by new granulation tissue (G), (3) distance between peaks of new granulation tissue (P-P), and (4) epithelial gap (EG). These variables were used to calculate the total new tissue volume (TNTV) by means of the following formula: $TNTV = \frac{1}{4}\pi \times SP \times TNG^2$, wherein SP represents superficial peaks ($[P_1 + P_2]/2$) and TNG is total new granulation tissue distance ($G_1 + G_2$). An alternative method of determining volume by a reticle method with a superimposed grid was also used for improved accuracy. **Figure 1** shows these methods schematically. Values reported are means ± SEs.

The primary end point was total new tissue produced during the process of healing, expressed as TNTV or as the 2-dimensional area of new granulation tissue and epithelium in cross-sectional histological slides. An additional end point in some studies was the fraction of wounds completely reepithelialized at the time of tissue collection. In any given rabbit, only 1 pair of treatments was evaluated. Statistical analysis was performed with the Student *t* test for epithelial gap, granulation tissue gap, and peak of granulation tissue. The Fisher exact test was used for comparison of the incidences of complete epithelialization between groups, and 1-way analysis of variance was used for comparison of dose-response characteristics among rabbits.

nucleosides accelerate wound healing may be related to regulatory roles of deoxyribonucleotide pools in cell proliferation and programmed cell death.

RESULTS

EFFECTS OF PN105 ON WOUND HEALING IN THE NORMAL RABBIT EAR ULCER MODEL

Complete epithelial closure (epithelial gap, 0 μm) was documented in 12 (67%) of the 18 PN105-treated wounds compared with only 7 (37%) of the 19 control wounds. The mean TNTV on day 7 was nearly 2-fold (191%) greater in the PN105-treated group than in controls (10.52 ± 1.55 mm^3 vs 5.52 ± 1.26 mm^3; $P<.01$) (**Figure 2**, A and B). A single treatment of wounds at the time of surgery did not significantly affect wound healing; multiple treatments (eg, every 2 days for 3 doses) were required for efficacy (**Figure 3**).

EFFECTS OF PN105 ON WOUND HEALING IN ISCHEMIC DERMAL ULCERS

Twenty-one ischemic control and 21 ischemic PN105-treated wounds were evaluated in 7 rabbits. The TNTV was significantly greater in the PN105-treated ischemic wounds than in vehicle-treated controls (2.66 ± 0.31 mm^3 vs 1.05 ± 0.21 mm^3; $P<.001$; 253% increase in TNTV).

WOUND HEALING EFFECTS OF DIFFERENT MIXTURES OF DEOXYRIBONUCLEOSIDES IN THE RABBIT EAR ULCER MODEL

Earlier experimental work in rats indicated that the individual deoxyribonucleosides (deoxyadenosine [dA], deoxycytidine [dC], deoxyguanosine [dG], and thymidine [dT]) applied singly to full-thickness dermal excision wounds had no effect on wound healing.[15] The key mixtures of 2 and 3 deoxyribonucleosides were tested and compared against the mixture of all 4 in the rabbit ear ulcer model. In the first study, the effects of PN105 were compared with those of dC + dG, dC + dG + dA, and dC + dG + dT. Each individual rabbit received treatment with PN105 (as a positive control) on 1 ear and 1 other mixture of deoxyribonucleosides on the other ear, to minimize effects of individual variation between animals (Figure 2, B and C). Treatment of wounds with PN105 resulted in significantly greater TNTV than any of the other tested mixtures of 2 or 3 of the constituent deoxyribonucleosides (**Table 1**).

In the second study, PN105 was compared with the mixtures of dA + dT and dC + dG. The methods used were the same as those in the first mixture study. The results show that PN105 treatment produced greater TNTV than did either pair, although statistical significance was not reached (**Table 2**). However, when taken together with the results of Table 1 and previous work with a rat model,[15]

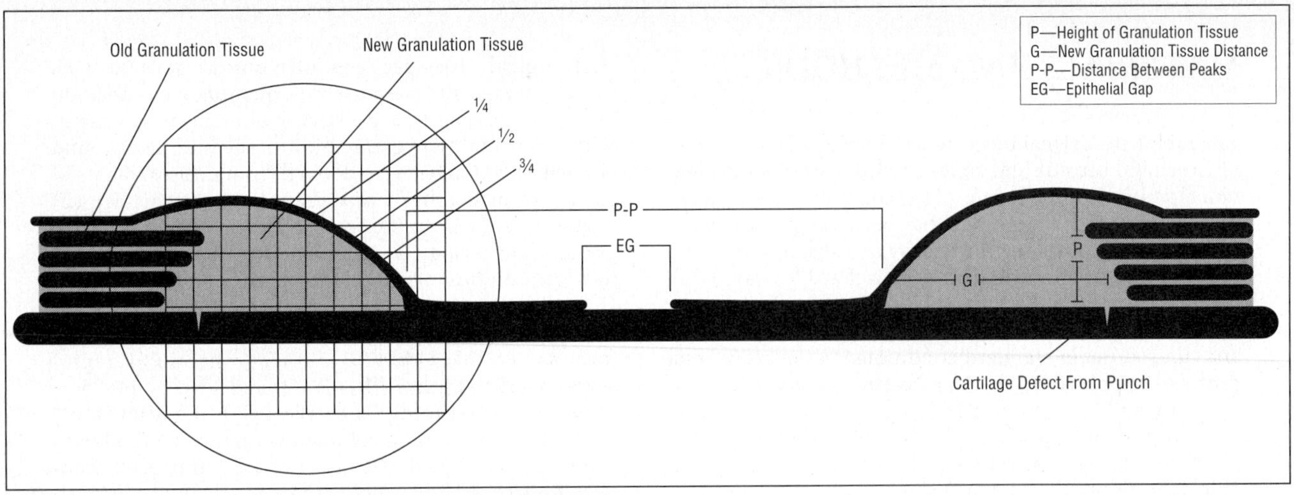

Figure 1. *Schematic diagram of the measurement points of wound healing.*

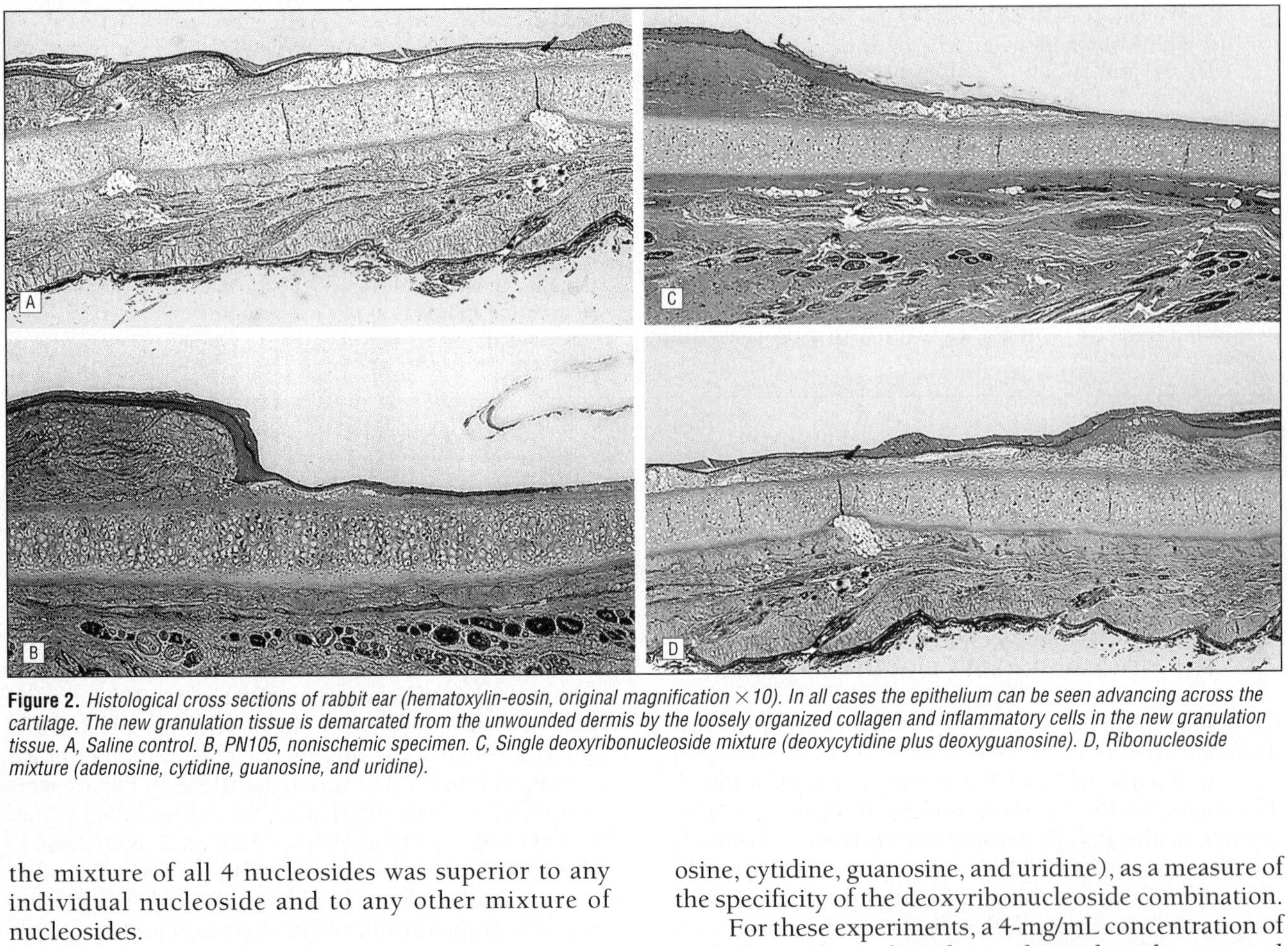

Figure 2. *Histological cross sections of rabbit ear (hematoxylin-eosin, original magnification × 10). In all cases the epithelium can be seen advancing across the cartilage. The new granulation tissue is demarcated from the unwounded dermis by the loosely organized collagen and inflammatory cells in the new granulation tissue. A, Saline control. B, PN105, nonischemic specimen. C, Single deoxyribonucleoside mixture (deoxycytidine plus deoxyguanosine). D, Ribonucleoside mixture (adenosine, cytidine, guanosine, and uridine).*

the mixture of all 4 nucleosides was superior to any individual nucleoside and to any other mixture of nucleosides.

EFFECTS OF DEOXYRIBONUCLEOSIDES VS RIBONUCLEOSIDES ON WOUND HEALING IN THE NORMAL RABBIT EAR ULCER MODEL

Since, chemically, RNA is a linear polymer of ribonucleosides joined by phosphodiester moieties and DNA is composed of 2′-deoxyribonucleosides otherwise linked identically, the relative effects of a mixture of deoxyribonucleosides were compared with those of a corresponding mixture of ribonucleoside nucleosides (adenosine, cytidine, guanosine, and uridine), as a measure of the specificity of the deoxyribonucleoside combination.

For these experiments, a 4-mg/mL concentration of each deoxyribonucleoside or ribonucleoside was used rather than the 10 mg/mL used in previous experiments, because this represents the solubility limit of the ribonucleosides. The TNTV was significantly greater in the deoxyribonucleoside-treated wounds (n = 16) than in controls (n = 15); there was no statistically significant difference between ribonucleoside-treated wounds (n = 14) and their respective controls (Figure 2, B and D, and **Figure 4**). The deoxyribonucleosides at a concentration of 4 mg/mL in this experiment produced about the same improvement as they did at 10 mg/mL, as de-

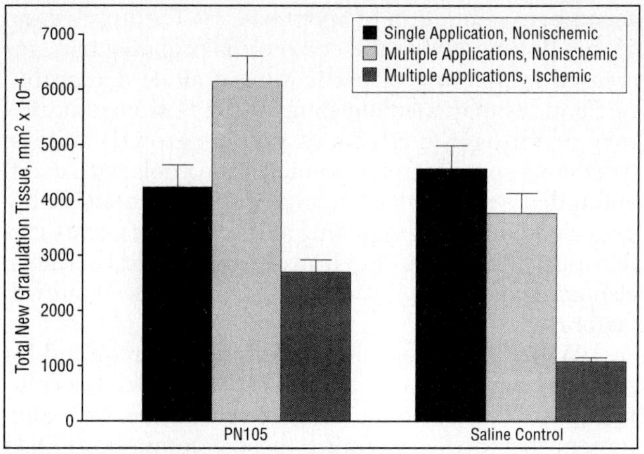

Figure 3. *Single vs multiple applications of PN105 on rabbit dermal ulcer model under nonischemic and ischemic conditions. Error bars indicate SEs.*

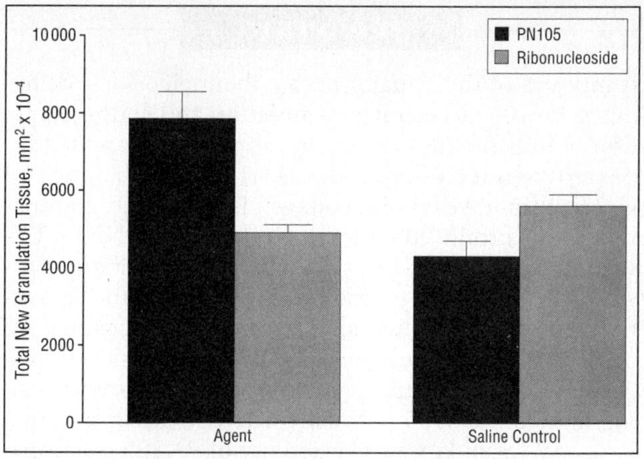

Figure 4. *Multiple applications of ribonucleoside mixture vs PN105 on rabbit dermal ulcer model under nonischemic conditions. Error bars indicate SEs.*

Table 1. Effects of PN105 and Mixtures of the Deoxyribonucleosides Containing dC and dG on TNTV*

TNTV, mm³				
PN105	**dC + dG**	**dC + dG + dA**	**dC + dG + dT**	***P***
8.20 ± 0.49	5.23 ± 0.95			.006
8.08 ± 0.55		5.82 ± 0.81		.03
7.74 ± 0.65			4.80 ± 0.64	.008

**Data are given as mean ± SEM. dC indicates deoxycytidine; dG, deoxyguanosine; TNTV, total new tissue volume; dA, deoxyadenosine; and dT, thymidine. PN105 is a mixture of the 4 deoxyribonucleosides.*

Table 2. Effects of PN105 and Other Mixtures of the Deoxyribonucleosides on TNTV*

TNTV, mm³			
PN105	**dC ± dG**	**dA ± dT**	***P***
5.81 ± 0.62	4.70 ± 0.60		.20
5.24 ± 0.57		3.87 ± 0.48	.07

**Data are given as mean ± SEM. See the footnote to Table 1 for explanation of abbreviations.*

Table 3. Experiments With PN105 in Carbomer-Based Gel*

	Total New Granulation, $\times 10^{-2}$ mm²	Total New Epithelium, $\times 10^{-2}$ mm²
PN105 in saline vs saline		
Saline	39.4 ± 4.2	24.4 ± 1.7
PN105	75.2 ± 3.7†	35.2 ± 1.8†
PN105 in gel vs gel		
Placebo gel	35.1 ± 4.1	25.4 ± 2.0
PN105 gel	68.3 ± 4.1†	38.7 ± 1.3†
Gel vs saline		
Saline	45.3 ± 6.0	26.7 ± 2.6
Placebo gel	43.0 ± 4.7‡	25.1 ± 1.8‡
PN105 in gel vs PN105 in saline		
PN105 saline	76.4 ± 7.3	34.8 ± 2.8
PN105 gel	71.2 ± 3.3‡	36.1 ± 2.2‡

**Data are given as mean ± SEM. PN105 is a combination of 4 deoxyribonucleosides (see the introduction section of the text).*
†$P<.001$.
‡*Not significant.*

scribed in the first experiment on normal wounds above (184% increase in new tissue at 4 mg/mL vs 191% at 10 mg/mL). The difference was not statistically significant.

EFFICACY OF A CARBOMER-BASED HYDROGEL FORMULATION OF PN105 IN THE RABBIT EAR ULCER WOUND HEALING MODEL

Control saline was demonstrated to have no effect on TNTV, and therefore PN105 (in the saline vehicle) was the active component in accelerating wound healing in the rabbit ear ulcer (Figure 2, A and B). For clinical use of PN105, a more viscous formulation with appropriate preservatives is preferable. Therefore, a carbomer-based hydrogel formulation was developed. The gel formulation contained each of the deoxyribonucleosides at 4 mg/mL, 0.625% Carbomer 934P (B. F. Goodrich Company, Cleveland, Ohio), 0.05% Quaternium-15 (Dow Chemical Company, Midland, Mich), 0.9% benzyl alcohol, and 0.05% EDTA in water (pH 6.9). A concentration of 4 mg/mL was selected on the basis of the observations that PN105 appears to be as effective at that dose as at the earlier tested concentration of 10 mg/mL and deoxyribonucleosides remain in solution in aqueous media at 4°C at 4 mg/mL but not at 10 mg/mL. Control wounds received either 0.9% saline alone or carbomer gel placebo. Sixteen wounds per group were evaluated except in the saline group used for comparison with the placebo gel group. In that case, 15 wounds were evaluable. Paired comparisons were made as before, with each ear being treated with 1 regimen, and thus 1 comparison being made with each group of rabbits. All permutations were tested, with the finding that the carbomer vehicle had no effect on healing, but that the PN105-carbomer combination was as effective as the PN105 in saline vehicle (**Table 3**). In addition, these separate experiments confirmed the efficacy of PN105 and demonstrated that they were not vehicle dependent.

COMMENT

A mixture of the 4 major deoxyribonucleosides, designated PN105, accelerates granulation and epithelialization of full-thickness ulcers in rabbits when applied repeatedly (once every 2 days). A normal balance of glycosaminoglycans and collagen is present in granulation tissue produced under the influence of PN105. The wound-healing activity is specific to deoxyribonucleosides (ie, in contrast to ribonucleosides), and the best activity is obtained when all 4 deoxyribonucleosides are present in the formulation together. PN105 is active in ischemic wounds, unlike some polypeptide wound healing factors.[16] PN105 is equally active in saline and in a hydrogel formulation. The activity of PN105 is comparable with that of platelet-derived growth factor or transforming growth factor β on total new wound healing tissue volume at day 7.[17]

Earlier literature suggested positive effects of topically applied DNA on formation of granulation tissue in excisional wounds.[18-20] The results presented herein support the validity of these results, and also suggest that the effect can be explained as a result of degradation of DNA to the level of deoxyribonucleosides (via the actions of ubiquitous nucleases and phosphatases), which are efficiently taken up by cells via carriers, in contrast to deoxynucleotides or oligodeoxyribonucleotides, which are restricted in their entry into cells by their anionic phosphate moieties.

When nucleosides are taken up by cells, they are rapidly phosphorylated to the level of nucleotides, which can then be used for nucleic acid synthesis or other purposes. It is generally assumed that deoxyribonucleotide availability is not normally limiting for cell proliferation, since cells have ribonucleotide reductase, which converts the relatively plentiful ribonucleotides (present in cells in nearly millimolar concentrations) to the much lower concentrations of deoxyribonucleotides (present in cells in low micromolar concentrations) required for DNA replication.

The mechanism of action of the mixture of deoxyribonucleosides in accelerating wound healing is more likely related to regulatory effects of deoxyribonucleotide pools on cell cycling and metabolic regulation than to simply the provision of limiting substrates for DNA synthesis. Cells must necessarily be capable of monitoring availability of deoxyribonucleotides (or their precursor ribonucleotides) as a check point signal in cell cycling, since a deficiency of 1 or more deoxyribonucleotides during DNA replication can lead to either mutations or incomplete replication, both of which can have deleterious consequences in multicellular organisms. This is the basis for the antineoplastic activity of inhibitors of deoxyribonucleotide synthesis such as thymidylate synthase inhibitors (eg, floxuridine [5-fluoro-2′-deoxyuridine]) or antifolates (eg, methotrexate); thymidine starvation is a signal for apoptosis (or active cell suicide) to prevent possible deleterious effects on genomic fidelity.[21,22]

In hematopoietic cells that undergo apoptosis in response to deprivation of growth factors such as interleukin 3, deoxyribonucleotide imbalances in response to interleukin 3 withdrawal are reported to mediate, not merely accompany, initiation of apoptosis.[23,24] The implication of this finding is that the converse is probably true; increased availability of particular (or all 4) deoxyribonucleotides may mediate some of the positive stimulatory or mitogenic effects of various growth factors. Augmentation of deoxyribonucleotide pools with exogenous deoxyribonucleosides may either potentiate or bypass elements of the signaling and metabolic events mediating stimulation of cell proliferation (or, perhaps, elaboration of extracellular matrix components) by growth factors.

While all 4 deoxyribonucleosides are required for maximal activity in the rabbit ear ulcer model, the combination of deoxycytidine and deoxyguanosine (or 3-component mixtures containing these 2 compounds) had some degree of efficacy. Nicander and Reichard[25] and Reichard[26,27] suggested that deoxycytidine nucleotides in particular have a regulatory role in cell proliferation, since deoxycytidine triphosphate concentrations in proliferating cells rise before initiation of DNA replication, whereas enhanced production of the other 3 deoxyribonucleotides during cell cycling coincides with DNA synthesis.

The enzyme ribonucleotide reductase, which provides the only pathway through which deoxyribonucleotides are synthesized de novo by cells, is directly regulated as a final common control point by a number of positive and negative regulators of cell division.[28] In the hematopoietic system, the inhibitory effect of several physiological agents on cell cycling can be overcome by providing exogenous deoxycytidine, thus bypassing the need for induction of ribonucleotide reductase, the activity of which rises and falls during cell cycling, reaching a peak just before and during DNA synthesis.[29,30]

Schwartz et al[31] reported that various pharmacological treatments that inhibit DNA synthesis specifically by depleting cellular pools of 1 or more of the precursor deoxyribonucleotides in keratinocytes induced their differentiation. While converse experiments investigating effects of superabundance of DNA precursors on keratinocyte differentiation were not discussed or reported, this finding again points toward an important role of deoxyribonucleotide pools in regulation of cell cycling and differentiation.

Determination of the details of the mechanism of action of the mixture of deoxyribonucleosides in accelerating healing may yield important insights into regulation of tissue repair and regeneration. It is striking that both granulation and epithelialization are enhanced by this agent, and that topical administration of the low-molecular-weight deoxyribonucleosides reproducibly accelerates healing in both normal and ischemic wounds to an extent equivalent to or greater than that reported for recombinant wound healing growth factors, ie, platelet-derived growth factor, insulinlike growth factor 1, insulinlike growth factor binding protein 1, keratinocyte growth factor, fibroblast growth factor, granulocyte-macrophage colony-stimulating factor, or transforming growth factor β1 in the rabbit ear ulcer model.[32-39] No other low-molecular-weight agents, whether endogenous metabolites or synthetic compounds, are known to display wound healing activity of this magnitude.

Deoxyribonucleosides are rapidly degraded by enzymes in plasma, erythrocytes, and the liver, so that systemic exposure to topically applied deoxyribonucleosides will be minimal.[40] Patients have received multiple grams of deoxycytidine and thymidine per day by intravenous infusion (for the purpose of modifying toxicity of antineoplastic antimetabolites) with no adverse effects.[41,42] Moreover, during maturation of erythrocytes, their enucleation releases approximately 1 g of DNA per day into the circulation (which is degraded to its constituent deoxyribonucleosides by serum enzymes), further indicating that exogenous deoxyribonucleosides applied to wounds are likely to be extremely safe. Furthermore, we have not seen scarring with multiple wound healing agents that are effective in accelerating healing in rabbits. Notably, platelet-derived growth factor does accelerate healing without scar on follow-up, which parallels the human situation for platelet-derived growth factor; no scarring was reported in human trials.[11,14,19] Therefore, in view of the safety, stability, and wound healing activity, these deoxyribonucleoside agents hold great therapeutic promise for improving treatment of chronic dermal ulcers and other varieties of wounds seen commonly in the clinic.

This work was supported by grant GM41303 from the National Institutes of Health, Bethesda, Md, and by funding from Pro-Neuron Inc, Gaithersburg, Md.

Reprints: Thomas Mustoe, MD, Division of Plastic Surgery, Northwestern Medical Center, 19th Floor, Ward Building, 333 E Chicago Ave, Chicago, IL 60611.

REFERENCES

1. Miescher F. Ueber die chemische Zusammensetsung der Eiterzellen. *Hoppe-Seyler's Medicinische-Chemische Untersuchunge.* 1871;4:441-460.
2. Dumont AE. Wound healing and extracellular deoxyribonucleic acid. *Ann Surg.* 1959;150:799-807.
3. Marshak A, Walker AC. Effect of a chromatin derivative on the healing of skin wounds. *Proc Soc Exp Biol Med.* 1945;58:62-63.
4. Nicolau SG, Badaniou A. Die stimulierende Wirkung der Desoxyribonucleinsaure bei der Vernarbung experimentell gesetzer Hautwunden. *Hautarzt.* 1966; 17:512-515.
5. Amellem O, Loffler M, Petterson EO. Regulation of cell proliferation under extreme and moderate hypoxia: the role of pyrimidine (deoxy)nucleotides. *Br J Cancer.* 1994;70:857-866.
6. Bjursell O, Reichard P. Effects of thymine on deoxyribonucleoside triphosphate pools and deoxyribonucleic acid synthesis in Chinese hamster ovary cells. *J Biol Chem.* 1973;248:3904-3909.
7. Ahn ST, Mustoe TA. Effects of ischemia on ulcer wound healing: a new model in the rabbit ear. *Ann Plast Surg.* 1990;24:17-23.
8. Mustoe TA, Pierce GF, Morishima C, Deuel TF. Growth factor-induced acceleration of tissue repair through direct and inductive activities in a rabbit dermal ulcer model. *J Clin Invest.* 1991;87:694-703.
9. Cromach DT, Pierce GF, Mustoe TA. TGF-β and PDGF mediated tissue repair: identifying mechanisms of action using impaired and normal models of wound healing. *Prog Clin Biol Res.* 1991;365:359-373.
10. Cromack DT, Porras-Reyes B, Purdy JA, Pierce GF, Mustoe TA. Acceleration of tissue repair by transforming growth factor β 1: identification of in vivo mechanism of action with radiotherapy-induced specific healing deficits. *Surgery.* 1993; 113:36-42.
11. Mustoe TA, Landes A, Cromack DT, et al. Differential acceleration of healing of surgical incisions in the rabbit gastrointestinal tract by platelet-derived growth factor and transforming growth factor, type β. *Surgery.* 1990;108:324-329.
12. Mustoe TA, Pierce GF, Thomason A, Oramates P, Sporn MB, Deuel TF. Accelerated healing of incisional wounds in rats induced by transforming growth factor-β. *Science.* 1987;237:1333-1336.
13. Wu L, Pierce GF, Galiano RD, Mustoe TA. Keratinocyte growth factor induces granulation tissue in ischemic dermal wounds: importance of epithelial-mesenchymal cell interactions. *Arch Surg.* 1996;131:660-666.
14. Wu L, Brucker M, Oruskin E, Roth S, Mustoe TA. Differential effects of platelet-derived growth factor BB in accelerating wound healing in aged versus young animals: the impact of tissue hypoxia. *Plast Reconstr Surg.* 1997;99:815-822.
15. von Borstel RW, Bamat MK, inventors; Pro-Neuron, Inc, assignee. Methods for promoting wound healing with deoxyribonucleosides. US patent 5 246 708. September 21, 1993.
16. Wu L, Pierce GF, Ladin DA, Zhao LL, Rogers D, Mustoe TA. Effects of oxygen on wound responses to growth factors: Kaposi's FGF, but not basic FGF stimulates repair in ischemic wounds. *Growth Factors.* 1995;12:29-35.
17. Galiano RD, Zhao LL, Clemmons DR, Roth SI, Lin X, Mustoe TA. Interaction between the insulin-like growth factor family and the integrin receptor family in tissue repair processes: evidence in a rabbit ear dermal ulcer model. *J Clin Invest.* 1996;98:2462-2468.
18. Pierce GF, Mustoe TA, Deuel TF. Transforming growth factor β induces increased directed cellular migration and tissue repair in rats. *Prog Clin Biol Res.* 1988;266:93-102.
19. Pierce GF, Tarpley JE, Yanagihara D, Mustoe TA, Fox GM, Thomason A. Platelet-derived growth factor (BB homodimer), transforming growth factor-β 1, and basic fibroblast growth factor in dermal wound healing: neovessel and matrix formation and cessation of repair. *Am J Pathol.* 1992;140:1375-1388.
20. Pierce GF, Mustoe TA, Lingelbach J, Masakowski VR, Oramates P, Deuel TF. Transforming growth factor-β reverses the glucocorticoid-induced wound-healing deficit in rats: possible regulation in macrophages by platelet-derived growth factor. *Proc Natl Acad Sci U S A.* 1989;86:2229-2233.
21. Greulich RC, Cameron IL, Thrasher JD, Stimulation of mitosis in adult mice by administration of thymidine. *Proc Natl Acad Sci U S A.* 1961;47:743-748.
22. Hiatt HH, Bojarski TB. The effects of thymidine administration on thymidylate kinase activity and on DNA synthesis in mammalian tissues. *Quant Biol.* 1961; 26:367-369.
23. Oliver FJ, Collin MKL, Lopez-Rivas A. Regulation of the salvage pathway of deoxynucleotides synthesis in apoptosis induced by growth factor deprivation. *Biochem J.* 1996;316:421-425.
24. Oliver FJ, Collins MK, Lopez-Rivas A. dNTP pools imbalance as a signal to initiate apoptosis. *Experientia.* 1996;52:995-1000.
25. Nicander B, Reichard P. Aphidicolin sensitivity of variant 3T6 cells selected for changes in ribonucleotide reductase. *Biochem Biophys Res Commun.* 1981;103: 148-155.
26. Reichard P. Interactions between deoxyribonucleotide and DNA synthesis. *Annu Rev Biochem.* 1988;57:349-374.
27. Reichard P. From deoxynucleotides to DNA synthesis. *Fed Proc.* 1978;37:9-14.
28. Albert DA, Rozengurt E. Synergistic and coordinate expression of the genes encoding ribonucleotide reductase subunits in Swiss 3T3 cells: effect of multiple signal-transduction pathways. *Proc Natl Acad Sci U S A.* 1992;89:1597-1601.
29. Schunk H, Schutt M, Langen P, Lord B, Laerum OD, Paukovits WR. Deoxycytidine, insulin, and epidermal growth factor overcome the effect of two natural inhibitors of the haematopoietic system. *APMIS Suppl.* 1988;2:120-129.
30. Wang J, Usami M, Yasuda I, et al. Effect of nucleosides and a nucleotide mixture on proliferation of human gastric cancer cells. *Kobe J Med Sci.* 1994;40:65-75.
31. Schwartz PM, Barnett SK, Milstone LM. Keratinocytes differentiate in response to inhibitors of deoxyribonucleotide synthesis. *J Dermatol Sci.* 1995;9:129-135.
32. Mustoe TA, Cutler NR, Allman RM, et al. A phase II study to evaluate recombinant platelet-derived growth factor-BB in the treatment of stage 3 and 4 pressure ulcers. *Arch Surg.* 1994;129:213-219.
33. Pierce GF, Mustoe TA, Altrock BW, Deuel T, Thomason A. Role of platelet-derived growth factor in wound healing. *J Cell Biochem.* 1991;45:319-326.
34. Jyung RW, Wu L, Pierce GF, Mustoe TA. Granulocyte-macrophage colony-stimulating factor and granulocyte colony-stimulating factor: differential action on incisional wound healing. *Surgery.* 1994;115:325-334.
35. Mustoe TA, Purdy J, Oramates P, Deuel TF, Thomason A, Pierce GF. Reversal of impaired wound healing in irradiated rats by platelet-derived growth factor-BB. *Am J Surg.* 1989;158:345-350.
36. Pierce GF, Brown D, Mustoe TA. Quantitative analysis of inflammatory cell influx, procollagen type I synthesis, and collagen cross-linking in incisional wounds: influence of PDGF-BB and TGF-β therapy. *J Lab Clin Med.* 1991;117:373-382.
37. Pierce GF, VandeBerg J, Rudolph R, Tarpley J, Mustoe TA. Platelet-derived growth factor-BB and transforming growth factor β 1 selectively modulate glycosaminoglycans, collagen, and myofibroblasts in excisional wounds. *Am J Pathol.* 1991; 138:629-646.
38. Wu L, Kumar SB, Porras-Reyes BH, Oramates PH, Mustoe TA. Platelet-derived growth factor BB accelerates wound closure in a new mesentery culture model without macrophages. *Ann Plast Surg.* 1994;33:155-161.
39. Pierce GF, Tarpley JE, Allman RM, et al. Tissue repair processes in healing chronic pressure ulcers treated with recombinant platelet-derived growth factor BB. *Am J Pathol.* 1994;145:1399-1410.
40. Beltz RE, Smith TR, Waters RN. Kinetics of the clearing of 14C-labeled deoxyribonucleosides from rat blood in vivo and in vitro. *Biochim Biophys Acta.* 1973; 279:258-267.
41. Bhalla K, Cole J, MacLaughlin W, et al. Deoxycytidine stimulates the in vitro growth of normal CFU-GM and reverses the negative regulatory effects of acidic isoferritin and prostaglandin E. *Blood.* 1986;68:1136-1141.
42. Zaharko DS, Bolten BJ, Chiuten D, Wiernik PH. Pharmacokinetic studies during phase I trials of high-dose thymidine infusions. *Cancer Res.* 1979;39:4777-4781.

ORIGINAL ARTICLE

Tumor of the Ampulla of Vater

Experience With Local or Radical Resection in 171 Consecutively Treated Patients

Hans G. Beger, MD; Frank Treitschke, MD; Frank Gansauge, MD; Nobuhiko Harada, MD; Naoki Hiki, MD; Torsten Mattfeldt, MD

Hypothesis: This study was designed to evaluate prospectively oncological factors determining survival after resection of tumors of the papilla, comparing local and radical oncological resection. We hypothesized that, in malignant lesions of the ampulla, the T and N stages are major determinants of the patient's long-term outcome.

Background Data: The frequency of malignant lesions in adenomas of the papilla is about 26%. Villous adenoma of the ampulla is considered a premalignant lesion. Local excision has been recommended for benign adenoma and pancreatoduodenectomy for malignant lesions.

Patients and Methods: From January 1, 1982, through June 30, 1997, 171 patients with tumors of the ampulla of Vater were surgically treated. Demographics, intraoperative factors, tumor pathological findings, and postoperative short- and long-term follow-up data were documented prospectively. Of the patients, 45 had adenoma of the papilla and 126 had malignant lesions of the ampulla.

Results: Local resection was performed in 40 of the 45 patients with adenoma. In 98 of the 126 patients with malignant lesions, a radical Kausch-Whipple resection or pylorus-preserving pancreatoduodenectomy was used. Of the patients with benign adenoma, 40 had local resection and 5 had pylorus-preserving pancreatic head resection, with a hospital mortality of 0%. Thirty of 35 patients had villous adenoma, 9 (30%) of the 30 with severe dysplasia. Of the 126 patients with malignant lesions, 98 had partial pancreatoduodenectomy and 10 had ampullectomy, with an overall hospital mortality of 3.1% for patients who underwent resection. Seventy-eight of the 98 patients had an R0 resection. The 5-year survival probability for all patients who underwent resection was 84% for cancer stage I, 70% for stage II, and 27% for stage III. In 8 patients with villous adenoma and carcinoma in situ and in 10 patients with cancer in the adenoma, ampullectomy with local lymph node dissection was performed. In 4 of the patients who had villous adenoma and a carcinoma in stage pT1 N0, an R0 resection was performed, resulting in cure of cancer. On the basis of a multivariate regression analysis, the prognosis after oncological resection of cancer of the ampulla is determined by the absence of lymph node metastasis ($P<.05$), the absence of infiltration into the pancreatic head tissue ($P<.05$), and the application of an R0 resection.

Conclusions: In patients with villous adenoma of the ampulla, ampullectomy was an adequate surgical treatment. In patients with a low-risk cancer in stages pTis and pT1 N0 M0, G1 or G2, a local resection with ampullectomy including local lymph node dissection is justified. An oncological resection of cancer of the ampulla by means of a pylorus-preserving partial pancreatoduodenectomy or the Kausch-Whipple resection is the surgical procedure of choice; the 3- and 5-year survival rates were 72% and 52%, respectively, in patients with R0 resections.

Arch Surg. 1999;134:526-532

From the Departments of General Surgery (Drs Beger, Treitschke, and Gansauge) and Pathology (Dr Mattfeldt), University of Ulm, Ulm, Germany; and the Departments of Gastroenterological Surgery (Dr Harada) and Surgery (Dr Hiki), Tokyo Women's Medical College, Tokyo, Japan.

CANCER of the ampulla or papilla of Vater is classified as periampullary cancer; 5% of all gastrointestinal tract malignant neoplasms are periampullary. Cancers of the ampulla are more frequent than common bile duct cancer; however, they are less frequent than pancreatic head cancer, with a ratio of 1:12. On the basis of autopsy investigations, the rate of neoplastic lesions of the ampulla was found to range between 0.063% and 0.21%.[1-4]

It has been suggested that survival of patients after resection of an ampullary tumor is most influenced by the origin of tumor epithelium. The anatomy of the ampulla of Vater is extremely complex. It consists of 3 epithelia—those of the bile duct, the pancreatic duct, and the duodenal mucosa—and it has 4 parts in 1 very narrow area of the ampulla including tissue of the periampullary pancreas.

Cattell and Pyrtek[5] first reported malignant transformation of an adenoma of the papilla. In more than 70% of the investigated carcinomas of the ampulla, tissue samples were found with severe dysplasia.[6-9] At present there are substantial arguments, including molecular biologi-

PATIENTS AND METHODS

Between January 1, 1982, and June 30, 1997, 171 patients with tumors of the ampulla of Vater were surgically treated. In the 15-year period, 45 patients with benign tumors of the papilla and 126 with cancer of the papilla were operated on. In the adenoma group, 20 (44%) of the patients were male and 25 (56%) were female; in the carcinoma group, 71 (56.3%) were male and 55 (43.7%) were female. The mean age of the adenoma patients was 59 years, ranging from 18 to 81 years; in the cancer group the mean age was 63 years, with a range of 33 to 89 years.

SURGICAL TECHNIQUES

Resection of the papilla was performed in 3 patients with benign lesions. Resection of the papilla included removal of the intraduodenal roof and the intraluminal common orifice of the papilla without the need for reinsertion of the common bile and pancreatic main duct entrance into the duodenal wall.[14]

An ampullectomy was performed in 37 patients with neoplastic lesions. The technique of ampullectomy is described elsewhere[14] and is based on the following principal surgical steps: (1) resection of biliopancreatic junction and of some pancreatic head tissue and (2) reinsertion of the common bile duct and the pancreatic main duct into the duodenal wall. In patients with severe dysplasia or a pT is cancer and in pT1 low-risk cancers, an additional lymph node dissection was performed, including the anterior and posterior lymph nodes of the pancreatic head and the supraduodenal lymph nodes along the foramen of Winslow.

Eighty-eight patients underwent major oncological resection by means of the Kausch-Whipple technique or a pylorus-preserving partial pancreatoduodenectomy (PPPD). The lymph node dissection in each patient included removal of the following lymph node regions: anterior and posterior head, supraduodenal, common and proper hepatic artery, hepatoduodenal ligament, and lymph nodes to the right of the superior mesenteric artery.

DEFINITION OF SURGICAL PRINCIPLES

Partial pancreatoduodenectomy was defined as resection of pancreatic head, duodenectomy, and resection of flexura duodenojejunalis; lymph node dissection, including anterior and posterior head, supraduodenal area, common and proper hepatic artery, hepatoduodenal ligament, and lymph nodes right of the superior mesenteric artery; resection of the lower common bile duct up to the common hepatic duct; and reconstruction with the first jejunal loop, pancreatojejunal anastomosis end to side, and hepaticojejunal anastomosis end to side. In patients with pylorus-preserving resection (PPPD), end-to-side anastomosis was performed, duodenum to jejunum. *Kausch-Whipple resection* (pPD) consisted of Billroth-II resection of the stomach and Braun enteroanastomosis. *R0 resection* indicates resection margins of the pancreas, common bile duct, duodenum, and retropancreatic tissue histologically free of carcinoma; *R1 resection*, histologically positive for carcinoma cells in a resection margin. *Radical resection* was partial pancreatoduodenectomy plus lymph node dissection plus retroportal, retropancreatic fatty tissue dissection.

FOLLOW-UP AND HISTOLOGICAL REEXAMINATION

The primary criterion of the prospective follow-up in the study was survival time; follow-up examinations took place at 3, 6, and 12 months; 2, 3, 4, and 5 years; and yearly after 5 years. Patient follow-up was completed August 31, 1997.

Histological examination of the operative specimens and biopsy material was performed twice and by 2 different pathological investigators. The first examination was done by a staff pathologist in charge of gastrointestinal tract histopathology. The second pathological investigator (T.M.) performed a blinded reexamination.

STATISTICAL ANALYSIS

Patient demographics, intraoperative factors, tumor pathology, and postoperative follow-up data were evaluated in both univariate and multivariate models to determine their impact on long-term survival. Survival analysis was done by the method of Kaplan-Meier. Differences in survival between subsets were compared by the log-rank test. Multivariate analysis was performed with the Cox proportional hazards model. Differences among subgroups of the cohort were evaluated with a 1-way analysis of variance. Results are reported as mean ± SD and median percentiles. Significance was accepted at the 5% level.

cal data, for the hypothesis of an adenoma-dysplasia-carcinoma sequence of neoplastic lesions of the ampulla of Vater.[8,10,11] A villous adenoma of the ampulla of Vater is considered a premalignant lesion, with the consequence of complete extirpation of the lesion to avoid development of cancer. The frequency of a malignant lesion in an adenoma of the papilla is around 26%.[6-13] Under these circumstances, oncological resection has been recommended.

To evaluate factors affecting survival, we prospectively documented and investigated 171 patients with neoplastic lesions of the ampulla of Vater who had been operated on for adenoma or carcinoma; we evaluated the preoperative clinical and histological data, the tumor stage, and the outcome after surgery with a long-term follow-up protocol.

RESULTS

Thirty-seven percent of the patients with a malignant tumor and 22% of those with a benign lesion of the ampulla were aged 70 years or older at the time of operation; 40% of the patients who had an ampullectomy for ampullary cancer and 68% of those who had only a biliary and/or gastric bypass procedure were aged 70 years or older when operated on. The median time of the patients' symptoms caused by the lesion of the papilla was 8 weeks in the adenoma group and 5 weeks in the patient group with carcinoma. The clinical manifestations in the patients with adenoma (n = 45) and carcinoma (n = 126) were as follows, respectively: epigastric pain, 25 (56%) and 59 (47%); jaundice, 13 (29%) and 93 (74%);

Table 1. Diagnostic Accuracy of Preoperative Histological Examination* in Neoplastic Lesions of the Ampulla of Vater in 90 Patients

	No. of Patients	No. False Positive	No. False Negative	Sensitivity, %
Adenoma	19	2	3	61
Adenoma and severe dysplasia	8	1	2	83
Adenoma and carcinoma	5	0	3	40
Carcinoma	58	3	15	69

*Endoscopy and multiple (2-11) biopsies.

Table 2. Surgical Treatment of Tumors of the Ampulla of Vater and Hospital Mortality

	Benign Lesion (n = 45)	Malignant Lesion (n = 126)
Resection of the papilla, No.	3	0
Ampullectomy, No.	37	10
Partial pancreatoduodenectomy, No.	5*	88†
Bypass procedure, biliary and/or gastric, No.	0	28
Hospital mortality (patients who underwent resection), %	0	3.2‡

*Five patients underwent pylorus-preserving resection.
†Fifty patients underwent pylorus-preserving resection, and 38 patients underwent Kausch-Whipple resection.
‡Without bypass procedure.

loss of body weight, 5 (11%) and 67 (53%); and nausea and vomiting, 19 (42%) and 79 (63%). Diabetes mellitus was observed in 8 (18%) of 45 patients with adenoma and in 23 (18%) of 126 patients with carcinoma.

The diagnostic accuracy in patients with an adenoma of the papilla was highest with the use of duodenoscopy and multiple biopsies, in terms of the diagnosis of tumor of the papilla. However, when the final histological diagnosis after surgical treatment was compared with the preoperative histological findings on biopsy, diagnostic accuracy was only 74%. In patients with cancer of the ampulla, the sensitivity of duodenoscopy and multiple biopsies was 40%, and the diagnostic accuracy was 78% (**Table 1**). The histological probes of the preoperative biopsy specimens and of the surgical specimens were reevaluated by a second, independent pathologist specializing in the gastrointestinal tract (T.M.).

Forty-five patients had benign tumors. In terms of the final histological findings, 35 patients had adenomas; 30 (86%) of these 35 patients demonstrated villous adenomas; 10 patients suffered from other types of lesions, eg, tumorlike adenomyosis and neurinoma. In patients with adenoma, final histological examination disclosed a tubular adenoma in 5, a villous adenoma in 14, and a tubulovillous adenoma in 16 cases. The dysplasia was graded mild in 20% (7 of 35 patients), moderate in 51% (18 of 35 patients), and severe in 29% (10 of 35 patients). Except for 5 patients, a local resection procedure was used in patients with benign tumors of the papilla. In 37 patients, ampullectomy was performed, with the need for reinsertion of the common bile duct and pancreatic main duct into the duodenal wall. Patients with a villous adenoma and a macroscopically based suspicion of malignant neoplasm (tumor >2 cm in maximum diameter, video documentation [since 1985] of ulcerations in adenoma) had an additional local lymph node dissection including the anterior and posterior lymph nodes of the pancreatic head and the supraduodenal lymph nodes. Five patients with suspected carcinoma underwent pylorus-preserving pancreatic head resection with lymph node dissection. No patient died of the surgical treatment. After surgery, the median follow-up of the patients with benign tumors was 43 months. Forty patients had no abdominal complaints or a local recurrence of the adenoma; 1 patient died at the age of 92 years of cardiac insufficiency. Median hospitalization time was 22 days for the whole group.

CANCER OF THE PAPILLA

One hundred twenty-six patients had malignant lesions of the papilla. Final histological diagnosis was carcinoma in 125 patients and carcinoid of the papilla in 1. When the patients were classified according to the pTNM staging (Union Internationale Contre le Cancer [UICC], 1993), 18% had stage I, 31% had stage II, 44% had stage III, and 7% had stage IV. The degree of cell differentiation was high in 3.1% (G1), moderate in 74.7% (G2), and low in 22.2% (G3). Fifty-seven patients (45.6%) showed no lymph node metastasis. Sixty-nine patients were pN positive; in these patients, a median of 18 lymph nodes (range, 5-35) were assessed. The resection rate was 77.8%. Seventy-eight patients had an R0 resection. Hospital mortality was 3.2% (3 of 93 patients) in patients with pancreatoduodenectomy and 0% in patients after ampullectomy for cancer. After radical resection, an intra-abdominal complication occurred in 25% of the patients; 6 of 88 patients had another operation, and in 2 patients a total pancreatectomy was completed during the second operation (**Table 2**).

pTNM STAGE AND PROGNOSIS

Among the patients with ampullary cancer in whom a local or radical resection was performed, none had a distant metastasis at operation. Considering the patients with an oncological radical resection (PPPD or Kausch-Whipple resection), the survival rate after 5 years was 84% for patients with stage I disease, decreasing to 70% for stage II and 27% for stage III; no patients with stage IV disease survived for more than 1 year after operation (**Figure 1**). The differences in survival rate between stage I and stage II ($P<.04$) and stage III and stage IV ($P<.006$) were highly significant.

EFFECT OF CANCER INVASION INTO THE PANCREAS ON PROGNOSIS

Cases of pT1 and pT2 cancer are considered on the basis of UICC definitions as cases without infiltration into pancreatic tissue, in comparison with pT3 and pT4, where tumor infiltration into the head of the pancreas has oc-

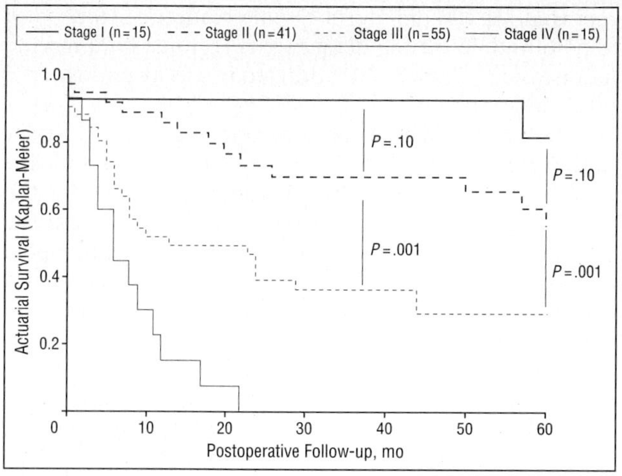

Figure 1. *Tumor stage and survival in 126 patients with cancer of the ampulla of Vater.*

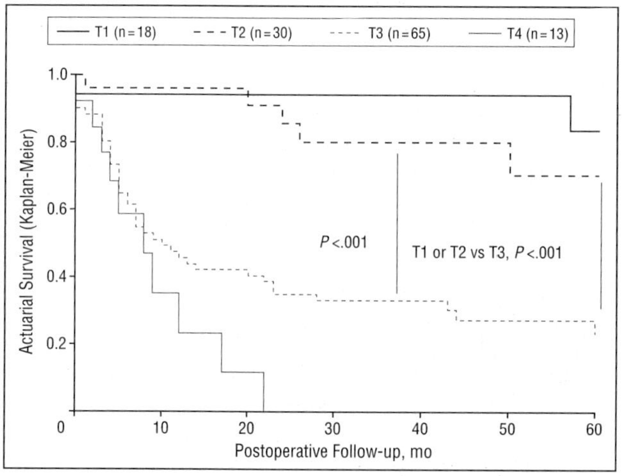

Figure 2. *Tumor stage and survival in 126 patients with cancer of the ampulla of Vater.*

curred. In the 50 patients without pancreatic invasion (pT1 and pT2), the survival rate was 87% at 3 years and 79% at 5 years. Among the 76 patients with cancer invasion into the pancreatic head, however, the 3- and 5-year survival was 40% and 24%, respectively (**Figure 2**). The differences in survival rates between these 2 groups were significant ($P<.002$).

LYMPH NODE METASTASIS AND PROGNOSIS

Fifty-seven (45%) of 126 patients had no lymph node metastasis and 69 patients had cancer cells in the lymph nodes on the basis of hematoxylin-eosin staining and histological examinations. The prognosis of the patients without lymph node metastasis was significantly better (3-year and 5-year survival, 72% and 63%, respectively) than that of the patients with lymph node metastasis (26% and 21%, respectively) (**Table 3** and **Figure 3**).

CORRELATION BETWEEN HISTOLOGICAL CELL DIFFERENTIATION AND PROGNOSIS

Patients who had a high or moderate degree of cell differentiation (G1 and G2) showed a significantly better

Table 3. Postsurgical Tumor Classification and Lymph Node Involvement in Patients With Cancer of the Ampulla of Vater

Classification	No. (%) of Patients (N = 98)	Positive Nodes, No. (%)
T1	18 (18)	4 (22)
T2	30 (31)	7 (23)
T3	43 (44)	20 (47)
T4	7 (7)	4 (57)

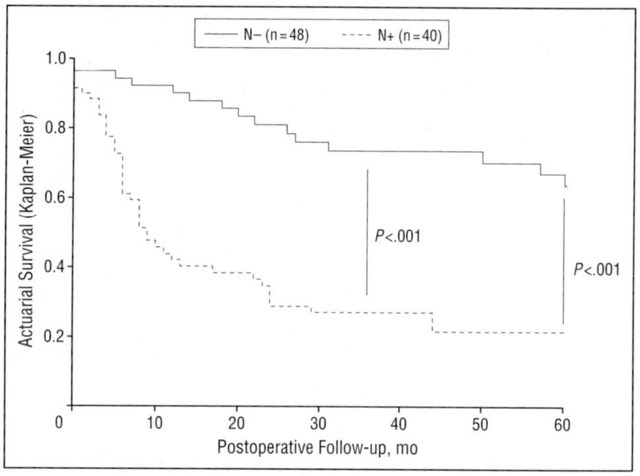

Figure 3. *Survival of patients with (N+) and without (N−) lymph node involvement in cancer of the ampulla of Vater.*

3- and 5-year survival than patients with a G3 degree of differentiation (**Figure 4**).

PROGNOSIS AFTER LOCAL RESECTION

In 10 patients a local resection was performed by means of ampullectomy completed by a local lymph node dissection. Four patients were operated on for villous adenoma, but on final histological examination they had carcinoma in the adenoma. In 6 patients a small adenocarcinoma was treated by ampullectomy; however, on the final histological examination this was an R1 resection. Because of the high degree of comorbidity and the high risk and advanced age of the patients (5 of the 6 were older than 70 years), an additional radical surgical procedure was not performed. After ampullectomy, no patient died; 3 of 4 patients after R0 ampullectomy were still alive at 7, 6, and 1.5 years; 1 patient died 6 years after resection following decompensation of liver cirrhosis without recurrence, but no patient with an R1 resection survived for 3 years (**Table 4** and **Figure 5**).

PROGNOSIS AFTER RADICAL RESECTION

Before 1990, a partial pancreatoduodenectomy by means of the Kausch-Whipple technique was the standard procedure for all patients with carcinoma of the ampulla of Vater. Since 1990, a PPPD was performed in most patients. The survival rate at 3 years was 72% in the patients with PPPD and 52% in those with Kausch-

Whipple resection, because the latter was applied more frequently in patients with advanced cancer stage.

COMMENT

There are substantial arguments for the hypothesis of an adenoma-dysplasia-carcinoma sequence of neoplastic lesions of the ampulla of Vater.[8-13] The frequency of a malignant lesion in a villous adenoma of the ampulla is observed to be 25% and higher.[8] In most of the carcinomas of the ampulla, tissue samples from adenomas were found in the stage of severe dysplasia. Of patients with a villous adenoma in this series, 16.6% finally displayed a cancer in the adenoma.

Recent advances in diagnostic techniques, such as duodenoscopy with multiple biopsies, and the use of endoscopic ultrasonography provide a precise preoperative diagnosis with regard to the nature and extent of the tumor. However, a single endoscopic biopsy has been reported to miss the diagnosis in 40% to 60% of cases.[12,15] Therefore, after the diagnosis of ampullary tumor is established, the most important diagnostic step is to assess the presence or absence of a carcinoma and the presence and extent of severe dysplasia. Most of the patients will have multiple endoscopic measures and multiple biopsies. Endoscopic ultrasonography has a particular advantage for the detection of invasion of the tumor into the duodenal wall and the pancreas and the occurrence of regional lymph node enlargement or metastases.[16,17] Accuracy rates of 78% to 87% have been reported for the diagnosis of pancreatic invasion[15] and of 54% to 83% for the diagnosis of regional lymph node metastasis,[18,19] with the additional use of endoscopic ultrasonography.

In patients with a carcinoma in situ or a T1 cancer in the villous adenoma, 6% to 10% have lymph node involvement.[20] Moreover, frozen section performed at the time of operation often fails to identify a cancer in the villous adenoma or cancer infiltration of the lymph node. Therefore, it seems to be nearly impossible to assess with certainty in each patient the presence of a carcinoma in situ or an infiltrating carcinoma in the adenomas without complete excision. Only in cases of a small tubular adenoma is an endoscopic snare excision justified; in all patients with a villous adenoma or a tubulovillous adenoma, surgical excision is mandatory because of the association with a carcinoma in situ or a pT1 cancer.[21-23]

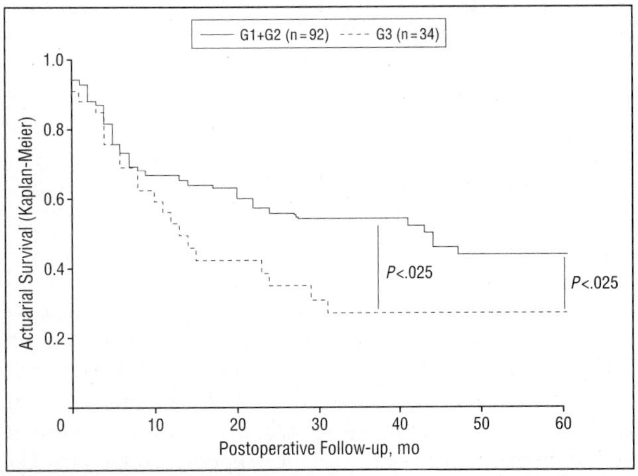

Figure 4. *Influence of grade of cell differentiation on survival of patients with cancer of the ampulla of Vater.*

LOCAL EXCISION OF pT1 CANCER OF THE AMPULLA

In 1899, Halsted[24] performed the first local extirpation of a carcinoma of the papilla. In patients with a pT1 cancer, local resection or ampullectomy has been advocated as being equal to or better than pancreatoduodenectomy.[25,26] The ampulla of Vater has a distinct pattern of lymphatic drainage and, in contrast to pancreatic tumors with a diffuse lymphatic spread, tumors of the papilla and ampulla tend to involve a local group of lymph nodes near the ampulla, even in advanced cases. These morphological features make ampullary lesions a distinct clinical entity, yielding a substantially superior prognosis if the infiltration does not include the pancreatic tissue. In case of an adenoma with a carcinoma in situ or a pT1 N0 M0 cancer of the ampulla, a local resection is indicated, except in patients who have a high-risk G3 or G4 cancer. Therefore, the low-risk group is defined as those with a carcinoma in situ and a pT1 N0 M0, G1 or G2 cancer.[20,27,28] If intraoperative findings show a cancer more advanced than T1 and a node-positive or higher G3 or G4 grade tumor, the procedure would have to be extended to a partial pancreatoduodenectomy, and this should even be true if postoperatively an adenoma or a T1 N0 cancer had to be reclassified by full histological evidence as pT2 N-positive, or if a poorly differentiated T1, G3 carcinoma was found. In this series of adenomatous lesions of the ampulla, treated surgically, an ampullectomy was performed in 8 patients with severe dysplasia consid-

Table 4. Local Resection of Villous Adenoma With Severe Dysplasia or Cancer Within Adenoma in 18 Patients

Procedure	Histological Findings	No. of Patients	Resection, No. (%) R0	Resection, No. (%) R1	Hospital Mortality, %	Alive Without Cancer, No.
Ampullectomy	Adenoma + severe dysplasia/cancer in situ*	8	8 (100)	0 (0)	0	7†
	Adenoma + pT1 cancer	10	4 (40)	6 (60)	0	R0: 3†; R1: 0‡
Partial pancreatoduodenectomy	Adenoma + pT1 cancer	5	5 (100)	0 (0)	0	5

*Severe dysplasia in a villous adenoma is classified as cancer in situ neoplasia.
†One patient died of cancer and treatment-unrelated disease.
‡Median survival, 18 months.

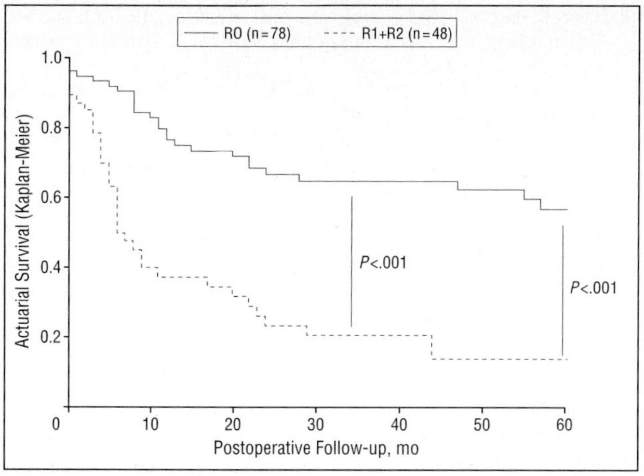

Figure 5. *Survival of patients with R0 and R1 + R2 resections in cancer of the ampulla of Vater.*

Table 5. Results of Univariate and Multivariate Analyses

	Univariate Analysis (N = 98)		Multivariate Regression Analysis (n = 88)	
	Patients, No.:No.	*P*	Risk Ratio	*P*
Node negative vs node positive	56:42	<.001	3.923	<.001
pT1 and pT2 vs pT3 and pT4	48:50	<.001	3.923	<.001
G1 and G2 vs G3	75:23	<.025	. . .*	.06*
R0 vs R1	82:16	<.001	. . .*	.05*

**Not significant.*

ered in situ carcinoma and in 4 patients with a villous adenoma in association with a pT1 cancer. All 4 patients were at an N0 stage. Local resection was justified, even in terms of curability from cancer lesions. According to the lower surgical morbidity and mortality, the use of ampullectomy has been recommended so far. In patients with a pTis or pT1 cancer, ampullectomy should be combined with a local lymph node dissection to ensure an oncological resection.

In 1912, Kausch reported the first successful 2-stage pancreatic head resection, to our knowledge, in a patient with carcinoma of the ampulla.[28,29] Today, the PPPD is the surgical procedure of choice in patients with cancer of the ampulla. The partial pancreatoduodenectomy includes resection of the duodenum, the distal common bile duct, and the head of the pancreas in combination with the lymph node dissection around the head of the pancreas, including N1 and N2 lymph nodes according to the Japanese classification of lymph node regions in cancer of the ampulla. Hospital mortality after PPPD is less than 5% in recently published series.[17,20,30,31] Patients with a UICC stage I or stage II cancer have a significantly better prognosis after partial pancreatoduodenectomy than patients with cancer stage III or IV. With respect to the results of PPPD in the present series, the survival rate at 3 years was 72% for patients who received a pylorus-preserving resection and 52% for those who received a partial pancreatoduodenectomy. While these findings are not strictly comparable because of differences between periods, the results demonstrate that, at least to date, PPPD has not had unfavorable effects on prognosis. Nakase et al[32] investigated the incidence of lymph node metastasis in 54 patients who had undergone partial pancreatoduodenectomy for carcinoma of the ampulla of Vater, finding the incidence of infrapyloric lymph node metastasis to be 3.7%. Accordingly, if no metastasis is confirmed in the infrapyloric lymph node by intraoperative frozen section examination, PPPD can be used for carcinoma of the ampulla of Vater.

ONCOLOGICAL FACTORS IN PROGNOSIS

The differences in survival rates after surgery between the 2 groups, classified on the basis of lymph node metastasis or extension of the cancer to the pancreatic head tissue, clearly reflect prognosis, and the 2 factors were significantly correlated (**Table 5**). Regional lymph node metastasis was seen in only 22% of the patients who had pT1 and pT2 cancer, whereas the proportion rose to 60% in patients with pT3 and pT4 cancer. These findings suggest that pancreatic invasion indirectly indicates the status of regional lymph node metastasis.[17,32,33] The prognostic significance of pancreatic invasion in carcinoma of the ampulla of Vater has been reported by other investigators. Kawarada et al[34] and others[35] reported the incidence of lymph node metastasis around the superior mesenteric artery to be 15.6% in carcinoma of the ampulla of Vater, and they showed the lymphatic pathways from posterior pancreatoduodenal lymph nodes to para-aortic lymph nodes via lymph nodes around the superior mesenteric artery.[34] In 1984, Hanyu[35] reported that extended lymph node dissection improved prognosis, showing a higher 5-year survival rate (81%) in patients who had undergone complete lymph node dissection around the superior mesenteric artery, compared with 40% in patients who had received incomplete tissue dissection around it. Therefore, an extended lymph node clearance should be considered as an additional procedure for patients with pancreatic invasion including the lymph nodes on both sides of the superior mesenteric artery. However, more controlled data are needed about the oncological impact of extended lymph node dissection.[36]

The chance of cure after the use of partial pancreatoduodenectomy including removal of the local lymph nodes is around 50%.[35] In recently published series, the 1-year survival is around 80%, the 3-year survival around 55% to 60%, and the 5-year survival around 35% to 50%.[33,35,36] The application of an R0 resection is the surgeon's contribution to increase 5-year survival. The median survival after R0 resection was around 45 months in this series. To improve the prognosis for patients with pancreatic invasion, further resection including extended lymph node removal is a recommended additional procedure.

Reprints: Hans G. Beger, MD, Department of General Surgery, University of Ulm, Steinhoevelstrasse 9, 89075 Ulm, Germany (e-mail: hans.beger@medizin.uni-ulm.de).

REFERENCES

1. Sobol S, Cooperman AM. Villous adenoma of the ampulla of Vater. *Gastroenterology.* 1978;75:107-109.
2. Oh C, Jemerin EE. Benign adenomatous polyps of the papilla of Vater. *Surgery.* 1965;57:495-503.
3. Perzin KH, Bridge MF. Adenomas of the small intestine: a clinicopathologic review of 51 cases and a study of their relationship to carcinoma. *Cancer.* 1981; 48:799-819.
4. Yamaguchi K, Enjoji M. Carcinoma of the ampulla of Vater: a clinicopathologic study and pathologic staging of 109 cases of carcinoma and 5 cases of adenoma. *Cancer.* 1987;59:506-515.
5. Cattell RB, Pyrtek LJ. Premalignant lesions of the ampulla of Vater. *Surg Gynecol Obstet.* 1950;90:21.
6. Hermanek P. Dysplasia in the gastrointestinal tract: definition and clinical significance. *Surg Endosc.* 1987;1:5-10.
7. Kozuka S, Tsubone M, Yamaguchi A, Hachisuka K. Adenomatous residue in cancerous papilla of Vater. *Gut.* 1981;22:1031-1034.
8. Baczako K, Büchler M, Kirkpatrick J, Haferkamp O, Beger HG. Morphogenesis and possible precursor lesions of invasive carcinoma of the papilla of Vater. *Hum Pathol.* 1985;16:305-310.
9. Sellner F, Jelinek R, Machacek E. Zur diagnostischen und therapeutischen Problematik der Adenome der Papilla Vateri. *Aktuelle Chir.* 1984;19:211-214.
10. Ryan PR, Schapiro RH, Warshaw AL. Villous tumor of the duodenum. *Ann Surg.* 1986;203:301-306.
11. Sellner F, Machacek E. Zur Entstehung der Karzinome der Papilla Vateri über eine Adenom-Karzinom-Sequenz: eine Analyse des eigenen Krankengutes und eine Literaturübersicht. *Wien Klin Wochenschr.* 1986;98:182-187.
12. Dupas JL, Marti R, Capron JP, Delamarre J. Villous adenoma of the duodenum: endoscopic diagnosis and resection. *Endoscopy.* 1977;9:245-247.
13. Seifert E, Schulte F, Stolte M. Adenoma and carcinoma of the duodenum and papilla of Vater: a clinicopathologic study. *Am J Gastroenterol.* 1992;87:37-42.
14. Beger HG, Staib L, Schoenberg MH. Ampullectomy for adenoma of the papilla and ampulla of Vater. *Langenbecks Arch Surg.* 1998;383:190-193.
15. Cubilla AL, Fitzgerald PJ. Surgical pathologic aspects of the ampulla-head-of-the-pancreas-region. In: Fitzgerald PJ, Morrison AB, eds. *The Pancreas.* Baltimore, Md: Williams & Wilkins; 1980:67-81.
16. Marty O, Aubertin JM, Bouillot JL, Hernigou A, Bloch F, Petite JP. Prospective comparison of ultrasound endoscopy and computed tomography in the assessment of locoregional invasiveness of malignant ampulla and pancreatic tumors verified surgically. *Gastroenterol Clin Biol.* 1995;19:197-203.
17. Farouk M, Niotis M, Branum GD, Cotton PB, Meyers WC. Indications for and the technique of local resection of tumors of the papilla of Vater. *Arch Surg.* 1991; 126:650-652.
18. Bittner R, Roscher R, Safi F, Dopfer HP, Schölzel E, Beger HG. Der Einfluß von Tumorgröße und Lymphknotenstatus auf die Prognose des Pankreaskarzinoms. *Chirurg.* 1989;60:240-245.
19. Fockens P, Huibregtse K. Staging of pancreatic and ampullary cancer by endoscopy. *Endoscopy.* 1993;25:52-57.
20. Klein P, Reingruber B, Kartl S, Dvorak O, Hohenberger W. Is local excision of pT1-ampullary carcinomas justified? *Eur J Surg Oncol.* 1996;22:366-371.
21. Jones TR, Nance FC. Periampullary malignancy in Gardner's syndrome. *Ann Surg.* 1977;185:565-573.
22. Schulten MF, Oyasu R, Beal JM. Villous adenoma of the duodenum: a case report and review of the literature. *Am J Surg.* 1976;132:90-96.
23. Martin FM, Rossi RL, Dorrucci V, Silverman ML, Braasch JW. Clinical and pathologic correlations in patients with periampullary tumors. *Arch Surg.* 1990;125: 723-726.
24. Halsted WS. Contributions to the surgery of the bile passages, especially of the common bile duct. *Boston Med Surg J.* 1899;141:645-652.
25. Asbun HJ, Rossi RL, Munson JL. Local resection for ampullary tumors: is there a place for it? *Arch Surg.* 1993;128:515-520.
26. Makipour H, Cooperman A, Danzi JT, Farmer RG. Carcinoma of the ampulla of Vater: review of 38 cases with emphasis on treatment and prognostic factors. *Ann Surg.* 1975;183:341-344.
27. Böttger TC, Boddin J, Heintz A, Junginger T. Clinicopathologic study for the assessment of resection for ampullary carcinoma. *World J Surg.* 1997;21:379-383.
28. Newman RJ, Pittam MR. Local excision in the treatment of carcinoma of the ampulla of Vater. *J R Coll Surg Edinb.* 1982;27:154-157.
29. Kausch W. Das Carcinom der Papilla duodeni und seine radikale Entfernung. *Beitr Klin Chir.* 1912;78:439-451.
30. Knox RA, Kingston RD. Carcinoma of the ampulla of Vater. *Br J Surg.* 1986;73: 72-73.
31. Goldberg M, Zamir O, Hadary Y, Nissan S. Wide local excision as an alternative treatment for periampullary carcinoma. *Am J Gastroenterol.* 1987;82:1169-1171.
32. Nakase A, Matsumuto Y, Uchida K, Honjo I. Surgical treatment of cancer of the pancreas and the periampullary region: cumulative results in 57 institutions in Japan. *Ann Surg.* 1977;185:52-57.
33. Harada N, Treitschke F, Imaizumi T, Beger HG. Pancreatic invasion is a prognostic indicator after radical resection for carcinoma of the ampulla of Vater. *J Hepato-Biliary-Pancreatic Surg.* 1997;4:215-219.
34. Kawarada Y, Takahashi K, Takata M, Isaji M, Ogura Y, Mizumoto R. Surgical treatment of carcinoma of the papilla of Vater. *J Hepato-Biliary-Pancreatic Surg.* 1993; 1:8-13.
35. Hanyu F, Imaizumi T, Nakamura M, Yoshikawa T. Proposed definition of early cancer of the papilla of Vater. *J Biliary Tract Pancreas.* 1984;5:847-852.
36. Willett CG, Warshaw AL, Convery K, Compton CC. Patterns of failure after pancreaticoduodenectomy for ampullary carcinoma. *Surg Gynecol Obstet.* 1993; 176:33-38.

ARCHIVES OF SURGERY

SUBSCRIPTION ORDER FORM

YES! Enter my personal subscription to ***Archives of Surgery*** at the special money saving rate checked below:

- ❑ AMA Member rate: One year (12 issues) — $95*.
- ❑ Individual non-member rate: One year (12 issues) — $145*.
- ❑ Corporate/Institutional rate: One year (12 issues) — $245.
- ❑ *My personal check in U.S. $ is enclosed. (Make check payable to *American Medical Association*).

❑ Charge my personal credit card: ❑ VISA ❑ MASTERCARD ❑ AMEX ❑ OPTIMA

Card No.__________ Exp. Date__________ Signature__________

Name (Please print) __________

Address __________

City__________ State/Province__________ Zip/Postal Code __________

Phone__________ Fax__________ e-mail __________

IMPORTANT: The individual non-member rate is available in the U.S. and Canada only. Payment must accompany order. Corporate/Institutional checks are not accepted for personal subscriptions. Canada residents add 7% GST. GST # (12622 5556 RT). I9X1DZ

ARCHIVES OF SURGERY

SUBSCRIPTION ORDER FORM

YES! Enter my personal subscription to ***Archives of Surgery*** at the special money saving rate checked below:

- ❑ AMA Member rate: One year (12 issues) — $95*.
- ❑ Individual non-member rate: One year (12 issues) — $145*.
- ❑ Corporate/Institutional rate: One year (12 issues) — $245.
- ❑ *My personal check in U.S. $ is enclosed. (Make check payable to *American Medical Association*).

❑ Charge my personal credit card: ❑ VISA ❑ MASTERCARD ❑ AMEX ❑ OPTIMA

Card No.__________ Exp. Date__________ Signature__________

Name (Please print) __________

Address __________

City__________ State/Province__________ Zip/Postal Code __________

Phone__________ Fax__________ e-mail __________

IMPORTANT: The individual non-member rate is available in the U.S. and Canada only. Payment must accompany order. Corporate/Institutional checks are not accepted for personal subscriptions. Canada residents add 7% GST. GST # (12622 5556 RT). I9X1DZ

NO POSTAGE NECESSARY IF MAILED IN THE UNITED STATES

BUSINESS REPLY MAIL
FIRST-CLASS MAIL PERMIT NO. 1376 CHICAGO IL

POSTAGE WILL BE PAID BY ADDRESSEE

SUBSCRIBER SERVICES CENTER
AMERICAN MEDICAL ASSOCIATION
PO BOX 10945
CHICAGO IL 60610-9902

NO POSTAGE NECESSARY IF MAILED IN THE UNITED STATES

BUSINESS REPLY MAIL
FIRST-CLASS MAIL PERMIT NO. 1376 CHICAGO IL

POSTAGE WILL BE PAID BY ADDRESSEE

SUBSCRIBER SERVICES CENTER
AMERICAN MEDICAL ASSOCIATION
PO BOX 10945
CHICAGO IL 60610-9902

Tolerance of the Liver to Intermittent Pringle Maneuver in Hepatectomy for Liver Tumors

Kwan Man, MB, PhD; Sheung-Tat Fan, MS, MD, FRCS(Glasg & Edin); Irene O. L. Ng, MD, FRCPath; Chung-Mau Lo, MBBS, MS, FRCS(Edin), FRACS; Chi-Leung Liu, MBBS, FRCS(Edin); Wan-Ching Yu, MB; John Wong, PhD, FRACS, FRCS(Edin)

Background: Hepatectomy can be performed with a low mortality rate, but massive hemorrhage during the operation remains a potentially lethal problem. The Pringle maneuver is traditionally used during hepatectomy to reduce blood loss, but the effect on the metabolic function of hepatocytes is potentially harmful. Although our randomized study showed that an intermittent Pringle maneuver is safe and effective during hepatectomy, the upper limit of the duration of the Pringle maneuver is not known.

Hypothesis: The liver can tolerate intermittent Pringle maneuver if the duration is not excessive.

Design: From July 20, 1995, to November 25, 1997, 112 patients underwent hepatectomy for liver tumors. The data of 50 patients who had hepatectomy without the Pringle maneuver were compared with those of 62 patients who had a liver transection using a Pringle maneuver for 20 minutes and a 5-minute clamp-free interval. The data were collected prospectively.

Main Outcome Measures: The surface area of liver transection was measured, and blood loss during liver transection per centimeter square of transection area was calculated. Routine liver biochemical tests, arterial ketone body ratio (AKBR), and plasma cytokine—interleukin (IL) 1α, 1β, 2, and 6, and tumor necrosis factor α—levels were measured before and after the operation. The morbidity and hospital mortality rates were also compared among the patients with different ischemic durations and those without an intermittent Pringle maneuver.

Setting: Tertiary referral center.

Results: The cutoff point of accumulated ischemic time that induced substantial liver damage, as shown by the postoperative recovery rate of the AKBR, was found to be 120 minutes. Compared with the control group, the patients whose accumulated ischemic time was shorter than 120 minutes had less blood loss related to transection area (10 mL/cm^2 vs 22 mL/cm^2; $P<.001$), less blood transfused (0 L vs 0.6 L; $P=.004$), a shorter transection time related to transection area (2.0 min/cm^2 vs 2.8 min/cm^2; $P=.002$), a significantly higher AKBR in the first 2 hours after liver transection, an equal recovery rate of the AKBR, and a comparable increase of the plasma level of IL-6 postoperatively. For the patients whose accumulated ischemic time was longer than 120 minutes, blood loss from the transection area was less than for the control group (14 mL/cm^2 vs 22 mL/cm^2; $P<.05$), but the transection time related to the transection area and the blood transfusion volume did not differ from those of the control group. Furthermore, they had a significantly lower recovery rate of the AKBR and higher plasma levels of IL-6 postoperatively than the control group.

Conclusion: The upper limit of tolerance of the liver to intermittent Pringle maneuver is 120 minutes.

Arch Surg. 1999;134:533-539

HEPATIC VASCULAR control is used by many surgeons to prevent massive hemorrhage during hepatectomy. The hepatic vascular inflow occlusion provides a relatively bloodless operative field and allows an unhurried, meticulous, and accurate intrahepatic dissection and hemostasis. There is always a risk of ischemic damage to the hepatocytes, however, especially in patients with chronic liver disease, the degree of which is likely to be accentuated with a prolonged period of vascular inflow occlusion. Within the period of ischemia that the liver can tolerate, the liver can recover from the operative and ischemic injury. Otherwise, a deterioration of liver function will ensue. The duration of the

From the Departments of Surgery (Drs Man, Fan, Lo, Liu, Yu, and Wong) and Pathology (Dr Ng), The University of Hong Kong, Queen Mary Hospital, Hong Kong, China.

PATIENTS AND METHODS

From July 20, 1995, to November 25, 1997, 112 patients (aged >18 years) undergoing hepatectomy were included in the study. The first 100 consecutive patients had been included in a randomized trial[1] for the evaluation of the Pringle maneuver (50 patients had hepatectomy under the Pringle maneuver, and 50 patients did not). The rest of the patients, seen from March 29 to November 25, 1997, received major hepatectomy with the use of an intermittent Pringle maneuver. The procedure of the intermittent Pringle maneuver was applied at the time of liver transection and consisted of cross-clamping the hepatoduodenal ligament (and the aberrant left hepatic artery, if that was present) for 20 minutes and releasing the clamp for 5 minutes until the liver transection was completed. Liver transection was performed in all patients by an ultrasonic dissector. Major hepatectomy was defined according to Goldsmith and Woodburne nomenclature[2] as the resection of 2 or more liver segments. For patients with a major hepatectomy, hilar dissection was done to ligate and divide the ipsilateral branch of the hepatic artery and portal vein. Minor hepatectomy was defined as the resection of only 1 or less than 1 segment. The study protocol was approved by the Ethics Committee of The University of Hong Kong, Hong Kong, China. Informed consent was obtained from every patient before the operation.

PREOPERATIVE ASSESSMENT

All patients had an indocyanine green clearance test[3]; measurement of the arterial ketone body ratio (acetoacetate to β-hydroxybutyrate [AKBR]) and serum transferrin, prealbumin, and retinol-binding protein levels; and routine liver and renal biochemical tests. The AKBR was performed by the method described by Ozawa,[4] using commercial kits (Ketorex; Sanwa Kagaku Kenkyusho Co, Nagoya, Japan) and a spectrophotometer[5] (Keto-340 II; Sanwa Kagaku Kenkyusho Co). Transferrin, prealbumin, and retinol-binding protein levels were measured by rate nephelometry using an array analyzer (Beckman Array Analyzer; Beckman Instruments Inc, Fullerton, Calif). Plasma levels of cytokines (interleukin [IL] 1α, IL-1β, IL-2, IL-6, and tumor necrosis factor α) were measured in 40 patients (24 patients in the group having the Pringle maneuver and 16 patients in the control group) in the latter part of the study. The levels of cytokines were measured by enzyme-linked immunosorbent assay (Quantikine kit; R&D Systems, Minneapolis, Minn), and the data were analyzed by commercial software (Softmax for Windows 95; Molecular Devices, Sunnyvale, Calif).

INTRAOPERATIVE ASSESSMENT

The AKBR and cytokine levels were measured before, during, and after liver transection and then hourly for 4 hours. The volume of blood loss was accurately measured before, during, and after liver transection from the weight of the soaked gauze, blood collected from the containers of suction apparatus, and an ultrasonic dissector. The volume of irrigation fluid was deducted accordingly. The blood loss was assessed in 3 phases of hepatectomy because the efficacy of the Pringle maneuver was measured mainly by the amount of blood loss during the transection phase. The duration of the liver transection was noted. After the liver transection was completed, the transection surface was marked on a piece of transparent plastic sheet. It was immediately transcribed to a piece of paper containing marks of square millimeter for the measurement of the area of liver transection surface. The blood loss during transection was expressed as milliliters per square centimeter of liver transection surface. Similarly, the liver transection time was expressed as minutes per square centimeter of liver transection surface. The liver transection time was measured from the beginning to the end of the liver transection. The ischemic time was the accumulated total duration of the application of the Pringle maneuver.

POSTOPERATIVE ASSESSMENT

The AKBR and cytokine levels were measured after the operation each day for the first 2 days. Serum transferrin, prealbumin, and retinol-binding protein levels were measured on postoperative days 1, 4, and 8. Routine hematologic tests and liver and renal biochemical tests were performed daily for 7 days. The indocyanine green clearance test was repeated on postoperative day 8. The recovery rate of the AKBR postoperatively was defined as follows: the AKBR minus the AKBR immediately after transection was divided by the AKBR immediately after transection.

STATISTICAL ANALYSIS

Results are expressed as medians and ranges. The Mann-Whitney *U* test was used to compare continuous variables. The χ^2 test was used to compare discrete variables. Significance was defined as $P<.05$. All the statistical analyses were made using a commercial statistical software package (SPSS for Windows; SPSS Inc, Chicago, Ill).

liver's tolerance to the Pringle maneuver remains the major concern of liver surgeons. We did this study to define the duration of Pringle maneuver that the liver can tolerate without substantial posthepatectomy injury.

RESULTS

The postoperative recovery rate of the AKBR was compared between the control group and the group having the Pringle maneuver with different accumulated ischemic times (**Figure 1**). The recovery rate for the group having the Pringle maneuver was significantly lower than that of the control group when the accumulated ischemic time exceeded 120 minutes in the third and fourth hours after liver transection and on the second day postoperatively. The upper limit of the Pringle maneuver was then set at 120 minutes. According to this upper limit of ischemic duration, the patients were categorized into Pringle group 1 (n = 50), whose accumulated ischemic time did not exceed 120 minutes; Pringle group 2 (n = 12), whose accumulated ischemic time exceeded 120 minutes; and a control group (n = 50) in whom hepatectomy was performed without a Pringle maneuver. The 3 groups of patients were comparable in terms of the hematologic status and liver biochemical test results, except the serum alanine aminotransferase (ALT) levels (**Table 1**). The tumor size, the proportion of patients with major hepatectomy, and the prevalence of chronic liver diseases were similar among the 3 groups (**Table 2**).

Compared with the control group, the benefit of Pringle maneuver was mainly seen in the patients in Pringle group 1 (Table 2). There was a reduction in blood loss per transection area, transection time per transection area, and blood transfusion requirement in the patients in Pringle group 1. In the patients in Pringle group 2, compared with those in the control group, there was a reduction only in blood loss per transection area, but their blood transfusion requirement and transection time per transection area were not reduced.

In the postoperative period, the AKBR recovery rate of the patients in Pringle group 1 was comparable with those in the control group. On the contrary, the patients in Pringle group 2 manifested a value of AKBR recovery rate less than 0 in the first 4 hours, indicating that their recovery was delayed (**Figure 2**, top).

Because of the higher preoperative serum ALT levels in the patients whose accumulated ischemic time exceeded 120 minutes, the difference between preoperative and postoperative levels of serum alanine aminotransferase was compared among the 3 groups to assess the degree of parenchymal injury. The increase of serum ALT levels of the patients in Pringle group 2 was significantly higher (*P*<.05) than that of the patients in the control group and Pringle group 1 throughout the first 6 postoperative days (**Figure 3**). The serum bilirubin levels of the patients in the 2 Pringle groups were lower than those of the control group, but compared with the control group, a significantly lower (*P*<.05) serum bilirubin level was found only in the patients in Pringle group 1 (**Figure 4**). A significantly higher (*P*<.05) level of increase of IL-6 postoperatively was seen in patients in Pringle 2 group than in those in the control group and Pringle group 1 (**Figure 5**, top).

Further analysis was made in the patients with chronic liver diseases (liver cirrhosis and chronic hepatitis). The analysis indicated similar findings as in the whole group of patients (**Table 3** and Figures 2 [bottom] and 5 [bottom]).

The levels of the plasma IL-1α and -1β, IL-2, and tumor necrosis factor α were very low before and after liver transection in patients in all 3 groups. The levels of 3 short-half-life carrier proteins and albumin and the degree of deterioration of indocyanine green clearance did not differ significantly between the 2 Pringle groups and the control group, whatever the liver status (*P*>.05).

Although morbidity among the 3 groups did not differ significantly (Table 2), whatever the liver status, there was a tendency of a higher postoperative complication rate in the patients whose accumulated ischemic duration exceeded 120 minutes, especially those with a cirrhotic liver (Tables 2 and 3). The details of the postoperative complications are listed in **Table 4**.

A subphrenic abscess developed in 1 patient with a normal liver in Pringle group 1 (accumulated ischemic

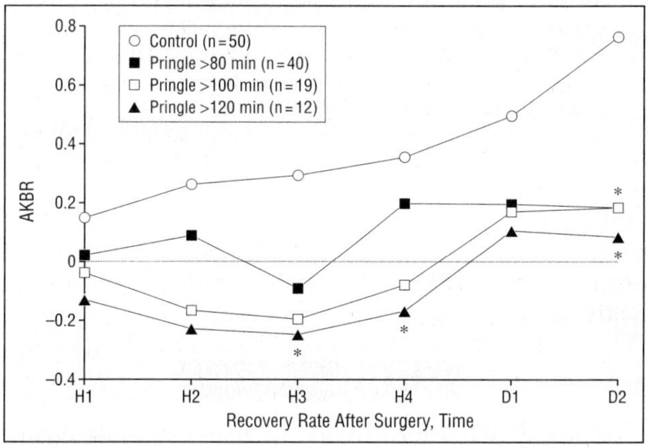

Figure 1. *The recovery rate of the arterial ketone body ratio (AKBR) in the patients undergoing a Pringle maneuver with different ischemic durations compared with the control group, as measured hourly (H) during the first 4 hours after surgery and days (D) 1 and 2. The recovery rate of the AKBR = (AKBR − AKBR immediately after transection)/AKBR immediately after transection. Pringle >80 minutes, Pringle >100 minutes, and Pringle >120 minutes indicate patients having the Pringle maneuver with accumulated ischemic durations longer than 80, 100, and 120 minutes, respectively; asterisk,* P<*.05, patients having the Pringle maneuver (various durations) vs control group.*

Table 1. Preoperative Data of Patients With Hepatectomy With the Pringle Maneuver and Control Patients*

Variable	Control Group (n = 50)	Pringle Group 1 (n = 50)	Pringle Group 2 (n = 12)
Age, y	52.5 (25-80)	52 (19-79)	50 (37-70)
Sex, M/F	41:9	39:11	10:2
Hemoglobin level, g/L	13.8 (8.6-16.5)	14.2 (8.7-16.6)	14.5 (11.0-17.0)
Platelet count, × 10^9/L	198.5 (65-421)	183.5 (52-479)	211.0 (82-317)
Prothrombin time, s	10.9 (9.4-13.9)	11.3 (9.5-15.3)	10.7 (9.8-11.7)
Serum levels			
Total bilirubin, µmol/L†	11.0 (5.0-27.0)	11.0 (3.0-29.0)	11.0 (4.0-34.0)
Aspartate aminotransferase, U/L	36 (16-227)	35 (10-148)	59 (10-283)
Alanine aminotransferase, U/L	34.0 (8-344)	38.0 (8-207)	67.5 (10-174)‡
Albumin, g/L	41 (23-50)	41 (30-50)	41 (35-48)
Arterial ketone body ratio	0.86 (0.15-3.20)	0.85 (0.18-3.10)	0.91 (0.35-1.82)
Indocyanine green retention at 15 min, %	8.4 (1.6-26.5)	8.7 (1.4-52.7)	9.2 (4.3-21.2)

**Pringle group 1 indicates patients with accumulated ischemic time <120 minutes; Pringle group 2, patients with accumulated ischemic time >120 minutes. Values are given as median (range).*

†*To convert bilirubin from micromoles per liter to milligrams per deciliter, divide micromoles per liter by 17.1.*

‡P<*.05, Pringle group 2 vs control group and Pringle group 1.*

Table 2. Intraoperative and Postoperative Data on All Patients Undergoing Hepatectomy With or Without Pringle Maneuver*

Variable	Control Group (n = 50)	Pringle Group 1 (n = 50)	Pringle Group 2 (n = 12)	P† Control Group vs Pringle Group 1	P† Control Group vs Pringle Group 2	P† Pringle Group 1 vs Pringle Group 2
Ischemia duration, min	0	83 (24-114)	134.5 (123-201)	. . .	. . .	**<.001**
Major hepatectomy, No. (%)	35 (70)	33 (66)	10 (83.3)	. . .	. . .	. . .
Cirrhosis, No. (%)	16 (32)	18 (36)	1 (8.3)	. . .	. . .	. . .
Chronic hepatitis, No. (%)	12 (24)	15 (30)	7 (58.3)	. . .	. . .	. . .
Normal liver, No. (%)	22 (44)	17 (34)	4 (33.3)	. . .	. . .	. . .
Tumor size, cm	6.4 (2-23)	5.0 (1-15)	8.0 (0.3-17.0)	.51	.59	.41
Transection area, cm^2	60.0 (16-155)	67.0 (22-130)	89.5 (58-115)	.42	**.004**	**.004**
Total blood loss, L	1.99 (0.26-13.90)	1.01 (0.23-9.02)	2.03 (0.56-9.42)	**<.001**	.74	.06
Blood loss during liver transection, L	1.41 (0.17-11.4)	0.56 (0.09-5.93)	1.36 (0.30-8.50)	**<.001**	.67	**.03**
Blood loss per transection area, mL/cm^2	22 (5-150)	10 (3-46)	14 (4-74)	**<.001**	**.05**	.23
Transection time, min	169.0 (40-463)	125.5 (33-245)	219.0 (174-300)	**.01**	**.01**	**<.001**
Transection time, min/cm^2	2.8 (0.2-6.0)	2.0 (0.9-4.2)	2.6 (1.8-3.6)	**.002**	.69	**.01**
Blood transfusion, L	0.6 (0-12.9)	0 (0-4.3)	0 (0-8.6)	**.002**	.44	.28
Blood transfusion, L‡	0.6 (0-9.9)	0 (0-4.3)	0 (0-8.6)	**.004**	.51	. . .
Postoperative complication, No. (%)	15 (30)	13 (26)	6 (50)	.66	.16	.10

*Values are given as median (range) except as otherwise noted. Ellipses indicate not applicable.

†Boldface values indicate statistical significance.

‡The comparison of blood transfusion among the 3 groups after excluding the patient in the control group whose blood transfusion was 12.9 L.

duration, 85 minutes), and the patient died of septicemia. Two patients in the control group with a normal liver died of liver failure (1 patient) and renal failure (1 patient).

COMMENT

The history of hepatic surgery is always a struggle against bleeding. Uncontrollable massive hemorrhage will lead to a deterioration of liver function and increased postoperative morbidity and mortality. Among all procedures of vascular control in hepatectomy, the Pringle maneuver is the simplest one to apply and was shown to be effective in reducing bleeding.[1] The limit of ischemic period that the liver can tolerate, however, remains the major concern of many surgeons. Elias et al[6] reported that an intermittent Pringle maneuver might be used for longer than 120 minutes without major complications, even in abnormal livers. Huguet et al[7] showed that patients with chronic liver diseases had increased postoperative morbidity and mortality rates after 60 minutes of continuous vascular exclusion. Kim et al[8] demonstrated that prolonged hepatic inflow occlusion could be used during hepatectomy for up to 60 minutes without serious complication in selected patients with active chronic liver disease. Wu et al[9] suggested that a cirrhotic liver could tolerate intermittent ischemia for up to 200 minutes without increased postoperative morbidity and mortality and serious long-term sequelae. All of these studies, however, were retrospective and focused on the clinical results and the levels of liver enzymes. A consistent result was not obtained from all these studies.

To find out the cutoff point of the ischemic duration during which the liver function is well preserved, we compared the postoperative recovery rate of the AKBR between the patients with a Pringle maneuver under different accumulated ischemic durations and the patients without a Pringle maneuver (Figure 1). The AKBR was chosen because it reflects the liver mitochondrial function, which is essential in maintaining liver cell viability under stress,[4,10] and is a useful marker for hepatic tolerance to portal triad cross-clamping in cirrhotic liver resection[11] and the energy status of the hepatic remnant.[12] The accuracy of the AKBR in reflecting liver function status was questioned by 2 recent studies[13,14] because the AKBR in these 2 studies varied greatly among individual patients for different periods. The difference may be explained by different extents of the use of the 2 types of ketone body, which probably depend on the blood glucose level and the adequacy of the perfusion of extrahepatic tissues. To reduce the effects of the differences among individual patients, we used the AKBR recovery rate, which was assessed only within a short time after hepatectomy, so that the variation in the condition that can affect the use of ketone bodies can be reduced. Unlike in other studies, the serum ALT level was not chosen because it happened that the patients in Pringle group 2 had a higher preoperative serum ALT level than did other patients.

The patients benefited from a Pringle maneuver and had a better preservation of liver function than the control group if the Pringle maneuver was used for less than 120 minutes. Within the 120 minutes' duration of ischemia, the recovery rate of the AKBR was well maintained even in the patients with cirrhosis. The delay of AKBR recovery in the patients whose accumulated ischemic time exceeded 120 minutes suggested that the liver was seriously injured and needed more time to recover from the acute stress (**Figure 6**). Furthermore, the increase of serum ALT levels was much higher in the patients whose ischemic time exceeded 120 minutes. Similarly, the lower level of bilirubin in the group having the Pringle maneuver was only contributed by the patients

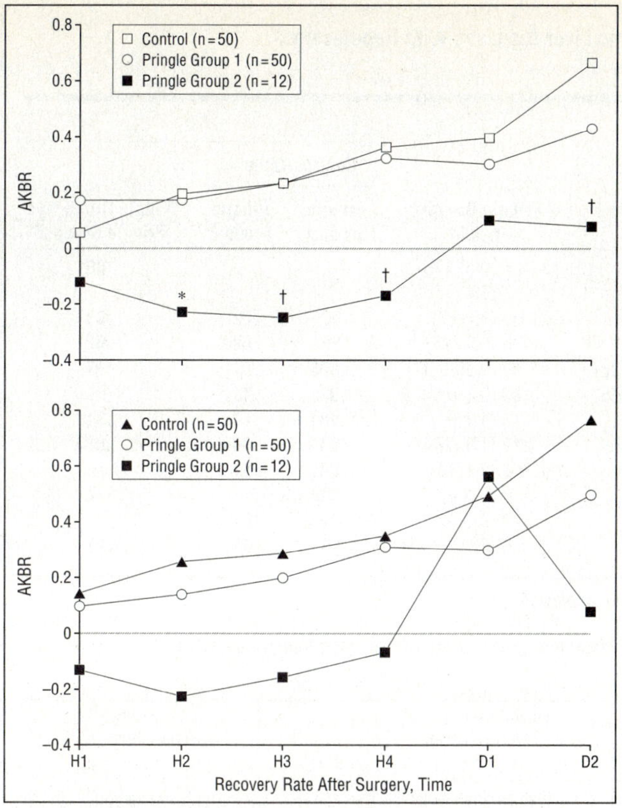

Figure 2. *The recovery rate of the arterial ketone body ratio (AKBR) of all patients (top) and patients with chronic liver diseases (bottom), as measured hourly (H) in the first 4 hours after liver transection and days (D) 1 and 2. Pringle group 1 indicates patients having an accumulated ischemic duration shorter than 120 minutes; Pringle group 2, patients with an accumulated ischemic duration longer than 120 minutes; asterisk, the difference between Pringle group 2 vs control group is significant; and dagger, the difference between Pringle group 2 vs Pringle group 1 is significant (*P*<.05 for both).*

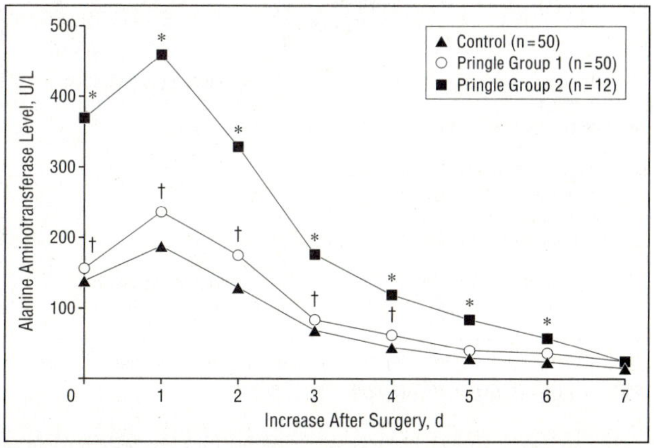

Figure 3. *Time of increase of serum alanine aminotransferase levels (compared with preoperative levels) of all patients postoperatively, by days measured. Asterisk indicates the difference between Pringle group 2 vs control group is significant; dagger, the difference between Pringle group 1 vs Pringle group 2 is significant (*P*<.05 for both).*

in Pringle group 1. The findings were further supported by the levels of IL-6, which is a response to ischemia-reperfusion injury[15] and correlates with complications and the mortality.[16] The levels of IL-6 were significantly higher in the patients whose ischemic time exceeded 120 minutes.

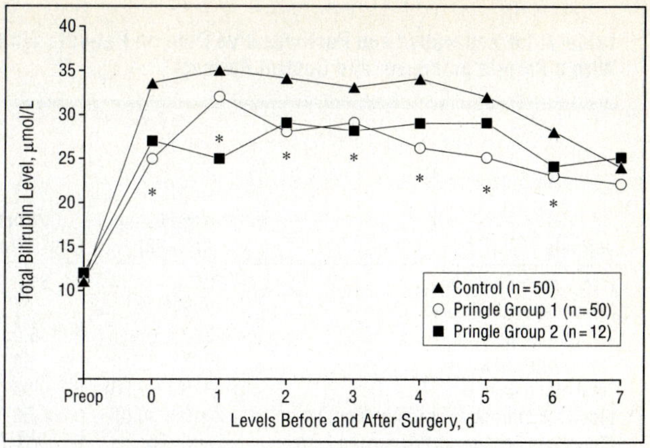

Figure 4. *Time of serum total bilirubin levels of all patients immediately before and after surgery, by days measured. Asterisk indicates the difference between Pringle group 1 vs control group is significant (*P*<.05).*

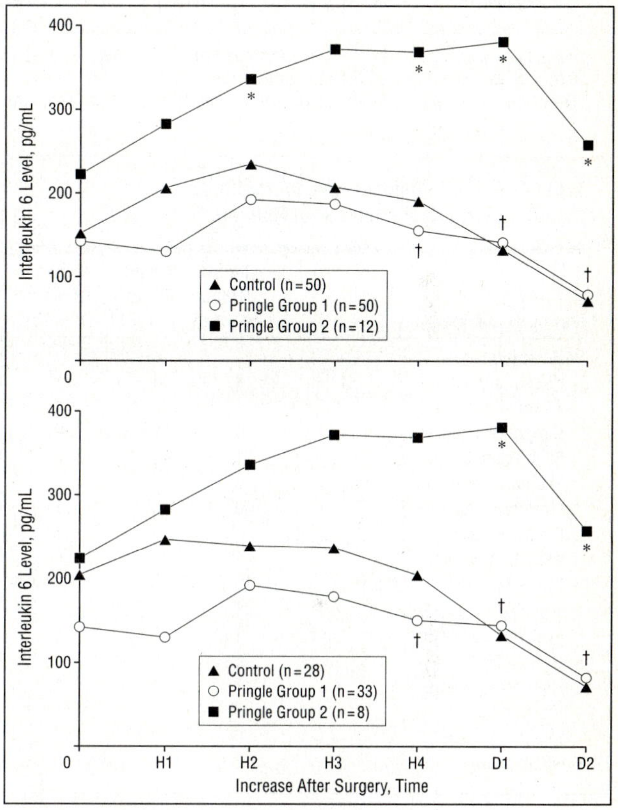

Figure 5. *The increase of plasma interleukin 6 (IL-6) levels (compared with preoperative IL-6 levels) in all patients (top) and patients with chronic liver disease (bottom), as measured immediately, hourly (H) the first 4 hours, and days (D) 1 and 2 after liver transection. Asterisk indicates the difference between Pringle group 2 vs control group is significant; dagger, the difference between Pringle group 2 vs Pringle group 1 is significant (*P*<.05 for both).*

Consistent with the experience of Japanese investigators,[17] tumor necrosis factor α, which is considered to be the main and the first wave of cytokine synthesis under stress[18] and is related to ischemia-reperfusion injury,[19] could not be found in the control and Pringle groups of our series. Contrary to previous experience,[20] IL-1α and IL-1β, the production of which should respond to stress promptly,[18,21] was found in low levels in all patients in the present study. The difference may be

Table 3. Intraoperative and Postoperative Data on Patients With Chronic Liver Diseases With Hepatectomy With a Pringle Maneuver and Control Patients*

				P†		
				Control Group vs		
Variable	**Control Group (n = 28)**	**Pringle Group 1 (n = 33)**	**Pringle Group 2 (n = 8)**	**Pringle Group 1**	**Pringle Group 2**	**Pringle Group 1 vs Pringle Group 2**
Ischemia duration, min	0	81.0 (24-112)	134.5 (126-175)	. . .	. . .	**<.001**
Major hepatectomy, No. (%)	19 (68)	21 (64)	7 (88)	. . .	. . .	. . .
Tumor size, cm	5.2 (2-13)	5.0 (1-15)	11.0 (3.1-17)	.90	**.02**	**.03**
Transection area, cm²	59 (35-155)	60 (22-107)	84.5 (58-115)	.68	**.004**	**.02**
Total blood loss, L	1.99 (0.79-9.36)	0.93 (0.23-3.26)	2.08 (0.56-9.42)	**.003**	.79	.13
Blood loss during liver transection, L	1.24 (0.31-6.0)	0.52 (0.09-2.55)	1.38 (0.3-8.5)	**<.001**	.73	.07
Blood loss per transection area, mL/cm²	23 (5-98)	10 (3-33)	13 (4-74)	**<.001**	.17	.34
Transection time, min	140 (89-260)	127 (33-244)	219 (175-264)	**.04**	**.006**	**.003**
Transection time, min/cm²	2.9 (1.1-5.3)	2.0 (0.9-4.2)	2.6 (2.1-3.5)	**.007**	.59	.70
Blood transfusion, L	0.3 (0-12.9)	0 (0-1.0)	0 (0-3.6)	**.003**	.45	.17
Blood transfusion, L‡	0 (0-9.0)	0 (0-1.0)	0 (0-3.6)	**.005**	.54	. . .
Postoperative complication, No. (%)	8 (29)	11 (33)	5 (62)	.69	.09	.13

Values are given as median (range) except as otherwise noted. Ellipses indicate not applicable.
†Boldface values indicate statistical significance.
‡The comparison of blood transfusion among the 3 groups after excluding the patient in the control group whose blood transfusion was 12.9 L.

Table 4. Overall Postoperative Morbidity and Hospital Mortality by Number of Patients*

Morbidity and Mortality	**Control Group (n = 50)**	**Pringle Group 1 (n = 50)**	**Pringle Group 2 (n = 12)**
Complication			
Pulmonary	8	4	1
Wound infection	4	2	1
Subphrenic abscess	0	1 (1)	0
Biliary fistula	1	1	0
Pseudomembranous colitis	0	1	0
Limb cellulitis	0	0	1
Pleural effusion	6	3	1
Wound dehiscence	1	0	0
Intra-abdominal bleeding	1	1	0
Bleeding peptic ulcer	1	1	1
Superior mesenteric vein thrombosis	1 (1)	0	0
Uremia	1 (1)	0	0
Pulmonary edema	1	1	1
Incision hernia	0	0	1
Infected ascites	0	0	1
Hospital death	**2**	**1**	**0**

The numbers in parentheses indicate patients who died of the complication.

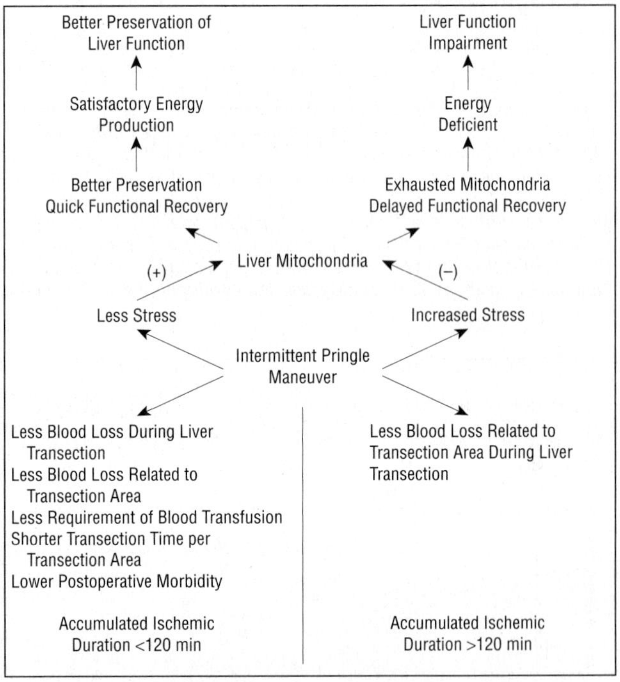

Figure 6. *Tolerance of the liver to an intermittent Pringle maneuver. Plus sign indicates protects; minus sign, compromises.*

because the Pringle maneuver was used in a continuous manner in the aforementioned studies, but in the present studies, it was used in an intermittent manner. Conceivably, an intermittent Pringle maneuver induces less stress and better preservation of liver sinusoidal cells, which are the major source of cytokine production.

The patients whose accumulated ischemic time exceeded 120 minutes had a larger transection area (Table 2). This is likely to be the case in patients who require the resection of middle segments of the liver, such as the right anterior segment or left medial segment. To avoid the prolongation of ischemia in such patients, the ipsilateral inflow pedicle may be clamped while transecting one side of liver segment.[22] When the ischemic duration exceeds 120 minutes and the liver transection is not yet completed, it may be advisable to continue the liver transection without the Pringle maneuver because the risk of liver failure negates the benefit of reducing blood loss. Fortunately, when the liver transection is nearly completed, the major source of bleeding is from the hepatic vein, and the need for the Pringle maneuver is diminished.

The liver is able to tolerate an intermittent Pringle maneuver within 120 minutes because it is not rendered totally ischemic.[23] The presence of hepatovenous back-perfusion plays a critical role during the Pringle maneuver. Tatsuma et al[24] showed that backflow from the hepatic veins could maintain liver adenosine triphosphate synthesis and, hence, liver viability during the Pringle maneuver. The perfusion of liver by hepatovenous backflow, however, is never perfect. In an animal experiment, continuous hepatic inflow interruption for 90 or 120 minutes resulted in severe injury to hepatic cells and liver sinusoids and in multiorgan failure.[25] In the present study, a tendency toward a higher incidence of postoperative complications was found in the patients whose accumulated ischemic duration exceeded 120 minutes. Therefore, liver transection using the Pringle maneuver has to be performed as expeditiously as possible.

CONCLUSION

Intermittent Pringle maneuver during liver transection is well tolerated within 120 minutes, whatever the liver status.

We thank Edward D. Janus, MD, PhD, and his staff in the Department of Clinical Biochemistry, The University of Hong Kong, Hong Kong, China, for performing the prealbumin, transferrin, and retinol-binding protein assays. Chun Yeung, MBBS, FRCS, Wai-Key Yuen, MBBS, and Chi-Ming Lam, MS, FRCS(Edin), participated in the operations.

Corresponding author: Sheung-Tat Fan, MS, MD, FRCS (Glasg & Edin), Department of Surgery, The University of Hong Kong, Queen Mary Hospital, 102 Pokfulam Rd, Hong Kong, China (e-mail: hrmsfst@hkucc.hku.hk).

REFERENCES

1. Man K, Fan ST, Ng IOL, Lo CM, Liu CL, Wong J. Prospective evaluation of Pringle maneuver in hepatectomy for liver tumors by a randomized study. *Ann Surg.* 1997;226:704-713.
2. Goldsmith NA, Woodburne RT. Surgical anatomy pertaining to liver resection. *Surg Gynecol Obstet.* 1957;195:310-318.
3. Caesar J, Shaldon S, Chiandussi L, et al. The use of indocyanine green in the measurement of hepatic blood flow and as a test of hepatic function. *Clin Sci.* 1961;21:43-57.
4. Ozawa K. The role of mitochondrial compensatory ability. In: *Liver Surgery Approached Through the Mitochondria: The Redox Theory in Revolution.* Tokyo, Japan: Medical Tribune Inc; 1992.
5. Tsuburaya A, Blumberg D, Burt M, Brennan MF. Energy depletion in the liver and in isolated hepatocytes of tumor-bearing animals. *J Surg Res.* 1995;59:421-427.
6. Elias D, Desruennes E, Lasser P. Prolonged intermittent clamping of the portal triad during hepatectomy. *Br J Surg.* 1991;78:42-44.
7. Huguet C, Gavelli A, Bona S. Hepatic resection with ischemia of the liver exceeding one hour. *J Am Coll Surg.* 1994;178:454-458.
8. Kim YI, Kobayashi M, Aramaki M, Nakashima K, Akizuki S. Liver resections performed under prolonged portal triad occlusion in patients with active chronic liver diseases. *Surg Today.* 1994;24:328-332.
9. Wu CC, Hwang CR, Liu TJ, Peng FK. Effects and limitations of prolonged intermittent ischemia for hepatic resection of the cirrhotic liver. *Br J Surg.* 1996;83:121-124.
10. Nakatani T, Spolter L, Kobayashi K. Arterial ketone body ratio as a parameter of hepatic mitochondrial redox state during and after hemorrhagic shock. *World J Surg.* 1995;19:592-596.
11. Yamaoka Y, Shimahara Y, Nakatani T, et al. Clinical role of blood ketone body ratio as an indicator evaluating hepatic tolerance for portal triad cross-clamping in cirrhotic liver resection. *Surg Res Commun.* 1988;3:87-93.
12. Ukikusa M, Ozawa K, Shimahara Y, Asano M, Nakatani T, Tobe T. Changes in blood ketone body ratio: their significance after major hepatic resection. *Arch Surg.* 1981;116:781-785.
13. Matsushita K, Kawasaki S, Makuuchi M. Arterial ketone body ratio in liver surgery. *Hepatology.* 1994;20:331-335.
14. Hanazaki K, Wakabayashi M, Sodeyama H, et al. Arterial ketone body ratio during hepatectomy. *Hepatogastroenterology.* 1997;44:1438-1444.
15. McCurry KR, Campbell DA Jr, Scales WE, Warren JS, Remick DG. Tumor necrosis factor, interleukin 6, and the acute phase response following hepatic ischemia/reperfusion. *J Surg Res.* 1993;55:49-54.
16. Biffl WL, Moore EE, Moore FA, Peterson VM. Interleukin-6 in the injured patient: marker of injury or mediator of inflammation? *Ann Surg.* 1996;224:647-664.
17. Kita Y, Sakon M, Yoshida T, Gotoh M, Monden M. Pringle maneuver during hepatic resection induces inflammatory cytokines. *Dig Dis Sci.* 1996;41:2459-2460.
18. Fey GH, Hocke GM, Wilson DR, et al. Cytokines and the acute phase response of the liver. In: Arias M, Boyer L, Fausto N, eds. *The Liver: Biology and Pathobiology.* 3rd ed. New York, NY: Raven Press; 1994:113-120.
19. Colletti LM, Remick DG, Burtch GD, Kunkel SL, Strieter RM, Campbell DA Jr. Role of tumor necrosis factor-α in the pathophysiologic alterations after hepatic ischemia/reperfusion injury in the rat. *J Clin Invest.* 1990;85:1936-1943.
20. Shito M, Wakabayashi G, Ueda M, et al. Interleukin 1 receptor blockade reduces tumor necrosis factor production, tissue injury, and mortality after hepatic ischemia-reperfusion in the rat. *Transplantation.* 1997;63:143-148.
21. Ito A, Takii T, Soji T, Onozaki K. Endotoxin-induced upregulation of type I interleukin-1 receptor mRNA expression in hepatocytes of mice: role of cytokines. *J Interferon Cytokine Res.* 1997;17:55-61.
22. Makuuchi M, Mori T, Gunven P, Yamazaki S, Hasegawa H. Safety of hemihepatic vascular occlusion during resection of the liver. *Surg Gynecol Obstet.* 1987;164:155-158.
23. Kim YI, Ishii T, Aramaki M, Nakashima K, Yoshida T, Kobayashi M. The Pringle maneuver induces only partial ischemia of the liver. *Hepatogastroenterology.* 1995;42:169-171.
24. Tatsuma T, Kim YI, Kai T, et al. Importance of hepatovenous back-perfusion for maintenance of liver viability during the Pringle maneuver. *Br J Surg.* 1995;82:1071-1075.
25. Liu DL, Jeppsson B, Hakansson CH, Odselius R. Multiple-system organ damage resulting from prolonged hepatic inflow interruption. *Arch Surg.* 1996;131:442-447.

ORIGINAL ARTICLE

Major Surgery Suppresses Maximal Production of Helper T-Cell Type 1 Cytokines Without Potentiating the Release of Helper T-Cell Type 2 Cytokines

Ramon Berguer, MD; Capt Normita Bravo, MS, USAF; Mark Bowyer, MD; Craig Egan, MD; Tom Knolmayer, MD; David Ferrick, PhD

Background: Major surgery is known to suppress T-cell function; however, its differential effects on the production of helper T-cell type 1 (T_H1) and type 2 (T_H2) cytokines remains unknown.

Objective: To measure the production patterns of T_H1 (interleukin 2 [IL-2] and interferon γ) and T_H2 (IL-4 and IL-10) cytokines following major surgery.

Design, Setting, and Patients: A cohort study of patients (both active and former members of the armed forces) at a military hospital.

Intervention: Aortic surgery or carotid endarterectomy and measurement of serum IL-6 levels by enzyme-linked immunosorbent assay.

Main Outcome Measures: Unstimulated and stimulated intracellular levels of IL-2, IL-4, IL-10, and interferon γ in $CD4^+$, $CD8^+$, and $\gamma\delta^+$ T cells and serum IL-6 levels immediately before and for 2 days after aortic surgery or carotid endarterectomy.

Results: No unstimulated production of T_H1 or T_H2 cytokines was detected. Stimulated intracellular levels of IL-2 and interferon γ were significantly depressed during the postoperative period in all T-cell subsets in both patient groups. There were no postoperative increases in stimulated IL-4 or IL-10 levels.

Conclusion: Major surgery suppresses the potential responses of T_H1 cytokines without enhancing production of T_H2 cytokines.

Arch Surg. 1999;134:540-544

DURING THE past 2 decades, clinicians and researchers have recognized that surgery results in an impaired immune response in the early postoperative period[1] and that this phenomenon may contribute to infectious complications[2] and cancer metastasis.[3] The immunosuppressive effect of surgery has been variously attributed to serum factors,[4] stress hormones,[4,5] the activation of suppressor cells,[5,6] decreased secretion of the cytokines interferon γ (IFN-γ) and interleukin 2 (IL-2),[7,8] and, most recently, to a shift in the balance of helper T-cell type 1 (T_H1) and type 2 (T_H2) cytokines from peripheral blood mononuclear cells.[9,10] A better understanding of perioperative immune function might enable clinicians to stratify patients as immunologically high risk before surgery and take appropriate preventive action or delay surgery. Alternatively, patients demonstrating substantial postoperative immune suppression could be considered for additional prophylactic treatment aimed at reducing the risk of infectious complication.

The present study used recently developed flow cytometry techniques for direct intracellular cytokine measurements along with current concepts of lymphocyte immunomodulation to arrive at a more precise understanding of the effects of surgical injury on immune function. The hypothesis was that surgical trauma suppresses cytokines through an increase in the production of T_H2 cytokines.

RESULTS

The patient characteristics for the 2 surgical groups are listed in the **Table**. Complete blood cell counts (**Figure 1**) demonstrated significant postoperative increases in the numbers of neutrophils in both groups compared with preoperative levels. Absolute lymphocyte counts decreased in both groups compared with preoperative levels. The postoperative platelet count decreased significantly in the aortic surgery group but not in the ca-

From the Departments of Surgery (Dr Berguer) and Pathology, Microbiology, and Immunology (Dr Ferrick), University of California, Davis; Clinical Investigation Facility (Capt Bravo) and Surgical Flight (Drs Bowyer, Egan, and Knolmayer), David Grant Medical Center, Travis Air Force Base; Surgical Service, Department of Veterans Affairs, Northern California Health Care System, Martinez (Dr Berguer); and Rigel Inc, Sunnyvale (Dr Ferrick), Calif.

PATIENTS AND METHODS

This study consisted of a cohort of 18 patients in the Veterans Affairs and US Department of Defense who underwent elective aortic surgery ($n = 10$) or carotid endarterectomy ($n = 8$). The study was approved by the Institutional Review Board at David Grant Medical Center, Travis Air Force Base, Calif, and all patients signed informed consent forms prior to participation in the study. Entry criteria excluded patients with diseases known to affect the immune system, such as acquired immunodeficiency syndrome, chronic hepatitis B and C, known active malignancy, and the use of immunosuppressive medications. Samples of peripheral venous blood (20 mL in EDTA for flow cytometry and 7-mL clot tube for serum assays) were obtained by venipuncture from each patient no more than 6 hours preoperatively and every morning after surgery until discharge from the hospital or for a maximum of 5 days. A group of 17 healthy volunteers were studied as reference subjects.

T-cell subsets and their intracellular cytokine production were identified by multiparametric flow cytometry.[11-13] Peripheral blood mononuclear cells were isolated from 20 mL of anticoagulated (EDTA) venous blood by density centrifugation and incubated at 37°C in a 5% carbon dioxide incubator for 4 hours in RPMI (Roswell Park Memorial Institute; Sigma-Aldrich Corp, St Louis, Mo) medium containing 10-µg/mL brefeldin A (Epicentre Technologies, Madison, Wis) to dissaggregate the Golgi complex and enable the intracellular accumulation of proteins.[14] During the incubation period, half the cells were separately stimulated with 20-ng/mL phorbolmystrateacetate (Sigma-Aldrich Corp) and 1-µg/mL ionomycin (Sigma-Aldrich Corp) to assess submaximal cytokine production, while the other half remained unstimulated. After incubation, cell suspensions were divided into 18 tubes with approximately 1×10^6 cells per tube corresponding to cell type ($CD4^+$, $CD8^+$, or $\gamma\delta^+$), cytokine combination (isotype control, IFN-γ/IL-4, or IL-2/IL-10), and stimulation category (unstimulated or stimulated). Cells were resuspended in buffer (phosphate-buffered saline plus 0.1% sodium azide plus 1% bovine serum albumin plus 5-mmol EDTA) and incubated for 15 minutes at 25°C with a 1:5 dilution of Tricolor-conjugated (a tandem conjugate of phycoerythrin and Cy-5; Caltag Laboratories, San Francisco, Calif) anti-γδ T-cell receptor, anti-CD4, or anti-CD8 monoclonal antibodies for phenotypic identification. After washing in phosphate-buffered saline, cells were fixed in 100 µL of solution A (cell permeabilization fixation; Caltag Laboratories) for 15 minutes at 25°C and washed again in phosphate-buffered saline. Intracellular cytokines were identified by resuspension in 50 µL of the permeabilization solution B (Caltag Laboratories) containing a 1:500 dilution of dinitrophenyl-conjugated anti–IFN-γ and a 1:100 dilution of biotin-conjugated anti–IL-4; or dinitrophenyl-conjugated anti–IL-10 and biotin-conjugated anti–IL-2; or dinitrophenyl-conjugated anti-mouse IgG1 and biotin-conjugated anti-mouse IgG2 for 15 minutes at 25°C. Specific intracellular cytokine identification was achieved by subsequent incubation (Strepavidin Red 670; Pharmingen Inc, San Diego, Calif) and fluorescein isothiocyanate–conjugated anti-dinitrophenyl antibody (Molecular Probes Inc, Eugene, Ore) for 15 minutes at 25°C. Finally, cells were resuspended in 0.5 mL of cytoflow buffer for analysis. Surface and intracellular fluorescence was measured using a flow cytometer (FACScan; Becton Dickinson Immunocytometry Systems, San Jose, Calif) and fluorescence data were analyzed with software (CellQuest; Becton Dickinson Immunocytometry Systems). After standard calibration of the flow cytometer, data were recorded until 5000 cells were acquired or the cell suspension volume of 0.5 mL was exhausted. The minimum number of cells was lowered to 2000 cells for $\gamma\delta^+$ T cells since these cells are much scarcer in the peripheral blood. Intracellular cytokine detection was performed by double gating each cell surface marker and a lymphocyte gate and measuring fluorescence channel 1 (fluorescein isothiocyanate) and fluorescence channel 3 (Strepavidin Red 670) fluorescence intensity. The data recorded included the total number of acquired cells, the percentage of total cells gated for each subset, and the number of cells positive for fluorescence channel 1 and fluorescence channel 3 internal fluorescence. Background fluorescence was measured using isotype-matched fluorochrome-conjugated IgG and arithmetically subtracted from the measured intracellular cytokine fluorescence to obtain the net detectable intracellular fluorescence. The average background fluorescence measured was less than 1%. Reference assays using fixed, but not permeabilized, cells demonstrated a reduction in the intracellular detection of IL-2 and IFN-γ by 99% and 98%, respectively. Preincubation with recombinant human cytokines before intracellular staining reduced intracellular detection of IL-2 and IFN-γ by 99% and 98%, respectively. Serum IL-6 levels were measured by enzyme-linked immunosorbent assay by the Clinical Investigation Facility at David Grant Medical Center.

A complete data set in both surgical groups was obtained for the preoperative point and the first 2 postoperative days. These data were analyzed using 2-way repeated-measures analysis of variance and Tukey post hoc test. Patient characteristics were compared using χ^2 analysis for proportional data and the Kolmogorov-Smirnov test for unpaired comparisons that were not normally distributed. All statistical analyses were performed with statistical software (STATISTICA; StatSoft, Tulsa, Okla) for Windows (version 5.0; Microsoft Corporation, Redmond, Wash).

rotid surgery group. Postoperative serum IL-6 levels were significantly elevated in the aortic surgery group only (Figure 1).

Unstimulated intracellular cytokine production was not detectable above nonspecific background activity in any T-cell subset. The stimulated production of the intracellular T_H1 cytokines IFN-γ and IL-2 was significantly decreased in the postoperative period in all T-cell subsets and in both surgical groups compared with preoperative values (**Figure 2** through **Figure 4**, C and D). There were no increases in T_H2 cytokine production after surgery. Small preoperative differences (<1.5%) in the stimulated production of IL-4 in $CD4^+$ and $CD8^+$ cells and IL-10 in γδ T cells between surgery groups were at the threshold of nonspecific background activity, although the differences were statistically significant (Figures 2-4, A and B). There were no significant differences in preoperative or postoperative stimulated

Patient Characteristics for the Surgical Groups*

Characteristic	Aortic Surgery† (n = 10)	Carotid Endarterectomy (n = 8)	*P*
Mean age, y	67.7	68.3	NS
Male/female	9/1	8/0	NS
Diabetes	10	13	NS
Coronary artery disease	50	25	NS
Smoker	60	38	NS
NSAID user	40	63	NS
Autologous donation	90	0	.002
Autologous transfusion	90	0	.002
Homologous transfusion	20	0	NS
Mean blood loss, mL	1685	147	<.001‡
Infectious complications	30	25	NS
Mean length of stay, d	8.6	5.4	<.005‡

**Values are expressed as percentages except where noted. NS indicates not significant (level of significance at* $P<.05$*); NSAID indicates nonsteroidal anti-inflammatory drug.*
†Seven patients underwent abdominal aortic aneurysmal repair and 3, aortic bifemoral grafting.
‡Kolmogorov-Smirnov test.

intracellular cytokine production between patients when grouped by operation type, preoperative cardiovascular risk factors (diabetes mellitus, history of coronary artery disease, and smoking), the presence of homologous or autologous transfusion, intraoperative blood loss, operating time, hospital stay, or the development of infectious complications.

COMMENT

There were no significant postoperative changes in unstimulated production of T_H1 or T_H2 cytokines after major vascular operations. These results suggest that major surgery does not trigger a systemic antigen-specific immune response. In contrast, stimulated (potential) production of T_H1 cytokines in $CD4^+$, $CD8^+$, and $\gamma\delta^+$ T cells significantly decreased in the postoperative period ($P<.05$). This effect persisted through the second postoperative day and was independent of the level of the type of operation performed. The decrease in stimulated production of T_H1 cytokines was not accompanied by a simultaneous postoperative increase in production of T_H2 cytokines. There were no differences in the cytokine responses when patients were stratified by preoperative medical diagnosis or by the presence of postoperative complications, although the small sample size limits the power of this observation.

The results of the present study are consistent with previous reports[15-20] that demonstrated that surgical trauma results in a depression of in vitro lymphocyte blastogenesis and proliferation during the early postoperative period. This effect has been attributed to stress-mediated decreases in the production of the T_H cytokines IL-2 and IFN-γ[8,21-23] when measured in bulk supernatants from in vitro cultures of peripheral blood mononuclear cells. More recently, immunosuppression in human disease has been attributed to a shift in cytokine production from a T_H1 (IL-2 and IFN-γ) to a T_H2 (IL-4 and IL-10) pattern.[24] The present study confirms a specific negative effect of surgical injury on the production of T_H1 cytokines without a simultaneous increase in the

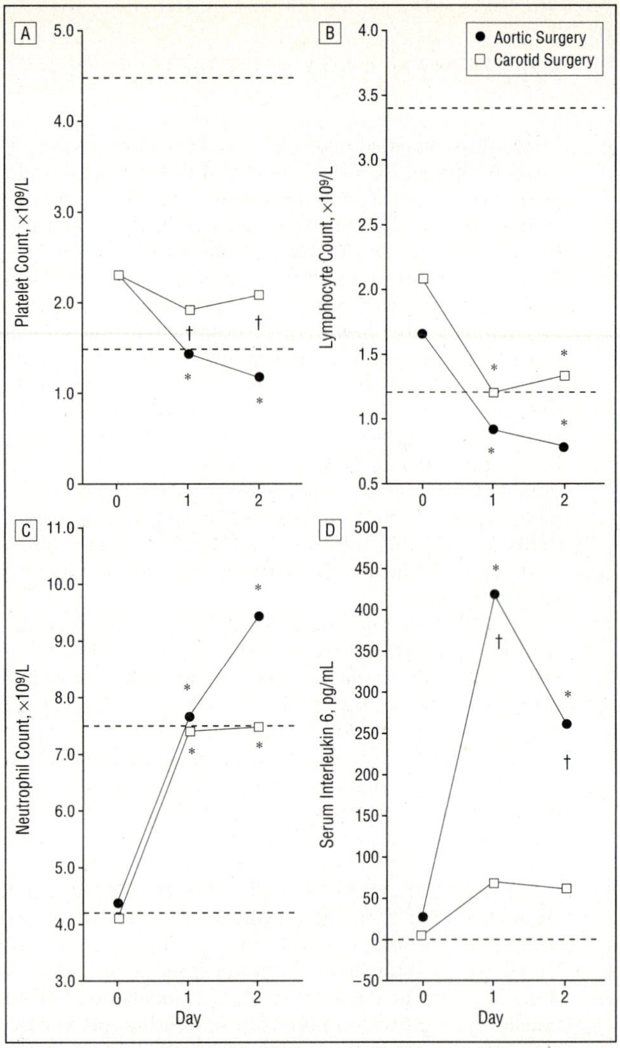

Figure 1. *Results of complete blood cell count and serum interleukin 6 measurements in 18 patients undergoing vascular surgery. Dashed lines represent the upper and lower 95% confidence intervals obtained from 17 reference subjects. Statistical analysis performed using analysis of variance and Tukey post hoc test. The asterisk indicates* $P<.05$ *vs preoperative levels; dagger,* $P<.05$ *aortic vs carotid surgery groups.*

production of T_H2 cytokines. These findings differ from recent reports by Decker et al[9,10] that suggested that postoperative suppression of T_H1 cytokine responses is associated with an increase in T_H2 cytokine production.

One explanation for the lack of an observed T_H2 cytokine response in the present study may be a high threshold of detection resulting from the use of a 2-step staining technique that might mask the expected 1% to 3% of T cells that produce IL-4 in response to phorbolmystrateacetate and ionomycin stimulation.[11] The determination of the exact patterns of postoperative cytokine production is also difficult because of the uncertainty of the precise timing of potential T_H2 responses after injury. The results of animal studies demonstrated that the T_H2 cytokine IL-4 is detectable in splenocytes within 24 hours of traumatic injury,[25] whereas the same cytokine is not measurable in splenic and peritoneal cavity T cells until 5 to 8 days after intraperitoneal infection with *Nippostrongylus brasiliensis*, a potent inducer of T_H2.[14] Therefore, it is possible that the first cytokine measurement at

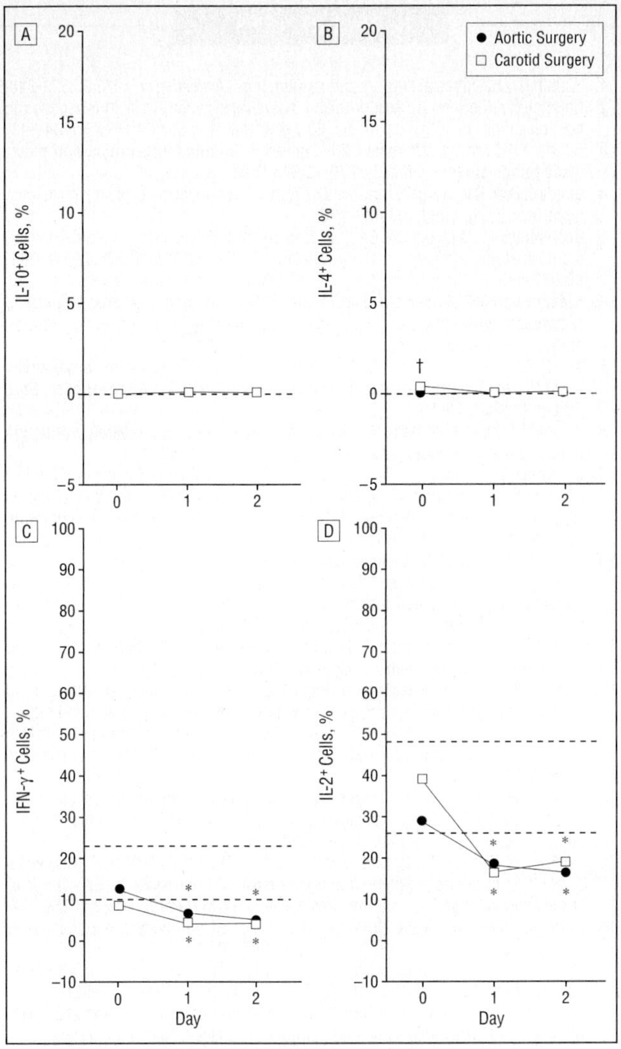

Figure 2. *Results of intracellular helper T-cell type 1 (T_H1) and type 2 (T_H2) cytokine measurements in CD4+ lymphocytes using multiparameter flow cytometry in 18 patients undergoing vascular surgery. IL indicates interleukin; plus sign, postive; and IFN, interferon. See legend for Figure 1 for definition of dashed lines, statistical analyses, asterisk, and dagger.*

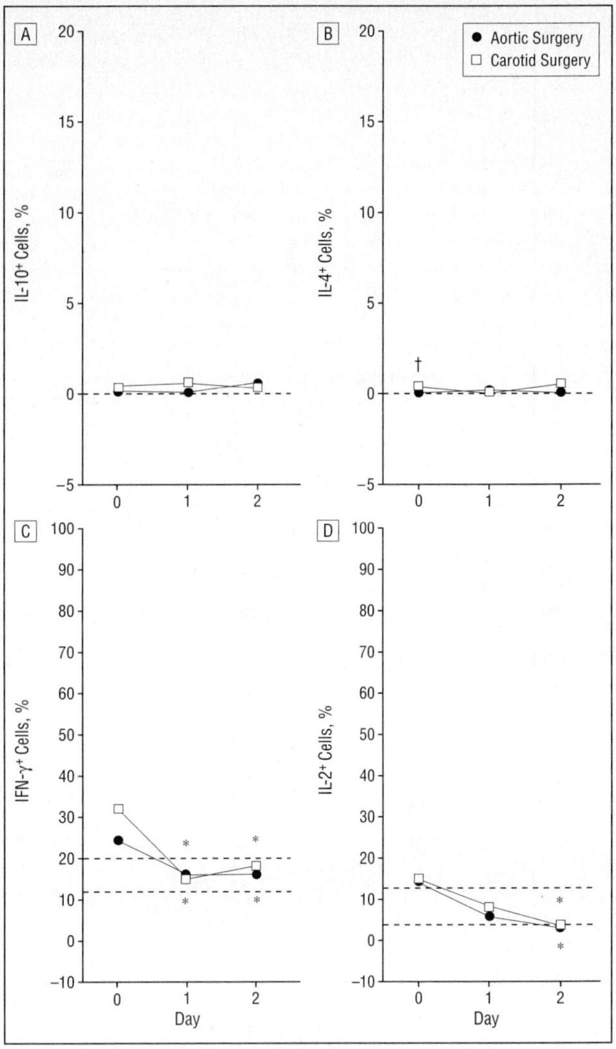

Figure 3. *Results of intracellular helper T-cell type 1 (T_H1) and type 2 (T_H2) cytokine measurements in CD8+ lymphocytes using multiparameter flow cytometry in 18 patients undergoing vascular surgery. IL indicates interleukin; plus sign, positive; and IFN, interferon. See legend for Figure 1 for definition of dashed lines, statistical analyses, asterisk, and dagger.*

24 hours postoperatively was too late to detect an early T_H2 response, which was reported by others.[10] It is also plausible that T_H2 responses developed in patients after the last measurement on postoperative day 2. However, a review of the limited data obtained in the present study between postoperative days 2 and 5 demonstrated no T_H2 cytokine production. Finally, cytokine production in the present study was only measured in T cells, not in other antigen-presenting cells or natural killer cells. These other cell types have been reported to produce T_H2 cytokines[24] in humans. Thus, T_H2 cytokine production by cells other than T cells may explain other reports[10] of postoperative elevations of T_H2 cytokine levels not seen in the present study. One study[24] suggested, however, that it would be unlikely to observe T_H2 cytokine responses in humans that do not involve CD4+ T cells.

The observation that the degree of postoperative suppression of T_H1 cytokine responses was the same after carotid endarterectomy and aortic surgery was surprising. This finding suggests the occurrence of a generalized suppression of T-cell function during the postoperative period that may be independent of the degree of tissue injury. Such a generalized immune suppression following surgical injury may change the immunological significance of what has been defined as major and minor surgery. An unexpected finding was the large variance in preoperative stimulated intracellular cytokine levels in the aortic surgery group; this variance was not present in the carotid endarterectomy group. The difference in preoperative immune reactivity between groups may reflect differences in the patient population, underlying vascular disease, or other unmeasured confounding factors. The potential correlation of decreased preoperative immune function in patients undergoing aortic surgery needs to be further investigated with respect to the risk of postoperative infectious complications.

The initial cytokine milieu is one of the main factors determining T_H1 and T_H2 differentiation in T cells. γδ T cells are an epithelial-associated lymphocyte subset that respond early to infection and cell injury.[26,27] These specialized lymphocytes can release T_H1 and T_H2 cytokines, which are thought to play a role in modulating the

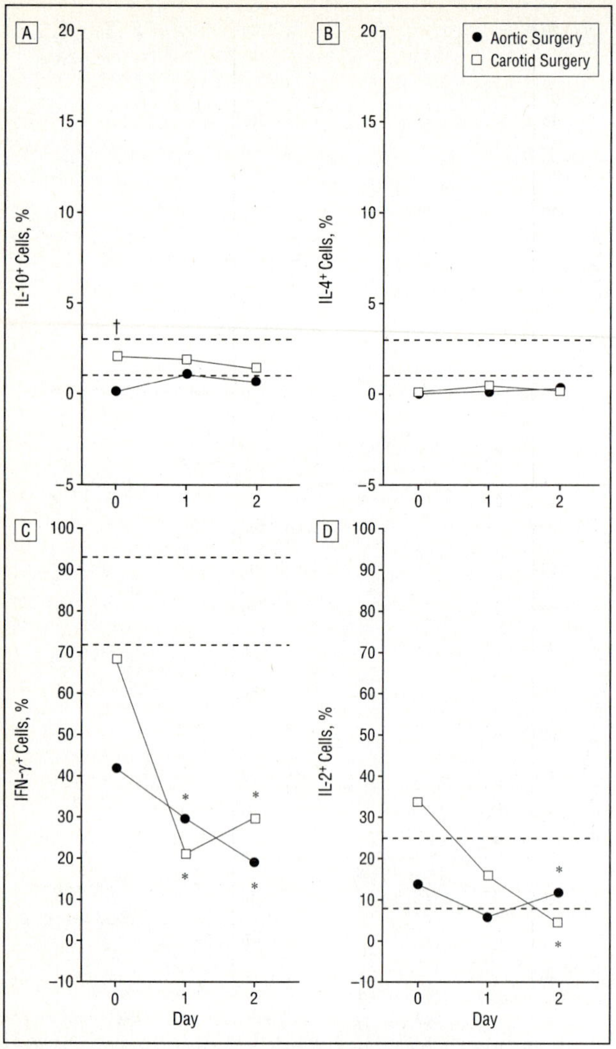

Figure 4. *Results of intracellular helper T-cell type 1 (T_H1) and type 2 (T_H2) cytokine measurements in T-cell receptor $\gamma\delta^+$ lymphocytes using multiparameter flow cytometry in 18 patients undergoing vascular surgery. IL indicates interleukin; plus sign, positive; and IFN, interferon. See legend for Figure 1 for definition of dashed lines, statistical analyses, asterisk, and dagger.*

functional differentiation of the T-cell response.[14] The present study demonstrates that γδ T cells are vigorous producers of IFN-γ, a finding reported by other investigators.[14,28,29] The finding that the responses of γδ T-cell T_H1 cytokines are significantly down-regulated after surgery merits further investigation in patients who have undergone surgery because γδ T cells play an important role in the epithelial barrier to bacterial infections,[30] in neutrophil recruitment[26,31] and the process of epithelial repair.[32]

In conclusion, the present study demonstrates that surgical trauma suppresses T_H1 cytokine responses without increasing T_H2 cytokine production. These results provide further information that may direct future treatments based on the T_H1 and T_H2 paradigm focused on decreasing the risk of postoperative infectious complications.

Reprints: Ramon Berguer, MD, Surgical Service, Department of Veterans Affairs Northern California Health Care System, 150 Muir Rd, Mail Code 112, Martinez, CA 94553 (e-mail: berguer.ramon@martinez.va.gov).

REFERENCES

1. Walton B. Anaesthesia, surgery and immunology. *Anaesthesia.* 1978;33:322-348.
2. Christou NV, Meakins JL, Gordon J, et al. The delayed hypersensitivity response and host resistance in surgical patients: 20 years later. *Ann Surg.* 1995;222:534-546.
3. Lundy J, Lovett EJ, Wolinsky SM, Conran P. Immune impairment and metastatic tumor growth. *Cancer.* 1979;43:945-951.
4. Lundy J, Ford CM. Surgery, trauma and immune suppression: evolving the mechanism. *Ann Surg.* 1983;197:434-438.
5. Berkenbosch F, Wolvers DA, Derijk R. Neuroendocrine and immunological mechanisms in stress-induced immunomodulation. *J Steroid Biochem Mol Biol.* 1991; 40:639-647.
6. Hansbrough JF, Bender EM, Zapata-Sirvent R, Anderson J. Altered helper and suppressor lymphocyte populations in surgical patients: a measure of postoperative immunosuppression. *Am J Surg.* 1984;148:303-307.
7. Abe Y, Miyake M, Horiuchc A, Kumori K, Kimura S. Changes in the productivity of cytokines and active-oxygen in peripheral blood cells following surgery. *Surg Today.* 1992;22:15-18.
8. Akiyoshi T, Koba F, Arinaga S, Miyazaki S, Wada T, Tsuji H. Impaired production of interleukin-2 after surgery. *Clin Exp Immunol.* 1985;59:45-49.
9. Decker D, Lindemann C, Decker P, Kania U, Hirner A, von Rucker A. Effect of endoscopic pre-peritoneal inguinal hernia repair and Shouldice inguinal hernia repair on T-cell differentiation [in German]. *Langenbecks Arch Chir Suppl Kongressbd.* 1997;114:261-265.
10. Decker D, Schondorf M, Bidlingmaier F, Hirner A, von Ruecker AA. Surgical stress induces a shift in the type-1/type-2 T-helper cell balance, suggesting down-regulation of cell-mediated and up-regulation of antibody-mediated immunity commensurate to the trauma. *Surgery.* 1996;119:316-325.
11. Jung T, Schauer U, Heusser C, Neumann C, Rieger C. Detection of intracellular cytokines by flow cytometry. *J Immunol Meth.* 1993;159:197-207.
12. Crucian B, Dunne P, Friedman H, Ragsdale R, Pross S, Widen R. Detection of altered T helper 1 and T helper 2 cytokine production by peripheral blood mononuclear cells in patients with multiple sclerosis utilizing intracellular cytokine detection by flow cytometry and surface marker analysis. *Clin Diagn Lab Immunol.* 1996;3:411-416.
13. Openshaw P, Murphy EE, Hosken NA, et al. Heterogeneity of intracellular cytokine synthesis at the single-cell level in polarized T helper 1 and T helper 2 populations. *J Exp Med.* 1995;182:1357-1367.
14. Ferrick DA, Schrenzel MD, Mulvania T, Hsieh B, Ferlin WG, Lepper H. Differential production of interferon-gamma and interleukin-4 in response to T_H1- and T_H2-stimulating pathogens by gamma delta T cells in vivo. *Nature.* 1995;373:255-257.
15. Berenbaum MC, Fluck PA, Hurst NP. Depression of lymphocyte responses after surgical trauma. *Br J Exp Pathol.* 1973;54:597-607.
16. Cullen BF, Belle GV. Lymphocyte transformation and changes in leukocyte count: effects of anesthesia and operation. *Anesthesiology.* 1975;43:563-569.
17. Vose BM, Moudgil GC. Post-operative depression of antiboty-dependent lymphocyte cytotoxicity following minor surgery and anaesthesia. *Immunology.* 1976; 30:123-128.
18. Park SK, Brody JI, Wallace HA, Blakemore WS. Immunosuppressive effect of surgery. *Lancet.* 1971;1:53-55.
19. Lennard JWJ, Shenton BK, Borzotta A, et al. The influence of surgical operations on components of the human immune system. *Br J Surg.* 1985;72:771-776.
20. Salo M. Effects of anesthesia and surgery on the immune response. *Acta Anesthesiol Scand.* 1992;36:201-220.
21. Hensler T, Hecker H, Heeg K, et al. Distinct mechanisms of immunosuppression as a consequence of major surgery. *Infect Immun.* 1997;65:2283-2291.
22. Deehan DJ, Heys SD, Simpson W, Broom J, McMillan DN, Eremin O. Modulation of the cytokine and acute-phase response to major surgery by recombinant interleukin-2. *Br J Surg.* 1995;82:86-90.
23. Chu SH, Hu RH, Lee YC, Chen KT. Changes of white blood cells, immunosuppressive acidic protein, and interleukin-2 receptor after open heart surgery. *Thorac Cardiovasc Surg.* 1995;43:94-98.
24. Lucey DR, Clerici M, Shearer GM. Type 1 and type 2 cytokine dysregulation in human infectious, neoplastic, and inflammatory diseases. *Clin Microbiol Rev.* 1996; 9:532-562.
25. Napolitano L, Campbell C, Bass B. Kinetics of splenocyte interleukin-4 production after injury and lethal endotoxin challenge. *J Surg Res.* 1997;67:33-39.
26. Ferrick D, Braun R, Lepper H, Schrenzel M. Gamma-delta T-cells in bacterial infections. *Res Immunol.* 1996;147:532-541.
27. Groh V, Steinle A, Bauer S, Spies T. Recognition of stress-induced MHC molecules by intestinal epithelial gamma delta T cells. *Science.* 1998;279:1737-1740.
28. Simpson SJ, Hollander GA, Mizoguchi E, et al. Expression of pro-inflammatory cytokines by TCR alpha beta+ and TCR gamma delta+ T cells in an experimental model of colitis. *Eur J Immunol.* 1997;27:17-25.
29. Berguer R, Ferrick DA. Differential production of intracellular γ-interferon in αβ and γδ T-cell subpopulations in response to peritonitis. *Infect Immun.* 1995;63:4957-4958.
30. Cheng SH, Cheng SH, Penninger JM, et al. Biology of murine gamma delta T cells. *Crit Rev Immunol.* 1991;11:145-166.
31. Boismenu R, Feng L, Xia YY, Chang JC, Havran WL. Chemokine expression by intraepithelial gamma delta T cells: implications for the recruitment of inflammatory cells to damaged epithelia. *J Immunol.* 1996;157:985-992.
32. Boismenu R, Havran WL. Modulation of epithelial cell growth by intraepithelial gamma delta T cells. *Science.* 1994;266:1253-1255.

Peritoneal Expansion by Artificially Produced Ascites During Perfusion Chemotherapy

Dimitris Tsiftsis, MD, PhD; Eelco de Bree, MD; John Romanos, MD; Anastasios Petrou, MD; Elias Sanidas, MD; John Askoxylakis, MD; Konstantinos Zervos, MD; Dimitris Michaloudis, MD

Hypothesis: In cases of peritoneal carcinomatosis, continuous hyperthermic peritoneal perfusion chemotherapy (CHPPC) accomplishes homogeneous distribution of the drug and heat to the entire peritoneal cavity and exposure of the visceral and parietal surfaces to the perfusate. A new closed technique for expansion that produces artificial ascites is safer for medical personnel because of less heat and drug loss and more efficacious in its hemodynamic effect on the patient.

Design: Prospective study.

Setting: University hospital.

Patients: Twenty-one patients with peritoneal carcinomatosis.

Interventions: We performed 23 continuous hyperthermic peritoneal perfusion chemotherapy (CHPPC) procedures with peritoneal cavity expansion to an intra-abdominal pressure up to 26 mm Hg, using artificially produced ascites with 4 to 9 L normal saline solution.

Main Outcome Measures: Intraoperative and postoperative complications and hemodynamic changes during CHPPC.

Results: No intraoperative complications were recorded. The artificially produced ascites did not cause significant hemodynamic changes. During the immediate postoperative period, 1 patient died of intra-abdominal hemorrhage and leakage of a colorectal anastomosis, resulting in a mortality rate of 4% in our series. Minor complications were seen in 14 patients. The complications were not attributable to the expansion technique.

Conclusions: Our proposed modification of closed-circuit CHPPC appears to be well tolerated and safe in patients with a high tumor load, as well as for the theater personnel. It remains to be investigated whether the theoretical advantages of the proposed technique will also lead to better long-term results.

Arch Surg. 1999;134:545-549

Continuous hyperthermic peritoneal perfusion chemotherapy (CHPPC) is a new mode of regional chemotherapy used for the treatment of malignant neoplasms with peritoneal dissemination. For optimal results, the temperature must be raised evenly in all compartments of the peritoneal cavity, and the entire serosal surface of the abdominal organs and the peritoneum must be exposed to the perfusate. To achieve this, many investigators have attempted the expansion of the peritoneal cavity using a peritoneal cavity expander.[1,2] We herein describe a new method of peritoneal cavity expansion, using artificially produced ascites intraoperatively in a closed system of continuous perfusion, and we report on the feasibility and safety of this technique tested in 23 cases.

See Invited Critique at end of article

From the Departments of Surgical Oncology (Drs Tsiftsis, de Bree, Romanos, Sanidas, Askoxylakis, and Zervos) and Anesthesiology (Drs Petrou and Michaloudis), Medical School, University of Crete, Hērákleion.

RESULTS

During most of the perfusion time, the temperatures measured at the mesenteric root and the outflow drain were equal, from 41°C to 43°C, and slightly lower than at the inflow drains, giving strong support to a homogeneous heat and drug exposure in a economically efficient model.

The hemodynamic effects of artificial ascites and hyperthermia on our patients are demonstrated in **Figure 2** and **Figure 3**.

There were no intraoperative complications. Minor postoperative complications were seen in 14 cases, including wound complications (n = 7), atrial fibrillation (n = 3), transient grade II acute renal insufficiency (n = 2), grades I and II

PATIENTS AND METHODS

From June 1, 1995, to November 30, 1997, 21 patients with peritoneal carcinomatosis with no evidence of extra-abdominal and parenchymal metastases were entered into a phase I study for cytoreductive surgery and intraperitoneal hyperthermic chemotherapy. The protocol was approved by the local ethics committee, and informed consent was obtained from all patients. Those 21 patients underwent 23 CHPPC procedures for peritoneal carcinomatosis caused mainly by gynecological malignant neoplasms. In 3 cases, the primary tumor was of colonic origin, whereas 1 treatment was for diffuse malignant mesothelioma. Twenty patients were women and 1 patient was a man, ranging in age from 42 to 80 years (mean, 65 years).

Our modification of the CHPPC technique is described below. The abdomen is approached through a median xyphoid-pubic incision. Comprehensive adhesiolysis is performed. The primary tumor is excised, if still present, and all visceral or parietal peritoneal surface tumor deposits are removed as completely as possible. If a deposit is infiltrating deeply into an organ, and it is impossible to peel the malignant neoplasm from the surface, the involved organ or a segment of it is excised.

The intraoperative hyperthermic chemotherapy is started immediately after surgery. Two 22F silicone arterial perfusion canulae (William Harvey R15600B; BARD, Tewksbury, Mass) are placed in the right and left subphrenic spaces for infusion, and 1 silicone-filtered sump drain catheter (Axiom Traum; Axiom Medical Inc, Rancho Dominiguez, Calif) is placed in the Douglas pouch for drainage of perfusion fluid through separate stump wounds. Through the air vents of the sump drain, 1 temperature probe and 1 pressure probe are introduced into the peritoneal cavity and placed at the root of the mesentery. Temperature is also recorded at the inflow and outflow catheters. A Swan-Ganz catheter is inserted to monitor core temperature and the hemodynamic parameters. We close the abdominal cavity temporarily using watertight continuous locking suture of the skin only. The inflow and outflow tubes are connected to the heat exchange and pump system, part of an extracorporeal pump and oxygenator machine (Sarns Inc, Ann Arbor, Mich) in which a filter is incorporated for elimination of free cancer cells. The patient is given adequate muscle relaxation. At the start of the CHPPC, the patient's core temperature is lowered to 33°C to 35°C using a cooling mattress, to avoid unwanted extreme increase of the core temperature during the hyperthermic perfusion. The closed perfusion system (**Figure 1**) is filled with 4 to 9 L isotonic sodium chloride solution, in most cases approximately 3.5 L/m^2 body surface area, resulting in a mean intra-abdominal pressure of 12 to 26 mm Hg. The pump system is started, and the circulating perfusate is heated. When the intraperitoneal temperature reaches 41°C, the chosen chemotherapeutic drugs are administered. Cisplatin, 80 to 120 mg/m^2 body surface area, was used in malignant neoplasms of the digestive tract and previously untreated gynecological malignant neoplasms, whereas docetaxel (Taxotere; Rhône-Poulenc Rorer, Collegeville, Pa), 75 mg/m^2 body surface area, was used in gynecological malignant neoplasms previously treated with chemotherapy. The intraperitoneal temperature is allowed to fluctuate from 41°C to 43°C, and the duration of the perfusion is 2 hours. To facilitate uniform temperature and drug distribution throughout the peritoneal cavity, vigorous agitation of the abdomen is performed continuously. The core temperature is kept below 38.5°C. After completion of the CHPPC, the abdomen is reopened, the canulae and probes are removed, and the excess fluid is dried from the abdominal cavity. The sump drain is left in place for postoperative drainage. The abdominal wall is closed in layers in the usual way.

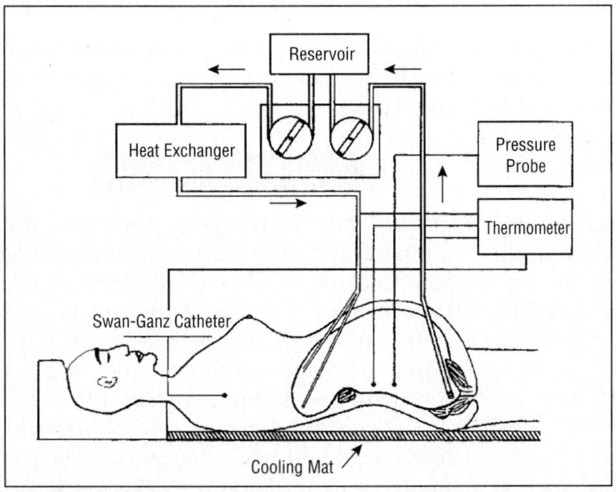

Figure 1. *The closed perfusion system.*

thrombocytopenia (n = 4), grade I leukopenia (n = 1), and intraperitoneal fluid collection (n = 1). The fluid collection was successfully drained under computed tomographic guidance. During the immediate postoperative period, 1 patient died of intra-abdominal hemorrhage and leakage of a colorectal anastomosis, resulting in a mortality rate of 4% in our series.

COMMENT

Chemotherapeutic agents are usually administered systemically. In recent years, regional administration of chemotherapy has been attempted in an effort to achieve high levels of the cytotoxic agent locally without systemic toxic effects. Regional chemotherapy is an established treatment in limb sarcomas and melanomas and in secondary liver and lung neoplasms using intra-arterial infusion or isolated perfusion of the extremity or organ. The perfusion technique for peritoneal carcinomatosis has not been standardized.

Four decades ago, intraperitoneal chemotherapy began with the instillation of the drug into a small volume of dialysate. The distribution of the dialysate in the peritoneal cavity was poor, and the method was abandoned.[3] To overcome the obstacle of incomplete seroperitoneal exposure, larger volumes were introduced in the abdominal cavity for 1 to 2 hours.[3,4] Since inadequate distribution of the drug to upper abdominal and small-bowel surfaces remained one of the most impor-

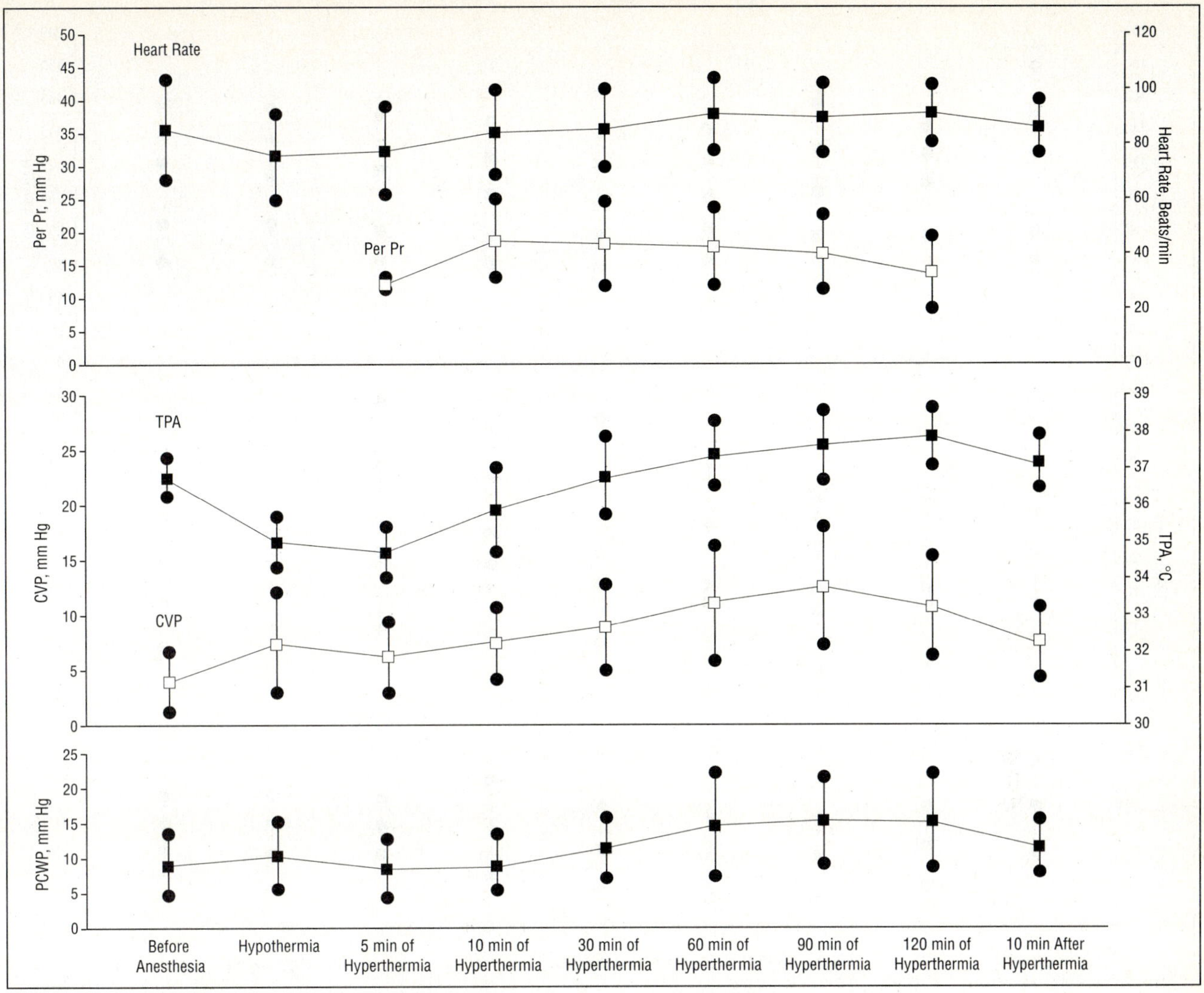

Figure 2. *Changes in hemodynamic variables and core temperature during hypothermia and subsequent intraperitoneal hyperthermia with artificial ascites during 23 continuous hyperthermic peritoneal perfusion chemotherapy procedures. Per Pr indicates peritoneal pressure; CVP, central venous pressure; TPA, pulmonary artery temperature; and PCWP, pulmonary capillary wedge pressure. All data are given as mean ± SD.*

tant causal factors for recurrence of peritoneal carcinomatosis, other treatment strategies were developed.[5]

Recently, CHPPC has been introduced with the heated perfusate circulating continuously through the peritoneal cavity. Hyperthermia is often used because it has a direct cytotoxic effect and amplifies the activity of most cytotoxic drugs.[6,7] The only limitation of the method is that it requires anesthetization, because intraperitoneal heat and chemotherapy are badly tolerated. Cytoreductive surgery always has to precede CHPPC during the same procedure, since the penetration depth of hyperthermic chemotherapy is estimated to be limited to 5 mm.[8,9]

Continuous peritoneal perfusion chemotherapy has certain advantages, such as the ability to wash out intraperitoneal free cancer cells, the combination with hyperthermia, direct exposure of the tumor to the drug, uniform distribution of the drug throughout the abdominal cavity, and the very high intraperitoneal drug concentration in relation to very low plasma levels.[6,7] The latter is attributed to the peritoneal-plasma barrier and the first-passage clearance of many drugs by the liver. Depending on their molecular weight, their affinity for lipids, and first-passage effect by the liver, the plasma concentration gradient of the drugs in the peritoneal cavity may be as high as 1000, as is the case with paclitaxel.[3] The disadvantages of the technique are the need for specialized personnel and apparatus as well as the prerequisite of an anesthetized patient to achieve maximal muscle relaxation and to tolerate the intraperitoneal heat and chemotherapy.

Continuous peritoneal perfusion can be performed using an open or a closed circuit.[6,7] Most surgeons prefer the closed-circuit model described by Spratt et al[10] in 1980, in which the perfusate circulates continuously. Their model is more economically efficient because of the lower drug level and lower heat loss.[11-14] To optimize the exposure of the serosal surface of the abdominal organs and the parietal peritoneum to the perfusate and to achieve a better distribution of heat and drug, Fujimara et al[1] introduced the concept of the "expanded peritoneal cavity" in an attempt to provide additional space for the peritoneal contents to float freely in the perfusate. They use an acrylic cylinder called a peritoneal cavity expander. The surgical wound is closed around the cylinder, and

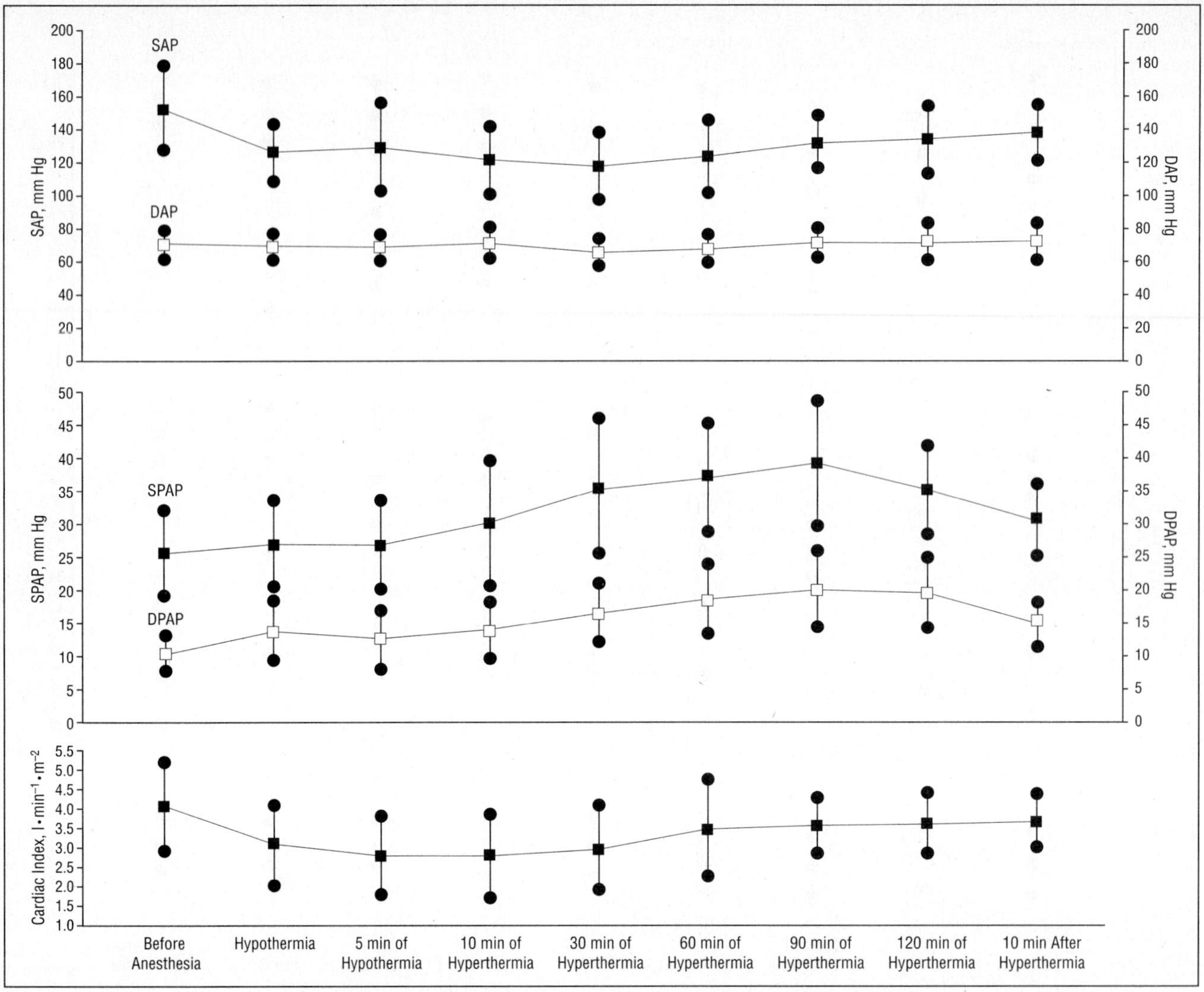

Figure 3. *Changes in hemodynamic variables and core temperature during hypothermia and subsequent intraperitoneal hyperthermia with artificial ascites during 23 continuous hyperthermic peritoneal perfusion chemotherapy procedures. SAP indicates systolic arterial pressure; DAP, diastolic arterial pressure; SPAP, systolic pulmonary arterial pressure; and DPAP, diastolic pulmonary arterial pressure. All data are given as mean ± SD.*

the abdominal cavity remains open through the cylinder. The intestine floats in the perfusate, and the surgeon's hand stirs the perfusate to secure even distribution.[1,2] In our proposed modification, satisfactory expansion of the peritoneal cavity is achieved by producing an artificial ascites with the abdominal cavity closed, in most cases infusing isotonic sodium chloride solution at approximately 3.5 L/m^2 body surface area. Since the total dose of the cytostatic drugs is calculated also per square meter of body surface area, the perfusate concentrations are expected to be nearly equal for all patients, to whom the same drug dose per square meter of body surface area is administered.

In comparison with the other techniques used, our modification is more efficient regarding heat loss; it prevents evaporation of the drug, decreases the risk for contamination, and maintains a tight surgical field. A significant leakage of perfusate at the base of the peritoneal cavity expander has been reported.[15] On this point, this closed-circuit technique is safer for the theater personnel by minimizing their exposure to the drug. In addition, a recent animal study demonstrated that raised intra-abdominal pressure may increase drug penetration into tissues.[16] Perfusion with an open abdominal cavity results in incomplete exposure of the intestine floating on the fluid surface and of the laparotomy wound to the perfusate. A high incidence of early wound recurrence has been reported after the use of the peritoneal cavity expander.[15]

As in other situations, patients tolerated increased intra-abdominal pressure very well. In patients with cirrhosis, a volume of 7 to 9 L ascites with an intra-abdominal pressure of 16 to 20 mm Hg is common.[17] In minimal invasive abdominal surgery, intra-abdominal pressure is raised to 14 mm Hg without any major adverse effects.[18]

The hemodynamic data show that there are no significant adverse effects on the patient's condition that cannot be handled (Figures 2 and 3). The cardiopressant effect of hypothermia during the period of extensive surgical maneuvering is significant, making the administration of vasoactive drugs mandatory in 14 of 23 cases. The stimulatory effect of the subsequent hyperthermia on the cardiovascular system usually diminished the need for these drugs. The increase in pulmonary artery and central venous pressure could be attributed to the sympathetic effect of hyperthermia or to the increased intra-abdominal pressure transmitted to the thoracic cavity. Cardiac preload probably decreases response to the increased intra-abdominal pressure.[18] It would therefore be prudent to observe these patients with extensive invasive monitoring during the whole procedure, because patients with marginal cardiovascular reserves might decompensate acutely.

One patient died within 1 month after the procedure, of intra-abdominal hemorrhage and leakage of a colorectal anastomosis, resulting in a mortality rate of 4% in our series. The mortality rate of our series is comparable with those reported by others, varying from 0% to 14%, regardless of the technique used.[11,19-23] Major complications from different techniques have been reported in up to 44% of the cases.[6,7,11,12,22,23] In our series, the remaining complications observed were minor and did not seem to be related to the expansion technique. The relatively high rate of wound complications may be attributed to the bad nutritional state of the patients, the systemic effect of the chemotherapeutic agent, and local exposure of the abdominal wound to hyperthermic chemotherapy. Transient renal insufficiency, observed in both cases in which higher doses (120 mg/m^2 body surface area) of cisplatin had been used, was probably related to the resorption of this intraperitoneally administered nephrotoxic drug. This had been reason to decrease the dose again to 100 mg/m^2. The other complications were not related to increased drug doses. The leukopenia and thrombocytopenia were other chemotherapy-related complications, although the extensive blood loss during operation also contributes to the latter. The episodes of atrial fibrillation in 3 patients may be attributed to fluid disturbances in the early postoperative period after CHPPC.

We have strong reason to believe that our proposed modification of closed-circuit CHPPC is efficient, safe, and effective and should be tried by other centers using this treatment method. It remains to be proved in multicenter trials whether the theoretical advantages of the proposed technique will also lead to better long-term results.

Corresponding author: Dimitris Tsiftsis, MD, PhD, Department of Surgical Oncology, University General Hospital, PO Box 1352, Hērákleion, Crete, 71110, Greece (e-mail: tsiftsis@cc.uch.gr).

REFERENCES

1. Fujimara T, Yonemura T, Fushida S, et al. Continuous hyperthermic peritoneal perfusion for the treatment of peritoneal dissemination in gastric cancers and subsequent second-look operation. *Cancer.* 1990;65:65-71.
2. Yonemura Y, Fujimara T, Fushida S, et al. Hyperthermo-chemotherapy combined with cytoreductive surgery for the treatment of gastric cancer with peritoneal dissemination. *World J Surg.* 1991;15:530-536.
3. Markman M. Intraperitoneal chemotherapy. *Semin Oncol.* 1991;18:248-254.
4. Sugarbaker PH, Jablonski KA. Prognostic features of 51 colorectal and 130 appendiceal cancer patients with peritoneal carcinomatosis treated by cytoreductive surgery and intraperitoneal chemotherapy. *Ann Surg.* 1995;221:124-132.
5. Zoetmulder FAN, Sugarbaker PH. Patterns of failure following treatment of pseudomyxoma peritonei of appendiceal origin. *Eur J Cancer.* 1996;32A:1727-1733.
6. Elias D, Detroz B , Debaene B, et al. Treatment of peritoneal carcinomatosis by intraperitoneal chemo-hyperthermia: reliable and unreliable concepts. *Hepatogastroenterology.* 1994;41:207-213.
7. Sayag AC, Gilly FN, Carry PY, et al. Intraoperative chemohyperthermia in the management of digestive cancers. *Oncology.* 1993;50:333-337.
8. Fujimoto S, Takahashi M, Kobayaski K, et al. Relation between clinical and histologic outcome of intraperitoneal hyperthermic perfusion for patients with gastric cancer and peritoneal metastasis. *Oncology.* 1993;50:338-343.
9. Van der Vaart PJM, van der Vange N, Zoetmulder FAN, et al. Intraperitoneal cisplatin with regional hyperthermia in advanced ovarian cancer: pharmokinetics and cisplatin-DNA adduct formation in patients and ovarian cancer cell lines. *Eur J Cancer.* 1998;34:148-154.
10. Spratt JS, Adcock RA, Muskovin M, Sherrill W, McKeown J. Clinical delivery system for intraperitoneal hyperthermic chemotherapy. *Cancer Res.* 1980;40:256-260.
11. Jacquet P, Stephens AD, Averbach AM, et al. Analysis of morbidity and mortality in 60 patients with peritoneal carcinomatosis treated by cytoreductive surgery and heated intraoperative intraperitoneal chemotherapy. *Cancer.* 1996;77:2622-2629.
12. Yonemura Y, Fujimara T, Nishimura G, et al. Effects of intraoperative chemohyperthermia in patients with gastric cancer with peritoneal dissemination. *Surgery.* 1996;119:437-444.
13. Fujimara T, Yonemura Y, Muraoka K, et al. Continuous hyperthermic peritoneal perfusion for the prevention of peritoneal recurrence of gastric cancer: randomized controlled study. *World J Surg.* 1994;18:150-155.
14. Fujimoto S, Shrestha RD, Kokobun M, et al. Positive results of combined therapy of surgery and intraperitoneal hyperthermic perfusion for far-advanced gastric cancer. *Ann Surg.* 1990;212:592-596.
15. Elias D, Damia E, Puizillout JM, et al. Thermic homogeneity and standardization of intraperitoneal chemohyperthermia for peritoneal carcinomatosis. *Reg Cancer Treat.* 1996;9:54-59.
16. Jacquet P, Stuart OA, Chang D, Sugarbaker PH. Effects of intra-abdominal pressure on pharmokinetics and tissue distribution of doxorubicin after intraperitoneal administration. *Anticancer Drugs.* 1996;7:596-603.
17. Kravetz D, Romero G, Argonz J, et al. Total volume paracentesis decreases variceal pressure, size and variceal wall tension in cirrhotic patients. *Hepatology.* 1997;25:59-62.
18. Gebhardt H, Bautz A, Ross M, Loose D, Wulf H, Schaube H. Pathophysiological and clinical aspects of the CO_2 pneumoperitoneum (CO_2-PP). *Surg Endosc.* 1997;11:864-867.
19. Koga S, Hamazoe R, Maeta M, Shimizu N, Murakami A, Wakatsuki T. Prophylactic therapy for peritoneal recurrence of gastric cancer by continuous hyperthermic peritoneal perfusion with mitomycin C. *Cancer.* 1988;61:232-237.
20. Ikeguchi M, Kondou A, Oka A, Tsujitani S, Maeta M, Kaibara N. Effects of continuous hyperthermic peritoneal perfusion on prognosis of gastric cancer with serosal invasion. *Eur J Surg.* 1995;161:581-586.
21. Yonemura Y, Ninomiya I, Kaiji M, et al. Prophylaxis with intraoperative chemohyperthermia against peritoneal recurrence of serosal invasion–positive gastric cancer. *World J Surg.* 1995;19:450-455.
22. Stephens AD, Averbach AM, Jacquet P, et al. Morbidity and mortality of cytoreductive surgery and hyperthermic intraoperative intraperitoneal chemotherapy with mitomycin C using the coliseum technique. *Reg Cancer Treat.* 1997;10 (suppl 1):52.
23. Piso P, Hiller WFA, Jaehne J, Schmoll E, Raab R. Do patients with peritoneal carcinomatosis benefit from cytoreductive surgery (CS) and hyperthermic intraperitoneal chemotherapy (HIC)? *Eur J Surg Oncol.* 1998;24:213.

Invited Critique

The authors provide a modification in technique of hyperthermic peritoneal perfusion for peritoneal adenocarcinomatosis that builds on earlier studies. However, there are technical and cytokinetic limitations to their approach. From the technical standpoint, their perfusion system would not avoid streaming of flow. Like the authors, my approach would be to resect the primary cancer, omentum, and as much of the peritoneal implants as possible. Afterward, I would copiously irrigate the peritoneal cavity with 5% dextrose in water heated on last wash to 55°C and leave it in for only 3 to 5 minutes before removing. This temperature for short exposure is as thermolethal as the lower temperature used by the authors for longer periods. There is some evidence that the mucopolysaccharides forming the viscous ascites in pseudomyxoma are miscible in 5% dextrose in water. Also, 5% dextrose in water has an osmolytic effect on cells. The solution is not removed, but will be absorbed into the circulation. From this point on, my chemotherapy technique, developed with Thomas Woodcock, MD (unpublished data, 1998) is influenced by the fact that many cases of peritoneal carcinomatosis are composed of cancer cells with very low proliferative indexes. With antiproliferative drugs only, cells that are in cycle will be affected by the drugs. This requires a more protracted course of chemotherapy, which is obtained by inserting a titanium peritoneal port (PORT-A-CATH [catalog No. 21-2000]; Pharmacia Deltech Inc, St Paul, Minn) before abdominal closure. Drugs are administered via the PORT-A-CATH at weekly intervals for 6 weeks, followed by a 2-week rest. The drugs are diluted in 2000 mL 5% dextrose in water. The solution is not removed but will be absorbed. This volume is necessary for diffusion to occur throughout the peritoneal cavity. The course continues for 1 year. In the case of bowel cancer, the weekly course consists of 750 mg of fluorouracil and 1000 mg of leucovorin calcium. This is very well tolerated. Lorazepam (Ativan) can be given before each treatment for the prevention of nausea.

Technically, the PORT-A-CATH is easier to manage and has less risk for complications than the intravenous route. If I were to design a clinical trial for the adjuvant therapy of bowel cancer, I would use this technique with some modification of the drugs as dictated by the cancer being treated. Many aspects of peritoneal carcinomatosis were reviewed in a monograph published in 1986.[1] These comments update that monograph.

John S. Spratt, MD
Louisville, Ky

1. Spratt JS, Edwards MJ, Kubota T, Lindberg R, Tseng MT. Peritoneal carcinomatosis: anatomy, physiology, diagnosis and management. *Curr Probl Cancer.* 1986;11:553-585.

IN OTHER AMA JOURNALS

ARCHIVES OF INTERNAL MEDICINE

Predictors of Survival After Deep Vein Thrombosis and Pulmonary Embolism: A Population-Based, Cohort Study

John A. Heit, MD; Marc D. Silverstein, MD; David N. Mohr, MD; Tanya M. Petterson, MS; W. Michael O'Fallon, PhD; L. Joseph Melton III, MD

Background: Because reported survival after venous thromboembolism (VTE) varies widely, we performed a population-based retrospective cohort study to estimate survival, compare observed with expected survival, and determine predictors of short-term (≤7 days) and long-term survival (>7 days) after VTE.
Methods: We followed the 25-year (1966-1990) inception cohort (n = 2218) of Olmsted County, Minnesota, patients with deep vein thrombosis alone (DVT) or pulmonary embolism with or without deep vein thrombosis (PE ± DVT) forward in time until death or the last clinical contact.
Results: During 14 629 person-years of follow-up, 1333 patients died. Seven-day, 30-day, and 1-year VTE survival rates were 74.8% (DVT, 96.2%; PE ± DVT, 59.1%), 72.0% (DVT, 94.5%; PE ± DVT, 55.6%), and 63.6% (DVT, 85.4%; PE ± DVT, 47.7%), respectively. Observed survival after DVT, PE ± DVT, and overall was significantly worse than expected for Minnesota whites of similar age and sex ($P<.001$). More than one third of deaths occurred on the date of onset or after VTE that was unrecognized during life. Short-term survival improved during the 25-year study period, while long-term survival was unchanged. After adjusting for comorbid conditions, PE ± DVT was an independent predictor of reduced survival for up to 3 months after onset compared with DVT alone. Other independent predictors of both short- and long-term survival included age, body mass index, patient location at onset, malignancy, congestive heart failure, neurologic disease, chronic lung disease, recent surgery, and hormone therapy. Additional independent predictors of long-term survival included tobacco smoking, other cardiac disease, and chronic renal disease.
Conclusions: Survival after VTE, and especially after PE ± DVT, is much worse than reported, and significantly less than expected survival. Compared with DVT alone, symptomatic PE ± DVT is an independent predictor of reduced survival for up to 3 months after onset, implying that treatment for the 2 disorders should be different. (*1999;159:445-453*)

Corresponding author: John A. Heit, MD, Hematology Research, Plummer 549, Mayo Clinic, 200 First St SW, Rochester, MN 55905 (e-mail: heit.john@mayo.edu).

Staging Investigations in Patients With Breast Cancer

The Role of Bone Scans and Liver Imaging

Rajiv Samant, MD; Pradip Ganguly, MD

Hypothesis: Metastatic workup for patients newly diagnosed as having breast cancer is variable, especially for early disease (T1-2 N0-1). Routine bone scans and liver imaging are often performed without any evidence to support their usefulness.

Design: A retrospective review of patients with breast cancer referred to our center during a 2-year period was performed to determine the value of staging investigations in detecting metastases.

Results: Of the total 250 patients referred to our center after initial diagnosis, 25 (10.0%) were diagnosed as having metastases, 23 of whom had either clinical symptoms or signs suggestive of metastatic disease or abnormalities on routine blood work or chest x-ray examinations. Only 2 patients with metastatic disease were diagnosed solely on bone scan results; none were diagnosed solely on liver imaging (either with an ultrasound or radionuclide isotope liver scan). Overall, 3% (5/161) of patients with pathologic T1-2 N0-1 disease had metastases diagnosed compared with 30% (18/61) of patients with pathologic stage T3-4 or N2 disease.

Conclusions: Our results confirm the low yield of routine bone scans and liver imaging among patients with asymptomatic, pathologically confirmed, early stage (T1-2 N0-1) breast cancer. Therefore, we do not recommend these tests for such patients, although intensive investigations are appropriate for more advanced (stage T3-4 or N2) tumors.

Arch Surg. 1999;134:551-553

MANY PATIENTS have extensive staging investigations to complete their metastatic workup following a diagnosis of breast cancer.[1-3] The goal of these tests is to identify those patients with incurable disease so that a more realistic prognosis can be given and their treatment can be tailored accordingly. Isotopic bone scans along with isotopic liver scans or liver ultrasound are still commonly used to detect subclinical metastatic disease at these sites.[4] The usefulness of these tests is debatable,[5-8] especially when one considers both their sensitivities and specificities.

See Invited Critique at end of article

Despite improvements in imaging modalities, clinical staging is still considered by many to be the most useful and cost-effective.[4,6] However, there is as yet no consensus on the most appropriate initial staging investigations. It remains to be determined whether tests apart from routine preoperative chest x-ray examination and blood work significantly improve the yield of a metastatic workup in asymptomatic patients.[6]

From the Department of Surgery, Faculty of Medicine, University of British Columbia, Vancouver (Dr Samant), and Department of Medicine, Faculty of Medicine, Memorial University of Newfoundland, St Johns (Dr Ganguly).

We have not previously had a standard policy regarding staging investigations for patients with breast cancer at our center, although extensive investigations are no longer routinely performed. Therefore, we decided to review the yield from the initial metastatic workup on our patients in previous years, specifically to see if routine liver and bone imaging done soon after diagnosis added much information once the patient's clinical status and surgical staging were taken into account.

RESULTS

Almost all patients had a chest x-ray examination and blood work performed (usually preoperatively) before their referral. Their subsequent investigations were at the discretion of the oncologist or referring physician, and at that time, our center did not have any specified guidelines regarding the staging workup. Of the 250 evaluable patients, 249 were women and 1 was a man, with ages ranging from 26 to 85 years. It was not possible to retrospectively determine the menopausal status, but 106 patients were 50 years or younger and 144 patients were older than 50 years. Below is the distribution of

METHODS

The medical records of patients with breast cancer referred to the Newfoundland Cancer Clinic in St Johns (recently renamed the Dr H. Bliss Murphy Cancer Centre) from January 1990 to December 1991 were retrieved for analysis. Initially, 329 charts were reviewed, but 79 were excluded for the following reasons: insufficient information in the chart (n = 5), no evidence of invasive disease (n = 17), bilateral or previous breast cancer (n = 8), unusual histological findings (n = 2), previous cancer excluding nonmelanoma skin cancer (n = 1), and referred more than 6 months after initial diagnosis (n = 46). A total of 250 patients referred to the Newfoundland Cancer Clinic after initial diagnosis of a pathologically confirmed, unilateral, invasive breast carcinoma and no previous malignant neoplasms (apart from nonmelanoma skin cancer) were evaluable. The investigations and staging performed on each patient as documented in the cancer clinic chart were retrospectively reviewed along with the clinical condition (ie, signs and symptoms of metastases). From these data, the incidence of metastatic disease along with the investigations performed were analyzed.

patients based on locoregional Union Internationale Contre le Cancer TNM classification.

Classification	Patients, No. (%)
T1-2 N0	86 (33.6)
T1-2 N1	75 (30.0)
T3 N0-1	20 (8.0)
T4 or N2	41 (16.4)
T1-2 Nx	6 (2.4)
Tx N0	6 (2.4)
Tx N1	16 (6.4)
Total	**250 (100)**

After the initial staging investigations, 25 patients (10% of our entire evaluable group) were diagnosed as having metastatic disease based on clinical and/or radiographic findings (a biopsy was not always necessary). As shown in the **Table**, 21 of the 25 patients appeared to have signs and/or symptoms suggestive of metastatic disease noted in the cancer clinic chart. Only 4 patients with metastatic disease were entirely asymptomatic at initial presentation. The **Figure** shows the distribution of metastases among the patients according to the TNM classification.[9] The T and N stage were based on pathologic criteria after surgery. Overall, only 5 (3%) of our 161 patients with early (T1-2 N0-1) breast cancer had documented metastases at initial presentation, regardless of tumor grade and other pathologic features, compared with 18 (30%) of our patients with locally advanced (T3-4 or N2) disease. Two (7%) of the 28 patients with incomplete locoregional staging (Tx N1) had metastases diagnosed after completion of staging investigations.

Most patients had at least a chest x-ray examination (anterior-posterior and lateral) and blood work (including a complete blood count; electrolytes, creatinine, calcium, and alkaline phosphatase levels; and liver function tests) performed. The use of more extensive investigations was somewhat variable. Radionuclide isotopic bone scans, liver scans, and liver ultrasounds were most commonly used to detect metastatic disease, although plain x-ray films, skeletal surveys, isotopic brain scans, and computed tomographic scans of the upper abdomen were occasionally used as well (although on a more sporadic basis).

Distribution of Patients With Metastases

	No. (%) of Patients	Entire Group, %
Symptomatic	21 (84)	8.40
Asymptomatic		
Normal preoperative investigation results	2 (8)	0.80
Abnormal preoperative investigation results	2 (8)	0.80
Total Group With Metastases	**25 (100)**	**10.00**

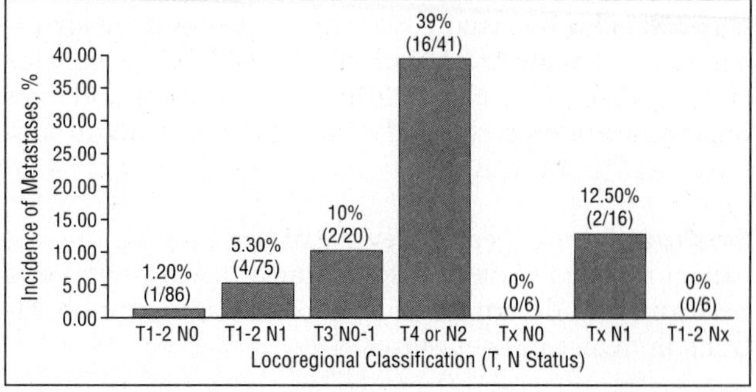

Distribution of metastatic disease identified according to locoregional classification (based on the Union Internationale Contre le Cancer TNM staging classification).

Of the 143 isotopic bone scans initially performed, 15 (10.5%) were considered positive for metastases, but only 2 (1.7%) of the 118 isotopic liver scans revealed metastases. Of the 4 asymptomatic patients found to have metastases, 2 had other abnormalities on either the chest x-ray film or liver function test results (specifically, an elevated alkaline phosphatase level). Only 2 patients (8% of those with metastases and 0.8% of the total evaluable group) were diagnosed as having metastatic disease based solely on routine bone scan results. Both these patients had stage TX N1 tumors. Four other patients had asymptomatic bone metastases noted on bone scans, but had clinical signs or symptoms suggestive of metastatic disease elsewhere. No patients were diagnosed as having metastases based solely on liver imaging (with either isotopic liver scans or ultrasound). The results of liver imaging were abnormal in 2 patients, but they had locally advanced disease (T3 or T4 tumors) and clinical evidence of metastases elsewhere. Other investigations, such as x-ray examinations and computed tomographic scans, did not improve the detection of metastases.

COMMENT

Traditionally, isotopic bone scans and liver imaging (with isotopic liver scans and, more recently, liver ultrasounds) have often been used to rule out bone and liver metastases and definitive-stage patients with breast cancer.[2] However, the overall yield of these investigations is reportedly low, especially with early (pathologic stage T1-2 N0-1) disease.[1,2,4,5] Often, fewer than 5% of patients with early breast cancers have bone metastases at presentation,[7,10] and the incidence of liver metastases is even lower.[4,11] With locally advanced breast cancer (pathologic stage T3-4 or N2), the incidence of metastases is much higher, and in such cases, more extensive investigations are justified.[1,2] Approximately 25% of patients with T3-4 tumors present with bone metastases at initial diagnosis.[4,12,13] The diagnostic accuracy of these tests is quite variable. Bone scans can be notoriously inaccurate, with more than 15% producing false-negative results and more than 30% producing false-positive results.[2,7] Isotopic liver scanning is associated with a 5% to 25% rate of false-negative and false-positive results.[3,14] Although ultrasound of the liver is more accurate than isotopic liver scanning, it is also not completely reliable.[4] In fact, we have found that some of our patients described as having normal staging investigations at presentation developed obvious metastases soon afterward. In retrospect, the results of their initial investigations (such as bone scans) were not entirely normal. This illustrates that, even with extensive investigations, it is not always possible to correctly identify patients with metastases.[2,4,7,15]

Our results show that 25 (10%) of the 250 patients with breast cancer had metastatic disease at initial presentation, which is probably because we had a large number of patients with locally advanced (T3-4 or N2) tumors. Actually, 61 (24%) of the 250 patients in our series had locally advanced disease, presumably due either to many patients in our province initially presenting with locally advanced breast cancer or to a significant number of patients with early cancers not being referred to our cancer center (resulting in proportionately more advanced tumors). However, only 3% of the patients with T1-2 N0-1 breast carcinoma had metastases diagnosed at initial presentation compared with 30% of patients with T3-4 or N2 breast carcinoma. These data are similar to other published reports.[1,2,4]

Our results confirm that most patients (84%) with metastases at presentation had clinical signs or symptoms suggestive of metastatic disease, and this has also been noted elsewhere.[5] Of the 4 patients diagnosed as having metastatic disease based on the bone scan results, 2 already had abnormalities on blood work results and/or chest x-ray films. Therefore, routine bone scans only picked up 2 additional patients with metastatic disease. Liver imaging by itself did not detect any patients with subclinical metastatic disease, although 2 patients with metastatic disease identified elsewhere were also found to have abnormalities suggestive of liver metastases after liver imaging.

Therefore, when one considers the sensitivities and specificities of bone scans and liver imaging, it remains doubtful whether these investigations should be performed routinely for patients with asymptomatic, pathologically confirmed, early-stage breast cancer if the results of the chest x-ray examination and blood work (including liver function tests and alkaline phosphatase levels) along with the clinical assessment are unremarkable. They are likely to be of low yield, yet time-consuming and expensive.[2,7]

CONCLUSIONS

Our results confirm the low yield of metastases at initial presentation of operable early (pathologic stage T1-2 N0-1) breast cancer and the relatively low yield of routine bone scans and liver imaging in asymptomatic patients. Therefore, we no longer recommend these investigations routinely unless the results of initial clinical assessment, chest x-ray examination, or blood work (including alkaline phosphatase levels and liver function tests) reveal abnormalities. However, in locally advanced (pathologic stage T3-4 or N2) breast cancer, the incidence of metastases is much higher, and more extensive investigations (with bone scans and liver ultrasound) are warranted. We believe this is the most efficient and cost-effective approach to staging patients with breast cancer.

Presented as a poster at the 19th Annual San Antonio Breast Cancer Symposium, San Antonio, Tex, December 11-14, 1996.

We thank Marilyn Paradis, Fraser Valley Cancer Centre, Surrey, British Columbia, and the Health Records Staff at the Dr H. Bliss Murphy Cancer Centre, St Johns, Newfoundland, for their secretarial and clerical assistance in the completion of this project.

Corresponding author: Rajiv Samant, MD, Northeastern Ontario Regional Cancer Centre, 41 Ramsey Lake Rd, Sudbury, Ontario P3E 5J1, Canada (e-mail: rsamant@neorcc.on.ca).

REFERENCES

1. Khansur TR, Haick A, Patel B, Balducci L, Vance R, Thigpen T. Evaluation of bone scan as a screening work-up in primary and loco-regional recurrence or breast cancer. *Am J Clin Oncol.* 1987;10:167-170.
2. Nomura Y, Kondo H, Yamagata J, et al. Evaluation of liver and bone scanning in patients with early breast cancer, based on results obtained from more advanced cancer patients. *Eur J Cancer.* 1978;14:1129-1136.
3. Weiner SN, Sachs SH. An assessment of routine liver scanning in patients with breast cancer. *Arch Surg.* 1978;113:126-127.
4. Baker RR. Preoperative assessment of the patient with breast cancer. *Surg Clin North Am.* 1984;64:1039-1050.
5. Berman CG, Clark RA. Diagnostic imaging in cancer. *Prim Care.* 1992;19:690-695.
6. Kinne DW. Staging and follow-up of breast cancer patients. *Cancer.* 1991;67:1196-1198.
7. Lee YN. Bone scanning in patients with early stage breast cancer: should it be a routine staging procedure? *Cancer.* 1982;47:486-495.
8. McNeil BJ. Value of bone scanning in neoplastic diseases. *Semin Nucl Med.* 1984;14:277-286.
9. Beahrs OH. *American Joint Committee on Cancer: Manual for Staging of Cancer.* 3rd ed. Philadelphia, Pa: JB Lippincott; 1988.
10. Wickerham L, Fisher B, Cronin W. The efficacy of bone scanning in the follow-up of patients with operable breast cancer. *Breast Cancer Res Treat.* 1984;4:303-307.
11. Sears HR, Gerber FH, Sturtz DC, et al. Liver scan and carcinoma of the breast. *Surg Gynecol Obstet.* 1975;140:409-411.
12. El-Domieri AA, Shroff S. Role of preoperative bone scanning in carcinoma of the breast. *Surg Gynecol Obstet.* 1976;142:722-724.
13. Gerber FH, Goodreau JJ, Kirchner PT, et al. Efficacy of preoperative and postoperative bone scanning in the management of breast carcinoma. *N Engl J Med.* 1977;297:300-303.
14. Castagna J, Benfield JR, Yamada H, Johnson DE. The reliability of liver scans and function tests in detecting metastases. *Surg Gynecol Obstet.* 1972;134:463-466.
15. Citrin DL, Bessent RG, Creig WR, et al. The application of the 99mTc-phosphate bone scan to the study of breast cancer. *Br J Surg.* 1975;62:201-204.

Invited Critique

I applaud the effort of the authors of this article to determine the value of bone scans and liver scans in the search for metastatic disease in patients who are newly diagnosed as having stage I or stage II breast cancer. This study demonstrated metastasis in only 0.8% of early stage breast cancer in 250 patients. In the 5 patients found to have unexpected metastatic disease, the therapeutic benefits are probably minimal in terms of overall survival. In addition, there are considerable disadvantages in the false-positive outcomes encountered with routine bone and liver scans. The false-positive rate reported in this article is 25% to 35%. The additional patient encounters resulting from false-positive test results and the exaggerated patient anxiety are not to be capriciously discounted. The elimination of nonproductive testing is essential to quality of care. This applies not only to evaluation at the time of initial breast cancer diagnosis but also to testing associated with long-term follow-up of patients with breast cancer.

Philip Z. Israel, MD
Marietta, Ga

IN OTHER AMA JOURNALS

ARCHIVES OF INTERNAL MEDICINE

Prediction of the Risk of Bleeding During Anticoagulant Treatment for Venous Thromboembolism

Philomeen M. M. Kuijer, MD, PhD; Barbara A. Hutten, MD; Martin H. Prins, MD, PhD; Harry R. Büller, MD, PhD

Objectives: To construct and validate the bleeding risk prediction score, which is based on variables identified in the literature that can be easily obtained before the institution of anticoagulant therapy, in a large independent cohort of patients who were treated with anticoagulant therapy for established venous thromboembolism to allow for quantitative assessment of the risks and benefits of the therapy and to adapt the patient's management accordingly.
Methods: We constructed a bleeding risk prediction score, based on variables and their odds ratios identified in the literature, which can be easily obtained before the institution of anticoagulant therapy (score = [1.6 × age] + [1.3 × sex] + [2.2 × malignancy]). Subsequently, we evaluated the score in a test group of 241 patients treated with anticoagulant therapy for venous thromboembolism to determine the optimal cutoff points for the prediction of hemorrhagic complications, using receiver operating characteristic curve analysis. We then validated this score in an independent cohort of 780 patients. A score of 3 or more points, 1 to 3 points, or 0 points represented a high, intermediate, or low bleeding risk, respectively.
Results: The score in about one fifth of the patients in the test group was classified as predicting high risk for bleeding complications. The risk of all bleeding complications was 26% in this group and the risk of major bleeding complications was 14%. The area under the curve was 0.75 (95% confidence interval, 0.64-0.84) and 0.82 (95% confidence interval, 0.66-0.98) for all bleeding complications and major bleeding complications, respectively. When validated, there was a moderate loss of predictive power of the score, but the categorization of the patients by the score remained clinically useful; 20% of the patients were classified as high risk, and the bleeding rate was 17% for all bleeding complications and 7% for major bleeding complications compared with 4% and 1%, respectively, in those categorized as low risk.
Conclusions: With the use of 3 easily obtainable, clinical variables in a prediction model, it is possible to identify a subgroup of patients at the start of anticoagulant therapy who have a high risk of developing hemorrhagic complications. Further studies should address whether additional measures to prevent bleeding decrease the bleeding incidence without compromising efficacy. *(1999;159:457-460)*

Reprints: Philomeen M. M. Kuijer, MD, PhD, Center for Haemostasis, Thrombosis, Atherosclerosis, and Inflammation Research, Academic Medical Center, University of Amsterdam, Meibergdreef 9, 1105 AZ Amsterdam, the Netherlands (e-mail: c.c.keyzers@amc.uva.nl).

Improved Continuity of Care in a Community Teaching Hospital Model

Vijay Mittal, MD; Whitney David, MD; Shun Young, MD; Alasdair McKendrick, MD; Thomas Gentile, Jr, MSA; Robert Casalou, MPH

Hypothesis: We created an ambulatory resident clinic in a community teaching hospital to improve the continuity of care in a surgery residency program.

Design: A retrospective chart review analysis.

Setting: A community hospital, general surgery residency training program, and its ambulatory practice.

Interventions: Providence Hospital, Southfield, Mich, has established a new model, the Surgical Associates of Michigan, which is an association comprising private practice physicians serving as full-time faculty in the Department of Surgery. In addition to clarification of teaching requirements and reimbursement for educational activities, the most dramatic feature is the relocation of private practice offices and the staff surgical office to one central location within the hospital. The proximity of the staff and private surgical offices facilitates closer interaction of attending physicians, residents, and patients.

Main Outcome Measures: Compliance rates of continuity of patient care provided by the same resident, as presented by the Surgery Residency Review Committee, including confirmation of diagnosis, provision of preoperative care, discussion with attending physician, selection and provision of intervention, direction of postoperative care, and postdischarge follow-up.

Results: Since the inception of this arrangement at our institution, surgical residents have seen 229 staff patients and 465 private patients in the offices under supervision. Compliance rate of continuity of care was defined as patient follow-up with the same senior surgical resident who performed an operation or evaluated the patient on initial presentation to the emergency department or offices. We achieved a compliance rate of 92.8% (169/182) in the staff surgical clinics. A compliance rate of 63.5% (205/323) for private general surgical patients and 70.4% (100/142) for vascular surgical patients was obtained. With the establishment of the teaching faculty group and the relocation of offices, we were able to achieve a dramatic improvement in continuity of care.

Conclusions: In addition to fulfilling the Surgery Residency Review Committee requirements, we believe our model facilitates broader education of surgical residents and improves risk management. We recommend further similar studies, greater involvement of primary care specialties in recruiting staff surgical referrals, and implementation of a specialized computer program to continue to improve continuity of care in surgery residency programs.

Arch Surg. 1999;134:555-558

From the Department of Surgery and Medical Education, Providence Hospital and Medical Centers, Southfield, Mich.

CONTINUITY of care is recognized as an important component of providing quality health care. The benefits of continuity of care include decreased hospital admissions, decreased length of stay, reduced duplication of diagnostic testing, enhanced patient satisfaction, more knowledgeable patients, and improved compliance with selected treatment regimens.[1] Historically, continuity of care has been emphasized only in the primary care setting.[2] The majority of studies analyzing methods to improve physicians in training experience with continuity of care have been performed in primary care residency programs. Recently, the Surgery Residency Review Committee (SRRC) emphasized that continuity of care should be an essential element in a surgery residency program. The 2 greatest obstacles to improving continuity of care have been lack of a specific definition of continuity of care and lack of adherence to a single structural model.[3,4]

The SRRC has provided the following definition of continuity of care, composed of 6 elements in which the same surgery resident is involved: (1) determine or confirm a diagnosis, (2) provide preoperative care, (3) discuss the case with the attending physician, (4) select and accomplish the appropriate procedure, (5) direct postoperative care, and (6) follow up after discharge.[5-7] Compliance with continuity of care is important at all levels of training but is essential at the senior resident level.[2]

PATIENTS AND METHODS

Beginning November 1996, Providence Hospital and Medical Centers, a community-based hospital, established a model for continuity of care for the general surgery residents. The intent of this model is to improve both resident continuity of care at the senior resident level and continuity of supervision by the surgical faculty. The hospital administrative faculty, in concert with the Department of Surgery, established the following plan:

1. Establish a corporate entity to facilitate the private practice surgeon participating as faculty in the residency training program.
2. Develop a contract with the hospital and the established corporate entity to pay faculty specifically for teaching duties and supervision of residents.
3. Establish qualification criteria and an agreed-on job description for the duties of the teaching faculty, who would be members of the corporate entity.
4. Provide a common patient office for teaching faculty that would also house the resident staff.
5. Establish enforcement policies to increase both resident and faculty physician compliance with continuity-of-care endeavors.
6. Relocate participating private practice and full-time salaried surgeons to a common area, with space allocated to the residency ambulatory care practice clinics (staff surgical offices) in a building adjacent and connected to the hospital (**Figure 1**).
7. Encourage residents to attend several different offices daily, rather than remain in one assigned office, to increase their percentage of patients seen after discharge.

The surgical residency program consists of 3 categorical residents per year and 6 preliminary positions that are distributed among first-, second-, and third-year residents, for an average total of 21 residents per year. More than half of these positions are designated. In addition, there are rotating residents from family practice, obstetrics-gynecology, and orthopedic surgery. There are no physician assistants or other "resident extenders" on any services, including away rotations. The only exception to this rule is the cardiothoracic surgery rotation, which has physician assistants. Each surgical service has 2 nonoperative days per week that are dedicated to attendance at surgical offices and research activities.

During the last 10 years, our parent institution has averaged 10 517 outpatient and 7635 inpatient surgical procedures per year. These figures include surgical subspecialties, such as cardiothoracic, plastic, and otolaryngological procedures. A total of 3975 general surgical procedures were performed last year. Each of our 3 chief residents (fifth year) perform an average of 1037 cases during their 5-year training period. This includes an average of 353 cases in the last year of training. Our institution averages 28 900 inpatient admissions, including 9400 "short stays" or less than 23-hour admissions per year. Outside rotations include trauma and transplant surgery at Wayne State University–affiliated hospitals, Detroit, Mich, during the fourth and third year, respectively. A pediatric surgery rotation is done at University of Michigan–affiliated hospitals, Lansing, during the third year of residency. At both these institutions residents are under direct supervision of full-time teaching faculty without any physician extenders. Our facilities provide all other surgery rotations, including outpatient, plastic, cardiothoracic, pulmonary, vascular, colorectal, and oncologic surgery.

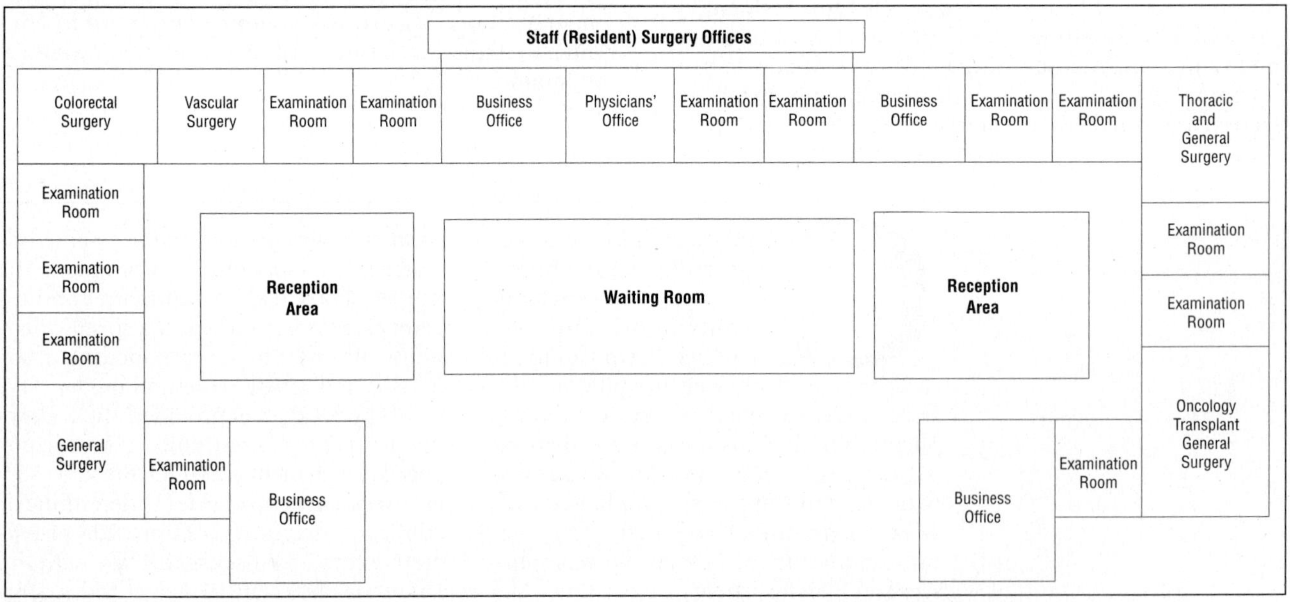

Figure 1. *Schematic diagram showing relocated staff offices in proximity to Surgical Associates of Michigan private faculty offices.*

Anderson et al[7] present, to our knowledge, the only study to date that closely analyzes compliance rates of surgery residents with each of the 6 phases of patient care. This study takes place in a university-based residency program. Although the compliance rates with each of the 6 components separately is higher, residents were able to complete all phases of care with the same patient in only 23.7% of cases. Involvement of the same resident with

The Surgical Association of Michigan (SAM) is the corporate name selected by the Department of Surgery and contracted as a teaching group by the hospital to supervise and teach in the residency training program. The SAM is composed of 16 teaching faculty members, including 10 general surgeons, 3 vascular surgeons, 1 thoracic surgeon, 1 colorectal surgeon, and 1 transplant surgeon. The faculty members of SAM supervise the staff surgical offices at all times. The residents also rotate to the private offices of the practicing surgeons who are faculty and members of SAM.

To coordinate the office practices of the faculty with the residents' time to participate in the office, the faculty are divided into 2 private service teams. Residents rotate on each of these team services and are able to see both preoperative and postdischarge patients in the private office together with the private practice faculty. Scheduling of the team service assignment permits the resident to arrange the postoperative patient office visit on a day the resident can be available for the private practice faculty office. Since the resident is assigned to the private practice faculty office, he or she also sees new patients with the faculty private practitioner and follows up these patients on the team service if admitted to the hospital. We have altered the resident office attendance requirements such that residents are encouraged to visit as many different offices as possible each day. The resident is encouraged to spend only a short time in any given office if this facilitates the greatest percentage of follow-up with the patients on whom that resident has performed an operation. Proximity of the staff and private surgical offices afforded by the relocation facilitates visiting a number of clinics in the most efficient manner (Figure 1). This structure is the basis for the continuity of supervision and continuity of care at Providence Hospital.

The third surgical service is the resident staff service, which is assigned to a senior resident and is supervised by an SAM member. The patients on the staff service are seen preoperatively and postoperatively in the staff surgical offices. Patients are also referred to the staff service from the emergency department and from other specialty resident ambulatory care practices. The staff service includes multiple trauma and other general surgical patients with acute conditions who are managed primarily by the senior resident through all phases of care under faculty supervision. The residents on the staff surgical service perform a variety of procedures, including exploratory laparotomies, laparoscopic cholecystectomies, appendectomies, mastectomies, breast biopsies, herniorrhaphies, colectomies, and gastric and esophageal operations.

Diligent record keeping was maintained by creating surgical office logs to be filled out by each resident. We created a clerical position dedicated specifically to updating patients' medical records with the name of the resident involved with each step of their care. Finally, residents receive repeated written and verbal reminders to follow up with patients and maintain their office and operative logs. Faculty aided compliance by allowing residents to attend various clinics as needed and in some cases notifying residents when patients they operated on would be coming to the clinic.

Our study monitors the experiences of the senior residents during the first 9 months since the inception of our model. We defined continuity of care as the same senior surgical resident having been involved with the same patient through all 6 phases of patient care as previously defined by the SRRC. We suspect our compliance rate with continuity of care before the implementation of our model fell way below the 23.7% rate discussed by Anderson et al.[7] However, we had no prior formal record-keeping system and thus no control group with which to generate a statistical analysis.

the same patient through all phases of care is said to reflect "perfect continuity." Attaining compliance with the requirements of continuity of care presents a challenge in the community hospital setting, where both private and full-time salaried surgeons participate as faculty.[7]

The objective of our study is to propose a model that will improve the rate of "perfect continuity" in a community-based hospital surgery residency training program.

RESULTS

In the first 9 months of this curriculum at Providence Hospital, 229 patients were seen in the staff surgery offices by senior residents. These included 167 patients referred from the emergency department and 89 patients referred from other specialty care resident ambulatory care practice offices. Of the 167 patients seen by the residents in the emergency department as staff patients, 27 did not return for follow-up. Of the 140 patients who did return for follow-up, 106 were followed up in the staff surgical offices but did not have any surgical procedures. A total of 102 of 106 patients managed nonoperatively were seen by the same resident, for a continuity-of-care rate of 96%. The 27 nonreturning patients were counted in this first calculation as a break in continuity of care. Of 34 patients who went to the operating room from the emergency department, 28 (82%) were seen for follow-up in the staff surgical office by the same senior resident who evaluated the patient initially and who performed the operation. Of the 89 patients who were directly referred to the clinic by other specialty clinics, 47 were nonsurgical patients and 42 underwent elective surgical procedures. The 47 nonsurgical patients were not included in continuity-of-care calculations since they were not required to return for a follow-up visit. Of the 42 patients who underwent elective surgical procedures, 39 were seen by the same operating resident for a continuity-of-care rate of 93% (**Figure 2**). Compilation of all the data from Figure 2 reveals an overall rate of complete continuity of care of 93% (169 of 182 possible patients seen) in the staff surgical offices (**Figure 3**).

A total of 465 patients were seen in the private attending surgeon's office by the senior resident during the 9 months of our study. A total of 142 patients were seen in the vascular surgery private offices before the operation. Of these, 100 patients (70%) were followed up by the same operating senior resident. A total of 323 patients were seen in the general surgery faculty offices, which includes colorectal, thoracic, and oncology patients in addition to general surgical patients. A total of 205 of 323 patients were followed up by the same resident after surgery and seen preoperatively in the surgeon faculty offices. A total of 142 patients were seen preoperatively in the vascular surgery private attending

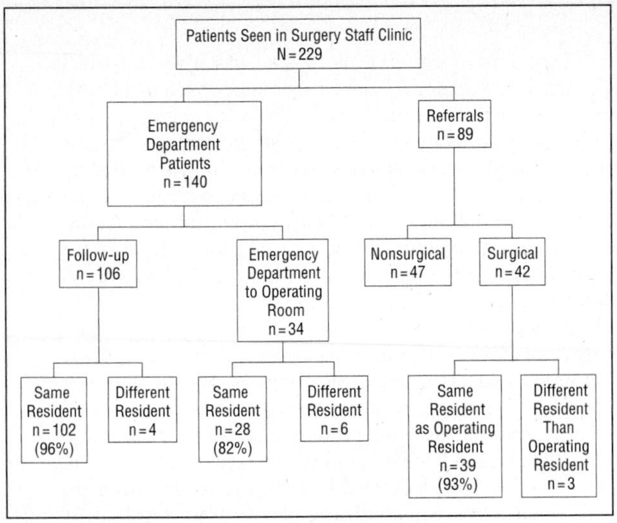

Figure 2. *The total number of patients seen in the surgery staff (chief resident) offices and their compliance with continuity of care.*

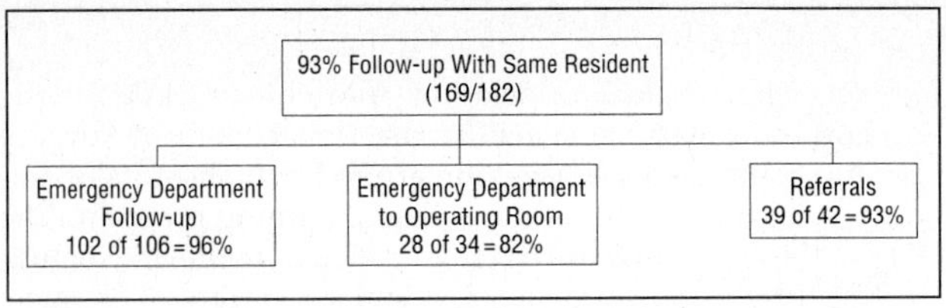

Figure 3. *Summary of compliance with continuity of care by chief residents in the staff surgery offices.*

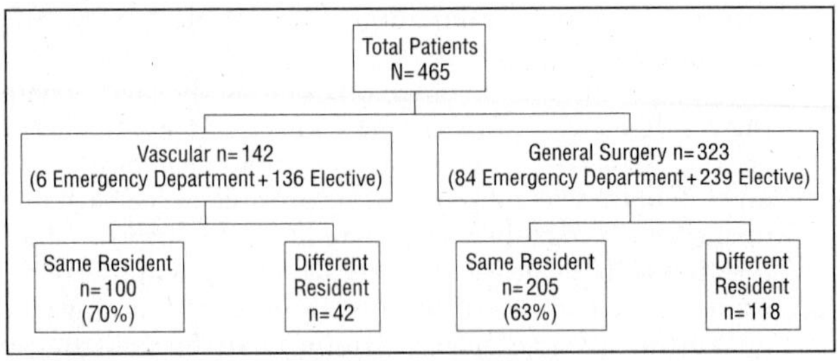

Figure 4. *Continuity-of-care compliance rate by chief residents in the teaching faculty private offices.*

offices. Of these, 100 patients were evaluated preoperatively and postoperatively in the private surgical offices for a continuity-of-care rate of 63% (**Figure 4**).

COMMENT

We believe this study demonstrates successful use of a model designed to improve continuity of care in surgery residency programs, with some limitations. The greatest limitation of this study is the lack of a control group. Like many surgery residency programs, our program allotted minimal attention to the details of continuity of care. Our efforts at tracking patient and resident follow-up before our model lack consistent documentation. However, we believe implementation of our model has facilitated dramatic improvement in continuity of care among senior surgical residents. Although we have no previous rate of continuity of care recorded, the consensus among residents and faculty in our institution is that residents are gaining much more exposure to all phases of management of the surgical patient. Undoubtedly, this broadened education produces a surgeon better equipped to deal with a multitude of surgical management decisions.

This model facilitates fulfillment of SRRC recommendations in a quantifiable manner. Studies examining the implementation of this model in other community-based as well as university-based surgery residency programs need to be performed to determine whether this or a similar model is a candidate for the single structural model sought by the SRRC to improve continuity of care. This model may at least serve as a template on which to make improvements on the path to creating a yardstick to compare all surgery residency programs' compliance with continuity of care.

During our study we noted that although all of our primary care residency programs have residency-run ambulatory care practices, there were minimal referrals between the primary care and surgical resident staff practices. Encouragement of greater consultation and referrals among the residency staff in the ambulatory arena would both increase the volume of patients encountered and grant experiences in referral patterns for residents of all specialties.

Although we examined only senior residents in this study, we suspect that, similar to many programs, continuity-of-care rates are decreased among junior residents. This is likely due to arrangement of call schedules and increased rotations outside the main hospital. Patient perception of continuity of care was not addressed in this study. This important issue may best be addressed by a separate study comparing patient perception to physician perception.

Finally, despite our diligent record-keeping efforts, our system lacks efficiency. Most of our record keeping is done by hand or with the aid of standard data processing computer programs. To maintain thorough documentation and increased accuracy, we are in the process of implementing a specialized computer program. The ideal program would be linked to residents' operative logs, allow patient information to be accessed by a number of different pathways, reveal patients' follow-up schedule in advance, and provide a patient notification system.

Reprints: Vijay Mittal, MD, Providence Hospital and Medical Centers, 16001 W Nine Mile Rd, Southfield, MI 48075 (e-mail: VMITTAL@providence-hospital.org).

REFERENCES

1. Rogers J, Curtis P. The achievement of continuity of care in a primary care training program. *Am J Public Health.* 1980;70:528-530.
2. Dumont-Driscoll M, Barbian L, Pollock B. Pediatric residents' continuity clinics: how are we really doing? *Pediatrics.* 1995;96:616-621.
3. Dent T. Meeting the rules of continuity of care. Paper presented at: Association of Program Directors in Surgery Annual Meeting; April 4, 1997; San Diego, Calif.
4. Friedman P. Meeting the requirements for continuity of care in a surgical residency program. *Curr Surg.* 1997;54:115-116.
5. Accreditation Council for Graduate Medical Education. *Graduate Medical Education Directory: Special Requirements for Residency Training in Surgery.* Chicago, Ill: Accreditation Council for Graduate Medical Education; 1993.
6. Accreditation Council for Graduate Medical Education. *Residency Review Committee for Surgery Newsletter.* Chicago, Ill: American Medical Association; July 19, 1993.
7. Anderson C, Albrecht RR, Anderson K, et al. Can continuity-of-care requirements for surgery residents be demonstrated in the current teaching environment? *Arch Surg.* 1996;131:915-921.

ORIGINAL ARTICLE

Laparoscopic Reoperation for Failed Antireflux Procedures

Myriam J. Curet, MD, FACS; Robert K. Josloff, MD; Othmar Schoeb, MD; Karl A. Zucker, MD

Background: Laparoscopic fundoplication has become the criterion standard for the surgical treatment of gastroesophageal reflux disease. Recently, several patients were referred with recurrent symptoms of gastroesophageal reflux disease or severe dysphagia following previous antireflux surgery for possible laparoscopic reoperation.

Hypothesis: To determine the safety and efficacy of this procedure.

Design: Case series, consecutive sample.

Setting: University-affiliated and community tertiary care hospitals.

Patients: Prospective study of 27 consecutive patients undergoing attempted laparoscopic reoperation for symptoms of recurrent gastroesophageal reflux disease or intractable dysphagia following antireflux surgery. Patients were available for follow-up for 1 to 60 months postoperatively.

Interventions: All patients underwent preoperative workup and attempted laparoscopic reoperation for treatment of symptoms.

Main Outcome Measures: Data were collected on preoperative symptoms and evaluation, operative time, blood loss, time to regular diet, length of hospitalization, morbidity, mortality, and long-term results.

Results: Twenty-six patients underwent successful laparoscopic operations, with no mortality and minimal morbidity. One patient underwent conversion to open laparotomy and then developed a proximal gastric leak, which was treated conservatively. Twenty-four patients began a liquid diet by postoperative day 1, and most were discharged from the hospital by postoperative day 3. One patient required dilation for postoperative dysphagia. The remaining patients are doing well and none have required treatment with acid-reducing medication.

Conclusions: Although technically challenging, laparoscopic reoperation for recurrent gastroesophageal reflux disease can be performed safely and with excellent results. In the hands of experienced endoscopic surgeons, patients who have undergone unsuccessful antireflux surgery should be offered laparoscopic reoperation.

Arch Surg. 1999;134:559-563

NISSEN fundoplication has long been a popular and successful procedure for the treatment of severe gastroesophageal reflux disease (GERD), with control of symptoms in 85% to 90% or more of patients undergoing fundoplication.[1-3] Recently, several prospective studies have demonstrated that the operation can be performed laparoscopically in more than 95% of patients.[4-7] These studies have indicated that when the operation is performed by experienced laparoscopic surgeons, excellent symptomatic and physiological results can be achieved with minimal mortality and morbidity rates that are comparable to conventional open antireflux procedures.[4-7] In addition, many of the benefits of minimally invasive techniques, such as decreased pain, a shorter hospital stay, and quicker return to regular activity, have been recognized.[4-7] An interesting subset of patients has been identified in our practice: patients referred for laparoscopic surgery who have undergone previous antireflux surgery and who then developed recurrent symptoms of GERD or intractable dysphagia. Reoperation for failed antireflux surgery performed prior to the era of minimally invasive surgery has been discussed thoroughly in the literature. Data concerning reoperative laparoscopic antireflux surgery have been sparse. After performing more than 100 primary laparoscopic operations for GERD, we believed that patients undergoing reoperative correction could also benefit from a minimally invasive approach to their disease. The purposes of this study were to evaluate closely 27 patients who developed recurrent symptoms of GERD or intractable dysphagia after primary antireflux surgery to determine which patients were appropriate candidates for a laparoscopic reoperation, to determine if reoperative antireflux surgery was technically

From the Department of Surgery, University of New Mexico School of Medicine, Albuquerque (Dr Curet); Abington Memorial Hospital, Abington, Pa (Dr Josloff); the Department of Surgery, University of Zurich, Zurich, Switzerland (Dr Schoeb); and the University of Arizona School of Medicine, Phoenix (Dr Zucker).

PATIENTS AND METHODS

From 1993 through 1998, our group evaluated 27 consecutive patients who had symptoms of recurrent GERD or intractable dysphagia after previous antireflux surgery. There were 14 women and 13 men ranging in age from 17 to 72 years (mean age, 46.2 years). Prior operations (**Table 1**) included 1 open Allison repair (anatomic), 1 open Allison repair with a concomitant truncal vagotomy and pyloroplasty, 21 Nissen fundoplications (13 open, 8 laparoscopic), 2 paraesophageal hernia repairs (1 laparoscopic, 1 open), 1 laparoscopic Toupet fundoplication, and 1 Heller myotomy and Belsey fundoplication done through a left thoracotomy. The initial antireflux operation had been performed 3 months to 30 years previously (mean, 7.2 years). Symptoms in all patients began 2 weeks to 25 years after the initial operation (mean, 2.3 years). Symptoms and preoperative evaluation are summarized in Table 1. Preoperative evaluation demonstrated a paraesophageal hernia in 4 patients, an excessively tight fundoplication in 2, a disrupted fundoplication in 9, a stricture in 2, a slipped wrap in 3 (1 of which had also herniated into the chest), an incomplete myotomy with a disrupted wrap in 1, and an intact fundoplication that had herniated into the chest in 2. We found no anatomic cause for the symptoms in 4 patients. It seemed that 3 patients simply had an inadequate fundoplication that now allowed for acid reflux, and 1 had severe gas bloating unresponsive to prokinetic agents or a laparoscopic pyloroplasty.

SURGICAL TECHNIQUE

A laparoscopic Nissen fundoplication was performed in 14 patients, while 12 patients underwent a laparoscopic Toupet fundoplication (270° wrap). The remaining patient had a partial wrap performed via an open laparotomy after conversion secondary to gastric perforation and poor visualization. A partial wrap was performed in 3 patients with paraesophageal hernias, in 1 patient with recurrent achalasia, in 2 patients with previous tight Nissen fundoplication, in 1 patient with a stricture, in 2 patients with disrupted fundoplications where preoperative manometry demonstrated severely impaired esophageal peristalsis, in 2 patients who had undergone previous laparoscopic Nissen fundoplications that developed wrap migration (1 of whom also had a slipped fundoplication), and in 1 patient with severe gas bloating (Table 1).

A 5-puncture technique as described by Weerts et al[4] and Pitcher et al[5] was used in all cases. The surgical technique previously described for primary antireflux surgery was followed as closely as possible.[5] In all cases, an open technique was used to enter the abdominal cavity with insertion of a Hasson trocar (Blunt Tip Trocar; Ethicon Endo-Surgery, Cincinnati, Ohio).[8] Usually, adhesions needed to be lysed prior to insertion of the accessory trocars. A 301-angled laparoscope was routinely used for optimal visualization. Two high-flow carbon dioxide insufflators, each set at a maximum pressure of 15 mm Hg, were used to maintain optimal distension and visualization of the peritoneal cavity. A flexible upper endoscope was introduced and positioned at the distal esophagus to transilluminate important landmarks with the lighted tip, thus facilitating identification of the distal esophagus. In all patients, there were numerous adhesions to the left lobe of the liver, proximal stomach, distal esophagus, and diaphragmatic crura that needed to be dissected. Elevation of the liver and retraction of the stomach caudad and to the left were performed in the usual fashion. Blunt and sharp dissection were then used in the area of the distal esophagus and gastroesophageal junction to free up adhesions in this area. The distal esophagus was mobilized, and in all patients, the right and left crus of the diaphragm and both vagi were identified. An opening was then made in the retroesophageal space under direct visualization by alternately dissecting on the left and right side of the esophagus. A Penrose drain was placed around the esophagus to help retract the gastroesophageal junction inferiorly and to the patient's left. In all patients, the retroesophageal window was enlarged (6 × 6 cm minimum) to allow for a tension-free wrap. A minimum length of 5 cm of intra-abdominal esophagus was mobilized to prevent postoperative slippage or disruption of the wrap. In several instances, this required dissection well above the diaphragm. In all cases, the crura were closed with several interrupted sutures. Short gastric vessels and any adhesions found between the fundus of the stomach and the spleen were divided to achieve a tension-free wrap in all patients. The posterolateral edge of the greater curvature was then brought posteriorly through the retroesophageal window to create the fundoplication. A 56F to 60F bougie dilator was passed orally through the gastroesophageal junction to calibrate the lumen to prevent postoperative dysphagia. In the 14 patients undergoing a 360° wrap, a 2- to 3-cm fundoplication was then created using 3 interrupted sutures. Each suture incorporated the anterior wall of the esophagus while avoiding the left vagus nerve.

In the 12 patients undergoing a laparoscopic Toupet fundoplication, the fundus of the stomach was secured to each crus of the diaphragm and to the esophagus with interrupted sutures (a total of 9 stitches). At the termination of the procedure, the flexible endoscope was reintroduced in all patients and the esophagus and stomach were carefully examined. The upper abdomen was covered with a saline solution while the esophageal and gastric lumens were distended with air so that any full-thickness injuries would be apparent. All fascial openings were closed with absorbable sutures and skin edges were approximated with staples.

POSTOPERATIVE MANAGEMENT

On termination of the procedure, the patients were taken to the floor and were not fed by mouth for the first night. The next day, an upper gastrointestinal gastrografin swallow procedure was performed, and if this demonstrated no leak or obstruction, patients were then fed clear liquids. Most patients were discharged from the hospital on day 2 or 3 and were allowed to return to their normal physical activities during the second postoperative week. The patients remained on full liquid diets for 2 to 3 weeks. All patients were seen in clinic within 2 weeks of discharge and were asked about symptoms of reflux and dysphagia. Patients were contacted by telephone at the time of this review and were questioned about use of acid-reducing medications or prokinetic agents. They were asked whether they were experiencing reflux symptoms, dysphagia, or other gastrointestinal symptoms. Finally, they were asked to rank their satisfaction with the results of the operation on a 3-point scale, where 1 indicated totally dissatisfied; 2, satisfied; and 3, very satisfied.

Table 1. Reoperative Laparoscopic Patients*

Symptoms	Previous Surgery	Workup	Cause	Repair
Dysphagia and reflux	Allison, V & P	EGD, UGI, Eman	Incompetent LES	LNF
Reflux	ONF	pH, Eman	Disrupted	LNF
Reflux	ONF	pH, Eman	Disrupted	LNF
Reflux	LNF	EGD, UGI	Slipped wrap	LNF
Reflux	Allison	EGD, pH, Eman	Incomplete LES	LNF
Reflux	ONF	UGI, pH, Eman	Disrupted	LNF
Reflux	ONF	UGI, pH, Eman	Disrupted	LNF
Reflux	ONF	EGD, UGI, pH, Eman	Disrupted	LT
Dysphagia	ONF	EGD, UGI, Eman	Stricture and Reflux	LNF
Dysphagia	LNF	EGD, UGI, Eman	Tight wrap	LT
Reflux	LNF	UGI, Eman	Wrap in chest	LNF
Dysphagia	LPEH	UGI	PEH (recurrent)	LT
Nausea/vomiting	ONF	UGI	PEH	LT
Reflux	ONF	EGD, UGI, Eman	Disrupted	LNF
Reflux	ONF	EGD, UGI, Eman	Disrupted	LNF
Reflux	ONF/HSV	EGD, UGI, Eman	Disrupted	LT
Reflux	LNF	EGD, UGI	Slipped wrap	LT
Reflux	LNF	EGD, UGI, Eman	Slipped wrap	OT
Dysphagia, chest pain	HM/Belsey	EGD, UGI, Eman	Incomplete myotomy, disrupted wrap	LT
Abdominal pain	LT	EGD, UGI, Eman, GES	PEH	LT
Reflux	ONF/HSV	EGD, UGI, pH, Eman	Disrupted wrap	LNF
Reflux	LNF	EGD, UGI, pH, Eman, GES	Wrap in chest	LT
Reflux	OPEH	EGD, pH, Eman	Incompetent LES	LNF
Dysphagia	ONF	EGD, UGI, Eman	Wrap too tight	LT
Dysphagia	LNF	EGD, UGI, GES	Stricture	LT
Dysphagia/gas bloating	LNF	EGD, UGI, GES	Gas bloating	LT
Abdominal pain	ONF	EGD, UGI, pH, Eman	PEH	LNF

**V & P indicates vagotomy and pyloroplasty; EGD, upper endoscopy; UGI, upper gastrointestinal tract series; Eman, esophageal manometry; LES, lower esophageal sphincter; L, laparoscopic; N, Nissen; F, fundoplication; O, open; T, Toupet; LPEH, laparoscopic paraesophageal hernia; PEH, paraesophageal hernia; HSV, highly selective vagotomy; HM, Heller myotomy; and GES, gastric emptying scan.*

feasible, and to evaluate the safety and efficacy of the procedure.

RESULTS

The fundoplication was completed laparoscopically in 26 patients. Mean operative time was 4.1 hours (range, 2.3-7.1 hours). Mean blood loss was 200 mL (range, 100-500 mL). No patient required perioperative transfusion. Complications are listed in **Table 2**. Five patients developed intraoperative pneumothoraces, which did not require a chest tube and did not interfere with completion of the laparoscopic fundoplication. One of these patients did require a Heimlich valve postoperatively. Another patient was noted to have an intraoperative lymph leak, which was controlled by clipping a branch of the thoracic duct. This patient experienced no postoperative problems. In 1 patient, the procedure was converted to open laparotomy because of poor visualization and 2 gastric perforations. The perforations were closed primarily after conversion. The patient later developed a proximal gastric leak that was treated successfully with closed suction catheter drainage. Four additional patients had either gastric or esophageal perforations, which were repaired intraoperatively. None of these patients developed a demonstrable postoperative leak, although 2 patients developed pleural effusions, 1 of whom eventually required a thoracotomy to treat an empyema.

The patient with the esophageal leak and 2 of the other 4 patients with an intestinal perforation were not fed by mouth postoperatively for 3 to 7 days. All other patients (including the other 2 patients with perforations) were given clear liquids on postoperative day 1 and were switched to a full liquid diet before discharge. Mean hospital stay was 3.7 days (range, 1-22 days). Three patients underwent prolonged hospitalization (>7 days). One patient, who had psychosis preoperatively, developed persistent nausea and vomiting following a Toupet fundoplication for a paraesophageal hernia. She eventually received biofeedback and was discharged from the hospital on postoperative day 9. The patient, whose operation had to be converted to open laparotomy and had a proximal gastric leak, was hospitalized for 22 days. A third patient with gastric perforation but no demonstrable leak postoperatively developed bilateral pleural effusions and respiratory distress. He was hospitalized for 9 days and was readmitted for surgical treatment of his left-sided thoracic empyema. Excluding these 3 patients, the mean length of hospital stay was 2.8 days (range, 1-6 days). The average time to return to normal activities after discharge was 9 days (range, 5-28 days). Follow-up data were available in all patients for a mean of 22 months (range, 1-60 months). All patients experienced complete relief of their reflux or obstructive symptoms. No patients are presently receiving acid-reducing medication. Four patients complained of transient gas bloating postoperatively, which resolved spontaneously 2 weeks to 4 months after surgery. One patient required dilation 5 weeks postoperatively for persistent dysphagia. One patient experienced delayed gastric emptying,

Table 2. Intraoperative and Postoperative Complications

Complication	No. of Patients
Pneumothorax	5
Lymph leak	1
Intestinal perforation	5
Intestinal leak	1
Pancreatitis	1
Pleural effusion	2
Empyema	1
Rectus sheath hematoma	1
Dysphagia	1
Delayed gastric emptying	1
Gas bloating	4
Trocar site hernia	1
Total	**24**

which was controlled with prokinetic agents. All patients were satisfied or very satisfied with their results.

COMMENT

Reports of open reoperation for failed antireflux procedures (including Nissen, Hill, Belsey, and Alison fundoplications) have been published previously.[9-16] Reports of laparoscopic reoperation have been anecdotal.[17-21] The failure rate of open fundoplications is estimated at 6% to 20%, with the most common symptoms being recurrent reflux (30%-60%) or dysphagia (10%-20%).[12,19,22-24] Most patients can be managed medically, with only 4% to 6% requiring reoperation.[12,18,23] Morbidity and mortality in these patients is higher than in primary antireflux surgery, with an average mortality rate of 3% (range, 2.5%-18%).[9-16,19,22,23] However, results are generally good, with success rates of 70% to 80% quoted for a first reoperation.[11,13,22,23] Analysis of failures of laparoscopic fundoplications is limited by the short follow-up times available. However, it appears that failure rates, reoperation rates, and presenting symptomatology are similar in patients who undergo unsuccessful antireflux surgery whether the initial fundoplication was open or laparoscopic.[18-21]

Reasons for failure have been well documented and generally are due to errors in technique, inexperience of surgeons, use of the wrong technique, or inappropriate patient selection.[18,19,22,23] Symptoms generally begin within the first 2 years postoperatively.[19,22] The most common cause for recurrent symptoms is breakdown of the wrap, which occurs in 25% to 35% of patients requiring reoperation. A wrap that is too tight or a stricture refractory to dilation leads to surgical revision 10% to 15% of the cases.[10,12,13,19-22] The wrap can herniate into the chest (5%-10%) or can slip down onto the stomach itself instead of staying around the gastroesophageal junction (10%-25%). Finally, patients can develop a paraesophageal hernia either because the crura were not closed or because they became disrupted (10%-15%).[18,19,20,21] Dallemagne et al[20] and Watson et al[21] found a higher incidence of early paraesophageal herniation in patients undergoing laparoscopic surgery (7%) than those undergoing open fundoplication (<2%), presumably due to poor or inadequate crural closure.

The reasons patients in our study required reoperation are similar to what has been reported previously: breakdown of the wrap, 37%; slipped wrap, 11%; paraesophageal hernia, 15%; too tight of a wrap or stricture that did not respond to dilation, 15%; and herniation of the intact wrap into the chest, 7%. In 3 patients (11%), an anatomic cause for recurrent reflux symptoms could not be found, but manometry studies demonstrated an incompetent lower esophageal sphincter.

Most patients with symptoms of recurrent GERD following antireflux surgery will not require reoperative surgery, as their symptoms can be effectively controlled with medications. Only patients with persistent, severe, refractory symptoms should be considered for reoperative exploration. We reoperated on 1 patient 3 months after his initial surgery because his workup demonstrated a clear technical problem that required surgical repair. Otherwise, we recommend aggressive long-term medical therapy prior to consideration of reoperation. In those patients selected for reoperative treatment, determination of the cause of failure of the original operation is critical to ensure that the patients receive the correct revision. Evaluation of the patient with symptoms that suggest failure of their antireflux surgery should include a combination of studies. Upper gastrointestinal tract series will rule out anatomic causes of failure such as paraesophageal hernia, wrap herniation into the chest, stricture, a wrap that is too tight, or a short esophagus. Endoscopy is helpful in determining if a wrap has been disrupted, or to document a recurrent hiatal hernia, poor gastric motility, or esophagitis. Manometry will confirm the presence of a wrap that is too tight, a disrupted wrap, an incompetent lower esophageal sphincter, missed achalasia, or poor esophageal motility. Patients with esophageal dysmotility will be candidates for a partial wrap because these patients experience an increased incidence of postoperative intractable dysphagia after a complete wrap. Studies of pH will confirm acid reflux and are especially important to obtain in patients with no demonstrable anatomic causes for their symptoms. Initially, if patients otherwise satisfied criteria for reoperation and demonstrated esophagitis on endoscopy, pH monitoring was not performed. However, performing full esophageal function tests including pH monitoring in all patients except those with paraesophageal hernias will lessen the chance of reoperation on patients for symptoms that are not due to their antireflux operation.

Most previous studies of reoperation after open antireflux surgery have used a Nissen fundoplication, although in large series, other gastric wraps and even esophagectomy with enteral interposition have been needed.[11,13,15] Some authors have recommended operation through the chest if the patient previously underwent an operation through the abdomen, but most surgeons perform the procedure they are comfortable with. We offered a laparoscopic approach to these patients, who came to us for treatment after failure of their initial antireflux procedure, because we believed they would benefit from a minimally invasive approach and would experience less pain, a shorter hospitalization, and an earlier return to regular activity compared with patients who undergo an open reoperation. Patients who had undergone an earlier open fundoplication confirmed that the laparoscopic approach resulted in an earlier discharge and a quicker recovery period. We performed a Nissen fundoplication on most of our patients. We recommend a posterior partial wrap 270° in patients with stricture, a wrap that was too tight or esophageal dysmotility to decrease the incidence of postoperative dysphagia. We also perform the Toupet fundoplication in patients with a paraesophageal hernia or herniation of the wrap into the chest, as the partial wrap anchors the wrap in the abdomen better than the full wrap does.

Our results are consistent with other reports of reoperative antireflux surgery, whether open or laparoscopic. The morbidity rate was higher than for primary surgery.[5] Operative times were significantly increased compared with patients undergoing a first time laparoscopic Nissen fundoplication.[5] Lack of progress in dissection leading to prolonged operative time (>5) should be considered an indication for conversion to open laparotomy. Neither hospital stay nor postoperative recovery was prolonged in most of our patients.[5] Symptomatic and clinical results were good to excellent in most patients.

Several technical points should be emphasized. Careful attention needs to be paid to dissection of the adhesions. Use of the endoscope will help identify the distal esophagus and prevent inadvertent gastric or esophageal perforation. If a perforation is identified, it should be repaired laparoscopically if possible. The fundoplication can cover the repaired perforation to help strengthen the repair. As with primary Nissen fundoplications, a tension-free wrap is important. This can be accomplished during the reoperation by dissecting out the retroesophageal space adequately. In addition, short gastrics must be taken down if they have not been ligated previously. Dissection of the stomach from the spleen may be necessary in patients who have had the short gastric vessels previously ligated. An adequate length of esophagus must be mobilized. This may necessitate dissection well up in the mediastinum. We have found that a 5- to 6-cm length of intra-abdominal esophagus should be mobilized. Closure of the crura is extremely important. In 3 of our patients, it appears that crural disruption with creation of a paraesophageal hernia was responsible for the recurrent reflux symptoms. It may be difficult to identify the crura or to close them without tension during the reoperation. In these cases, a patch can be sutured or stapled over the crural closure to reinforce it.

Alexander et al[17] recently reported their experience with 2 patients who underwent successful reoperation laparoscopically. Average hospitalization was 3.5 days. Average operating time was 148 minutes. Both patients are free of symptoms. Croce et al[18] described 5 patients who had recurrent symptoms of GERD following previous primary surgical therapy. Four of their patients underwent reoperation laparoscopically. The fifth required conversion to open laparotomy to manage a short esophagus and perform a total duodenal diversion. Clinical results were excellent in all patients undergoing laparoscopic reoperation. These studies, combined with our results, show that laparoscopic reoperation on patients who have had previous antireflux surgery for GERD can be done safely, with minimal morbidity and no mortality. Clearly, the advantages of laparoscopic surgery, including decreased pain, earlier discharge, and quicker return to regular activity, can be applied to this group of patients.

CONCLUSIONS

Laparoscopic reoperative surgery for previous failed antireflux procedures is technically possible and can be completed safely with good symptomatic results and improved recovery. Patients with this problem should be evaluated and treated only by an experienced laparoscopic surgeon. An appropriate preoperative workup to determine the cause of symptoms should be undertaken. The appropriate surgical technique should be applied. These patients need to be informed that there is a high risk of conversion and an increased risk of complications compared with a primary laparoscopic fundoplication.

Corresponding author: Myriam J. Curet, MD, FACS, Department of Surgery, University of New Mexico Health Sciences Center, ACC-Second Floor, 2211 Lomas Blvd NE, Albuquerque, NM 87131 (e-mail: mjcuret@unm.edu).

REFERENCES

1. DeMeester TR, Bonavina L, Albertucci M. Nissen fundoplication for gastroesophageal reflux disease. *Ann Surg.* 1986;204:9-20.
2. Spechler SJ, for the VA Gastroesophageal Reflux Disease Study Group. Comparison of medical and surgical therapy for complication gastroesophageal reflux disease in veterans. *N Engl J Med.* 1992;326:786-792.
3. DeMeester TR, Stein HJ. Surgical treatment of gastroesophageal reflux disease. In: Castell DO, ed. *The Esophagus.* Boston, Mass: Little Brown & Co Inc; 1992: 579-625.
4. Weerts JM, Dallemagne B, Hanoir E, et al. Laparoscopic nissen fundoplication: detailed analysis of 132 patients. *Surg Laparosc Endosc.* 1993;3:359-364.
5. Pitcher DE, Curet MJ, Martin DT, Castle RR, Gerstenberger PD, Vogt D, Zucker KA. Successful management of severe gastroesophageal reflux disease with laparoscopic Nissen fundoplication. *Am J Surg.* 1994;168:547-554.
6. Hinder RA. Laparoscopic nissen fundoplication. In: Condon RE, ed. *Current Techniques in General Surgery.* Milwaukee, Wis: Lawrence DellaCorte Publications; 1993;2:2-7.
7. Bagnato VJ. Laparoscopic Nissen fundoplication. *Surg Laparosc Endosc.* 1882; 2:188-190.
8. Fitzgibbons RJ, Salerno GM, Filipi CJ. Open laparoscopy. In: Zucker KA, ed. *Surgical Laparoscopy.* St Louis, Mo: Quality Medical Publishing Inc; 1991:87-100.
9. Zucker KA, Peskin GW, Saik RP. Recurrent hiatal hernia repair. *Arch Surg.* 1982; 117:413-414.
10. Stein HJ, Feussner H, Siewart JR. Failure of anti-reflux surgery: causes and management strategies. *Am J Surg.* 1996;171:36-40.
11. Skinner DB. Surgical management after failed anti-reflux operations. *World J Surg.* 1992;16:359-363.
12. O'Hanrahan T, Marples M, Bancewicz J. Recurrent reflux and wrap disruption after Nissen fundoplication: detection, incidence and timing. *Br J Surg.* 1990; 77:544-547.
13. Little AG, Ferguson MK, Skinner DB. Reoperation for failed anti-reflux operations. *J Thorac Cardiovasc Surg.* 1986;91:511-517.
14. Luostarinen ME, Isolauri JO, Koskinen MO, Laitinen JO, Matikainen MJ, Lindholm TS. Refundoplication for recurrent gastroesophageal reflux. *World J Surg.* 1993;17:587-594.
15. Hatton PD, Selinkoff PM, Harford FJ. Surgical management of the failed Nissen fundoplication. *Am J Surg.* 1984;148:760-763.
16. Siewert JR, Isolauri J, Feussner H. Reoperation following failed fundoplication. *World J Surg.* 1989;13:791-797.
17. Alexander HC, Hendler RS. Laparoscopic reoperation on failed anti-reflux procedures: report of two patients. *Surg Laparosc Endosc.* 1996;6:147-149.
18. Croce E, Azzola M, Russo R, Golia M, Olmi S. Laparoscopic re-operation from gastro-oesophageal reflux. *Hepatogastroenterology.* 1997;44:912-917.
19. Hinder RA, Klingler PJ, Perdikis G, Smith SL. Management of the failed antireflux operation: surgery of the esophagus. *Surg Clin North Am.* 1997;77:1083-1098.
20. Dallemagne B, Weerts JM, Jehaes C, Markiewicz S. Causes of failures of laparoscopic antireflux operations. *Surg Endosc.* 1996;10:305-310.
21. Watson DI, Jamieson GG, Devitt PG, Mitchell PC, Game PA. Paraesophageal hiatus hernia: an important complication of laparoscopic Nissen fundoplication. *Br J Surg.* 1995;82:521-523.
22. Reiger NA, Jamieson GG, Britten-Jones R, Tew S. Reoperation after failed antireflux surgery. *Br J Surg.* 1994;81:1159-1161.
23. Jamieson GG. The results of anti-reflux surgery and re-operative anti-reflux surgery. *Gullet.* 1993;3:41-45.
24. Martin CJ, Crookes PF. Reoperation for failed antireflux surgery. *Aust N Z J Surg.* 1990;60:773-778.

ORIGINAL ARTICLE

Reasons Why Trauma Surgeons Fail to Screen for Alcohol Problems

Per E. Danielsson, MD; Frederick P. Rivara, MD, MPH; Larry M. Gentilello, MD; Ronald V. Maier, MD

Background: Alcohol screening and intervention have been recommended as routine components of trauma care but are rarely performed.

Hypothesis: An association exists between current screening and counseling practices and the trauma surgeon's knowledge, attitude, and perceived role and responsibility toward alcohol problems.

Participants: Random-sample survey (n = 241) of members of the American Association for the Surgery of Trauma.

Main Outcome Measures: Reported screening and counseling practices.

Results: Fifty-four percent of respondents screened 25% or fewer patients, while only 29% screened most patients. The most common reason for not screening was "lack of time." Most (76%) were not familiar with the most common clinically used screening questionnaires, and 83% reported no training in alcohol screening. Screening was more likely if attending physicians perceived a major responsibility for screening ($P<.001$). Nonscreeners were twice as likely to state screening was "not what I was trained to do" and more frequently believed screening offends patients ($P = .001$). Independent predictors of screening were perceived major role responsibility (odds ratio [OR], 2.35; 95% confidence interval [CI], 1.38-4.01) and confidence in screening ability (OR, 1.96; 95% CI, 1.05-3.67) and counseling ability (OR, 2.27; 95% CI, 1.34-3.85). Eighty-eight percent of respondents would be willing to devote time to training if shown that counseling is effective.

Conclusions: Lack of screening and counseling appears to be due to cognitive factors, not lack of motivation. Skills on how to screen and counsel for alcohol abuse should be taught to trauma surgeons, because a strong correlation exists between screening and confidence in skills. There is a need for education regarding results of effective intervention trials in medical settings.

Arch Surg. 1999;134:564-568

From the Harborview Injury Prevention and Research Center (Drs Danielsson, Rivara, Gentilello, and Maier) and the Departments of Pediatrics (Dr Rivara), Surgery (Dr Gentilello), and Epidemiology (Dr Maier), University of Washington, Seattle.

THE NATIONAL Institute on Alcohol Abuse and Alcoholism has suggested that trauma surgeons should become more involved in the identification and referral of trauma patients with alcohol problems for counseling and not just in the treatment of their injuries.[1] This recommendation is based on increasing evidence that demonstrates the effectiveness of relatively brief alcohol interventions that are capable of being conducted within the time, staffing, and financial constraints typical of a busy trauma center.[2-10]

Currently, most trauma centers do not screen patients for alcohol problems, and the provision of counseling is even more rare. If recommendations to integrate alcohol screening and counseling into trauma care are to be implemented, a better understanding of the reasons why trauma surgeons are currently not doing so is required.[11-14] Surgeons may feel that it is not their role (responsibility), they may not be aware of literature supporting screening and intervention (knowledge), they may have inadequate skills (confidence), or they may believe that screening is intrusive or upsetting (attitudes).[15]

The specific hypothesis tested in this study was that there is an association between current screening practices and the perceived role, responsibility, knowledge, confidence, and attitudes of trauma surgeons toward alcohol screening and intervention. To our knowledge, this is the first study of trauma surgeons that has examined the reasons why screening and counseling for alcohol problems are so infrequent in trauma centers.

MATERIALS AND METHODS

The study was performed at the University of Washington School of Medicine, Seattle. The study population was the membership of the American Association for the Surgery of Trauma, the leading academic society dedicated to the advancement of the care of the injured patient. A survey was sent to a random sample of 50% of the association's membership (n = 419) in April 1996, and a second mailing was sent to nonresponders 6 weeks later. Anonymity was provided to enhance validity of the responses and increase the response rate.

The questionnaire consisted of 29 items and incorporated principles derived from prior surveys of physician knowledge of screening techniques, attitudes toward screening, and active screening patterns.[16,17] It was pilot tested on a separate group of physicians (the surgical faculty, residents, and fellows at the University of Washington), then revised and mailed to the random sample of trauma surgeons. Data analysis was performed using χ^2 tests for categorical data and logistic regression analysis for examination of potential confounding factors.

RESULTS

A total of 241 surveys were returned, a response rate similar to most published mail survey reports involving trauma surgeons.[18-20] Of these, 38 were eliminated: 7 because the respondents were retired and 31 because they worked primarily in pediatric trauma centers. A total of 203 (48.4%) of 419 surveys sent were completed by physicians actively working in adult trauma centers and were therefore included in the analysis. Men constituted 93.0% of respondents, and the median year of graduation from medical school was 1974. Most respondents (80.3%) practiced in an academic setting; 16.3% listed community hospitals as their primary practiced setting and 3.4% of surgeons practiced in both settings.

Eighty-three percent of respondents stated they had had no prior training in screening or diagnosing patients with alcohol problems. Another indicator of a lack of knowledge of screening for alcoholism was the finding that 76.4% of the trauma surgeons responding were unfamiliar with the most common clinically used alcohol screening instrument, the CAGE questionnaire (**Table 1**).

Only 18.7% of respondents reported routinely screening all trauma patients. Screening for alcohol abuse was performed often (defined as screening >75% of patients) by only 29.0% (58/200) of respondents. This group is henceforth referred to as *screeners*. More than half, 53.5% (107/200) reported screening 25% or fewer trauma patients, and this group is referred to as *nonscreeners*. To determine the predictors of screening, we compared the responses of screeners and nonscreeners. A total of 16.7% of trauma surgeons stated they screen approximately 50% of trauma patients, and we did not include this intermediate group in this analysis.

Table 1. Attitude Toward and Knowledge of Commonly Used Alcohol Screening Tools Among Trauma Surgeons

Screening Instrument*	Useful, %	Not Useful, %	Not Familiar With, %
BAC	81.1	5.6	13.3
SMAST	16.1	3.4	80.5
CAGE	21.3	2.3	76.4
AUDIT	7.5	4.0	88.5
TWEAK	3.5	2.3	94.2

*BAC indicates blood alcohol concentration; SMAST, Short Michigan Alcoholism Screening Test; CAGE, Have you ever tried to Cut down on your drinking? Are you Annoyed when people complain about your drinking? Do you ever feel Guilty about your drinking? Do you ever drink Eye-openers? AUDIT, Alcohol Use Disorders Identification Test; and TWEAK, Tolerance, Worry, Eye-openers, Anger, Cutting-down.

Table 2. Main Reasons Why Trauma Surgeons Do Not Screen Trauma Patients for Alcohol Abuse or Dependence

Reasons for Not Screening	Screeners, % (n = 58)	Nonscreeners, % (n = 107)	P
Too busy	28.2	46.6	.04
Not feasible	30.7	27.3	.49
Not necessary	7.7	12.5	.51
Only needs to be done selectively	30.7	30.7	.95
Don't know how	10.2	21.6	.12
Doesn't do any good	20.5	22.7	.86
Not what I was trained to do	10.2	22.7	.07
Not interested	10.2	22.7	.09
Not my responsibility	10.2	6.8	.42
Not enough treatment resources	46.2	45.4	.89

Table 3. Health Care Provider Group With Major Responsibility for Screening Patients With Alcohol Problems as Perceived by Surgeons

Major Responsibility*	Screeners†, % (n = 58)	Nonscreeners†, % (n = 107)	P
Attending	54.5	25.5	<.001
Chief resident	40.4	22.6	.03
Resident	37.7	30.7	.49
Nurse	29.2	17.5	.15
Social worker	39.2	36.6	.54
Psychologist	16.7	14.4	.92
Trauma nurse coordinator	36.5	20.8	.06

*Respondents were instructed to rate responsibility of each group as none, minor, moderate, or major.

†For an explanation of screeners and nonscreeners, see the "Results" section.

The most common reason cited by nonscreeners for failure to screen was "too busy" (46.6%). In contrast, only 28.2% of screeners reported being "too busy" to screen (P = .04, **Table 2**). The survey specifically asked trauma surgeons who they believed should be responsible for screening. The attending physician was felt to have major responsibility for screening by 54.5% of screeners compared with 25.5% of nonscreeners ($P<.001$, **Table 3**). A significantly greater percentage of screeners (40.4%) also stated the chief resident has major responsibility for screening compared with 22.6% of nonscreeners ($P=.03$). No single group of health professionals was consistently cited as being responsible for screening by nonscreeners.

Screeners (54.4%) were significantly more confident in their screening skills than nonscreeners (25.4%) ($P=.02$). The most common test used to screen for alcohol problems was the admission blood alcohol concentration, which 89.1% of screeners reported using in 75% to 100% of patients (**Table 4**). Asking questions about alcohol-related behavior was used with intermediate frequency; 55.0% of screeners reported asking most patients questions about alcohol use and about the quantity of alcohol they consume but rarely used formal questionnaires or substance abuse consultations.

The perceived efficacy of screening tests at identifying problem drinkers was high in both groups but was higher in screeners (94.8%) than in nonscreeners (83.2%) ($P=.06$). In contrast, the perceived efficacy of alcohol treatment was relatively low; only 34.5% of screeners and 24.3% of nonscreeners rated brief interventions as being at least moderately effective ($P=.23$, **Table 5**). Almost half of both screeners and nonscreeners also believed that there were "not enough treatment resources available to make screening worthwhile." A significantly greater proportion of nonscreeners (29.9%) vs screeners (10.3%) thought that screening patients for alcohol problems was intrusive and offends patients ($P=.008$).

Table 4. Methods Used by Screeners to Detect Alcohol Problems

	Reported Frequency of Use, %		
Method or Question	<25% of Patients	50% of Patients	>75% of Patients
Blood alcohol concentration	7.3	3.6	89.1
Questionnaires	79.6	6.1	14.3
Behavioral observations	27.4	17.6	55.0
Psychiatry or social work consult	47.1	19.6	33.3
Asking about quantity of alcohol consumed	10.3	12.1	77.6
Asking about maximum quantity of alcohol consumed on average drinking day	14.0	19.3	66.7

Logistic regression was used to examine predictors of screening while controlling for other factors, and the results are shown in **Table 6**. Belief that the attending physician has major responsibility for screening, confidence in the ability to diagnose alcohol problems, and confidence in the ability to personally counsel patients were the 3 significant predictors of alcohol screening. Each factor roughly doubled the likelihood of screening for alcohol abuse. No other factors were significant predictors of screening in the multivariate model.

COMMENT

The scientific justification for routine alcohol screening and counseling in trauma centers has been established, as documented by reports from the Institute of Medicine and the National Institute of Alcohol Abuse and Alcoholism.[1,21] In this survey of members of the American Association for the Surgery of Trauma, most trauma surgeons reported that they screen less than one quarter of their patients for alcohol problems. We attempted to determine why current recommendations for alcohol screening and intervention in trauma centers have largely been ignored.

This survey revealed that trauma surgeons' knowledge and confidence toward alcohol screening are relatively poor, and these factors are significant predictors of screening behavior. The most common reason provided for failure to screen was "too busy." Screening for alcohol problems can easily be performed by obtaining an admission blood alcohol concentration in the emergency department when blood is drawn for other diagnostic tests. An intoxicating blood alcohol concentration has a high correlation with a subsequent positive result on screening questionnaires. The use of a Breathalyzer or passive nasal breath test is another rapid and inexpensive means of determining blood alcohol concentration.[22]

Screening questionnaires can also be incorporated into trauma center routines with minimal expense and disruption. The CAGE test is a simple 4-item screening questionnaire with its name derived from key words in each of the 4 questions that can easily be incorporated into an admission history or interview: Have you ever tried to *C*ut down on your drinking? Are you *A*nnoyed when people complain about your drinking? Do you ever feel *G*uilty about your drinking? Do you ever drink *E*ye-openers?[23] The CAGE

Table 5. Beliefs About Alcohol Screening and Treatment Among Trauma Surgeons (n = 203)

	Proportion Agreeing With Statement,* %		
Statement	Screeners (n = 58)	Nonscreeners (n = 107)	*P*
Screening does identify problem drinkers	94.8	83.2	.06
Screening does not offend patients	89.7	70.1	.001
Alcoholism is a treatable illness	87.9	90.6	.78
Brief interventions are at least somewhat effective in reducing alcohol abuse	34.5	24.3	.23
Compared to diabetes, treatment of alcohol abuse is at least somewhat effective	34.5	47.2	.16

For an explanation of screeners and nonscreener, see the "Results" section.

Table 6. Independent Predictors of Screening for Alcohol Use Disorders

Variable	Adjusted OR (95% CI)*
Belief that attending physician has major responsibility for screening	2.35 (1.38-4.01)
Confidence in ability to diagnoses alcohol problems	1.96 (1.05-3.67)
Confidence in ability to counsel patients	2.27 (1.34-3.85)

**OR indicates odds ratio; CI, confidence interval.*

test has been extensively tested in trauma patients and has been shown to have a high rate of agreement with the admission blood alcohol concentration and with more lengthy screening instruments.[24,25]

Most surgeons indicated that they have had no training in screening or recognition of alcohol problems and have little confidence in their ability to interview patients with respect to their alcohol problems. Three of 4 surgeons were not familiar with the CAGE questionnaire, and 4 of 5 were not familiar with the Michigan Alcoholism Screening Test, another commonly used screening instrument.

Nearly 30% of trauma surgeons also responded that screening "only needs to be done selectively." However, the ability to clinically detect acute alcohol intoxication using clinical suspicion or physical examination is poor.[26] The false-negative rate has been reported to be as high as 23% and increases to more than one third when patients are severely injured, chemically paralyzed, brain injured, or intubated.[27]

Many trauma surgeons responded that there were inadequate treatment resources available to make screening worthwhile. Studies[10,27] (also L. M. Gentilello, MD; A. Villaveces, MD; R. R. Ries, MD; unpublished data, 1998) on the use of brief interventions capable of being delivered within 1 or 2 counseling sessions have demonstrated a significant reduction in alcohol intake in patients who are not severely dependent, which characterizes the alcohol use characteristics of most of the trauma patient population. A recent review of 32 randomized controlled trials of brief interventions revealed a consistent 20% to 50% reduction in alcohol intake in treated compared with control patients.[2]

Most patients reduce or stop their drinking for a period after treatment. Comparisons reveal that patients who abuse substances have compliance rates comparable with patients receiving treatment for diabetes, asthma, or hypertension, and the likelihood of requiring additional treatment due to relapse within a 12-month period is generally higher for these conditions than for alcoholism.[28,29] If interventions are routinely provided to patients who access the health care system, the cumulative quantity of alcohol consumed and the number of symptom-free periods can be significantly reduced. This is the approach recommended by the Institute of Medicine's report *Broadening the Base of Treatment for Alcohol Problems*, which recommends using nonspecialists to provide brief counseling for patients with mild to moderate alcohol problems in a variety of health care settings.[21]

One encouraging finding of this survey was that trauma surgeons appeared to have a belief in their primary roles in the identification and treatment of alcohol problems in their patients, since most did not believe that screening should only be done by specialists in the field. Trauma surgeons also appeared to be motivated to learn about addressing alcohol problems. Nearly all respondents were willing to devote at least 1 hour to learn brief intervention techniques if they could be convinced they are effective.

This article has documented that the lack of alcohol screening and counseling in trauma centers seems to be due to cognitive factors and not to a lack of motivation or sense of responsibility on the part of trauma surgeons. There appears to be an urgent need for training in alcohol-related issues, because alcoholism is the most common cause of injuries and their recurrence. Thus, addressing alcohol problems is vital to successful injury prevention programs. We recommend training of surgical residents and established trauma surgeons on screening methods for alcoholism, since there was a strong correlation between screening practices and confidence in screening skills. Because surgeons also appear to lack knowledge about the success rate of alcohol treatment, there is also a compelling need for education regarding the successful results of brief intervention programs in health care settings that have been documented in the alcohol treatment literature.

Injuries should no longer be considered the "neglected disease of modern society" but, rather, the neglected symptom of alcoholism. Knowledge about alcohol screening and treatment should be considered part of the skills required to care for injured patients and should be taught in surgical residencies, advanced trauma life support programs, and continuing medical education courses.

This study was supported by grant R40-CCR-00-2750 from the Centers for Disease Control and Prevention, Atlanta, Ga, and grant RO1-AA09045 from the National Institutes of Health/National Institute on Alcohol Abuse and Alcoholism, Bethesda, Md.

Corresponding author: Frederick P. Rivara, MD, Harborview Injury Prevention and Research Center, Box 359960, 325 Ninth Ave, Seattle, WA 98104 (e-mail: FPR@u.washington.edu).

REFERENCES

1. National Institute on Alcohol Abuse and Alcoholism. *Eighth Special Report to the US Congress on Alcohol and Health.* Rockvill, Miss: US Department of Health and Human Services; 1993.
2. Bien TH, Miller WR, Tonigan JS. Brief interventions for alcohol problems: a review. *Addiction.* 1993;88:315-335.
3. Babor TF, Grant M. *Program on Substance Abuse: Project on Identification and Management of Alcohol Related Problems: Report on Phase II: A Randomized Clinical Trial of Brief Interventions in Primary Health Care.* Geneva, Switzerland: World Health Organization; 1992.
4. World Health Organization Brief Intervention Study Group. A cross national trial of brief intervention with heavy drinkers. *Am J Public Health.* 1996;86:948-955.

5. Fuller MG, Diamond DL, Jordan ML, et al. The role of a substance abuse consultation team in a trauma center. *J Stud Alcohol.* 1995;56:267-271.
6. Greber RA, Allen DM, Soeken KL, et al. Outcome of trauma patients after brief intervention by a substance abuse consultation service. *Am J Addict.* 1997;6: 38-47.
7. Wilk AI, Jensen NM, Havighurst TC. Meta-analysis of randomized control trials addressing brief interventions in heavy alcohol drinkers. *J Gen Intern Med.* 1997; 12:274-283.
8. Holder H, Longabaugh R, Miller WR, et al. The cost effectiveness of treatment for alcoholism: a first approximation. *J Stud Alcohol.* 1991;52:517-540.
9. Fleming MF, Barry KL, Maxwell LB, Johnson K, London R. Brief physician advice for problem alcohol drinkers: a randomized controlled trial in community based primary care practices. *JAMA.* 1997;277:1039-1045.
10. Project MATCH Research Group. Matching alcoholism treatments to client heterogeneity: Project MATCH posttreatment drinking outcomes. *J Stud Alcohol.* 1997;58:7-29.
11. Soderstrom CA, Daily JT, Kerns TJ. Alcohol and other drugs: an assessment of testing and clinical practices in US trauma centers. *J Trauma.* 1994;36: 68-73.
12. Soderstrom CA, Smith GS, Dischinger PC, et al. Psychoactive substance use disorders among seriously injured trauma center patients. *JAMA.* 1997;277: 1769-1774.
13. Gentilello LM, Donovan DM, Dunn C, Rivara FP. Alcohol interventions in level 1 trauma centers: current practice, future directions. *JAMA.* 1995;274:1043-1048.
14. Gentilello LM, Duggan P, Drummond D, et al. Major injury as a unique opportunity to initiate treatment in the alcoholic. *Am J Surg.* 1988;156:558-561.
15. Dunn C, Donovan D, Gentilello LM. Practical guidelines for performing alcohol interventions in trauma centers. *J Trauma.* 1997;42:299-304.
16. Geller G, Levine DM, Mamon JA, et al. Knowledge, attitudes, and reported practices of medical students and house staff regarding the diagnosis and treatment of alcoholism. *JAMA.* 1989;261:3115-3120.
17. Bradley KA, Curry SJ, Koepsell TD, et al. Primary and secondary prevention of alcohol problems: US internist attitudes and practices. *J Gen Intern Med.* 1995; 10:67-72.
18. Esposito TJ, Kuby A, Unfred C, et al. General surgeons and the Advanced Trauma Life Support course: is it time to refocus? *J Trauma.* 1995;39:929-933.
19. Esposito TJ, Kuby AM, Unfred C, et al. Perception of differences between trauma care and other surgical emergencies: results from a national survey of surgeons. *J Trauma.* 1994;37:996-1002.
20. Esposito TJ, Maier RV, Rivara FP, et al. Why surgeons prefer not to care for trauma patients. *Arch Surg.* 1991;12:292-297.
21. Institute of Medicine, Committee for the Study of Treatment and Rehabilitation Services for Alcoholism and Alcohol Abuse. *Broadening the Base of Treatment for Alcohol Problems.* Washington, DC: National Academy Press; 1990.
22. Gerberich SG, Gerberich BK, Fife D, Cicero JJ, Lilja GP, Van Berkom LC. Analyses of the relationship between blood alcohol and nasal breath alcohol concentrations: implications for assessment of trauma cases. *J Trauma.* 1989;29: 338-342.
23. Mayfield D, McLeod G, Hall P. The CAGE questionnaire: validation of a new alcoholism screening instrument. *Am J Psychol.* 1974;131:1121-1123.
24. Nilssen O, Ries RK, Rivara FP, Gurney JG, Jurkovich GJ. The CAGE questionnaire and the Short Michigan Alcohol Screening Test in trauma patients: comparison of their correlations with biological markers. *J Trauma.* 1994;36: 784-788.
25. Soderstrom CA, Smith GS, Kufera JA, et al. The accuracy of the CAGE, the Brief Michigan Alcoholism Screening Test, and the Alcohol Use Disorders Identification Test in screening trauma center patients for alcoholism. *J Trauma.* 1997; 43:962-969.
26. Grossman DC, Mueller BA, Kenaston T, et al. The validity of police assessment of driver intoxication in motor vehicle crashes leading to hospitalization. *Accid Anal Prev.* 1996;28:435-442.
27. Kristenson H, Ohlin H, Hulten-Nosslin MB, et al. Identification and intervention of heavy drinking in middle-aged men: results and follow-up of 24-60 months of long-term study with randomized control. *Alcohol Clin Exp Res.* 1983;7:203-208.
28. McLellan AT, Woody GE, Metzger D, et al. Evaluating the effectiveness of addiction treatments: reasonable expectations, appropriate comparisons. *Milbank Q.* 1996;74:51-85.
29. O'Brien CP, McLellan AT. Myths about the treatment of addiction. *Lancet.* 1996; 347:237-240.

IN OTHER AMA JOURNALS

ARCHIVES OF INTERNAL MEDICINE

Screening for *Helicobacter pylori* and Nonsteroidal Anti-inflammatory Drug Use in Medicare Patients Hospitalized With Peptic Ulcer Disease

Hugh M. Hood, MD; Cynthia Wark, RN, MSN; Patricia A. Burgess, RN, BSN; David Nicewander, MS; Michael W. Scott, RN, BSN

Background: Peptic ulcer disease has well-defined causes, with most cases related to *Helicobacter pylori* infection and nonsteroidal anti-inflammatory drug use.

Objectives: To report performance rates on measures of care related to peptic ulcer disease in hospitalized Medicare patients and to identify improvement opportunities.

Methods: Retrospective study of 2267 Medicare beneficiaries hospitalized with peptic ulcer disease. Data were obtained from 2 sources: medical records (n = 1580) from 80 hospitals—16 hospitals in each of 5 states (Alabama, Florida, Louisiana, Tennessee, and Texas)—and a national random sample (n = 687). Three measures of care were evaluated: (1) rate of diagnostic screening or treatment for *H pylori* infection, (2) rate of screening for nonsteroidal anti-inflammatory drug use on admission to the hospital, and (3) rate of assessment of risk factors for recurrence.

Results: The rate of screening or treatment for *H pylori* infection was 52.9% to 59.8% among the 5 states and 55.6% in the national random sample. The rate of screening for nonsteroidal anti-inflammatory drug use was 64.6% to 75.4% among the states and 73.4% in the national random sample. The rate of assessment at discharge from the hospital for additional risks for ulcer recurrence was 66.1% to 73.6% among the states and 70.9% in the national random sample.

Conclusions: Based on hospital records, slightly more than half of the Medicare patients admitted with diagnoses studied are being considered for *H pylori* eradication. If recurrence of this disease is to be reduced, physicians must adopt current screening and treatment recommendations. *(1999;159:149-154)*

Reprints: Hugh Hood, MD, Alabama Quality Assurance Foundation, One Perimeter Park, Suite 200, Birmingham, AL 35243-2354 (e-mail: Hhood@AQAF.com).

Surgery in Belgium

Pierre Mendes da Costa, MD; Roger Detry, MD; Jacques Gruwez, MD; Luc Harper, MD; Patrick Rutten, MD

To fully understand the present state of surgery in Belgium, it is necessary to know the structure of the Belgian State, the type of education, the statutory health insurance system, and the professional bodies representing surgeons. One of the most important problems is the excessive number of physicians, which recently led to the establishment of limits on the number of candidates receiving medical certification. Surgical training modalities are described and the results of a retrospective study concerning the quality of training are detailed. The continuing medical education and peer-review system (accreditation) is presented. *Arch Surg. 1999;134:569-574*

THE STRUCTURE OF THE BELGIAN STATE

In 1993, the unitary Belgian State was transformed into a federal state. The opening lines of Article 1 of the Belgian constitution read, "Belgium is a federal state, composed of communities and regions." The communities are empowered with regard to the so-called personalized matters and culture, which include education.

Recent developments affect the health care system, training, and the accreditation program of surgeons. The federal kingdom is composed of 3 geographic regions (Flanders, Wallonia, and Brussels) and 3 cultural communities (Flemish, French, and German). The federal government and the regions and communities have their specific responsibilities in regard to health care. The regions and communities have responsibilities concerning provision of health care for the population; at the federal level, the Ministry of Public Health is responsible for health insurance and hospital legislation.

Educational matters are the concern of the communities, so it is the Ministry of Education of each community that regulates the undergraduate education of medical students, whereas specialist training is regulated at the federal level. Thus, the health system in Belgium is a complex entity, and health planning and programming are difficult.

From the Departments of Surgery, Centre Hospitalier Universitaire Brugmann, Université Libre de Bruxelles, Brussels (Drs Mendes da Costa and Harper), Cliniques Universitaires Saint-Luc, Université Catholique de Louvain, Louvain (Dr Detry), Universitaire Ziekenhuizen Leuven, Katolieke Universiteit Leuven, Louvain (Dr Gruwez), and Centre Hospitalier de L'Ardenne, Libramont (Dr Rutten), Belgium.

EDUCATION IN BELGIUM

For Belgian boys and girls, basic education starts at the age of 3 years and continues through 12 years of age. After basic education, youngsters attend secondary school up to the age of 18 years, after which they may enroll in the medical faculty of 1 of the 7 universities (Université Libre de Bruxelles, Brussels; Université Catholique de Louvain, Louvain; Université d'Etat de Liège, Liège; Katolieke Universiteit Leuven, Louvain; Vrij Universiteit van Brussel, Brussels; Rijksuniversiteit Gent, Ghent; and Universitaire Instelling Antwerpen, Antwerp).

Until recently, for entry into a medical school, only a diploma of secondary education was compulsory for Belgians, an analogous national certification for other European citizens, or a certificate recognized as equivalent by law, decree, a European directive, or an international treaty.

The medical curriculum is composed of 2 cycles, consisting of 3 and 4 years, respectively. During the first year, students study a survey of philosophy, basics of mathematics, physics, chemistry, and biology. The normal human is the major subject of

Table 1. Surgeons in Belgium as of January 1, 1997

Surgical Discipline	No. of Recognized Surgeons	No. (%) Who Were Trainee Surgeons
General surgery	1402	348 (24.8)
Orthopedic surgery	730	173 (23.7)
Urology	293	48 (16.4)
Plastic surgery	120	23 (19.2)
Neurosurgery	102	24 (23.5)
Total	**2647**	**616** (23.3)

study in the second and third years, although some pathology subjects are dealt with during the third year. In these candidatures, a nursing course is compulsory. The second cycle of 4 years prepares the student in the knowledge of the sick person. Theory and practice of human health care appear in the fourth and fifth years. The sixth year is devoted to a housemanship. In the seventh year, the medical student has the opportunity to choose 1 of 4 branches: general practice, prespecialization, public health, or research. At this stage, he or she is graduated with the degree MD and can embark on training as a specialist or in general practice.

THE STATUTORY HEALTH INSURANCE SYSTEM

Compulsory health insurance for employees was introduced in Belgium by law in 1945 as part of a statutory sickness and invalidity scheme, operated through a reorganized structure of mutual benefit societies.[1] These organizations have existed for many decades, providing health insurance on a voluntary basis to people of various political and occupational affinities. In 1945, when health insurance became compulsory for all employees, it was decided to preserve these societies and use them to run state health insurance. At a national level, they were grouped together into 5 confederations with specific affiliations: Christian, socialist, liberal, professional, and neutral. A sixth independent state carrier, the National Sickness and Invalidity Insurance Fund, was created to care for insured persons who wanted to join a society without political or philosophical connotation. Unlike this national fund, the mutual benefit societies are private organizations selected by the patient, but they operate under identical rules for benefits, contributions, and refunds. The management, at a national level, belongs to the National Institute for Sickness and Invalidity Insurance. This institute collects the money from the taxpayer and passes it on to the mutual benefit societies and to the national fund.

Medical care coverage was progressively extended through the years, the most important being the addition of a scheme for the self-employed in 1963. Today almost the whole population is protected by an insurance system managed by the National Institute for Sickness and Invalidity Insurance. One of the main features of this health system is the important place occupied in it by the private sector.

The dispensing of medical care is monitored by the Central Medical Control Service of the National Institute for Sickness and Invalidity Insurance, which oversees the control functions exercised by the advisory medical officers of the societies. In this way medical practitioners are supervised by their peers.

Private medicine has an important place in the health care system. Free choice of medical practitioner and a fee-for-service scale for reimbursing medical care expenses are important features of health care in this country.

MEDICINE AND SURGERY IN BELGIUM AS OF JANUARY 1, 1997

From 1956 to 1997, we observed an increase in the number of physicians from 9937 to 38 690.[2] As of January 1, 1997, 91% of physicians were in clinical practice, 46.5% were specialists, 43.7% were general practitioners, and 9.9% were specialist candidates. From 1987 to 1997, there was an increase of 35% for specialist candidates and 10% for general practitioners. **Table 1** gives the surgical situation in Belgium as of January 1, 1997.

In all surgical specialties, the percentage of women among trainee surgeons is increasing. When the age distribution among surgeons is examined, the youngest practitioners are found in plastic surgery, then urology and orthopedics, while the oldest are in neurosurgery and general surgery.

THE PLETHORA OF PHYSICIANS

In Belgium the number of physicians is at present 38 690, representing an almost 4-fold increase during the last 40 years. The number of inhabitants per physician decreased from 850 to 262 in the same period (3.4 times fewer). The number of physicians per 100 000 inhabitants was 387 as of 1997.[3] This number has increased from 120 in 1966. Belgium ranked third (behind Italy and Spain) among European countries in the number of physicians per 100 000 inhabitants in 1989, and it has maintained this position. Belgium has more than twice as many physicians per 100 000 inhabitants than Ireland; Italy is at the top of the European rank, with 3 times more physicians per 100 000 than in Ireland.[3]

The increase in Belgium is steady and more pronounced for specialists than for general practitioners, as can be seen from the Belgian figures for 1990 through 1993: an increase of 8% among specialists and 2% among general practitioners.[3]

With the Act of April 26, 1996, Belgian authorities finally accepted the principle of limiting the number of physicians. A federal commission was established to examine the needs in terms of medical personnel and to suggest quotas accordingly. The present number of 1064 new physicians certified per year will be reduced to 700 in 2004, 650 in 2005, and 600 in 2006.

The second part of the new regulation concerns the implementation of a mechanism to achieve this reduction. However, since education is no longer a federal matter, but a responsibility of the communities, 2 approaches emerge. In Flanders a decree on July 24, 1996, introduced, as of the academic year 1997-1998, a compulsory interuniversity entrance examination as a condition of entry to the medical school. The entrance examination aims at testing the competence of the students to round off successfully a medical or dental education.

The examination consists of 2 parts: (1) knowledge and understanding in sciences, namely, physics, chemistry, mathematics, and biology; and (2) the capacity of acquiring and processing information relating to the professional practice of physicians or dentists. The examination will be held twice a year and students will be allowed to compete twice.

The French-speaking community introduced a totally different system. The students will not be selected at entry into medical studies, but 3 years later, at the end of the first cycle. A jury in every French-speaking university will evaluate the candidates during the 3 candidatures, taking into account their academic results, their capacity to practice medicine, their participation in academic activities, contacts with patients, and the integration of basic science in clinical activity. A certificate will be granted to the successful candidates, which will be a mandatory condition to proceed to training as general practitioner or specialist after obtaining the physicians' diploma (at the end of the second cycle).

THE SETTING FOR THE SURGICAL PLAY

It is clear that one of the more dramatic changes we are confronted with in Europe, and especially in Belgium, is the excess of physicians and medical specialists.[4]

Not only are we much more numerous, but the specialist's practice has become much more complex. The training includes a multitude of requirements, a massive administration (logbook, audit, etc), in-training examination, final assessment, scientific papers, etc. The specialist practice implies continuous efforts and stress from the daily confrontation with the hospital management, the problems surrounding up-to-date instrumentation and its rising costs, the subtle distinction between aggressive therapy and a less efficient but safer attitude, the fear of litigation, the rising insurance fees, and the medical or surgical audit, not to mention the neglected family.

The surgical or specialist's work has been transformed. In one single career, therapeutic approaches, anesthesia, indications, and techniques have changed more than during the previous whole century, eg, the revival of local anesthesia, the disappearance of ulcer or conventional reflux surgery, the boom in laparoscopic surgery, and endovascular procedures. Our surgical strategies have to be modified constantly. Adaptability has become a major requirement for the modern surgeon.

In 1997, there were 1402 surgeons in Belgium; if a limit on the number is not instituted, there will be 1834 surgeons in the year 2017 and 2167 in 2042. This medical plethora is, however, balanced by aging and feminization, 2 factors linked with less activity. This means that in specialties where there are fewer women, the excess of physicians is all the more deeply felt (eg, orthopedics and urology).

The number of surgeons practicing is a factor that influences individual surgical activity. A sufficient level of activity is a guarantee of sufficient experience and good professional practice. Decrease of individual activity decreases professional experience. To avoid increasing the excess, it will be necessary to limit the number of trainee surgeons to 33 per year.

THE STRUCTURES

On the national level, 4 types of representative surgical groupings exist: (1) the scientific ones: Royal Belgian Society for Surgery, Belgian Association of Cardiothoracic Surgery, Belgian Association of Surgical Oncology, Belgian Association of Surgical Trainees, Belgian Association of Vascular Surgery, Belgian Group of Endoscopic Surgery, Belgian Trauma Society, and Belgian Association of Pediatric Surgery; (2) the professional one: Professional Union of Belgian Surgeons; (3) the Consilium Chirurgicum Belgicum; and (4) the ministerial ones: High Council for Medical Specialists and General Practitioners, and the French and Flemish Commission for Recognition.

Royal Belgian Society for Surgery

The Royal Belgian Society for Surgery was created in 1893 and celebrated its first centenary in 1993. The aim of the society is study, progress, teaching, and the promotion of surgical meetings. It organizes 3 scientific meetings each year, 2 postgraduate trainee courses, and a national congress. It publishes a journal, *Acta Chirurgica Belgica*.

The society awards 3 prizes:

1. An annual prize (prize of the Royal Belgian Society for Surgery; André Duprez Prize) in memory of a late former general secretary who proposed its creation. This prize of BF 100 000 rewards the first author (corresponding member younger than 40 years) of the best article published in *Acta Chirurgica Belgica* in the past year.

2. A triennial prize (prize of the president of the Royal Belgian Society for Surgery; René Kiekens Prize) in memory of a former president who died during his term. This prize is worth BF 150 000 and rewards a clinical or experimental study leading to an advance in surgery.

3. An annual prize called "Award of Young Surgeon's Publication," worth BF 50 000, for the best article published by a trainee during the previous year in *Acta Chirurgica Belgica*.

The Royal Belgian Society for Surgery has in recent years initiated various scientific associations (Belgian Association of Surgical Oncology, Belgian Association of Surgical Trainees, Belgian Trauma Society). It also collaborates with other scientific societies (Belgian Association of Cardiothoracic Surgery, Belgian Association of Vascular Surgery, Belgian Group of Endoscopic Surgery, Belgian Society for Pediatric Surgery). It participates in the work of the Professional Union and the Consilium Chirurgicum Belgicum.

Belgian Surgeons Professional Union

In defense of the individual rights of its members and without prejudice to the rights of these to act directly themselves, the union can go to court either to defend the members concerned or to request to join the action or participate in the proceedings.

The union represents its members before any authority in matters of training, protection of the status, and conditions of practice as well as before hospital administration institutions where surgery is performed.

Consilium Chirurgicum Belgicum

In view of the forthcoming governmental regulations of the health care system and taking into account the urgent need for unity and strength of Belgian surgery, the Consilium Chirurgicum Belgicum was founded in 1991, assembling representatives of the responsible authority for training and certification, the Royal Belgian Society of Surgery, the Professional Association of Belgian Surgeons, and the Academic Surgical Units. The aim of this board is to foster the development of surgery in Belgium. The Consilium Chirurgicum Belgicum offers the surgical community a body in which the problems of the profession, necessitating a common approach, can be discussed. This body is meant to be a brainstorming unit, playing a federating, coordinating, and eventually arbitrarial role.

Matters of interest that the Consilium share with the surgical community are as follows: (1) the quality of surgical training; (2) the access to specialization determined by the needs of the population and the capacity for training; (3) surgical audit and peer review; (4) subspecialization in surgery; (5) intratraining and final evaluation of the surgical trainees (this has proved to be an important step toward controlling the acquisition of the knowledge and skills to be mastered by the surgeon); (6) dialogue with other specialties concerning common matters; and (7) dialogue and deliberation at a European level.

Another objective of the Consilium is to harmonize training and educational programs of Belgian surgeons with the surgical curricula of the other European countries, a must since the opening of frontiers to free exchange.

SURGICAL TRAINING MODALITIES IN BELGIUM

Before 1953, no regulations concerning surgical training existed. In 1955, the Professional Union of Belgian Surgeons established criteria for surgical recognition by the surgeons. In the 1960s, the government, through the Ministry of Public Health, issued regulations concerning the accreditation of 25 medical specialties. The scope of training in each of these specialties is set by law on the advice of the High Council for Medical Specialists and General Practitioners, whose members are appointed by the Minister of Health. For each specialty, a commission for accreditation monitors training and gives advice to the Minister of Health as to the issue of a certificate of completion of training. Each commission is composed of 2 chambers, one for each linguistic community.[5]

Surgery as a whole has been divided into 5 official surgical specialties: surgery, orthopedic surgery, plastic surgery, urology, and neurosurgery. The possibility for the commissions to issue additional certificates for particular competences in the different fields of each specialty has also been incorporated in its mission.

The requisites with regard to the quality of the training, the trainers, and the training centers were fixed by law on July 18, 1979. A distinction is made between basic surgical training of variable length (4 years in general surgery; 2 or 3 years in orthopedic surgery, urology, and plastic surgery; and 1 year in neurosurgery) and a higher surgical training (2 years in general surgery, 5 years in neurosurgery, and 3-4 years in the other cutting specialties). It should be noted that the 4-year basic training in general surgery represents more than a rudimentary exposure to general surgery, and must be considered as a valid training of such length in this field. One year of surgical training abroad is allowed. The majority of candidates for a surgical career are selected at the end of the medical curriculum (7 years) in the 7 medical schools, but a freelance training program is possible.

The criteria for the trainers are 8 years of surgical experience, responsibility for the organization of weekly seminars, supervision of the activities of the trainee, the provision of the possibility of scientific work, an annual report concerning each trainee, the allocation of 25 beds per 1 to 3 trainees, a clinic and an emergency department, and a minimum of 1 coworker per 50 beds.

For complete training, training centers must be able to offer a staff meeting room, a medical library, a sufficient administrative infrastructure, a broad activity in the various surgical areas, 100 beds, a minimum of 1500 operations per year, a clinic with 2000 new cases per year, and involvement in emergency and intensive care. For partial training, the center must offer 50 beds, 750 operations per year, and 1000 new patients at the clinic, together with facilities similar to those of the above training centers. Patient registration and operative notes are compulsory.

Training is controlled by the 2 Commissions of Recognition (Flemish and French). The commissions are composed of a parity of university professors and representatives of the professional organization.

The commission verifies the training program of each candidate (which must be provided before the training is started), an annual logbook, and the annual reports written by both the trainer and the trainee. At the end of the training, all the documents of the candidate (opinion of the coordinating trainer, original article or paper delivered in a scientific meeting as first author, fulfillment of the conditions of the catalog of interventions, passing of the theory examination at the end of the course) are verified by the commission for certification.

During the whole 6-year training period, the trainee is gradually given increased responsibility and performs operations of increasing difficulty under the close supervision of the full-time staff members. Trainees must keep logbooks in which they note all the operations they perform themselves or assist with. They must also note all the meetings, courses, and seminars they attend.

Trainees must present at least 1 paper in a scientific meeting or publish an article in a peer-reviewed medical journal during the training period. The training must be pursued on a full-time basis in a Belgian surgical department. On special request, the specialty board may al-

Table 2. Number of Surgical Procedures Performed by a Trainee Surgeon During 6 Years of Training

	Average	Range
No. of procedures in which trainee surgeon participates	2969	2235-3582
No. of procedures carried out as leader by trainee surgeon	987	513-1902
Minor interventions, No. (INAMI* nomenclature: <K180 or N400)	806	423-1539
% of total	27.1 (806/2969)	25.2-29.9
% of "personal activity"	81.6 (806/987)	69.2-90.2
Major interventions, No. (INAMI nomenclature: ≥K180 or N400)	181	67-363
% of total	6.1 (181/2969)	4.3-7.6
% of "personal activity"	18.4 (181/987)	9.8-30.8

Belgian health insurance system.

Table 3. Activity of Trainee Surgeons During 6 Years of Training

Surgical Discipline	Average, %*	Range, %
Digestive	37.9	32.9-51.2
Orthopedics-traumatology	19.7	10.9-24.3
Vascular	11.7	10.8-12.8
Thoracic	7.5	4.4-10.2
Urology	6.0	4.1-9.5
Gynecology	0.8	0.8-0.9
Others (plastic, ENT†, stomatology, etc)	16.2	11.1-21.8

**Percentage of the total procedures in which the surgeon has participated.*
†ENT indicates ear, nose, and throat.

Table 4. Number of Procedures to Be Carried Out as Leader by a Trainee Surgeon in 6 Years According to Surgical Discipline

Surgical Discipline	Total No.
Digestive	280
Vascular	**100**
Venous	70
Arterial	30
Bone surgery	**100**
Traumatology	70
Orthopedics	30
Cardiothoracic	50
Urology-gynecology	50
Endocrinology	20
Breast surgery	20
Others	130
Total	**750***

**Minor interventions, 625; major interventions, 125.*

Table 5. Number of Procedures to Be Carried Out as Leader by the Trainee Surgeon According to Year of Training

Year of Training	No. of Procedures as Leader	% of Procedures in Which Trainee Participated
1	45	15
2	80	20
3	100	25
4	155	40
5	170	45
6	200	50

low a training period of maximum 1 year in a foreign department, provided this department is accredited as a training center.

The specialty board supervises the training period by annual inspection of the trainee's logbook and by approval instructor's report, controlling the progress in education and the distribution of the training among surgical subspecialties.

Eventually, the board may modify the training schedule and even propose to prolong the training period. The trainee may appeal against this resolution to the supervising high council. At the end of the training period, the specialty board certifies that the trainee is "apt to practice surgery, independently, under his own responsibility." The Ministry of Health confers on the trainee a Certificate of Specialist in General Surgery after his or her 6-year training program has been successfully completed.

To summarize, after graduating as a doctor of medicine, a candidate for training in general surgery submits a training program to the specialty board for general surgery. This program must be pursued in approved surgical departments under the direction of approved instructors. The candidate contacts the instructors, and the application is accepted or rejected by an individual instructor or by a local committee of instructors after an interview of all candidates for the post.

From the time of Billroth until 4 decades ago, the surgeon practiced the whole scale of surgical treatments, including visceral and fracture surgery, urology, neurosurgery, orthopedics, and thoracic surgery. Presently, our young colleagues are almost compelled to acquire a very specialized profile if they want to seize a position in one of our hospitals.

STUDY CONDUCTED IN THE FRENCH-SPEAKING PART OF THE COUNTRY

We conducted a retrospective study of the files of 16 trainee surgeons who obtained their degree in surgery after 6 years of training in the French-speaking part of the country. The results are given in **Table 2** and **Table 3**.

The catalog currently used by the French-Speaking Community Recognition Commission (**Table 4** and **Table 5**) will soon be used by the Flemish Community Recognition Commission. Currently the data of each new recognition are recorded to update annually the catalog. The catalog is eventually adapted according to new techniques (eg, celioscopy or endovascular surgery).

Training centers are visited every 5 years by a commission composed of 3 members of the Recognition Commission and 2 members of the High Council. These departments are revisited at each renewal of the responsible trainer.

According to a survey conducted within the Ministry of Health,[6] the average number of working hours of a trainee surgeon is 9.93 hours a day. Trainee surgeons spend approximately 25.6 hours on duty per week. The average salary of a trainee surgeon is BF 46 925 per month. Of trainee surgeons, 97.5% of those who qualify find work; 26% do part of their training abroad.

A new bill has been drafted that proposes to limit the working hours of a trainee surgeon to 44 hours a week with a 24-hour recuperation period after 24 hours on duty and allowing 4 hours per week for scientific work. If this bill is passed, it is likely that the training period of a surgeon will have to be prolonged to 7, 8, 9, or even 10 years.

ACCREDITATION AND RECERTIFICATION

A continuing medical education system was adopted in 1994. It is managed by the Accreditation Steering Group, which has equal representation of physicians from the professional organizations and the sick funds, supplemented by experts from medical faculties and scientific societies. The role of the Accreditation Steering Group is to approve the continuing medical education programs proposed by the joint committees and to define the basic requirements for continuing medical education and the proportion of ethics, health economy, and use and quality of health care. Moreover, the Accreditation Steering Group decides on the minimal level of medical activity, the guidelines for quality evaluation and peer review, and directives concerning medical records and the local peer review groups.

The Joint Committee (*Comité paritaire*) for each discipline is composed of equal numbers of physicians representing the professional associations and physicians delegated by the universities and the scientific societies. The task of this committee is to evaluate the continuing medical education program, to monitor implementation, and to propose a minimal level of activity. The individual physician or specialist can apply for accreditation by submitting an accreditation attestation and the attendance certificate. A mechanism of appeal is provided, as well as a moderate preferential honorarium and a financial compensation for the cost of continuing medical education.

On January 31, 1997, there were 9097 accredited general practitioners and 11 242 accredited specialists.

THE FUTURE

Explosion of new technologies, such as 3-dimensional visualization of anatomy, virtual reality, surgical simulations, and virtual prototyping of surgical equipment and operating rooms, will modify the surgeon's environment (preoperative diagnosis, surgical procedure, and surgeon's education) in the year 2000.

Preoperative 3-dimensional reconstruction, telerobotics (computer-guided robot, voice-controlled robot) in operating theaters, ultrasound stereoimaging, teleoperation, computer-assisted surgical procedures, telemanipulation, and image-guided surgery will represent a revolution in the development of surgery. These combined technologies and the miniaturization of surgical instruments will increase the quality of minimally invasive surgical procedures.

New surgical approaches will certainly appear. Examples include development of multidisciplinary treatments in digestive surgery (preoperative, intraoperative, and postoperative radiochemotherapy); in utero video surgery; endoscopic lifting, cutaneous substitutes for burn therapy, and laser therapy in plastic surgery; tissue engineering, biomaterials, and computer applications in orthopedic surgery; intracerebral embryonic cell grafts, stereotactic surgery, radiosurgery, and computer-aided navigation in neurosurgery; transperitoneal celioscopic resection of suprarenal tumors and video-assisted cervicotomy in endocrine surgery; an increase in ambulatory surgery; endoprosthesis in vascular surgery; video-assisted thoracoscopy, phototherapy, and brachytherapy in thoracic surgery; coronary bypass on the beating heart, minimally invasive surgery for valvular abnormalities and simple congenital defects, and intracardiac video-assisted surgery in cardiac surgery; and in the field of transplantation, artificial liver, lung, and heart, venotransplantation, and celioscopy for kidney live donors.

The dawn of the third millennium brings exciting times for surgeons, with more problems of ethics, competence, and responsibility and an increasing importance of the patient's informed consent.

Dr Mendes da Costa is past-president of the Royal Belgian Society of Surgery; Dr Detry, president of the Consilium Chirurgicum Belgicum; Dr Gruwez, president of the Professional Union of Belgian Surgeons; Dr Harper, trainee's surgeon; and Dr Rutten, president of the Recognition Commission for General Surgery.

Reprints: Pierre Mendes da Costa, MD, Digestive Surgery and Coelioscopy, CHU Brugmann–ULB, Place A. Van Gehuchten, 4, B-1020 Brussels, Belgium.

REFERENCES

1. Hubens A, Van Hee R. Surgical training in a statutory health insurance system: Belgian experience. *World J Surg.* 1994;18:667-670.
2. Moens M. La médecine spécialisée en Belgique; de specialistische geneeskunde in België. In: Moens M, ed. Annuaire 1997 jaarboek Groupement des Unions Professionnelles Belges de Médecines Spécialisées (G.B.S.): Verbond der belgische beroepsverenigingen van geneesheren: specialisten (V.B.S.). Brussels, Belgium: Poot SA; 1997.
3. Gruwez JA. Criteria for entry to medical school in Belgium. *Acta Chir Belg.* 1997;97:271-272.
4. Mendes da Costa P. La responsabilité des maîtres de stage vis-à-vis des malades et vis-à-vis des chirurgiens en voie de formation. *Acta Chir Belg.* 1987;87:52-59.
5. Gruwez JA. The Belgian surgical specialist in Europe. *Acta Chir Belg.* 1996;96:99-103.
6. Dercq JP, Somer A, Valckenaers J, Nowak JP, Baert E, Ministère des Affaires Sociales de la Santé Publique et de l'Environnement. Direction de l'Art de Guérir: enquête sur la formation des médecins spécialites. *J Med.* 1995;suppl:1-72.

The Value of Physician Assistants in the Modern Surgical Setting

Dr McMillen's comments on the value of surgical residents compared with surgical physician assistants in the October 1998 ARCHIVES[1] displayed a misunderstanding of the strengths of the physician assistant profession and underestimated some of the inherent weaknesses of residency programs.

Dr McMillen points out that residents work "80 to 100 hours per week." Surgical physician assistants, on the other hand, work an average of 48.7 hours per week for their primary employer (excluding on-call hours), according to the 1998 American Academy of Physician Assistants Physician Assistant Census Survey.[2] Residents may be gone in a few years; physician assistants, as staff, are there as employees. From the perspectives of a hospital interested in providing continuity of quality care, a patient interested in an alert staff, and a surgeon interested in having a team player who knows to place late-night telephone calls when a case is beyond his or her experience or education, physician assistants make sense.

The physician assistant profession has existed for more than 30 years, during which time the percentage of physician assistants working in general and subspecialty surgical settings has increased. If these quality health-care professionals were not cost-effective, one would think fewer hospitals and surgeons would be hiring physician assistants. The services physician assistants provide are reimbursed by Medicare and by third-party payers. According to the 1998 American Academy of Physician Assistants Physician Assistant Census Survey, the median total annual income from primary employers for surgical physician assistants was $67 288. In its *Physician Compensation and Production Survey: 1998 Report Based on 1997 Data*,[3] the Medical Group Management Association estimated that the mean ratio of compensation to gross charges was 0.418 for physician assistants in a surgical practice.

Surgical physician assistants will never replace surgical residents. This is because good surgeons are still essential to the delivery of quality medical care in the United States, and good surgeons are the outcome of good residency programs. Patients need experienced surgeons and surgeons need a strong medical team working with them—one that includes physician assistants.

Stephan C. Crane, PhD, MPH
Alexandria, Va

1. McMillen MA. The value of surgical residencies to community teaching hospitals. *Arch Surg*. 1998;133:1039-1040.
2. American Academy of Physician Assistants. *1998 AAPA Physician Assistants Census Report*. Available at: http://www.aapa.org/98pacr.htm. Accessed March 16, 1999.
3. Medical Group Management Association. *Physician Compensation and Production Survey: 1998 Report Based on 1997 Data*. Englewood, Colo: Medical Group Management Association; 1998.

In reply

I am unsure that Dr Crane and I are really in disagreement. The point of the commentary was that properly supported surgical education at community hospitals is a valuable part of surgical education, and that the expenses of supporting surgical residency education are justified in that it is an asset to the community teaching hospital, not a liability. My underlying personal concern is that surgical educators and the surgical educational establishment have perhaps focused too much on the 17% of health care provided at university and major teaching hospitals, and underemphasized the 83% of American health care provided at community hospitals and community teaching hospitals. This may help to explain why the expertise of many of our organizations is underappreciated by policymakers concerned about the comprehensive delivery of health care—we are too little concerned about how our recommendations "will play in Peoria."

It is my personal bias that physician assistants are the best solution to provide surgical assistance at community hospitals and to ensure that surgical residencies at teaching hospitals stay focused on education as their first priority, by helping control the service load and providing the continuity described in Dr Crane's letter. It is interesting that on the same day I received Dr Crane's letter, I was contacted by the American College of Surgeons about my recommendations for surgical assistants in nonteaching hospitals. I unequivocally recommended physician assistants as the optimal assistants, based on my experience of their high educational qualifications, their involvement in comprehensive patient care both in and outside the operating room, and their demanding professional standards.

Marvin A. McMillen, MD
Chicago, Ill

Somatostatin Receptor Scintigraphy and Endoscopic Ultrasonography for Occult Carcinoid Tumor

We read with interest the report by Rubio et al[1] on "Carcinoid Tumor Metastatic to the Breast" in the October 1998 ARCHIVES. We agree that the presentation is consistent with carcinoid tumor metastatic to the breast; however, consideration should be given to the addition of serum chromogranin

A, the somatostatin receptor for scintigraphy, and endoscopic ultrasonography to elucidate the occult primary carcinoid tumor. Chromogranin A is a valuable serum marker for neuroendocrine tumors, with the highest values found in patients with metastatic carcinoids of unknown primary sites. A correlation has been demonstrated between serum chromogranin A levels and somatostatin receptor positivity for midgut carcinoids.[2] Evaluation for occult foregut carcinoid tumor should include endoscopic ultrasonography, which has a sensitivity of approximately 90% for tumors smaller than 2 cm.[3] Scintigraphy combines the advantage of whole-body imaging with sensitivity of 75% to 100% and specificity of 90% to 100% to detect the unknown primary tumor and other sites of metastasis.[4] Following external scintigraphy, gamma-detection probes can be employed intraoperatively to assist in the detection of nonpalpable (<5 mm), surgically occult lesions.[5]

Finally, positive somatostatin uptake on scintigraphy predicts the efficacy of future somatostatin analog therapy, a possible conduit for radiation treatment and posttreatment follow-up.[6]

Carmine Volpe, MD
Ralph J. Doerr, MD
Buffalo, NY

1. Rubio IT, Korourian S, Brown H, Cowan C, Klimberg VS. Carcinoid tumor metastatic to the breast. *Arch Surg*. 1998;133:1117-1119.
2. Wiedemann B, Bader M, Scherubl H, et al. Gastroenteropancreatic tumor imaging with somatostatin receptor scintigraphy. *Semin Oncol*. 1994;21(suppl 13):29-32.
3. Zimmer T, Ziegler K, Bader M, et al. Localisation of neuroendocrine tumors of the upper gastrointestinal tract. *Gut*. 1994;35:471-475.
4. Hoegertle S, Nitzsche EU, Stumpf A, et al. Incidental appendix carcinoid: value of somatostatin receptor imaging. *Clin Nucl Med*. 1997;22:467-469.
5. Ohrvall U, Westlin JE, Nilsson S, et al. Intraoperative gamma detection reveals abdominal endocrine tumors more efficiently than somatostatin receptor scintigraphy. *Cancer*. 1997;80(suppl 12):290-294.
6. Nilsson O, Kolby L, Wangberg B, et al. Comparative studies on the expression of somatostatin receptor subtypes, outcome of octreotide scintigraphy and response to octreotide treatment in patients with carcinoid tumours. *Br J Cancer*. 1998;77:632-637.

IN OTHER AMA JOURNALS

JAMA

Improved Prognosis of Thoracic Aortic Aneurysms: A Population Based Study

William Darrin Clouse, MD; John W. Halley, Jr, MD; Hartzell V. Schaff, MD; Michelle M. Gayari, BS; Duane M. Ilstrup, MS; L. Joseph Melton III, MD

Context.—Managing thoracic aortic aneurysms identified incidentally by increased use of computed tomography, echocardiography, and magnetic resonance imaging is problematic, especially in the elderly.
Objective.—To ascertain whether the previously reported poor prognosis for individuals with thoracic aortic aneurysms has changed with better medical therapies and improved surgical techniques that can now be applied to aneurysm management.
Design.—Population-based cohort study.
Setting and Patients.—All 133 patients with the diagnosis of degenerative thoracic aortic aneurysms among Olmsted County, Minnesota, residents between 1980 and 1994 compared with a previously reported cohort of similar patients between 1951 and 1980.
Main Outcome Measures.—The primary clinical end points were incidence, cumulative rupture risk, rupture risk as a function of aneurysm size, and survival.
Results.—In contrast to abdominal aortic aneurysms, for which men are affected predominately, 51% of thoracic aortic aneurysms were identified in women who were considerably older at recognition than men (mean age, 75.9 vs 62.8 years, respectively; $P = .01$). The overall incidence rate of 10.4 per 100 000 person-years (95% confidence interval [CI], 8.6-12.2) between 1980 and 1994 was more than 3-fold higher than the rate from 1951 to 1980. The cumulative risk of rupture was 20% after 5 years. Seventy-nine percent of ruptures occurred in women ($P = .01$). The 5-year risk of rupture as a function of aneurysm size at recognition was 0% for aneurysms less than 4 cm in diameter, 16% (95% CI, 4%-28%) for those 4 to 5.9 cm, and 31% (95% CI, 5%-56%) for aneurysms 6 cm or more. Overall 5-year survival improved to 56% (95% CI, 48%-66%) between 1980 and 1994 compared with only 19% between 1951 and 1980 ($P < .01$).
Conclusions.—In this population, elderly women represent an increasing portion of all patients with clinically recognized thoracic aortic aneurysms and constitute the majority of patients whose aneurysm eventually ruptures. Overall survival for thoracic aortic aneurysms has improved significantly in the past 15 years. *(1998;280:1926-1929)*

Reprints: John W. Hallett, Jr, MD, Division of Vascular Surgery, Mayo Clinic, 200 First St, SW, Rochester, MN 55905 (e-mail: hallett.john@mayo.edu).

Cattell and Surgical Technique

RICHARD Bartley Cattell (**Figure 1**), surgeon-in-chief (1935-1960) of the Lahey Clinic, Burlington, Mass, was arguably the finest technical surgeon of his day. He made complicated surgical procedures look easy, with a precise, unhurried style that made the clock seem motionless. This proficiency was maintained despite an illness in later years that made the use of his left hand difficult. Opinions concerning his greatness were supported by his excellent operative results and outstanding worldwide reputation in an era when surgical technique was of major importance.

His typical morning list included 4 to 5 cases, most of which were major, such as Whipple procedure (2½ to 3 hours), cholecystectomy with common duct exploration (¾ hour), thyroidectomy (¾ hour), and Miles abdominoperineal resection (1¼ hours).

These procedures were usually done in 1 operating theatre, so coordination of support personnel was essential (**Figure 2**). These involved 2 or 3 residents or fellows, a scrub nurse (Lucy Williamson) who worked with him for many years and handed him the proper instruments without request, and other operating room personnel who adapted their schedule to the operative list.

One procedure in which he excelled was Miles resection, which he almost always finished in 1 hour, 15 minutes. This procedure was the subject of a Cine Clinic for the American College of Surgeons, and the general opinion was that the film speed was increased at the viewing, but this was not true. The time of 1 hour 15 minutes included the colostomy, abdominal closure, turning the patient, preparing the perineum, and applying the perineal dressing. Routinely the perineal prep was the personal domain of the operating suite supervisor (hard to find today), who lurked outside the door and entered immediately after the patient was turned. All of this was known by the resident staff as "the hour of charm."

One particular morning, during which a full schedule was in progress and during a Miles resection, there was a group of visiting surgeons on the operating room floor, who stood on platforms and looked over the surgeons' shoulders. The perineal outer dressing and binder were customarily attached to the room wall by 2-sided tape in readiness for instant application, but when they looked for it, it was missing and seen attached to the back of a visitor who was departing the room. Perfection had not been achieved, but it was one of life's lesser catastrophes.

Cattell liked to tell a story of 3 Boston surgeons, a senior and 2 assistants, who had a flat tire while traveling to perform some itinerant surgery (allowed years ago). While the tire was being changed, the senior queried his assistants by asking, "Why am I such a good surgeon?" Their replies mentioned his good judgment and wonderfully gentle touch, both of which were denied by the senior. He then declared that the real reason was "I get patients." His use of this story is somewhat out of character for a man who worked hard at his craft, refined his techniques, discarded hesitancies and false moves, and had a capacity for hard work that was legendary. Perhaps he felt that young surgeons needed instruction in areas not ordinarily considered.

It is important to recall some of these details of earlier times when excellence in patient care and surgical technique was of prime importance and the advantage of experience in complicated surgery was widely recognized.

John W. Braasch, MD
Burlington, Mass

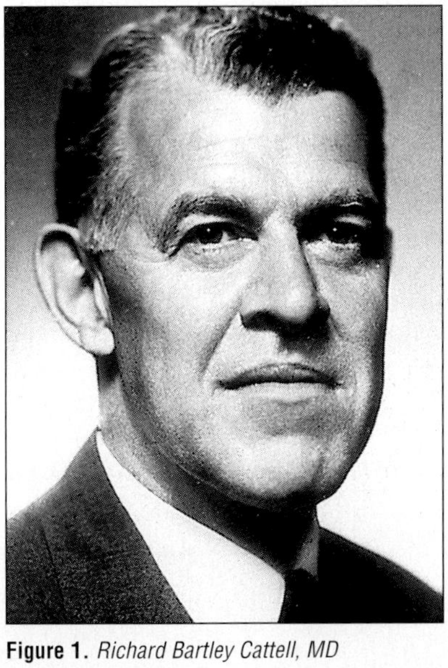

Figure 1. *Richard Bartley Cattell, MD*

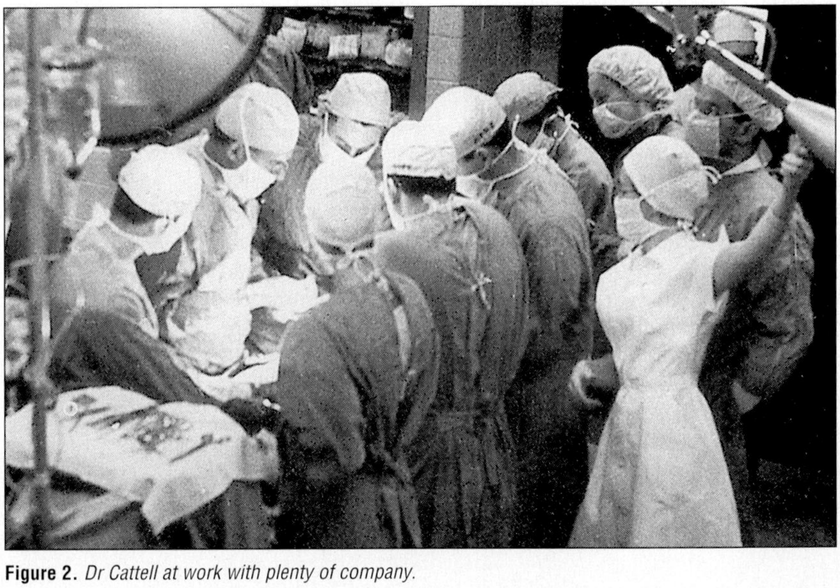

Figure 2. *Dr Cattell at work with plenty of company.*

Crawford Williamson Long

SEVEN AMERICAN surgeons, including Ephraim McDowell, Charles and William Mayo, Charles Drew, Mary Walker, and Harvey Cushing have been honored by having their likenesses placed on US postage stamps. However, it was Crawford Long who became the country's first scalpel bearer so memorialized some 6 decades ago. Such lasting "first-time" esteem stands in contradistinction to earlier events in his life. Long was born in Danielsville, Ga, in 1815, was graduated from that state's university (1835), and then spent 1 year working under a medical preceptor at Transylvania University, Lexington, Ky. Moving to Philadelphia, he received a medical degree from the University of Pennsylvania in 1839, and immediately relocated to New York City where he worked for the next 18 months furthering his medical education and training in various hospitals and almshouses. Family commitments caused him to return to his native state, where he begana small-town practice in the village of Jefferson, Ga.

While a medical student, Long had become familiar with nitrous oxide "frolics" at which the chemical compound was inhaled to achieve a high. In January 1842, a group of his friends induced him to have such a frolic in his home. Long could find no readily available nitrous oxide in the town and did not have the necessary laboratory equipment to prepare the compound. He suggested to his friends that sulfuric ether might produce similar mind-altering results. His acquaintances proceeded to inhale the ether and during their antics received various bruises and cuts. None of these injuries had been felt, and Long rightfully concluded that ether must abolish pain.

Attempting to prove the value of his observation, in March 1842, Long successfully removed a small cyst from the neck of James Venable, who had been etherized. The gentleman underwent a second such procedure that June. By September 1846, Long had performed 8 surgical operations involving the administration of sulfuric ether and was convinced that people rendered unconscious by the influence of this particular gas felt no pain. However, Long, a retiring and shy sort, did not detail his experiments with any other members of the medical profession, written or otherwise.

Only after he had become aware of the countrywide controversy surrounding the conflicting claims of Charles Jackson (1805-1880), Horace Wells (1815-1848), and William Morton (1819-1868) regarding their "invention" and first-time use of ether anesthesia in 1846, did Long publish his results in the *Southern Medical and Surgical Journal* (1849). Consequently, although Long's use of sulfuric ether for surgical anesthesia certainly antedates that of Morton et al by more than 4 years, it is also true that his actions did not encourage other physicians or surgeons to follow his example. Although it would be incorrect to withhold from Long the credit for independent observation and scientific experimentation, he cannot be assigned any distinctive influence on the historical development of surgical anesthesia. In 1850, Long moved to Athens, Ga, home of the state's university and a celebrated center of Southern culture. He continued in the private practice of medicine and surgery and died there in 1878.

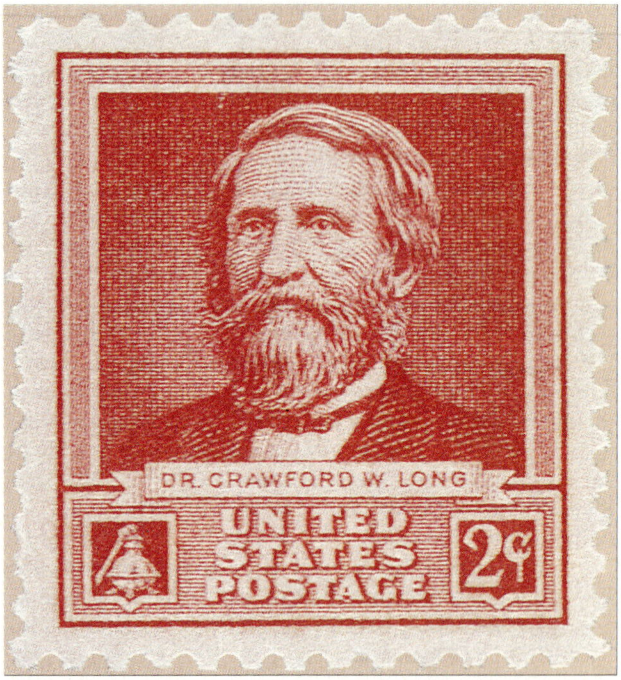

Crawford Williamson Long, depicted in 1940, as part of the "Famous American" series of US postage stamps.

Ira M. Rutkow, MD, MPH, DrPH

PRODUCTS & SERVICES

The information given here is supplied by the companies cited. Publication of these notices does not imply endorsement or warranty by the American Medical Association, publishers of the *Archives of Surgery*.

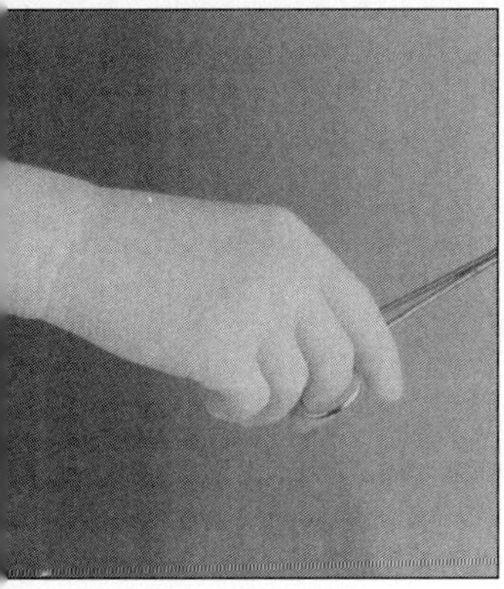

JRGICAL PRODUCT —

Sales of the Duraprene™ Synthetic Surgical Glove from Allegiance Healthcare Corporation have grown more than 300% over the past two years, making Allegiance the new market leader in non-latex surgical gloves.

Duraprene™ gloves, available powdered and powder-free, feature a patented synthetic formulation that provides fit, feel and performance comparable to a natural rubber latex glove.

The Powder-Free Duraprene™ Glove is also the first in the industry to be sterilized by Allegiance's Ster-E-Beam™ process that enhances the physical performance of surgical gloves.

This revolutionary technology offers significant benefits over traditional sterilization processes, including improvements in glove tensile strength, softness, durability and coloration.

For information write

ALLEGIANCE HEALTHCARE CORP.
Attn: Debra Schotz
1430 Waukegan Road
McGaw Park, IL 60085-6787

Phone

847-578-2212

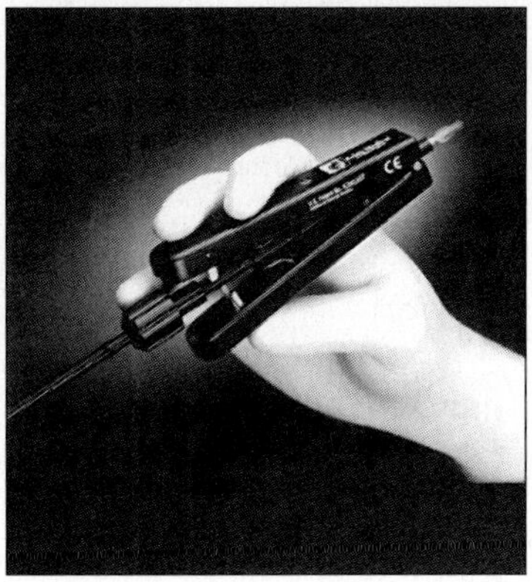

SURGICAL PRODUCT —

Aslan Medical Technologies has introduced the Sensor™ handle for its new line of VersaLap™ surgical instruments. The in-line handle is designed for optimum sensitivity and control with less hand fatigue during minimally invasive surgery.

The Sensor™ handle is available in locking and non-locking styles. Both models are insulated and electrocautery-capable. Construction is of lightweight surgical stainless steel and durable autoclavable ULTEM® for multiple re-use with the VersaLap™ system's dozens of quickly interchangeable tips.

For information write

ASLAN MEDICAL TECHNOLOGIES
Attn: Robert Sheldon
4110 South 9th Street
Kalamazoo, MI 49009

Call toll free

800-551-4561

Phone

612-338-5098

Fax

616-372-9639

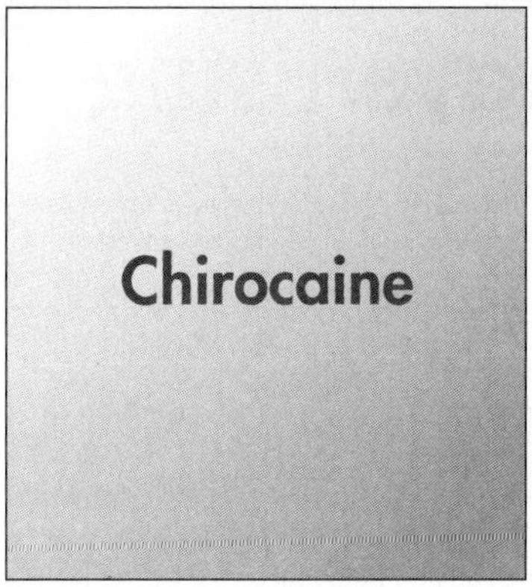

SURGICAL ANESTHETIC —

Chiroscience Group plc announces that, at the meeting of the Anesthetics and Life Support Drugs Advisory Committee of the United States Food and Drug Administration, the Committee voted unanimously in favor of recommending to the FDA that Chirocaine would not need to carry a "black-boxed" warning on the label. Also, during the meeting, the FDA indicated that Chirocaine is approvable.

Chirocaine is the long acting local anesthetic developed by Chiroscience for use in a wide range of surgical procedures and in pain management, both in adults and in children. Chirocaine received approval by the Medical Products Agency in Sweden in December 1998.

Chirocaine is a new drug derived from the established anesthetic bupivacaine. Pre-clinical studies have shown that Chirocaine is as potent as bupivacaine, but has a superior safety profile in its action on the heart and central nervous system. Its efficacy and safety profiles have been confirmed in over 25 clinical trials which have been completed in the UK, USA, Australia, New Zealand, Denmark and the Netherlands.

For information contact

Dr John Padfield, Chief Executive
Christine Soden, Finance Director
Chiroscience Group plc
44-1223-420-430

Web site

www.chiroscience.com

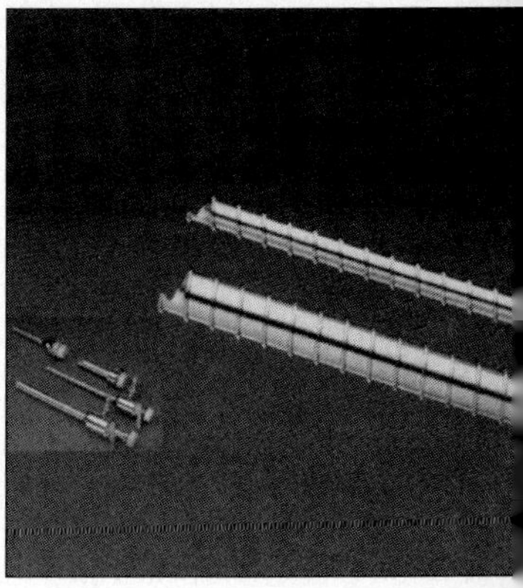

INFORMATIONAL CD-ROM

In an effort to promote awareness of its latest laparoscopic innovation, Karl Storz Endoscopy-America, Inc has created an educational CD-ROM to demonstrate the clinical application of the EndoTIP™ cannula system. This reusable access device provides visualization and control when entering the peritoneal cavity.

The CD-ROM incorporates two-dimensional animation, OR footage and narration to detail the minimally invasive use of the instrument and its unique features. Inventor Art Ternamian, MD, guides users through a case, offering recommendations on technique and commentary about the benefits of using EndoTIP™.

Free CD-ROMs will be given away at the Society of American Gastrointestinal Endoscopic Surgeons (SAGES) meeting March 25-27. Physicians may also contact their local Karl Storz representative for a copy.

For information write

KS ENDOSCOPY-AMERICA, INC
600 Corporate Pointe
Culver City, CA 90230-7600

Call toll free

800-421-0837

Web site

www.karlstorz.com

Classified Advertising

Academic/Faculty
Cardiovascular/Thoracic Surgery
CME Corner
Chiefs/Department Heads/Directors
Courses/Symposia/Seminars
Facial Plastic Surgery
Graduate Training/Residencies/Fellowships
Locum Tenens Wanted
Neurosurgery
Multiple Specialties/Group Practice
Notices
Othopedic Surgery
Pediatric Surgery
Plastic Surgery
Practices For Sale
Surgical Specialities
Thoracic Surgery
Vascular Surgery

Sales Information

1999 CLASSIFIED ADVERTISING RATES

Regular	1x 1.65/wd	*3x 1.55/wd
Bold	1x 1.85/wd	*3x 1.75/wd

*In order to receive the 3-time frequency price, the request must be made upon initial placement. The minimum charge is 20 words. A word consists of one or more letters surrounded by space on each side. For information on display advertising and our network buys contact an account representative.

POLICY

Orders for classified advertising must be submitted in writing. Although the American Medical Association believes the classified advertisements in these pages to be from reputable sources, the Association does not investigate the offers made and assumes no liability concerning them. Acceptance of advertising is restricted to professional opportunities, practices for sale, and medical office space available. The Association reserves the right to decline, withdraw, or edit advertisements at its discretion. Every care is taken to avoid mistakes but responsibility cannot be accepted by the Association for clerical or printer's errors.

REPLY BOX SERVICE

Confidential box numbers are available for an additional $25 per issue, plus the words: Box ________, c/o SUR. When responding to a box number, please send to Archives of Surgery, Box ________, c/o SUR, 515 N State St, Chicago, IL 60610.

CANCELLATIONS/CHANGES

Cancellations/changes must be received in writing at least 25 days prior to the date of the issue. In order to expedite, please fax to 312-464-5909 to the attention of your account representative.

GENERAL INFORMATION

To contact a Classified Advertising account representative, call 312-464-2475/2490/2491/4485 or 800-AMA-2260. Or fax your insertion order to 312-464-5909. Mail your materials to AMA Classified Advertising, 12th Floor, 515 N State St, Chicago, IL 60610.

ACADEMIC/FACULTY

SPARTANBURG REGIONAL HEALTHCARE SYSTEM. SURGICAL EDUCATION. SOUTH CAROLINA - GENERAL SURGERY RESIDENCY PROGRAM: An exceptional opportunity for a board-certified Surgeon with an emphasis in general surgery and critical care medicine to join the Surgical Education Faculty at Spartanburg Regional Medical Center. The physician will be responsible for teaching general surgery residents as well as conducting a limited private practice. Affiliated with the Medical University of South Carolina and the University of South Carolina. Exceptional call coverage arrangement. A previous academic appointment will be a plus. Trauma experience is necessary, as Spartanburg Regional Medical Center is one of four Level I Trauma facilities in the state of South Carolina. Outstanding salary based upon background and experience, as well as an excellent comprehensive benefits package including relocation expenses, CME and professional liability insurance. Research opportunities are also available. For confidential consideration please contact Cathy K. Benson, CMSR, Spartanburg Regional Medical Center, 800-890-0138 or Fax your CV: 864-560-7472. Cbenson@srhs.com EOE.

HEMATOLOGY & ONCOLOGY

SPARTANBURG REGIONAL HEALTHCARE SYSTEM. SURGICAL EDUCATION. SURGICAL ONCOLOGIST: South Carolina - General Surgery Residency Program: An exceptional opportunity for a board-certified Surgical Oncologist to join the Surgical Education Faculty at Spartanburg Regional Medical Center. The physician will be responsible for teaching general surgery residents as well as conducting a limited private practice. Affiliated with the Medical University of South Carolina and the University of South Carolina. Exceptional call coverage arrangement. A previous academic appointment will be a plus. Trauma experience is necessary, as Spartanburg Regional Medical Center is one of four Level I Trauma facilities in the state of South Carolina. The system offers a range of specialized healthcare services that is unrivaled in its five-county service region, featuring world-class specialty centers, including the Regional Cancer Center, a 100,000+ square foot state-of-the-art facility scheduled to open in June of 1999. Outstanding salary based upon background and experience, as well as an excellent comprehensive benefits package including relocation expenses, CME and professional liability insurance. Research opportunities are also available. For confidential consideration please contact Cathy K. Benson, CMSR, Spartanburg Regional Medical Center, 800-890-0138 or Fax your CV: 864-560-7472. Cbenson@srhs.com EOE.

LEGAL SERVICES

MALPRACTICE CASE EVALUATION
Board-certified medical experts needed. All specialties. All locations. Defense and plaintiff cases. Excellent remuneration. Send CVs to:
Barry Gustin, MD, MPH, FACEP
AMERICAN MEDICAL FORENSIC SPECIALISTS, Inc
2991 Shattuck Ave, Ste 302
Berkeley, CA 94705

LOCUM TENENS WANTED

LOCUM TENENS OPPORTUNITIES: are available throughout the US for Physicians of all specialties. Please Fax CV to Staff Exchange @ 770-751-6695 or call: 888-842-4049.

HKA LOCUM TENENS is looking for quality surgical specialty physicians to do Locum Tenens. We have opportunities coast-to-coast. We furnish Occurrence Malpractice Insurance (no tail necessary). Please call **HKA LOCUM TENENS** at (800) 226-6347, Extension AM7.1.

PRACTICES FOR SALE

SENIOR SOLO: General Surgeon in Atlanta area wishes to sell practice totally. FAX inquires to 770-739-2803.

TEXAS: Take over lucrative, highly successful practice with 70-member multispecialty group. Extremely well-managed group with incomes in the top 99th percentile nationwide. 1 in 4 call. Community of 80,000 just over 2 hours from Dallas. Exceptional real estate values, gorgeous homes and country clubs. Contact Todd Dillon: 800-883-7345, ID# 6439AR, Fax; 810-603-2942, E-mail: tdillon@cejka.com Visit our website: www.cejka.com

SURGERY: GENERAL

ADVANTAGE HEALTHCARE STAFFING: has permanent placement opportunities for BC/BE General Surgeon, Orthopedic Surgeon & Vascular Surgeon. Excellent salary and benefits! Call: 888-446-8586.

ALASKA, KETCHIKAN: Seeking recent or impending graduate of approved surgical residency program to join busy, rural, 2 physician hospital based practice in scenic southeast Alaska. Ketchikan is located 1 1/2 hours by jet from Seattle. Excellent opportunity, long term commitment. Little to no managed care. Must be comfortable dealing with wide spectrum of clinical problems. BC or BE. Excellent salary and benefits package. No J-1 Visa opportunities available. Send CV to Ketchikan General Hospital, 3100 Tongass Ave, Ketchikan, AK 99901. Fax: 907-228-8322. E-mail: Panslinger@Peacehealth.org or contact Patti Anslinger: 907-228-8300 ext 389.

BE/BC GENERAL SURGEON: Six surgeon group expanding to meet growth. The practice is located near beautiful Orlando, Florida. This metropolitan area offers all of the amenities of a big city as well as the beautiful weather and environment associated with Florida living. The practice has been in operation for over 25 years and is well established at two of the three hospital system in the area. This is a career opportunity for the right individual to join an established practice. The full range of general surgery is provided and there is a thriving referral base. No vascular. Send CV to Surgical Associates, Attn: Administrator, 1181 Orange Ave, Winter Park, FL 32789 or Fax to 407-647-2710.

EVANSVILLE, IN: A prestigious clinic needs an additional General Surgeon. Call 1:5. Competitive income guarantee package. Live in a safe, family oriented community. Two universities. Cultural activities: music, theatre and dance. Numerous parks & recreational centers offer everything from ice hockey to golf courses. Call Anne Sheahan: 800-678-7858, x3478. Fax CV to 314-726-0026 or E-mail asheahan@cejka.com ID#6345AR; Visit our website at www.cejka.com

---

FLORIDA - WEST CENTRAL: BC/BE general surgeon to join 5 surgeons in busy practice which includes endoscopy, vascular and chest surgery. Competitive salary with incentive leads to full partnership at 18 months. Excellent hospital in rural county of 110,000. 70 miles from two major metropolitan areas. Best rated schools in Florida. Unlimited year round recreation. Prefer recent graduate of university training program. Inquiries - 352-344-4452 - ask for Lynn.

GENERAL SURGERY, ACADEMIC POSITION: Immediate opening for a General Surgeon at Scott & White Clinic and Texas A&M University Health Science Center at the assistant-associate professor level. Scott & White is the largest multispecialty clinic in the Southwest with over 500 physicians and boasts over a century of patient care. Our not-for-profit HMO, which currently contributes about 30% of our business, has over 165,000 members and has been ranked as one of the best in the nation. Interested candidates should have an academic background and a strong interest in teaching residents and medical students. The operative case load is 500+ per year and includes general and advanced laparoscopic surgery. No vascular, thoracic or endoscopic experience is required. Call is 1/6. Please respond with curriculum vitae and three letters of reference to Mike Nichols, Director of Physician Recruitment, Scott & White Clinic, 2401 S 31st St, Temple, TX 76508, or Fax: 254-724-4974. For more information about Scott & White, please visit our web site at http://www.sw.org Scott & White is an equal opportunity employer. Women & minority candidates are encouraged to apply. No J-1 opportunities available.

GENERAL SURGICAL GROUP seeking Board Certified surgeon with Trauma and ICU experience. Please send Curriculum Vitae to Flint Surgical Specialists, PC, 5210 Lapeer Rd, Burton, MI 48509.

LOGAN, UTAH: One BE/BC general surgeon needed for an outstanding practice opportunity. Employment position in a multi-specialty clinic within Intermountain Health Care's Physician Division. Practice in an area where many people visit to ski, fish, hike, camp and enjoy the beauty of the area. A low crime rate and family oriented culture makes this an ideal place in which to live. A negotiable salary and generous benefits package are offered with moving costs negotiable. For more information, send/Fax a CV to IHC Physician Services, Attn: Wilf Rudert, 36 S State St, 20th Fl, Salt Lake City, UT 84111. 800-888-3134 #1. Fax: 801-442-2999. E-mail: comdixon@ihc.com Internet: http://www.ihc.com/phys_recruit

---

MERITCARE MEDICAL GROUP: is seeking a BC/BE general surgeon interested in a practice of General/Laparoscopic, cesarean sections, gyn, and endoscopy surgeries. Join a group of six primary care physicians, an orthopedic surgeon and additional support staff. Detroit Lakes is a resort community of about 15,000 in the heart of western Minnesota Lake country and forty-five miles from a tri-college metropolitan area. The local Hospital is a modern 87-bed acute care facility. Physician will share call and the practice with a partner 20 miles away supported by 6 family physicians in a 29 bed hospital facility. Tertiary Center with 40+ specialists represented is located less than an hour away. For more information please contact Kathleen McKittrick Toft at 800-437-4010 or Fax vitae to 701-234-2316. E-mail: kathetoft@meritcare.com or see www.meritcare.com

---

NEW YORK - LONG ISLAND: $200,000. General/Vascular surgeon to join expanding single specialty group practice. Magnificent waterfront location. Early partnership. "Carriage trade" patient population. Fax CV Dr Jacobs: 914-833-1711; voice: 914-833-1700; ejmsearch@aol.com; #6265c

NORTHWESTERN GENERAL SURGERY PRACTICE: Seeks fourth surgeon for established group. This is a lifestyle practice. Enjoy four-season climate with spectacular mountains and ocean near by. Strong referral base. Four-day workweek and partnership potential are some of the outstanding professional components of this opportunity. $170K salary with production and great benefits. Call Kendrick McLaughlin @ 800-347-7987, ext 8-160 or Fax your CV to her @ 800-254-8233. E-mail address: kmcl@hkainc.com

---

OKLAHOMA: General/Vascular Surgeon. $250,000. Fax CV to Jack Gingold: 914-833-1711. Tel: 914-833-1700; 800-333-2999. ejmsearch@aol.com #6457C.

OPPORTUNITY IN NORTHEASTERN OKLAHOMA LAKE COUNTRY: Strong 70 bed JCAHO accredited not-for-profit hospital has an opportunity for 1 general surgeon. General surgery service area of 60,000+. 12 BC physicians on staff including an anesthesiologist. 40 minutes from Tulsa. Negotiable financial arrangements. Call Stan Schuermann at INTEGRIS Baptist Medical Center at 800-332-8663.

PIEDMONT NORTH CAROLINA: General Surgeon. Ideal candidate should have a strong vascular interest. You would be co-located with a solo general surgeon who has built a tremendous practice since moving here from residency nearly three years ago. This position will offer a guaranteed salary for the first year and a partnership tract. Candidates should have completed medical school at the LCME-accredited program and residency at a ACGME-accredited program. Safe, family-oriented community enjoys excellent school system, low crime, 97%+ employment, and many recreational activities in the beautiful rolling hills of NC. Mail CV to Randy Mitchell, Randolph Hospital, 364 White Oak St, Asheboro, NC 27203. Or Fax: 336-626-7664. Or call: 336-633-7777. E-mail: rlm@atomic.net Visit our website at www.randolphhospital.org

---

SOUTH TEXAS – GENERAL SURGERY: If you enjoy "Quality of Life" issues such as, low crime, excellent schools, no state income tax, clean air, and a low cost of living, then this practice opportunity is for you. A brand new hospital with a medical service area of 78,000 needs additional general surgery coverage. A generous income guarantee, no managed care, and an established referral system, are all excellent reasons why you should call to get additional information. This is a predominantly Hispanic community. If you're looking for unlimited income potential and a family oriented community, then please call for further details. For more information, call Robert Overfield: 800-839-4728. E-mail: overfield@beck-field.com Fax: 210-651-4338.

THREE PHYSICIAN GENERAL/VASCULAR PRACTICE: seeking surgeon with expert skills in breast and laparoscopic surgery. Board certified or Board eligible. Fax resume to 908-722-8676.

TRAUMA SURGERY IN BEAUTIFUL SUNNY CALIFORNIA: Just one and a half-hours from San Francisco. Very busy multispecialty group is seeking trauma surgeons to cover their hospital contract. $200,000 plus production and an excellent benefits package make this a can not miss opportunity. Call Robert Evans at 800-866-7987 ref #9-005 or Fax your CV to 800-428-2520. E-mail: hkaphoenix@mindspring.com or visit us at our website at www.medopps-hka.com No J-1 visa opportunities available.

SURGERY: ORTHOPEDIC

OPPORTUNITY IN NORTHEASTERN OKLAHOMA LAKE COUNTRY: Strong not-for-profit hospital has an opportunity for 1 orthopedic surgeon. Orthopedic surgery service area of 60,000+. 70 bed JCAHO accredited hospital with 12 BC physicians on staff including an anesthesiologist. 40 minutes from Tulsa. Negotiable financial arrangements. Call Stan Schuermann at INTEGRIS Baptist Medical Center at 800-332-8663.

SURGERY: SURGICAL SPECIALTIES

TWO-SURGEON PRACTICE, located in central New York, seeks general surgeon with laparoscopic, vascular, and/or thoracic capabilities. Recent fellowship training desirable. Based in the scenic and cosmopolitan home of Cornell University. The practice serves two progressive medical centers. Excellent lifestyle opportunities abound in housing, education, and recreation. Reply to Box 323, c/o SUR, 515 N State St, 12th Fl, Chicago, IL 60610.

SURGERY: VASCULAR

SPARTANBURG REGIONAL HEALTHCARE SYSTEM: SURGICAL EDUCATION. VASCULAR SURGEON: South Carolina - General Surgery Residency Program: An Exceptional opportunity for a board-certified Vascular Surgeon to join the Surgical Education Faculty at Spartanburg Regional Medical Center. The physician will be responsible for teaching general surgery residents as well as conducting a limited private practice. Affiliated with the Medical University of South Carolina and the University of South Carolina. Exceptional call coverage arrangement. A previous academic appointment will be a plus. Trauma experience is necessary, as Spartanburg Regional Medical Center is one of four Level I Trauma facilities in the state of South Carolina. The system offers a range of specialized healthcare services that is unrivaled in its five-county service region, featuring world-class specialty centers, including the Regional Heart Center. Outstanding salary based upon background and experience, as well as an excellent comprehensive benefits package including relocation expenses, CME and professional liability insurance. Research opportunities are also available. For confidential consideration please contact Cathy K. Benson, CMSR, Spartanburg Regional Medical Center, 800-890-0138 or Fax your CV: 864-560-7472. Cbenson@srhs.com EOE.

VASCULAR SURGEON: Beautiful Central Florida. Easy access to Orlando and Tampa. Moss-draped oak trees line hundred year old streets in our beautiful city. Practice vascular surgery and some general surgery as the third surgeon in a busy practice. Affiliate with two hospitals with more than 550 beds in the community. Call Robert Estes at 800-321-2460. FAX CV to 407-253-9055.

ANNOUNCEMENT

Travel Grants for Research

The Burroughs Wellcome Fund (BWF) is accepting applications for 3 types of research travel grants, which enable US and Canadian scientists and medical historians to work for brief periods (2 weeks to 6 months) in the United Kingdom or the Republic of Ireland. The BWF annually makes approximately 50 research travel grants, including 10 grants in the history of medicine. The grants cover travel and subsistence expenses and range from $1000 to $15 000. Candidates must be citizens or permanent residents of the United States or Canada. Scientific investigators and medical historians must have a MD or PhD degree and hold an academic appointment at the assistant professor level or above at a degree-granting institution. Postdoctoral fellows must be early in their careers, and graduate students must be within a year of receiving their doctorates.

There are 3 application deadlines per year: March 1, July 1, and November 1. For information contact Rolly Simpson, Program Associate, telephone (919) 991-5110, e-mail: mailback@bwfund.org, or visit the Web site at http://www.bwfund.org.

ANNOUNCEMENT

Grants for Cancer Research

The American Cancer Society is accepting applications for its research project grants. Submitted proposals must focus on poor and underserved populations but may address a variety of behavioral, epidemiologic, policy, health delivery, clinical, and basic science issues. Interdisciplinary collaborations are encouraged and the novelty and uniqueness of the proposed projects will be an important aspect in the evaluation process. Grants will be for 3 years, up to $250 000 per year, including 25% indirect costs.

The first application deadline is April 1, 1999. The next date will be October 15, 1999, and the same dates in subsequent years.

For further information, contact Donella Wilson, PhD at (404) 329-7717 or e-mail: dwilson@cancer.org. Applications materials can be downloaded at www.cancer.org.

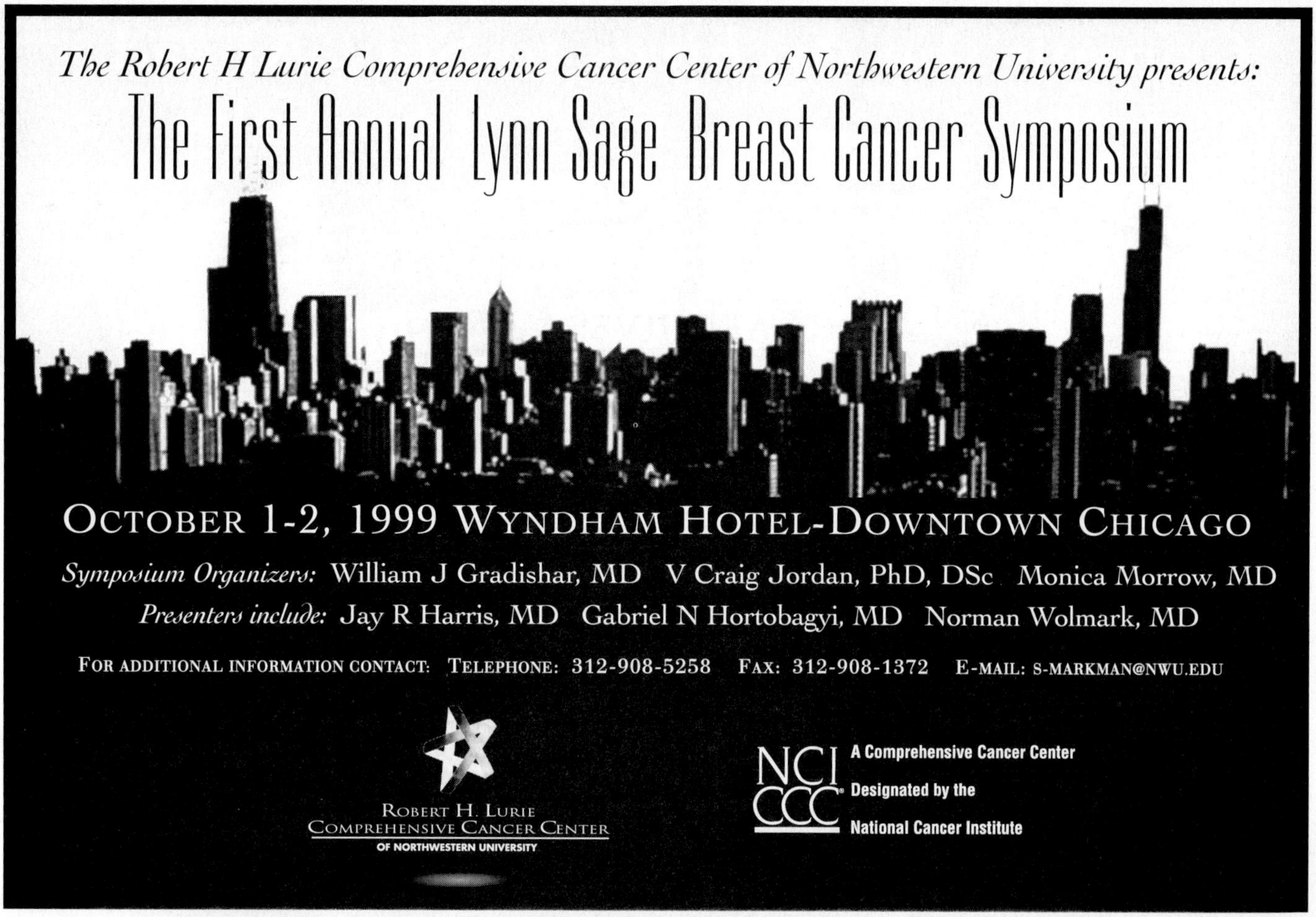
The Robert H Lurie Comprehensive Cancer Center of Northwestern University presents:
The First Annual Lynn Sage Breast Cancer Symposium
OCTOBER 1-2, 1999 WYNDHAM HOTEL-DOWNTOWN CHICAGO
Symposium Organizers: William J Gradishar, MD V Craig Jordan, PhD, DSc Monica Morrow, MD
Presenters include: Jay R Harris, MD Gabriel N Hortobagyi, MD Norman Wolmark, MD
FOR ADDITIONAL INFORMATION CONTACT: TELEPHONE: 312-908-5258 FAX: 312-908-1372 E-MAIL: S-MARKMAN@NWU.EDU
ROBERT H. LURIE COMPREHENSIVE CANCER CENTER OF NORTHWESTERN UNIVERSITY
NCI CCC
A Comprehensive Cancer Center Designated by the National Cancer Institute

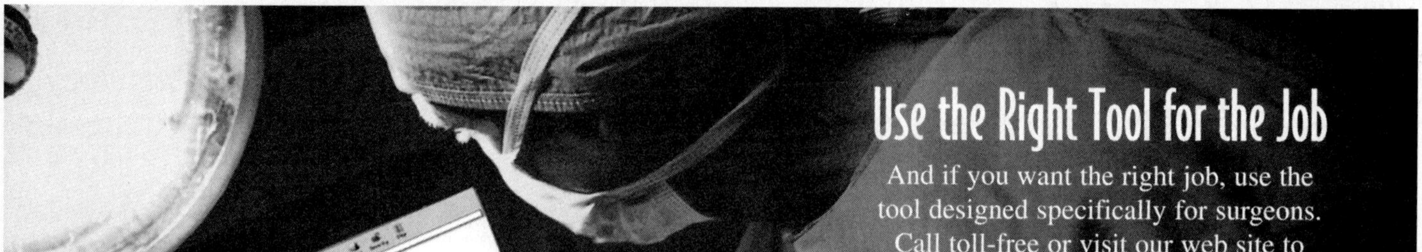
THE ASGS SURGICAL OPPORTUNITY PROGRAM
CANDIDATES
EMPLOYERS
Use the Right Tool for the Job
And if you want the right job, use the tool designed specifically for surgeons. Call toll-free or visit our web site to research the opportunity market at your convenience, 24 hours a day.
You can also register in a 'position wanted' database that is browsed frequently by participating employers.
This cutting edge service is brought to you by the American Society of General Surgeons.
www.theasgs.org
or call toll-free
877-700-ASGS(2747)
To post an opportunity call 877-700-0370
Powered By ART

Index of Advertisers

BRAINTREE LABORATORIES
Nulytely ..... Cover 3

CLASSIFIED ADVERTISING 580-584
http://www.ama-assn.org

ETHICON INC
Suture Assist 470

GLAXO WELLCOME
Panorex 476

NOVARTIS PHARMACEUTICALS CORP
http://www.norvartis.com
Apligraf 465-466

PFIZER, US PHARMACEUTICAL GROUP
http://www.pfizer.com
Diflucan ..... Cover 2-462

While every precaution is taken to ensure accuracy, we cannot guarantee against the possibility of an occasional change or omission in the preparation of this index.

Document Delivery Information

Copies of individual articles are available from the following:

UnCover
Tel: 800-787-7979
303-758-3030
Fax: 303-758-5946
URL: http://uncweb.carl.org
e-mail: uncover@carl.org

Institute for Scientific Information (ISI)
Tel: 800-336-4474
215-386-0100
Fax: 215-386-6362
URL: http://www.isinet.com

American Medical Association Alliance Inc. 1999 Annual Session Chicago

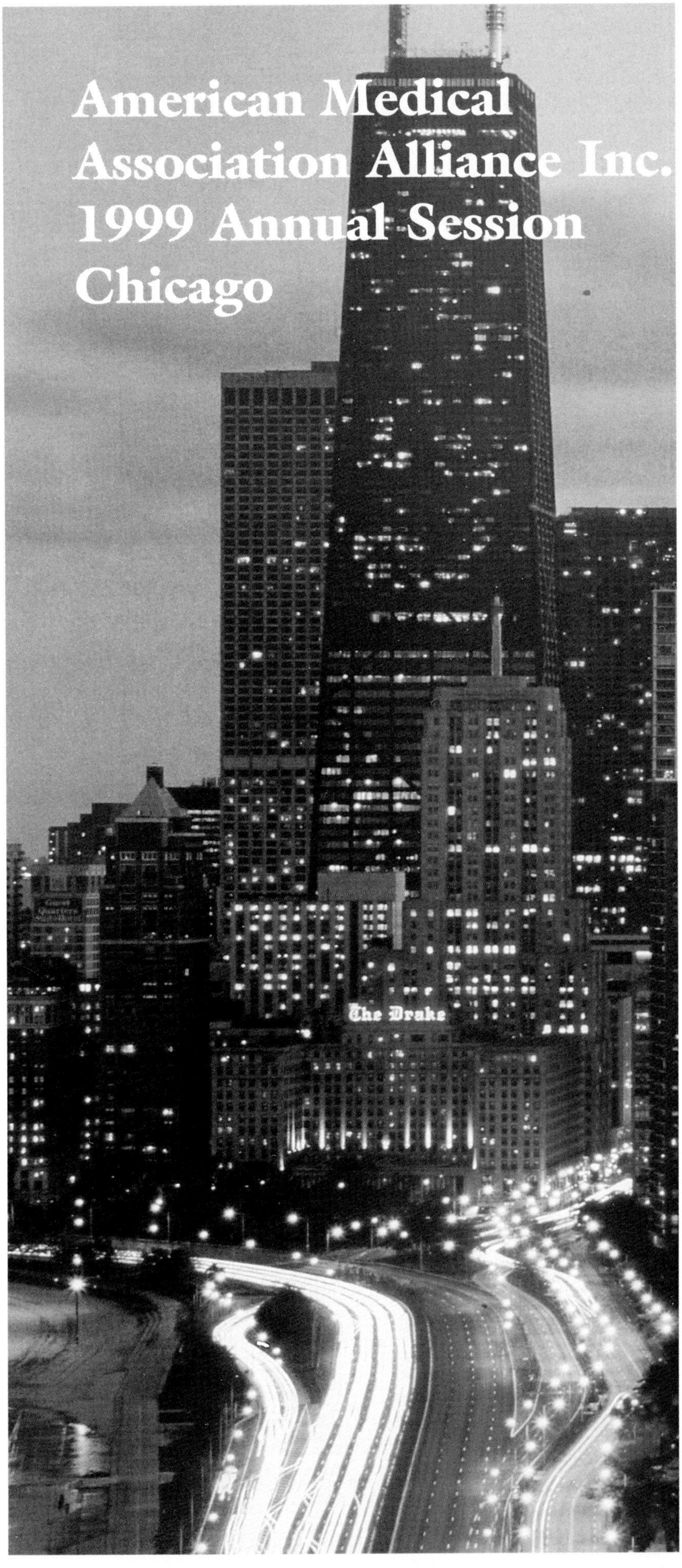

Special Events

Complimentary shuttle service will be provided for these events from the Hilton Chicago and Towers to The Drake.
All AMA Alliance members and physicians' spouses are invited to these special events:

The Second City
Special AMA Alliance Revue
Mon., June 21, 11:30 a.m. - 1:30 p.m.

The Second City comedy troupe is always original, always daring and always hilarious. Join your friends and colleagues for lunch at The Drake and then be entertained by this unique group of performers. Don't miss this one-time performance by The Second City Troupe written and performed especially for the AMA Alliance. $40.00 (AMA Alliance member) $42.50 (non-member)

Morton Kondracke — A Washington perspective
Tues., June 22, 11:30 a.m. - 1:30 p.m.

A journalist for nearly 35 years, Morton Kondracke has covered nearly every phase of American politics and foreign policy. He is the executive editor and columnist for Roll Call, Capitol Hill's feisty, independent, twice-weekly newspaper. The AMA Alliance is fortunate to have Mr. Kondracke as the luncheon speaker at The Drake telling the latest from the beltway. $40.00 (AMA Alliance member) $42.50 (non-member)

House and Garden Tour — Everything old is new again
Wed. June 23, 9:00 a.m. - 12:15 p.m.

Planned especially for the AMA Alliance, this tour shouldn't be missed. Sheffield, a national historic district located in the Lincoln Park neighborhood, is one of Chicago's most interesting, distinctive neighborhoods and also is known for its award-winning gardens. You will take a walking tour of the area to visit the gardens and interior of a Victorian-era home. Buses will depart from and return to both The Drake and the Hilton Chicago and Towers. Note when registering at which hotel you are staying so proper arrangements can be made. $27.50 (AMA Alliance member) $30.00 (non-member)

To register or for more information, contact the AMA Alliance. Phone: (312)464-4470, fax: (312)464-5020, E-mail: AMAA@ama-assn.org.

American Medical Association Alliance

WOW! ONLY 1 PREP HAS...

52% LESS SALT & NO SODIUM SULFATE

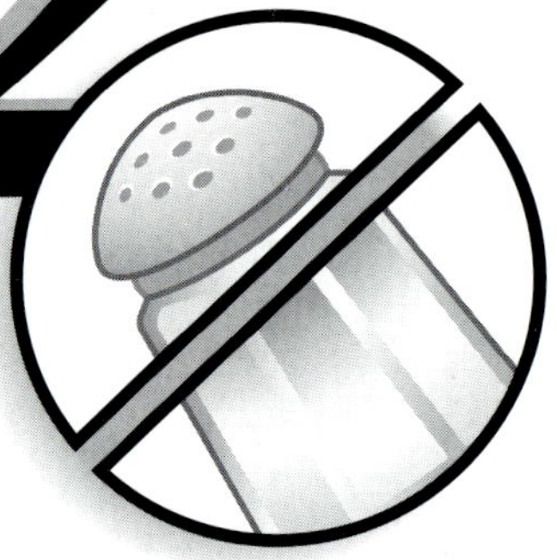

FOR GREAT TASTE

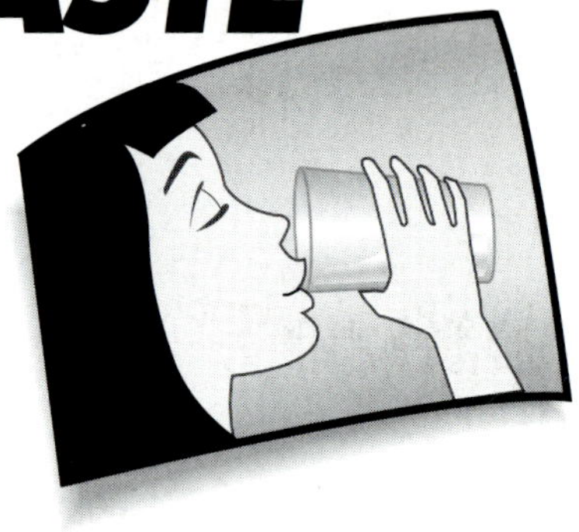

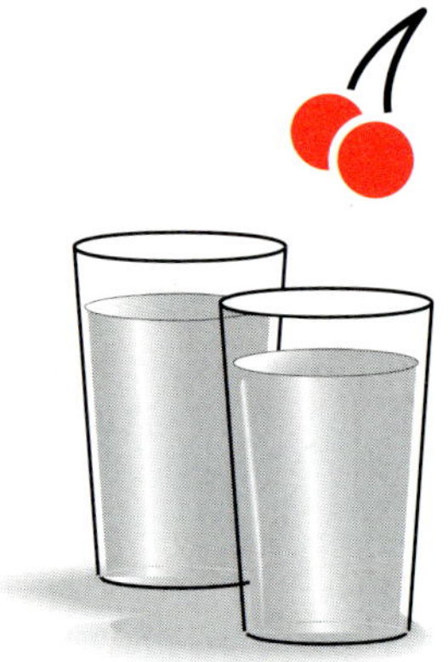

NuLYTELY®

and

CHERRY FLAVOR NuLYTELY®

PEG 3350, Sodium Chloride, Sodium Bicarbonate and Potassium Chloride for Oral Solution

This UNIQUE FORMULA eliminates sodium sulfate and reduces total salt by 52%[1] ... your patients get a bowel prep with improved taste

Patients have a choice: Cherry Flavor NuLYTELY or Regular NuLYTELY with a pleasant mineral-water taste

Cherry Flavor NuLYTELY is the #1 prescribed flavored bowel prep[2]

Contraindicated in patients with gastrointestinal obstruction, gastric retention, bowel perforation, toxic colitis or toxic megacolon

Brief summary: Before prescribing, please see full prescribing information.

Indications and Usage: NuLYTELY is indicated for bowel cleansing prior to colonoscopy. **Contraindications:** NuLYTELY is contraindicated in patients with gastrointestinal obstruction, gastric retention, bowel perforation, toxic colitis or toxic megacolon. **Warnings:** No additional ingredients, e.g. flavoring, should be added to the solution. NuLYTELY should be used with caution in patients with severe ulcerative colitis. Use of NuLYTELY in children younger than 2 years of age should be carefully monitored for occurrence of possible hypoglycemia, as this solution has no caloric substrate. Dehydration has been reported in 1 child and hypokalemia has been reported in 3 children. **Precautions: General:** Patients with impaired gag reflex, unconscious, or semiconscious patients, and patients prone to regurgitation or aspiration should be observed during the administration of NuLYTELY, especially if it is administered via nasogastric tube. If a patient experiences severe bloating, distention or abdominal pain, administration should be slowed or temporarily discontinued until the symptoms abate. If gastrointestinal obstruction or perforation is suspected, appropriate studies should be performed to rule out these conditions before administration of NuLYTELY. **Adverse Reactions:** Nausea, abdominal fullness and bloating are the most common adverse reactions (occurring in up to 50% of patients) to administration of NuLYTELY. Abdominal cramps, vomiting and anal irritation occur less frequently. These adverse reactions are transient and subside rapidly. Isolated cases of urticaria, rhinorrhea, dermatitis and (rarely) anaphylactic reaction have been reported which may represent allergic reactions. **Oral Administration, Pediatric Patients:** (aged 6 months or greater): At a rate of 25 mL/kg/hour, until the rectal effluent is clear or 4 liters are consumed. Rapid drinking of each portion is preferred to drinking small amounts continuously. **Storage:** Store in sealed container at 25°C. When reconstituted, keep solution refrigerated. Use within 48 hours. Discard unused portion. NDC 52268-301-01. ℞ **only.** Distributed by Braintree Laboratories, Inc., Braintree, MA 02185. Revised 9/97

References: **1.** Fordtran JS, Santa Ana CA, Cleveland MvB. *Gastroenterology.* 1990;98:11-16. **2.** Data on file, Braintree Laboratories, Inc.

BRAINTREE LABORATORIES·IN

The Leader in Lavage

ARCHIVES OF SURGERY

JUNE 1999

PAPERS PRESENTED AT THE 106TH SCIENTIFIC SESSION OF THE WESTERN SURGICAL ASSOCIATION, INDIANAPOLIS, IND, NOVEMBER 16-18, 1998

VISIONS: MEDICAL EDUCATION AND SURGICAL TRAINING IN EVOLUTION

LONG-TERM RESULTS OF BILIARY RECONSTRUCTION AFTER LAPAROSCOPIC BILE DUCT INJURIES

PROPHYLACTIC ANTIBIOTICS FOR ELECTIVE LAPAROSCOPIC CHOLECYSTECTOMY

LAPAROSCOPIC VS OPEN ADRENALECTOMY FOR THE TREATMENT OF PRIMARY HYPERALDOSTERONISM

ENDOSCOPIC ULTRASOUND AND FINE NEEDLE ASPIRATION FOR THE EVALUATION OF PANCREATIC MASSES

SPORADIC PRIMARY HYPERPARATHYROIDISM IN YOUNG PATIENTS

COMPLETE TABLE OF CONTENTS INSIDE

American Medical Association
Physicians dedicated to the health of America

www.ama-assn.org/surgery

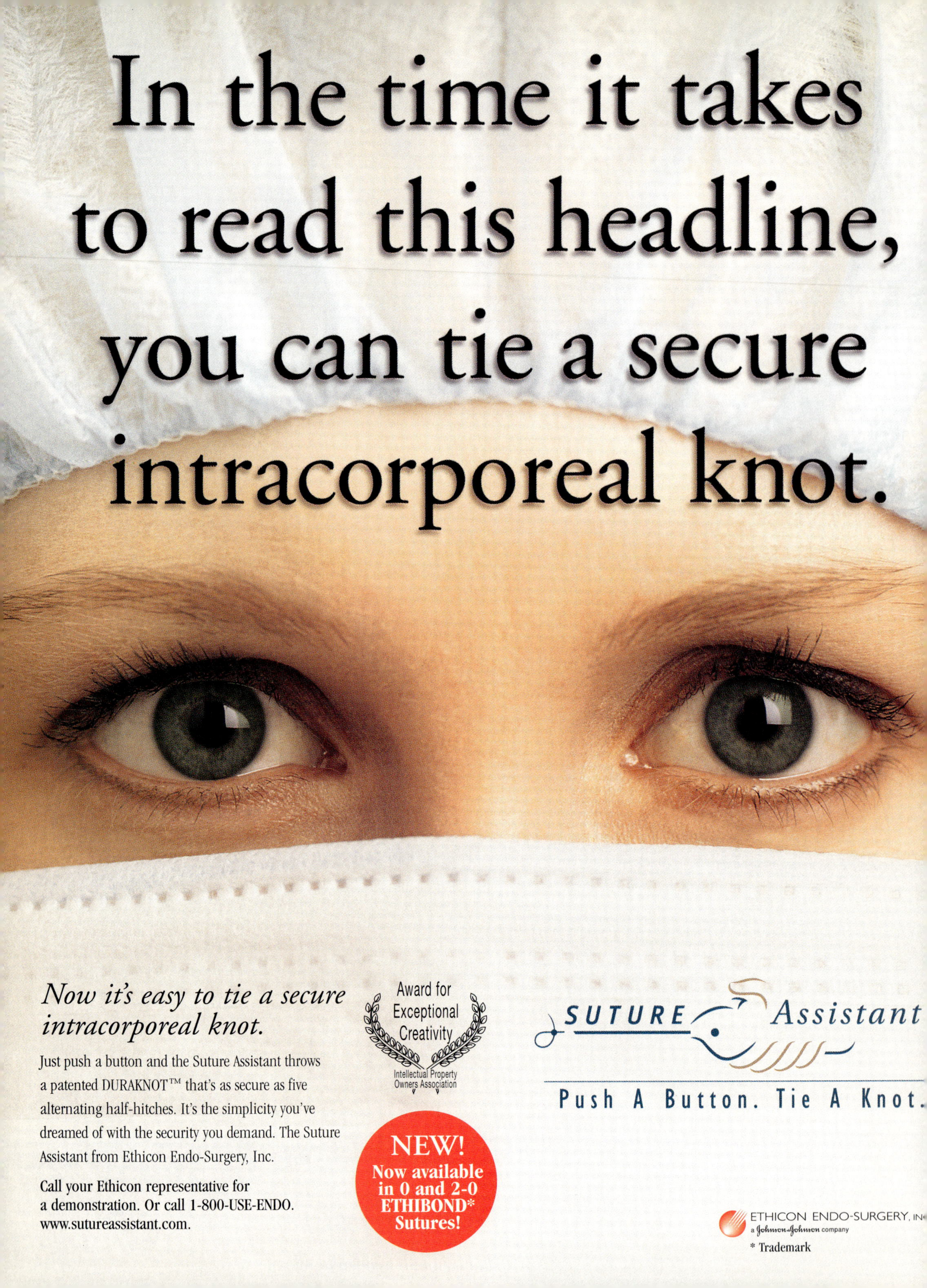

In the time it takes to read this headline, you can tie a secure intracorporeal knot.
Now it's easy to tie a secure intracorporeal knot.
Just push a button and the Suture Assistant throws a patented DURAKNOT™ that's as secure as five alternating half-hitches. It's the simplicity you've dreamed of with the security you demand. The Suture Assistant from Ethicon Endo-Surgery, Inc.
Call your Ethicon representative for a demonstration. Or call 1-800-USE-ENDO.
www.sutureassistant.com.
Award for Exceptional Creativity
Intellectual Property Owners Association
NEW! Now available in 0 and 2-0 ETHIBOND* Sutures!
SUTURE Assistant
Push A Button. Tie A Knot.
ETHICON ENDO-SURGERY, INC.
a Johnson & Johnson company
* Trademark

ARCHIVES OF SURGERY

The ARCHIVES OF SURGERY is a member of the consortium of AMA journals listed below. The complete text of all AMA journals is available online from Dialog Information Services and Ovid Technologies, Inc.

The Journal of the American Medical Association (JAMA)
Archives of Dermatology
Archives of Facial Plastic Surgery
Archives of Family Medicine
Archives of General Psychiatry
Archives of Internal Medicine
Archives of Neurology
Archives of Ophthalmology
Archives of Otolaryngology–Head & Neck Surgery
Archives of Pathology & Laboratory Medicine
Archives of Pediatrics & Adolescent Medicine
Archives of Surgery

The ARCHIVES OF SURGERY (ISSN 0004-0010) is published monthly by the American Medical Association, 515 N State St, Chicago, IL 60610, and is an official publication of the Association. The ARCHIVES OF SURGERY reaches more than 19 000 readers in over 69 countries each month. Periodicals postage paid at Chicago, IL, and at additional mailing offices. GST registration number 12622 5556 RT. Canada Post International Publications Mail (Canadian Distribution) Sales Agreement No. 319309. Printed in the USA.

Official Publication of the New England Surgical Society, Pacific Coast Surgical Association, Surgical Infection Society, Western Surgical Association.

SUBSCRIPTION RATES—The personal subscription rates for the ARCHIVES OF SURGERY are $145 for 1 year (12 issues) in the United States and US possessions; $195 in the Americas; £125 outside the Americas. The institution rates for 1 year are $245 in the US; $345 in the Americas; £195 outside the Americas. Special rates for residents and medical students are available. Address all subscription communications to: Subscriber Services Center, American Medical Association, PO Box 10946, Chicago, IL 60610-0946. Phone: (800) 262-2350. Fax: (312) 464-5831. E-mail: ama-subs@ama-assn.org. For mailing addresses outside the United States and US possessions, see International Subscription Information.

CHANGE OF ADDRESS—POSTMASTER, send all address changes to ARCHIVES OF SURGERY, c/o Subscriber Services, American Medical Association, 515 N State St, Chicago, IL 60610. Please notify us of address change at least 6 weeks in advance to ensure uninterrupted service. Include both old and new addresses, a recent mailing label, and new ZIP code. For mailing addresses outside the United States and US possessions, see International Subscription Information.

SUBSCRIBER SERVICES—For information about subscribing to any of the AMA publications, change of address, missing issues, or purchasing back issues, please contact Subscriber Services Center, American Medical Association, PO Box 10946, Chicago, IL 60610-0946, or call (800) 262-2350 or (312) 670-SUBS (670-7827) between 8:30 AM and 4:30 PM CST. Fax: (312) 464-5831. E-mail: ama-subs@ama-assn.org. For mailing addresses outside the United States and US possessions, see International Subscription Information.

INTERNATIONAL SUBSCRIPTION INFORMATION—Subscriptions outside the United States and US possessions are served according to geographic region. Please address correspondence to the following 2 offices based on delivery address: (1) For delivery in North America, Central America, and South America, contact Subscriber Services, AMA, PO Box 10946, Chicago, IL 60610-0946. Phone: (312) 670-7827. Fax: (312) 464-5831. E-mail: ama-subs@ama-assn.org. (2) For delivery outside the Americas contact JAMA & Archives Journals, Reader Services Centre, PO Box 299, London WC1H 9TD, England. Phone: +44 (0)171-383-6270. Fax: +44 (0)171-383-6402. E-mail: jama-archives@dial.pipex.com.

REPRINTS—Authors place their reprint order at the time the edited typescript is reviewed and should allow 4 to 6 weeks for delivery following publication. Requests for individual reprints should be sent directly to the author at the address shown in the article.

For bulk reprint orders for distribution by commercial organizations, please contact Wanda Bartolotta, 500 Fifth Ave, #2210, New York, NY 10110. Phone: (212) 354-0050. Fax: (212) 354-1169. E-mail: wanda_bartolotta@ama-assn.org. For reprint orders in limited quantities for distribution by educational organizations and for author reprints, please contact Reprint Coordinator, 515 N State St, Chicago, IL 60610. Phone: (312) 464-4594. Fax: (312) 464-4849.

PERMISSIONS—Contact Rhonda Bailey, Permissions Assistant, 515 N State St, Chicago, IL 60610. Phone: (312) 464-2513.

WORLD WIDE WEB ADDRESS—http://www.ama-assn.org.
SURGERY HOME PAGE—http://www.ama-assn.org/surgery.

ARCHIVES OF SURGERY

www.ama-assn.org/surgery

VOL 134 NO. 6, JUNE 1999

MISSION STATEMENT

To promote the art and science of surgery by publishing relevant peer-reviewed clinical and basic science information to assist the surgeon in optimizing patient care. The *Archives of Surgery* will also serve as a forum for the discussion of issues that involve ethics, teaching, surgical history, and socioeconomic concerns.

*Approved by the Editorial Board, *Archives of Surgery*, July 19, 1996.

PRESIDENTIAL ADDRESS

Visions: Medical Education and Surgical Training in Evolution 590
Jay L. Grosfeld, MD

PAPERS

Adenosquamous Carcinoma of the Pancreas 599
James A. Madura, MD; Benjamin T. Jarman; Michael G. Doherty; Moo-Nahm Yum, MD; Thomas J. Howard, MD

Long-term Results of Biliary Reconstruction After Laparoscopic Bile Duct Injuries 604
Michel M. Murr, MD; François Gigot, MD; David M. Nagorney, MD; William S. Harmsen, MS; Duane M. Ilstrup, MS; Michael B. Farnell, MD

Prophylactic Antibiotics for Elective Laparoscopic Cholecystectomy: Are They Necessary? 611
Andrew Higgins, MD; Jeremy London, MD; Scott Charland, PharmD; Erick Ratzer, MD; Jeffrey Clark, MD; William Haun, MD; D. Patrick Maher, MD

Complex Aortofemoral Prosthetic Infections: The Role of Autogenous Superficial Femoropopliteal Vein Reconstruction 615
Lori L. Gordon, MD; Ryan T. Hagino, MD; Mark R. Jackson, MD; J. Gregory Modrall, MD; R. James Valentine, MD; G. Patrick Clagett, MD

Oral Contrast Solution and Computed Tomography for Blunt Abdominal Trauma: A Randomized Study 622
Renae E. Stafford, MD; Michael D. McGonigal, MD; John A. Weigelt, MD; Thomas J. Johnson, MD

American Medical Association

Physicians dedicated to the health of America

All articles published, including editorials, letters, and book reviews, represent the opinions of the authors and do not reflect the policy of the American Medical Association, the Editorial Board, or the institution with which the author is affiliated, unless this is clearly specified.

Laparoscopic vs Open Adrenalectomy for the Treatment of Primary Hyperaldosteronism 628
Wen T. Shen, MD; Robert C. Lim, MD; Allan E. Siperstein, MD; Orlo H. Clark, MD; William P. Schecter, MD; Thomas K. Hunt, MD; Jan K. Horn, MD; Quan-Yang Duh, MD

Short Esophagus: Analysis of Predictors and Clinical Implications 633
Otávio L. Gastal, MD; Jeffrey A. Hagen, MD; Jeffrey H. Peters, MD; Guilherme M. R. Campos, MD; Majid Hashemi, MD; Jörg Theisen, MD; Cedric G. Bremner, MD; Tom R. DeMeester, MD

Endoscopic Ultrasound and Fine Needle Aspiration for the Evaluation of Pancreatic Masses 639
Jason Suits, BS; Richard Frazee, MD; Richard A. Erickson, MD

Image-Guided Surgery: Preliminary Feasibility Studies of Frameless Stereotactic Liver Surgery 644
Alan J. Herline, MD; James D. Stefansic, MS; Jacob P. Debelak, MS; Steven L. Hartmann, BS; C. Wright Pinson, MD; Robert L. Galloway, PhD; William C. Chapman, MD

Sporadic Primary Hyperparathyroidism in Young Patients: A Separate Disease Entity? 651
C. Richard Harman, MD; Jon A. van Heerden, MD; David R. Farley, MD; Clive S. Grant, MD; Geoffrey B. Thompson, MD; Kathleen Curlee, RN

***Candida* Infections in Critically Ill Trauma Patients: A Retrospective Case-Control Study** 657
Anthony P. Borzotta, MD; Kathleen Beardsley, RN, MS

BASIC SCIENCE FOR SURGEONS

The Acute Inflammatory Response and Its Regulation 666
Peter A. Ward, MD; Alex B. Lentsch, PhD

OPERATIVE TECHNIQUES

Proctectomy and Coloanal Anastomosis for Rectal Cancer 670
Thomas E. Read, MD; Ira J. Kodner, MD

ARCHIVES OF SURGERY

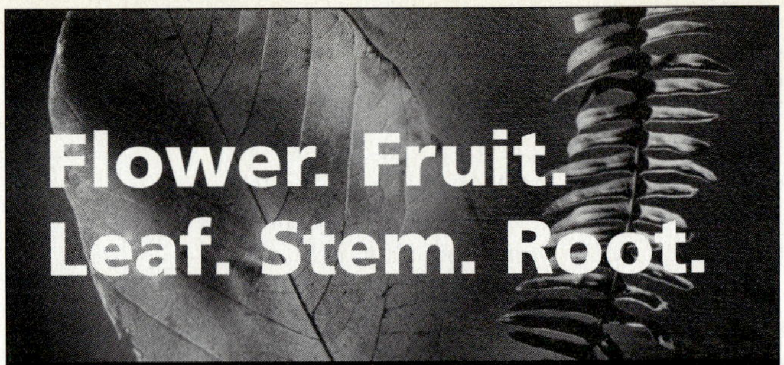
Flower. Fruit.
Leaf. Stem. Root.

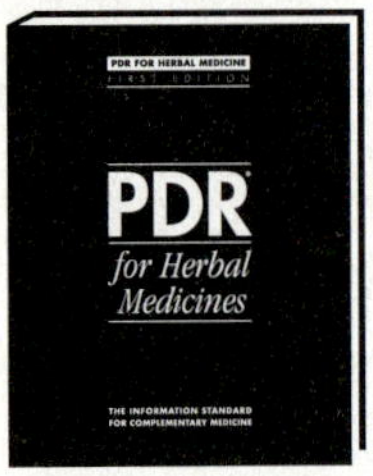
PDR
for Herbal
Medicines

ARCHIVES
OF
SURGERY

SURGICAL REMINISCENCES

George W. Stephenson, MD, FACS (1902-1998): A Personal Remembrance 678
Gerald O. Strauch, MD, FACS

MOMENTS IN SURGICAL HISTORY

Anesthesia During the Civil War 680
Ira M. Rutkow, MD, MPH, DrPH

CORRECTION

Enteral Nutrition Prevents Bacterial Translocation but Does Not Improve Survival During Acute Pancreatitis 643
Joji Kotani, MD; Makoto Usami, MD; Hideaki Nomura, MD; Atsunori Iso, MD; Hiroshi Kasahara, MD; Yoshikazu Kuroda, MD; Harumasa Oyanagi, MD; Yoichi Saitoh, MD

DEPARTMENTS

Surgical Anatomy 679

Products & Services 681

Classified Advertising 683

Index to Advertisers 688

Instructions for Authors—
See January 1999 issue, page 107, or visit the Web site at http://www.ama-assn.org/surgery.

Visions

Medical Education and Surgical Training in Evolution

Jay L. Grosfeld, MD

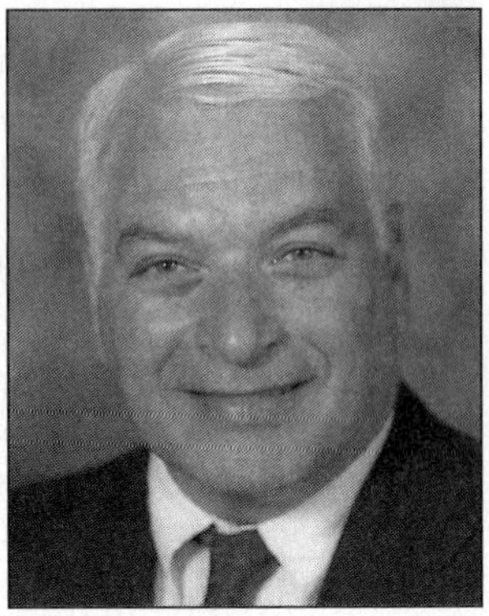

Jay L. Grosfeld, MD

I sincerely appreciate the support and confidence of the Western Surgical Association for allowing me to serve as your president; this has been one of the highlights of my professional career. I am extremely grateful, and thank you for giving me this opportunity. In reflecting about this event, it is clear that I have been fortunate to have been nurtured by some very special people who were outstanding educators and had the rare gift of stimulating a young resident's intellectual curiosity and desire to learn. Frank C. Spencer, MD, chairman of the Department of Surgery at New York University, New York, NY, aroused my interest in an academic career when I was a general surgery resident and gave me my first job as a member of the faculty. H. William Clatworthy, Jr, MD, professor of Pediatric Surgery at Ohio State University and the Children's Hospital in Columbus, was my mentor, who not only taught me the "nuts and bolts" of pediatric surgery but also asked the questions for which there were no answers and pushed the thought process to the limit. He taught a very special, unique philosophy of caring for infants and children. The late John E. Jesseph, MD, my predecessor as chairman of the Department of Surgery at Indiana University, recruited me to Indianapolis as a pediatric surgeon. Jack was a steady influence, a good friend, and a great patriot who gave me a chance to "run with the ball" and allowed me to be that person who was in the right place at the right time. He also was my sponsor for membership in the Western Surgical Association.

I was also fortunate to come from a loving, intact family with supportive parents who taught me the foundations and lessons of life.

There are my 5 children—Alicia, Denise, Janice, Jeff, and Mark—who have always rallied around me and given me their love, support, and understanding, despite the fact that they had to share their father on a daily basis with many other infants and children who were total strangers. Alicia and her husband, Bruce Thorne; Denise and her husband, Jean Philippe Maheu; and Janice and her husband, Martin Kaefer, MD, have each given my wife and me 2 of our 6 grandchildren—Julian, Ian, Jack, Peter, Sam, and Anna Elena. Most of all, however, I want to thank my dear wife, Margie, who, right from the start with her unselfish, steadfast commitment, embraced my goals and aspirations as her own. She has been a great resource of strength, a stabilizing force, a loving companion, my strongest advocate, and at times, a magnificent single parent who performed all of those other duties that allowed me the opportunity to follow my star. She has truly been a ray of light, even on the darkest day, and has been the wind beneath my wings, and I thank the Good Lord for bringing her into my life.

I want to thank the surgical faculty at Indiana University for being understanding, and my secretarial staff, led by Sandy Davis and Cindy Smith, who have made this very busy year run smoothly. I

From the Section of Pediatric Surgery, Department of Surgery, Indiana University School of Medicine, Indianapolis.

also want to thank our hardworking secretary, David Richardson, MD, who has been the backbone of the Western Surgical Association and has made my year as president practically problem-free.

MEDICAL EDUCATION AND SURGICAL TRAINING IN EVOLUTION

During the past 2 centuries, a number of outstanding individuals have developed a vision regarding the concepts of professional education. One of the most innovative minds was Thomas Jefferson, the draftsman of the Constitution and third president of the United States. His vision was to create an institution of higher learning, a comprehensive university with unusual versatility that embodied novel and far-reaching educational concepts, ie, the "academical village," where students and faculty worked and lived closely together in a community of learning.[1] Jefferson considered the founding of the University of Virginia, Charlottesville, the noblest work of his life. The educational principles he promoted became a reality when the University of Virginia opened its doors in 1825. Jefferson struggled to establish this goal under mounting personal, political, and financial pressures. He purchased the land, planned the grounds, designed the buildings, supervised the construction, hired the professors, and devised a curriculum while serving as the chief executive officer, secretary, and architect. He imported faculty from overseas. The first was Robley Dunglison from Cambridge University, who was a writer of medical subjects and would instruct at the School of Medicine. The first degree offered at the University of Virginia was a Doctor of Medicine, with the first diploma issued in 1828. Students lived and dined together in a plan worked out by Jefferson to promote student self-government, as he believed that young men from the best families could be counted on to govern themselves and remain well behaved. He was promptly disillusioned. Given such complete freedom, the students became disorderly, and incidents of rebellion against authority occurred. The faculty threatened to resign their positions if effective policing was not put into effect, and Jefferson responded. Strict regulations were adopted, and the riot leaders were expelled. A curfew was placed at 9 PM, and gambling, smoking, and drinking were outlawed. Despite this, the students continued to periodically rebel, and 2 students shot and mortally wounded the chairman of the faculty in 1840. By 1842, order had been restored, and an honor system had been introduced to prevent cheating on examinations. Faculty and student relations improved, and each year the professors would give a ball for the students and provide an annual supper. Although the university was founded on the principle of separation of church and state, Jefferson recognized the importance of spirituality and set aside a room in the rotunda for religious services and made provisions for a chaplain, with the salary paid by private funds but not by the university. Although Jefferson's vision eventually produced a fine university, there were many unexpected obstacles in the path of its development, and the need for proper discipline and order became apparent.

William Stewart Halsted, MD, was born in New York City in 1852. He attended the College of Physicians and Surgeons and graduated in 1877. His surgical practice was in New York City at Bellevue Hospital, where he attempted to develop a form of anesthesia using cocaine, to which he subsequently became addicted. In 1886 he joined a group of distinguished professors, including Sir William Osler, William Welch, and H. A. Kelley, becoming the first professor of surgery at the Johns Hopkins University School of Medicine, Baltimore, Md.[2] The availability of anesthesia changed Halsted's vision of how surgery should be performed and had a great impact on his developing a system of surgical education. Careful operative technique characterized by gentle handling of tissue and limiting blood loss became the hallmark of his training. Although Thomas Watson first described surgical gloves in 1842, it was Halsted's use of rubber gloves in the operating room that popularized this concept.[3] Physicians and nurses were required to use gloves, but masks were not yet in vogue. Osler and Halsted were firm advocates of bedside training for medical students. At Johns Hopkins, the interests of the medical school and the hospital were noted to be inseparable. Halsted's vision laid the basis for the future training of surgeons.

Abraham Flexner graduated from Johns Hopkins University in 1886. He was not a physician, but served as a secondary school teacher and principal. In 1908 he joined the research staff of the Carnegie Foundation for the Advancement of Teaching, Pittsburgh, Pa. At the time, leaders of American medicine were chagrined at the quality of medical training offered throughout this country and the lack of a structured curriculum and appropriate standards. The initial length of training in American medical schools in the 19th century was up to 6 months and, in some instances, less. Raising the entrance requirements and lengthening the school year or increasing the amount of work resulted in many schools losing students to medical schools with easier requirements. Flexner was given the responsibility to evaluate American medical education, which resulted in his famous report of 1910 on *Medical Education in the United States and Canada*.[4] Flexner's report hastened the much-needed reforms, standards, and organization of curricula of American medical schools. Flexner's vision of developing proper medical education led to the demise of proprietary medical schools with inadequate supervision and training. The reshaping of American medical education at Johns Hopkins was of great importance, since the medical school required a college degree as a prerequisite for admission and provided a 4-year graded curriculum, using the laboratories for teaching purposes and integrating the hospital and college facilities to provide clinical training. Surgical education varied widely throughout the next 30 years in structure and quality. The American College of Surgeons (ACS) was established in 1913. J. T. H. Finney was the first president of the ACS. Advances in anesthesia, operative techniques, and research continued to serve as powerful catalysts for the development of the field. In 1928, the American Medical Association (AMA) House of Delegates developed "The Essentials of Approved Residencies and Fellowships."[5] In 1937, the ACS published its own set of standards, "The Fundamental Requirements for Graduate Training in Surgery," and in 1939 published its first list of hospitals approved for postgraduate training. The American Board of Surgery (ABS)

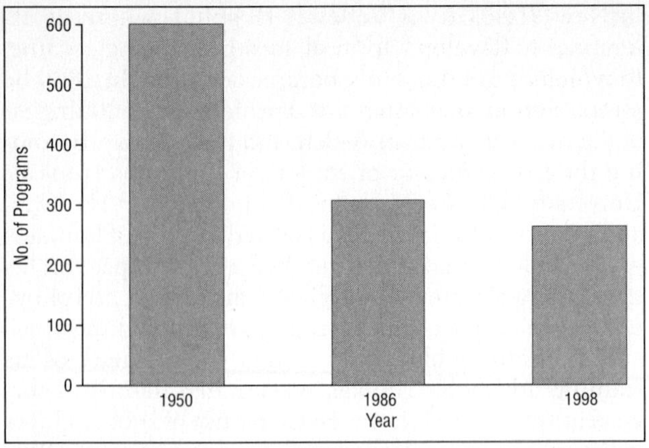

Figure 1. *Number of surgical training programs.*

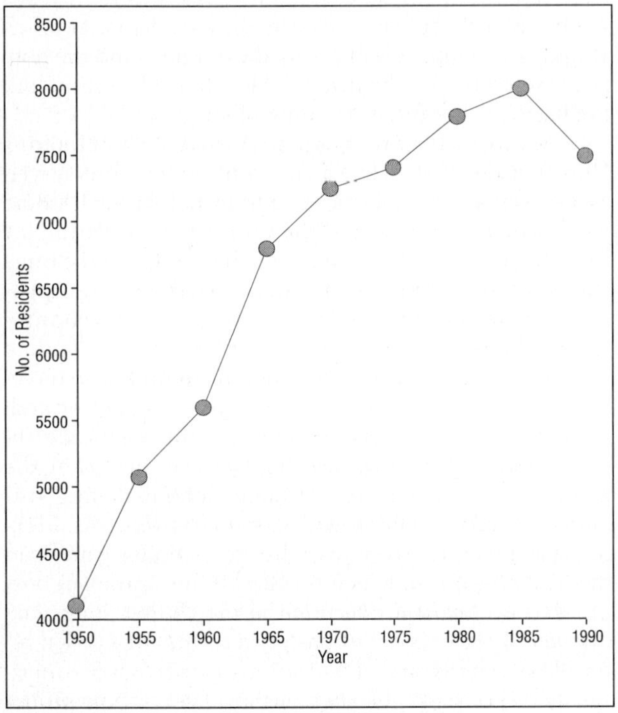

Figure 2. *Number of general surgery residents (from Boberg[5]).*

was established in 1937.[5] Evarts Graham, MD, of St Louis, Mo, was the first chairman of the board.[5] John Gibbon, MD, of Philadelphia, Pa, developed the first heart-lung machine (1937), and Robert E. Gross, MD, of Boston, Mass, began treating children with patent ductus arteriosus and coarctation of the aorta (1938).[6] In 1942, the AMA and the Association of American Medical Colleges formed the Liaison Committee on Medical Education that accredited medical schools. One should recall it was not until the end of World War II that antibiotics were readily available. In 1945, many surgeons returned from the war, and a new phase of surgical training began to evolve: the modern era of residency training in the United States.[6]

POST–WORLD WAR II

Before 1950, the ACS and the AMA published separate lists of hospitals approved for surgical training. The AMA approved 2-year programs of preliminary nature, whereas the ACS approved 3- and 4-year programs. At the time, more than 600 programs were listed.[5] With time, the residents in the 2-year programs became nondesignated residents. Programs were often pyramidal in structure, and the number of junior residents far exceeded the number of senior resident positions available. First the Conference Committee on Graduate Training in Surgery (1949)—sponsored by the AMA, ACS, and ABS—became the body that accredited surgery residencies. This Committee was replaced by the Residency Review Committee (RRC) for Surgery, which was established in 1950.[3] Frederick A. Coller, MD, of Ann Arbor, Mich, was the first chairman of the RRC, and E. H. Leveroos, MD, the first executive secretary. The RRC for Surgery was responsible for establishing educational criteria and curricula and accrediting surgical training programs based on observations made at special site visits to the training centers. The 12 RRC members were appointed by the AMA, ACS, and ABS. In 1972, the Liaison Committee for Graduate Medical Education became the coordinator of education and was to oversee the RRCs for all specialties. By 1975, all 3-year programs were changed to 4-year programs. Medical school graduates who previously obtained rotating internships were shifted to straight surgical internships extending training in surgery to 4 or 5 years. In 1980, the Liaison Committee for Graduate Medical Education was replaced by the Accrediting Council for Graduate Medical Education. By 1980, all training programs were at least 5 years in length. Some residents spent additional time in the research laboratory from 1 to 3 years. Based on more stringent institutional and training program requirements, the RRC for Surgery reduced the number of training programs to 303 by 1986, the year that John T. Boberg, PhD, became the executive secretary[5] (**Figure 1**). During the past 12 years, a further reduction to 260 accredited training programs in general surgery has occurred. However, the actual number of surgery residents completing training each year has remained rather steady (925-1000 per year), suggesting consolidation of residency training programs, with residents being absorbed from one program into another (**Figure 2**). The ABS certifies surgeons who have completed training in an accredited program by administering written qualifying and oral certifying examinations. The ABS belongs to a larger body, the American Board of Medical Specialties, that supports the activities of individual boards and their efforts to develop and use professional educational standards for the evaluation and certification of specialists. The ACS, the ABS, and the RRC for Surgery, often working in concert, have created a surgical troika that has served American surgery well.

After World War II, the inclusion of laboratory and clinical research into the training experience of young surgeons was spearheaded by leaders with vision such as Owen Wangensteen, MD, at the University of Minnesota, Minneapolis, Francis Moore, MD, at Harvard University, Boston, Alfred Blalock, MD, at Johns Hopkins University, Isidore Ravdin, MD, and Jonathan Rhoades, MD, at the University of Pennsylvania, Philadelphia, and Henry Harkins, MD, at the University of Washington, Seattle, as well as many others.[6] The establishment of Medicare in 1965 changed the method of payment to physicians and hospitals for the care of the elderly and all patients with end-stage renal disease; Medicare also paid hospitals to host medical education and stipends to residents. The formula to disburse direct and indirect medical expenses varied widely from city to city and state to state. During this era, the number of US medical schools increased from 80 to 126, and the schools increased the size of their classes because of enhanced governmental support per student and a perceived shortage of physicians. American medical schools now graduate more than 16 000 students annually. In 1965, there were 56 000 residents in training in all specialties. This increased to 106 000 residents by 1995. The size of medical school faculties also increased dramatically. The research effort grew into a productive enterprise that was funded by grants, gifts, and especially physician reimbursement for clinical services rendered by members of the faculty. New frontiers of surgical science were developed in the fields of cardiovascular surgery, organ transplantation, surgical oncology, trauma and surgical critical care, burn care, hepatobiliary disease, alimentary tract disorders, endocrine surgery, pediatric surgery, peripheral vascular surgery, and the like that became part of the training curriculum of future practicing surgeons and ushered in the age of specialization. Approximately half of the general surgical graduates obtained further training in other surgical subspecialties.

The training of surgeons continued to evolve with the establishment of more structured training standards and criteria to enhance the resident's cognitive knowledge by integrating basic science, as it has an impact on clinical management, as well as their clinical and operative skills. Pyramidal training programs essentially disappeared, and almost all programs became rectangular in nature for categorical surgical residents. Preliminary positions in the training programs were constant for trainees designated for future training in specialties such as urology, otolaryngology, neurosurgery, orthopedic surgery, and anesthesia; however, the number of nondesignated preliminary positions, once excessive, became strictly controlled. Led by the vision of Ward Griffen, MD, PhD, the executive director of the ABS, and subsequently his successor, Wallace P. Ritchie, Jr, MD, PhD, the training scope was more clearly identified by establishing primary and secondary components of general surgery and requiring a specified case experience in various designated surgical categories.[7] Standardized annual in-training examinations sponsored by the ABS were developed to monitor an individual resident's progress compared with that of peers across the country at the same training level and to identify gaps in the knowledge base.

TRANSFORMATION OF AMERICAN MEDICINE AND IMPACT OF MANAGED CARE ON TRAINING

Advances in surgical science that started with bench and laboratory research efforts and were then translated to the clinical setting became expensive treatments that required significant resources. This coincided almost simultaneously with the development of new and extremely expensive medical technology (eg, ultrasonography, magnetic resonance imaging, computed tomography, advanced nuclear scintigraphy, mass spectrometry, laser development) that drove the cost of medical care up until it reached a zenith of greater than 15% of the gross national product in 1995.[8] The government response to escalating health care costs was initiated in 1983 with the advent of the diagnostic related groups (DRGs) as a method to reduce hospital payments. In contrast to its expected goals, the DRG system actually resulted in an increased payment to hospitals, especially the teaching hospitals. In 1990, the government attempted to redistribute health care payments from procedural specialists to cognitive physicians using the resourced-based relative value scale system for Medicare patients. At the same time, the Joint Commission for Accreditation of Hospitals implemented processes such as quality assurance, quality improvement, utilization review, and risk management. Although these were worthy endeavors, implementing them proved to be very costly, as they required significant increases in hospital administrative staff to perform and skyrocketed the administrative overhead of almost every hospital in the country. The Clinton administration attempted to enact a new health care program just after the 1992 election. Failure to enact health care reform helped usher in the current managed care era controlled mainly by big business, major insurers, and hospital administrators. Cost-control measures (managed cost) were implemented at the expense of quality care to drive corporate and shareholder profit. Managed care converted the physician mind-set to provide only essential care. The primary care initiative was established in medical schools, where new curriculum changes were set in place to teach population-based health care, public health, preventive medicine, alternative medicine, and holistic medicine and to produce more primary care physicians and fewer specialists.[9-13] Managed care programs in which the provider accepts the responsibility for a collection of patients for a fixed fee became very popular. The managed care group had to share financial risk with the hospital in capitated risk-based contracts. Unfortunately, managed care programs sponsored by health maintenance organizations have neither achieved their goals regarding quality of care and patient satisfaction nor addressed the care of the uninsured and inner-city indigent populations that have historically been underserved.[14] Health maintenance organizations cannot seem to manage and do not seem to care. Numerous preferred provider insurance networks appeared and determined which hospital and physician would treat patients at a significantly reduced reimbursement rate. Primary care physician networks have generally not fared well financially, and hospitals and specialist groups that hired their own primary care physicians have for the most part experienced considerable financial loss. This frantic reorganization of health care services led to hospital and group mergers and consolidations, often bringing together former rivals with clashing cultures attempting to maintain a patient base and avoid potential takeovers by large national insurer groups. These organizations are often driven by business ideology that places the educational and research missions of academic training programs at risk.[15-17] Few new business ventures desire to divert funds toward these noble goals. Academic medical centers have entered into such relationships through the process of "mergermania," driven by fears of nonsurvival. Some academic institutions have been purchased by major health care insurers and have lost control of the distribution of dollars, have little input into decision making, and are threatened by loss of departmental structure through the development of facsimiles of industrial product service lines organized to respond to market forces that treat patients with systemic conditions as consumers and urge horizontal integration of physician groups.[8,15,17] As one might anticipate, not all of these relationships are successful. The recent chapter 11 bankruptcy of the Allegheny University of the Health Care Sciences, Philadelphia, involving the Pennsylvania Medical College–Hahnemann Medical School merger is a good example.[18] Nine hospitals are being auctioned off for $502 million to help offset a loss of more than $1.3 billion. The medical school is a major cost center and may not survive, and even if it does, elimination of academic programs, decreased class size, and consolidation of research efforts is likely. Two separate faculty study reports suggest that the medical school at the University of Hawaii, Honolulu, is suffering from such a severe fiscal crisis that closure of the school has been recommended.[19] In other teaching institutions, managed care has resulted in downsizing of faculty (including the firing of academic leaders by chief executive officers) and reduction of teaching activity by deploying faculty to remote sites to perform ambulatory procedures. A decrease in the number of patients at some training program centers has led to a reduction in the number of residency positions because of an inadequate caseload available for training. Amid all this turmoil, the Budget Reconciliation Act of 1997 by the US Congress will further the woes of many teaching hospitals by gradually reducing the indirect medical education payments from 7.7% in 1997 to 5.5% by the year 2001. The actual number of residents is capped at the total number of resident positions existing at an institution on December 31, 1996, which affects direct graduate medical education payments. Hospitals that make voluntary reductions of residents can apply for incentive payments, but these no doubt will be short-lived. Teaching hospitals that have traditionally cared for the indigent population and the uninsured can also expect a reduction in disproportionate share payments of 1% per year until a level of 5% is reached in 2002. Payments to hospitals for their bad debt related to Medicare will also be reduced by 25% in 1998, 40% in 1999, and 45% thereafter. The relatively lucrative overpayments that were formula-driven for ambulatory surgery, radiology, and diagnostic procedures will be replaced by a far less attractive prospective payment system for hospital outpatient services in 1999.

RESIDENT CONCERNS

These observations have led to a growing list of resident concerns regarding fewer hospital beds, patients, and teaching faculty; dilution of faculty who operate at off-campus ambulatory sites; anticipated change in the resident funding mechanism; less contact with patients and less opportunity to develop physician-patient relationships because of shorter length of hospital stay; availability and funding for protected research time; heavy workload due to increased severity of illness for inpatients; debt; lack of family time; changing lifestyles; and the availability of fellowships and job opportunities at the completion of training. Approximately 20% of categorical residents in general surgery drop out of training.[20,21]

Another nagging question that has surfaced is the status of residents during their training and whether residents are considered students or employees. For the past 30 years, residents' activities have been service-driven through graduate medical education funded by Medicare. Recent allegations from the public concerning excess working hours and inadequate supervision and that residents are cheap labor cloud the residency training system. Anxious residents become a target of opportunity for unions. We believe the entire purpose of residency training is an educational process. Resident selection is quite different than hiring employees for their services, and the stipends received by residents are not determined by the value of their service, their skill, or an hourly rate. Resident activity depends on the level of graduate training and experience. The resident's participation in patient care is to achieve advancement in training. Unfortunately, in the present system Medicare will only pay for residents who are working on clinical services taking care of patients. Residents who have educational opportunities in the laboratory are not covered by Medicare funds.

During the next few months, the National Labor Relations Board will attempt to answer the question of whether residents should be considered students or employees. If residents are considered employees, there would be a schism in the future teacher-learner relationship. Allegations of unfair labor practices, binding arbitration, grievances, the right to strike, and union control of rotations, work hours, duty assignments, pay scales, methods of evaluation, and whether promotion, termination, or mediation is required for any specific trainee could disrupt training considerably. Actions such as this would threaten the current training scheme.

FACULTY CONCERNS

The faculty morale at many teaching centers is also at a low ebb. Practicing in an unstable health care market, having less time to teach and conduct research, facing the threat of downsizing and an increased call schedule, being accountable for systems that they do not control, lacking input into contracting, and using most of their energy to perform procedural activity to generate enough income to sustain their own salary and continue to subsidize research and development are pressures that have an adverse impact on morale.[22]

The dilemmas faced by surgery department chairmen in the corporate managed care era are also considerable.[22-24] In past years, the chairman of the Department of Surgery was expected to be a charismatic teacher; an excellent surgeon with solid leadership, organizational, and administrative skills; and a research scientist who attracted grant support or at least strongly supported the research mission of the department. At present, time for those aspects of the position that were once considered of paramount importance have shifted to other responsibilities in a new paradigm of leadership. Many teaching hospitals may indeed require partnering with nonacademic hospital groups to survive the financial crisis that is likely imminent. Choosing the right partner is of obvious importance. True integration is often difficult to achieve and may not be in the best interest of the department and its faculty.[17,25-28] Integration requires some compatibility among the cultures, a share in the governance and power structure, maintenance of some degree of autonomy, and a scenario where dollars do not blur judgment. Active participation in the administrative activities of merged programs, hospitals, and health systems by attendance at an endless number of committee meetings that often begin early with breakfast and end late with dinner have become the routine of the day. The contemporary chairman must be a strategic planner and persuasive communicator and become financially astute regarding the market forces in an evolving health care environment that affect the department's clinical, educational, and research efforts. The chairman must be able to negotiate aggressively and be part of the decision-making process. In the present era, it has become more difficult for the chairman to be "the man or woman for all seasons." It is therefore imperative to develop a core of faculty who embrace the goals of a well-conceived and thoughtful department plan and are willing to step up to the plate and actively participate in seeing the plan succeed. An academic "cabinet" of advisors who participate in the planning process and assume responsible physician leadership roles throughout the newly merged organization is essential.

Departments must develop sound economic management practices to remain productive and not overspend their budgets. Jordan Cohen, MD, the president of the American Association of Medical Colleges, has suggested the concept of mission-based management be implemented at academic medical centers to identify and to account for costs associated with each medical school function (eg, teaching, research, patient care, community service, and administration) and to match those costs with the various revenue streams available.[26] The American Association of Medical Colleges has requested that the federal government develop a shared-responsibility mechanism to replace those teaching hospitals and medical school revenues formerly embedded in payments received from third-party payers for clinical services. Cohen further suggests that mission-based management and federally shared responsibility are complementary, as neither alone can brace the financially challenging future.[26] We agree with the necessity of demonstrating fiscal responsibility, but doubt whether the federal government is willing to share that responsibility at this time. On the other hand, it is essential that the public and the federal government (ie, Congress) be made aware and be convinced that graduate medical education is a valuable public resource that must be supported ultimately for the benefit of the people. Until that unassailable message becomes reality, we must seek alternative funding methods, including gifts and grant acquisitions, and consider partnering with industry to maintain the research enterprise and to support resident activity in the laboratory. Developing strategies for establishing centers of excellence within departments and schools will facilitate the vision of a successful clinical and scholarly environment to train future residents. Full-time and volunteer surgical faculty can play important roles in the evolution of the surgical training program of the future.

THE VISION FOR SURGICAL EDUCATION IN THE NEXT MILLENNIUM

In addition to describing the historical development, I have tried to paint the picture of the present forces and evolving trends affecting surgical training. Although some of the following comments regarding surgical training represent my own personal bias, many aspects are derived from my participation as a director of the ABS for 8 years and as a member of the RRC for Surgery for the past 2 years. It has been an honor and privilege to serve on both of these fine organizations, along with many dedicated surgical leaders who receive no compensation for their enormous time commitment, effort, and vital service to the public.

The optimal environment for training remains a very important component of the equation for success. The relationship of hospitals, medical schools, and departments of surgery are sometimes complex; however, these interrelationships are inseparable and directly affect residency training.[27]

As the elderly represent a larger proportion of patients requiring health care, institutions that have a strong cardiovascular disease presence and an active cancer detection and oncology treatment center will have the best opportunity to fill beds, maintain financial stability, and ensure surgical trainees adequate exposure and experience. A gastrointestinal tract disease center managing motility disturbances, inflammatory bowel disease, peptic disorders, and hepatobiliary and pancreatic disease is an asset for training. Logistically available ambulatory offices and surgical facilities for continuity of care and outpatient surgical experience will also be necessary. The presence of a thriving solid organ transplantation program will ensure access to patients with end-stage organ failure of the liver, kidneys, pancreas, heart, and lungs and the additional spin-off of those patients who do not require transplantation but other types of medical and surgical care. The presence of an ACS-approved level I trauma center (with a top-flight ground and air transport service), a burn center, and ample surgical critical care experience are also key components of a successful facility for training. As 1 of every 4 operations are performed on children, housing or affiliating with a busy children's hospital with a pediatric surgical service is a valued asset. We believe that general surgical training should remain a 5-year clinical experience dedicated to the following broadly based primary components of the field[7]: breast, skin, and soft tissue; head and neck; ailmentary tract; abdomen and its contents; trauma; vascular system; endocrine system; surgical critical care; and surgical oncology. Experience in the secondary components of cardiovascular thoracic surgery, plastic surgery, neurosurgery, transplantation, and pediatric surgery should also remain a required part of training. Rotations in orthopedic surgery and urology are still preferred, but anesthesia and gynecology experience are more optional and perhaps designed more for trainees planning to practice in rural locations. Similarly, elective rotations in surgical pathology can be tailored to trainees interested in an academic career. Exposure to the emergency department will require thoughtful consideration and flexibility if the facility has a residency program in emergency medicine in place. In the latter instance, adequate emergency department experience can be obtained by participating in trauma care and on a consultative basis. Flexibility for unique elective rotations should also be available. Although some surgical subspecialty leaders desire to reduce the number of years of general surgery required before entry into their area of expertise, I firmly believe the best subspecialist surgeons are those who have completed a good general surgery program.

ASIDE FROM the tumultuous changes in health care provision, the past decade has been characterized by an explosion of exciting new scientific information and advances in medical and information technology. Molecular genetics, cell biology, growth factors, immune modulators, and the expanding fields of antiangiogenesis and gene therapy will no doubt be integrated into management schemes, with trainees introduced to these topics in an expanded and upgraded surgical basic science curriculum. The other major teaching conferences vital to training, such as the morbidity and mortality conference, surgery grand rounds, tumor board, trauma conference, gastrointestinal tract disease conference, journal club, and numerous subspecialty conferences should be maintained. Residents should be free from service responsibilities to attend educational meetings.

Emerging technologies that prove durable and useful must also be included in the surgical training curriculum. These include, for example, minimally invasive surgical techniques (eg, laparoscopy, thoracoscopy), endoscopy, stereotactic breast biopsy, laser technology, electrosurgery, vascular stenting, use of ultrasonography for trauma and emergency care, and scintigraphic sentinel lymph node identification and biopsy as it relates to breast cancer and melanoma management. These are best taught to residents during a period of years when they ideally acquire such experience in surgical technology centers with inanimate and animate skill laboratories, including surgical simulation that has clinical application and research capability to study outcomes, procedural durability, patient satisfaction, and cost-effectiveness. These centers of technology learning should be available on-site at the training facility, avoiding unnecessary travel to distant corporate centers to acquire limited sporadic learning. Development of these centers may require partnering with industry, but will result in training excellence under faculty supervision, which competent graduating surgical residents can take to their practice communities and use to positively influence the future care of patients. Ultimately this will also obviate the need for verification after a less-than-desirable weekend course presently being supplied to practicing physicians trying to become accredited in the new technologies.

Another vital addition to the surgical trainee's curriculum is information technology, which has become fundamental to the teaching, learning, and scholarship mission of modern universities and departments. Information technology can enhance the teaching and learning process and is an essential tool for access to information, network resources, computing, research, and communication (including telecommunication and telemedicine) for faculty, residents, and students. Surgical departments should have their own Web sites, and all residents should be given an e-mail address. Residents and faculty should have reliable network access from the office, on-call, at home, in the clinical setting, and while traveling. Telemedicine libraries should be available for grand rounds presentations and other conferences for residents, students, and faculty to review or catch up if a session is missed. Every resident must develop computer skills and be able to use interactive technology and informatics effectively. Computerized learning also has the advantage of being learner paced and controlled.

Residents must also learn modern practice skills to deal with managed care using evidence-based learning and cost-effective quality care. Residents must become familiar with regulatory requirements such as quality assurance, quality initiatives, utilization review, risk management, malpractice, and other medicolegal considerations. Surgery residents must also receive instruction in bioethics and issues concerning death, dying, and living wills and become familiar with quality-of-life issues as an important part of clinical care.[28] Residents must learn how to develop a personal involvement with their patients, serve as their advocate, and place their well-being as the highest priority. House staff must learn to consider the importance of pain and suffering, social interaction, physical function and autonomy, intellectual function, and the emotional well-being of their patient as they decide on clinical interventions.[28] Faculty must continue to remind house staff of the importance of retaining professional values regarding morality, altruism, service, and integrity in meeting their patients' needs and public expectations.[29,30] These principles influence the development of character in trainees and must be addressed, as cognitive and moral development may be quite separate.[31] This is especially important in the present era of managed health care, where a clash of values characterized by consumerism, response to market forces, profit, and responsibilities to stockholders takes precedence over the patients' best interests.[28-30]

Teaching students and residents about spirituality may also enhance the physician-patient relationship.[32,33] Spirituality has been shown to help patients cope with serious illness. Prayer can complement medical care rather than compete with it. People tend to become more religious as they get older, and many elderly patients see health and illness as being partly attributable to God and to some extent godly intervention. Many patients want spiritual issues addressed, especially when they are dealing with chronic or serious illness and death. Patients expect their physician to be compassionate to their needs and to give them nonjudgmental respect as well as provide optimum care. Physicians must regain the confidence and respect of their patients and the public to be able to influence decisions regarding support of the missions of research and professional education. Including these items in the curriculum prepares the resident to do this more effectively.

At least one dedicated year devoted to research (preferably between the second and third clinical year) is an essential part of the scholarly environment required for training. Residents planning an academic career and desiring a second year of research should be accommodated when possible. This remains one of the most rewarding experiences in a training program. Residents must be taught to design research projects, to interpret data, and to prepare abstracts and manuscripts and be given instruction in biostatistics. This unique opportunity allows the resident to develop intellectual curiosity, critical thinking, and grant-writing skills; to pursue laboratory investigation; to explore new horizons of discovery; and to recognize the value of professional enlightenment and the need for lifelong learning.[23,27] The laboratory must be supported by appropriate personnel (technicians and doctors of philosophy), modern equipment, and adequate funding to perform the research projects. Advanced planning and careful supervision by a faculty mentor are helpful in getting the research year off to a fast start. The area of research should be the resident's choice.

In addition to these curricula, probably the most sought-after instruction in a surgical training program is faculty teaching at the bedside, in the clinic, and in the operating theater. Training in an environment with shoulder-to-shoulder faculty-to-resident instruction and the right balance of supervision and independence results in the development of a well-informed, experienced, and confident resident. It is imperative for new residents to have early clinical and technical skills assessment. Changes in medical school curricula toward generalism may have reduced the opportunity for some students to develop adequate physical examination skills, such as detecting a breast mass, and to perform relatively simple tasks such as venapuncture, nasogastric tube insertion, and bladder catheterization.[34-36] Early close supervision and instruction may be an invaluable beginning. The availability of skills laboratories previously mentioned will also serve as an important learning resource to the novice surgeon.

Maintaining a chain of command and having an established supervisory reporting structure is a useful method of communication and support. The concept of surgery being a team sport, with students, residents, and faculty all participating together in the care of patients, has served training programs quite well in the past and should continue to do so in the future. On some services, however, a one-on-one preceptorial relationship between faculty and residents may also have a place in training. Faculty and residents should treat each other with mutual respect. Faculty must be sensitive to the current diversity of surgery residents regarding gender, ethnicity, and cultural differences. Similarly, residents are in close contact with medical students and should be supportive rather than abusive and willing to teach them in the clinical setting. Residents should be nurtured, but discipline is important, and trainees should be reprimanded when necessary—always in a private setting and never in public. Residents must be made aware of what is expected of them (goals and objectives) and should be kept responsible and accountable for their actions and maintain the academic and professional standards of the department. Developing the right attitude toward learning, establishing a strong work ethic, acquiring good communication skills, preparing for operative procedures, and demonstrating the desire to be the best they can be on a daily basis are attributes that serve residents well. Faculty should be the teachers of and advocates for the residents and strive to serve as their role models. Residents require and desire feedback concerning their performance to improve. By working in the trenches, residents have a unique opportunity to assess the training program in regard to the curriculum, quality of education, and faculty participation and to make valuable suggestions to improve the program. Resident critiques should be submitted anonymously to avoid the fear of potential retribution. The training center should provide residents with a safe, clean on-call environment with proper nutrition and separate sleeping and bathroom facilities for women residents. The present system requirements of every third night call and a 24-hour period each week free from duty should allow time to rest, study, and be with family.

The void in the present training system is the need to establish guidelines to measure an individual physician's competence. Until this time it was the training program director who determined whether a surgical resident completing training was competent to practice by signing training certificates and applications for admissibility to the ABS examination for certification. The ABS and the American Board of Medical Specialties are presently studying the relationship of certification and diplomate recertification to competence. The American Board of Medical Specialties suggests that general competence for all physicians encompasses medical knowledge, clinical skills, medical ethics, interpersonal skills, professionalism, understanding of systems-based practice, medical informatics, and continuous quality improvement. The ABS is considering measuring competence by evaluating the following 4 major areas: (1) intellectual tools and abilities, (2) motor and technical skills, (3) attitudes and habits, and (4) interpersonal skills. For example, intellectual abilities would include observation, knowledge, organization, synthesis, and judgment. Although these efforts have merit, it is difficult to understand how competence can be accurately measured. The measurement of outcomes may be the best measure of competence by evaluating mortality and complication rates, diagnostic accuracy, patient satisfaction, and overall cost. The goal is to certify to the public that surgeons are competent to practice their specialty.

In many ways, a good surgical residency has a close resemblance to Jefferson's vision of the academical village. Residents join a department and work alongside their professors for 5 to 7 years. This includes working together sometimes day and night, often under stress, sharing knowledge and episodes of adversity and success, occasionally dining together, and having some social exchange that includes family, in a learning community dedicated to the missions of quality patient care, education, and research. Despite the mounting pressures of the present health care environment, I firmly believe that preservation of this training model with necessary additions to the educational curriculum as outlined will maintain the international leadership of the American surgical residency system, which is the envy of surgeons throughout the world.[27] This also will assure the public that knowledgeable, well-trained, highly qualified, confident, and competent surgeons will be available to provide for their surgical care in the future.

Presented at the 106th Scientific Session of the Western Surgical Association, Indianapolis, Ind, November 16, 1998.

Reprints: Jay L. Grosfeld, MD, 545 Barnhill Dr, EH 205, Indianapolis, IN 46202 (e-mail: jgrosfel@iupui.edu).

REFERENCES

1. Dabney V. *Mr. Jefferson's University: A History.* Charlottesville: University of Virginia Press; 1981:1-60.
2. Cameron JL. William Stewart Halsted: our surgical heritage. *Ann Surg.* 1997; 225:445-458.
3. Lyons AS, Petrucelli RJ. *Medicine: An Illustrated History.* New York, NY: Harry N Abrams Inc; 1987:550-554.
4. Flexner A. *Medical Education in the United States and Canada: A Report to the Carnegie Foundation for the Advance of Teaching.* Boston, Mass: Updyke; 1910. Bulletin 4.
5. Boberg JT. Accreditation: procedures and staff support for the Surgery Residency Review Committee. *Arch Surg.* 1990;125:1246-1251.
6. Wangensteen OH, Wangensteen SD. *The Rise of Surgery.* Minneapolis: University of Minnesota Press; 1978.
7. Ritchie WP Jr. What the future may hold for general surgery. *J Am Coll Surg.* 1995;180:481-484.
8. Grosfeld JL. The challenge of a new decade: a surgeon's perspective of the 1990s. *Surgery.* 1990;108:595-600.
9. University of California Commission on the future of medical education. *West J Med.* 1998;168:445-482.
10. Cohen JJ. Generalism in medical education: the next steps. *Acad Med.* 1995;70 (suppl 1):57-59.
11. Bondurant S. Health care reform: theme for academic medicine. *Acad Med.* 1995; 70:93-97.
12. Lurie N. Preparing physicians for practice in managed care environment. *Acad Med.* 1996;71:1044-1049.
13. Greenlick MR. Educating physicians for the twenty-first century. *Acad Med.* 1995; 70:179-185.
14. McCart PM. Rearranging the deck chairs on the *Titanic. Am J Surg.* 1998;176: 88-91.
15. Buchwald H. A clash of cultures: personal autonomy versus corporate bondage. *Surgery.* 1998;124:595-603.
16. Korn D. Re-engineering academic medical centers: re-engineering academic values? *Acad Med.* 1996;71:1033-1043.
17. Kataria S. The turmoil of academic physicians: what AMCs can do to ease their pain. *Acad Med.* 1998;73:728-730.
18. Diago S. Faculty group has plan for bankrupt medical school. *American Medical News.* October 10, 1998:10-12.
19. Reports suggest closure of Hawaii Medical School. *American Medical News.* October 5, 1998:7.
20. Griffen WO Jr, Schwartz RW. Life style as a factor in choosing a medical career. *Am J Surg.* 1990;159:89-90.
21. Aufses AH Jr, Slater GI, Hollier LH. The nature and fate of categorical surgical residents who "drop out." *Am J Surg.* 1998;175:236-239.
22. Conter RL. The death of academic surgery? *J Surg Res.* 1998;76:1-6.
23. Wells SA Jr. Transitions. *Ann Surg.* 1998;227:607-617.
24. Organ C. The future of general surgery. *Acad Surg.* 1990;125:845-846.
25. Krauss K, Smith J. Rejecting conventional wisdom: how academic medical centers can regain their leadership positions. *Acad Med.* 1997;72:571-575.
26. Cohen JJ. Mission based management: lessons from the real world. *Acad Med.* 1998;73:982.
27. Walt A. The uniqueness of American surgical education and its preservation. *Bull Am Coll Surg.* 1994;79:8-20.
28. Tanaka T, Gotay CC. Physicians' and medical students' perspectives on patients' quality of life. *Acad Med.* 1998;73:1003-1005.
29. Hensel WA, Dickey NW. Teaching professionalism: passing the torch. *Acad Med.* 1998;73:865-870.
30. Swick H. Academic medicine must deal with the clash of business and professional values. *Acad Med.* 1998;73:751-755.
31. Coles R. *The Moral Intelligence of Children.* New York, NY: Random House Inc; 1997:1-218.
32. Polchalski CM, Larson DB. Developing curricula in spirituality and medicine. *Acad Med.* 1998;73:970-974.
33. Pargament KI, Ensing DS, Falgout K, et al. Religious coping efforts as predictors of the outcomes to significant negative life events. *Am J Community Psychol.* 1990;18:793-824.
34. Lee KC, Dunlop D, Dolan NC. Do clinical breast examinations improve during medical school? *Acad Med.* 1998;73:1013-1019.
35. Wray NP, Friedland JA. Detection and correction of house staff experience in physical diagnosis. *JAMA.* 1983;249:1035-1037.
36. Wiener S, Nathanson M. Physical examination: frequently observed errors. *JAMA.* 1976;236:852-855.

Announcement

The *Archives of Surgery* will give priority review and early publication to seminal works. This policy will include basic science advancements in surgery and critically performed clinical research.

PAPER

Adenosquamous Carcinoma of the Pancreas

James A. Madura, MD; Benjamin T. Jarman; Michael G. Doherty; Moo-Nahm Yum, MD; Thomas J. Howard, MD

Hypothesis: Adenosquamous carcinoma of the pancreas is a rare but particularly virulent variant of invasive ductal carcinoma. This review will demonstrate the aggressive biologic activity, histopathologic features, and DNA flow cytometric characteristics of this aggressive lesion. In addition, the outcome is less favorable than in other pancreatic neoplasms, in spite of aggressive surgical and postoperative adjuvant therapy.

Design: A retrospective review of 6 patients treated during an 8-year period.

Setting: A major urban university tertiary referral hospital.

Patients: There were 6 patients with this unusual tumor seen between 1990 and 1998. There were 4 men and 2 women, all white, with a mean ± SD age of 63.5 ± 14.7 years. Symptoms were similar to those in patients with more common pancreatic malignant neoplasms.

Results: Four patients with tumors in the head of the pancreas had pancreatoduodenectomy, and 2 with body and or tail lesions had distal pancreatectomy and splenectomy. Pathologically, all the tumors were poorly differentiated and aneuploid, and 5 of the 6 were locally metastatic. All but 1 patient had postoperative complications, but there were no operative deaths. One half of the patients received postoperative adjuvant chemotherapy and radiation therapy. Only 1 patient is still alive at 9 months after surgery, but has known residual cancer around his portal vein noted during palliative distal pancreatectomy.

Conclusions: Adenosquamous carcinoma of the pancreas is an uncommon variant of exocrine pancreatic neoplasm. It is characterized by an admixture of adenomatous and squamous cell elements and demonstrates aggressive biologic behavior. This series of 6 patients is similar to the 134 cases reported since 1907, in that survival is short despite aggressive surgical therapy. Few patients with this disease live more than 1 year. Aggressive therapy should be tempered by the realization of the uniform poor prognosis associated with this malignant neoplasm.

Arch Surg. 1999;134:599-603

INVASIVE DUCTAL carcinoma accounts for the majority of pancreatic malignant neoplasms and has a poor prognosis with the exception of a series of highly selected patients undergoing radical surgical therapy for cure. Adenosquamous carcinoma of the pancreas is an unusual variant of pancreatic neoplasm. It has been variously referred to as adenoacanthoma, mixed squamous and adenocarcinoma, and mucoepidermoid carcinoma. These tumors are histologically characterized by adenomatous cell populations mixed with varying amounts of keratinized squamous cell elements. Major institutional reviews of autopsy and/or surgical specimens suggest an incidence of approximately 4% of all pancreatic neoplasms; however, only 134 cases have been reported in the accessible world's literature. Most of the reports have been small series or single case reports, and, of the large autopsy or surgical tissue reviews, only a few reports detail clinical, histopathologic, and patient outcome data. Survival times have been short in those patients found to have unresectable tumors, as well as in those who have undergone aggressive resection for attempted cure. The prognosis of this uncommon lesion appears to be even less favorable than the invasive ductal tumor, with only a few patients surviving more than 1 year. Because of its rarity, only anecdotal studies of adjunctive radiation or chemotherapy are available.

This series of 6 cases over an 8-year period demonstrates the aggressiveness of this tumor, and its rapid course from discovery to death, despite aggressive surgical treatment.

From the Departments of Surgery (Drs Madura and Howard and Messrs Jarman and Doherty) and Pathology (Dr Yum), Indiana University School of Medicine, Indianapolis.

PATIENTS AND METHODS

Between 1990 and 1998, six patients were diagnosed as having adenosquamous carcinoma of the pancreas and treated at the Indiana University Medical Center Hospitals, Indianapolis. There were 4 men and 2 women, all white, whose mean ± SD age was 63.5 ± 14.7 years. The duration of symptoms prior to presentation was 4.3 ± 3.9 months, and symptoms included abdominal pain and weight loss in 5 of the 6 patients, nausea and vomiting in 3 patients, and anorexia and jaundice in 2 patients. A single patient with a large tumor invading the duodenum presented with upper gastrointestinal tract bleeding and anemia. Physical findings included upper abdominal tenderness in 4 patients, jaundice in 2 patients with tumors in the head of the pancreas, and a palpable abdominal mass in 1 patient. Laboratory studies were unremarkable with the exception of elevated bilirubin and alkaline phosphatase levels in the 2 patients with jaundice and moderately elevated serum carbohydrate antigen 19-9 (Ca 19-9) of 200 U/mL (reference value, ≤70 U/mL) in 1 patient. Computed tomography and endoscopic ultrasound both accurately demonstrated and localized a pancreatic mass in all 6 patients (**Figure 1**). Endoscopic retrograde cholangiopancreatography was performed in 5 patients and demonstrated pancreatic ductal obstruction by tumor in the head or body, which corresponded with the tumor location on the imaging studies (**Figure 2**). Three patients had preoperative fine-needle aspiration biopsy of the tumor mass but none of the specimens were diagnostic of adenosquamous carcinoma. All 3 of the patients with tumors in the head of the pancreas underwent pancreatoduodenectomy, and those with tumors in the body and/or tail of the pancreas were treated by distal pancreatectomy and splenectomy.

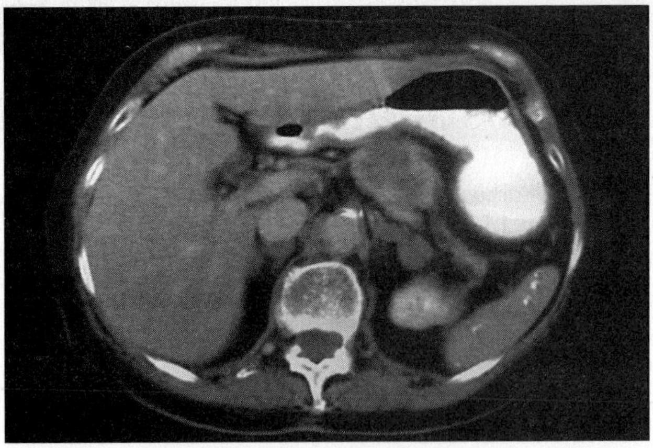

Figure 1. *Computed tomographic scan of a patient with large adenosquamous carcinoma of the mid-body of the pancreas.*

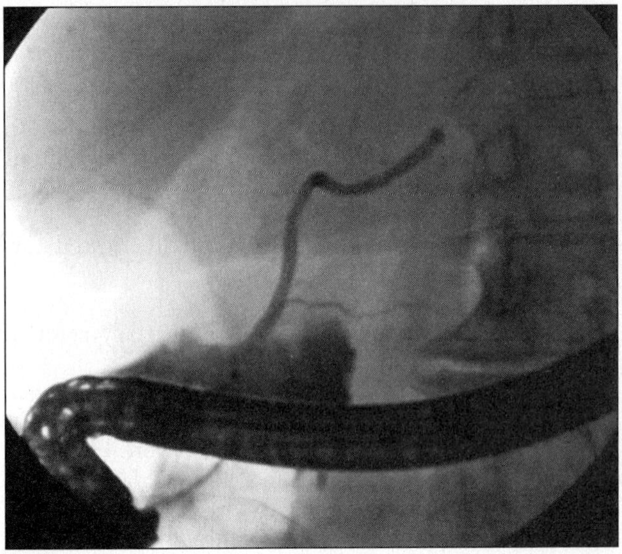

Figure 2. *The endoscopic retrograde cholangiopancreatogram of the patient in Figure 1, demonstrating pancreatic ductal cutoff in the mid-body of the pancreas.*

RESULTS

There were no postoperative deaths, but 5 of the 6 patients had postoperative complications, including 3 with ventilator dependence and 2 with pancreatic fistulas that responded to nonoperative management. Postoperatively, survival was short, with a mean ± SD survival of 5.04 ± 3.58 months. Three of the patients received adjuvant chemoradiation therapy, but this did not result in significant prolongation of survival. One of the patients who had previously undergone pulmonary resection for lung carcinoma committed suicide at 4 months postoperatively. Four patients died of their malignancy at 1, 3, 5, and 12 months postoperatively. One patient with known residual tumor surrounding the portal vein is alive at 8 months and has undergone radiation therapy along with gemcitabine therapy.

Four tumors were located in the head of the pancreas and 2 were in the body and tail. Tumor size ranged from 1.2 to 6.5 cm, with a mean size of 4.2 cm. Grossly, the lesions were firm with a light tan to yellowish color and merged imperceptibly with the surrounding pancreatic parenchyma. Histologically, the tumors all displayed a mixture of ductal adenocarcinoma and squamous cell carcinoma, with the latter comprising more than 30% of the lesion. In a single case, the squamous cell component exceeded the glandular component by a 9:1 ratio. The adenocarcinoma consisted of ductlike structures lined by columnar cells having large vesicular nuclei and prominent nucleoli. Most of these cells had pale to clear cytoplasm with occasional mucin vacuoles. The malignant squamous cells were large and polygonal, having large hyperchromatic nuclei and eosinophilic cytoplasm with intercellular bridges and occasional squamous pearls. They were arranged in diffuse sheets and lobules. These squamous and glandular components were for the most part intimately admixed (**Figure 3**). The tumors elicited a desmoplastic response, which accounted for the firmness appreciated on gross examination.

Peripancreatic fat and neural invasion was present in all 6 cases. Lymphatic invasion was noted in 4 cases and the duodenal wall was invaded by tumor in 3 of the 4 tumors located in the head of the pancreas. Lymph node metastases were found in 5 of the 6 patients. DNA flow cytometry demonstrated aneuploidy in 5 patients with S-phase determination between 5.2% and 30.0% (**Table 1**).

COMMENT

Exocrine tumors of the pancreas have been classified histologically in several large institutional reviews.[1-4] The majority of cases are recognized as invasive ductal carcinomas. Other recognized variants include the mucinous tumors; pleomorphic, anaplastic, and large cell types; acinar cell carcinoma; spindle cell tumors; microadenocarcinomas; and oncocytic cancers.[5] Adenosquamous and squamous cell carcinomas are recognized much less frequently and probably account for 1% to 4% of all reported tumors.

The first known report of adenosquamous carcinoma in the literature is credited to Herxheimer[6] in 1907 in which he referred to this lesion as "cancroide." Subsequently, other authors have referred to this tumor of mixed columnar adenocarcinoma and keratin-containing squamous cell elements as mixed squamous and adenocarcinoma, mucoepidermoid carcinoma, and adenoacanthoma. This admixed tumor has been seen more commonly in other organ systems, such as the lungs, esophagus, colon, stomach, salivary glands, and the female reproductive organs. Several reports describe pancreatic tumors with a more unicellular squamous appearance without the glandular component.[7-9] Most pure squamous lesions of the pancreas are thought to represent metastatic disease, and it is suggested that in the absence of another primary lesion the squamous pancreatic lesion will usually be found to have a glandular component with more careful histological inspection.[10] Since the pancreas does not normally contain any squamous cell elements, it has been proposed that squamous metaplasia occurs as a result of ductal inflammation due to chronic pancreatitis or obstruction by an adenomatous tumor. Currently, there are several theories, none well proven, of the origin of the adenosquamous tumor. The most favored theory is that of squamous metaplasia occurring as a result of obstruction and inflammation and differentiating into a malignant form.[11] The "collision theory" suggests that 2 histologically different tumors arise independently and join or coalesce. No reports have proven this transition phenomenon, but rather have demonstrated squamous cell components intermingled in the body of the predominantly adenocarcinoma. Electron microscopy has demonstrated 2 clearly different cell types. The adenocarcinoma cell demonstrates abundant endoplasmic reticulum and well-developed Golgi apparatus and secretory vesicles. The other cell has scant amounts of endoplasmic reticulum but prominent bundles of tonofilaments, similar to cells seen in other squamous cell tumors.[10] A final theory is that of malignant differentiation by a pluripotential duct cell into the 2 histological types.[12] This theory has received support by an immunocytochemical study demonstrating positive stains for Ca 19-9, ST 439, and keratin in varying degrees in both the squamous and adenomatous cells.[13] There is a report demonstrating carcinoma in situ in squamous metaplasia.[14] In addition, there is a single report of an adenosquamous tumor focus in an equally unusual mucinous cystic neoplasm.[15]

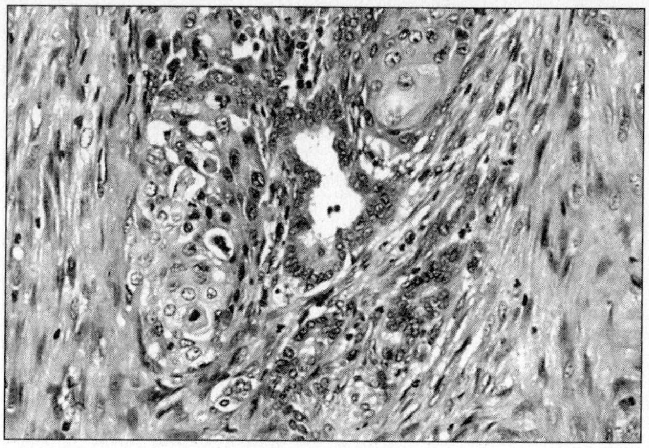

Figure 3. *Histopathologic specimen in a patient with adenosquamous carcinoma of the pancreas. There is desmoplastic stroma with spindly fibroblasts and nests of squamous cell carcinoma and a malignant glandular adenocarcinoma focus in the center (hematoxylin-eosin, original magnification ×250).*

Table 1. Histopathological Characteristics and Flow Cytometric Data in 6 Patients With Adenosquamous Carcinoma of the Pancreas*

Patient No.	Tumor Size, cm	Nodes, No. Positive/ Total	DNA Cytometry	S-Phase, %	DNA Index
1	1.2 × 0.8 × 0.3	0/15	Aneuploid	30	1.45
2	4.6	1/1	Diploid	15	1.00
3	5.0 × 2.5 × 1.7	1/3	Aneuploid	15	1.74
4	6.0	3/5	Aneuploid	20	1.52
5	6.5 × 5.0 × 3.0	2/2	Aneuploid	13	1.86
6	2.0	6/9	Aneuploid	6	1.00

**All tumors were poorly differentiated.*

The incidence of this unusual lesion is really not known, but estimates from review and classification of pancreatic tumors from autopsy and/or surgically resected specimens have been demonstrated to be approximately 4% (**Table 2**). Of the reported series, the incidence ranges from 0.9% to 11.1%, but this latter estimate was from a series of 27 surgical specimens.[17] A number of reports suggest that many of these lesions are large and inoperable; therefore, analysis limited to surgical cases may not be totally indicative of the true incidence since many of these patients have not undergone subsequent surgery or autopsy.

A comprehensive review of 31 available reports between 1907 and 1997 identified 134 patients with adenosquamous tumors[1-36] (**Table 3**). From those reports with detailed clinical data, there were 69 men and 45 women, a ratio of 1.53:1. The mean age of these patients was 62.4 ± 11.7 years, with a range of 33 to 86 years. The major symptoms were no different than those of the usual invasive ductal lesions of the pancreas, and included abdominal and back pain, weight loss, anorexia, and jaundice in patients with lesions in the head of the

Table 2. Incidence of Adenosquamous Carcinoma in Major Retrospective Autopsy and Surgical Studies

Source, y	No. of Specimens		No. (%) of Adenosquamous Carcinomas
	Autopsy	Surgical	
Halpert et al,[16] 1965	120	0	5 (4.2)
Cihak et al,[11] 1972	90	0	4 (4.4)
Baylor and Berg,[1] 1973	5075	0	46 (0.9)
Kissane,[3] 1975	205	0	6 (2.9)
Cubilla and Fitzgerald,[2] 1980	525	120	20 (3.1)
Ishikawa et al,[17] 1980	0	27	3 (11.1)
Morohoshi et al,[4] 1983	167	97	10 (3.8)
Chen and Baithun,[5] 1985	275	116	13 (3.4)
Motojima et al,[13] 1992	145	57	6 (3.0)

Table 3. Details of Reported Patients With Adenosquamous Carcinoma of the Pancreas*

	Literature Review	Present Series
Total No. of reported patients, 1907-1997[1-36]	134	6
M/F ratio	69:45	4:2
Age, mean ± SD, y	62.4 ± 11.7	63.5 ± 14.7
Location in pancreas, No.		
Head	31	4
Head and body	4	0
Body	7	0
Body and tail	8	2
Tail	5	0
Diffuse	4	0
Survival, mo		
Mean ± SD	5.7 ± 4.1	5.0 ± 3.6
Range	0.06-18	1.03-12.03

**Not all reports contained complete data about each patient.*

pancreas. Tumor location was in the head of the pancreas in 31 patients, head and body in 4, body in 7, body and tail in 6, and tail in 8. It was diffuse in 4.

Whether or not surgical resection was attempted, survival was short, averaging 5.7 ± 4.1 months in 72 patients for whom survival data were available. Few studies report tumor marker data or flow cytometry results, but the present series provides evidence that these lesions are poorly differentiated, metastatic, and have aneuploid DNA characteristics. Because of the small numbers of reported cases, only anecdotal reports of adjunctive therapy are available and none of the therapies seem to prolong survival in this aggressive lesion.[20]

Accurate preoperative diagnosis of this lesion is difficult. There are no characteristics on imaging studies to differentiate it from the more common exocrine neoplasms of the pancreas. A recent report by Kuji et al[21] suggests that these lesions may selectively take up gallium 67 and be visualized by nuclear scanning. In several recent case reports, preoperative percutaneous and intraoperative cytologic studies have been diagnostically correct, but this did not alter treatment decisions or survival.[22-25]

Once these lesions are identified, with or without accurate preoperative or intraoperative cytologic diagnosis, the question arises as to the extent of treatment. Since survival appears to be uniformly poor, should aggressive resection be undertaken, even if it appears potentially curative at the time of operation? From the review of the literature, there are only 5 known patients who have survived 1 year or longer, in contrast to reported series of highly selected patients with invasive ductal carcinomas in whom 5-year survival rates of 20% to 30% have been reported. In addition, mean survival with or without resection is less than 6 months in the present series, as well as those accumulated cases in the literature. One has to consider the risk and complications of major resective surgery in light of this rather short postoperative survival. If these lesions are small and there is no intraoperative evidence of nodal or distant metastasis, should these patients be denied an attempt at curative resection? Since pancreatoduodenectomy and distal pancreatectomy can currently be done with acceptably low morbidity and mortality, these procedures are probably the best palliative procedures available. In the near future, more effective chemotherapy combined with radiation may allow better survival with an acceptable quality of life.

Presented at the 106th Scientific Session of the Western Surgical Association, Indianapolis, Ind, November 18, 1998.

Reprints: James A. Madura, MD, Department of Surgery, Indiana University School of Medicine, 545 Barnhill Dr, EM 244, Indianapolis, IN 46202-5125.

REFERENCES

1. Baylor SM, Berg JW. Cross-classification and survival characteristics of 5,000 cases of cancer of the pancreas. *J Surg Oncol.* 1973;5:335-358.
2. Cubilla A, Fitzgerald P. Surgical pathology of tumors of the exocrine pancreas. In: Moosa AR, ed. *Tumors of the Pancreas.* Baltimore, Md: Williams & Wilkins; 1980:159-193.
3. Kissane JM. Carcinoma of the exocrine pancreas: pathologic aspects. *J Surg Oncol.* 1975;7:167-174.
4. Morohoshi T, Held G, Klöppel G. Exocrine pancreatic tumors and their histological classification: a study based on 167 autopsy and 97 surgical cases. *Histopathology.* 1983;7:167-174.
5. Chen J, Baithun S. Morphologic study of 391 cases of exocrine pancreatic tumours with special reference to the classification of exocrine pancreatic carcinoma. *J Pathol.* 1985;146:17-29.
6. Herxheimer G. Über heterologe Cancroide. *Beitr Pathol Anat.* 1907;41:348-412.
7. Lawrence DH Jr. Squamous cell carcinoma of the pancreas. *Colo Med.* 1934; 31:172-175.
8. Case records of the Massachusetts General Hospital. *N Engl J Med.* 1953;249: 74-76. Case 39282.
9. Lowry C, Whitaker HJ, Greiner D. Squamous cell carcinoma of the pancreas. *South Med J.* 1949;42:753-757.
10. Kovi J. Adenosquamous carcinoma of the pancreas: a light and electron microscopic study. *Ultrastruct Pathol.* 1982;3:17-23.
11. Cihak RW, Kawashima T, Steer A. Adenoacanthoma (adenosquamous carcinoma) of the pancreas. *Cancer.* 1972;29:1133-1140.
12. Jamieson JD, Ingber DE, Mureson V, et al. Cell surface properties of normal, differentiating, and neoplastic pancreatic acinar cells. *Cancer.* 1981;47:1516-1525.
13. Motojima K, Tomioka T, Kohara N, et al. Immunohistochemical characteristics of adenosquamous carcinoma of the pancreas. *J Surg Oncol.* 1992;49:58-62.
14. Hartsock RJ, Fisher EJ. Cancer-in-situ in pancreatic squamous metaplasia. *Arch Surg.* 1961;82:674-677.
15. Campman SC, Fajardo MA, Rippon MB, et al. Adenosquamous carcinoma arising in a mucinous cystadenoma of the pancreas. *J Surg Oncol.* 1997;64: 159-162.
16. Halpert B, Makk L, Jordan GLJ. A retrospective study of 120 patients with carcinoma of the pancreas. *Surg Gynecol Obstetr.* 1965;121:91-96.
17. Ishikawa O, Matsui Y, Aoki I, Iwanga T, Terasawa T, Wada A. Adenosquamous carcinoma of the pancreas: a clinicopathologic study and report of three cases. *Cancer.* 1980;46:1192-1196.

18. Sommers SC, Meissner WA. Unusual carcinomas of the pancreas. *Arch Pathol.* 1954;58:101-111.
19. Cubilla AJ, Fitzgerald PJ. Morphological patterns of primary nonendocrine human pancreas carcinoma. *Cancer Res.* 1975;35:2234-2248.
20. Onoda N, Kang S-M, Sugano S, Yamashita Y, Chung Y-S, Sowa M. Mucoepidermoid carcinoma of the pancreas: report of a case. *Surg Today.* 1995;25:843-847.
21. Kuji I, Sumiya H, Taki J, et al. Intense Ga-67 uptake in adenosquamous carcinoma of the pancreas. *Ann Nucl Med.* 1997;11:41-43.
22. Smit W, Mathy J-P, Donaldson E. Pancreatic cytology and adenosquamous carcinoma of the pancreas: a case report. *Pathology.* 1993;25:420-422.
23. Wilczynski SP, Valente PT, Atkinson BF. Cytodiagnosis of adenosquamous carcinoma of the pancreas: use of intraoperative fine needle aspiration. *Acta Cytol.* 1984;28:733-736.
24. Leiman G, Markowitz S, Svensson LG. Intraoperative cytodiagnosis of pancreatic adenosquamous carcinoma: a case report. *Diagn Cytopathol.* 1986;2:72-75.
25. Gupta RK, Wakefield SJ, Fauck R, Stewart RJ. Immunocytochemical ultrastructural findings in a case of rare carcinoma of pancreas with predominance of malignant squamous cells in an intraoperative needle aspirate. *Acta Cytol.* 1989;33:153-156.
26. Case records of the Massachusetts General Hospital (case #31222). *N Engl J Med.* 1945;232:657-659.
27. Frantz VK. *Atlas of Tumor Pathology: Tumors of the Pancreas.* Washington, DC: Armed Forces Institute of Pathology; 1959. Section VII, fascicles 27 and 28. American Registry of Pathology.
28. Elias E. Carcinoma of the pancreas. *Arch Surg.* 1969;98:138-140.
29. Sasaki J, Ito S, Kashiwagi T, Imamura T, Iwashita A. Adenosquamous carcinoma of the pancreas. *Naika Intern Med.* 1977;39:337-341.
30. Weitzner S. Adenoacanthoma of the pancreas: report of 4 cases and literature review. *Am Surg.* 1978;44:206-209.
31. Sears HF, Kim Y, Strawitz J. Squamous cell carcinoma of the pancreas. *J Surg Oncol.* 1980;14:261-265.
32. Yamaguchi K. Adenosquamous carcinoma of the pancreas: a clinicopathologic study. *J Surg Oncol.* 1991;47:109-116.
33. Yamaguchi K. Carcinoma of the uncinate process of the pancreas with a peculiar clinical manifestation. *Am J Gastroenterol.* 1992;87:1046-1050.
34. Beyer KL, Marshall JB, Metzler MH, Poulter JS, Seger RM, Diaz-Arias AA. Squamous cell carcinoma of the pancreas: report of an unusual case and review of the literature. *Digest Dis Sci.* 1992;37:312-318.
35. O'Connor DS, Ruchman R. Adenosquamous carcinoma of the pancreas. *N J Med.* 1993;90:527-529.
36. Makiyama K, Takuma K, Zea-Iriarte W, et al. Adenosquamous carcinoma of the pancreas. *J Gastroent.* 1995;30:798-802.

DISCUSSION

Gerard V. Aranha, MD, Maywood, Ill: Dr Madura has presented us with 6 cases of adenosquamous carcinoma of the pancreas, a very rare variant of the usual adenocarcinoma. There were 4 patients with head lesions and 2 with lesions in the body; all were resected, but none survived more than 12 months, suggesting also a poorer prognosis than patients with adenocarcinoma. The pathology evaluation revealed that 5 of the 6 patients had peripancreatic or perineural invasion as well as lymph node metastasis and that 5 of the 6 had aneuploid tumors, all harbingers of poor prognosis. As far as theories go, there are many, but the one that makes the most sense is the one that you first alluded to—the one that says that there may be squamous metaplasia in an adenocarcinoma that leads to 2 pathologic entities in one tumor.

In your lymph node metastasis, which of the elements metastasized, was it the glandular type or the squamous type? Can you conjecture why the prognosis was so bad in these patients? Is it possible that squamous metaplasia occurs more often in adenocarcinoma and that we do not find it because we do not search enough for it? The incidence of this tumor you said was 4%, but in a Japanese study, it was 11%. If this variant occurs more, should we be reconsidering our adjunctive therapy? Our therapy now is geared toward adenocarcinoma. Should we be changing the chemotherapy or combining it with something geared toward squamous, let's say, platinum-based therapy?

You talked about ERCP (endoscopic retrograde cholangiopancreatography). If you had these patients first and you saw a CT scan clearly showing you a mass, would you put them through an ERCP?

Finally, one other question about biopsy. Because you saw 6 cases of this variant with bad prognosis, are you going to change your philosophy? I suspect you are like me and do not do a biopsy preoperatively or intraoperatively. Would you change your philosophy based on these 6 patients?

Dr Madura: Dr Aranha, your first question was about the cellular pattern of the lymph node metastases. We reviewed all of the lymph nodes in the 5 patients with metastases. Three of these patients had mixed adenocarcinoma and squamous cell carcinoma in the nodes, while 2 patients, interestingly, had only squamous cell elements. We also evaluated the pancreatic lesions for total content of each of the 2 specific cell types and found that 5 of the patients had 30% squamous cell cancer in their tumor, while 1 patient had more than 90% squamous cells in his tumor. You asked whether these patients should be treated with a chemotherapeutic regimen more suited for the squamous cell element. Unfortunately, these lesions are very unusual, and there are no series of patients treated with such an approach. Our sole survivor at this point has known residual disease but has survived nearly 9 months and he has been treated with gemcitabine and irradiation. I am not sure of this agent's efficacy with squamous cell tumors, but it does have some advantage in adenocarcinomas. I think your concept may be correct and in the future, we might change our adjuvant therapeutic approach.

You asked if we had diagnosed any of these lesions ahead of time, and, with the exception of those patients arriving with previous biopsy, we do not attempt a preoperative aspiration nor do we do any tissue sampling in the operating room. If the lesion looks amenable to removal on preoperative assessment and in the operating room, we go ahead with the resection. One of these patients gave us no choice since her tumor had eroded into the duodenum and was bleeding. I do not think that a diagnosis of adenosquamous carcinoma preoperatively would change our approach. It would give us an opportunity to inform the patient and their family about the prognosis, and perhaps allow us to stimulate our oncologic colleagues to consider a different postoperative regimen.

PAPER

Long-term Results of Biliary Reconstruction After Laparoscopic Bile Duct Injuries

Michel M. Murr, MD; Jean-François Gigot, MD; David M. Nagorney, MD; William S. Harmsen, MS; Duane M. Ilstrup, MS; Michael B. Farnell, MD

Hypothesis: The Hepp-Couinaud approach to biliary enteric reconstruction for laparoscopic bile duct injuries provides a durable, long-term result in most patients.

Design: Retrospective study of patients who underwent operative repair of laparoscopic bile duct injuries from January 1990 through December 1997.

Setting: Academic tertiary referral center.

Main Outcome Measures: Outcome was assessed using a grading system based on clinical symptoms, liver function tests, and need for reintervention for anastomotic stricture. The Kaplan-Meier method was employed to estimate stricture-free survival.

Results: Fifty-nine consecutive patients underwent operative repair of the following laparoscopic bile duct injuries (Strasberg classification): B: n = 2 (3%), C: n = 1 (1%), D: n = 2 (3%), E_1: n = 5 (8%), E_2: n = 16 (27%), E_3: n = 25 (42%), E_4: n = 5 (8%), and E_5: n = 3 (5%). Forty-seven patients (80%) had 1 or more interventions prior to the index repair. The extrahepatic left bile duct (Hepp-Couinaud approach) was used in 46 of 53 patients who underwent a Roux-en-Y hepaticojejunostomy. Follow-up (mean ± SEM, 3.7 ± 0.3 years) was complete in 54 of the 57 patients still alive. Five patients developed subsequent anastomotic strictures and were treated with percutaneous transhepatic dilation (n = 3), endoscopic dilation (n = 1), and operative revision (n = 1). Excellent to good long-term results were achieved in the remaining 49 patients (91%). Life-table analysis yielded 95% and 88% chances of stricture-free survival at 2 and 5 years, respectively.

Conclusions: Complex iatrogenic proximal bile duct injuries and strictures are amenable to operative repair using the extrahepatic left bile duct. The Hepp-Couinaud approach offers a durable result in more than 90% of patients, even after previous interventions have failed.

Arch Surg. 1999;134:604-610

IATROGENIC INJURIES to the bile ducts are uncommon entities in clinical practice that have been encountered more frequently after the advent of laparoscopic surgery.[1,2] The pattern of bile duct injuries occurring during laparoscopic cholecystectomy seems to differ from those injuries sustained during an open procedure; many occur in a more proximal location and the resultant strictures are more extensive. The fact that as many as 15% of such operative repairs for bile duct injuries had to be revised[3] underscores the complexity of these injuries and the need for long-term follow-up.

The long-term success of repairing iatrogenic laparoscopic bile duct injuries is difficult to assess because many of the reports in the literature contain a small number of patients or have a short follow-up period. A previous report from our institution[4] outlined the pattern of the initial wave of complications from laparoscopic cholecystectomy and their treatment. That experience was reported expediently to alert surgeons to the increasing incidence of serious bile duct injury, and hence a long follow-up period was not practical.

The aim of this study was to report the long-term results of biliary reconstruction for laparoscopic duct injuries using the Hepp-Couinaud approach,[5] which incorporates the extrahepatic portion of the left main hepatic duct (**Figure 1**).

From the Departments of Surgery (Drs Murr, Gigot, Nagorney, and Farnell) and Health Sciences Research (Messrs Harmsen and Ilstrup), Mayo Clinic and Foundation, Rochester, Minn; Dr Murr is now with the Department of Surgery, University of South Florida, Tampa. Dr Gigot is now with the St Luc University Hospital, Louvain Medical School, Brussels, Belgium.

RESULTS

PATIENT CHARACTERISTICS

Fifty-nine patients (8 men and 51 women aged 45±2 years) underwent repair of iatrogenic laparoscopic bile duct injuries at the Mayo Clinic (January 1990–December 1997). All patients were referred from other institutions at variable periods after sus-

MATERIALS AND METHODS

The medical records of all 59 consecutive patients (January 1990 through December 1997) who underwent operative repair of laparoscopic bile duct injuries at the Mayo Clinic, Rochester, Minn, were reviewed. The records were abstracted for demographic information; preoperative and postoperative clinical characteristics, including symptoms, laboratory values, and imaging studies; and subjective assessment of the quality of life. Due to the nature of our tertiary practice, it was not practical for some patients who reside in different states and countries to have long-term follow-up at our center. Hence, postoperative follow-up was arranged with local physicians who communicated results of laboratory and imaging studies to us. In this subset of patients, critical aspects of postoperative care, such as removal of transanastomotic biliary stents, were determined by our surgeons after review of pertinent contrast studies obtained at local facilities. A detailed questionnaire was mailed to all patients by a dedicated survey research center at our institution. Nonresponders were subsequently contacted by telephone. Follow-up information was pooled from postoperative visits at our center, contacts from referring physicians, and the results of the follow-up survey.

STRICTURE CLASSIFICATION

All pertinent imaging studies were reviewed by 2 of us (M.M.M. and M.B.F.), and strictures were classified according to Strasberg et al[6] (**Figure 2**). The classification of strictures was primarily based on ductal anatomy as it appeared on percutaneous transhepatic cholangiography. When percutaneous transhepatic cholangiography was not done or not available for review, strictures were classified based on other imaging studies, such as endoscopic retrograde cholangiopancreatography, and the impression of our attending surgeon at the time of the index repair as documented in our operative records. In 5 patients whose original contrast studies were not available for review, the injuries were classified based on reports in the medical record and operative description at the time of index repair.

OUTCOME MEASUREMENTS

Outcomes of operative repair of bile duct injury were graded according to a classification that accounts for both subjective criteria (symptoms of pain, jaundice, and cholangitis) and objective criteria (serum liver function tests, need for reintervention).[7,8] Patients were graded as excellent (asymptomatic and normal serum liver function test results), good (asymptomatic, mildly abnormal liver function test results), or poor (symptomatic and abnormal liver function test results). Patients who required postoperative intervention for management of recurrent strictures were considered to have treatment failure(s).

DATA ANALYSIS

Life-table analysis using the Kaplan-Meier method was employed to estimate the stricture-free survival in patients who underwent reconstruction using the Hepp-Couinaud approach. The 95% confidence intervals were plotted on all survival curves. For the purposes of calculating the duration of follow-up, intervention for a postoperative stricture was considered an end point. Data are reported as mean ± SEM, unless otherwise indicated.

taining the injury (median, 5 months; range, 4 days to 6 years). Details about the conduct of the laparoscopic cholecystectomy were available from operative notes and from hospitalization records of 24 patients. The indications for cholecystectomy were cholelithiasis (86% [n = 51]), chronic cholecystitis (20% [n = 12]), acute cholecystitis (15% [n = 9]), and pancreatitis (2% [n = 1]). Clinical presentation after bile duct injury included pain (66% [n = 39]), jaundice (54% [n = 32]), cholangitis (37% [n = 22]), pruritus (32% [n = 19]), weight loss (18% [n = 11]), biliary fistula (10% [n = 6]), and ascites (8% [n = 5]). Six patients (10%) had minimal or no symptoms at the time of referral.

Forty-seven patients (80%) had at least 1 or a combination of therapeutic percutaneous (n = 13), endoscopic (n = 20), or operative (n = 34) interventions prior to referral to our institution. Two patients with active intraperitoneal biliary leak or sepsis at the time of referral to our institution underwent percutaneous or operative placement of drains prior to definitive repair to optimize the local conditions and allow the inflammatory reaction to subside.

STRICTURES

Most commonly, strictures were proximal in the biliary tree. More than 50% involved the confluence or extended to the bifurcation of the right and left bile ducts (E_3: 25 [42%], E_4: 5 [8%], E_5: 3 [5%]) (**Table 1**). Isolated injuries to the right sectoral ducts were rare (class B and C: 3 patients). Lateral injury (class D) occurred in only 2 patients.

DIAGNOSTIC STUDIES

A combination of preoperative diagnostic radiological tests were employed. Most commonly, percutaneous transhepatic cholangiography (37 [63%]) and endoscopic retrograde cholangiopancreatography (29 [49%]) provided enough information to secure the diagnosis. Computed tomographic scan and ultrasonography were performed in 28 (47%) and 12 (20%) patients, respectively, to evaluate fluid collections and hepatic atrophy/hypertrophy. Four patients with suspected vascular injury underwent mesenteric angiography.

INDEX BILIARY REPAIR

The Hepp-Couinaud technique was used to incorporate the extrahepatic segment of the left hepatic duct into the repair in 46 of the 53 patients who underwent a Roux-en-Y hepaticojejunostomy (**Table 2**). The Hepp-Couinaud approach was not used as part of a Roux-en-Y

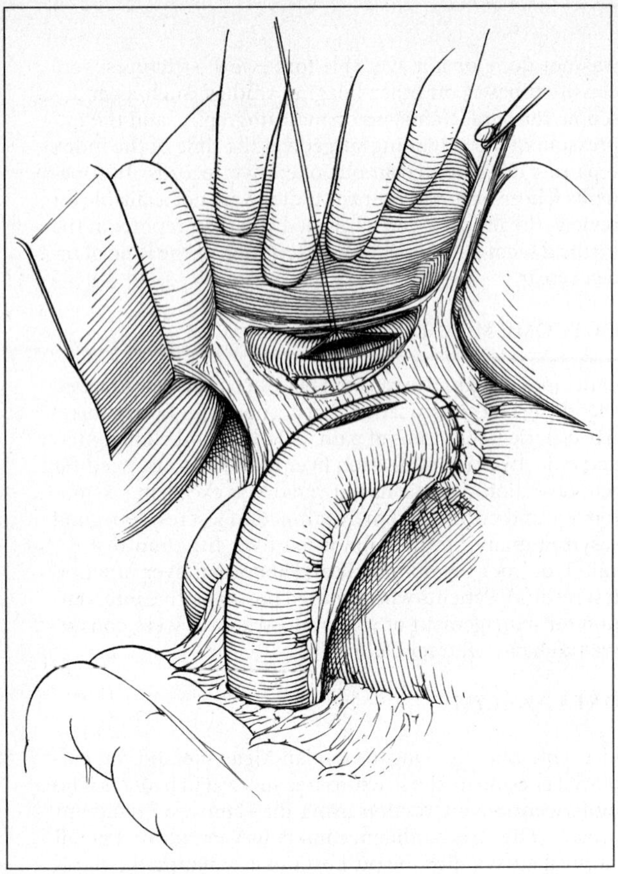

Figure 1. *The origin of the main hepatic duct, confluence, and left main hepatic duct are exposed by incising the Glisson capsule at the base of segment IV. We then retract the segment IV cephalad and incise the vasculobiliary sheath overlying the proximal extrahepatic biliary system. Roux-en-Y loop is carried through the right transverse mesocolon in preparation for a 2- to 3-cm, side-to-side, biliary enteric anastomosis (drawing by D. Factor, Mayo Clinic, Rochester, Minn, copyright 1995).*

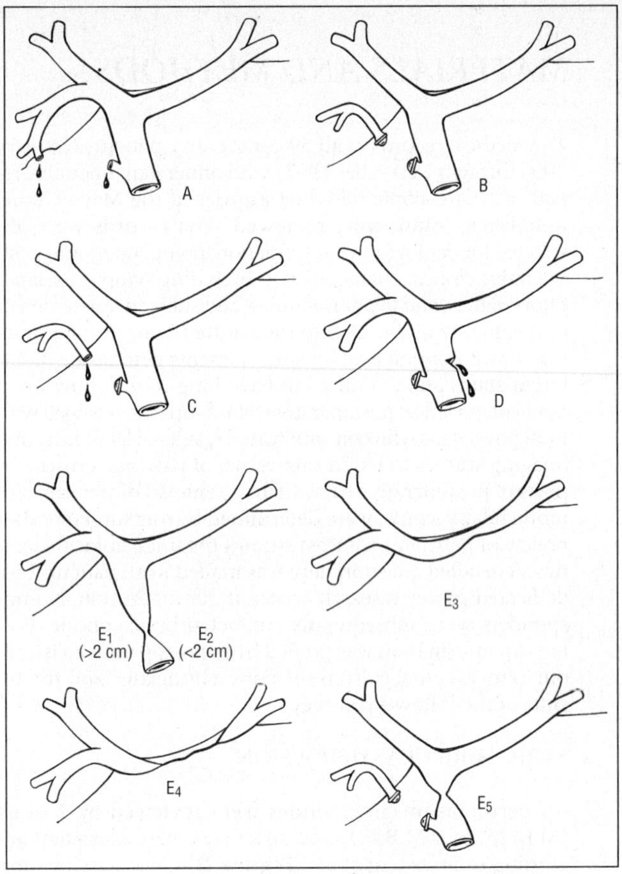

Figure 2. *Strasberg classification of bile duct injuries and strictures.[6] Class A, Injury to small ducts in continuity with the biliary system, with a leak in the duct of Luschka or the cystic duct. Class B, Injury to a sectoral duct, with resultant obstruction of part of the biliary system. Class C, Injury to a sectoral duct with bile leak; bile leakage occurs from a duct not continuous with the biliary system. Class D, Lateral injury to the extrahepatic biliary ducts. Class E_1, Stricture more than 2 cm from the bifurcation of the right and left bile ducts. Class E_2, Stricture less than 2 cm from the bifurcation of the right and left bile ducts. Class E_3, Stricture at the bifurcation of the right and left bile ducts. Class E_4, Stricture involving the right and left bile ducts; the left and right ducts are not continuous. Class E_5, Complete occlusion of all bile ducts, including sectoral ducts (Mayo Clinic, Rochester, Minn, copyright 1998).*

hepaticojejunostomy in 7 patients who had E_1 (n = 2), E_2 (n = 4), and E_3 (n = 1) strictures. The remaining 6 patients had a Roux-en-Y cholangiojejunostomy (n = 3), choledochorraphy (n = 2), and hepaticoduodenostomy (n = 1). Transanastomotic stents were used in 43 patients for 45±3 days postoperatively. The length of stay was 9±0.5 days.

COMPLICATIONS

One patient died 13 days postoperatively from pancreatitis and renal insufficiency that progressed to multisystem organ failure. She had 2 prior interventions and was in respiratory failure when transferred to our center.

Fifty-two patients (88%) had no postoperative complications. Ten complications developed in 7 patients: intra-abdominal abscesses (n = 3), wound infection (n = 3), cholangitis (n = 2), hemobilia (n = 1), and pancreatitis (n = 1). One of the abscesses was the result of an anastomotic leak; all abscesses were treated successfully with percutaneous drainage. At the time of last follow-up, none of these patients had developed any postoperative strictures. In all patients with wound infection, the condition responded to wound drainage and antibiotic treatment.

FOLLOW-UP

At the time of the study, 2 patients had died. One patient, mentioned above, died of multisystem organ failure, and another died at home of myocardial ischemia 42 days postoperatively. Fifty-seven patients were available for follow-up, 50 of whom responded to the survey in 1998. Four patients did not respond in 1998 but had responded to our earlier survey in 1995. Three patients (5%) were lost to follow-up (no current or forwarding address or international patients). Mean follow-up was 3.7 ± 0.3 years. The longest follow-up period was 7.3 years.

OUTCOMES

Final outcome was graded in 54 patients (2 died and 3 were lost to follow-up). Forty-six patients (85%) had excellent results, 3 patients (6%) had good results, and 5 patients (9%) subsequently developed anastomotic strictures that required intervention. These patients were con-

Table 1. Classification of Laparoscopic Bile Duct Injuries in 59 Patients*

Class	No. (%) of Patients
B	2 (3)
C	1 (1)
D	2 (3)
E_1	5 (8)
E_2	16 (27)
E_3	25 (42)
E_4	5 (8)
E_5	3 (5)

*According to Strasberg et al.[6]

sidered to have treatment failure (**Table 3**). Four patients were treated at our center with percutaneous transhepatic (n = 3) or endoscopic (n = 1) dilation. The fifth patient had operative revision of the biliary-enteric anastomosis at another facility 4.5 years after the index operation at our center. Life-table analysis predicts 95% and 88% chances of stricture-free survival, respectively, at 2 and 5 years when the Hepp-Couinaud approach is used (**Figure 3**).

COMMENT

The incidence of laparoscopic bile duct injuries has recently been observed to plateau.[9] It is estimated that major bile duct injury occurs in approximately 0.5% to 0.6% of patients undergoing laparoscopic cholecystectomy as opposed to 0.2% to 0.4% during open cholecystectomy.[2,10,11]

Injuries to bile ducts can be avoided by meticulous attention to the anatomical variants in the hepatocystic triangle and adherence to principles of safe dissection in that area. Information about the conduct of laparoscopic cholecystectomy was available for our review in only 24 patients, making it difficult to classify the mechanisms of injury (eg, avulsion, transection, or electrocautery) with an acceptable and reliable degree of certainty. Invariably, when the injury was recognized intraoperatively, the surgeon's note indicated the presence of "biliary anomaly." In other cases, when an intraoperative cholangiogram was obtained, the imaging study was interpreted as normal by the operating surgeon at the time of cholecystectomy.

We have adopted a modification of the Bismuth classification of bile duct strictures advocated by Strasberg et al[6] to account for injuries that occur during laparoscopic cholecystectomy with or without the subsequent development of strictures (Figure 1). We have found that the modified classification allows uniform reporting and communication among hepatobiliary surgeons. This classification allows reporting of injuries that can be treated by nonoperative means, such as endoscopic stenting in the case of lateral injuries (class D) or cystic duct or duct of Luschka leaks (class A).

Prior to referral to our institution, an attempt to correct the injury after it was recognized was undertaken in 80% of patients, with one or a combination of operative, endoscopic, or percutaneous procedures. Immediate surgery may fail because of both the small size and thin wall of the ducts. In addition, concomitant bile leak, perianastomotic infection, and inflammation are unfavorable conditions for immediate repair. We believe that the final extent of injury and strictures evolves over time as the ischemic ductal tissue is replaced with fibrotic scar tissue. This may result in underestimation of the extent of the stricture and may explain why so many immediate repairs have a propensity to fail.

Precise diagnosis is crucial and all intrahepatic ducts must be visualized; hence, percutaneous tranhepatic

Table 2. Operation Used for Repair of Laparoscopic Bile Duct Injury in 59 Patients

Operation	Injury Classification*	No. of Patients	Hepp-Couinaud Approach†
Hepaticoduodenostomy	E_2	1	NA
T-tube choledochorrhaphy	D	1	NA
	E_1	1	NA
Roux-en-Y cholangiojejunostomy	B	2	NA
	C	1	NA
Roux-en-Y hepaticojejunostomy	D	1	Yes
	E_1	2	No
	E_1	2	Yes
	E_2	4	No
	E_2	11	Yes
	E_3	1	No
	E_3	24	Yes
	E_4	5	Yes
	E_5	3	Yes

*According to Strasberg et al.[6]
†NA indicates not applicable.

Table 3. Outcome of Operative Treatment for Laparoscopic Bile Duct Injuries in 54 Patients*

Outcome	No. (%) of Patients
Excellent	46 (85)
Good	3 (6)
Poor	0 (0)
Failure	5 (9)

*Mean ± SEM follow-up was 3.7 ± 0.3 years; 2 patients died and 3 patients were lost to follow-up.

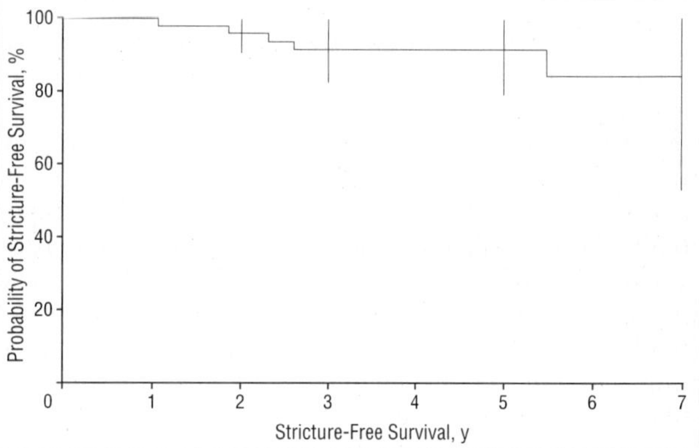

Figure 3. *Stricture-free survival in 46 patients after repair of laparoscopic bile duct injury using the Hepp-Couinaud approach.*

Table 4. Characteristics of 5 Patients With Treatment Failures*

Injury Classification†	Bile Leak	Prior Interventions	Stent, d	Time to Postoperative Stricture, y	Treatment of Postoperative Stricture
E_2	Yes	Operative (×1)	None	2	Endoscopic (×1)
E_3	Yes	Operative (×2)	43	5.5	Operative (×1)
E_3	No	Operative (×1)	22	2.5	TH (×3)
E_4	Yes	None	35	1	TH (×4)
E_4, RHA	Yes	Operative (×1), endoscopic (×1)	99	2.5	TH (×1)

**TH indicates percutaneous transhepatic dilation; RHA, injury to right hepatic artery. The index repair was Roux-en-Y hepaticojejunostomy and the Hepp-Couinaud approach. There was no postoperative morbidity.*
†According to Strasberg et al.[6]

cholangiography is our modality of choice to delineate biliary anatomy and the proximal extent of the stricture. Other useful modalities, such as endoscopic retrograde cholangiopancreatography, may not visualize the proximal extent of the stricture in the case of complete or near complete obstruction, or in injuries that involve accessory or sectoral ducts that do not communicate with the rest of the intrahepatic bile ducts. Although preoperative decompression of the bile ducts is a matter of debate in obstruction secondary to malignant neoplasms, we regard it as a useful adjunct in intraoperative localization of bile ducts and postoperative stenting of the anastomosis. Our practice in limiting the duration of postoperative stenting differs from that of others,[12] who have used stents up to 14 months as an integral part of biliary-enteric anastomoses. We used stents both to decompress the biliary tree in the immediate postoperative period and to obtain postoperative contrast studies. The contrast studies are obtained to assess the integrity of the anastomosis and confirm drainage of all components of the intrahepatic biliary tree.

The optimal timing of repair following injury has not been clearly established. We have based our approach on clinical characteristics. In patients presenting with complete occlusion and no bile leak, the definitive repair can be undertaken when the bile ducts become dilated. Percutaneous tubes can be intermittently clamped to allow dilation up to a diameter of 10 mm. Operation can be undertaken within 2 to 3 weeks of injury in this instance. In patients with evidence of bile leak, biliary fistula, or bile peritonitis, we delay repair to allow the inflammation to subside and also to allow the ducts to dilate, typically 3 to 6 months later.

We believe that the proper use of operative techniques may be the most important predictor of success in biliary reconstruction. We initially became familiar with the Hepp-Couinaud technique in 1982, were encouraged by our initial experience[8] with the technique for benign strictures, and have used it exclusively for proximal strictures since then. In that report,[8] 45 patients had iatrogenic strictures, most of which (n = 26) followed open cholecystectomy. The Hepp-Couinaud technique was used in 21 patients and was compared with standard techniques for the remaining 24 patients. With a median follow-up of 4.6 years, 95% (n = 20) of the patients treated with the Hepp-Couinaud technique achieved excellent or good results. At the time of last follow-up, none of those patients had required reintervention.

The Hepp-Couinaud technique capitalizes on the extrahepatic course of the left main hepatic duct. Incising the investing fascia that condenses around the porta hepatis and forms the "hilar plate" allows easy exposure of the extrahepatic left hepatic duct. The left hepatic duct is an excellent choice for repair of proximal stricture because its location at the base of segment IV and its investing fascia protect it from iatrogenic injury and the inflammatory reaction engendered by bile leakage and infection. In addition, it has a rich blood supply that is not affected by the iatrogenic event, in contrast to the tenuous axial blood supply of the common hepatic and bile ducts.

While most patients who had hepaticojejunostomy in the present study, 46 (87%) of 53 patients, underwent repair using the Hepp-Couinaud technique, for patients with more distal injuries (class E_1 and selected class E_2), the presence of pliable, well-vascularized duct below the confluens may allow repair without the necessity for elevation of the hilar plate and incision along the left main duct. Six patients, 2 with class E_1 and 4 with class E_2 injuries, were treated in this manner, and all were graded as excellent at follow-up.

Excellent to good results in most patients (>85%) have been achieved by others using Roux-en-Y hepaticojejunostomy.[13-15] However, these reports do not stratify results by whether the Hepp-Couinaud approach was used, and they include patients with injuries secondary to heterogeneous causes, such as cholecystectomy, pancreatitis, trauma, or choledochal cysts. In sharp contrast, in 1 recent report[16] in which the authors did not use the Hepp-Couinaud technique, all 4 patients with E_3 and E_4 (Bismuth class III and IV) strictures were symptomatic at follow-up. In addition, the authors' claim that longer follow-up will improve their results is unfounded because the narrowed diameter of such anastomoses will not increase over time.

Excellent or good results were obtained in 33 of 38 and 48 of 52 patients treated for laparoscopic bile duct injuries in 2 centers with substantial expertise in biliary surgery.[3,12] The authors do not indicate when the Hepp-Couinaud approach was used. However, judging from the distribution of injuries, it is likely that the Hepp-Couinaud approach was used to repair the more proximal strictures. The results in the present study for repair using the Hepp-Couinaud approach parallel our previously reported results with benign strictures[8] and compare favorably with other reported series.[3,12]

Four of 5 patients in the present study in whom the index repair failed share common characteristics

(**Table 4**): failed previous attempts at repair prior to referral, bile leaks, proximal location of the stricture (class E_3 and E_4), and transanastomotic stenting. All 5 patients became symptomatic more than 1 year after the index biliary repair, underscoring the importance of long-term follow-up. We have noted the propensity, after the Hepp-Couinaud technique has been used, for recurrent strictures to occur almost invariably at the right hepatic duct orifice, and we have elected to treat these anastomotic recurrences nonoperatively by means of percutaneous or endoscopic balloon dilation and stenting. One patient who was known to have a poor result underwent an operative revision at another institution 4.5 years after the index repair at our center. All of these patients had minimal or no symptoms at the time of follow-up.

Although the true incidence of bile duct injuries and successful repairs in nontertiary centers is not known, the case against repair of these complex injuries outside centers with special interest in biliary surgery is illustrated by the 25% postoperative stricture rate in a national multi-institutional report from the Netherlands.[17] In our opinion, expert repair of these complex injuries provides optimal patient outcome; thus, we advocate reconstruction by surgeons with special expertise and interest in biliary surgery.

The financial ramifications of iatrogenic bile duct injuries are well documented.[18] All our patients except 2 have alleged negligence and sought compensation for their bile duct injury.

CONCLUSION

Iatrogenic bile duct injuries and strictures are a complex challenge to the treating physician. Operative treatment of complex proximal strictures achieved excellent to good long-term results in more than 90% of patients. The Hepp-Couinaud approach of using the extrahepatic left bile duct offers durable results even in patients for whom previous repairs failed. These operations are best undertaken by surgeons experienced in biliary surgery after the sequelae of bile leakage have subsided. Treatment outcomes should take quality of life issues into consideration.

Presented at the 106th Scientific Session of the Western Surgical Association, Indianapolis, Ind, November 16, 1998.

Corresponding author: Michael B. Farnell, MD, Department of Surgery, Mayo Clinic, Rochester, MN 55905 (e-mail: mfarnell@mayo.edu).

REFERENCES

1. Gouma DJ, Go PM. Bile duct injury during laparoscopic and conventional cholecystectomy. *J Am Coll Surg.* 1994;178:229-233.
2. Deziel DJ, Millikan KW, Economou SG, Doolas A, Ko ST, Airan C. Complications of laparoscopic cholecystectomy: a national survey of 4,292 hospitals and an analysis of 77,604 cases. *Am J Surg.* 1993;165:9-14.
3. Branum G, Schmitt C, Baillie J, et al. Management of major biliary complications after laparoscopic cholecystectomy. *Ann Surg.* 1993;217:532-541.
4. Ress AM, Sarr MG, Nagorney DM, Farnell MB, Donohue JH, McIlrath DC. Spectrum and management of major complications of laparoscopic cholecystectomy. *Am J Surg.* 1993;165:655-662.
5. Hepp J. Hepaticojejunostomy using the left biliary trunk for iatrogenic biliary lesions: the French connection. *World J Surg.* 1985;9:507-511.
6. Strasberg SM, Hertl M, Soper NJ. An analysis of the problem of biliary injury during laparoscopic cholecystectomy. *J Am Coll Surg.* 1995;180:101-125.
7. Terblanche J, Worthley CS, Spence RAJ, Krige JEJ. High or low hepaticojejunostomy for bile duct strictures? *Surgery.* 1990;108:828-834.
8. McDonald ML, Farnell MB, Nagorney DM, Ilstrup DM, Kutch JM. Benign biliary strictures: repair and outcome with a contemporary approach. *Surgery.* 1995; 118:582-591.
9. Woods, MS, Traverso W, Kozarek RA, et al. Characteristics of biliary tract complications during laparoscopic cholecystectomy: a multi-institutional study. *Am J Surg.* 1994;167:27-34.
10. Adamsen S, Hansen OH, Funch-Jensen P, Schulze S, Stage JG, Wara P. Bile duct injury during laparoscopic cholecystectomy: a prospective nationwide series. *J Am Coll Surg.* 1997;184:571-578.
11. Shea JA, Healey MJ, Berlin JA, et al. Mortality and complications associated with laparoscopic cholecystectomy: a meta-analysis. *Ann Surg.* 1996;224:609-620.
12. Lillermoe KD, Martin SA, Cameron JL, et al. Major bile duct injuries during laparoscopic cholecystectomy: follow-up after combined surgical and radiologic management. *Ann Surg.* 1997;225:459-471.
13. Tocchi A, Costa G, Lepre L, Liotta G, Mazzoni G, Sita A. The long-term outcome of hepaticojejunostomy in the treatment of benign bile duct strictures. *Ann Surg.* 1996;224:162-167.
14. Nealon WH, Urrutia F. Long-term follow-up after bilioenteric anastomosis for benign bile duct stricture. *Ann Surg.* 1996;223:639-648.
15. Myburgh JA. The Hepp-Couinaud approach to strictures of the bile ducts: injuries, choledochal cysts, and pancreatitis. *Ann Surg.* 1993;218:615-620.
16. Bauer TW, Morris JB, Lowenstein A, Wolferth C, Rosato FE, Rosato EF. The consequences of a major bile duct injury during laparoscopic cholecystectomy. *J Gastrointest Surg.* 1998;2:61-66.
17. Schol FPG, Go PM, Gouma DJ. Outcome of 49 repairs of bile duct injuries after laparoscopic cholecystectomy. *World J Surg.* 1995;19:753-757.
18. Savader SJ, Lillemoe KD, Prescott CA, et al. Laparoscopic cholecystectomy-related bile duct injuries: a health and financial disaster. *Ann Surg.* 1997;225: 268-273.

DISCUSSION

Robert Rege, MD, Dallas, Tex: Currently, the rate of bile duct injury with laparoscopic cholecystectomy is reported to be about 0.2%, or 1 in 500. The incidence is high enough to make it of concern to surgeons in the surgical community, but not high enough that any given surgeon will develop a large series of patients. Though this patient series is quite extensive, the outcome in these patients was deemed to be good and excellent in 90% of the patients despite the fact that 80% of the patients had previous intervention before their index repair. The results in these series compare very favorably with the best results reported in the literature. The authors attribute their success to the Hepp-Couinaud approach, in which a 2- to 3-cm anastomosis is constructed between a Roux-en-Y jejunal loop and the extrahepatic left bile duct. This approach was used in 46 of 53 patients requiring a hepaticojejunal reconstruction. During a mean follow-up period of 3.7 years, 5 of these patients developed a late postoperative stricture. Four of the patients required therapy that was nonoperative, and 1 had operative therapy at another institution. These strictures are considered their failures. Therefore, the failure rate for the Hepp-Couinaud approach was about 10% to 11%. It is important to understand that the patients who developed strictures developed them between 1 and 5.5 years after the reconstruction, showing that these patients are always at risk for developing late postoperative strictures.

I would like to ask several questions. Seven of the patients underwent a Roux-en-Y hepaticojejunostomy without the Hepp-Couinaud technique and none developed late stricture. Why and when was an approach used other than the Hepp-Couinaud approach? Is the Hepp-Couinaud approach what the authors would use in patients who had primary duct repairs, as opposed to the ones referred later, after they have had a failed procedure? The patients were rated as excellent if they were asymptomatic and had normal liver function tests. Three patients were rated as good, and they had abnormal liver function tests but were asymptomatic. How many of the failures developed abnormal liver function tests and were asymptomatic before the stricture was found? To ask this question another way, are the 6% of patients in the good category likely to develop strictures in the future?

The study deals largely with repairs at a tertiary center in patients who had previous procedures that failed. Based on their experience, could the authors recommend their approach for the surgeon who recognizes an injury at the time of surgery, or shortly thereafter? I would also like the authors to expound on the need for postoperative stenting and the duration of stenting when it was used. In their study, they used stenting in most of their patients, but it was discontinued earlier than in some of the other series in the literature. My question is, is stenting necessary, and how long would that stenting be recommended? What was the course of the patients after the percutaneous dilation for their late stricture? In those 4 patients, did they require repeat dilatations? Are they symptomatic now and do they have abnormal liver function tests?

Frank Moody, MD, Houston, Tex: I also want to congratulate the authors on their success but ask the question about the 3 people who seem to have disappeared from the face of the earth. Have you found them since you put together the paper? Shouldn't they be included as maybe questionable in terms of their outcome?

You might expand a little bit on how you did the anastomosis. Is it as Blumgart tells us, with a single layer and sort of parachute it down?

Maybe you could tell us whether the 5 people who have obviously failed had a little bit more difficult time in getting the intestine to the bile duct.

Finally, tell us about the deaths; while it was not 30 days for 1 death to occur, it was 42 days, and from a myocardial infarction. Was this one of these early discharges to Houston possibly, or some other place, in which the patient really was having some problems in the hospital at the time of discharge, but the significance was unrecognized?

Lawrence Koep, MD, Phoenix, Ariz: Do you have any concomitant hepatic artery injuries? If so, did you see that as correlating with the failure rate?

Dr Farnell: There was a question concerning why the Hepp technique was not used in 7 patients. There were 2 reasons: first, many of those patients had injuries that were very distal in the bile duct and thus it was not necessary to get up to the confluence to do the repair, and secondly, by surgeon preference. I must point out that there were a number of surgeons performing these repairs and not all of the surgeons perhaps embraced the Hepp technique.

Dr Rege asked what advice we would give a surgeon who recognizes an injury at the time of surgery. This is a difficult question to answer and it depends greatly on the expertise of the surgeon involved. We often will receive a call while the surgeon is in the operating room telling us that they have attempted a laparoscopic cholecystectomy, have opened, and they see bile issuing forth from the confluence from more than 1 duct. Our advice in that situation generally is to drain, close, and refer the patient. What we will do when we receive the patient is to gain control of the biliary tree, drain any collections, and defer operation. We have been pleased with the technical aspects of the Hepp-Couinaud technique in terms of the results that are reflected here, but the timing of the operation is particularly critical. For those patients who have occlusion without contamination or peritonitis, early reconstruction within a few days or a week or so is technically feasible. For those patients who have injury associated with leakage, it is our preference to gain control, allow them to convalesce and allow the inflammatory process to settle down, and then do an elective reconstruction. Operation is delayed approximately 3 months to allow for optimal local conditions for reconstruction.

What about stenting? It has been our practice to stent the majority of these patients. Our preference is to place stents preoperatively. These are typically pigtail-type catheters. When we perform the reconstruction, we leave the transhepatic and transanastomotic stent in place, primarily for 2 reasons. One is to decompress the anastomosis in the immediate perioperative period and secondly to perform cholangiography prior to removal of the stent. We feel that the decompression is helpful and cholangiography is useful in confirming the integrity of the anastomosis. It allows us to prognosticate, if you will, with regard to the quality of the anastomosis and allows us to perhaps anticipate problems. Our usual practice is to remove the stents approximately 21 days postoperatively. In the manuscript the average was about 45 days, so obviously there are some patients who for extenuating circumstances have the tubes in for longer periods of time.

There was a question about the failures and Dr Koep asked about hepatic artery injury. To our knowledge, there was only 1 patient in the series who had a right hepatic artery injury, and that patient did fail. The slide illustrates the therapies that were used in these 5 patients (Table 4). There were 3 patients who had transhepatic dilatations. There was 1 patient who had the native bile duct still in continuity, and there was a partial occlusion distal to the anastomosis, and endoscopic dilatation was possible in that patient. Lastly, there was 1 patient who had surgery at another institution. At the time of follow-up all of these patients were salvaged and were doing well.

Dr Moody asked about the technical aspects of the anastomosis, and indeed, we do perform it very much as Blumgart has described. We use a single layer of absorbable suture, typically a 4.0 or 5.0, and perform the anastomosis end-to-side. We are extremely careful to try to obtain supple, pliable bile duct proximal to the level of inflammation. The Achilles heel of this operation is the orifice of the right duct. In patients we have operated on with type E_3 and type E_4 injuries, those at or near the confluence, one can usually obtain excellent left main duct to work with. If the stricture extends to the orifice of the right duct, this is the area that is difficult to get a technically satisfactory anastomosis. Indeed, in those patients who failed, the site of failure was at the orifice of the right main duct. Accordingly, the dilatation required was not of the left main duct, but of the orifice of the right anterior or posterior duct.

Dr Moody also asked about the patients who died. I should comment that 1 patient died in the early postoperative period, and that patient was operated on not only because the patient had a bile duct injury, but primarily because an endoscopic sphincterotomy, which had been performed prior to referral, resulted in retroperitoneal necrosis. The operation was done because of sepsis. The patient who died 42 days postoperatively after discharge from the hospital had been seen in consultation preoperatively by our cardiac surgeons on 2 occasions in an effort to consider revascularization prior to planned biliary surgery. It was determined by the cardiac surgeon that operation was not indicated. Unfortunately, in spite of an uneventful postoperative course, after dismissal the patient developed an inferior myocardial infarction and bradycardia and died.

Dr Moody also asked and commented about the patients lost to follow-up. Unfortunately, some of those patients are international and we have not to date been able to find them. Even if one were to ascribe the patients lost to follow-up to a poor outcome, we still feel that on the whole, this technique and this approach give us good results.

PAPER

Prophylactic Antibiotics for Elective Laparoscopic Cholecystectomy

Are They Necessary?

Andrew Higgins, MD; Jeremy London, MD; Scott Charland, PharmD; Erick Ratzer, MD; Jeffrey Clark, MD; William Haun, MD; D. Patrick Maher, MD

Hypothesis: Prophylactic antibiotic treatment in elective laparoscopic cholecystectomy does not lower the already low infection rate associated with this procedure.

Design and Setting: Prospective double-blind randomized trial at a community-based training hospital.

Patients: Four hundred fifty patients undergoing elective laparoscopic cholecystectomy were randomized into 1 of 3 treatment arms: (1) preoperative cefotetan disodium, 1 g intravenously; (2) preoperative cefazolin, 1 g intravenously; and (3) intravenous placebo. There were no demographic differences between groups in age, smoking history, American Society of Anesthesiologists score, infection risk class, time of antibiotic administration prior to surgery, and type of skin preparation.

Interventions: Laparoscopic cholecystectomy was attempted in all cases; however, 10 patients required conversion to an open cholecystectomy and they were included in the statistical analysis. Preoperatively, all patients were randomized in a blinded manner and received cefotetan, cefazolin, or placebo intravenously.

Results: There were 10 postoperative infections. In the cefotetan group, there were 3 cases of superficial surgical site infections. In the cefazolin group, there were 2 superficial surgical site infections—1 pneumonia and 1 rhinosinusitis. In the placebo group, there were 2 superficial surgical site infections and 1 urinary tract infection. The overall infection rate in this series was 2.4%. Follow-up was performed at routine postoperative visits and by telephone contact. Data were evaluated using the χ^2 test and analysis of variance with Duncan post hoc test ($P<.05$).

Conclusion: Based on our data, use of prophylactic antibiotics does not decrease the rate of wound infections in elective laparoscopic cholecystectomy.

Arch Surg. 1999;134:611-614

From Exempla Saint Joseph Hospital (Drs Higgins, London, Ratzer, Clark, Haun, and Maher), Roche Pharmaceuticals (Dr Charland), and Kaiser Permanente (Dr Maher), Denver, Colo.

THE USE OF prophylactic antibiotics reduces wound infections in elective open cholecystectomies.[1-3] Targarona et al[4] found no difference in the rate of infections with the prophylactic use of broad-spectrum penicillins vs cephalosporins. They reported a wound infection rate of 6.5% in low-risk patients undergoing open cholecystectomy without prophylactic antibiotics.[4]

Elective laparoscopic cholecystectomy has a low risk for infection, but many surgeons still use prophylactic antibiotics. We postulated that use of prophylactic antibiotics in elective laparoscopic cholecystectomy would not lower its already low infection rate. This study was designed to determine the infection rate in patients undergoing elective laparoscopic cholecystectomy. This controlled study was conducted comparing cefotetan or cefazolin with placebo.

RESULTS

In the 25-month study period, 450 patients were selected for the study protocol. Four hundred twelve patients were evaluable after randomization into 1 of 3 arms. A total of 137 patients received cefotetan; 140 received cefazolin; and 135 received placebo. The 3 groups were well matched for the demographics listed in the "Patients and Methods" section (**Table 1**). Thirty-eight patients were excluded from the statistical analysis for protocol violations. The cefotetan group excluded 13 patients, the cefazolin group excluded 11, and the placebo group excluded 14 (**Table 2**). Seventy-eight percent of study patients received their study medication within 60 minutes of surgery.

There was no statistical difference between the 3 groups for superficial, deep, or distant infections ($P>.05$). The cefotetan group (137 patients) had 3 superficial surgical site infections for a 2.2%

PATIENTS AND METHODS

PATIENTS

Following institutional review board approval of the protocol, all patients undergoing elective laparoscopic cholecystectomy at Exempla Saint Joseph Hospital, Denver, Colo, from January 1, 1995, to February 2, 1997, were evaluated for the protocol. Four hundred fifty patients having elective laparoscopic cholecystectomy were selected for a double-blind randomized prospective study. Group 1 received cefotetan disodium, 1 g intravenously; group 2 received cefazolin, 1 g intravenously; and group 3 received 50 mL of isotonic sodium chloride solution.

When the patient was confirmed for the study, the Saint Joseph Pharmacy randomly selected a sealed envelope and delivered the appropriate solution to the preoperative holding area. The medical staff and the patient were unaware of the identity of the solution. Patients were given the study medication by the anesthesiologist or operating room nurse prior to surgery.

Laparoscopic cholecystectomy was planned for all patients. The only allowed variables were number and location of port sites, disposable or nondisposable trocars, intraoperative cholangiograms, port site used for gallbladder removal, and method of skin preparation and closure.

The following data were collected on each patient: age, sex, skin preparation technique, times of antibiotic administration, time of skin incision, number and location of ports, disposable or nondisposable trocars, type of skin closure, duration of operation, American Society of Anesthesiologists classification, wound infection risk classification,[5] intraoperative cholangiogram, bile spillage, gallbladder histological findings, conversion to open cholecystectomy, length of hospital stay, body mass index, and evidence of infection.

All patients were examined by an attending surgeon 7 to 10 days after surgery and were followed up for 30 days after the procedure. Infections were classified as superficial surgical site, deep surgical site, and distant. A superficial surgical site infection is defined as erythema and/or purulent drainage at the surgical site above the fascia. A deep surgical site infection is defined as purulent material deep to the fascia or near the gallbladder fossa. A distant infection is defined as any infection remote to the surgical site. The attending surgeon obtained cultures at his or her discretion.

Inclusion criteria in the protocol were all patients scheduled for elective laparoscopic cholecystectomy aged between 18 and 80 years with biliary colic and meeting no exclusion criteria.

Exclusion criteria were patients younger than 18 years and older than 80 years; pregnant or lactating women; β-lactam or cephalosporin allergy, sensitivity, or anaphylaxis; antibiotic therapy within 48 hours prior to surgery; evidence of acute cholecystitis, cholangitis, or obstructive jaundice; previous biliary tract surgery; evidence of choledocholithiasis; history of prosthetic valves or joints; contraindication to laparoscopic cholecystectomy as determined by the attending surgeon; and patients determined to be at increased risk of infection secondary to their medical condition.

DATA ANALYSIS

A sample size of 450 patients (150 patients per treatment arm) was predicted to detect a significant difference in the wound infection rate between the 3 arms. The sample size was based on the following: a χ^2 value of 2.35, an α error of .05 (2-tailed), a power of 0.80, and an overall wound infection rate of 6.5% in low-risk patients receiving no prophylactic antibiotics. Data were analyzed using the Power and Precision statistical computer program.[6] The 6.5% wound infection rate is historical data from patients undergoing open cholecystectomy without prophylactic antibiotics.[4] It was believed that the infection rate would be lower in patients undergoing elective laparoscopic cholecystectomy; therefore, a poststudy power analysis was planned.

STATISTICAL ANALYSIS

Continuous data were compared using 1-way analysis of variance with a Duncan post hoc test. All frequency data were compared using χ^2 analysis by means of the Stat Most statistical package.[7] Correlation was determined by calculating the Spearman rank correlation. An interim analysis was performed after 225 patients (75 per arm) had completed the protocol and no significant difference had been obtained, so the study continued. $P<.05$ was considered significant.

wound infection rate. The cefazolin group (140 patients) had 2 superficial surgical site infections and 2 distant infections for a wound infection rate of 1.4% and an overall infection rate of 2.9%. The placebo group (135 patients) had 2 superficial surgical site infections and 1 distant infection for a wound infection rate of 1.5% and an overall infection rate of 2.2%. There was no correlation between pathologic findings, bile spillage, and wound infection rate. None of the 22% of patients who received their study medication more than 60 minutes prior to surgery had an infectious complication.

Ten patients underwent conversions to open cholecystectomy: 2 from the cefotetan group, 6 from the cefazolin group, and 2 from the placebo group. All patients remained in the study because of "intention to treat." One patient from the cefazolin group who underwent conversion to an open procedure had both a superficial surgical site infection and pneumonia. Nine of the 10 patients who were converted to open cholecystectomy received intraoperative and/or postoperative antibiotics, including the patients with the infectious complications. Another 10 patients without evidence of infection received antibiotics postoperatively: 7 from the cefotetan group, 2 from the cefazolin group, and 1 from the placebo group. All of these patients were included in the statistical analysis.

COMMENT

Several reviews have demonstrated a significant decrease in wound infections in open cholecystectomy with the use of prophylactic antibiotics.[1-3] These data cannot

Table 1. Demographic Data*

	Cefotetan Group (n = 137)	Cefazolin Group (n = 140)	Placebo Group (n = 135)
Age, y	48.2 ± 13.6	48.1 ± 15.4	47.1 ± 12.6
BMI, kg/m²	28.7 ± 6.4	28.9 ± 5.9	29.0 ± 7.1
ASA score			
1	37	37	35
2	89	91	81
3	10	12	18
NR	1	0	1
Length of operation, min	68.9 ± 31.2	64.0 ± 28.8	63.5 ± 25.2
Risk class			
0	116	122	110
1	20	16	22
2	0	1	0
NR	1	1	3
Antibiotic administration prior to incision, min	52.9 ± 52.6	49.7 ± 32.7	44.9 ± 30.5

**Data are given as mean ± SD or number of patients. BMI indicates body mass index; ASA, American Society of Anesthesiologists; and NR, not recorded.*

Table 2. Protocol Violations

	Treatment Group, No. of Patients		
	Cefotetan	Cefazolin	Placebo
Antibiotic administration not documented	10	8	11
Operation cancelled	2	1	3
Missing chart	1	1	0
Other	0	1	0

be extrapolated to elective laparoscopic cholecystectomy.

Some antibiotics that are used are very expensive and are no more effective than less expensive antibiotics.[4] We selected cefotetan and cefazolin as they were widely used by surgeons at our institution. However, there is a marked cost difference, with cefazolin costing $2.41 per gram vs cefotetan at $8.80 per gram. This translates to a charge of $9.25 per gram of cefazolin and $24.40 per gram of cefotetan. Cefotetan was most commonly given in a 2-g dose, which doubled this amount. It was estimated that use of cefazolin only could result in a $24 362 savings per year. If no antibiotic is needed, this results in a savings of $30 060 per year. These estimates are for our institution.

Our data demonstrated no lowering of infection rates with a single dose of prophylactic antibiotics in elective laparoscopic cholecystectomy. Illig et al[8] had similar results in a prospective randomized study. They compared use of 3 perioperative doses of cefazolin with no use of antibiotics in elective laparoscopic cholecystectomy. This study was published in April 1997, well after our study started. It should be noted that in their study, patient enrollment was halted at 250 patients "because of the paucity of major infectious complications, the primary end point." The authors concluded that their study suffered from "relative small sample in relation to a relatively rare event." We continued our study out to a sample size that was predicted to detect a significant difference in wound infection rates between the 3 arms. Using a power analysis, we now estimate that a sample size of 5444 patients would be necessary to detect significant differences between the 3 arms of this study, because of the rarity of wound infection. Illig et al have studied an additional 108 "low-risk" patients undergoing elective laparoscopic cholecystectomy in the 12 months following their study and they have found no infectious complications without the use of prophylactic antibiotics. Frantzides and Sykes[9] had similar results in a prospective nonrandomized study comparing preoperative cefotetan with preoperative chlorhexidine gluconate scrub without preoperative antibiotics. In fact, they reported more infections in the group of patients receiving cefotetan (n = 14) than in the group of patients who received only a scrub (n = 0). Frantzides and Sykes believed that in properly selected, low-risk patients, a well-performed surgical scrub was all that was needed. One question that can be asked is: does the use of prophylactic antibiotics create a false sense of security in the operating team and lead to careless technique? If this is true, we need better technique not more antibiotics.

Our study consisted of a preselected group of patients who had no evidence of acute cholecystitis, choledocholithiasis, or gallstone pancreatitis. In these high-risk patients, we support the use of prophylactic antibiotics.

Elective laparoscopic cholecystectomy carries a low risk of wound infection. Use of prophylactic antibiotics is not justified in patients undergoing elective, uncomplicated laparoscopic cholecystectomy.

Presented at the 106th Scientific Session of the Western Surgical Association, Indianapolis, Ind, November 16, 1998.

Corresponding author: D. Patrick Maher, MD, Kaiser Permanente, Department of General Surgery, 2045 Franklin St, Denver, CO 80205.

REFERENCES

1. Ulualp K, Condon RE. Antibiotic prophylaxis for scheduled operative procedures. *Infect Dis Clin North Am.* 1992;6:613-625.
2. Kellum JM, Duam RJ, Gorbach SL, et al. Single-dose antibiotic prophylaxis for biliary surgery. *Arch Surg.* 1987;122:918-922.
3. Meijer WS, Schmitz PIM, Jeekel J. Meta-analysis of randomised, controlled clinical trials of antibiotic prophylaxis in biliary tract surgery. *Br J Surg.* 1990;77:283-290.
4. Targarona EM, Garau J, Muños-Ramos C, et al. Single dose antibiotic prophylaxis in patients at high risk for infection in biliary surgery: a prospective and randomized study comparing cefonicid with mezlocillin. *Surgery.* 1990;107:327-334.
5. Culver DH, Horan TC, Gaynes RP, et al. Surgical wound infection rate by wound class, operative procedure, and patient risk index. *Am J Med.* 1991;91(3B):152s-157s.
6. Borenstein M, Rothstein H, Cohen J. *Power and Precision® Version 1.0.* Los Angeles, Calif: Dataxiom Software Inc; 1997.
7. *Stat Most® Version 1995.* Los Angeles, Calif: Dataxiom Software Inc; 1995.
8. Illig KA, Schmidt E, Cavanaugh J, Krusch D, Sax HC. Are prophylactic antibiotics required for elective laparoscopic cholecystectomy? *J Am Coll Surg.* 1997;184:353-356.
9. Frantzides CT, Sykes A. A reevaluation of antibiotic prophylaxis in laparoscopic cholecystectomy. *J Laparoendosc Surg.* 1994;4:375-378.

DISCUSSION

Mitchel P. Byrne, MD, Evanston, Ill: This is the authors' second prospective study from St Joseph's Hospital in Denver presented to the Western Surgical Association over the last few years. It questions the value of antibiotics in low-risk patients undergoing elective laparoscopic cholecystectomy. Their study is a blinded perspective one, done with hospital institutional review board review and involvement of the clinical pharmacy staff. The study compared 3 equal groups: cefazolin, cefotetan, and a placebo group. Excluded were patients younger than 18, older than 80, and those with evidence of acute cholecystitis, common bile duct stones, or gallstone pancreatitis, and those considered at increased risk of infection secondary to medical condition. Results confirm as one other paper in the literature in the last year that in these low-risk gallbladder patients antibiotics are not needed. Obviously, if all low-risk patients undergoing laparoscopic cholecystectomy stop getting antibiotics, there is a big potential reduction in cost as well as avoidance of a variety of antibiotic problems. I have 3 questions. Who do you consider a high-risk patient, and could you comment on some of these such as diabetics, renal failure patients, and others? What about common bile duct procedures that are necessary that are found based on intraoperative cholangiogram? Do you begin antibiotics at that point; do you consider doing that? Have you at St Joseph's Hospital stopped using antibiotics for these routine cases of laparoscopic cholecystectomy? What are your estimates of cost savings in this group?

Hiram C. Polk, Jr, MD, Louisville, Ky: I rise to endorse this meticulous paper and hope that you will take it home and practice it. It has been generally gratifying about the appropriate use of prophylactic antibiotics. It is the most common use of antibiotics in the world today, but it is also the most common misuse. This study puts that in very good perspective. Many surgeons, thinking that drugs are totally safe, use antibiotics when the chance of an adverse effect from the drug is greater than the chance for infection in the patient. This report did not address drug complications, but they are numerous. I wanted to suggest one other thing that I thought the authors did especially well and that was to include the principles of Elliott and Chetlin in this study in which patients who get the best advantage from antibiotic prophylaxis are those who have their common bile duct manipulated, are elderly, or have subsiding acute cholecystitis. All of the rest of the biliary patients do not. This is just an exceptional study. It is a big challenge to the membership to see whether you have the courage of their convictions to begin to implement this practice. The gain for your individual patients is probably going to be small, but in the long run, it will be substantial. This is a first-class paper.

Daniel Elliott, MD, Dayton, Ill: In the 1960s the infection rate in a clean operating room environment was exactly the same as reported here, 1.5%. In a clean environment, almost all wound infections are the result of internal contamination from the patient's own bacteria. Very large series of gallbladder cultures taken at routine cholecystectomies are almost uniformly negative. Less than 1% grow bacteria. In contrast, in acute cholecystitis the incidence of bacteria is 40%, and with common bile duct stones, 60%. These bacteria are in concentrations roughly equivalent to feces when cultured quantitatively. Because there is no internal contamination at uncomplicated cholecystectomies, prophylactic antibiotics are of no value. On the other hand, if you are operating in the third world, or in some of the older hospitals in Europe, from which many statistics on infection rates have been published, there is a different situation. Where operating room contamination is a threat, prophylactic antibiotics may help.

Dr Clark: Who do we consider a high-risk patient? Anyone who had any evidence of common duct stones, presented in an acute fashion with an elevated white cell count, fever, or tenderness in the right upper quadrant would be a high-risk patient and were excluded from our study. Do we consider diabetes and chronic renal failure to be high risk? I do not know the number of diabetic patients in this series. There were, however, no patients with chronic renal failure on dialysis, but those groups have been shown in other studies to be high risk. Diabetics were not excluded in our study. I suspect that it would be a surgeon's discretion whether or not to use antibiotics in these situations. We do not perform routine cholangiography for elective cholecystectomy; most of our surgeons use that technique selectively. Twenty-four surgeons contributed cases to the study. No common bile duct injuries occurred in the study. If we do have an intraoperative cholangiogram that is positive and we do explore the duct, then I think most surgeons would use antibiotics in that situation as that throws the patient out of this low-risk elective situation that we studied.

Our definition of infection was very liberal. In fact, only 1 patient required opening of the incision; the rest were given oral antibiotics only for localized cellulitis and resolved without further intervention.

The cost savings were going to be studied prospectively, but it turned out to be too much of a problem with the logistics of getting the costs and charges on all of these patients. We estimate retrospectively that we could save between $24 000 and $30 000 a year at our institution by not using antibiotics in this group. That cost savings is based on approximately 600 laparoscopic cholecystectomies that are electively done at our institution per year.

As a result of this study, have we stopped using antibiotics on these low-risk elective laparoscopic cholecystectomies? We finished the study just a few months ago and actually we would like to know that information as well. Since we have done about 3 prospective randomized controlled studies at our hospital, we want to do a retrospective analysis of whether or not the surgeons believe the very studies that were done at their own institution. So, we are actually going to do a retrospective analysis of that data to see if practice patterns were changed.

Complex Aortofemoral Prosthetic Infections

The Role of Autogenous Superficial Femoropopliteal Vein Reconstruction

Lori L. Gordon, MD; Ryan T. Hagino, MD; Mark R. Jackson, MD; J. Gregory Modrall, MD; R. James Valentine, MD; G. Patrick Clagett, MD

Background: With increasing experience, we have encountered patients with complex aortofemoral prosthetic infections in whom extra-anatomic bypass (EAB) is not an option.

Hypothesis: Autogenous superficial femoropopliteal vein (SFPV) aortic reconstruction provides a limb-saving and lifesaving alternative with acceptable morbidity and mortality.

Design: Retrospective review.

Setting: University-based county, private, and Veterans Affairs hospitals.

Patients: Seventeen patients with infected aortofemoral bypasses in whom conventional EAB was impossible because of infection of previously placed EAB, massive groin and/or thigh sepsis, or both.

Main Outcome Measures: Morbidity and mortality.

Results: Multiple previous operations were common (mean, 4 per patient) and included EAB (n = 11), replacement aortofemoral bypass (n = 4), prosthetic femoropopliteal bypass (n = 7), and thoracobifemoral bypass (n = 1); all bypasses became infected. Overall, 11 patients had sepsis at the time of presentation. Of the patients with massive groin infection, 7 had extensive deep infections involving most of the proximal thighs or retroperitoneum, 4 had enterocutaneous fistulae, and 2 had necrotizing fasciitis of the lower abdomen and thigh. Polymicrobial infections were common (n = 9). Four patients (24%) died in the perioperative period, 8 (47%) suffered major complications, and 4 (24%) underwent major amputations. Mortality in this group of patients was 3 times that of all other patients undergoing autogenous SFPV aortic reconstruction for prosthetic infection (8%). Amputation rates were also increased (24% vs 6%). The mean ± SD follow-up time is 23 ± 21 months. All patients maintained patent SFPV reconstructions.

Conclusions: In the setting of complex aortofemoral prosthetic infections, autogenous SFPV aortic reconstruction is a useful option for patients in whom EAB is impossible and limb loss and/or death would be inevitable without revascularization.

Arch Surg 1999;134:615-621

Autogenous superficial femoropopliteal vein (SFPV) reconstruction has successfully been used as an alternative to extra-anatomic bypass (EAB) in the treatment of infected aortic prostheses.[1-4] Superficial femoropopliteal vein reconstruction offers many advantages including resistance to reinfection, durability, excellent long-term patency in the face of compromised outflow, low amputation rates, minimal lower extremity venous morbidity, and no risk for aortic stump blowout.[2,5] In earlier reports from our group, all patients underwent SFPV reconstruction regardless of their eligibility for EAB.[1,2] As experience has accrued, we have encountered patients with more complex and advanced disease in whom EAB was not feasible, leaving autogenous SFPV aortic replacement as the only solution. These patients presented with infection of previously placed EABs or massive lower abdominal, groin, and thigh infection that precluded safe EAB. This subgroup of desperately ill patients with aortic prosthetic infection treated using autogenous SFPV aortic reconstruction is the subject of our report. Our purpose is to determine the feasibility and usefulness of SFPV reconstruction in this unusual circumstance.

From the Division of Vascular Surgery, University of Texas Southwestern Medical Center, Dallas (Drs Gordon, Jackson, Modrall, Valentine, and Clagett), and the Vascular Surgery Section, Wilford Hall Medical Center, Lackland Air Force Base, San Antonio, Tex (Dr Hagino).

RESULTS

PATIENT DEMOGRAPHICS AND CLINICAL PRESENTATION

Included in this study were 12 men and 5 women with a mean age of 58 ± 10 years (range, 40-70 years). Fifteen (94%) of 16 patients were past or present cigarette smokers with a mean of 54 ± 31 pack-years. Other pertinent risk factors included coronary ar-

PATIENTS AND METHODS

Data were collected on all patients undergoing SFPV reconstruction for aortic prosthetic infection since January 1, 1990. We identified 17 patients in whom conventional EAB was impossible because of infection of previously placed EAB (n = 11) and/or massive groin and/or thigh sepsis (n = 9). Three patients had both conditions. Six of the 11 patients with infected EABs had concomitant graft occlusion.

Eighteen procedures were performed in 17 patients. All patients underwent single-staged procedures consisting of SFPV harvest, infected graft removal, and SFPV aortofemoral reconstruction. Using a 2-team approach, 1 team to harvest SFPV and 1 team to expose the aorta, the time of operation is greatly reduced. The SFPV harvest is performed through an incision placed along the lateral border of the sartorius muscle. Reflection of the sartorius muscle medially exposes the SFPV. The proximal transection should be placed flush with the profunda femoris–common femoral vein junction to prevent significant venous hypertension. The length of required reconstruction determines the extent of distal dissection. Valvulotomy is necessary to allow placement of the vein graft in a nonreversed direction. All infected prosthetic material is removed, septic tissue is debrided, and aortofemoral reconstruction is performed.[1] Surviving patients were observed at 6-month intervals with clinical examination and noninvasive testing that included ankle-brachial indexes, toe pressures, and duplex studies of the SFPV reconstruction and remaining deep venous system.

Continuous data are expressed as mean ±SD. The Society for Vascular Surgery/International Society for Cardiovascular Surgery (SVS/ISCVS) standards were used to calculate runoff scores to assess extent of distal disease.[6]

tery disease (n = 8, 47%), hypertension (n = 11, 65%), diabetes mellitus (n = 2, 12%), hyperlipidemia (n = 4, 24%), obesity (n = 4, 24%), chronic obstructive pulmonary disease (n = 3, 18%), and renal disease (creatinine level, >176.8 μmol/L [2.0 mg/dL]) (n = 2, 12%).

Information on individual patients is presented in the **Table**. The original indication for operation was aortoiliac occlusive disease in 12 patients (71%), aortoiliac aneurysmal disease in 3 (18%), and unknown in 2 (12%). Initial operations consisted of 11 aortobifemoral bypasses (AFBs), 3 AFBs with simultaneous femoropopliteal bypasses (14 total AFBs), and 3 axillobifemoral bypasses. All AFBs had been performed with Dacron prostheses; 2 axillobifemoral and all femoropopliteal bypasses had been performed using expanded polytetrafluoroethylene (ePTFE) prostheses. One axillobifemoral bypass was a Dacron implant. In addition, 4 patients underwent subsequent femoropopliteal bypasses, 3 of these with ePTFE and 1 with in situ greater saphenous vein (GSV).

A mean of 52 ± 59 months (range, 2 weeks to 216 months) elapsed between primary revascularization and documentation of prosthetic infection. Once prosthetic infection was diagnosed, 13 patients underwent multiple procedures in an attempt to eradicate infection and/or restore graft patency (Table). The mean number of operations (excluding primary procedure) for these 13 patients was 4.3 ± 2.6 (range, 1-9) and included abscess drainage and wound debridement with local and systemic antibiotics (n = 9), EAB with removal of infected AFB (n = 8), prosthetic AFB replacement (n = 4), thrombectomy (n = 5), repair of femoral false aneurysms (n = 4), and thrombolytic therapy followed by thrombectomy (n = 1). Prosthetic AFB replacements were performed after EAB failure.

Presenting signs and symptoms exemplified the severity of disease. Eleven patients had sepsis at the time of presentation as defined by elevated white blood cell count, fever, and tachycardia. The 5 blood cultures performed yielded positive results; 1 of these patients had diabetic ketoacidosis. In the 9 patients with massive groin infection, 7 had extensive deep infections involving most of the proximal thighs or retroperitoneum; 4 had enterocutaneous fistulae, 2 had necrotizing fasciitis of the lower abdomen and thigh, and 2 had large, expanding, and cellulitic femoral false aneurysms. All 4 patients with enterocutaneous fistulae had contiguous involvement of their aortic prosthesis. Two of these patients had fistulae of the duodenum; 1 patient, of the jejunum; and 1 patient, of the colon. All 4 had gastrointestinal tract fluid and pus draining from the groin. Other presenting factors included rest pain (n = 7), gastrointestinal tract bleeding (n = 1), exposed prosthetic material (n = 2), and psoas abscess (n = 1).

Overall, infection of previously placed EABs developed in 11 patients, and 6 of these had coexistent thrombosis. Three axillobifemoral bypasses were performed as primary revascularization procedures in 3 patients with rest pain and/or impending tissue loss; all 3 patients had had a documented myocardial infarction within the previous 6 months. Nine EABs were performed in 8 patients as secondary procedures for treatment of aortic prosthetic infections. These 9 procedures included 4 bilateral axillofemoral bypasses, 1 axillobifemoral bypass, 1 thoracobifemoral bypass, 1 unilateral transobturator iliopopliteal bypass, 1 unilateral axilloprofunda bypass, and 1 unilateral axillopopliteal bypass. In addition, all 7 patients with prosthetic femoropopliteal bypasses had contiguous involvement with infection.

At the time of autogenous SFPV aortic reconstruction, polymicrobial infections were common (n = 9), as seen in the following tabulation:

Patient No.	Organisms
1	*Staphylococcus epidermidis, Enterococcus*
2	*Staphylococcus aureus, Bacteroides fragilis, Streptococcus*
4	*Bacteroides distasonis, Prerotella oris*
7	Methicillin-resistant *S aureus,* group B streptococci, *Klebsiella, Pseudomonas*
8	*Escherichia coli, Enterococcus, Klebsiella oxytoca, Acinetobacter baumanii*
12	*Pseudomonas,* diphtheroids
13	Methicillin-resistant *S aureus, Enterococcus, Pseudomonas, B fragilis*
16	*S epidermidis, Saccharomyces cerevisni* (yeast)
17	*Klebsiella, Candida albicans, Candida glabrata*

Cultures from 6 patients yielded single organisms only. Final cultures yielded no growth in 2 patients, but clinical signs of graft infection were seen at the time of operation, including nonincorporation of the graft with surrounding turbid fluid. All organisms are listed in the following tabulation:

Organism	No. of Patients
S aureus (methicillin-resistant *S aureus*)	5 (2)
S epidermidis	3
Pseudomonas aeruginosa	3
Enterococcus species	3
Bacteroides species	3
Klebsiella species	3
Streptococcus species	2
E coli	2
C albicans and C glabrata	2
Enterobacter cloacae	1
Propionibacterium acnes	1
A baumanii	1
P oris	1
S cerevisni	1
No growth	2

SFPV RECONSTRUCTION

Bilateral SFPV was harvested simultaneously in 12 patients and sequentially in the 1 patient who underwent 2 separate procedures. Unilateral SFPV was harvested in the remaining 4 patients. Greater saphenous vein was also harvested for supplemental procedures in 7 patients; 1 patient underwent bilateral harvest of SFPV and GSV; 1 patient, contralateral harvest of GSV; and all others, harvest of SFPV and GSV in an ipsilateral lower extremity.

Reconstructions consisted of 7 unilateral SFPV aortofemoral bypasses (6 SFPV femoral crossovers and 1 GSV femoral crossover), 6 SFPV AFBs, 1 SFPV aortofemoral and contralateral aortoiliac bypass with GSV, 1 unilateral aortofemoral bypass, 2 SFPV from prosthetic AFB limb to femoral bypasses, and 1 aortoiliac bypass with iliofemoral crossover bypass (**Figure**).

Fifteen proximal anastomoses were performed in an end-to-end fashion and 2 in an end-to-side fashion. One proximal anastomosis required splicing 2 SFPVs together to fit end-to-end to a large native aorta. Another proximal anastomosis was fashioned by partitioning an aneurysmal native aorta into 2 orifices for separate SFPV end-to-end anastomoses. The supraceliac aorta was the site of 1 proximal anastomosis, whereas all others were located in an infrarenal position.

There were a total of 33 distal anastomoses. Most were to the common femoral arteries (n = 13, 39%) or profunda femoris arteries (n = 8, 24%). Twenty (61%) of all distal anastomoses were performed in an end-to-side fashion. The mean SVS/ISCVS runoff score was 4.7 ± 2.5, with a minimum value of 1 (normal runoff) and a maximum value of 10 (no runoff).

PERIOPERATIVE MORBIDITY AND MORTALITY

Within the first 30 days of operation, there were 3 deaths. Two patients died secondary to myocardial infarction and the third patient of respiratory failure. One patient died in the hospital after 30 days due to multiple-system organ failure, for an overall in-hospital mortality of 24%. Eight patients (47%) had significant postoperative complications. Four patients (24%) required 5 amputations (3 above-knee and 1 below-knee amputations and 1 hip disarticulation due to preexisting irreversible ischemia at the time of SFPV reconstruction). Six patients (35%) underwent fasciotomies, with 4 being prophylactic and 2 for compartment syndrome. One patient experienced a postoperative myocardial infarction and acute renal failure requiring dialysis. Acute renal failure that did not require dialysis developed in another patient. Wound infections requiring debridement developed in 4 patients (24%), and 1 of these required gracilis muscle flap for wound closure. Unilateral lower-extremity paresis secondary to distal spinal cord and/or nerve root ischemia developed in 1 patient (6%). One patient (6%) ruptured a pseudoaneurysm at the site of GSV-to-SFPV anastomosis, necessitating ligation of the SFPV reconstruction and above-knee amputation. Multiple-system organ failure developed in this patient, who died 2 months postoperatively. Other complications included pneumonia and respiratory failure in 2 additional patients and graft thrombosis in 1 patient.

FOLLOW-UP

Mean follow-up among the 13 surviving patients was 23 ± 21 months. The crude primary patency rate was 92%, with 100% secondary patency rate. Two patients died of comorbid factors greater than 1 year after autogenous SFPV aortic reconstruction. One patient experienced unilateral SFPV limb occlusion at 49 months due to an anastomotic stenosis at an end-to-end anastomosis to the superficial femoral artery. Patency was successfully restored with thrombectomy and anastomotic revision.

There have been no notable long-term venous morbidities, although 6 patients (35%) had transient mild-to-moderate lower-extremity edema treated with compression stockings. Results of physiologic testing demonstrated mild venous outflow obstruction, rich collateral development, and valvular competence in donor limbs.[5] No chronic venous insufficiency was seen, as evidenced by the lack of increased skin pigmentation, venous claudication, and venous ulceration.

COMMENT

The patients in this series represent the most desperately ill of those presenting with vascular prosthetic infections. Most had sepsis at the time of presentation; failure due to infection, with or without concomitant thrombosis, of secondary and tertiary procedures; or massive groin, thigh, and lower-abdominal soft tissue infections with deep extension into the thigh along supplementary prosthetic infrainguinal bypasses. Extra-anatomic bypass with staged removal of infected vascular prostheses would be the preferred approach, offering the prospect of less physiologic stress and improved morbidity and mortality.[7] However, EAB was not an option in these patients because of previous failure of EABs and the lack of clean, uninfected tissue planes.

Patient Details*

Age, y/Sex	Primary Operation	Secondary and Tertiary Operations to Treat Infection	Presentation	Reason EAB Not Feasible
67/M	Axillobifemoral bypass	Bilateral groin I and D; removal EAB	Infected, open groin wounds; rest pain	Failed EAB; groin sepsis
70/M	AFB	Groin I and D; axillobifemoral bypass; removal AFB	Groin abscess; infected EAB	Failed EAB; groin sepsis
63/M	AFB plus femoropopliteal bypass	None	Diabetic ketoacidosis; septicemia; multiple groin and thigh abcesses	Massive groin and thigh sepsis
70/M	AFB	None	Groin abscess; perforated sigmoid diverticulitis; necrotizing fasciitis; colo-groin cutaneous fistula	Massive groin and thigh sepsis
49/F	AFB	Bilateral axillofemoral bypasses; removal AFB; multiple thrombectomies; replacement AFB with bilateral femoropopliteal bypasses	Bilateral draining groin sinuses	Failed EAB; groin and thigh sepsis
58/M	AFB plus bilateral femoropopliteal bypasses	None	Ruptured, infected femoral false aneurysm	Massive groin and thigh sepsis
69/M	AFB	Repair ruptured femoral false aneurysm; 2 axillofemoral bypasses; multiple thrombectomies	Groin abscesses; infected, thrombosed EAB	Failed EAB; groin sepsis
56/M	AFB plus femoropopliteal bypass	None	Septicemia; draining groin abscess	Massive groin and thigh sepsis
55/F	AFB	Repair ruptured, infected femoral false aneurysm; axillobifemoral bypass; removal AFB	Septicemia; draining groin abscess	Failed EAB; groin sepsis
40/M	AFB	Removal AFB; bilateral axillofemoral bypasses; replacement AFB	Jejunal-groin cutaneous fistula; septicemia; thrombosed EAB; rest pain	Failed EAB; massive groin and thigh sepsis
51/M	AFB	Repair femoral false aneurysms 3 times; prosthetic iliofemoral EAB; bilateral axillofemoral bypasses; removal AFB; multiple thrombectomies; thoracobifemoral EAB	Bilateral draining groin abscesses	Failed EAB; massive groin and thigh sepsis
52/M	AFB	Prosthetic femoropopliteal bypass became infected, requiring in situ vein femoral tibial bypass	Ruptured, infected femoral false aneurysm	Massive groin and thigh sepsis
49/F	Axillobifemoral bypass	I and D groin abscesses	Rest pain; occluded EAB	Failed EAB; groin sepsis
39/M	AFB	AFB limb thrombectomies 3 times; replacement AFB and femoropopliteal bypass; repair femoral false aneurysms 3 times; obturator bypass	AFB occlusion; rest pain; groin abscess	Failed EAB; groin sepsis
66/M	AFB	Axillobifemoral bypass; removal AFB; thrombectomy; replacement AFB; I and D groin abscess	Septicemia; aortoenteric fistula	Failed EAB; groin sepsis
69/F	AFB	I and D groin abcess; removal AFB limb; saphenous vein femoral crossover bypass; above-knee amputation	Duodenal-groin cutaneous fistula	Massive groin and thigh sepsis
66/F	Axillobifemoral bypass	Multiple thrombectomies; AFB and femoropopliteal bypass; groin I and D 2 times	Draining groin abscess	Failed EAB; groin sepsis

**AFB indicates aortobifemoral bypass; I and D, incision and drainage; and EAB, extra-anatomic bypass.*

Autogenous aortofemoral reconstruction remains the only reasonable option in dealing with this problem.[8] We have championed the use of SFPVs for aortofemoral reconstruction because of their resistance to infection from a wide variety of gram-positive and gram-negative bacteria and fungal organisms, their durability and lack of long-term deterioration or aneurysm formation, and their excellent patency in the face of multiple-level occlusive disease and poor runoff.[1,2] In a larger series, the 5-year cumulative patency of autogenous aortofemoral SFPV reconstruction was 83% for primary patency and 100% for secondary or assisted patency.[2] Other autogenous reconstructions include those fashioned from endarterectomized arterial segments and GSV. We and others have found these reconstructions to be less desirable because their high failure rates due to progressive neointimal hyperplasia.[1,2,9]

Aortic allograft replacement is another option and has been used successfully to treat aortic prosthetic infections.[10-12] The main advantages of this approach include convenience and a decreased operating time, ob-

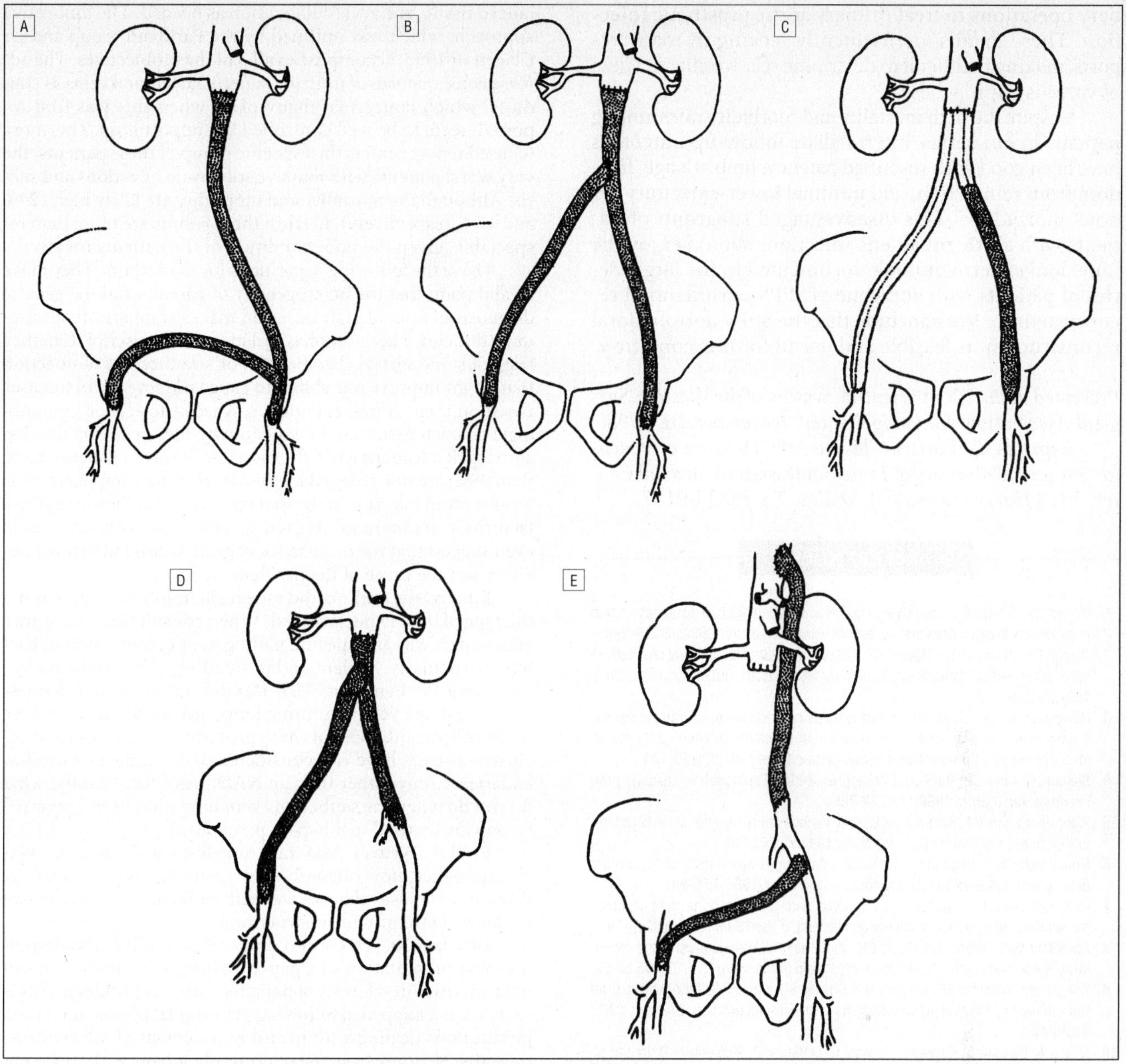

Superficial femoropopliteal vein (SFPV) aortofemoral reconstructions. A, Unilateral SFPV aortofemoral bypass with femoral crossover (n = 7); B, SFPV aortobifemoral bypasses (n = 6); C, SFPV from prosthetic aortofemoral bypass limb to femoral bypass (n = 2); D, Unilateral SFPV aortofemoral bypass with contralateral aortoiliac bypass (n = 1); and E, SFPV aortoiliac bypass with iliofemoral crossover (n = 1). Unilateral SFPV aortofemoral bypass (n = 1) is not shown.

viating the need to harvest and prepare autogenous conduits. However, allografts are subject to reinfection and short-term and long-term deterioration, often with disastrous consequences. Many consider autogenous allograft replacement to be a "bridge" procedure until a more definitive reconstruction can be undertaken.[9,11]

Five patients in this study were included in a larger, previous report.[2] Data from these 5 patients were removed from the larger group for analysis of morbidity and mortality comparisons between the groups. The in-hospital mortality in our present subgroup was 24%, 3 times the mortality of 8% in the larger series of autogenous SFPV aortofemoral reconstructions, usually performed as a secondary procedure after infection or failure of a primary AFB.[2] In addition, the acute amputation rate was also higher, 24% vs 6%, and other major complications were common in our present subgroup. This is not surprising, given the severity of illness of these patients at the time of presentation and the fact that most had already undergone multiple secondary and tertiary operations to treat aortic prosthetic infection.

This raises another issue relative to reporting vascular prosthetic infections. A wide range of incidences for mortalities and other outcomes have been reported with multiple operative approaches.[13] These are heterogeneous patients with varying levels of illness dependent on extent and virulence of infection, severity of underlying occlusive disease, presence and types of medical comorbidities, types of initial aortic reconstruction, presence of additional prosthetic infrainguinal bypasses involved with infection, presence of aortoenteric erosion or fistula, and performance of previous secondary or tertiary operations to treat primary aortic prosthetic infection. These details are frequently lacking in many reports, making it difficult to determine relative effectiveness of various approaches.

Despite the high mortality and morbidity rates among patients in our series, intermediate follow-up outcomes have been good with sustained patency, limb salvage, freedom from reinfection, and minimal lower-extremity venous morbidity.[5] This disadvantaged subgroup of patients with aortic prosthetic infections should enjoy the same longer-term outlook documented in the larger series of patients with autogenous SFPV aortofemoral reconstruction.[2] We conclude that the SFPV aortofemoral reconstruction is feasible and useful for this condition.

Presented at the 106th Scientific Session of the Western Surgical Association, Indianapolis, Ind, November 16, 1998.

Reprints: G. Patrick Clagett, MD, Division of Vascular Surgery, University of Texas Southwestern Medical Center, 5323 Harry Hines Blvd, Dallas, TX 75235-9157.

REFERENCES

1. Clagett GP, Bowers BL, Lopez-Viego MA, et al. Creation of a neo-aortoiliac system from lower extremity deep and superficial veins. *Ann Surg.* 1993;218:239-249.
2. Clagett GP, Valentine RJ, Hagino RT. Autogenous aortoiliac/femoral reconstruction from superficial femoral-popliteal veins: feasibility and durability. *J Vasc Surg.* 1997;25:255-270.
3. Nevelsteen A, Lacroix H, Suy R. Autogenous reconstruction with the lower extremity deep veins: an alternative treatment of prosthetic infection after reconstructive surgery for aortoiliac disease. *J Vasc Surg.* 1995;22:129-134.
4. Sladen JG, Chen JC, Reid JDS. An aggressive local approach to vascular graft infection. *Am J Surg.* 1998;176:222-225.
5. Wells JK, Hagino RT, Bargmann KM, et al. Venous morbidity after superficial femoral-popliteal vein harvest. *J Vasc Surg.* 1998;29:282-291.
6. Rutherford RB, Flanigan DP, Gupta SK, et al. Suggested standards for reports dealing with lower extremity ischemia. *J Vasc Surg.* 1986;4:80-94.
7. Reilly LM, Stoney RJ, Goldstone J. Improved management of aortic graft infection: the influence of operation sequence and staging. *J Vasc Surg.* 1987;5:421-429.
8. Ehrenfeld WK, Wilbur BG, Olcott CN IV, Stoney RJ. Autogenous tissue reconstruction in management of infected prosthetic grafts. *Surgery.* 1979;85:82-92.
9. Seeger JM, Wheeler JR, Gregory RT, Snyder SO, Gayle RG. Autogenous graft replacement of infected prosthetic grafts in the femoral position. *Surgery.* 1983; 93:39-45.
10. Keiffer E, Bahnini A, Koskas F, Ruotolo C, LeBlevec D, Plissonnier D. In situ allograft replacement of infected infrarenal aortic prosthetic grafts: results in forty-three patients. *J Vasc Surg.* 1993;17:349-356.
11. Bahnini A, Ruotolo C, Koskas F, Kieffer E. In situ fresh allograft replacement of an infected aortic prosthetic graft: eighteen months' follow-up. *J Vasc Surg.* 1991; 14:98-102.
12. Nevelsteen A, Feryn T, Lacroix H, Suy R, Goffin J. Experience with cryopreserved arterial allografts in the treatment of prosthetic graft infections. *Cardiovasc Surg.* 1998;6:378-383.
13. Bunt TJ. Treatment options for graft infections. In: Bunt TJ, ed. *Vascular Graft Infections.* Armonk, NY: Futura Publishing Co Inc; 1994:175-204.

DISCUSSION

Bruce L. Gewertz, MD, Chicago, Ill: I approach this podium with some trepidation. Bill Fry, a terrific surgeon, member of the Western Surgical, as well as father of Will Fry, a new member here today, had the mixed blessing of training both Pat Clagett and me. Bill Fry taught me many things, but one thing he taught me that I have remembered and up to this day have adhered to is never give a paper or a discussion on infected grafts.

The time-tested principles of management of arterial graft infections are very well delineated in this nice presentation. They include removal of prosthetic material, debridement of devitalized tissue, and revascularization as needed. The innovative approach, which was outlined by the Parkland group and Dr Clagett in 1993, accomplishes all 3 of these objectives. The adverse consequences of utilizing superficial femoral veins as conduits, which concerned many of us when this was first reported, seem to be well controlled by support hose. This more focused report centers on a specific group of these patients, the very worst patients with massive soft tissue infections and sepsis. Although the mortality and morbidity are fairly high (24% and 47%, respectively), in truth these results are more than respectable, given the poor condition of the patients involved.

I have the following 3 questions for the authors. They make a valid point that the heterogeneity of patients and the general diagnosis of arterial graft infection makes comparison of series quite difficult. This is emphasized in their manuscript. Can they suggest some sort of classification or stratification of infection that might improve our ability to gauge the severity of disease? Based on their overall experience, what historical or immunologic characteristics might explain why these patients develop aortic graft infections when the vast majority of our patients, more than 98%, are unburdened by this devastating complication? Is groin wound infection at the first operation still the greatest risk factor? Or, are more subtle predispositions at work? One could even suggest that the occurrence of groin wound infection is an effect, not the cause of the problem.

Finally, the authors did an excellent job of documenting the type of organisms involved. When considering their entire experience, was any specific pathogen or combination of bacteria particularly virulent and portending of bad outcome?

Gary W. Lemmon, MD, Dayton, Ohio: I have 3 questions. First, are you continuing long-term antibiotics for these patients? Second, most of these procedures were done for occlusive disease; have you considered performing an aortoiliac endarterectomy rather than an NAIS procedure? Lastly, what do you do when the saphenous vein has either been harvested or previously used in a bypass procedure?

Fred A. Weaver, MD, Los Angeles, Calif: In your overall experience, how often do these grafts develop the intrinsic vein graft stenoses that we see with saphenous vein bypasses for lower-extremity reconstruction?

Dr Claggett: Dr Gewertz reiterates Dr Bill Fry's admonition that presentation of a paper on infected grafts will result in an increase in referrals of patients with this problem. This is exactly what happened following our original presentations and publications dealing with in situ replacement of infected aortic grafts. Not only have the referrals of patients with this problem increased, they have become more complex. We are no longer seeing straightforward patients (if there is such a thing) with aortic graft infections. Most of the patients we now see have very advanced disease and complex situations, and this, in part, spurred us to develop this series.

Dr Gewertz raises the issue of stratification of these patients and whether or not this might be helpful in determining prognoses. This is a very important point. If one looks at the literature on this topic, one is impressed with the heterogeneity of patients in various series as well as the wide variance in morbidity and mortality. Comparing patients in different series and outcomes from these series is like comparing apples and oranges. There are several factors that portend a poor outcome, such as the presence of aortoenteric fistula or erosion, sepsis at the time of initial presentation, extent of prosthetic involvement, status of runoff, the numbers and types of previous vascular operations, and medical comorbidities. All of these are important factors in determining outcomes, and the more risk factors present, the worse the outcome will be. We definitely need a system to stratify these patients. We have reporting standards in other areas in vascular surgery, and we need to also develop reporting standards for this problem.

Dr Gewertz asked if these patients with advanced disease were immunologically disadvantaged. Some of these patients had obvious comorbidities that predisposed them to severe and virulent infections. These included diabetes mellitus, malnourishment, and, in one case, chronic steroid use because of chronic obstructive pulmonary disease. In many patients, it is difficult to sort out whether the patients' multiple operations disadvantaged them and predisposed them to further complications, or whether they had some underlying condition that led to the multiple operations. Dr Gewertz also asked whether distal gangrene or wound infections at the time of primary operation may have predisposed these patients to problems. Most of these patients were referred patients, and information with regard to their primary operations was somewhat sketchy, so I can't answer this question with completeness.

As far as pathogens are concerned, gram-negative infections are generally considered to be more virulent and serious. Some of the gram-negative organisms secrete exoproteases that can actually dissolve autogenous tissue, and this has been a particular concern of ours in developing this reconstruction. However, we have noted no difference in outcomes among the many different types of organisms that we have encountered. Many of the patients in our original series had *S epidermidis* infections, and these infections are easier to control and eradicate by removal of prosthetic material. However, we have also had many gram-negative infections, including *Pseudomonas* species. In the present series, most patients had polymicrobial infections with mixed gram-negative and gram-positive organisms.

Dr Lemmon asked about long-term antibiotics. We keep these patients on antibiotics for as long as invasive lines are in, and this is approximately 4 to 5 days. He also asked about the possibility of endarterectomizing arterial segments, such as the native aortoiliac system, and using this for reconstruction. In my experience, the retroperitoneum of these patients is like concrete, and it is almost impossible to dig out the old aortoiliac system intact. Others have reported using endarterectomized vascular segments but have experienced a high incidence of occlusion from neointimal hyperplasia.

The other question deals with the potential problem of harvesting the deep vein when the saphenous vein is absent. In many of our patients, the saphenous vein had been harvested previously, or we have had to use it at the time of this reconstruction for an additional reconstruction such as a distal bypass. We do not hesitate to harvest the saphenous vein when we need it. It is interesting that the venous morbidity is minimal in these patients. We have followed up to 60 patients prospectively for short- and long-term venous morbidity after harvesting the deep vein, and it does not appear to make any difference whether or not the ipsilateral saphenous vein is present. Some of these patients have transient swelling that is controlled with compression stockings, but in fact very few of them need long-term compression stocking treatment.

Dr Weaver asked whether or not these large vein grafts were predisposed to neointimal hyperplasia. They certainly can develop neointimal hyperplasia, but this is less likely to lead to occlusion or failure in comparison with saphenous vein grafts and other smaller conduits. The difference is that these are large conduits, and a little bit of neointimal hyperplasia really makes no difference in patency. We have had significant neointimal hyperplasia at anastomotic sites, and we have had to revise anastomoses in 2 of our patients on long-term follow-up. We do not get the problem of neointimal hyperplasia at valve sites such as one sees with saphenous veins.

IN OTHER AMA JOURNALS

ARCHIVES OF INTERNAL MEDICINE

Use of Nonsteroidal Anti-inflammatory Drugs and Incidence of Colorectal Cancer: A Population-Based Study

Walter Smalley, MD, MPH; Wayne A. Ray, PhD; James Daugherty, MS; Marie R. Griffin, MD, MPH

Background: Previous observational studies have provided limited information on the effect of specific nonsteroidal anti-inflammatory drugs (NSAIDs) and different patterns of use (duration and dose) on the incidence of colorectal cancer.
Objective: To determine how patterns of use (duration, dose, and specific drug) of NSAIDs affect incidence of colorectal cancer.
Design: Population-based retrospective cohort study.
Setting: Tennessee Medicaid Program, 1985-1992.
Subjects: Enrollees (n = 104 217) aged 65 years or older with at least 5 years of enrollment.
Main Outcome Measures: Incident histologically confirmed colorectal cancer.
Results: Users of nonaspirin NSAIDs for at least 48 months of the previous 5 years had a relative risk (RR) of 0.49 (95% confidence interval [CI], 0.24-1.00) for colon cancer when compared with those with no use of NSAIDs. Among those with more than 12 months of cumulative use, those using NSAIDs in the past year (recent users) had an RR of 0.61 (95% CI, 0.48-0.77), whereas those with no recent use had an RR of 0.76 (95% CI, 0.50-1.15). No specific NSAID offered a unique protective effect and low doses of NSAIDs appeared to be at least as effective as higher doses. Protection was most pronounced for right-sided lesions. The RR among recent users with more than 12 months of cumulative use was 0.81 (95% CI, 0.49-1.32) for rectal cancer, 0.77 (95% CI, 0.55-1.08) for left-sided colon cancer, and 0.48 (95% CI, 0.34-0.68) for right-sided colon cancer.
Conclusions: In this elderly population, long-term use of nonaspirin NSAIDs nearly halved the risk of colon cancer. This study was consistent with previous studies that suggest that duration of use but not daily dose of NSAIDs is an important factor for chemoprevention. Our data also suggest that the protective effect is shared by most NSAIDs, and not confined to a small number of these drugs. (*1999;159:161-166*)

Reprints: Walter E. Smalley, MD, MPH, A-1129 MCN, Vanderbilt University Medical Center, Nashville, TN 37232.

Oral Contrast Solution and Computed Tomography for Blunt Abdominal Trauma

A Randomized Study

Renae E. Stafford, MD; Michael D. McGonigal, MD; John A. Weigelt, MD; Thomas J. Johnson, MD

Hypothesis: Oral contrast solution (OC) is unnecessary in the acute computed tomographic (CT) evaluation of the patient with blunt abdominal trauma.

Design: Randomized controlled clinical trial.

Setting: Level I trauma center at a university-affiliated teaching hospital.

Patients: Five hundred adult patients sustaining blunt abdominal trauma and requiring urgent resuscitation and CT evaluation of the abdomen were eligible for the study. Those patients who were younger than 18 years, pregnant, or in police custody were excluded. One hundred six patients were excluded from the analysis (15 for inappropriate enrollment, 9 because a CT scan had not been performed, 1 owing to inability to accept a nasogastric tube, and 81 owing to missing or incomplete records). Three hundred ninety-four patients with an average age of 36 years, an average Revised Trauma Score of 10, and an average Glasgow Coma Scale score of 12 are included in the analysis.

Interventions: Patients were randomized via computer-generated assignment to 1 of 2 groups either receiving OC or not receiving OC (no OC) after placement of a nasogastric tube. All patients received intravenous contrast solution and then underwent helical CT scan of the abdomen and pelvis using the GE HiSpeed Advantage CT scanner (GE Medical Systems, Milwaukee, Wis).

Main Outcome Measures: Abnormal CT results, need for laparotomy, missed gastrointestinal tract and solid organ injuries, nausea, and vomiting.

Results: There were 199 patients in the OC group and 195 patients in the no OC group. Vomiting occurred in 12.9% of patients and the incidence was not different between groups. One hundred five abnormal scans (50 OC and 55 no OC) were obtained and 33 patients with abnormal scans (19 OC and 14 no OC) underwent laparotomy. There was 1 nontherapeutic laparotomy in each group. There was 1 missed small-bowel injury in the OC group (sensitivity, 86%) and no missed small-bowel injuries in the no OC group (sensitivity, 100%). Six bowel injuries were identified at laparotomy in the OC group. Two of the injuries were perforations without contrast extravasation but with pneumoperitoneum in 1. Three bowel injuries were identified in the no OC group, none of which were perforations. Seven of the 9 patients with bowel injury at laparotomy had associated intra-abdominal injury. Specificity for solid organ injury was 94% in the OC group and 57.1% in the no OC group. Sensitivity for solid organ injury was 84.2% in the OC group and 88.9% in the no OC group. The average time to abdominal CT scanning after placement of a nasogastric tube was 39.02 ± 18.73 minutes in the no OC group and 45.92 ± 24.17 minutes in the OC group ($P = .008$).

Conclusion: The addition of OC to the acute CT protocol for the evaluation of the patient with blunt abdominal trauma is unnecessary and delays time to CT scanning.

Arch Surg. 1999;134:622-627

From the Departments of Surgery at Regions Hospital (Drs McGonigal and Johnson) and the University of Minnesota (Drs Stafford and Weigelt), St Paul.

ORAL CONTRAST solution (OC) is recommended by both surgeons and radiologists when computed tomography (CT) is used for evaluation of the abdomen in patients with blunt abdominal trauma.[1-8] Oral contrast aids in the identification of bowel loops, helps delineate bowel mesentery, and distinguishes opacified intestine from hematoma, hemorrhage, and pancreatic pathologic findings.[5-7,9-11] Finally, extravasation of OC is a specific finding for the diagnosis of hollow viscus perforation.[3,8,11] The use of OC for blunt abdominal trauma CT scans does have potential disadvantages. These include vomiting with pulmonary aspiration and interference with subsequent angiographic studies.[4,9,12] The effective use of OC also requires additional time for gut opacification, which may delay definitive treatment of injuries.[1,13,14] The value of OC for CT scans in patients with blunt trauma has

PATIENTS, MATERIALS, AND METHODS

All adult trauma patients presenting to the St Paul Ramsey Medical Center, St Paul, Minn, a level I trauma center, who required urgent resuscitation and CT evaluation of the abdomen for blunt abdominal trauma between June 1993 and October 1996 were eligible for entry into the study.

Patients who were younger than 18 years, pregnant, or in police custody were excluded from the study. Eligible patients were prospectively randomized to either the OC group or the group not receiving OC (no OC). Randomization was implemented by computer-generated assignment. The study was approved by our institutional review board.

All patients had a nasogastric tube placed prior to randomization. Patients in the OC group received 30 mL of diatrizoate meglumine (Gastrografin Oral; Bracco Diagnostics, Princeton, NJ) mixed with 700 mL of tap water, which was administered via the nasogastric tube in the emergency department. All patients received intravenous contrast by a mechanical injector at 2 mL/s at a maximum dose of 2 mL/kg. Intravenous contrast agents were either diatrizoate sodium (Renografin 76; Bracco Diagnostics) or iopromide (Ultravist; Berlex, Wayne, NJ). Computed tomographic scans were performed using the GE HiSpeed Advantage helical scanner (GE Medical Systems, Milwaukee, Wis). Scans were obtained using 7-mm cuts from the dome of the diaphragm to the pelvic crest and 10-mm cuts from the pelvic crest to the symphysis pubis. Scans were immediately examined by an attending radiologist, staff trauma surgeon, and chief surgical resident. Initial management decisions were based on this reading. Data collected at the time of CT scanning included demographic data, mechanism of injury, Glasgow Coma Scale score, Revised Trauma Score, and a history of aspiration or vomiting. The length of time in minutes for travel from the emergency department to the CT scanner, for scanning of the abdomen and pelvis, and for travel from the CT scanner to the ward, intensive care unit, or operating room was recorded. Patient records were reviewed for abnormal CT results on the final staff radiologist reading, need for laparotomy, and missed gastrointestinal tract injuries and complications. Laparotomy findings were compared with both initial and final preoperative CT results. Statistical analysis was performed using the χ^2 test, t test, and Fisher exact test where appropriate. $P \leq .05$ was considered statistically significant.

been questioned.[2,13,15] Despite many reports of the accuracy of CT scans with OC in patients with blunt abdominal trauma, the necessity of OC as part of the CT scanning protocol has never been assessed in a randomized prospective fashion.

To evaluate the necessity of OC in CT evaluation of the patient with blunt abdominal trauma and to assess possible disadvantages of its use, we evaluated 500 consecutive patients who required CT evaluation of the abdomen for blunt abdominal trauma in a randomized prospective study.

RESULTS

Five hundred consecutive patients who fit eligibility criteria were enrolled in the study (**Figure**). One hundred six patients were excluded from the analysis. Of these 106 patients, 15 patients were inappropriately enrolled in the study, 9 patients required immediate laparotomy obviating the need for abdominal CT scan, 1 patient was excluded because of the inability to pass a nasogastric tube, and the remaining 81 patients had incomplete or missing records. These 81 patients were prospectively identified and had initial data points collected, but final data could not be collated because their medical records could not be retrieved from our institution. Thus, 394 patients are included in the final analysis. There were 278 men (70%) and 116 women (30%). Their average ages were 35.6 and 37.8 years, respectively. Motor vehicle crashes accounted for 60.4% of the injuries; pedestrian vs auto accidents, 9.9%; falls, 9.6%; motorcycle crashes, 7.6%; and other mechanisms, 12.5%. The overall average Revised Trauma Score was 10 (range, 4-12) and the overall average Glasgow Coma Scale score was 12.0 (range, 3-15). These variables were not significantly different between the OC and no OC groups.

There were 199 patients in the OC group and 195 patients in the no OC group. There were 105 abnormal CT scans (50 OC and 55 no OC). Of those patients with abnormal CT scans, 33 (31%) underwent laparotomy. Of the 33 laparotomies performed, 19 were OC patients and 14 were no OC patients. There was 1 nontherapeutic laparotomy in each group. One missed small-bowel injury occurred in an OC patient and there were no missed small-bowel injuries in the no OC patients. Vomiting occurred in 27 OC patients (13.6%) and 24 no OC patients (12.3%). There were 2 witnessed aspiration episodes; however, neither of these were related to administration of OC therapy. None of these differences between the patient groups were statistically significant.

There were 6 bowel injuries confirmed at laparotomy in the OC group (**Table 1**). Thickening of the bowel wall was noted on CT in 3 of the patients in this group, and free fluid was noted in 2. Two of the injuries involved perforations. Only 1 of the perforations was associated with a pneumoperitoneum. There was no contrast extravasation seen on CT scan in either of the patients who had a perforation. The nontherapeutic laparotomy in this group occurred in a patient who had an initial CT scan that was read as negative except for an acetabular fracture. Because of persistent ileus, a second CT scan was performed that showed free fluid in the pelvis. No injury was found at laparotomy.

In the no OC group, there were 3 bowel injuries identified at laparotomy (Table 1). Two patients had free fluid and 1 patient had a thickened bowel as seen on the preoperative CT scan. There were no perforations in this group. Nontherapeutic laparotomy was performed on a patient who had been in a motor vehicle crash and sustained a pancreatic laceration with peripancreatic fluid

Table 1. Patients With Abnormal CT Scan and Bowel Injury at Laparotomy*

CT Scan	Laparotomy
OC Group	
Small amount of peritoneal fluid	Ileal mesenteric tear, hematoma
Small-bowel thickening, pneumoperitoneum perforations†	Ileal and cecal
Thickening of the mid small bowel‡	Midjejunal perforation
Free fluid in pelvis	Mesenteric tears midileum
Soft tissue density in mesenteric fat near tail of pancreas and thickened bowel wall, soft tissue density at hepatic flexure	Mesenteric tears, hepatic flexure, bowel wall hematoma
Free intraperitoneal fluid	Serosal tears descending colon, bladder perforation
No OC Group	
Free fluid in pelvis, soft tissue stranding adjacent to pancreas	Mesenteric and serosal tears in midjejunum and sigmoid
Free fluid in pelvis	Mesenteric jejunal hematoma
Thickened, dilated duodenum	Duodenal hematoma

*CT indicates computed tomographic; OC, oral contrast solution; and no OC, no oral contrast solution.
†This patient had no contrast extravasation seen on CT scan.
‡This patient had no contrast extravasation or pneumoperitoneum seen on CT scan.

Table 2. Associated Findings in Patients With Bowel Injury*

CT Scan	Laparotomy
OC Group	
Small amount of pelvic fluid	Bilateral pelvic wall lacerations
Splenic laceration, rupture of the abdominal wall	Abdominal wall disruption, transsected rectus muscle, splenic laceration
Transverse process fracture L5	None
Intraparenchymal splenic fluid	Splenic laceration with active bleeding
Soft tissue density in mesenteric fat near tail of pancreas and thickened bowel wall, soft tissue density at hepatic flexure	Splenic laceration with active bleeding
Sacral fractures with pelvic hematoma	Retroperitoneal hematoma, bladder rupture
No OC Group	
Left femur fracture	None
Free peritoneal fluid, deflated bladder	Bladder rupture
Enlarged head of pancreas with peripancreatic fluid	Pancreatic hematoma

*CT indicates computed tomographic; OC, oral contrast solution; L5, fifth lumbar vertebra; and no OC, no oral contrast solution.

and a liver laceration as seen on CT scan. At laparotomy, no liver or pancreatic injuries were noted, although retroperitoneal edema was seen. The patient was discharged from the hospital 8 days after the injury.

A missed small-bowel injury occurred in 1 patient in the OC group who sustained multiple orthopedic injuries by attempting suicide by jumping from a bridge. An abdominal and pelvic CT scan done at admission was read by an attending radiologist as negative for hollow viscus or solid organ injury, although the patient did have multiple pelvic fractures. The hospital stay was marked by an ileus, fever, and urinary tract infection. Despite treatment of the urinary tract infection, the patient remained febrile and subsequent workup revealed free air on a chest x-ray film. An exploratory laparotomy was performed on hospital day 20. At laparotomy, bowel content was noted in the peritoneal cavity. A perforation on the antimesenteric border of the midjejunum was found. The postoperative course was complicated by an anastomotic leak and the patient was discharged 60 days after injury.

Of those patients with bowel injury found at laparotomy, 7 had associated intra-abdominal injuries (**Table 2**). Most had solid organ injuries, and there were 2 bladder ruptures. Solid organ injury, most commonly of the spleen, was the most prevalent finding at laparotomy in those patients without bowel injury.

There were 11 patients who underwent laparotomy in the OC group who were suspected of having 17 solid organ injuries on the basis of preoperative CT scan. Sixteen injuries were confirmed at laparotomy (specificity, 94%). However, 3 injuries (liver, spleen, and pancreas) were identified at laparotomy that were not identified on the preoperative CT scan (sensitivity, 84.2%). In the no OC group, 12 patients were suspected of having 14 solid organ injuries on the basis of the preoperative CT scan results. Eight injuries were confirmed at laparotomy (specificity, 57.1%). One solid organ injury was found at laparotomy that was missed by the CT scan (sensitivity, 88.9%).

Accurate time data were available for 282 (138 no OC and 144 OC) patients. The average time from placement of a nasogastric tube or orogastric tube to abdominal CT scan was 39.02 ± 18.73 minutes in the no OC patients and 45.92 ± 24.17 minutes in the OC patients ($P = .008$).

COMMENT

Computed tomography has become the radiographic technique of choice in many trauma centers for the evaluation of the hemodynamically normal patient with blunt abdominal trauma.[8,9] While many authors and investigators have advocated the use of OC in addition to intravenous contrast as part of the abdominal trauma CT scanning regimen,[1-8,16] considerable controversy remains regarding its necessity.[9,13,15] In particular, there is concern regarding time delay to diagnosis of potentially lethal injuries, aspiration of gastric contents and contrast with subsequent pulmonary toxic effects, interference with evaluation of angiographic studies, and whether OC actually adds information to make the diagnosis of a critical bowel injury.[4,9,12,13,15] In addition, there are pediatric and adult trauma centers where OC is not routinely used as part of the blunt abdominal CT scan protocol.[15,17,18]

The rationale for the use of OC in trauma CT of the abdomen is well delineated in the literature. One of the most commonly cited diagnostic signs of bowel perforation is the extravasation of OC.[3,8,11,16] However, this is a rare event.[8] In fact, the incidence ranges from 0% to 19% in patients who received OC for CT evaluation of blunt abdominal trauma and who had bowel perforation documented at laparotomy.[3,11,13,16,19] Unfortunately, current data sets do not address a possible time bias for contrast extravasation as a positive finding. In a series of 24 patients seen in a 5-year period who had signs of bowel injury on CT, the CT scans were performed anywhere from 1 hour to as many as 6 weeks after injury.[11] Rizzo et al[3] reported 59% undergoing CT within 6 hours of injury and the remainder at varying times after admission and after discharge from the emergency department. There was no contrast extravasation in the 2 patients in this study who had bowel perforations. Both patients underwent scanning within 1 hour after injury and were in the OC group. All of our patients were studied on admission and all except 3 were done within 2 hours after admission, making our data pertinent to the immediate use of OC for diagnosis of bowel injuries.

The optimal use of OC also requires adequate transit time for gut opacification.[1,13,14] Theoretically, opacification enables the gut to be distinguished from solid organs and omentum. Recommendations for the optimal length of time between administration of contrast and starting the abdominal CT scan vary. There are few studies where the amount of contrast in the gut has been quantified or addressed. Tsang et al[13] evaluated 70 CT scans of patients with blunt abdominal trauma and found that only 59% of the scans had adequate small-bowel opacification despite an average time from OC administration to performance of the CT scan of 144 ± 5.9 minutes. Given that many patients with blunt trauma have a history of alcohol use and/or may have associated head injuries and lumbar fractures that can be associated with delayed gastric emptying and ileus, this is not a surprising finding.[15,20] If adequate gut opacification cannot be achieved in a reasonable amount of time, the delay to diagnosis of potentially lethal injuries becomes a larger problem and patients are subjected to the administration of an agent that may be potentially harmful. In fact, we did find that the average time to abdominal CT scanning in those patients who received OC was longer than in the no OC patients and this was significantly different. We did not attempt to assess adequacy of gut opacification or radiologic interpretation between the 2 groups since we considered this subjective data not amenable to explicit review.

Pneumoperitoneum is considered to be another diagnostic sign of hollow viscus rupture.[7,10,11] While this may be seen in up to 50% of patients with blunt abdominal trauma, a significant number of patients with perforation will not have pneumoperitoneum.[10,11,15] Donohue et al[11] reported pneumoperitoneum seen on CT scan in only 3 of 8 patients with documented bowel perforation at laparotomy. This was seen in only 1 of 2 patients in our series who had bowel perforation. It may be that the time interval from perforation to CT scan completion is an important factor in this determination.[10] Small perforations may seal quickly and prevent extravasation of contrast and/or air that could then be detected by CT scan.[10,18]

The sensitivity of CT scan with OC for the diagnosis of blunt bowel injury ranges from 80% and 100% depending on the criteria used.[14,19,21] Kearney et al[14] reported a sensitivity of only 80% for detection of bowel injury by CT scan with OC, while Sherck et al[19] reported a sensitivity of 92%. In a center where OC is not used in the protocol for blunt abdominal trauma CT scans, 6 patients with small-bowel injury at laparotomy all had findings on CT that were suggestive of bowel injury and 2 of these only had bowel wall thickening and free peritoneal fluid.[18] Other investigators have determined that OC was unnecessary for the diagnosis of small-bowel injury.[13,15] In those patients who had bowel injury at laparotomy, we identified 6 of 7 patients in the OC group (sensitivity 86%) and 100% in the no OC group by using the presence of free fluid not explained by solid organ injury and/or thickened bowel wall in addition to pneumoperitoneum and contrast extravasation as criteria for bowel injury. This difference was not statistically significant. Other investigators have found that the addition of these factors increases the sensitivity for detection of bowel injury.[11,19,22,23] Thus, it seems that the sensitivity of CT scan for the detection of bowel injury at centers that use OC does not differ significantly from those centers that do not use OC, and our data concur.

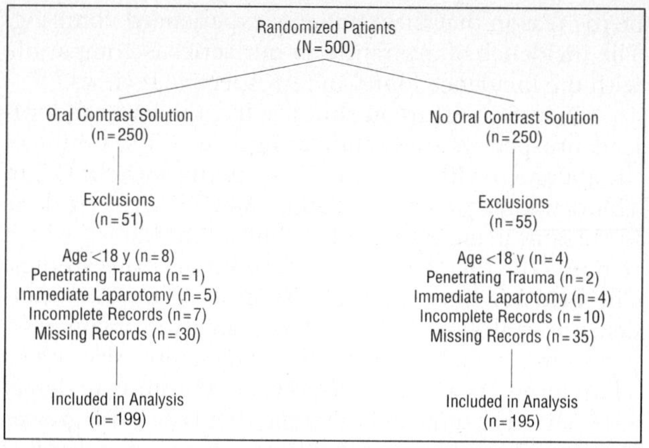

Flow diagram.

The sensitivity of CT scan with OC varies between 90% and 100% for the diagnosis of solid organ injury. Our data, for both OC and no OC CT scans, is within this range. The significant number of false-positive CT results in the no OC group may be the result of "overreading" by the radiologist because no contrast was used. However, only 1 patient in this false-positive group had a nontherapeutic laparotomy. While the specificity was low, there was only 1 nontherapeutic laparotomy because of concurrent intra-abdominal injuries that were identified on the same no OC CT scans.

While vomiting and aspiration have been discussed in the literature as potential disadvantages to the use of OC, the incidence of these events and their temporal relationship to OC administration is not always easy to identify. Our study design required placing a nasogastric or orogastric tube in each patient before the administration of OC. Aspiration of gastric contents was also done before OC was given. These steps would explain the 12.9% incidence of vomiting that we saw, which is less than that in a previous report.[13] Our low incidence and no difference between the groups could be related to nasogastric tube or orogastric tube placement. That contrast material was added to a full stomach may be the reason that these patients experienced vomiting. The incidence of aspiration in our series is compatible with the incidence found in retrospective reviews.[9,13]

Our study is, to our knowledge, the first randomized, prospective study comparing acute CT scanning of the abdomen with OC with CT scanning without OC in a blunt trauma patient population. All CT scans were done in the same manner and within similar time frames, which removes the time bias associated with previous studies. The primary limitation of this study is the low incidence of small-bowel injuries. Our inability to obtain missing records, which decreases the study sample size, is also a limitation. As a result, the power of the study to detect a statistically significant difference between the 2 groups is limited. Therefore, a true difference between the groups may exist that was not detected by this study. This is also a limitation of all retrospective studies.[3,7,19] Given the low prevalence of hollow viscus injury, a large number of injured patients would be needed in each arm of a similarly randomized study to prove that there is no difference in outcomes between the groups. This would require a multicenter trial.

A high index of suspicion for hollow viscus and solid organ injury remains necessary when evaluating the patient with blunt abdominal trauma. Clinical signs and symptoms of peritonitis in addition to CT findings of unexplained free intraperitoneal fluid or pneumoperitoneum, extravasation of OC, streaking of the mesentery, and thickened bowel wall are suggestive of hollow viscus injury. The addition of OC to the acute CT protocol for the patient with blunt abdominal trauma is unnecessary and actually delays time to CT scanning. Our prospective findings are consistent with retrospective reports and we believe this correlation warrants our conclusion until a larger prospective study can refute this growing body of evidence. Subsequent CT examinations of the abdomen and pelvis in this population may not require OC either; however, this issue is not addressed in this study and requires further evaluation.

Presented at the 106th Scientific Session of the Western Surgical Association, Indianapolis, Ind, November 16, 1998.

Corresponding author: John A. Weigelt, MD, Department of Surgery, Regions Hospital, 640 Jackson St, St Paul, MN 55101 (e-mail: John.A.Weigelt@HealthPartners.com).

REFERENCES

1. Meyer DM, Thal ER, Weigelt JA, Redman HC. Evaluation of computed tomography and diagnostic peritoneal lavage in blunt abdominal trauma. *J Trauma.* 1989; 29:1168-1172.
2. Marx JA, Moore EE, Jorden RC, Eule J. Limitations of computed tomography in the evaluation of acute abdominal trauma: a prospective comparison with diagnostic peritoneal lavage. *J Trauma.* 1985;25:933-937.
3. Rizzo MJ, Federle MP, Griffiths BG. Bowel and mesenteric injury following blunt abdominal trauma: evaluation with CT. *Radiology.* 1989;173:143-148.
4. Toombs BD, Lester RG, Ben-Menachem YB, Sandler CM. Computed tomography in blunt trauma. *Radiol Clin North Am.* 1981;19:17-35.
5. Hofer GA, Cohen AJ. CT signs of duodenal perforation secondary to blunt abdominal trauma. *J Comput Assist Tomogr.* 1989;13:430-432.
6. Cox TD, Kuhn JP. CT scan of bowel trauma in the pediatric patient. *Radiol Clin North Am.* 1996;34:807-818.
7. Nghiem HV, Jeffrey RB, Mindelzun RE. CT of blunt trauma to the bowel and mesentery. *AJR Am J Roentgenol.* 1993;160:53-58.
8. Wolfman NT, Bechtold RE, Scharling ES, Meredith JW. Blunt upper abdominal trauma: evaluation by CT. *AJR Am J Roentgenol.* 1992;158:493-501.
9. Federle MP, Peitzman A, Krugh J. Use of oral contrast material in abdominal CT scans: is it dangerous? *J Trauma.* 1995;38:51-53.
10. Cook DE, Walsh JW, Vick CW, Brewer WH. Upper abdominal trauma: pitfalls in diagnosis. *Radiology.* 1986;159:65-69.
11. Donohue JH, Federle MP, Griffiths BG, Trunkey, DD. Computed tomography in the diagnosis of blunt intestinal and mesenteric injuries. *J Trauma.* 1987;27:11-17.
12. Davis RA, Shayne JP, Max MH, Woolfitt RA, Schwab W. The use of computerized axial tomography versus peritoneal lavage in the evaluation of blunt abdominal trauma: a prospective study. *Surgery.* 1985;98:845-849.
13. Tsang BD, Panacek EA, Brant WE, Wisner DH. Effect of oral contrast administration for abdominal computed tomography in the evaluation of acute blunt trauma. *Ann Emerg Med.* 1997;30:7-13.
14. Kearney PA Jr, Vahey T, Burney RE, Glazer G. Computed tomography and diagnostic peritoneal lavage in blunt abdominal trauma. *Arch Surg.* 1989;124:344-347.
15. Clancy TV, Ragozzino MW, Ramshaw D, Churchill MP, Covington DL, Maxwell JG. Oral contrast is not necessary in the evaluation of blunt abdominal trauma by computed tomography. *Am J Surg.* 1993;166:680-685.
16. Sherck JP, Oakes DD. Intestinal injuries missed by computed tomography. *J Trauma.* 1990;30:1-7.
17. Taylor GA, Fallat ME, Potter BM, Eichelberger MR. The role of computed tomography in blunt abdominal trauma in children. *J Trauma.* 1988;28:1660-1664.
18. Bulas DI, Taylor GA, Eichelberger MR. The value of CT in detecting bowel perforation in children after blunt abdominal trauma. *AJR Am J Roentgenol.* 1983; 153:561-564.
19. Sherck J, Shatney C, Sensaki K, Selivanov V. The accuracy of computed tomography in the diagnosis of blunt small-bowel perforation. *Am J Surg.* 1994;168: 670-675.
20. Feliciano DV. Diagnostic modalities in abdominal trauma. *Surg Clin North Am.* 1991;71:241-255.
21. Fabian TC, Mangiante EC, White TJ, Patterson CR, Boldreghini S, Britt L. A prospective study of 91 patients undergoing both computed tomography and peritoneal lavage following blunt abdominal trauma. *J Trauma.* 1986;26:602-608.
22. Kunin JR, Korobkin M, Ellis JH, Francis IR, Kane NM, Siegel SE. Duodenal injuries caused by blunt abdominal trauma: value of CT in differentiating perforation from hematoma. *AJR Am J Roentgenol.* 1993;160:1221-1223.
23. Mirvis SE, Gens DR, Shanmuganathan K. Rupture of the bowel after blunt abdominal trauma: diagnosis with CT. *AJR Am J Roentgenol.* 1992;159:1217-1221.

DISCUSSION

Cleon W. Goodwin, Jr, MD, Fort Sam Houston, Tex: Dr Stafford and her associates have convincingly demonstrated that adding OC agent to intravenous contrast for CT evaluation of blunt abdominal trauma patients has no positive benefit and at best is a nuisance in the management of such patients. This certainly is my experience sitting beside these patients in the CT room as they vomited throughout the procedure. This is a huge and deceptively difficult study carried out in a 3-year period. I have a few questions on how you made this study work.

I know that you had institutional review board clearance. Did you have to obtain informed consent from these patients? I suspect you did not because historically up to 50% of such patients choose not to participate in clinical trials. Who carried out the randomization? It seems you had a specific coordinator for this prospective study and, if so, how did you end up with incomplete records from 81 patients presumably with prospectively collected data?

I think you have settled the issue of whether OC must be used with these patients.

Richard E. Burney, MD, Ann Arbor, Mich: One of the areas that is hard to see by CT after trauma is the pancreaticoduodenal area, and contrast frequently helps to differentiate duodenal and pancreatic injuries. I wondered how many patients had pancreatic or duodenal injury, and did you have any problem in visualizing those injuries?

John Barrett, MD, Chicago, Ill: I wonder if you could expand on the point that you made in your presentation that the total number of patients who have gastrointestinal injuries in the study is extremely small. All of these patients had small-bowel injuries and none had duodenal injuries. Since these are the patients who would most commonly benefit from OC, I wondered how you can justify your conclusions.

J. David Richardson, MD, Louisville, Ky: Do your radiologists agree with your findings? We have had very similar results, but our radiologists simply refuse to interpret the CT scan without OC making this point moot for us. We agree with your results and interpretation of them.

Dr Weigelt: Dr Goodwin, as far as our consent issue, we convinced the institutional review board that both methods were standard of care and so we did not have to obtain consent before we enrolled the patient, as long as we approached the patient afterwards. At that time the patient usually agreed to participate.

The randomization was done by our computer. We had envelopes in the room, and once the nasogastric tube was placed, we essentially drew an envelope that assigned the patient to receive OC or not to receive it.

The 81 records that are not available is deceptive. We have the records on those patients from this prospective study. What is not available is basically their medical records, which could not be retrieved from our medical records department. Since our study design demanded these records to be reviewed, we had to exclude these patients. I know anybody who has tried to get a record out of a medical record department realizes that sometimes that is an impossible feat.

Both Dr Burney and Dr Barrett talked about the duodenal injuries. We have very few duodenal injuries in this group but do not believe this detracts from our conclusions. We can say pretty conclusively that there is no difference between the two given the limitations of the injuries that you saw in the study.

As far as the question about will the radiologist agree with this approach, presently we have some enlightened radiologists who do agree with it. We have some others who are still resistant to approach this as our standard. However, Dr McGonigal and the group is working on a practice guideline currently that will include the radiologists. It seems that we have the better data set than they do so we may actually be able to persuade them.

IN OTHER AMA JOURNALS

JAMA

Accuracy of Data in Abstracts of Published Research Articles

Roy M. Pitkin, MD; Mary Ann Branagan; Leon F. Burmeister, PhD

Context The section of a research article most likely to be read is the abstract, and therefore it is particularly important that the abstract reflect the article faithfully.

Objective To assess abstracts accompanying research articles published in 6 medical journals with respect to whether data in the abstract could be verified in the article itself.

Design Analysis of simple random samples of 44 articles and their accompanying abstracts published during 1 year (July 1, 1996-June 30, 1997) in each of 5 major general medical journals (*Annals of Internal Medicine, BMJ, JAMA, Lancet,* and *New England Journal of Medicine*) and a consecutive sample of 44 articles published during 15 months (July 1, 1996-August 15, 1997) in the *CMAJ*.

Main Outcome Measure Abstracts were considered deficient if they contained data that were either inconsistent with corresponding data in the article's body (including tables and figures) or not found in the body at all.

Results The proportion of deficient abstracts varied widely (18%-68%) and to a statistically significant degree ($P<.001$) among the 6 journals studied.

Conclusions Data in the abstract that are inconsistent with or absent from the article's body are common, even in large-circulation general medical journals.(*1999;281:1110-1111*) www.jama.com

Corresponding author: Roy M. Pitkin, MD, 10921 Wilshire Blvd, Suite 403, Los Angeles, CA 90024-3908 (e-mail: rpitkin@greenjournal.org).

PAPER

Laparoscopic vs Open Adrenalectomy for the Treatment of Primary Hyperaldosteronism

Wen T. Shen, MD; Robert C. Lim, MD; Allan E. Siperstein, MD; Orlo H. Clark, MD; William P. Schecter, MD; Thomas K. Hunt, MD; Jan K. Horn, MD; Quan-Yang Duh, MD

Hypothesis: That the clinical presentations, biochemical profiles, and surgical outcomes of patients treated with laparoscopic vs open adrenalectomy for primary hyperaldosteronism are different.

Design, Settings, Patients, and Interventions: The medical records of 80 patients with primary hyperaldosteronism who underwent open adrenalectomy between 1975 and 1986 or laparoscopic adrenalectomy between 1993 and 1998 at the University of California–San Francisco were reviewed by a single unblinded researcher (W.T.S.).

Main Outcome Measures: Severity of hypertension and hypokalemia at diagnosis, their improvement after adrenalectomy, and operative complications.

Results: Thirty-eight patients underwent open adrenalectomy and 42 patients underwent laparoscopic adrenalectomy. The patients who underwent open adrenalectomy had documented hypertension for a median of 5 years before surgery; all had diastolic blood pressures greater than 100 mm Hg. Laparoscopically treated patients had documented hypertension for a median of 2.5 years preoperatively, and 20 (48%) had diastolic blood pressures greater than 100 mm Hg. The median preoperative serum potassium levels for the open and laparoscopic groups were 2.6 mmol/L and 3.3 mmol/L, respectively; the mean serum aldosterone levels were 1.47 nmol/L and 1.30 nmol/L. Thirty-two (84%) of the 38 patients who underwent open surgery and 41 (98%) of the 42 patients treated laparoscopically had adrenal adenomas. The sensitivity of preoperative computed tomographic scanning for adenomas was 83% for the patients treated with open adrenalectomy and 93% for those treated laparoscopically. There were 4 postoperative complications in the open surgery group and none in the laparoscopic group. Postoperatively, 30 (81%) of 37 patients (excluding 1 patient who died of adrenocortical carcinoma) in the open surgery group and 37 (88%) of 42 patients treated laparoscopically were normotensive. Postoperative values were 3.6 to 5.0 of serum potassium per liter and 3.5 to 4.9 of serum potassium per liter in the open and laparoscopic groups, respectively.

Conclusions: Patients who are treated with laparoscopic adrenalectomy for primary hyperaldosteronism are being referred with less severe hypertension and hypokalemia than patients formerly treated with open adrenalectomy. Patients treated laparoscopically had fewer postoperative complications and were equally likely to improve in blood pressure and hypokalemia. Laparoscopic adrenalectomy has become the treatment of choice for patients with primary hyperaldosteronism because of lower morbidity.

Arch Surg. 1999;134:628-632

From the Department of Surgery, University of California–San Francisco (Drs Shen, Lim, and Hunt); UCSF/Mt Zion Medical Center (Drs Siperstein and Clark); San Francisco Veterans Affairs Medical Center (Dr Duh); and San Francisco General Hospital (Drs Schecter and Horn).

PRIMARY hyperaldosteronism is an uncommon but surgically correctable disease that affects approximately 1 in every 200 hypertensive patients.[1] First described by Jerome Conn in 1954, primary hyperaldosteronism is characterized by hypertension, hypokalemia, elevated plasma aldosterone, and low plasma renin activity. The most common underlying pathology for this syndrome is an aldosterone-producing adrenal adenoma. Primary hyperaldosteronism can also be caused by bilateral adrenal hyperplasia and other rarer diseases such as primary unilateral adrenal hyperplasia, glucocorticoid-responsive hyperaldosteronism, and adrenocortical carcinoma.

The surgical treatment of choice for primary hyperaldosteronism caused by an aldosterone-secreting adenoma is unilateral adrenalectomy.[2-10] Until recently, this operation required an open surgical procedure, usually through a posterior "Hugh-Young" incision. We have previously reported our experience with open adrenalectomy for the treatment of primary hyperaldosteronism in the 1970s and 1980s.[11] Since that time, however, several technological advancements have been made in the diagnosis and treatment of this condition. Improvements in the sensitivity of

MATERIALS AND METHODS

We retrospectively analyzed the medical records of 80 patients who underwent adrenalectomy for primary hyperaldosteronism at University of California–San Francisco between 1975 and 1998. Open adrenalectomy was performed in 38 patients between 1975 and 1986. Thirty-four patients underwent unilateral open adrenalectomy, while 4 patients underwent bilateral open adrenal exploration with removal of 1 adrenal tumor. The patient profiles and results of operation from these 38 patients have been previously reported.[11] Laparoscopic adrenalectomy was performed in 42 patients between 1993 and 1998; all 42 patients underwent unilateral exploration and adrenalectomy.

Several biochemical and clinical parameters were measured in the preoperative evaluation of patients in this study. Serial blood pressure measurements were obtained, along with preoperative serum potassium levels, plasma aldosterone levels, and plasma renin activity. Plasma aldosterone levels were measured with the patient in the supine and upright positions, whenever possible. We also recorded the duration of documented preoperative hypertension. Preoperative localization of the aldosterone-secreting adenomas was done using CT scanning; 5-mm to 1-cm sections were used in 29 (76%) of the 38 patients treated with open adrenalectomy and 3-mm sections were used in all patients who underwent laparoscopic adrenalectomy. Other methods of localization included selective adrenal vein catheterization to measure the gradient of plasma aldosterone levels, iodocholesterol I 131 adrenal scintigraphy, and NP-59 (^{131}I-6β-iodomethyl-19-norcholesterol) scanning.

We also studied operative approach (posterior or lateral), complication rates, and tumor pathology. Postoperatively, we documented blood pressures and serum potassium levels as indications of cure. The duration of follow-up ranged from 6 months to 6 years for the patients who underwent open adrenalectomy and from 4 months to 3 years for the laparoscopically treated patients.

computed tomographic (CT) scanning have facilitated the imaging of the adrenal glands.[12,13] In addition, the introduction of laparoscopic adrenalectomy has dramatically altered the approach to surgical treatment of patients with primary hyperaldosteronism.

Within the past decade, laparoscopic adrenalectomy has become an increasingly popular surgical treatment for patients with primary hyperaldosteronism, Cushing syndrome, and pheochromocytoma.[4,5,7,9,10] Since 1993 we have performed more than 150 laparoscopic adrenalectomies, including 42 laparoscopic adrenalectomies for primary hyperaldosteronism. Few publications have compared the clinical profiles and outcomes of patients treated with laparoscopic vs open adrenalectomy for primary hyperaldosteronism. We therefore decided to analyze our experience with patients with primary hyperaldosteronism and to determine whether there were differences in demographics, biochemical and clinical presentations, and postoperative outcomes between patients treated with laparoscopic adrenalectomy and those treated with open adrenalectomy.

RESULTS

The 38 patients treated with open adrenalectomy included 6 men and 32 women, with a median age of 35 years. The 42 patients who underwent laparoscopic adrenalectomy included 29 men and 13 women, with a median age of 50 years. There were statistically significant differences in age ($P<.05$, t test) and sex ($P<.05$, χ^2 analysis) between the 2 groups. All patients had documented hypertension on serial blood pressure measurements. The median duration of documented hypertension was 5 years for the patients who underwent open adrenalectomy and 2.5 years for the laparoscopically treated patients. All of the patients treated with open adrenalectomy had a diastolic blood pressure of greater than 100 mm Hg without antihypertensive medications, whereas only 20 (48%) of the 42 patients treated laparoscopically had diastolic blood pressures of greater than 100 mm Hg with no medications.

Preoperative laboratory evaluation included serum potassium levels, plasma renin activity, and plasma aldosterone levels, usually measured with the patient in the supine and upright positions. The median serum potassium level was 2.6 mmol/L in the patients who underwent open adrenalectomy and 3.3 mmol/L in patients treated laparoscopically. There was a statistically significant difference in median serum potassium levels between the 2 groups ($P<.05$, t test). Spironolactone, potassium supplements and, occasionally, amiloride were used to correct preoperative hypokalemia. The mean plasma aldosterone level in patients who underwent open adrenalectomy was 1.47 nmol/L (reference range, <0.86 nmol/L); the mean plasma aldosterone level in laparoscopically treated patients was 1.33 nmol/L. There was no statistical difference in the mean plasma aldosterone levels in the 2 groups. Supine and upright plasma aldosterone levels were measured in 35 patients treated with open adrenalectomy; 34 (97%) exhibited abnormal postural responses (paradoxical decrease or minimal change) in serum aldosterone levels. Abnormal postural responses in plasma aldosterone levels were noted in 14 (93%) of 15 patients who were treated laparoscopically. Plasma renin activity was decreased in all 38 patients who underwent open adrenalectomy and in 39 (93%) of the 42 laparoscopically treated patients.

Preoperative imaging studies differed according to the period during which the operation was performed. The 38 patients treated with open adrenalectomy underwent CT scanning (29 patients), iodocholesterol I 131 adrenal scanning (16 patients), or selective adrenal vein catheterization (11 patients). Iodocholesterol I 131 scanning correctly identified the adenoma in 9 (56%) of 16 patients. Computed tomographic scanning correctly identified the adenoma in 22 (83%) of 29 patients. Selective venous catheterization was conclusive in 9 (82%) of 11 patients and inconclusive in the remaining 2 patients. All of the 42 patients who underwent laparoscopic adrenalectomy were studied with preoperative high-resolution CT scanning using 3-mm sections (as opposed to the 5-mm to 1-cm sections used in the CT scans of the open adrenalectomy patients). Computed tomographic scanning correctly identified the adenoma in 39 (93%) of these 42 patients. Selective venous catheterization was performed in 2 patients who underwent laparoscopic adrenalectomy; both of these studies correctly localized the adenoma. Scanning with NP-59 was used in 1 patient treated with laparoscopic adrenalectomy and correctly identified the adenoma. Of note, none of the adrenal tumors were identified incidentally ("incidentaloma").

Of the 38 patients who underwent adrenalectomy via the open approach, 34 underwent unilateral exploration and adrenalectomy, while 4 patients underwent bilateral adrenal exploration and resection of one adrenal tumor. These 4 bilateral explorations were performed because of equivocal localizing studies, and all occurred between 1975 and 1977, which were the first years of our experience included in this study. The 42 laparoscopically treated patients all underwent unilateral exploration and adrenalectomy.

Twenty-eight (74%) of the patients treated with open adrenalectomy were operated on through a posterior approach, 6 (16%) underwent lateral exploration, and 4 (10%) underwent exploration bilaterally through an anterior approach. The 42 laparoscopically treated patients included 28 (67%) who underwent lateral transabdominal exploration and 14 (33%) who underwent posterior retroperitoneal exploration.

Of the 38 patients who underwent open exploration, 32 had aldosterone-secreting adenomas, 5 had bilateral adrenal hyperplasia, and 1 had adrenocortical carcinoma. The five patients with bilateral adrenal hyperplasia were all thought to have adenomas prior to operation; 2 had false-positive CT scans (showing adenomas that were not found in the pathologic specimen) and 3 had negative CT scans (showing no abnormalities). Two patients with hyperplasia achieved normalization of blood pressure following unilateral adrenalectomy. The 1 patient with adrenocortical carcinoma exhibited all of the preoperative biochemical and symptomatic criteria for an aldosterone-producing adrenal adenoma. He died of disseminated adrenocortical carcinoma 2 years after surgery.

Forty-one (98%) of the 42 patients who underwent laparoscopic adrenalectomy had histologically confirmed adenomas. The one exception in this group was a patient who had a preoperative CT scan that showed a 2-cm left adrenal adenoma and a possible smaller mass in the right adrenal gland. A laparoscopic unilateral left adrenalectomy was performed with removal of a 2-cm adenoma within a hyperplastic cortex; however, the patient continued to be hypokalemic and hypertensive following operation. In retrospect, we found that this patient had bilateral adrenal hyperplasia and a nonfunctioning left adrenal adenoma that could have been diagnosed if a preoperative selective venous catheterization had been performed based on the CT scan showing possible bilateral abnormalities.

Postoperative complications occurred in 4 (11%) of the 38 patients who underwent open adrenal exploration and adrenalectomy. Two patients developed postoperative hypotension and anemia; they required vigorous fluid replacement but no transfusions. Two other patients developed postoperative persistent acidosis and hyperkalemia due to mineralocorticoid deficiency. As mentioned, 1 patient with adrenocortical carcinoma died 2 years after the adrenalectomy. No postoperative complications occurred in the patients who underwent laparoscopic adrenalectomy; the difference in postoperative complication rates between the 2 groups was statistically significant ($P<.05$, Fisher exact test).

Postoperatively, 30 (81%) of the 37 patients who underwent open adrenalectomy for benign disease became normotensive and no longer required postoperative blood pressure medications. Thirty-seven (88%) of the 42 laparoscopically treated patients became normotensive and did not require medications postoperatively. The postoperative serum potassium levels ranged from 3.6 to 5.0 mmol/L in the open adrenalectomy group and from 3.5 to 4.9 mmol/L in the laparoscopic adrenalectomy group. The differences in postoperative blood pressures and serum potassium values were not statistically significant.

COMMENT

The results of this retrospective review document that laparoscopic adrenalectomy is a safe and effective treatment for primary hyperaldosteronism. Laparoscopically treated patients had fewer postoperative complications and were equally likely to improve in blood pressure and hypokalemia when compared with patients treated with open adrenalectomy. Additional benefits of laparoscopic adrenalectomy that were not addressed in this study include smaller incisions, decreased postoperative pain, and shorter hospitalizations, as reported by others.[4,5,7,9,10] All of these factors have contributed to the increasing popularity of laparoscopic adrenalectomy for the treatment of patients with primary hyperaldosteronism and, in many medical centers (including our own), the laparoscopic technique has replaced open surgery as the treatment of choice for this condition and other benign adrenal gland tumors.

Besides providing information regarding the safety and efficacy of laparoscopic vs open adrenalectomy for primary hyperaldosteronism, this study also allows us to comment on changes that have occurred during the past decade in both the diagnosis and clinical presentation at the time of referral of patients with this disease. All of the patients in this study who underwent laparoscopic adrenalectomy were operated on after 1993, whereas patients who were treated with open adrenalectomy underwent surgery between 1975 and 1986. An important technological advancement during the past decade has been the improvement of CT scanning. All patients treated laparoscopically were studied with high-resolution CT scanning (3-mm sections), with an overall sensitivity of 93%. In contrast, the patients treated with open adrenalectomy underwent CT scanning (5-mm to 1-cm sections) or other imaging studies, including iodocholesterol I 131 adrenal scanning and selective adrenal vein catheterization; the sensitivity of CT scanning in this group was 83%. When used in conjunction with the appropriate laboratory tests, high-resolution CT scanning has helped endocrinologists and surgeons to differentiate more accurately between an adrenal adenoma and bilateral adrenal hyperplasia. This observation is supported by the fact that 32 of 38 patients in the open adrenalectomy group and 41 of 42 laparoscopically treated patients were correctly identified preoperatively as having adrenal adenomas; the differentiation between adenoma and hyperplasia in patients with primary hyperaldosteronism is crucial because patients with adenomas are almost always responsive to surgery while those with hyperplasia are best managed medically.[1,13,14]

There were statistically significant differences in the demographic and clinical profiles of patients between the laparoscopic and open groups. Patients who underwent laparoscopic adrenalectomy were older and had been hypertensive for a shorter period of time than patients who were treated with open surgery; in addition, there were more men than women in the laparoscopic group (29 men, 13 women), while the opposite was true in the open surgery group (6 men, 32 women). These differences between the 2 groups lead us to believe that we are currently operating on a different population of patients with primary hyperaldosteronism than we were in previous decades. We offer 2 reasons for this change in patient populations. First, improvements in CT scanning have resulted in the earlier detection of aldosterone-secreting adenomas and have therefore facilitated the diagnosis of patients with less severe disease, including patients whose tumors may have been missed in the decades prior to improved CT scanning. Second, it is possible that the introduction of laparoscopic adrenalectomy has altered the referral patterns of primary care physicians and endocrinologists; these physicians may be referring older patients and patients with less severe disease for surgical treatment because they perceive the laparoscopic procedure to be less invasive and therefore having less morbidity for patients.

In conclusion, the improved sensitivity of CT scanning during the laparoscopic era has improved the diagnosis and localization of adrenal adenomas in patients with primary hyperaldosteronism. Patients who underwent laparoscopic adrenalectomy for primary hyperaldosteronism had less severe hypertension and hypokalemia than patients treated with open adrenalectomy. In addition, patients treated laparoscopically suffered fewer postoperative complications and were equally likely to improve in blood pressure and hypokalemia. As reported in other series, laparoscopic adrenalectomy causes less pain than open adrenalectomy and usually requires only an overnight hospital admission. It has therefore become the procedure of choice for the treatment of patients with primary hyperaldosteronism caused by an aldosterone-secreting adenoma.

Supported in part by UCSF/Mt Zion Health Systems, San Francisco, Calif.

Presented at the 106th Scientific Session of the Western Surgical Association, Indianapolis, Ind, November 18, 1998.

We thank the endocrinologists who have helped us care for these patients: J. B. Tyrrell, MD; P. A. Fitzgerald, MD; M. Schambelan, MD; and E. G. Biglieri, MD.

Corresponding author: Quan-Yang Duh, MD, Surgical Service 112, 4150 Clement St, San Francisco, CA 94121 (e-mail: Quan-Yang.Duh@med.va.gov).

REFERENCES

1. Blumenfeld JD, Sealey JE, Schlussel Y, et al. Diagnosis and treatment of primary hyperaldosteronism. *Ann Intern Med.* 1994;121:877-885.
2. Lo CY, Tam PC, Kung AWC, Lam KS, Wong JW. Primary aldosteronism: results of surgical treatment. *Ann Surg.* 1996;224:125-130.
3. Weigel RJ, Wells SA, Gunnells JC, Leight GS. Surgical treatment of primary hyperaldosteronism. *Ann Surg.* 1994;219:347-352.
4. Staren ED, Prinz RA. Adrenalectomy in the era of laparoscopy. *Surgery.* 1996;120:706-711.
5. Duh QY, Siperstein AE, Clark OH. Laparoscopic adrenalectomy: comparison of the lateral and posterior approaches. *Arch Surg.* 1996;131:870-876.
6. Go H, Takeda M, Imai T, et al. Laparoscopic adrenalectomy for Cushing's syndrome: comparison with primary aldosteronism. *Surgery.* 1995;117:11-17.
7. Korman JE, Ho T, Hiatt JR, Phillips EH. Comparison of laparoscopic and open adrenalectomy. *Am J Surg.* 1997;63:908-912.
8. Celen O, O'Brien MJ, Melby JC, Beazley RM. Factors influencing outcome of surgery for primary aldosteronism. *Arch Surg.* 1996;131:646-650.
9. Stuart RC, Chung SCS, Lau JYW, et al. Laparoscopic adrenalectomy. *Br J Surg.* 1995;82:1498-1499.
10. Takeda, M, Go H, Imai T, Nishiyama T, Morishita H. Laparoscopic adrenalectomy for primary aldosteronism: report of initial ten cases. *Surgery.* 1994;115:621-625.
11. Lim RC, Nakayama DK, Biglieri EG, Schambelan M, Hunt TK. Primary aldosteronism: changing concepts in diagnosis and management. *Am J Surg.* 1986;152:116-121.
12. Sheaves R, Goldin J, Reznek RH, et al. Relative value of computed tomography scanning and venous sampling in establishing the cause of primary hyperaldosteronism. *Eur J Endocrinol.* 1996;134:308-313.
13. Gleason PE, Weinberger MH, Pratt JH, et al. Evaluation of diagnostic tests in the differential diagnosis of primary aldosteronism: unilateral adenoma versus bilateral micronodular hyperplasia. *J Urol.* 1993;150:1365-1368.
14. Feltynowski T, Ignatowska-Switalska H, Wocial B, et al. Postural stimulation test in patients with aldosterone producing adenomas. *Clin Endocrinol.* 1994;41:309-314.

DISCUSSION

Richard A. Prinz, MD, Chicago, Ill: I want to compliment the San Francisco group for continuing to unfold the story of the surgical management of primary hyperaldosteronism for us. This problem, when due to a small, benign unilateral adenoma, is ideally suited for laparoscopic management. The hypertension that these patients have can be reversed with minimal morbidity and risk from the operation. The authors have confirmed the safety and efficacy of the laparoscopic approach in comparison with open adrenalectomy. I was struck by the patient demographic differences in their 2 groups.

First, it seems that the 38 open operations were accumulated during an 11-year period from 1975 to 1986. The laparoscopic patients have all been treated in the last 5 to 6 years. I wonder why there is this hiatus in between the 2 groups? Are you reporting all of the patients treated with primary hyperaldosteronism by the surgeons at UCSF? Clearly, you are seeing more patients now. I think you would have access to your referral sources to tell us if these have widened to explain the increased number of patients? Do you think that, much like laparoscopic cholecystectomy, there has been a loosening of indications for this operation in patients with suspected hyperaldosteronism? The gender and age of the 2 groups are significantly different, with the laparoscopic patients being much older and more commonly male. Is this actually the same disease that you are seeing? It is hard to explain such a change in gender and age characteristics. You would think that you would be diagnosing patients at an earlier age today, rather than a later age.

I would like to touch on your preoperative evaluation. Three of your laparoscopic adrenalectomy patients did not have suppressed plasma renin activity. This is supposed to be one of the hallmarks of this disease. I would like to know, what was the outcome in these 3 patients? Was one of these the patient that you noted as having hyperplasia? More importantly, what is your laboratory criteria for diagnosis of primary hyperaldosteronism? Computed tomographic scanning was used throughout the study. More recently with the laparoscopic patients, 3-mm cuts were used to identify the tumor, and you did so in 39 of the 42 laparoscopically treated patients.

I would ask about the use of NP-59 scanning and selective venous catheterization and how you use these studies in your current practice. Keeping in mind that as many as 2% of patients undergoing CT scanning will have an incidental adrenal nodule identified, do you use these functional localizing studies to rule out an incidental adrenocortical nodule and do you think that the patient who remained hypokalemic and hypertensive after your unilateral laparoscopic adrenalectomy actually had an incidental adrenal cortical adenoma that you initially removed? Both the lateral and posterior retroperitoneal approaches were used in two thirds and one third of the laparoscopically treated patients, respectively. I know a subsequent paper will deal with this issue, but can you comment on the specific advantages of each approach for primary hyperaldosteronism? I would also like to ask you why your follow-up is short for the open adrenalectomy patients. This group offers a unique opportunity for studying the long-term outcome in primary hyperaldosteronism, and I think it would be important for you to share that with us.

Norman Thompson, MD, Ann Arbor, Mich: Mr Shen mentioned that the first patient with an aldosteronoma was operated on at the University of Michigan. I think I am the only person in this room who actually helped to take care of that patient. That was 44 years ago when I was a medical student. She had one of the complications that you mentioned, anemia. However, her anemia was due to the fact that she was in the hospital for 6 months preoperatively and 1 month postoperatively and had blood drawn every day. That was before we had HMOs. Her exploration occurred on December 14, 1954. Jerry Conn was in attendance with William Baum, the urologist who explored her. He was the most junior attending surgeon on the urology service. Reed Nesbitt, who was chief, was not very enthusiastic at that time in this new entity that was proposed by Jerry Conn. The operation proposed was a bilateral adrenalectomy because hyperplasia was the suspected diagnosis. No one had ever described an aldosterone-secreting adenoma before. On exploration, a 4-cm tumor was found in the right adrenal and removed. The first paper on aldosteronism was published 2 months later, almost record time. It was part of Jerry Conn's presidential address to the Society of Clinical Investigation given in October 1954 but included an addendum about this first patient and operation. Looking into the reason for that, the *Journal of Laboratory and Clinical Medicine* was edited by William Robinson, who was chairman of the Department of Internal Medicine at the University of Michigan. With that background, I would like to make a few comments about this particular paper. It is very surprising that you found so many males when in most series 3 of 4 are females. It makes me wonder whether in the era before laparoscopic surgery, males were afraid to be operated on. Could that be the explanation?

The other point is related to early diagnosis. Again, it is hard to understand that patients with a mean age of 50 years compared with those with a mean age of 35 years would suggest earlier diagnosis. There is some discrepancy. You make note that diagnosis of an adenoma was established or suspected by CT scanning. Fortunately, you did point out that CT scanning might detect an incidentaloma rather than an aldosteronoma. I would warn everyone that one can be misled to remove an incidentaloma on the side opposite a small adenoma. Subsequently you could end up with a bilateral adrenalectomy, which would be a real tragedy. We have emphasized the use of NP-59 scintiscanning which, incidentally, was also developed at the University of Michigan. We do that in every patient because we do not want to take out an adrenal that may not have the small adenoma. About 10% of patients have adenomas that are too small to be detected even by either the type of CT you are using or NP-59 scans. In those cases, I think there is a place for selective venous sampling. Dr Clark, tell us what you actually do. Are you taking a risk in not obtaining substantiating localization studies in patients who could have incidentalomas?

Steven DeJong, MD, Maywood, Ill: I have 2 brief questions. Could you give us some information about operative time and pain medication required in your patients as this experience is evolving into the operation of choice or the route of choice for treating patients with surgical hypertension from excess aldosterone production.

Did you use any other technology, such as intra-abdominal laparoscopic ultrasonography, when operating on these patients? Was it helpful? These are relatively small tumors compared with some of the other adrenal tumors that we deal with and some have reported that this technology might be helpful.

Dr Clark: One weakness of our study is that we compared our laparoscopically treated patients with patients who had previously been treated by open adrenalectomy at our medical center and were previously reported by Dr Robert Lim. This difference certainly contributed to the variation in patient profiles in the 2 groups. The short-term follow-up in our open group was because no one has done a long-term outlook study in these patients. During the period we did open adrenalectomies, it was more difficult to make the diagnosis of primary hyperaldosteronism as assays for aldosterone and renin were not as accurate as they are today and localization tests were not as sensitive. Thus, for almost all of our initial (open) group of patients, a referring endocrinologist would send his patients to another endocrinologist at UCSF who specialized in adrenal tumors and hypertension.

Dr Prinz asked if there is a loosening of indications for laparoscopic adrenalectomy similar to that observed for cholecystectomy, and the answer we believe is yes. He also asked why the change in demographics? We are not sure. In the laparoscopic group, 9 operations were done at the VA Medical Center in San Francisco, but this would not completely account for the predominance of men in our laparoscopic group since most endocrine diseases are more common in women. Has the disease changed? I do not think so. We make the diagnosis the same way it was done previously, that is, by documenting an increased aldosterone level in a patient with a low renin level. More postural studies were done in our open group. In patients with an adrenocortical adenoma the aldosterone levels would paradoxically fall or fail to increase with standing whereas in normal patients and in those with hyperplasia, the aldosterone levels usually increased with standing.

Dr Thompson asked a very important question regarding the possibility of an adrenal "incidentaloma" in patients with primary hyperaldosteronism. This is a real possibility since adrenal incidentalomas occur in about 1.5% of the population. For example, a patient with primary hyperaldosteronism could have a coexisting nonfunctioning adrenocortical adenoma. Our one failure in our laparoscopic group might have been prevented if we had done postural studies or adrenal vein catheterization studies for aldosterone and cortical levels preoperatively. I would strongly recommend that such studies be done for any patient when hyperplasia (bilateral disease) is a possibility. Scanning with NP-59 might also be useful in such patients as suggested by Dr Norman Thompson, but we have limited experience with this study.

In this retrospective study, we did not compare duration of hospitalization, postoperative pain, or time taken to return to work. These data have been reported by others and after laparoscopic adrenalectomy, patients can be hospitalized for a shorter time, experience less pain, and return to work sooner. However, after an open Hugh-Young (posterior) approach, most patients could also go home within 24 hours.

Dr DeJong, our duration of operation was initially about 3 hours, but now takes less time. These procedures are done with our surgical residents and most have been directed by Dr Siperstein and Dr Duh. Intraoperative ultrasound is quite useful, especially in some of the heavier patients. Most adrenocortical adenomas that cause primary hyperaldosteronism are small (<2-cm) tumors. Intraoperative ultrasound certainly helps identify these tumors.

ARCHIVES OF SURGERY

SUBSCRIPTION ORDER FORM

YES! Enter my personal subscription to ***Archives of Surgery*** at the special money saving rate checked below:

- ❑ AMA Member rate: One year (12 issues) — $95*.
- ❑ Individual non-member rate: One year (12 issues) — $145*.
- ❑ Corporate/Institutional rate: One year (12 issues) — $245.
- ❑ *My personal check in U.S. $ is enclosed. (Make check payable to *American Medical Association*).
- ❑ Charge my personal credit card: ❑ VISA ❑ MASTERCARD ❑ AMEX ❑ OPTIMA

Card No.________ Exp. Date______ Signature________

Name (Please print) ________

Address ________

City________ State/Province______ Zip/Postal Code ______

Phone________ Fax________ e-mail ________

IMPORTANT: The individual non-member rate is available in the U.S. and Canada only. Payment must accompany order. Corporate/ Institutional checks are not accepted for personal subscriptions. Canada residents add 7% GST. GST # (12622 5556 RT). **I9X2DZ**

ARCHIVES OF SURGERY

SUBSCRIPTION ORDER FORM

YES! Enter my personal subscription to ***Archives of Surgery*** at the special money saving rate checked below:

- ❑ AMA Member rate: One year (12 issues) — $95*.
- ❑ Individual non-member rate: One year (12 issues) — $145*.
- ❑ Corporate/Institutional rate: One year (12 issues) — $245.
- ❑ *My personal check in U.S. $ is enclosed. (Make check payable to *American Medical Association*).
- ❑ Charge my personal credit card: ❑ VISA ❑ MASTERCARD ❑ AMEX ❑ OPTIMA

Card No.________ Exp. Date______ Signature________

Name (Please print) ________

Address ________

City________ State/Province______ Zip/Postal Code ______

Phone________ Fax________ e-mail ________

IMPORTANT: The individual non-member rate is available in the U.S. and Canada only. Payment must accompany order. Corporate/ Institutional checks are not accepted for personal subscriptions. Canada residents add 7% GST. GST # (12622 5556 RT). **I9X2DZ**

NO POSTAGE
NECESSARY
IF MAILED
IN THE
UNITED STATES

BUSINESS REPLY MAIL
FIRST-CLASS MAIL PERMIT NO. 1376 CHICAGO IL

POSTAGE WILL BE PAID BY ADDRESSEE

SUBSCRIBER SERVICES CENTER
AMERICAN MEDICAL ASSOCIATION
PO BOX 10945
CHICAGO IL 60610-9902

NO POSTAGE
NECESSARY
IF MAILED
IN THE
UNITED STATES

BUSINESS REPLY MAIL
FIRST-CLASS MAIL PERMIT NO. 1376 CHICAGO IL

POSTAGE WILL BE PAID BY ADDRESSEE

SUBSCRIBER SERVICES CENTER
AMERICAN MEDICAL ASSOCIATION
PO BOX 10945
CHICAGO IL 60610-9902

NO POSTAGE
NECESSARY
IF MAILED
IN THE
UNITED STATES

BUSINESS REPLY MAIL
FIRST-CLASS MAIL PERMIT NO. 1376 CHICAGO IL

POSTAGE WILL BE PAID BY ADDRESSEE

SUBSCRIBER SERVICES CENTER
AMERICAN MEDICAL ASSOCIATION
PO BOX 10945
CHICAGO IL 60610-9902

ARCHIVES OF SURGERY

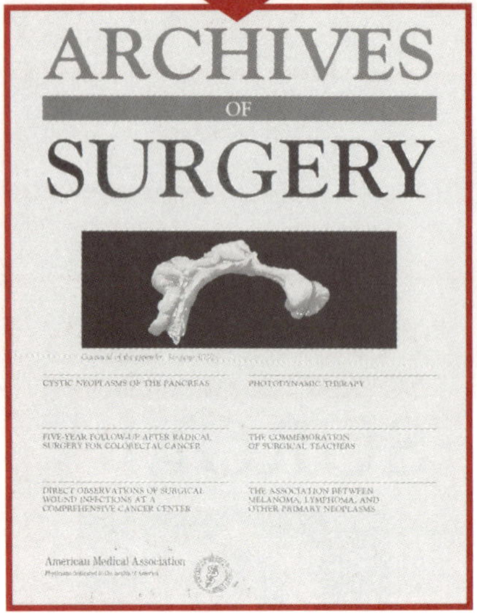

Essential reading to stay on the cutting-edge of clinical developments...

SUBSCRIBE NOW!

NO RISK GUARANTEE:

If you are not completely satisfied with your first issue, you may cancel and receive a full refund of your subscription payment. Or, if at any time, *Archives of Surgery* stops meeting your needs, you may cancel and receive a full refund of all unmailed issues.

PAPER

Short Esophagus

Analysis of Predictors and Clinical Implications

Otávio L. Gastal, MD; Jeffrey A. Hagen, MD; Jeffrey H. Peters, MD; Guilherme M. R. Campos, MD; Majid Hashemi, MD; Jörg Theisen, MD; Cedric G. Bremner, MD; Tom R. DeMeester, MD

Hypothesis: Preoperative assessment can identify the predictors of esophageal shortening in patients with gastroesophageal reflux disease.

Design and Setting: Patient comparison study in a university-based tertiary care center.

Patients: A total of 236 patients with gastroesophageal reflux disease underwent primary antireflux procedures. Sixty-five patients were suspected of having a short esophagus and underwent a transthoracic approach. In 37 patients, a lengthening procedure was necessary to avoid tension on the repair. The remaining 28 patients were thought—after complete esophageal mobilization—to have sufficient length for a repair without needing a gastroplasty. An abdominal approach (laparoscopic Nissen fundoplication) was performed on 171 patients judged to have normal esophageal length.

Main Outcome Measures: Univariate and multivariate analyses of preoperative variables were performed to identify predictors of a short esophagus.

Results: On univariate analysis, manometric esophageal length below the fifth percentile of normal was associated with esophageal shortening. On multivariate analysis, only the presence of an esophageal stricture predicted the need for a Collis gastroplasty (odds ratio, 7.5). The presence of Barrett's esophagus of 3 cm or greater identified patients in whom the transthoracic esophageal mobilization alone was sufficient (odds ratio, 3.4).

Conclusions: The presence of a stricture was associated with esophageal shortening sufficient to require a gastroplasty. Transthoracic esophageal mobilization alone was usually sufficient to perform a safe repair without tension in patients with a Barrett's esophagus of 3 cm or greater.

Arch Surg. 1999;134:633-638

THE INCREASING popularity of laparoscopic antireflux repairs with associated shorter recovery time and greater patient acceptability has increased the number of patients referred for surgical therapy. The 2 most common causes of technical failure in these patients are the low placement of the fundoplication and herniation of the fundoplication into the chest.[1] Such complications are likely to occur when the esophagus is short or when mobilization is inadequate.[2]

Esophageal shortening occurs most commonly in patients with advanced reflux disease due to acid-related inflammatory changes in the muscular wall of the esophagus. On healing, this results in contracture.[3] Although severe degrees of esophageal shortening are obvious on a contrast esophagogram, subtler degrees of acquired shortening are difficult to detect. As a result, acquired esophageal shortening remains a potential cause of treatment failure with the laparoscopic approach. The purpose of this study was to identify clinical markers of a short esophagus in patients with gastroesophageal reflux disease (GERD) to avoid failure of laparoscopic antireflux surgery.

RESULTS

Of the 236 patients with GERD and adequate esophageal peristalsis who underwent fundoplication, 37 (15.7%) had objective evidence of esophageal shortening. In these patients, esophageal lengthening was required, despite complete esophageal mobilization at thoracotomy, to reduce the gastroesophageal junction without tension. In an additional 28 patients (11.9%), extensive esophageal mobilization by the transthoracic approach was sufficient. The remaining 171 patients were judged clinically to have an esophagus of normal length. All of these

From the Departments of Surgery (Drs Gastal, Peters, Campos, Hashemi, Theisen, Bremner, and DeMeester) and Cardiothoracic Surgery (Dr Hagen), University of Southern California School of Medicine, Los Angeles.

POPULATION AND METHODS

STUDY POPULATION

From January 1992 to December 1997, 248 patients with symptomatic GERD underwent primary antireflux procedures at the University of Southern California University Hospital. There were 162 males and 86 females, with a median age of 51 years (range, 15-81 years). All had increased esophageal acid exposure, confirmed by 24-hour pH monitoring using a glass electrode (Ingold Inc, Urdorf, Switzerland) positioned 5 cm above the upper border of the lower esophageal sphincter determined on manometry. Increased esophageal acid exposure was defined when the DeMeester composite acid score was above 14.7.[4,5] Preoperative evaluation included a video-contrast esophagogram, upper endoscopy with routine biopsies of the gastroesophageal junction and lower esophagus, and stationary esophageal motility.

SELECTION OF OPERATIVE PROCEDURE

Our previously published selection algorithm[6] determined the operative procedure performed (**Figure 1**). Patients who appeared on clinical grounds to have normal esophageal length underwent laparoscopic Nissen fundoplication according to our previously published technique,[7] including complete mobilization of the fundus with division of the short gastric vessels and crural closure. Esophageal shortening was suspected preoperatively in patients with a hiatal hernia of 5 cm or larger, a nonreducible hernia, or an esophageal stricture. The presence of 1 or more of these features excluded the laparoscopic approach and directed a transthoracic antireflux procedure.[8]

For patients who underwent a transthoracic procedure, the length of their esophagus was assessed after it had been mobilized from the diaphragmatic hiatus up to the aortic arch. The gastroesophageal junction was marked with a stitch. If the length of the esophagus after mobilization did not allow the stitch to be placed without tension in the abdomen, a Collis gastroplasty and Belsey partial fundoplication were performed.[9] Patients who were judged after mobilization to have sufficient esophageal length to allow a tension-free repair underwent a transthoracic Nissen fundoplication.[10]

Based on preoperative manometric, endoscopic, and radiologic evaluation, 12 patients were identified as having ineffective esophageal body motility. These patients underwent a partial fundoplication without gastroplasty and were excluded from analysis, as were those with type II or III paraesophageal hernias. Of the remaining 236 patients with effective esophageal motility, 65 were suspected of having a short esophagus on clinical grounds and had an antireflux procedure performed using a transthoracic approach. Of these patients, 28 were judged intraoperatively to have sufficient esophageal length, whereas 37 required an additional lengthening procedure (Collis gastroplasty). During the same period, 171 patients judged to have normal esophageal length on clinical grounds underwent a laparoscopic antireflux procedure and were included as a comparison group.

STUDY VARIABLES

The following variables were submitted to multivariate analyses to identify factors associated with the procedures performed: age, sex, height, weight, obesity, radiologic stricture, size and reducibility of hiatal hernia, esophagitis, presence and length of Barrett's esophagus, and manometric esophageal length. Obesity was defined by a body mass index (a measure of weight in kilograms divided by the square of height in meters) of 28 or more. Radiologic stricture was defined as any nonneoplastic segmental narrowing of the esophagus, excluding esophageal rings and webs. Size of a hiatal hernia, when present, was assessed radiologically using 5 liquid barium swallows in the prone position. Reducibility of the hiatal hernia was assessed on assumption of the upright position at the time of esophagram. Esophagitis was defined as the presence of linear or confluent erosions in the distal esophagus (Savary grades II and III) on preoperative endoscopy. Length of Barrett's columnar-lined esophagus was measured by endoscopy and confirmed by histologic biopsy. Manometric esophageal length was measured from the lower border of the upper esophageal sphincter to the upper border of the lower esophageal sphincter. A diagnosis of manometric esophageal shortening was made when measurements fell below the fifth percentile value of 95 asymptomatic volunteers (males, 19.1 cm; females, 18.3 cm).

A physician other than the responsible surgeon assessed symptomatic outcome in all patients by means of a standardized questionnaire. Outcome was considered excellent if the patient was asymptomatic, good if symptoms were relieved but minor gastrointestinal complaints (eg, bloating or flatulence) persisted, fair if the symptoms were improved but medical therapy was necessary for complete relief, and poor if the symptoms were not improved. Particular attention was made to determine whether the primary symptom responsible for surgical referral was relieved. Whenever possible, patients who had an unsatisfactory outcome underwent endoscopy and/or video esophagogram to determine the cause of failure.

STATISTICS

Stepwise logistic regression was performed to identify independent associations with the different surgical procedures. The Fisher exact test was used to compare proportions. Manometric esophageal length in patients and volunteers was compared by analysis of variance. Statistical significance was considered at $\alpha < .05$ for all analyses.

patients were found to have adequate esophageal length at the time of operation and had a laparoscopic Nissen fundoplication performed. Patient characteristics in the 3 treatment groups are shown in **Table 1**.

Average manometric esophageal length for the 3 treatment groups and in normal subjects is shown in **Figure 2**. All reflux patients had a shorter esophagus on average than normal subjects. Furthermore, patients who underwent a transthoracic procedure had a shorter mean esophageal length than the laparoscopic Nissen group and normal subjects. However, individual variability in the treatment groups did not allow the identi-

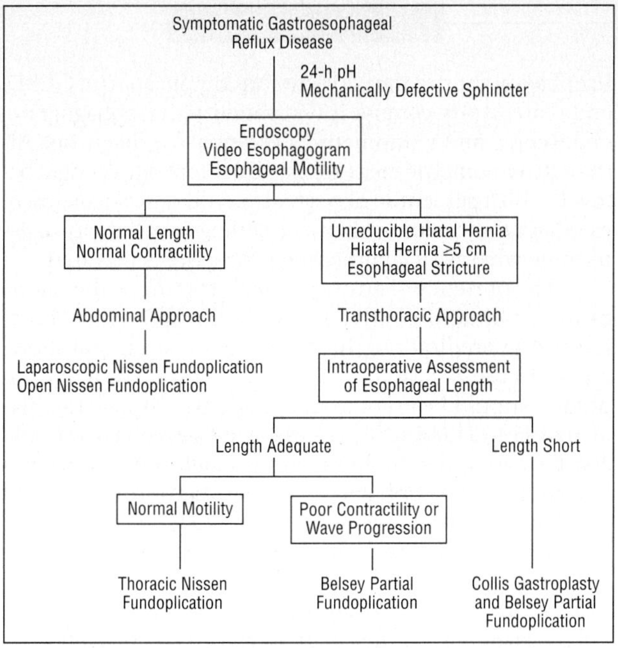

Figure 1. *Algorithm for the selection of antireflux procedures on the basis of clinical and functional evaluation.*

fication of a threshold value below which a short esophagus can be reliably determined to exist.

The prevalence of hiatal hernia, Barrett's esophagus, and strictures in the treatment groups is shown in **Table 2**. On multivariate analysis of patients who had a transthoracic procedure, the presence of an esophageal stricture identified those in whom a gastroplasty was likely to be required after esophageal mobilization (odds ratio, 7.5). Transthoracic esophageal mobilization alone appeared to be sufficient for patients with a long segment (≥3 cm) of Barrett's esophagus (odds ratio, 3.4) (**Table 3**). The combined presence of a hiatal hernia of 5 cm or greater and an esophageal stricture was strongly associated with the need for a gastroplasty ($P<.001$). This was not so for the combination of a 5-cm or longer hiatal hernia and a 3-cm or longer Barrett's esophagus.

An excellent or good outcome was achieved in 89% of patients in the gastroplasty group, 93% in the esophageal mobilization group, and 91% in the laparoscopic group. There were no significant differences in outcome between treatment groups.

In patients with fair or poor outcome, objective documentation of the cause of failure was identified in 9 of 15 in the laparoscopic Nissen group and in all 8 patients in the transthoracic groups. Of the 9 patients who underwent laparoscopic Nissen fundoplication with a fair or poor outcome who also underwent diagnostic studies, 6 had technical failure of the fundoplication (wrap disruption with or without herniation). In contrast, there were no technical failures in the 8 patients with unsatisfactory outcome in the transthoracic groups. Rather, 5 had persistent difficulty with stricture, 2 had excessive bloating and diarrhea, and 1 had postthoracotomy pain. The likelihood of technical failure as the cause of an unsatisfactory outcome was significantly different (6 of 9 vs 0 of 8; $P=.01$).

Table 1. Patient Characteristics

Variables	Collis Gastroplasty	Esophageal Mobilization	Laparoscopic Procedure	*P*
Sex, M/F	25/12	13/15	116/55	.08
Age ≥50 y	25/37	20/28	82/171	.01
Obesity	14/37	15/28	73/151	.43

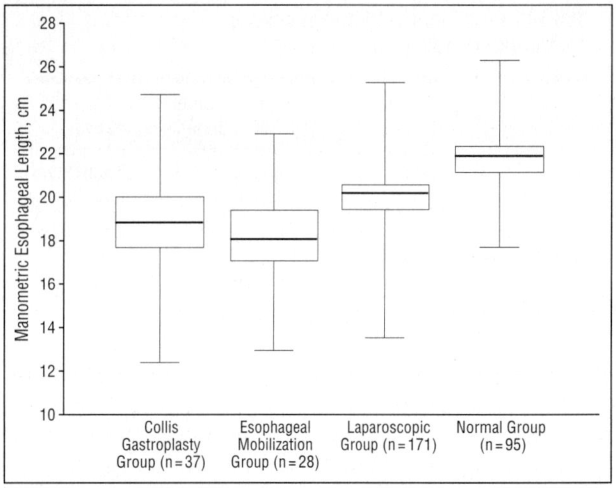

Figure 2. *Mean manometric esophageal length in patients and volunteers. Error bars indicate 2 SEMs. For the Collis gastroplasty and esophageal mobilization groups,* $P=.39$. *For the laparoscopic group,* $P<.001$ *for comparison with the Collis gastroplasty and mobilization groups. For the normal group,* $P<.001$ *for comparison with all other groups.*

COMMENT

Acquired esophageal shortening, when unrecognized, remains a threat to the success of transabdominal or laparoscopic antireflux procedures. Although severe esophageal shortening may be easily detected on a contrast esophagram, the diagnosis of milder degrees of esophageal shortening remains subjective. In an attempt to define objective criteria for the preoperative identification of the short esophagus, we used the need for a gastroplasty for esophageal lengthening as the defining criteria for the existence of a short esophagus. The results of our study suggest that a combination of preoperative findings can be used to identify patients at risk for the presence of esophageal shortening in whom a transthoracic procedure is advisable.

Overall, 28% of our study population had evidence suggesting esophageal shortening. In 16% of patients, there was unequivocal esophageal shortening, despite complete esophageal mobilization at thoracotomy; in 12%, tension-free reduction of the hiatal hernia could be accomplished after thorough transthoracic esophageal mobilization. A similar high prevalence of esophageal shortening was reported by Swanstrom et al[11] in patients with GERD who underwent laparoscopic antireflux surgery. Since a short esophagus may be the most important factor resulting in the 2 most common causes of failure,[1,2] preoperative recognition of a short esophagus is critical to the successful outcome of laparoscopic fundoplication.

Pearson et al[9] first suggested that patients with esophageal strictures may also have longitudinal shortening of

Table 2. Preoperative Assessment

Variables	Collis Gastroplasty	Esophageal Mobilization	*P*
Hiatal hernia ≥5 cm	18/37	17/28	.45
Barrett's esophagus ≥3 cm	3/37	10/28	.01
Obesity	17/37	7/28	.12

Table 3. Predictors of Short Esophagus on Multivariate Analysis

Variables	Odds Ratio (95% Confidence Interval)	
	Collis Gastroplasty	Esophageal Mobilization
Stricture	7.5 (3.3-16.7)	1.6 (0.6-4.4)
Barrett's esophagus ≥3 cm	0.3 (0.06-1.0)	3.4 (1.4-8.6)

the esophagus. They and others[12] suggest that partial fundoplication in combination with Collis gastroplasty is the treatment of choice for such patients. Our results support this approach in that to perform a tension-free repair, transthoracic esophageal mobilization was necessary in the presence of a long segment of Barrett's esophagus, but true esophageal shortening requiring a gastroplasty was likely in the presence of an esophageal stricture.

The association between severe esophagitis, stricture formation, and esophageal shortening is supported by previously published experimental findings.[13,14] In these studies, reflux composed of acid, biliary, and pancreatic secretions has been shown to allow penetration of H^+ ions into the deeper layers of the esophageal wall, resulting in fibrosis. This fibrotic reaction leads to retraction of the esophagus and shortening.

We have shown that, in patients with GERD and clinical evidence of esophageal shortening, esophageal length on manometry was shorter and differed significantly from normal subjects. However, there was considerable individual variability. As a consequence, there was no threshold value below which esophageal shortening could be identified reliably.

Our results suggest that the presence of a short esophagus should be suspected in patients with a hiatal hernia of 5 cm or more, either alone or in combination with a stricture or long-segment Barrett's esophagus. In the presence of these factors, esophageal shortening sufficient to require a gastroplasty was found in more than 58%. Whether these patients can be effectively managed by laparoscopy and extensive transhiatal esophageal mobilization remains to be determined. However, the fact that treatment failed in 6 of the 9 patients in the laparoscopy group because of technical reasons related to unrecognized shortening—despite our conservative approach to patient selection—would suggest that the liberal use of transthoracic antireflux procedures may be advisable. Whether the recently described techniques of laparoscopic gastroplasty will reduce the need for the more invasive transthoracic approach awaits further study.

CONCLUSIONS

Esophageal shortening is a common complication of GERD, and a careful preoperative investigation with esophagogram, endoscopy, and manometry is essential for diagnosis. Although manometric measurements of esophageal length below the fifth percentile of normal should raise suspicion of esophageal shortening, they lack sufficient specificity to determine whether a lengthening procedure is required.

The presence of an esophageal stricture, either alone or in combination with a hiatal hernia of 5 cm or more, is a strong predictor of the presence of esophageal shortening. In these patients, the need for a transthoracic approach should be emphasized. Patients with a large hiatal hernia and long segments of Barrett's esophagus should also be managed with thoracotomy to allow complete mobilization of the esophagus and an evaluation of the esophageal length to achieve the goal of a tension-free antireflux repair in patients with advanced disease.

Presented at the 106th Scientific Session of the Western Surgical Association, Indianapolis, Ind, November 17, 1998.

Corresponding author: Jeffrey A. Hagen, MD, Department of Surgery, University of Southern California School of Medicine, 1441 Eastlake Ave, Suite 7418, Los Angeles, CA 90033-4612 (e-mail: hagen@hsc.usc.edu).

REFERENCES

1. Law SYK, Hagen JA, Kauer WK, DeMeester TR. Reoperation for failed antireflux procedures. In: Bremner CG, DeMeester TR, Peracchia A, eds. *Modern Approach to Benign Esophageal Disease.* St Louis, Mo: Quality Medical Publishing Inc; 1995:183-190.
2. Peters JH, DeMeester TR. The lessons of failed antireflux repairs. In: Peters JH, DeMeester TR, eds. *Minimally Invasive Surgery of the Foregut.* St Louis, Mo: Quality Medical Publishers Inc; 1994:188-196.
3. Pearson FG. Hiatus hernia and gastroesophageal reflux: indications for surgery and selection of operation. *Semin Thorac Cardiovasc Surg.* 1997;9:163-168.
4. DeMeester TR, Wang CI, Wernly JA, et al. Technique, indications, and clinical use of 24-hour esophageal pH monitoring. *J Thorac Cardiovasc Surg.* 1980;79:656-670.
5. Johnson LF, DeMeester TR. Development of the 24-hour intraesophageal pH monitoring composite scoring system. *J Clin Gastroenterol.* 1986;8(suppl 1):52-58.
6. Kauer WK, Peters JH, DeMeester TR, Heimbucher J, Ireland AP, Bremner CG. A tailored approach to antireflux surgery. *J Thorac Cardiovasc Surg.* 1995;110:141-146.
7. Peters JH, DeMeester TR, Crookes P, et al. The treatment of gastroesophageal reflux disease with laparoscopic Nissen fundoplication: prospective evaluation of 100 patients with "typical" symptoms. *Ann Surg.* 1998;228:40-50.
8. Peters JH, DeMeester TR. Indications, principles of procedure selection, and technique of laparoscopic Nissen fundoplication. *Semin Laparoscopic Surg.* 1995;2:27-44.
9. Pearson FG, Langer B, Henderson RD. Gastroplasty and Belsey hiatus hernia repair: an operation for the management of peptic stricture with acquired short esophagus. *J Thorac Cardiovasc Surg.* 1971;61:50-63.
10. DeMeester TR. Nissen fundoplication for gastroesophageal reflux disease: the "DeMeester" modification—technique and results. *Dis Esophagus.* 1996;9:263-271.
11. Swanstrom LL, Marcus DR, Galloway GQ. Laparoscopic Collis gastroplasty is the treatment of choice for the shortened esophagus [see comments]. *Am J Surg.* 1996;171:477-481.
12. Bonavina L, Fontebasso V, Bardini R, Baessato M, Peracchia A. Surgical treatment of reflux stricture of the oesophagus. *Br J Surg.* 1993;80:317-320.
13. Lillemoe KD, Johnson LF, Harmon JW. Taurodeoxycholate modulates the effects of pepsin and trypsin in experimental esophagitis. *Surgery.* 1985;97:662-667.
14. Gozzetti G, Pilotti V, Spangaro M, et al. Pathophysiology and natural history of acquired short esophagus. *Surgery.* 1987;102:507-514.

DISCUSSION

Richard C. Thirlby, MD, Seattle, Wash: This presentation of a manuscript typifies the strength of previous work from the USC group. This study looks at surgery for GERD as a complex disease entity that requires flexibility in the evaluation of surgical treatment. Most operations that we perform are anatomic. We relieve obstructions, close holes, or remove diseased organs.

Surgery for GERD is unique in that it requires repair of altered physiology. Unfortunately, too many operations for GERD are being performed by surgeons with little or no formal training in the physiologic management of GERD, with only one surgical approach to the whole patient population: the laparoscopic Nissen. Perhaps in no other current area of general surgery could our specialty be subject to the valid criticism of the adage, "If all you have is a hammer, everything looks like a nail." The USC group exemplifies the ideal. Each patient is studied carefully and surgical treatment is individualized. For that reason, they are to be congratulated.

However, at this point, my agreement with the work presented today ceases. I must confess, I reviewed the abstract with Luke Hill and Don Low at the Mason Clinic last week. Since I am a politically correct kind of guy, I cannot repeat their assessment of this study. I can paraphrase their thoughts, however. In a nutshell, we disagree with most of the conclusions presented today. First and foremost, we believe the term *short esophagus* is misleading. Sliding hiatal hernias no more shorten the esophagus than sliding groin hernias shorten the colon. The stomach migrates into the chest, and the esophagus contracts. Reduction of the hernia will restore esophageal length in all cases. The combined experience at the Mason Clinic by Luke Hill and Don Low now exceeds 3500 operations for GERD, with no cases of short esophagus requiring Collis gastroplasty. In all cases, the stomach was reduced and the esophagus anchored in the abdomen. Good-to-excellent results are achieved in 80% to 90% of patients at 15 to 20-year follow-up. Clearly, the contention that a 5 cm hiatal hernia implies a short esophagus is simply not true.

What about strictures? In patients with GERD and esophageal strictures, primary Hill repairs result in good-to-excellent results in about 90% of cases, with patients requiring only 1 or 2 perioperative dilatations. Patients requiring multiple dilatations during the years prior to presentation to the surgeon do poorly, yet only about half report good results in long-term follow-up. All strictures therefore are not alike. Most patients with GERD and strictures can be handled with standard operative procedures combined with perioperative dilatation. On the other hand, the patient with strictures who has been dilated every month for years will not do well with any simple operation, whether it be the Hill, the Nissen, or the Collis gastroplasty.

My first question for the authors relates to the management of patients with strictures. What is your recommendation for the treatment of patients with strictures who have been dilated innumerable times? Impaired motility in this segment will likely result in poor results after any procedure. We believe that many of these patients are best served with up-front resections.

What are your criteria for resection and reconstruction? Similarly, what are your recommendations for open abdominal procedures? Getting back to my original suggestion that not all patients are best treated with a laparoscopic Nissen procedure, we believe that some patients with large hernias are best treated with open, abdominal procedures facilitating anchoring of the abdomen.

And what about the Collis gastroplasty? I find it puzzling that Dr DeMeester's group would, on the one hand, operate on patients and publish papers devoted to the elimination of the Barrett's esophagus and then, on the other hand, tell us today to surgically create an iatrogenic Barrett's esophagus. The Collis gastroplasty creates an aperistaltic neoesophagus lined with acid-secreting parietal cell mucosa. Over one third of these patients will have esophagitis at follow-up, and nearly one half will have an aperistaltic neoesophagus. In both theory and practice, this is a bad operation.

With regard to the other conclusions presented today, I have a few problems. The abstract states that on multivariate analysis, the presence of a hiatal hernia greater than 5 cm remains strongly associated with transthoracic approach. I thought they chose the transthoracic approach when there was a long hiatal hernia. In other words, the conclusions were predetermined. With respect to the conclusion that when a stricture is present, a lengthening procedure is likely to be required, I have an alternate conclusion. Thirty-seven of 65 patients operated on via the transthoracic approach required a Collis gastroplasty, whereas none of 171 patients undergoing the abdominal approach required a Collis gastroplasty. I believe the most accurate conclusion one can reach from these data is that the transthoracic approach limits the ability to mobilize and adequately anchor the esophagus in the abdomen and therefore, increases the chance of needing to perform the Collis procedure. In other words, I believe the correct take-home message from the data presented today is, "Don't operate through the chest if the patient has a large hiatal hernia."

My final question relates to perhaps the most notable deficiency in the presentation: the lack of good outcomes data. What is the duration of follow-up? The bottom line should always be, "how are the patients doing?" Can the authors tell us more about the patients who had the iatrogenic Barrett's or Collis procedure? Is there any endoscopic or manometric follow-up in these patients? Have there been any problems with esophageal ulcers, poor motility, etc?

In closing, Luke Hill and Don Low asked me to repeat to all of you their standing offer: If any of you have a patient with an apparent short esophagus that you anticipate being unable to reduce, send the patient to Seattle, and they will fix it free of charge.

Ronald A. Hinder, MD, Jacksonville, Fla: I also believe that the short esophagus is extremely rare, and speak for many surgeons with a large experience in this disease. I would estimate that a truly short esophagus exists in less than 1% of patients who are operated on for GERD. I also wish to ask the authors why they subject 20% or 30% of their patients to a thoracotomy when a laparoscopy is so simple. A very small proportion of patients will fail due to a short esophagus; and in those patients, more extensive surgery can take place as a redo. Why should we subject 12% of patients to an unnecessary thoracotomy?

Philip E. Donahue, MD, Chicago, Ill: Ten percent of the patients with either operation fail, laparoscopic or the transthoracic. I wonder if you could say a word about patterns of failure. Was reflux a problem, or are you talking about other problems such as mechanical slippage of the wrap into the chest?

Jay L. Grosfeld, MD, Indianapolis, Ind: Were any of these patients reoperative candidates, and would you ever perform a Collis gastroplasty on someone who has had previous antireflux surgery?

Dr Peters: I also thank Dr Hinder and the other discussants, particularly Dr Thirlby for his kind comments. I am grateful for the fact that Dr Hill and perhaps the remainder of the Mason Clinic group are not here as well.

The discussants certainly highlight the controversy surrounding the short esophagus, which is why we felt the need and the importance of putting together our paper. As you heard, the very existence of the short esophagus is controversial, let alone how to identify it once it exists. We believe firmly that it does exist. Dr Gastal's lead slide pointed out that the major reasons for failure of antireflux procedures were reherniation and/or slippage of the wrap. Both are a likely consequence of the short esophagus. I note that Dr Hinder has a paper tomorrow with similar findings.

Dr Thirlby questions the problem of stricture management. Patients with strictures are indeed a very difficult population, particularly those, as you pointed out, who require repeated dilatations. Primary resection is a consideration in these patients, although the need is relatively rare. Generally, an attempt at an antireflux repair of some sort is warranted unless the esophagus is completely failed. We've performed 7 or 8 primary resections in some 10 years of practice in our group for reflux disease. This is relatively new, but it *does* exist.

You asked whether there is an indication for an open transabdominal approach. I don't think so these days, with the exception of patients who may have extensive previous abdominal surgery or perhaps, with Dr Hinder's paper in mind tomorrow, the population of redo patients. Most abdominal procedures can now be performed laparoscopically, and I don't think there is a great advantage to reducing the hernia or lengthening the esophagus by performing the procedure open abdominally rather than laparoscopically.

Is a Collis gastroplasty an iatrogenic Barrett's esophagus? That's not entirely correct. Remember, Barrett's esophagus is colonic tissue, not gastric tissue by the way we define it today. Its major risk is the development of adenocarcinoma, and it is non-acid--secreting tissue. I think that is stretching the discussion a bit unrealistically.

All of these were primary procedures. At last year's Western Surgical, we presented our series of primary Collis gastroplasties with an 85% to 90% success rate, and I refer you to that paper for the results of our primary gastroplasty group.

Have we used circular reasoning with regard to how we selected our patients? No. As you may have noticed in the presentation, variables such as criteria, a large and/or a fixed hiatal hernia which we used as criteria for procedure selection, were removed from analysis. The study variables that were significant, that is, Barrett's esophagus greater than 3 cm or the presence or absence of a stricture, were not criteria for procedure selection.

Does the transthoracic approach limit mobilization? Of course not. It is clear that you can mobilize the esophagus more transthoracically than you can transabdominally without injury to the vagus. This fact is self-evident to those performing both transabdominal and transthoracic procedures.

Mean follow-up time was 36 months, and was slightly longer for the open group than for the laparoscopic group.

Dr Hinder brought up the point that shortening of the esophagus and esophageal mobilization should be rare, less than 1% of the patients. This gets back to the controversy of whether the short esophagus even exists. Again, we feel that it does. I point out, Dr Hinder, that Lee Swanstrom has found a 16% incidence of esophageal shortening defined by the need for a Collis gastroplasty in his laparoscopic group. It seems others are also seeing this.

I don't think that we should take the approach of doing laparoscopic procedures on everyone and falling back on a second operation on those who fail. The long-term results of second antireflux procedures are clearly not as good.

Dr Donahue points out that 10% of these patients fail, no matter what we do. It is true that there is an incidence of failure with anti-reflux surgery. It is around 10% if you do it well. Most of this tailored concept comes out of the fact that, in the early days, the incidence of failure in patients with severe disease, ie, those with strictures and large hernias, was in the range of 50%. We think we are doing better than that now.

Dr Grosfeld, none of these were reoperative procedures, but we do do Collis procedures for the reoperative population.

PAPER

Endoscopic Ultrasound and Fine Needle Aspiration for the Evaluation of Pancreatic Masses

Jason Suits, BS; Richard Frazee, MD; Richard A. Erickson, MD

Hypothesis: Endoscopic ultrasound (EUS) and endoscopic ultrasound–guided fine needle aspiration (EUS-FNA) are accurate for the preoperative staging of pancreatic ductal carcinoma.

Design: Retrospective medical record review.

Patients: A prospective registry of 98 patients having EUS-FNA for peripancreatic masses from April 1994 to April 1998 was analyzed.

Main Outcome Measure: The accuracy of EUS-FNA for preoperative diagnosis and staging of peripancreatic neoplasms.

Results: Ninety-eight patients, aged 41 to 91 years (mean age, 67 years) with peripancreatic masses were evaluated by EUS-FNA. All patients had initial computed tomography scanning with a mass seen in 49 patients, "fullness" to the pancreas in 28 patients, and no mass seen in 21 patients. Evaluation with EUS-FNA revealed 22 benign lesions, 18 T2 masses, 37 T3 masses, 1 T4 mass, and 20 masses representing nonpancreatic tumors. Results of EUS-FNA of adjacent lymph nodes were positive in 27 patients. Twenty-seven patients had surgical resection or palliation permitting operative and pathologic staging. On comparison of EUS-FNA staging with surgical staging, 12 patients were the same stage, 14 patients were upstaged, and 1 patient was downstaged. The remaining patients who did not have surgery have been followed up for a mean of 15 months. Overall accuracy of EUS-FNA for differentiating benign from malignant masses was 96%.

Conclusions: Endoscopic ultrasound–guided fine needle aspiration is a useful technique for the evaluation of pancreatic masses. It is highly accurate for differentiating between benign and malignant lesions and for predicting T stage, but is limited for predicting nodal status.

Arch Surg. 1999;134:639-643

From the Departments of Surgery (Mr Suits and Dr Frazee) and Medicine (Dr Erickson), Scott & White Clinic and Memorial Hospital, Scott, Sherwood and Brindley Foundation, Texas A&M University Health Science Center, College of Medicine, Temple.

THE PREOPERATIVE diagnosis and staging of pancreatic masses is limited with standard radiographic techniques. Conventional computed tomography (CT) and transabdominal ultrasound do not reliably detect pancreatic tumors of less than 3 cm.[1-4] Early detection is important as tumor size is an independent predictor of improved prognosis.[5-8]

Endoscopic ultrasound (EUS) represents a newer imaging modality that provides excellent visualization of the pancreas and the adjacent structures.[9-12] It also allows fine needle aspiration (FNA) biopsy of the pancreatic mass and regional lymph nodes to give preoperative cytologic diagnosis of the primary tumor and to determine involvement of adjacent lymph nodes. Since the introduction of EUS and endoscopic ultrasound–guided fine needle aspiration (EUS-FNA), there has been considerable debate as to its use as a diagnostic and staging tool. Several reports comparing results of endoscopic ultrasound alone with computed tomography, angiography, and transabdominal ultrasound for preoperative diagnosis and staging have been published, but little has been written about the use of EUS-FNA for suspected pancreatic neoplasms. We present our data on EUS and EUS-FNA for the preoperative evaluation of patients with a suspected pancreatic neoplasm.

RESULTS

Ninety-eight patients, aged 41 to 91 years (mean age, 67 years) were evaluated by EUS-FNA. There were 56 men and 42 women. One patient underwent the procedure twice for a total of 99 EUS-FNA diagnoses. All patients with the exception of one had initial conventional CT. The CT findings included a mass in 49 patients (50%), "fullness" to the pancreas in 28 patients (29%), and no mass seen in 21 patients (21%). Patients with no mass seen on CT had pancreatic ductal dilatation, common bile duct dilatation, or continued clini-

PATIENTS AND METHODS

Ninety-eight patients with suspected peripancreatic malignant neoplasms were evaluated by EUS and EUS-FNA at Scott & White Clinic and Memorial Hospital, Temple, Tex, from April 1995 to April 1998. Patients were identified from a prospective registry of patients undergoing EUS-FNA evaluation, and their medical records reviewed in a retrospective fashion. All procedures were done under the direction of a single endoscopist (R.A.E.) in the endoscopy suite. All patients with the exception of one had an initial CT evaluation. All patients had masses or pancreatic or bile duct dilatation demonstrated on CT scan or otherwise had continued clinical suspicion for a pancreatic malignancy.

Endoscopic ultrasound was performed as previously described.[13] After conscious sedation with medazolam and meperidine hydrochloride, upper endoscopy was performed prior to EUS to rule out any unsuspected mucosal abnormality. A diagnostic EUS examination was then performed using a radial scanning echoendoscope (Olympus GF-UM20; Olympus America, Inc, Lake Success, NY). This device produces 360° live images of surrounding structures at 7.5 or 12 mHz with a range of up to 12 cm. If a pancreatic mass, lymph node, or liver lesion requiring FNA was visualized, the radial scanning instrument was removed, and a curved linear array scanning echoendoscope (Pentax/Hitachi FG-32UA or FG-36UX, Pentax Precision Instrument Corporation, Orangeburg, NY) was inserted. This instrument allows for real-time visualization of the fine needle exiting the biopsy channel and entering the lesion of interest. It scans at 5 or 7.5 mHz and has color flow and Doppler capabilities, which allow for distinguishing vessels from other echolucent structures. The lesion was then located by linear array EUS, and a path for FNA, whereby no major vascular structures were traversed in aspirating the lesion, was found using color flow and/or Doppler ultrasonography. Fine needle aspiration was performed using either the Mediglobe (GIP-Medi-Globe, Grassau, Germany) or the Wilson-Cook EchoTip (Wilson-Cook, Medical, Inc, Winston-Salem, NC) 22-gauge aspiration needles. A reusable aluminum handle controls the insertion of the aspiration needle with a plunger that can extend the needle up to 12 cm from the tip of the echoendoscope. A cytopathologist was present for all EUS-FNA procedures. Aspiration specimens were stained with Diff-Quik (Stat Lab Medial Products, Lewisville, Tex), as well as rapid Papanicolaou stain. Aspiration sampling was continued until the cytopathologist examining the slides reported that adequate tissue had been obtained for diagnosis of the lesion. The mean number of FNA passes was 3.5 (range, 1-10 passes). After the EUS-FNA, the patient recovered for 30 to 60 minutes and was discharged from the endoscopy suite.

Results of the EUS evaluations were compared with operative and pathologic findings in the patients who underwent surgery and with the clinical course in those patients who did not undergo surgery.

cal suspicion of pancreatic neoplasm as an indication for further evaluation.

Results of EUS-FNA were pancreatic adenocarcinoma in 56 patients (57%), a benign mass or fluid collection in 23 patients (23%), and nonpancreatic ductal tumors in 20 patients (20%). The nonpancreatic tumors included cholangiocarcinoma, lymphoma, islet cell tumors, gastric adenocarcinoma, gallbladder carcinoma, paraganglioma, metastatic breast cancer, leiomyosarcoma of the inferior vena cava, duodenal carcinoma, and cancer of unknown origin. For patients with ductal adenocarcinoma, 45 occurred in the head (80%), 6 in the neck (10%), and 6 in the body and tail (10%). Using TMN criteria, 18 masses were graded as T2, 37 masses as T3, and 1 mass as T4. One recurrent lesion was diagnosed at the margin of the gastric anastomosis 3 years after resection. The size of the carcinomas averaged 3.9 cm, with a range of 1.7 to 8 cm.

Assessment with EUS and EUS-FNA of adjacent lymph nodes determined that 18 patients (32% of patients with pancreatic adenocarcinoma) had positive lymph nodes. Node positivity was determined by EUS alone in 11 patients and node negativity was determined by EUS alone in 34 patients. Node positivity was confirmed by EUS-FNA in 7 patients, negative node status was diagnosed by EUS-FNA in 4 patients, and hepatic metastases were diagnosed by EUS-FNA in 2 patients.

Twenty-seven patients with pancreatic adenocarcinoma underwent operative intervention for resection or palliation. Findings of EUS were correlated with operative findings. Twelve patients (44%) were the same stage, 14 patients (52%) were upstaged, and 1 patient (4%) was downstaged. The upstaged patients had nodal metastasis (8 patients), increase in T stage (1 patient), distant metastasis (2 patients), and T and N stage (1 patient); 2 patients whose masses were diagnosed as benign were found to have carcinoma at celiotomy. One patient was downstaged from T3 to T1b at surgery owing to the surgeon's ability to peel the tumor away from the portal vein.

Nonoperative patients have been followed up for a mean of 15 months (range, 4-36 months). Two patients determined to have benign masses by EUS-FNA were subsequently diagnosed as having carcinoma. This translates to a false-negative rate for adenocarcinoma of 7%. Three of the 4 patients with false-negative cytologic diagnosis had chronic pancreatitis. The overall accuracy of EUS-FNA for differentiating benign from malignant masses was 96%.

COMMENT

Pancreatic adenocarcinoma carries a poor prognosis with fewer than 20% of affected individuals surviving more than 1 year and only 3% remaining alive at 5 years after diagnosis.[6,14] Currently, complete resection offers the only hope for long-term survival. In the past, radical pancreaticoduodenectomy has had an unacceptably high operative mortality rate. Several recent series, however, have shown operative mortality of less than 5% for the Whipple procedure.[5,15,16] Survival following resection has improved in recent years with 5-year survival rates ranging from 14% to 33%. This increase in survival probably reflects improved patient selection as much as improvements in treatment.

The preoperative diagnosis and staging of peripancreatic neoplasms has been difficult. Transabdominal ultrasound and CT are commonly used but can fail to image cancers of less than 3 cm in up to 40% of cases. In addition, a mass lesion of the pancreas can occur from inflammatory disease and mimic carcinoma. False-positive diagnoses by ultrasound and CT may occur as a result of common bile duct dilatation that occurs from causes other than malignant obstruction. Endoscopic retrograde cholangiopancreatography is another imaging option, but relies on indirect signs of ductal obstruction and is therefore less accurate.

Endoscopic ultrasound represents a new imaging modality for lesions in the upper gastrointestinal tract. It utilizes high-frequency ultrasound (5-12 MHz), which provides excellent resolution and detailed visualization of the pancreas and surrounding structures. Computed tomography detected a mass in 79% of our patients, but no mass was seen in 21% by CT. The masses seen on CT scan averaged 3.7 cm in diameter, whereas the masses measured 2.9 cm in the 21 patients with "negative" CT. Endoscopic ultrasound has previously been compared with transabdominal ultrasound and CT. Palazzo et al[17] compared EUS with ultrasound and CT in 64 patients with suspected pancreatic adenocarcinoma. Endoscopic ultrasound was more accurate (91%) than CT (66%) and ultrasound (64%) for the diagnosis of pancreatic cancer. Endoscopic ultrasound was also more accurate for detecting lymph node metastases than CT and ultrasound (74% vs 42% and 37%, respectively). Nakaizumi et al[2] analyzed 232 patients for pancreatic carcinoma by EUS, CT, and ultrasound. They reported accuracy of 96% for EUS compared with 88% for CT and ultrasound.

Helical CT offers advantages over conventional CT in that it has faster scanning times, dynamic injection of contrast, and reconstruction of images for multiplanar depictions of anatomy.[18] This has led to higher-quality images. Helical CT has been compared with EUS and found to produce similar results with the exception of small tumors. For tumors less than 3 cm, EUS carries a greater sensitivity than helical CT.[3,4]

Endosonography alone can be used to predict lymph node metastasis. The endosonographic features of lymph node metastasis include size greater than 10 mm, rounded contour, sharply demarcated borders, and hypoechoic structure. Catalano et al[19] found that EUS had a sensitivity of 89% and a specificity of 92% when lymph nodes were imaged endosonographically. They also found that, regardless of specific sonographic features, the likelihood of N1 disease was 86% in patients who had lymph nodes imaged. In patients who did not have lymph nodes identified, the chance of N0 disease was 79%.

Endoscopic ultrasound–guided fine needle aspiration is another application of echoendoscopy and was first reported in 1992.[3] It permits cytologic biopsy of the pancreas and areas of metastatic disease. It is performed using the curved linear array echoendoscope so that the biopsy needle passes within the view of the ultrasound imaging. The presence of a cytopathologist during aspiration avoids the problem of inadequate cellularity of the FNA specimen. In our experience, a mean of 3.5 passes of the biopsy needle was required to achieve a diagnosis. The morbidity associated with EUS-FNA is less than 2% for solid lesions, with bleeding, infection, and pancreatitis as the main concerns. The risk of malignant seeding along the needle biopsy tract has been expressed as a concern, but this complication has not been reported with use of EUS-FNA. In patients with resectable disease, the course of the needle tract will be resected at the time of pancreatic resection.

The accuracy of EUS-FNA has been reported by other investigators. A collaborative multicenter study of 164 consecutive cases showed a sensitivity of 83% and a specificity of 90%.[20] Sensitivities and specificities in other reports range from 85% to 90% and 85% to 100%, respectively. Sensitivity in our series was 96% and specificity was 100%. Four patients in our series had false-negative biopsy results. Three of these 4 patients had coexistent pancreatitis. Other authors have reported similar difficulty in patients with chronic pancreatitis. In this setting, surgical exploration may be warranted, even with a negative FNA result.

Although EUS-FNA was highly accurate for differentiating between benign and malignant masses, it was less accurate for preoperative staging of malignancy. Staging by EUS-FNA of patients in our series who had surgery for pancreatic carcinoma showed that 44% were the same TMN stage after surgery. Fourteen patients were upstaged because of undetected nodal metastasis (8 patients), an increase in T stage (1 patient), distant metastasis (2 patients), and an increase in T and N stage (1 patient); and 2 patients originally diagnosed as having benign masses had carcinoma at exploration. In addition, 1 patient was downstaged from T3 to T1b at surgery owing to the surgeon's ability to peel the tumor away from the portal vein at surgery.

Use of EUS-FNA has several potential applications in clinical practice. It is useful in differentiating between benign and malignant masses, it delineates the relationship of the pancreatic cancer with the portal vein, and, finally, it allows detection of lymphatic metastasis in a significant number of patients. These latter patients could be entered into neoadjuvant therapy protocols for advanced disease. With improved preoperative diagnosis and staging, patients can be better selected for potentially curative resection vs palliative care.

Presented at the 106th Scientific Session of the Western Surgical Association, Indianapolis, Ind, November 17, 1998.

Reprints: Richard Frazee, MD, 6200 Regional Plaza, Suite 1400, Abilene, TX 79606.

REFERENCES

1. Muller MF, Meyenberger C, Bertschinger P, Schaer R, Marincek B. Pancreatic tumors: evaluation with endoscopic ultrasound, computed tomography, and magnetic resonance imaging. *Radiology.* 1994;190:745-751.
2. Nakaizumi H, Uehara H, Iishi H, et al. Endoscopic ultrasonography in the diagnosis and staging of pancreatic cancer. *Dig Dis Sci.* 1995;40:696-700.
3. Legmann KP, Vignauz OP, Dousset B, et al. Pancreatic tumors: comparison of dual-

phase helical CT and endoscopic sonography. *Am J Radiol.* 1998;170:1315-1322.
4. Howard TJ, Chin AC, Streib EW, Kopecky KK, Wiebke EA. Value of helical computed tomography, angiography, and endoscopic ultrasound in determining resectability of periampullary carcinoma. *Am J Surg.* 1997;174:237-241.
5. Yeo CJ, Cameron JL, Lillemoe KD, et al. Pancreaticoduodenectomy for cancer of the head of the pancreas. *Ann Surg.* 1995;221:721-731.
6. Geer RJ, Brennan MF. Prognostic indicators for survival after resection of pancreatic adenocarcinoma. *Am J Surg.* 1993;165:68-73.
7. Fortner JG, Klimstra DS, Senie RT, Maclean BJ. Tumor size is the primary prognosticator for pancreatic cancer after regional pancreatectomy. *Ann Surg.* 1996; 233:147-153.
8. Sperti C, Pasquali C, Piccoli A, Pedrazzoli S. Survival after resection for ductal adenocarcinoma of the pancreas. *Br J Surg.* 1996;85:625-631.
9. Chang KJ, Albers CG, Erickson RA, Butler JA, Wuerer RB, Lin F. Endoscopic ultrasound guided fine needle aspiration of pancreatic carcinoma. *Am J Gastroenterol.* 1994;89:263-266.
10. Bhutani MS. Endoscopic ultrasound in pancreatic disease. *Semin Gastrointest Dis.* 1998;9:51-60.
11. Erickson RA, Sayage-Rabie L, Avots-Avotins A. Clinical utility of endoscopic ultrasound guided fine needle aspiration. *Acta Cytol.* 1997;41:1647-1653.
12. Cahn M, Chang K, Nguyen P, Butler J. Impact of endoscopic ultrasound with fine needle aspiration on the surgical management of pancreatic cancer. *Am J Surg.* 1996;172:470-472.
13. Frazee RC, Singh H, Erickson RA. Endoscopic ultrasound and fine needle aspiration of peripancreatic masses. *Am J Surg.* 1997;174:596-599.
14. Delcore R, Rodriguez FJ, Forster J, Hermreck AS, Thomas JH. Significance of lymph node metastasis in patients with pancreatic cancer undergoing curative resection. *Am J Surg.* 1996;172:463-468.
15. Stephens J, Kuhn J, O'Brien J, et al. Surgical morbidity, mortality, and long term survival in patients with peripancreatic cancer following pancreaticoduodenectomy. *Am J Surg.* 1997;174:600-603.
16. Sung JP, Stewart RD, O'Hara VS, Westpal KF, Wilkinson JE, Hill J. A study of forty-nine consecutive Whipple procedures for periampullary carcinoma. *Am J Surg.* 1997;174:6-10.
17. Palazzo L, Roseau G, Gayet B, et al. Endoscopic ultrasonography in the diagnosis and staging of pancreatic adenocarcinoma. *Endoscopy.* 1993;25:143-150.
18. Zeman RK, Cooper C, Zeiberg AS, et al. TMN staging of pancreatic carcinoma using helical CT. *Am J Radiol.* 1997;169:459-464.
19. Catalano MF, Sivak MV, Toce T, Gragg LA, Van Dam J. Endosonographic features predictive of lymph node metastasis. *Gastrointest Endosc.* 1994;40:442-446.
20. Chang KJ, Wiersema M, Giovanni M, et al. Multicenter collaborative study on endoscopic ultrasound guided fine needle aspiration of the pancreas [abstract]. *Gastrointest Endosc.* 1996;43:417.

DISCUSSION

Fabrizio Michelassi, MD, Chicago, Ill: I am here to read the discussion prepared by Dr Daniel Deziel, who could not be here because of a family medical emergency. Dr Deziel was kind enough to contact me and fax his discussion which follows. Mr Suits and his colleagues have presented their experience with EUS for the evaluation of peripancreatic masses with an appropriate emphasis on ductal carcinoma of the pancreas. In general, our therapeutic strategy for pancreatic cancer will be improved by earlier diagnosis to increase resectability and by more accurate staging to minimize unnecessary interventions in patients who are not likely to benefit. High-resolution ultrasound performed by endoscopic, laparoscopic, or intraoperative approaches, has inherent advantages over any conventional external imaging techniques.

From the standpoint of early diagnosis, we would be interested in knowing how useful EUS was for identifying tumors that were not detected otherwise. There were 49 patients without a definite mass on CT scan. Can you tell us first how often EUS discovered a pancreatic lesion in this group? Second, tell us whether cancers only discovered by EUS were potentially more curable based on stage and resectability?

As a cautionary note regarding diagnosis, 4 of the 22 patients felt to have benign lesions by ultrasound and FNA actually turned out to have pancreatic cancer. The distinction between benign and malignant was particularly difficult in patients with chronic pancreatitis when the sonographic diagnosis should not obviate the need for an operation.

As far as staging is concerned, there are a number of current modalities at our disposal including CT and MRI [magnetic resonance imaging], laparoscopy, and endoscopic or laparoscopic ultrasonography. The utility of any particular staging strategy is determined by a comparative evaluation of its accuracy and cost and by an assessment of how it influences therapy by increasing resectability rates, or by decreasing the rate of nontherapeutic operation. Results of this report show a poor correlation (44%) between operative staging and the findings on EUS; over one half of patients had higher stage tumors than ultrasound suggested. The main discrepancy was in regard to lymph node status where, in general, the sensitivity of ultrasound is more limited since one of the primary criteria it depends on is the lymph node size and small nodes can still be malignant. How often, however, did this change in stage affect your treatment or decision to resect?

Finally, how does laparoscopy with laparoscopic ultrasound fit into your current approach for staging pancreatic cancer? In many centers this has become an important tool for staging a variety of intra-abdominal malignancies. Experience with pancreatic cancer has demonstrated about a 90% accuracy in predicting resectability and has allowed about 25% of patients deemed resectable by other imaging techniques to avoid laparotomy. Laparoscopic staging with laparoscopic ultrasound is capable of detecting occult liver and peritoneal metastases that other modalities, including EUS cannot. It has a positive predicted value for vascular invasion that exceeds 90%. How useful did you find EUS for assessing the peripancreatic vessels?

Gerald Aranha, MD, Maywood, Ill: It took me many years to convince the residents and some of my colleagues. A preoperative biopsy is unnecessary in patients who had resectable mass in the head of the pancreas with obstructive jaundice. Now comes a test which some of our colleagues may use, not to operate on patients with pancreatic cancer and avoid giving them the only chance they have at cure. My questions to you are the following: (1) Do you think it is important to get a biopsy in those patients who present with pancreatic mass, obstructive jaundice and for all purposes on CT have a resectable lesion? (2) Did you do peritoneal cytology on your patients whom you operated on for cancer? Dr Warshaw has shown that in patients with peritoneal cytology washings, 75% of those who had preoperative biopsy had a positive peritoneal cytology. (3) How do you think that this test will ultimately be used? Would it be for those who will receive neoadjuvant therapy and for those whose tumors appear unresectable?

Richard Thirlby, MD, Seattle, Wash: For the most part, I agree with the concept of EUS with biopsy. This technology is very expensive, but provides true potential gains for our patients. One is to confirm the diagnosis of cancer more safely in patients who do not have resectable disease. The issue raised by the previous discussant regarding concern for seeding with percutaneous biopsies is not a problem with the technology since it is transduodenal biopsy.

The distressing finding in the paper to me, however, was the downstaging at operation. One patient was felt to have portal vein invasion on EUS, but this was found not to be the case in the operating room. It is very distressing if patients are potentially denied curative operation based on this test. Can the authors tell us how many patients went to the operating room with the EUS suggesting venous invasion?

Dilip Parekh, MD, Los Angeles, Calif: This paper reflects a series of papers now published largely in the medical literature emphasizing the role of EUS for staging pancreatic cancer. There is one problem with most of the papers that I have seen so far including this one—the quality of CT scanning that is utilized in these studies is not state of the art. Did the authors use double-spiral CT scanning? We currently have an NIH [National Institutes of Health]–funded study whereby we are comparing CT scanning, laparoscopic ultrasound, and laparoscopy for staging these patients which we are in the process of completing. We found that the diagnostic accuracy for staging vascular involvement with a state of the art, double-spiral CT is about 85% to 90%. In this study, only 40% of the patients were accurately staged with CT. So, clearly the problem here was not the value of EUS as much as the fact that the quality of CT scanning that was utilized in this study was poor. Endoscopic ultrasound is very much operator dependent. Our experience at USC [University of Southern California] has found that in about one third of the patients, the endoscopist is unable to make the determination of vascular involvement. There are 2 critical factors for resectability of pancreatic cancer: vascular involvement and metastatic disease. Very little data are present on this in this paper and correlated with accuracy of EUS. There are 2 specific questions that I would like the authors to address. What type of CT scanning technique was used in this study? How accurate was ultrasound assessment for identifying vascular involvement? Did the authors use intraoperative laparoscopy to rule out small metastatic deposits?

Richard Prinz, MD, Chicago: I also wonder about the need for preoperative biopsy in patients with resectable pancreatic lesions. My question concerns the fact that more than half of the patients in this study did not undergo operation. I would like to know the reasons why these patients were not explored, and whether patients with resectable lesions were denied pancreaticoduodenectomy?

Steven Stain, MD, Los Angeles: Did you actually compare your sensitivity of CT scan in predicting portal vein involvement?

Dr Frazee: Dr Michelassi, you asked, does ultrasound lead to an earlier diagnosis? This is one of the advantages of EUS in that it is very sensitive for detecting small tumors. That is one factor that has been shown to be an independent predictor of survival, and is one of the potential advantages of EUS over the other modalities.

The other questions pertain to cost-effectiveness. The importance of EUS in this area is by eliminating a variety of other diagnostic procedures. By going straight to the EUS examination with FNA, a number of adjuvant tests that have been done in the past, including ERCP [endoscopic retrograde cholangiopancreatography] and angiography, can be eliminated as part of the diagnostic workup and leads to a more cost-effective evaluation. The other area where it leads to cost-effectiveness is identifying patients who would not benefit from surgical therapy. We will then avoid the cost and the morbidity to the patient of unnecessary abdominal exploration.

You asked about laparoscopic ultrasound. We are just initiating that process in the evaluation of our patients with pancreatic tumors, so we do not have enough data to comment on that at this point.

Several of the discussants asked about EUS and its use for vascular invasion. Actually, this is one of the benefits of EUS. It is very accurate for detecting the relationship of the pancreatic mass to the portal and superior mesenteric veins. We had 1 patient in whom EUS overpredicted the portal vein invasion. This was out of a total of 10 patients shown to have vascular invasion. Three patients in our series had portal venous resection as part of their operation. It helps to identify preoperatively those patients who you are considering for portal venous resection. We used a criteria of 1.5 cm of interface between the mass and the portal vein as a prediction of portal venous invasion.

Dr Aranha, you brought up the issue of preoperative biopsy in the patient with a pancreatic mass. In the past, my philosophy regarding operative biopsy of a pancreatic mass in the patient who clinically presents with carcinoma has been similar to your own. I based the decision to perform resection upon clinical criteria and suspicion for a carcinoma. Because EUS-FNA can be done with such minimal morbidity, and gives a tissue diagnosis, I have now changed my philosophy in regards to preoperative biopsy. It is also very useful in those patients who are not candidates for surgical therapy. It is a very safe way to obtain a cytologic diagnosis and then put those patients in the category of palliative care or enter them into neoadjuvant therapy protocols in the hopes of performing later resection.

You mentioned the concern of peritoneal cytology and, as Dr Thirlby mentioned, the path of the needle is transduodenal and so it does not traverse the peritoneal cavity. In theory, this should not create problems with peritoneal seeding, but again, this is something that needs further study.

You also asked, does this open the door to neoadjuvant therapy, and indeed it does. If we can identify the patients who have metastatic lymph node involvement who do not have distant disease preoperatively, it opens the door for entering those patients into neoadjuvant therapy protocols and then offer them later resective therapy.

One of the discussants brought up the use of double-phase helical CT and the majority of the CT scans in this series were standard CT. The purpose of our paper was not to compare those, but other authors have done that and have shown similar results in delineating the relationship of the tumor in relationship to the vascular structures. Helical CT, however, was not as sensitive in detecting small tumors measuring less than 3 cm. So, for the tumor size, 3 cm and under, EUS is more accurate.

Dr Prinz, you asked why half the patients were not explored. A significant number of the patients had benign disease and therefore did not receive exploration. The others had disease that was not amenable to resective therapy. They were entered into palliative care at that stage.

Correction

Error in References. In the original article by Kotani et al titled "Enteral Nutrition Prevents Bacterial Translocation but Does Not Improve Survival During Acute Pancreatitis," published in the March issue of the ARCHIVES (1999;134:287-292), reference 30 was missing from the list of references on page 292. Reference 30 should have been listed as "Keith RG. Effect of a low fat elemental diet on pancreatic secretion during pancreatitis. *Surg Gynecol Obstet.* 1980;151:337-343." The journal regrets the error.

PAPER

Image-Guided Surgery

Preliminary Feasibility Studies of Frameless Stereotactic Liver Surgery

Alan J. Herline, MD; James D. Stefansic, MS; Jacob P. Debelak, MS; Steven L. Hartmann, BS; C. Wright Pinson, MD; Robert L. Galloway, PhD; William C. Chapman, MD

Background: Liver surgery can be difficult because there are few external landmarks defining hepatic anatomy and because the liver has significant vascularity. Although preoperative tomographic imaging (computed tomography or magnetic resonance imaging) provides essential anatomical information for operative planning, at present it cannot be used actively for precise localization during surgery. Interactive image-guided surgery involves the simultaneous real-time display of intraoperative instrument location on preoperative images (computed or positron-emission tomography or magnetic resonance imaging). Interactive image-guided surgery has been described for tumor localization in the brain (frameless stereotactic surgery) and allows for interactive use of preoperative images during resections or biopsies.

Hypothesis: The application of interactive image-guided surgery (IIGS) is feasible for hepatic procedures from a biomedical engineering standpoint.

Methods: We developed an interactive image-guided surgery system for liver surgery and tested a porcine liver model for tracking liver motion during insufflation; liver motion during respiration in open procedures in patients undergoing hepatic resection; and tracking accuracy of general surgical instruments, including a laparoscope and an ultrasound probe.

Results: Liver motion due to insufflation can be quantified; average motion was 2.5 ± 1.4 mm. Average total liver motion secondary to respiration in patients was 10.8 ± 2.5 mm. Instruments of varying lengths, including a laparoscope, can be tracked to accuracies ranging from 1.4 to 2.1 mm within a 27-m^3 (3 × 3 × 3-m) space.

Conclusion: Interactive image-guided surgery appears to be feasible for open and laparoscopic hepatic procedures and may enhance future operative localization.

Arch Surg. 1999;134:644-650

THE ANATOMICAL location of hepatic tumors is usually determined preoperatively using tomographic imaging (computed tomography [CT] or magnetic resonance imaging [MRI]). This allows critical assessment of tumor resectability and assists in operative planning. However, this preoperative information at present cannot be actively used during surgery to guide resections and probe placements for ablative therapies (eg, cryoablation or radiofrequency ablation). Intraoperative ultrasonography (IOUS) can provide intraoperative imaging information regarding tumor location and surrounding vascular anatomy,[1] but it requires special expertise to perform and to interpret properly. In addition, there are the following inherent technical limitations regarding its use for operative guidance in hepatic procedures: it is 2-dimensional in its present format; there can be significant interuser variation in results; and image obliteration occurs after resection or ablative therapy is initiated.

One suggested method to provide tomographic information for surgical guidance involves operating room placement of scanners.[2,3] However, these systems have substantial barriers to broad acceptance. First, these units are expensive, based on installation cost, cost per procedure, and intraoperative modification of instruments to avoid magnetic interference. Second, these systems are large and can make standard operations more difficult because of space occupied by imaging equipment. Third, there is an image lag-time delay (up to 8 seconds), and, compared with MRI units placed in radiology suites

From the Departments of Hepatobiliary Surgery and Liver Transplantation (Drs Herline, Pinson, and Chapman and Mr Debelak) and Biomedical Engineering (Drs Herline and Galloway and Messrs Stefansic and Hartmann), Vanderbilt University, Nashville, Tenn.

This article is also available on our Web site: www.ama-assn.org/surgery.

MATERIALS AND METHODS

EXPERIMENTS TO DEFINE LIVER MOTION

Porcine Model

A porcine model was developed to quantify liver motion due to pneumoperitoneum. Pigs weighing 25 kg underwent initial laparotomy and had 8 to 10 radiopaque markers placed throughout the liver. The markers were placed on the surface as well as intraparenchymally. Surface markers were hollow plastic cylinders (inner diameter, 7 mm; height, 5 mm) filled with an aqueous solution of combined 165 mg/mL of iodinated CT contrast (Conray; Mallinckrodt Medical, Inc, St Louis, Mo) and 0.5-mmol/L magnetic resonance contrast agent (Magnevist; Berlex Laboratories, Wayne, NJ), and parenchymal markers were conical cylinders filled with iodinated CT contrast (Omnipaque; Nycomed Inc, Princeton, NJ) (inner diameter, 5 mm; height, 10 mm).

Following midline laparotomy, insertional markers were placed within the liver. Surface markers were applied using polypropylene mesh and cyanoacrylate. The animal's midline wound was closed using a single layer of running suture. The animals were awakened and returned to their holding area.

After 7 days of recovery, a 5-mm laparoscopic trocar was placed in the left lower quadrant, and the animals were transported directly to the radiology suite. Helical CT scanning with 3-mm slices was performed on a helical CT scanner (Picker PQ 5000; Picker, Cleveland, Ohio). Diaphragmatic motion was controlled using an end-inspiration breath-hold technique at 20 to 25 cm H_2O. Following the initial scan, the abdomen was insufflated with carbon dioxide using a standard laparoscopy insufflator to 13 cm pressure and immediately rescanned using the same technique.

Image registration was performed using a mutual information algorithm on a Sun Workstation (Sun Microsystems Inc, Palo Alto, Calif).[12,13] Coordinates (x, y, z) for each marker in each scan were recorded. Marker movement between preinsufflation and postinsufflation scans was determined using the Euclidean distance formula, as follows:

$$d = (x_1 - x_2)^2 + (y_1 - y_2)^2 + (z_1 - z_2)^2$$

where d is the distance in millimeters between preinsufflation and postinsufflation scans; x_1, y_1, z_1, the 3-dimensional CT space position of the marker before insufflation; and x_2, y_2, z_2, the 3-dimensional CT space position of the marker after insufflation.

Human Liver Motion With Respiratory Changes

During open exploration for planned hepatic resection in patients with liver tumors ($n = 2$), points on the liver surface were tracked to determine respiratory-associated hepatic movement. After standard chevron incision and placement of a Bookwalter retractor (Codman and Shutleff, New Brunswick, NJ), an operative probe was placed on 3 points on the liver (falciform ligament at point of entry into the liver, lateral-most tip of left lobe, and the central portion of the gallbladder fossa). Approximately 950 localization points (x, y, z) were continuously collected using the optical camera and localization pointer with IREDs from each location. Both patients had more than 2800 localization points collected during continuous respiratory cycles with standard continuous mandatory ventilator cycling

Continued on next page

solely for scanning purposes, operating room units are underused during the procedure when image localization is not required.

We have initiated studies investigating alternative methods of intraoperative guidance for liver surgery that we believe will provide more tomographic data and be much more cost-effective than placing scanners in the operating room. An operative guidance system must be accurate and display images in a format that is user-friendly for the surgeon. Interactive image-guided surgery (IIGS) is a method of intraoperative localization that provides for the synchronous display of surgical position on preoperative or intraoperative images during an operation.[4,5] This method of intraoperative localization and surgical guidance has been used in neurosurgical and ear, nose, and throat procedures,[6-10] but has not been reported for use in general surgical procedures, including hepatic surgery.

Stereotactic frames function by defining a space (x_f, y_f, z_f) in the frame surrounding the patient's skull. Images obtained with the frame in place define each point of interest in the brain with coordinates (x_i, y_i, z_i) in an image (CT or MRI) space. A mathematical relationship between the image space and frame space can be calculated so that a target (eg, tumor) could be determined in the image and then assigned coordinates in frame space. This process is known as mapping or registration. However, frames are uncomfortable to patients, must be applied immediately before imaging and procedures, and are cumbersome in the operating room. These factors led to the development of frameless stereotaxy systems that use a variety of methods to register the tomographic images to patient physical space and intraoperative localization devices capable of tracking surgical instruments within an operating room.[6]

Any IIGS system must have the following 3 components: a registration process that will map the location of a point in the patient onto the same point in an image, an instrument whose location may be tracked in the operating room, and a method for displaying the physical location of the instrument onto an image and updating the images or location in real time. Once a registration is completed, it remains reliable as long as the object (eg, skull) is not moved. The liver or any other nonrigid organ does not follow this constraint. It seems intuitive that the liver moves, but the quantity of movement is unknown and crucial to determining the potential application of IIGS to liver surgery.

The first experiments presented explore liver motion with standard insufflation associated with laparoscopy and with respiratory-associated diaphragmatic movement. The second experiments investigated our ability to track newly developed instruments for application in open and laparoscopic applications. The

(**Figure 2**). The change in position of the tracked points with respiration is calculated relative to the resting base position of the liver.

INSTRUMENT TRACKING

We tested the reliability of intraoperative localization and tracking of various lengths of operative probes, an ultrasound probe, and a laparoscope. The conventional neurosurgical probe is 20 cm in length and has 24 IREDs that spiral around a handle (Figure 1). Because the diameter is small compared with its length, it is relatively insensitive to roll; in addition, a "dead spot" exists if the shaft is pointed directly at the infrared camera. In laparoscopic applications, however, many complex manipulations are performed, so it is important to have created a rigid body that is sensitive to roll and minimizes dead spots. A rigid body (**Figure 3**) to account for these problems was designed and constructed containing 24 IREDs. An active optical position sensor (Optotrak 3020; Northern Digital, Waterloo, Ontario) was used to track instruments.[12] The process of calibrating each instrument involves the following: A 3-mm diameter spherical ball is firmly attached to the tip of the probe or endoscope and placed in a corresponding cup, allowing rotation but no translation. The assembly is rotated about the tip of the scope until the position sensor has captured approximately 1000 frames of data. Once this rigid-body space is defined, the IREDs on the rigid body are mapped into that space and define the instrument tip relative to the IREDs.

The following experiment was conducted using a 20 × 20 × 20-cm cube machined with 52 divot points whose coordinates (*x, y, z*) in and distances relative to the other points are precisely defined. A spherical tip (1 mm) on the instrument is placed into each of 7 points on the cube (**Figure 4**). The computer collects the location (*x, y,* and *z*) of the tip in a divot as determined by the optical camera. Of the 7 collected points, 3 are required to perform a point-based registration. These points are referred to as fiducials. The other 4 points are referred to as targets. All 35 possible combinations of fiducials and targets were used to calculate an average fiducial registration error (FRE) and target registration error (TRE). The FRE is the measure of accuracy in locating points used for calculating the point-based registration. The TRE is a measure of accuracy in locating points (targets) not used in the registration and a better assessment of clinical accuracy. It is a function of the number of fiducials used and the ability to determine the location of the points used for registration. Because of the registration process, FRE is almost always less than TRE, but TRE is a more exacting measure of error.[11]

The above process was performed with 8 instrument sizes (3.5-49 cm). Three trials of 7 collection points per trial were performed for each instrument length. The 49-cm instrument trial was performed with the "gearshift knob" attached to a telecam endoscopic camera (telecam-20210130; Karl Storz GmbH & Co, Tuttlingen, Germany) with a 0° Olympus scope (Olympus America, Melville, NY). The gearshift knob attaches to all the instruments and camera via a bayonet device (Figure 3) that allows for rigid nonpermanent attachment to an instrument or laparoscope.[13,14]

Registration and error calculations were performed on software written in our laboratory using Borland C. Graphs (Inprise Corp, Scotts Valley, Calif) of marker position and instrument length vs error were performed on a PC workstation using a commercially available statistical package (SPSS 8.0, SPSS Inc, Chicago, Ill). Results are presented as mean ± SD.

instruments we have assembled for the present IIGS system have attached infrared-emitting diodes (IREDs) (**Figure 1**), which fire sequentially and are localized by 3 infrared cameras. If 3 or more of the IREDs are detected, the tip of the instrument can be localized by triangulation in physical space (x_s, y_s, z_s) with an error of 0.3 mm.[11] After the instruments are registered to the images, the IIGS process provides continuous, real-time 3-dimensional guidance using standard tomographic images (CT or MRI). We varied the lengths of the instruments to make them suitable for open hepatic procedures and constructed new tracked instruments of laparoscopic length. The goal of our present study is to develop necessary technical instrumentation and test the feasibility of IIGS from a biomedical standpoint for hepatic surgical applications.

RESULTS

PORCINE LIVER MOTION MODEL

Two pigs with an average of 9 markers each placed on or in the liver had preinsufflation and postinsufflation scans analyzed for individual marker movement. The x position change is an anatomical left-to-right change; the y position change, an anatomical anterior-to-posterior change. The z position change is on the craniocaudad axis of the animal. Average marker movement after pneumoperitoneum in the x, y, and z dimensions was 1.8 ± 12, 4.1 ± 6.4, and 0.1 ± 0.4 mm, respectively. The axial movement (z) is extremely small relative to slice thickness (3 mm). Total average marker movement for the animals was 2.5 ± 1.4 mm.

LIVER MOTION WITH RESPIRATORY CHANGES

Base resting liver position was calculated as the average coordinate (x, y, and z) for all points collected from the liver. Average change in position from the base is reported as a change in x, y, z relative to a reference emitter on the operative field. Liver motion is sinusoidal, and average liver position change is calculated by interpolating the peak inspiratory and expiratory position (Figure 2). Average motion with respiration was 10.3 ± 2.5 mm.

INSTRUMENT TRACKING

Eight instruments ranging from 3.5 to 49 cm were calibrated, tracked, and localized. Each length's error represents more than 1000 data points collected for calibration and 280 points collected for fiducial and target registration. Five instruments ranging in lengths from 3.5 to 22.5 cm were considered open instruments. Three instruments ranging in lengths from 26 to 49 cm were considered laparoscopic instruments.

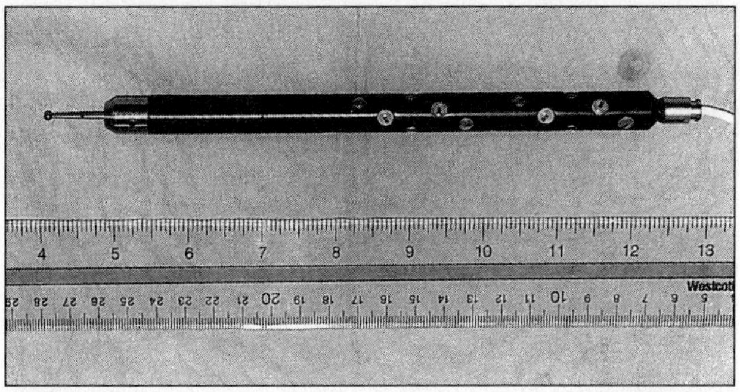

Figure 1. *A surgical probe used for neurosurgery with 24 infrared-emitting diodes that fire sequentially, allowing for detection and localization by the infrared cameras. The ruler indicates inches.*

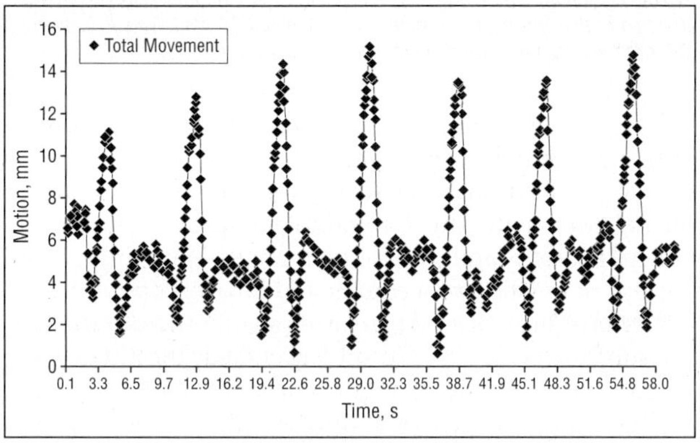

Figure 2. *A recording of liver movement with respiration by the interactive image-guided surgery system during an open hepatic procedure. This sinusoidal pattern of liver motion can be modeled and used for motion correction in the future.*

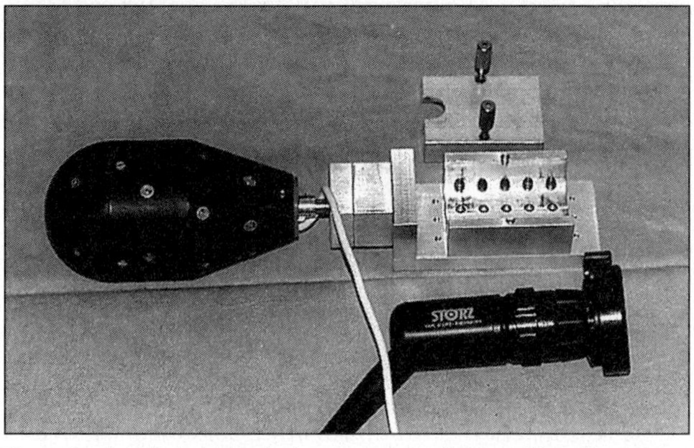

Figure 3. *Rigid body design for laparoscopic applications. The oblong shape accounts for "roll" and removes "dead spots" for any position. A rigid but nonpermanent attachment to the laparoscopic camera is used.*

Average TRE for all instruments ranged from 1.2 to 3.2 mm, with an overall average of 1.7 ± 0.1 mm. A comparison of FRE, TRE, and the error locating a target using the worst set of fiducials in one's registration (TRE_{max}) is presented in **Figure 5**.

COMMENT

Surgical guidance during hepatic resection or ablative procedures is currently performed with previous review of tomographic scans, tactile sensation, and IOUS. Due to intrahepatic location of large vascular structures, variability of the internal anatomy of the liver, and paucity of external anatomical landmarks, preoperative imaging not only is valuable for diagnostic purposes, but is essential for operative planning and guidance.[8,14] Ablative procedures, eg, cryoablation and radiofrequency ablation, are especially dependent on precise probe placement and tissue destruction from the tumor's volumetric center to reduce local failure. This is particularly important, since tissue margins cannot be assessed pathologically after ablation, as is done following standard hepatic resection. The IOUS can provide this guidance, but is affected by its 2-dimensional nature, by the sonographer's skill, and by image ablation once resections or tumor ablations are initiated.[1]

Laparoscopy combined with laparoscopic IOUS has been used as another method to optimize patient selection for liver resection.[15,16] Although laparoscopy has the potential to decrease procedure-associated morbidity, it reduces the surgeon's ability to palpate and visualize the liver and therefore to localize tumors.[15] Interactive image-guided surgery has the potential to combine these separate modalities (preoperative tomographic imaging, IOUS, and laparoscopy) and to provide an active imaging process using preoperative and intraoperative information.

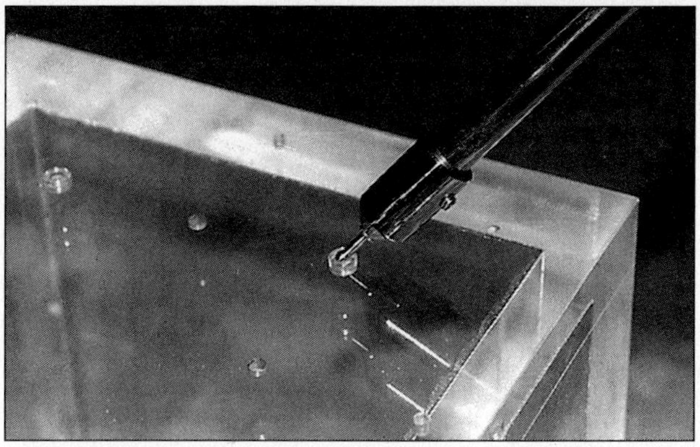

Figure 4. *Collection of divot locations from a precisely defined cube using the tracked laparoscope. Shown is an enlargement of the "ball and cup" fit of the probe into the cube's divots.*

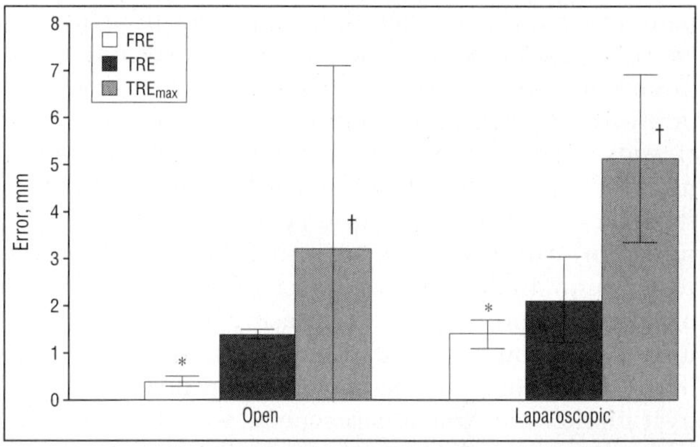

Figure 5. *Instrument localization comparing fiducial registration error (FRE), target registration error (TRE), and the error locating a target using the worst set of fiducials in one's registration (TRE_{max}) for open (3.5-22.5 cm) and laparoscopic instruments (26.5-49 cm). The FRE is a measure of the ability to localize points used for registration; the TRE, all other known points. Asterisk indicates* $P<.05$ *for FRE, open vs laparoscopic instruments; dagger,* $P<.05$ *for TRE_{max}, open vs laparoscopic instruments.*

The combination of intraoperative and preoperative information may significantly improve laparoscopic guidance and/or allow liver procedures to be performed laparoscopically. Toward this end, we have accomplished registration of a mobile organ and developed tracked instruments for use in open or laparoscopic procedures.

Image-guided techniques have been developed and applied for neurosurgical operative procedures for several years, and our group has had significant involvement in this area.[5,6,7,11,13] However, there are several technical limitations to the application of IIGS for hepatic surgery that have prevented an immediate use in this new area. First, unlike the skull, the abdominal wall is not rigid but moves with respiration, and markers are not easily attached to the liver preoperatively, as can be done for the skull. In addition, the liver is normally mobilized away from the diaphragm and abdominal wall in most hepatic procedures, further altering the relationship between the abdominal wall and the liver. To overcome these limitations, we are using a combination of surface and point-based registration techniques to remove the constraints of point-to-point registration and eliminate the need for extrinsic marker placement. Intrinsic points on the liver (eg, edge of falciform ligament, portal vein bifurcation) can be used as intrinsic fiducial markers for registration. In the current project, markers were placed on and in the porcine liver to measure how well the preinsufflation and postinsufflation CT scans are mapped, but were not used in the registration process. Average liver marker movement is presumed to represent overall liver movement. Our average marker movement before and during laparoscopic insufflation was 2.5 mm, using an end-inspiration breath-hold technique, and occurred in an anterior-to-posterior direction.

Tracking of liver motion due to respiratory changes has been of interest in the field of radiology, particularly for interventional procedures. To our knowledge, no other work has physically tracked an intra-abdominal organ's motion during the respiratory cycle (Figure 2). These data are useful in our project as a means of testing system reliability. It will also be useful to model motion of the liver as we develop constraints for the IIGS system.[17]

The instruments developed and used in our study all can be localized and tracked with a high degree of accuracy. The TRE_{max} is a measure of the worst combination of fiducials used for the registration process. With any surgical navigation system, it is important to know expected accuracies as well as worst-case scenarios.

No association between instrument length and error was demonstrated in these experiments. This is valuable as one evaluates the use of IIGS in laparoscopy. The 49-cm instrument (actual laparoscope) demonstrated an average TRE of 1.2 mm. Some additional error in our study is likely present due to the rigid, nonpermanent attachment of the gearshift knob to the camera in the laparoscopic tracking. Error related to a loose fit could be eliminated with a camera that has IREDs directly attached. We emphasize the importance of defining one's measure of error in evaluating image-guidance systems.

Our experiments are preliminary work in the feasibility of IIGS in the field of general surgery and specifically for hepatic applications. The results answer basic engineering questions with regard to the feasibility of image-guided liver surgery.

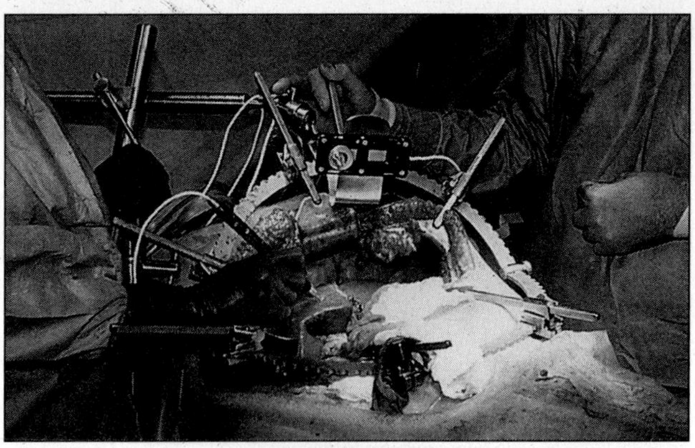

Figure 6. *The interactive image-guided surgery system in use in an open hepatic resection. Pictured are the 6 infrared-emitting diode reference body attached to the Bookwalter retractor (Codman and Shutleff, New Brunswick, NJ) and the operative probe being used on the liver surface.*

We believe that this technology has applicability in the field of hepatic surgery and may improve definition of normal anatomy and pathologic changes. With the increasing use of ablative procedures and laparoscopy, intraoperative imaging will hold increasing significance for the general surgeon. Being able to display accurately the intrahepatic position of instruments (eg, cryoprobes, radiofrequency probes) on CT images could improve placement of probes, margins of resection or ablation, and evaluation of resectability (**Figure 6**). We have demonstrated that liver motion with pneumoperitoneum is small (<5 mm), and we have developed an accurate method to register the liver in a porcine model. We have demonstrated that we can track and localize a laparoscopic instrument to within 2 mm of accuracy in an operating room. This seems sufficient for hepatic IIGS, and the accuracy may improve as the equipment being used is attached directly to the localization devices. Interactive image-guided liver surgery appears to be feasible, and further investigation is warranted into the intraoperative use of image-guided systems.

This work was supported by grant BES-9703714 from the National Science Foundation, Arlington, Va, and grants NIGMS GM52798 and NRSA 1 F32 DK 09671-01 SB from the National Institutes of Health, Bethesda, Md.

Presented at the 106th Scientific Session of the Western Surgical Association, Indianapolis, Ind, November 17, 1998.

We acknowledge Odie Lawrence for his machining and corrections of our designs, Cindy Duncan and Tina Herron for their help with collection of computed tomographic images, and Karl-Storz GmbH & Co, Tuttlingen, Germany, for the loan of laparoscopic equipment.

Reprints: William C. Chapman, MD, Vanderbilt University Medical Center, 801 Oxford House, Nashville, TN 37232-4753 (e-mail: will.chapman@surgery.mc.vanderbilt.edu).

REFERENCES

1. Rafaelsen SR, Kronborg O, Larsen C, Fenger C. Intra-operative ultrasonography in detection of hepatic metastases from colorectal cancer. *Dis Colon Rectum.* 1995;38:355-360.

2. Klotz HP, Flury R, Erhart P, et al. Magnetic resonance-guided laparoscopic interstitial laser therapy of the liver. *Am J Surg.* 1997;174:448-451.
3. Wilson DL, Carrillo A, Zheng L, Genc A, Duerk JL, Lewin JS. Evaluation of 3D image registration as applied to MR-guided thermal treatment of liver cancer. *J Magn Reson Imaging.* 1998;8:77-84.
4. Fried MP, Kleefield J, Gopal H, et al. Image-guided endoscopic surgery: results of accuracy and performance in a multicenter clinical study using an electromagnetic tracking system. *Laryngoscope.* 1997;107:594-600.
5. Galloway RL. Stereotactic frame systems and intraoperative localization devices. In: Maciunas RJ, ed. *Interactive Image-Guided Neurosurgery.* Park Ridge, Ill: Neurosurgical Topics, American Association of Neurological Surgeons Publications Committee; 1993:9-16.
6. Galloway RL, Maciunas RJ, Edwards CA. Interactive, image-guided neurosurgery. *IEEE Trans Biomed Eng.* 1992;39:1226-1231.
7. Galloway RL, Maciunas RJ, Bass WA, Carpini WJ. Optical localization for interactive image-guided neurosurgery. *Proc SPIE.* 1994;2164:137-145.
8. Gao L, Heath DG, Kuszyk BS, Fishman EK. Automatic liver segmentation technique for 3-dimensional visualization of CT data. *Radiology.* 1996;201:359-364.
9. John TG, Greig JD, Crosbie JL, Miles WFA, Garden OJ. Superior staging of liver tumors with laparoscopy and laparoscopic ultrasound. *Ann Surg.* 1994;220:711-719.
10. Waner A, Ploder O, Enislidis G, Truppe M, Ewers R. Virtual image guided navigation in tumor surgery: technical innovation. *J Craniomaxillofac Surg.* 1995; 23:271-273.
11. Maurer CM, Fitzpatrick JM, Wang MY, Galloway RL, Macinuas RJ, Allen GS. Registration of head volume images using implantable fiducial markers. *IEEE Trans Med Imaging.* 1997;16:447-462.
12. Maciunas RJ, ed. *Interactive Image-Guided Neurosurgery.* Park Ridge, Ill: Neurosurgical Topics, American Association of Neurological Surgeons Publications Committee; 1993.
13. Stefansic JD, Herline AJ, Chapman WC, Galloway RL. Endoscopic tracking for use in interactive, image-guided surgery. *Proc SPIE Med Imaging Image Display.* 1998;3335:208-218.
14. Bennett WF, Bova JG, Petty L, Martin EW. Preoperative rendering of MR imaging in liver metastases. *J Comput Assist Tomogr.* 1991;15:979-984.
15. Katkhouda N, Mouiel J. Laparoscopic surgery of the liver. In: Arregui ME, ed. *Principles of Laparoscopic Surgery: Basic and Advanced Techniques.* New York, NY: Springer-Verlag YN Inc; 1996:345-355.
16. Hoh CK, Dahlbom M, Harris G, Choi Y, Hawkins A. Automated iterative 3-dimensional registration of positron emission tomography. *J Nucl Med.* 1993;34:2009-2018.
17. Davies SC, Hill AL, Holmes RB, Halliwell M, Jackson PC. Ultrasound quantitation of respiratory organ motion in the upper abdomen. *Br J Radiol.* 1994;67: 1096-1102.

DISCUSSION

James E. Goodnight, Jr, MD, PhD, Sacramento, Calif: I will open this discussion with an anecdote which underscores the point that Dr Grosfeld made yesterday about our need to be on top of technology and the fact that we share this technology with multiple disciplines. When I received Dr Chapman's manuscript, I realized it was a technology that our neurosurgeons had recently begun to use, and so I went to them to get a perspective and information. The first person I encountered was their RN, who sets up their equipment in the OR and who makes things go smoothly. She said, "Oh, yes, I know about that. You put these infrared diodes on the scalp and that allows you to register those points on an image that is already contained in the machine." Well, I was duly impressed. The first time I had ever heard registration used in this context was when I read Dr Chapman's manuscript. She went on to explain the technology about superimposing it on images and so forth and then stopped at one point and looked at me earnestly and said, "You know, this is really cool stuff." And that was my reaction exactly. This is really cool stuff. Our neurosurgeons are indeed using this optotrack system. Currently it is most effective for spine work. They take their fiducial registration points, if you will, the base registration points, directly from the bony spine after they open. Neither the bony skeleton nor the spinal cord moves very much, and therefore this system provides superb localization for operation or probe placement. The system is equally effective for localizing lesions in the brain, except that the brain shifts, particularly once they turn a flap and begin to work on the brain. They use intraoperative ultrasound to test the positions (once again fiducial registration and target registration), and the software of the system utilizes the ultrasound information to update the preoperative MRI that has been incorporated into the system. This to me is a fairly dramatic process, that you can use these preoperative static images and then update them with a computer and with the probe at the time of operation. They were quite intrigued with Dr Chapman's efforts to correct for motion and apply this technique to liver surgery. They are not as fully trusting of the localization in the brain as they are in the spine. So Dr Chapman's work on motion is right on. In addition, they thought the low FRE (fiducial registration error and target registration error) which Dr Chapman is reporting to be very good tolerances.

I also discussed this paper with my colleague, Dr Phil Schneider, who is using radiofrequency probes to ablate liver lesions. He echoes the sentiments that Dr Chapman expresses in the manuscript, that ultrasound can be tricky for precise localization of these probes, particularly if one is looking inferiorly at the liver up toward the dome.

As all of us know, a surgeon sees with more than his or her eyes. Tactile stimuli are a critical part of the composite image our brains form of the operative field. Both tactile stimuli and depth are lost with current laparoscopic techniques. Dr Chapman and his colleagues offer us a highly innovative means by which we may be able to see in a composite fashion to do liver surgery, either by laparoscopic techniques or in fact to extend our range with open procedures. It is a beginning to be sure, as Dr Chapman points out, and much remains to be done to bring it to prime time. But I am certainly indebted to him and his colleagues for bringing this technique to our attention and the possible clinical use.

I have 4 questions. The first is a relatively obvious question, but I will ask it for clarification. Am I correct that our ability with this technique to determine the margins of a tumor or an interface with blood vessels in the liver is dependent on the quality of the CT or MRI images, or, for that matter, the resolution of the intraoperative ultrasound? Second, I think perhaps a very important question of this study is, as I move the liver at operation, can I still accurately localize the probe or, for that matter, the position of the tumor despite bleeding or tissue resection or the movement that I have created?

Then, particularly as I watched the video, what is the learning curve or user variation of this technique, perhaps compared to IOUS? And of course this is obviously a system under development. Could you give us some idea of the likely commercial cost—$25 000, $50 000, $300 000?

Steven C. Stain, MD, Los Angeles, Calif: I think the importance of this work is that it will allow us to utilize images, CT or MRI, in the operating room more precisely. I have 2 questions. How important do you believe it is to be able to place an instrument or a probe within 3 mm of its intended location? Most of the work that we do operatively does not allow us to place sutures or a cryoprobe within that amount of precision.

Second, with the current ablative procedures, which require a half centimeter or a centimeter of margin, is a 3-mm accuracy in placement really important?

Jeffrey H. Peters, MD, Los Angeles: A quick question. The CT image of course provides dichotomous rather than continuous data collection, that is, images at centimeter or half-centimeter intervals. How does the computer manage the space in between when you are working with a continuous image?

John A. Weigelt, MD, St Paul, Minn: This is an exciting technology. I have 1 question. Have you thought to explore the possibility of changing your anesthetic technique with this device to either using a high-frequency or an oscillation technique, which would then decrease the liver motion?

Dr Chapman: One of the major reasons this project has been successful is that we have had one of our surgical residents, who has training and experience as a biomedical engineer, working on this project, Dr Allen Herline, who is here for this meeting.

Dr Herline has been able to help us learn the biomedical techniques and engineering background that we have to have to make this project successful. He has been a key part of making this project develop to the point where we are, although we do have a ways yet to go to demonstrate clinical utility.

Dr Goodnight, in response to your specific questions, the issue of imaging resolution and tumor margins in resections or ablative procedures, you are right on the mark. This technique can only be as good as the imaging which is acquired and utilized in the process, so this is only able to show you information that you gained from your prior imaging studies.

As far as the issue of mobilization of the liver during hepatic procedures, that is an issue, and this is something we are having to work with to determine what our most optimal registration methods will be. In the interest of time and because we are not as far along in this area, I didn't get into the other methods for registration, but another technique involves surface registration where we can actually use our IRED probes to outline the surface of the liver, generate a surface rendering that can then be matched to CT-generated surface renderings, and allow for matching of the location and position of preoperative images with our operative localization procedure. This will allow us to work around the mobilization issues.

Will there be user variation? We hope that this will be minimized once this technique is fully developed. When a registration is performed, you are able to immediately get a targeting accuracy so that you can generate a fiducial error in your registration immediately, and you know what your accuracy is. There will be a threshold cutoff that we would all use, and whether that is 2 mm or 3 mm or 5 mm of accuracy in your registration, I think that will be variable. But if the registration is not a good fit, you exclude that information and start again until you do have accurate targeting. I do think there will be a learning curve with this technology. How difficult that will be remains to be seen.

You asked about cost. It's hard to know that for certain. Right now the major costs involve the infrared camera. That camera costs between $25 000 and $50 000 in its early-development phase. The PC is a standard PC system like any of us would use in our offices that costs around $3000. The probes can be manufactured relatively inexpensively. So I would estimate the system costs to be between $35 000 and $50 000 at the present time. These costs may come down in the future. This is much more cost-efficient than an alternative concept, which involves putting imagers, for example, MR scanners, actually in the operating room.

Dr Stain asked about accuracy placement, and do we really need 3-mm accuracy? We don't think we do need 3-mm accuracy. In the neurosurgical applications, the accuracy has been generally within 0.5 mm to 1.0 mm for the actual targeting and tumor biopsies. We have room for some error. The smallest accuracy we could achieve would be most ideal.

The other point I would mention is that in certain areas like tumor ablations, the more you are away from the volumetric center at the time an ablation is begun, the bigger your ultimate error once that tumor volume is encompassed. It is helpful to be as accurate as possible.

The issues regarding the variations in anesthetic management will require some investigation and whether or not imaging and procedure manipulations will be done at a set time in the ventilatory cycle, for example, at end-inspiration, or whether we alter ventilatory techniques to use high-flow ventilation, are issues we will have to look into and address. But certainly we believe the technique allows us to measure movement and our errors so that we will be able to control for hepatic movement during the procedures.

IN OTHER AMA JOURNALS

ARCHIVES OF GENERAL PSYCHIATRY

Education and Peer Discussion Group Interventions and Adjustment to Breast Cancer

Vicki S. Helgeson, PhD; Sheldon Cohen, PhD; Richard Schulz, PhD; Joyce Yasko, PhD, FAAN

Background: We report a clinical trial comparing the effectiveness of education-based and peer discussion–based group interventions on adjustment to breast cancer.
Methods: Women with stage I, II, or III breast cancer (n = 312) were randomly assigned to 1 of 4 group conditions: control, education, peer discussion, or education plus peer discussion (combination). Seven groups (each comprising 8-12 women) were conducted in each of the 4 conditions (28 groups total). Adjustment was measured before the intervention, immediately after the intervention, and 6 months after the intervention.
Results: Consistently positive effects on adjustment were seen in the education groups both immediately follow-ing and 6 months after the intervention. There were no benefits of participation in peer discussion groups, and some indications of adverse effects on adjustment at both follow-up examinations. The effects could be explained by changes in self-esteem, body image, and intrusive thoughts about the illness.
Conclusions: Education-based group interventions facilitated the initial adjustment of women diagnosed with early stage breast cancer. There was no evidence of benefits from peer discussion group interventions. *(1999;56:340-347)*

Reprints: Vicki S. Helgeson, PhD, Psychology Department, Carnegie Mellon University, Pittsburgh, PA 15213.

PAPER

Sporadic Primary Hyperparathyroidism in Young Patients

A Separate Disease Entity?

C. Richard Harman, MD; Jon A. van Heerden, MD; David R. Farley, MD; Clive S. Grant, MD; Geoffrey B. Thompson, MD; Kathleen Curlee, RN

Hypothesis: Sporadic primary hyperparathyroidism (1 HPT) in young persons is thought to be extremely rare. The exact incidence is unknown and little is known of the characteristics of the disease.

Methods: From 1976 to 1998, 33 patients aged 19 years or younger underwent operation for sporadic 1 HPT at a single institution. Data were recorded regarding the clinical, surgical, pathologic, and biochemical aspects, as well as long-term patient follow-up.

Results: There were 17 male subjects and 16 female subjects ranging in age from 9 to 19 years (median age, 17 years). Thirty-one (94%) were symptomatic: 14 (42%) had renal stones, 9 (27%) had bone disease, 1 (3%) had pancreatitis, and 7 (21%) had vague nonspecific symptoms alone. The high incidence of symptoms was matched by correspondingly high biochemical values (mean serum calcium level, 3.02 mmol/L [12.1 mg/dL]) and large adenomas (mean weight, 967 mg). Five patients (15%) underwent exploration for persistent/recurrent 1 HPT. Thirty-one patients (94%) were normocalcemic postoperatively. One patient was temporarily hypocalcemic. No patient had vocal cord paralysis or paresis. Two patients developed recurrent disease in the mean follow-up period of 10.3 years. None have shown evidence of an inherited disorder.

Conclusions: It appears that 1 HPT in young patients presents as a more severe disease, in terms of symptoms, biochemistry, and extent of pathologic findings. Physicians should be aware that 1 HPT does occur in young persons in a nonfamilial setting and that it may be responsible for a wide spectrum of symptoms. As in the adult population, 1 HPT is safely and effectively treated with surgical intervention.

Arch Surg. 1999;134:651-656

From the Department of Surgery, Mayo Clinic and Mayo Foundation, Rochester, Minn.

SPORADIC PRIMARY hyperparathyroidism (1 HPT) in young persons is thought to be extremely rare, although the exact incidence is unknown.[1-3] The surgical literature regarding the disease is limited to case reports and a few small series of cases. In 1982, Allo et al[1] described 53 young patients with 1 HPT, only 18 of whom were younger than 18 years and half of whom had chief cell hyperplasia. Ten of the 53 patients had an inherited multiple endocrine neoplasia syndrome. Rapaport et al[4] documented a series of 7 patients younger than 17 years with sporadic 1 HPT. In this series, the disease appeared different than that in adults in that all patients were symptomatic with a high incidence of bone disease and nephrolithiasis. It was also noted that there was a higher incidence of the disease found in young male subjects, which is in sharp contrast to the preponderance of the disease in female subjects in the adult population.

We have compiled a database of 33 patients with sporadic 1 HPT presenting to our institution at age 19 years or younger. By comparing these patients with a large adult population of patients with 1 HPT,[5] we have identified several areas in which the disease differs significantly between the 2 groups.

RESULTS

DEMOGRAPHICS

There were 17 male subjects and 16 female subjects who ranged in age from 9

PATIENTS AND METHODS

From a total of 49 patients aged 19 years or younger with 1 HPT (1976-1998) at the Mayo Clinic in Rochester, Minn, 33 patients underwent an operation for sporadic 1 HPT. Patients with multiple endocrine neoplasia or any associated non–multiple endocrine neoplasia familial diseases were excluded (n = 16).

We examined the patient demographics, preoperative symptoms and complications of the disease, laboratory values, localization techniques, operative procedure and postoperative complications, pathologic findings, and immediate and long-term disease status. Follow-up was obtained by review of the medical records and direct contact with the patient and/or home physician.

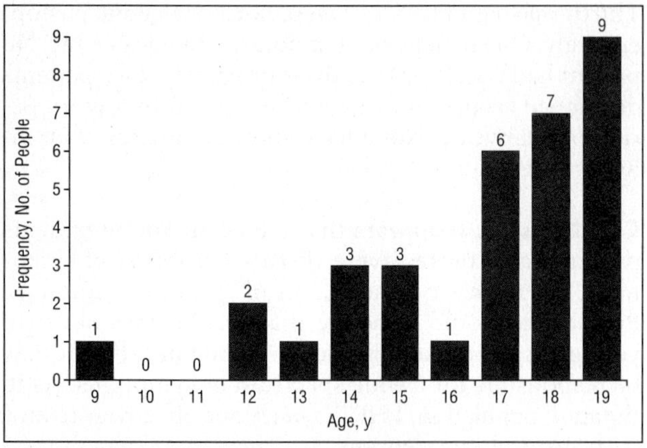

Figure 1. *Age histogram of young patients with primary hyperparathyroidism.*

to 19 years (median age, 17 years) at presentation (**Figure 1**). Five patients (15%) had persistent disease, having undergone unsuccessful exploration elsewhere prior to our evaluation.

SYMPTOMS AT PRESENTATION

Eighty-two percent (n = 27) of the patients were symptomatic, with 20 patients having major symptoms attributable to 1 HPT: renal stones, bone disease, or pancreatitis. Twenty-one percent (n = 7) had symptoms that were categorized as nonspecific (**Table 1**).

The most common finding was renal colic, defined as pain attributed to the documented history of the passage of a kidney stone or the presence of kidney stones on radiologic examination. Of the 14 patients (42%) presenting with kidney stones, all but 2 had symptoms and 5 had required surgical intervention. Bone disease, which was present in 9 patients (27%), implied bone pain, typical x-ray film changes, diminished bone densitometry, or actual fractures. Two patients had lytic lesions in their long bones, the most severe case being a 14-year-old girl who had been healthy until the age of 11 years when she developed genu valgum requiring orthopedic intervention. In addition, multiple lytic lesions (brown tumors) were present in her metacarpal bones (**Figure 2**, top and bottom).

One patient presented with acute pancreatitis and required hospitalization for 10 days. This 11-year-old girl

Table 1. Symptoms in 33 Young Patients With Primary Hyperparathyroidism

Symptoms	No. (%)*
Major symptoms from	20 (61)
Kidney stones	14 (42)
Bone disease	9 (27)
Pancreatitis	1 (3)
Nonspecific symptoms alone	7 (21)
Severe fatigue	4 (12)
Depression	1 (3)
Fatigue, anorexia, and weight loss	1 (3)
Severe fatigue, polydipsia, polyuria, and hypertension	1 (3)
Asymptomatic	6 (18)
Total	**33 (100)**

**Some patients had more than 1 symptom.*

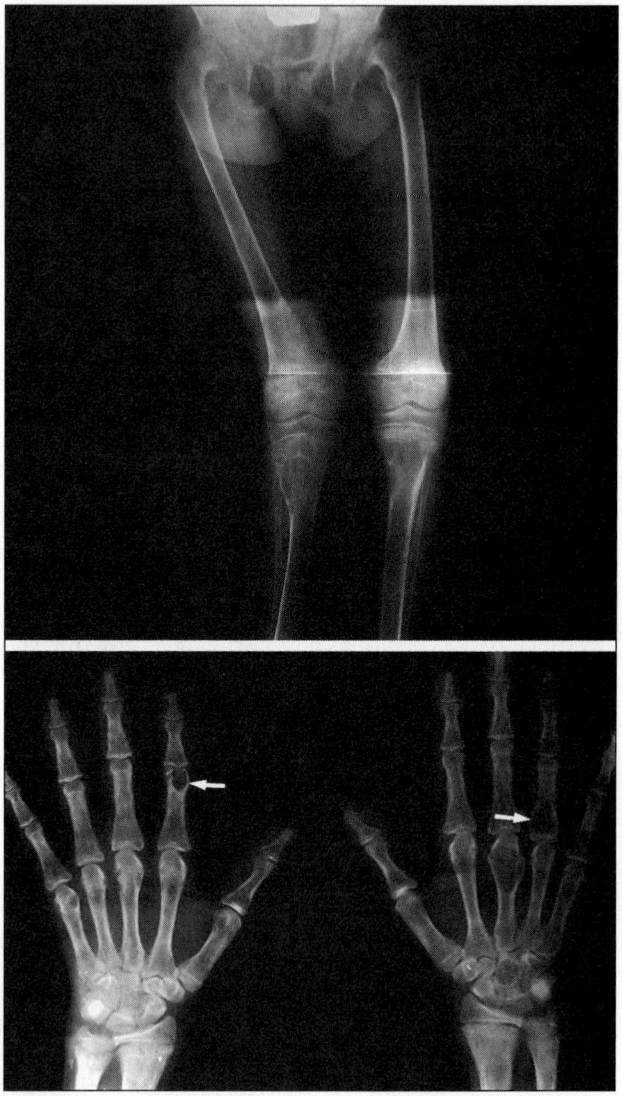

Figure 2. *Top, Severe genu valgum. Bottom, Multiple brown tumors (arrows).*

Table 2. Biochemical Data of 33 Young Patients With Primary Hyperparathyroidism*

Biochemical Value and Unit	No. of Patients Undergoing Test	Mean	Range	Reference Range
Serum calcium, mmol/L (mg/dL)	100	3.02 (12.1)	2.55-4.55 (10.2-18.2)	2.22-2.52 (8.9-10.1)
Serum phosphorus, mmol/L (mg/dL)	100	0.93 (2.9)	0.61-1.32 (1.9-4.1)	0.81-1.45 (2.5-4.5)
Urinary calcium, mmol/d (mg/24 h)	100	99.25 (397)	29.75-282.50 (119-1370)	0-62.50 (0-250)
ICMA, pmol/L	36	9.9	2.7-34	1-5.2
PTH, pmol/L	64	22.1	2.7-170	1.0-5.2

**ICMA indicates immunochemiluminescent assay; PTH, parathyroid hormone.*

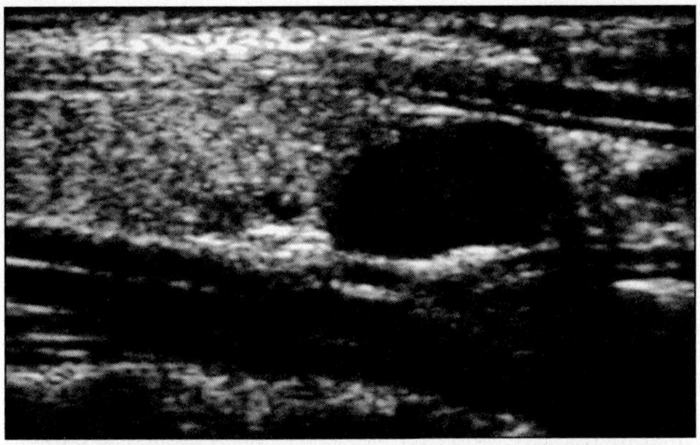

Figure 3. *An ultrasound view of a 400-mg adenoma in an 11-year-old girl who presented with pancreatitis, renal stones, lethargy, and weight loss.*

also had a history of renal stones, bone disease, a weight loss of 44.1 kg, anorexia, and severe fatigue. In those patients classified as having major symptoms, 7 also had associated nonspecific symptoms (4 with fatigue, 4 with polydipsia and polyuria, 3 with weight loss, 1 with headache, and 1 with anxiety). In the remaining asymptomatic group (n = 6), the disease was discovered coincidentally during the evaluation of an unrelated medical problem.

Three patients presented with a serum calcium level greater than 3.87 mmol/L (>15.5 mg/dL). One patient presented with hypercalcemic crisis and had a serum calcium level of 4.55 mmol/L (18.2 mg/dL). This patient required large-volume intravenous saline infusion and both mithramycin and calcitonin preoperatively and a semiurgent operative procedure with excision of a 1.6-g parathyroid adenoma.

BIOCHEMISTRY

All patients in the study were hypercalcemic. The relevant biochemical details are listed in **Table 2**.

LOCALIZATION

Prior to their operation, 17 patients had preoperative localization studies. Small-part ultrasonography was the most common modality employed (n = 16), with a sensitivity of 70% and an accuracy of 70%. **Figure 3** shows the typical ultrasound image of a parathyroid adenoma. Other localization studies employed were computed tomographic (CT) scanning (n = 3), thallium-technetium sestamibi scanning (n = 2), and magnetic resonance imaging (n = 1). Three such studies clearly identified the adenoma (CT, 1; thallium-technetium scanning 1; and magnetic resonance imaging, 1). The indications for preoperative localization in those who had not had previous surgery were young age and disease severity at presentation.

Three of the 5 patients who had persistent disease had preoperative localization. Findings from half of these localizing studies (CT, 2; ultrasonography, 1; and thallium-technetium scanning, 1) were normal, while the other half were abnormal (CT, 1; ultrasonography, 2; and thallium technetium scanning, 1). The 2 patients who did not have preoperative localization were thought to have had an inadequate exploration elsewhere and were operated on in 1977 prior to currently established localization techniques.

SURGERY AND PATHOLOGIC EXAMINATION

All patients underwent operative intervention. Thirty-one patients had cervical exploration and 2 had combined cervical-mediastinal exploration requiring sternotomy. Chief cell adenomas were removed in 31 patients (mean weight, 967 mg; median, 410 mg; range, 100-9760 mg). No patient was found to have parathyroid hyperplasia. In 2 patients, no abnormal parathyroid tissue was removed. Both sides of the neck were routinely explored and additional normal glands were identified in all but 1 patient, who had a thymic adenoma. Sixteen patients had all 4 glands identified, 7 had 3, 7 had 2, 2 had 1, and in 1 patient, no parathyroid glands were identified.

COMPLICATIONS

There was no long-term morbidity. One patient was rendered temporarily hypocalcemic and required calcium supplementation for 6 months; this patient had 2 remaining normal glands (after removal of a 1450-mg adenoma) on which biopsies were performed, which likely resulted in some degree of parathyroid devascularization. Two patients had small superficial hematomas that did not require drainage. One patient had an area of superficial skin necrosis on the superior skin flap of the cervical incision. No patient had either temporary or permanent recurrent laryngeal nerve dysfunction.

FOLLOW-UP

Long-term follow-up via telephone interview was possible in 29 of the 33 patients. In the 4 patients whom we were unable to contact, documented 1-month postoperative serum calcium levels were normal. Long-term follow-up ranged from 1 to 266 months, with a mean of 123 months (10.3 years).

Thirty-one patients were initially cured (rendered normocalcemic) after removal of a parathyroid adenoma. Two patients in whom no abnormal tissue was removed remained hypercalcemic postoperatively. One of these patients, an 18-year-old woman, underwent an unsuccessful reoperation after a negative exploration elsewhere. Postoperatively, a CT scan of the neck and chest was normal and the patient declined a third exploration. Her serum calcium level remained elevated for 6 years, after which the level spontaneously returned to normal.

The other patient who was not cured had 2 normal superior glands identified at cervical exploration. Both inferior glands could not be identified. A diagnosis of mediastinal adenoma was pursued. The patient had a normal thallium-technetium scan. Because the original biochemical diagnosis of 1 HPT was equivocal, the diagnosis was questioned. She was discharged from the study, but 4 years after her unsuccessful surgery she remains hypercalcemic (serum calcium level, 2.92 mmol/L [11.7 mg/dL]) with renal stones.

Two patients who initially recovered have developed recurrent disease. One of them underwent the removal of a 1240-mg adenoma from the left superior position. A normal left inferior gland was seen, but no glands were identified on the right side. This patient developed hypercalcemia and renal stones 17 years later. A 2½ gland parathyroidectomy for hyperplasia resulted in normocalcemia. The other patient had a hypercalcemic crisis (serum calcium level, 3.42 mmol/L [13.7 mg/dL]) 9 years after his original operation (a 1550-mg adenoma excised). At the time of the second exploration, a 910 mg second adenoma was excised, and the the patient's serum calcium level has since remained normal for 11 years.

At long-term follow up, 32 of patients (97%) remain surgically cured of 1 HPT. No patients have developed features of associated endocrinopathies or have offspring with parathyroid disease that might suggest familial disease.

COMMENT

Sporadic 1 HPT in young patients is thought to be extremely rare. The exact incidence is unknown and little is known of the characteristics of the disease.[1-4,6-8] The prevalence of 1 HPT has been suggested as being approximately between 1 and 3 in 1000 adolescents.[9] This study represents the largest group of patients younger than 20 years with sporadic 1 HPT evaluated and treated at a single institution. During the study period, 4919 patients were operated on at our institution for 1 HPT. These 33 patients, therefore, represent 0.7% of such patients, emphasizing the extreme rarity of 1 HPT in the young. Several differences between the adult group and this group are apparent. Comparing the results of this study with a previous study from this institution of all patients with 1 HPT in a 2-year period[5] highlights the differences (**Table 3**).

In contrast to our adult population, 1 HPT in young patients seems to be at least as common in males; others report that 1 HPT is even more common in young men than in young women.[1,3,6,8] The preponderance of 1 HPT in women is attributed to an increase in the incidence of 1 HPT in postmenopausal women.[10]

Table 3. Comparison of Young and Adult Patients With Primary Hyperparathyroidism

Variable	Adult Patients (n = 379)	Young Patients (n = 33)
Female patients, %	74	48
Patients with symptoms, %	44	79
Mean serum calcium level, mmol/L (mg/dL)	2.82 (11.3)	3.02 (12.1)
Mean weight of adenoma, mg	948	967

Most of the patients (82%) in this series had symptoms that could be directly attributable to 1 HPT. This is in contrast to our adult series, where only 44% had overt symptoms and most patients were diagnosed from routine blood screening. Some of our young patients had severe symptoms, which at times were life threatening. In fact, 3 patients had serum calcium levels higher than 3.87 mmol/L (>15.5 mg/dL), which is tantamount to a hypercalcemic crisis in the adult population.[11,12]

One of the striking findings of this study was the severity of the young patients' symptoms. Most patients with renal stones were symptomatic, and 5 had required surgical intervention for nephrolithiasis. Three of the 10 patients with bone disease had severe changes on x-ray films, and 1 patient had genu valgum, had stopped growing, and required orthopedic surgical intervention.

While others have noted an increase in incidence of both renal (in children with nephrolithiasis, approximately 6% have 1 HPT) and bone disease,[1,13] to our knowledge, none have commented on the generalized severity of symptoms identified in this study group. On the contrary, some authors[3,14,15] have suggested that the incidence of renal involvement is less than that of their adult counterparts. There are reports of severe bone disease in which the patients developed genu valgum.[6] The changes seen are similar to the changes seen in rickets, and the association with 1 HPT is not well reported.[4] A single patient in this series presented with acute pancreatitis. As in the adult population, this is a rare complication of the disease, but it has been reported previously.[16,17]

The severity of symptoms may be reflected in the magnitude of the serum calcium level and the large size and weight of the glands removed, which were both as high as those in the adult population. Does this mean that it is a different disease than the one in the adult population? Probably not; it is more likely that a biased sector of patients with this disease is seen, and that the patients being identified are the ones with severe disease who have become symptomatic. Only 18% of our patients were diagnosed incidentally, in contrast to our adult series,[5] where the asymptomatic patients made up 56% of the group. This is a trend that is historically well known. In the 1930s, half of the patients had renal stones and severe bone disease, whereas most patients are now diagnosed even before they become symptomatic. The younger patients are much less likely to undergo a serum calcium level screening than their adult counterparts; thus, 1 HPT may be a more common entity in young people than previously thought.[8] Physicians should be aware that this disease does exist in the young and may be a cause of nonspecific symptoms such as lethargy, failure to thrive, growing problems, headaches, and the more well-known symptoms of renal stones, bone pain and deformities, and pancreatitis. Delay in diagnosis of this disease can be associated with long-term renal dysfunction.[18] While only 1 patient in this study underwent thallium-technetium sestamibi scanning, 3 of the 33 patients had a mediastinal adenoma excised (2 via sternotomy). We were similarly struck by the high incidence (15%) of failed initial operation in this group of patients and would suggest that all young patients have a thallium-technetium sestamibi scan prior to surgery to help localize the tumor and to exclude a mediastinal adenoma to prevent unsuccessful surgery in these young patients.

The surgery for this disease in the sporadic form can be performed as safely as in adults despite the fact that many patients had serum calcium levels that were dangerously high (as long as the patients are well-hydrated preoperatively). None of the patients in this study developed postoperative problems secondary to their hypercalcemia, and most of the operations can be performed electively.

Allo et al[1] stated that hyperplasia was common in these younger patients, although she included all patients with 1 HPT, including those with multiple endocrine neoplasia. This was not the case in our study. We excluded patients with multiple endocrine neoplasia, and only 1 of our patients had 4-gland hyperplasia identified with operative intervention and long-term follow-up. Huang et al[8] studied 100 young patients with HPT reported in the literature. While 30 had hyperplasia, 87% of those with hyperplasia were neonates. Neonates should be considered a different group and characteristically do have hyperplasia.[19-22] We have identified only 1 patient with definite hyperplasia and 1 with a double adenoma, both identified many years after their initial curative surgery. This emphasizes 2 points: (1) although hyperplasia is rare in young patients, these patients need to be screened for the disease as in adults, and (2) young patients need long-term follow-up.

One of the 2 patients who were not cured by operation underwent "spontaneous" normalization of her serum calcium level 6 years after cervical exploration. Although this is a rare event, it is well documented and is most likely due to partial or total devascularization of the abnormal gland during cervical exploration.[23]

CONCLUSION

We have demonstrated several differences in the presentation of sporadic 1 HPT in the young patients compared with adult patients. It is likely that 1 HPT is only diagnosed when the symptoms are severe and that we may actually greatly underestimate the number of young people with this disorder. Physicians should be aware that 1 HPT may be responsible for a wide spectrum of symptoms. A serum calcium level test is useful to screen the young patient presenting with constitutional or vague symptoms potentially attributable to renal stones, bone disease, or pancreatitis. The disease is usually due to a single adenoma, and surgery is an extremely safe and effective method of preventing complications of this disease.

Presented at the 106th Scientific Session of the Western Surgical Association, Indianapolis, Ind, November 16, 1998.

Corresponding author: Jon A. van Heerden, MD, Department of Surgery Mayo Clinic, 200 First St SW, Rochester, MN 55905.

REFERENCES

1. Allo M, Thompson NW, Harness JK, Nishiyama RH. Primary hyperparathyroidism in children, adolscents, and young adults. *World J Surg.* 1982;6:771-776.
2. Girard RM, Belanger A, Hazel B. Primary hyperparathyroidism in children. *Can J Surg.* 1982;25:11-32.
3. Bjernulf A, Hall K, Spogren I, et al. Primary hyperparathyroidism in children. *Acta Pediatr Scand.* 1970;59:249-258.
4. Rapaport D, Ziv Y, Rubin M, Huminer D, Dintsman M. Primary hyperparathyroidism in children. *J Pediatr Surg.* 1986;21:395-397.
5. van Heerden JA, Grant CS. Surgical treatment of primary hyperparathyroidism: an institutional perspective. *World J Surg.* 1991;15:688-692.
6. Heath H, Hodgson SF, Kennedy MA. Primary hyperparathyroidism: incidence, morbidity and potential economic impact in a community. *N Engl J Med.* 1980; 302:189-193.
7. Makhdoomi KR, Chalmers J, Campbell IW, Browning GGP. Delayed diagnosis of juvenile primary hyperparathyroidism. *J R Coll Surg Edinb.* 1996;41:351-353.
8. Huang C-B, Huang S-C, Chou F-F, Chen W-J. Primary hyperparathryoidism in children: report of a case and a brief review of the literature. *J Formos Med Assoc.* 1993;92:1095-1098.
9. Horowitz M, Nordin BEC. Primary hyperparathyroidism. In: Norbin BEC, Need AG, Morris HA, eds. *Metabolic Bone and Stone Disease*, 3rd ed. London, England: Churchill Livingstone Inc; 1993:119-131.
10. Muller H. Sex, age and hyperparathyrodism. *Lancet.* 1969;1:449-450.
11. Allo MD. Hypercalcemic crisis. In: van Heerden JA, ed. *Common Problems in Endocrine Surgery.* Chicago, Ill: Year Book Medical Publishers Inc; 1989:151-155.
12. Grossman RF, Jossart GH. Hypercalcemic crisis. In: Clark OH, Duh Q-Y, eds. *Textbook of Endocrine Surgery.* Philadelphia, Pa: WB Saunders Co; 1997:432-438.
13. Malek RS, Panayotis PK. Urologic manifestations of hyperparathyrodism in childhood. *J Urol.* 1976;15:717-719.
14. Mannix HJ. Primary hyperparathyroidism in children. *Am J Surg.* 1975;29: 528-531.
15. Vazquez AM. Nephrocalcinosis and hypertenesion in juvenile primary hyperparathyroidism. *AJDC.* 1973;125:104-106.
16. Daum F, Rosen JF, Boley S. Parathyroid adenoma, parathyroid crisis and acute pancreatitis in an adolescent. *J Pediatr.* 1973;83:275-277.
17. Karitzky D. Akute Pankreatitis Als Erstmanifesttion Einer Hypercalcamie Bei Primarem Hyperparathyroidism Im Kindersalter. *Monatsschr Kinderheilkd.* 1989; 137:225-227.
18. Palmer M, Bergstrom R, Akerstrom G, et al. Survival and renal function in untreated hypercalcaemia: population-based cohort study with 14 years of follow-up. *Lancet.* 1987;I:59.
19. Hillman DA, Seriver CR, Pedvis S, et al. Neonatal familial primary hyperparathyroidism. *N Engl J Med.* 1960;270:483-490.
20. Thompson NW, Carpenter LC, Kessler DL, et al. Hereditary neonatal hyperparathyroidism. *Arch Surg.* 1978;113:100-103.
21. Spiegel AM, Harrison HE, Stephen JM, et al. Neonatal primary hyperparathyroidism with autosomal dominant inheritance. *J Pediatr.* 1977;90:269-272.
22. Goldbloom RB, Gillis DA, Prasad M. Hereditary parathyroid hyperplasia: a surgical emergency of early infancy. *Pediatrics.* 1972;49:514-523.
23. Mir R, Gerold T, Khan S, Weitz J. Spontaneous infarction of parathyroid adenoma: case report and literature review. *Head Neck.* 1993;15:566-568.

DISCUSSION

Norman W. Thompson, MD, Ann Arbor, Mich: First I would like to congratulate Dr Harman, Dr van Heerden, and colleagues for an excellent presentation, sharp, concise, beautiful slides, and conclusions that I can agree with. I was the coauthor of one of the papers that you initially mentioned with Drs Maria Allo and Jay Harness. We reviewed our experience in 1982, and it was published in the *World Journal of Surgery*. At that time it was the largest series in the world, but once again, the Mayo Clinic has outdone us. The truth is that we had 53 patients in contrast to the 33 in this group, but the difference was that we included patients up to the age of 30 because many of those patients had symptoms that had gone undetected, as far as hyperparathyroidism was concerned, for as long as 10 years. Actually, 27 of those patients had symptoms before the age of 18. We also included patients with familial disease because it was frequently diagnosed only in retrospect. In fact, there were 4 previously unrecognized MEN type 1 patients in that group who have, in the ensuing 16-year period, all had distal pancreatectomies for neuroendocrine disease. None of those were known to have MEN type 1 at the time of exploration. I know from the article that during this same period, the Mayo Clinic had 16 patients with parathyroid hyperplasia due to MEN type 1 or MEN type 2 who were not included in this paper. I would like to point out that some of these patients present just like any other patient with sporadic hyperparathyroidism. I would ask Dr van Heerden, who is going to close, what he would do today when he encounters a patient with no family history and 4-gland hyperplasia such as that seen in 1 of your patients. What kind of follow-up studies would be necessary?

As the authors pointed out, what is striking about the young patients is that they basically have the same disease as the adults, but it is apparently more advanced. Fifty percent of their patients had kidney stones and 50% of our patients had kidney stones when they first presented. Many of them had other symptoms that represented advanced disease, such as brown tumors or von Recklinghausen's bone disease. Your series had a considerably higher incidence of bone disease than ours.

These diagnosed cases may represent only the tip of the iceberg. I would ask you at the Mayo Clinic, do the pediatricians screen their patients as adults are screened with serum calcium levels? Until we reviewed our experience, our pediatricians did not, but now do so and in the ensuing 16 years we've had an increasing incidence of children in whom the disease is detected at an earlier stage.

Another striking point is that in this series of 33 patients, 3, or 9%, actually had a deep mediastinal adenoma. That is much higher than in adults. In the article, the question was raised whether all children should have a thallium-technetium sestamibi scan or other localization study before their procedure. I think this consideration was based on that higher incidence of deep mediastinal disease. In our series, we had 2 out of 53 who had deep mediastinal tumors. I personally don't think that possibility alone is a reasonable justification. I would ask the authors whether they would address that issue and whether they really feel that localization studies are indicated in children. Identification of 1 tumor does not rule out a second tumor or multiple gland disease merely on the basis of a localization study.

Finally, there is a technical point that I think is worth emphasizing in which children differ from adults. I will show 1 slide to illustrate the point. When you explore a young patient who has a serum calcium level of 13 or 14 mg/dL, as some of your patients did, I think the objective should be to cure the disease with 1 operative procedure. In children, even with deep mediastinal adenomas, you can usually do that. If you find 3 glands that are normal, the fourth gland is likely to be in the deep mediastinum. The difference in children and young adults as in this patient is that the mediastinal tumor can be extracted from a cervical incision, as shown in this picture, showing an adenoma within the thymus 13 cm below the level of the sternal notch. In children with thymuses that are not atrophic, one can usually extract the deep mediastinal tumor within the thymus with the exclusion of those in the aortopulmonary window. The other thymic point is that some of these children have thymic tissue around all 4 parathyroid glands. We recently saw a patient who had 3 normal parathyroid glands removed because the surgeon, with all due respect to our President, who was a pediatric surgeon at another institution, mistakenly thought they were enlarged glands. The fourth gland was in the chest and was an adenoma that had been missed on a preoperative thallium-technetium sestamibi scan because the scan had not been done low enough to show a deep mediastinal tumor.

Orlo H. Clark, MD, San Francisco, Calif: I have 2 questions. Is there a different cause than that found in older individuals? Have you ruled out benign familial hypocalciuric hypercalcemia, and did all of these children have urinary calcium levels determined? Also, did any of them have radiation exposure that, as you know, can increase the frequency of parathyroid disease? What were the final pathologic findings in these patients? Were the distribution of parathyroid pathologic findings the same as in your adult population, such as about 80%, with solitary adenomas?

Dr van Heerden: To answer Dr Clark's questions first: (1) All of these children were screened for benign familial hypocalciuric hypercalcemia and none of these children had benign familial hypocalciuric hypercalcemia. We believe very strongly in urine calcium level screening in these patients to rule out that rare but very troublesome misdiagnosis. (2) None of these children had had previous radiotherapy, which is interesting. (3) The pathological distribution was exactly the same. In adults, we know that 90% have adenomas, 9% hyperplasia, and 1% cancer. We had no cancers in this study, 1 patient was subsequently found to have hyperplasia, but of these 33 patients, 31 had solitary adenomas and 1 had dual adenomas.

Norman Thompson raised 4 issues. First, thymectomy. I think this comes from a lot of experience, Norman. Thymectomy in children is much easier than the adult, isn't it? And one mustn't necessarily feel that because the child has a low anterior mediastinal tumor that a median sternotomy is required. It can be removed transcervically.

Secondly, as Dr Farley said, I think this disease is probably underdiagnosed in the pediatric population. Routine calcium levels are not obtained as a screening modality worldwide. We are probably seeing the tip of the iceberg only, and we need to think of this diagnosis more often in the pediatric age group.

Dr Thompson asked what would we do if we found a child with multiple gland disease. I think whenever you find multiple gland disease, you need to think of familial non-MEN disease or MEN type 1, which sets a definite protocol into operation. Today we have the genetic screening for MEN type 1 and that should certainly be done, not only in the child but in the family members. Secondly, long-term follow-up is vitally important.

Thirdly, Norman raised the issue of thallium-technetium sestamibi scanning. We continue not to advise routine preoperative localizing modalities, be it ultrasound, CT, or thallium-technetium sestamibi in the nonoperated adult neck. We have suggested in this paper, though, that in these patients perhaps we should, and I think when we can make a point for routine localization in the pediatric age group only. I don't feel we need to start with a thallium-technetium sestamibi scan, which is expensive, but perhaps we should start with a cervical ultrasound and if that is unequivocally positive, I don't think you need any other localizing modalities. The very fact that 12% of these children had mediastinal tumors behooves us to think about localizing modalities.

In summary, what our group has shown is that this diagnosis is delayed and therefore the pathologic findings are more advanced and there was a high failure rate. If you take our failure rate (2 patients), plus the 5 patients who came to us as failures, that adds up to a failure rate of almost 20%, which is in contrast to 1% in the adult population. That is unacceptable. Because of that we feel localization is justifiable.

Thirdly and somewhat anecdotally, in our large experience with patients with primary hyperparathyroidism, I have only seen 2 patients with pancreatitis whose pancreatitis could be directly attributable to primary hyperparathyroidism. I think there is something different about these kids. Two patients in my experience were both pediatric patients, and they both had severe primary hyperparathyroidism. I have never seen an adult patient in whom I could unequivocally attribute the pancreatitis to primary hyperparathyroidism.

PAPER

Candida Infections in Critically Ill Trauma Patients

A Retrospective Case-Control Study

Anthony P. Borzotta, MD; Kathleen Beardsley, RN, MS

Hypothesis: We sought to determine whether the usual risk factors for fungal infections are applied to trauma patients.

Design: Case-control study.

Setting: American College of Surgeons Committee on Trauma–certified Level I trauma center in a tertiary care community hospital.

Patients: Screening of medical records of a consecutive sample of 459 patients aged 16 years or older admitted to an intensive care unit for 4 days or more from 1993 through 1996 identified 20 patients infected with *Candida* species. Two case controls for each were selected from the remaining patients using sex, age within 5 years, mechanism of injury, and best fit of first 4 Abbreviated Injury Scale scores; the Injury Severity Score and intensive care unit length of stay were also used if needed.

Interventions: None.

Results: Univariate analyses by t and χ^2 tests showed significance ($P<.05$) for number of units of blood transfused in the first 24 hours after injury, gastrointestinal perforation, hemodialysis, and total parenteral nutrition. Steroids, fungal colonization, use of central venous catheters, Acute Physiology and Chronic Health Evaluation II score, mechanical ventilation for 3 days or more, and the number and duration of antibiotics were not significantly different. Logistic regression analysis showed that only total parenteral nutrition was an independent risk factor in this trauma population.

Conclusion: Many of the classic risk factors for fungal infection in other populations are actually concomitants of injury severity and its requisite level of care in trauma patients. Hyperalimentation in persistently critically ill trauma patients significantly increases the risk of *Candida* infection.

Arch Surg. 1999;134:657-665

THE CRITICALLY ill injured patient is immunosuppressed, invasively monitored, and exposed to microbial pathogens at the time of injury and while residing in the intensive care unit (ICU). The incidence of nosocomial infections by *Candida* species has surged over the past decade, from the eighth to the fourth most common cause of nosocomial bloodstream infection[1] in the general hospital population. In surgical patients, the incidence of *Candida* infections has increased from 2.5 to 5.6 per 1000 discharges, with mortality rates of 30% to 75%.[2-4] The mortality rate due to candidemia is 38%, with almost half of the deaths occuring in the first week after diagnosis.[5]

Most reports are drawn from general hospital populations,[6,7] or general surgery,[3] burn,[8] and oncology services.[9] In these reports, the predisposing factors include hematological malignancy and myelosuppression, solid organ tumors, neutropenia, intravascular devices and hyperalimentation, skin damage, gastrointestinal surgery, infancy, antimicrobial therapy, and adrenal corticosteroid therapy.[10] Few reports specifically concern the trauma patient population.[11,12] Isolates of *Candida* species were recovered in up to 22% of trauma patients who did not respond to antibiotics while in the critical care unit[11] and more than 18% of patients who stayed in a surgical ICU for more than 3 days.[13] Reports of increasing infection rates combined with the frequent presence of such risk factors in critically ill trauma patients has led to recommendations for both prophylactic and early presumptive use of antifungal therapy.[2,14-17] However, one result of widespread use of powerful antifungal drugs administered for increasingly broader indications has been a dramatic increase in the isolation of non*albicans*

From the Trauma Service, Legacy Emanuel Hospital, Portland, Ore.

MATERIALS AND METHODS

CASE FINDING

This investigation was carried out as a retrospective, case-control study. The trauma registry at the Legacy Emanuel Hospital Level I trauma center, Portland, Ore, was used to search all admissions from January 1, 1993, through December 31, 1996. There were 4631 admissions of patients aged 16 years or older, and 1746 spent at least 1 day in the ICU. All patients admitted to the ICU for 4 or more days were eligible for the study. Of 464 such patients, 460 medical records were found and screened by trained reviewers for any evidence of fungal infection or treatment. All positive records were also reviewed by us. Using predetermined definitions, infected patients were identified and their medical records were abstracted in detail.

Case controls were selected at a 2:1 ratio from the remaining sample population using the following characteristics in a stepwise fashion: sex, mechanism (blunt or penetrating), age within 5 years, and best fit of the first 4 Abbreviated Injury Scale scores.[19] The latter is a unique approach that accounts not only for specific areas of injury, but also for multiple injuries in a given body area, patterns obscured when using only the final Injury Severity Score. Body area of injury was believed to be an important potential confounding variable for risk for fungal infection and it was thought that using the Abbreviated Injury Scale score would best control for this variable. For example, abdominal surgery has been cited as a specific risk factor for yeast infections.[2,3] Length of stay in the ICU and final Injury Severity Score[20] were secondary considerations for matching. Third controls were sometimes chosen to balance injury patterns or length of stay. The control patients were selected without knowledge of their outcome.

RISK FACTORS

Previously defined risk factors were abstracted from medical records. Risk factors recorded as yes (factor present or treatment delivered) or no (not present) included steroids, dialysis, burns, gastrointestinal tract perforation, and hyperglycemia (a blood glucose level >9.99 mmol/L [>180 mg/dL] for 48 hours or longer). Continuous variables included colonization with yeast (as the number of sites), the Acute Physiology and Chronic Health Evaluation (APACHE) II score on the first injury day, and the number of units of packed red blood cells transfused in the first 24 hours after injury. The number of days of exposure was obtained for the following: total parenteral nutrition (TPN), central venous devices, and mechanical ventilation, all of which were also analyzed as yes/no variables.

Antibiotic therapy was counted in terms of days of exposure to treatment and number of antibiotics given for 24 hours or longer, including those given prophylactically. The number of antibiotics were further categorized as none to 2 or 3 or more. A broad-spectrum drug was defined as second- or third-generation cephalosporins, lactamase-resistant forms of drugs, or combinations of narrower-spectrum drugs used simultaneously. All specimens obtained for culture were recorded by site and microbe, if any.

DEFINITIONS

Candidemia was defined by the isolation of yeast in at least 1 blood culture.[21] Catheter-related candidemia occurred when the same species of *Candida* was isolated in the blood and if more than 15 colony-forming units were found in semiquantitative culture of an intravascular device. Yeast isolated from any sterile area such as the pleura, peritoneum, or other site was considered a pathogen, including specimens with concurrent bacterial isolates. Funguria was considered evidence of systemic infection regardless of whether a bladder catheter was in place if the patient had signs of sepsis and no bacterial pathogen at the same or a remote site and if there were 10^5 colonies or more per milliliter; if all of these criteria were not met, the bladder was considered colonized.[16] Patients with any amount of *Candida* growth from 2 or more sites who had a fever (temperature >38.5°C), a white blood cell count greater than 12×10^9/L,

Candida species, and resistant forms of *Candida*.[18,12] We hypothesize that the commonly stated risk factors for fungal infections also apply to trauma patients, and that the presence of multiple risk factors requires routine antifungal prophylaxis in this population.

RESULTS

Age, sex, and mortality rates were not significantly different among the entire ICU cohort and the infected and control patient groups (**Table 1**). Significantly more infected patients incurred penetrating injuries than the entire population (there is a 12:88 ratio of penetrating to blunt injuries at this center). Length of stay in the ICU and hospital were significantly longer for the infected patients, but not between controls and the total population. In 9 patients, the isolation of yeast was within 8 days of injury (4 in the peritoneum, 3 in the pleura, and 1 each in the bloodstream or wound), which is typically associated with penetrating trauma. Eleven patients developed infections between 11 and 55 days following injury, mainly in the bloodstream and at pulmonary sites.

Three (15%) of 20 infected patients died: one 79-year-old woman owing to candidemia, *Pseudomonas pneumonia,* and *Enterococcus bacteremia* infection; a 27-year-old man owing to multiple organ failure due to progressive peritonitis; and a 55-year-old man from whom support was withdrawn when renal failure added to respiratory failure, thereby complicating steroid-dependent chronic obstructive pulmonary disease. Three patients (6.7%) died in the control group: a 73-year-old woman owing to multiple organ failure; a 38-year-old man owing to anoxic brain injury, renal failure, and pneumonia; and a 54-year-old man owing to pulmonary embolus. All 20 infected patients received fluconazole in doses ranging from 100 to 400 mg/d for 4 to 35 days. Five received amphotericin B for 2 to 21 days.

Mucosal and skin colonization occured in 152 patients (32.8%): 108 at a single site, 35 at 2 sites, and 9 at 3 sites. The sites from which yeasts were cultured are listed and no coexisting bacterial isolates from clinical specimens within 48 hours of the fungal isolate were considered to have yeast sepsis.[22]

For the purpose of the initial screening of the medical records, colonization was broadly defined as cultures growing yeast, a clinical narrative report of typical yeast colonization (thrush, vulvovaginal, intertrigenous skin), and/or the use of topical antifungal drugs. An empiric course of intravenous antifungal therapy with no demonstrated yeast isolates in any specimen was not considered to represent a *Candida* infection. No patient demonstrated disseminated candidiasis marked by embolic cutaneous, ocular, or deep tissue invasion with or without candidemia.

MICROBIOLOGIC STUDIES

Blood cultures were drawn by the nursing staff using the standard broth blood culture system (Bactec; Johnston Laboratories, Towson, Md). Blood cultures are reported in this article as growth in a set; that is, as growth in either or both of 1 aerobic and 1 anaerobic bottle. Body fluids were plated onto Sabouraud agar and colonies were identified using the Vitek method (Vitek Systems, Hazelwood, Miss) and assimilation of carbohydrate and nitrogen and fermentation of carbohydrates. This system was in use throughout the review.

CLINICAL PRACTICES

The ICU in which these patients resided is a mixed surgical specialty ICU with an open staffing pattern, although trauma patients are cared for by the trauma surgery service. Sucralfate is preferred for gastritis prophylaxis over histamine$_2$ blockers. Routine surveillance cultures of patients in the ICU are not done. All cultures are obtained for the usual clinical reasons: to speciate the cause of purulence or to search for a cause of fever and leukocytosis. Indwelling, thermistor-equipped urinary bladder catheters are routinely used in all patients. Only urine specimens suggestive of infection by urinalysis are fully cultured.

Total parenteral nutrition is delivered through 1 dedicated lumen of multilumen, antiseptic-impregnated central venous catheters (CVCs) (Arrowgard; Arrow International Inc, Reading, Pa), and occasionally through 1 lumen of a pulmonary artery catheter. These are our standard CVCs, which are left in place until no longer needed (up to 3 weeks) or are removed as part of a sepsis workup. Combined solutions of protein, carbohydrate, and lipid emulsion, prepared daily by the pharmacy infusion service, are routinely used. Intravascular device site care is done by the unit nurses according to hospital policies.

Antibiotic use is defined by trauma service protocols for certain prophylactic purposes: cefazolin for the duration of use of chest tubes, intracranial pressure monitors or ventriculostomies; cefazolin and gentamicin for 48 hours for compound long-bone fractures; and cefotaxime for 5 days for compound facial fractures. Prophylactic antifungal therapy is not used. First-choice therapeutic antibiotics include ampicillin-sulbactam, cefazolin, cefotetan, gentamycin, metronidazole, nafcillin, and vancomycin. Other agents are used very sporadically, or when sensitivities or organ dysfunction requires them. If there is any general philosophy, it is to treat specific infections, not fever and leukocytosis.

STATISTICAL METHODS

Data are presented as mean ± SEM. Univariate analyses were done by applying the Levene test for equality of variances for each paired variable, and then by using the 2-tailed Student *t* test for equality of means, with significance set at $P<.05$. Pearson χ^2 tests with a continuity correction for small numbers in a cell were performed on categorical data, using the Fisher exact test for significance set at $P<.05$. A stepwise logistic regression analysis was carried out on significantly different variables between the infected and case-control groups. All tests were done using the SPSS statistical software on a desktop computer (SPSS Graduate Pack Advanced Version 7.5.1; SPSS Inc, Chicago, Ill).

by species in **Table 2**. *Candida albicans* was the most commonly identified pathogen in this series (73%), with an almost equal distribution of other species, including *Candida glabrata*. There are insufficient numbers of non-albicans species to draw any conclusions concerning characteristic sites of infection.

Seven cases of candidemia occurred (36.8% in the infected group, or 1.5% in the entire study population) and the mortality rate was 28%. Five catheters had 15 or more colony-forming units of *Candida* species, and none of the 7 catheters were infected or colonized with bacteria. There were 3 concurrent bacteremias (15%) in the infected group (of 59 paired sets of blood cultures in 17 patients, with 3 contaminated sets). One control patient (2%) had persistent *Staphylococcus aureus* bacteremia for 6 days (of 109 sets in 21 patients, with 4 contaminated sets).

In addition to the risk factors listed in **Table 3**, all patients had indwelling urinary bladder catheters, only 1 patient was burned, and no patients had malignant neoplasms, neutropenia, human immunodeficiency virus infection, or were receiving chemotherapy. Steroid use, colonization with *candida*, the presence of a CVC, the initial 24-hour APACHE II score, and mechanical ventilation for 3 or more days were not significantly different between the 2 groups. Risk factors significantly greater among infected patients than controls by univariate analysis include the number of units of blood transfused in the first 24 hours after injury, gastrointestinal perforation at any time during the ICU course, hemodialysis, and the use of central parenteral nutrition.

The infected patients required more invasive support for longer periods than the controls, as presented in **Table 4**. Significant differences occured in total hospital days of CVC use (infected patients, 23.6±2.9 vs controls, 10.5±1.2), of TPN administration (infected patients, 16.6 ± 3.0 vs controls, 10.0±5.6), and mechanical ventilation (infected patients, 21.5±5.4 vs controls, 9.6 ± 1.7). However, when these last 3 variables are mea-

Table 1. Patient Characteristics

Variable	All*	Control	Infected
No. of patients	**459**	45	20
Sex, % men	70.2	56.8	60
Mean ± SEM age, y	42.9 ± 1.0	39.2 ± 2.5	38.6 ± 3.4
Mechanism of injury, %			
Blunt	91.6	84.1	75
Penetrating	8.4	15.9	25
Mean ± SEM Injury Severity Score	29.2 ± 0.6	32.4 ± 1.8	29.1 ± 2.5
Mean ± SEM length of stay, d			
Hospital	21.5 ± 1.9†	20.0 ± 1.7†	39.8 ± 4.0
Intensive care unit	9.7 ± 0.4†	9.9 ± 1.1†	20.4 ± 2.4
Mortality, %	10.8	6.7	15

*All indicates entire sample of patients in the intensive care unit for 4 days or more.

†P<.001 compared with infected cases.

Table 2. *Candida* Species in Both Infected and Colonized Sites in Infected Patients*

	Species				
Site	*Candida albicans*	*Candida parapsilosis*	*Candida kruseii*	*Candida lusitania*	*Candida glabrata*
Blood	6	1	...	...	...
Central venous catheter	4	1	...	...	...
Peritoneum	6	...	...	...	...
Respiratory†	2	...	...	...	1
Urine	2	...	...	1	1
Pleura	1	...	1	...	1
Sinus	1	...	...	...	...
Wound	1	...	...	...	...
Abscess	...	...	1	1	...
Total	**23**	**2**	**2**	**2**	**3**

*Ellipses indicate data not available.

†Respiratory indicates tracheal or bronchoscopic aspirates, not tissue culture.

sured in the infected patients as the duration of exposure to the risk factor prior to the isolation of a yeast, there is no difference compared with the controls. The total time actually reflects the severity of illness rather than the exposure to the risk factor. The proper value for comparison of risk factors between the 2 groups is the preisolation time.

The number and duration of antibiotics used prior to fungal isolation are not significantly different compared with control patients (Table 3). No difference was found when the number of antibiotics was dichotomized into categories of 2 or less or 3 or more drugs. Throughout their hospital course, infected patients received significantly more antibiotics (exclusive of antifungal agents) (5.2 ± 0.5) given for significantly longer (22.8 ± 2.0 days) than control patients (2.4 ± 0.3 and 10.5 ± 1.3 days, respectively).

Microbiological findings of the infected and control cases are presented in **Table 5**. Concomitant bacterial infections were considered clinically relevant isolates from any site within 48 hours of a candidal isolate.

Table 3. Case-Control Statistical Analysis of Risk Factors for *Candida* Infections in Trauma Patients*

Variable and Group	Result	χ^2	*t* Test	95% CI
Antibiotics, d				
Infected	8.9 ± 1.5	...	.44	−2.44 to 5.54
Control	10.4 ± 1.3	...	...	...
Antibiotics, No.				
Infected	2.3 ± 0.3	...	.77	−0.651 to 0.869
Control	2.4 ± 0.3	...	...	...
≥2 Antibiotics, %				
Infected	35	1.00	...	−0.232 to 0.304
Control	38.6	...	...	...
APACHE II score				
Infected	16.7 ± 1.9	...	.09	−7.85 to 0.615
Control	14.2 ± 0.9	...	...	...
Colony, %				
Infected	78.9	...	.16	−0.622 to 0.109
Control	53.3	...	...	...
CVC, %				
Infected	100	.31	...	−0.254 to 0.032
Control	89	...	...	...
Dialysis, %				
Infected	20	.03	...	−0.316 to −0.040
Control	2.2	...	...	...
Enteral nutrition, %				
Infected	85	...	...	−0.367 to 0.118
Control	70.4	...	...	...
GI perforation, %				
Infected	55	.02	...	−0.376 to 0.118
Control	15.6	...	...	...
PRBC, No.				
Infected	15.2 ± 3.4	...	.02	−13.18 to −1.36
Control	7.9 ± 1.3	...	...	...
Steroids, %				
Infected	20.0	.17	...	−0.299 to 0.032
Control	6.7	...	...	...
Glucose >9.99 mmol/L (>180 mg/dL), %				
Infected	26.3	...	...	...
Control	22.2	...	...	...
TPN, d				
Infected	17 ± 2.5	...	<.001	...
Control	10 ± 1.8	...	...	...
TPN, %				
Infected	85	<.001	...	−0.891 to −0.498
Control	15.6	...	...	...
Mechanical ventilation ≥3 d, %				
Infected	85	1.00	...	−0.230 to 0.175
Control	82.2	...	...	...

*Data are reported as mean ± SEM unless otherwise indicated. Colony indicates number of body sites colonized; APACHE II, Acute Physiology and Chronic Health Evaluation II; CVC, central venous catheter; dialysis, use of hemodialysis; GI perforation, gastrointestinal perforation at any time during the hospital stay; PRBC, number of packed red blood cell transfusions given in the first 24 hours; steriods, any mineralocorticoid; TPN, total parenteral nutrition; and ellipses, data not available.

Three patients with sustained fever and leukocytosis and signs of sepsis had *Candida* alone isolated as a pathogen: 1 with budding, mycelial forms in the upper respiratory tract; a quadriplegic patient with candiduria who had an indwelling bladder catheter; and 1 with CVC-related candidemia. Six patients had candidal isolates with simultaneous bacterial pathogens at anatomically remote sites. Eleven patients had mixed yeast and bacterial infections, including peritonitis (6 patients), pneumonia/

Table 4. Days of Exposure to Risk Factors in the Hospital

Variable	Control Cases, Total Days	Index Cases	
		Total Days	Prefungal Days
Antibiotics	10.5 ± 1.3 (45)	22.8 ± 2.8† (20)	8.8 ± 1.6 (20)
Central venous catheters	10.5 ± 1.2 (37)	23.6 ± 2.9† (20)	10.2 ± 2.0 (18)
Enteral feeding	11.4 ± 1.6 (40)	18.7 ± 3.8 (15)	4.9 ± 1.7† (12)
Total parenteral nutrition	10.0 ± 5.6 (5)	17.0 ± 2.5 (17)	5.4 ± 1.6 (15)
Mechanical ventilation	9.6 ± 1.7 (43)	21.5 ± 5.4† (20)	10.6 ± 2.8 (19)

*Data are presented as mean ± SEM (number of patients).
†$P<.05$, t test.

tracheobronchitis (4 patients), empyema (1 patient), bacteremia (1 patient), sinusitis (1 patient), and deep-wound infection (1 patient). If more restrictive definitions are applied to the same population (that is, *Candida* infection defined as fungemia or exclusive isolation of yeast from a usually sterile site in a septic host), only 8 cases occured in 459 patients housed in the ICU for longer than 3 days, an incidence of 1.7%.

A forward conditional logistic regression was performed using categorical (yes/no) variables of TPN, CVC, steroids, hemodialysis, gatrointestinal tract perforation, and the number of antibiotics used as a single continuous variable (throughout the hospital course in the control group but only prior to yeast isolation in the infected group). Only TPN ($P<.001$) was independently associated with fungal infections.

Table 5. Microbiological Findings in Patients Infected With *Candida* and in Control Patients*

Site	Infected		Control, Total
	Concomitant	Total Episodes	
Bacteremia	4	6	1
Central catheter			
>15 CFU/TIP	1	2	8
No growth	6	24	17
Respiratory	9	17	47
Pleura	2	2 (5 patients)	2 (6 patients)
Sinuses	2	2	1
Urine	0	3	6 (23 patients)
Peritoneum	6	7	1 (2 patients)
Other			
Wound/drains	...	4	...
Kidney	...	1	...
Orthopedic	...	...	2
Biliary	...	...	1
Otitis	...	...	1
Gram-positive bacteria	...	46	30
Gram-negative bacteria	...	69	34
Anaerobes	...	11	1
No bacterial isolates	...	0	16

*CFU indicates colony-forming units; TIP, tip of catheter; ellipses, data not available.

COMMENT

A powerful finding in this study is the low rate of fungal infections in a large group of badly injured, critically ill trauma patients who do not receive antifungal prophylaxis. The infection rate is 4.4%, compared with 18% to 22% in other centers.[11-13] This rate may be elevated by the definitions of infection used in the study design. A few of the usual risk factors for *Candida* infection were found to pertain to trauma patients in the ICU, and only the use of TPN is independently correlated. A complex set of interactions is necessary for these ubiquitous commensal organisms to become pathogenic. Failures of local or systemic immunity are implicit in fungal infections. In this sense, risk factors can be considered predisposing conditions that alter host defenses (chemotherapy, immunosuppressive drugs, corticosteroids, or acquired immunodeficiency syndrome) or actions that breach them (open wounds, gut perforations, intravascular devices, or hemodialysis). Prior treatment with broad-spectrum antibiotics may be an important factor in altering colonization and permitting yeast numbers to increase to a concentration at which they become pathogenic.

The presence of a CVC was not significant as a risk factor, although the duration of use was significantly greater in the index than the control group. Central venous catheter use is a risk factor for candidemia in some,[3,4,7,23] but not all,[24] previous studies. For Marsh et al,[25] catheters, TPN, and antibiotics increased risk, but only conjointly and not as independent variables. The administration of fluids and medications in very ill patients for long periods often requires CVCs, reflected by the presence of CVCs in 85% to 100% of patients in many studies of candidemia[2,4,7,24]; however, when use is controlled for by multivariate analysis, CVCs are not independent risk factors.[6] Further, in a prospective cohort study of routine surveillance cultures in a surgical ICU, CVCs were not a risk factor for fungal infections.[24]

Central venous catheter infections are associated with the site of placement, local site care, and the composition of the devices themselves. Careful attention to the mechanics of skin preparation and routine site care are beneficial, and risk increases with the degree of difficulty at the time of insertion.[26] Safety increases with the use of antiseptic-impregnated catheters[27] (such as the ones used in our center), subdermally inserted cuffs impregnated with slowly released silver compounds,[28] or catheters manufactured with antibiotics.[29] Pulmonary artery catheters can be used safely to deliver TPN in the critical-care unit,[30] at least for brief periods, but multilumen CVCs create an increased risk for infection compared with single-lumen devices, particularly when used to deliver TPN.[31] Removal of any intravascular device associated with candidemia is generally recommended.[4]

Total parenteral nutrition was significantly and independently associated with fungal infections here and in other studies,[3,7,23] and remained an independently associated variable using logistic regression analysis. Four possible mechanisms are described.[32] One is that hyperalimentation fluid is an excellent medium, with in vitro growth curves showing a selective advantage of *Candida* species over bacteria.[33] Another is that frequent entry into a TPN delivery system increases the likelihood of contamination.[33] Although our hospital's policy is not to invade TPN delivery systems, it is quite likely that this happens in the ICU.

A third mechanism is the immunosuppressive effect of long-chain unsaturated fatty acids used in intravenous lipid emulsions. Linoleic and linolenic acids inhibit several immune responses in human and murine cells.[34] When trauma patients were randomized to receive intravenous glucose plus fat emulsions or glucose only during TPN, the lipid group had more infections.[35] Nevertheless, there is conflicting evidence that lipids impair polymorphonuclear cells, macrophage or reticuloendothelial system function, or have a clearly adverse clinical effect.[36,37]

A fourth mechanism may be TPN-induced hyperglycemia, which in turn alters host defenses. Although no significant difference in the frequency of hyperglycemia existed between the index group (20%) and controls (26.7%) in the current study, Hostetter[38] showed that a blood glucose level higher than 11.1 mmol/L [>200 mg/dL] within 3 days of isolation of *Candida* was the most common risk factor for hospitalized patients. Overett et al[39] found that CVC infections were 5 times more frequent in diabetic patients compared with nondiabetic patients given the same TPN solution.

This article suggests another mechanism by which TPN may be linked to candidiasis: via its opposite relationship to enteral nutrition. Three quarters of the index cases received TPN for at least 5 days prior to fungal isolation, compared with only 11% of control patients. The difference was not owing to surgeon preference for the parenteral route, but was related to gut dysfunction, even with jejunal feeding. The gut was not so much rested as it was unusable for nutritional support, and TPN was the only alternative. Total parenteral nutrition is associated with increased bacterial translocation in animal models,[2] with decreased peritoneal macrophage superoxide production and *Candida* phagocytosis[40] and similar impairments in alveolar macrophages.[41] In small-animal models, infusion of lipids shifts the distribution of injected bacteria from splenic sequestration to accumulation in the lungs.[37] That this phenomenon may occur in humans is suggestd by trials comparing enteral to TPN support in trauma patients. Enteral nutrition reduces infection rates, particularly due to pneumonia, but also from intra-abdominal abscesses.[42,43]

Several factors enhance translocation of microbes across the intestinal barrier. *Candida* species are commonly found in the oropharynx, esophagus, and rectum of humans, and will increase in density owing to antibiotic suppression of competing bacteria.[44] At high concentrations, yeast will pass across even the intact, healthy gut,[45] which occurs more easily when the intestinal barrier is disrupted by operation, trauma, or disuse atrophy associated with TPN. Some *Candida* species, such as *Candida tropicalis*, are more invasive of the gastrointestinal tract than *C albicans*.[46] Once the mucosal barrier is breached, immune defects associated with the host response to severe injury and to blood tranfusions may predispose patients to disseminated infection.

Colonization is associated with increased rates of hematogenous candidiasis in patients with cancer and neutropenia,[47] and was an independent risk factor for candidemia in a university hospital population.[6] Positive surveillance cultures were predictive of systemic infection,[48] and severity of illness and the intensity of colonization independently increased risk for later candidal infection in a surgical ICU population. However, we could identify no increased risk for candidemia, disseminated disease, or mortality associated with colonization in our study. Colonization occurred in 152 trauma patients (33.1%), 12 of whom died (7.9%), compared with 35 deaths (11.4%) in 307 noncolonized patients (χ^2 test, $P>.10$). It is possible that a microbiological laboratory-based definition of colonization, rather than the less precise one used here, may have led to findings similar to previous reports. However, the low intensity of growth in the clinical specimens (usually described as "scant" or "light") suggests that a lower burden of candidal growth may account for the failure to identify colonization as a risk factor. Although Solomkin and Anaissie[14] recommend prophylactic fluconazole in ICU patients with *Candida* colonization, this practice does not lower the yeast sepsis rate[15] and is associated with a significant frequency of secondary mycoses, which have a 38% suspected infectious mortality rate.[12] This phenomenon occurred in 2 patients in this series. One patient was treated for 35 days with fluconazole for persistent *C albicans* as indicated by peritoneal and wound drain cultures, which evolved to *Candida kruseii* on day 29. A second patient began with *Candida albicans* in the peritoneum, and after a course of fluconazole had *Torulopsis glabrata* in the pleura.

Candida species are frequently cultured from intra-abdominal abscess or peritoneal fluid, but rarely result in disseminated candidiasis except in immunocompromised patients.[49] Their isolation requires only routine drainage and treatment of the bacterial infection. The presence of yeast may put a debilitated patient at risk of serious infection rather than act as a commensal organism.[50] Patients who go on to develop systemic *Candida* infections have recurrent intra-abdominal infections and/or extensive communication with the external environment through drains or fistulas. The study by Solomkin et al[51] dealing with purulent peritonitis in 55 patients lowered a 70% mortality rate to 33% if amphotericin B was administered prior to candidemia, but it excluded patients with acute peritoneal contamination by yeast-containing enteric contents, as in this study.

Rutledge et al[49] found no localized intraperitoneal or systemic complications in the peritoneal fluid or in 24 intra-abdominal abscesses in 39 patients with *Candida* who were not given antifungal therapy. All 6 patients with peritoneal *Candida* isolates in this study had polymicrobial infections, and all underwent drainage and received antibacterial and antifungal therapy. Three also had *Candida* in the urine, pleura, mouth, or skin. Two had persistent fungal isolates from abscesses, drains, or wounds, and 1 died of multiple organ failure despite amphotericin B therapy. Patients with repeated isolation of *Candida* species from peritoneum or drains or with multiple risk factors can be treated with antifungal agents.[14]

To our knowledge, this is the first report of an association between candidiasis and red blood cell transfusions. During the first 24 hours of hospitalization, 7 index cases (35%) had fewer than 5 blood transfusions and 65% received 23.1 ± 3.6 U, compared with 26 (58%) of control patients with fewer than 5 and the remainder given 13.9 ± 1.6 U ($P<.05$). Rosemurgy et al[52] reported an average of 18 ± 3 U of blood transfused per person in a review of 33 trauma patients with candidiasis, but had no control group for comparison. Blood transfusions have immunomodulatory effects that may lead to an increased frequency of postoperative infections.[53] Aside from any immunologic influences of blood transfusion itself, hemorrhage and resuscitation produce immunosuppression due to increased prostaglandin E_2 production, suppressor-soluble serum factors, suppressor cell appearance, decreased cellular adenosine triphosphate level, and altered calcium homeostasis.[54] Thus, the severity of hemorrhage and/or the magnitude of red blood cell transfusions may be risk factors for candidiasis particular to trauma patients.

The role of corticosteroid therapy as a risk factor is repeatedly found in studies involving preterm infants,[55] leukemic children,[56] surgical patients,[2] and in a case-control study of a general hospital population.[6] But Karabinis et al[9] did not identify steroids as a risk factor using multivariate analysis in a case-control study of patients with cancer, nor was their use a prognostic indicator of mortality in fungemic surgical patients.[57] Steroids were not statistically important in our population, most likely owing to too few examples for reliable statistical analysis.

Severity of illness defined by an APACHE II score greater than 10 has been reported as a risk factor,[15] and independently predicted *Candida* infections in a multivariate analysis by Pittet et al.[24] When coupled with candiduria, an elevated APACHE II score predicted disseminated disease, and was considered an indicator for early empiric antifungal therapy.[16] The APACHE II scores were no different in control and infected cases in the present study, whether considered as continuous variables or as a categorical variable (score >10). Most likely, it is the excessive weight of the Glasgow Coma Scale component of APACHE II in trauma patients, as opposed to general surgical or medical patients, that may account for this disparity with earlier reports.

This population of critically ill ICU patients with *Candida* infections is characterized by a high incidence of gut perforations and a sustained need for TPN, implying prolonged dysfunction of the gastrointestinal tract. The use of corticosteroids or hemodialysis is simultaneously a sign of progressively deteriorating physiology and indicates an abrogation of immune defenses. Our finding that neither number of antibiotics nor duration of antibiotic use were significant risk factors for candidiasis is of particular interest. Although many studies have associated antimicrobials with increased risk, most of the studied patients also had severe deficiencies in host defenses.[58] In immunosuppressed patients with leukemia, candidiasis was more closely associated with the duration of leukopenia and steroid therapy than with antimicrobial therapy.[59] It may be that restrictive antibiotic ordering practices and a policy of early enteral nutritional support combine to minimize multiplication of a common enteric commensal organism into numbers sufficient to overcome local host defenses. As a result, we cannot support recommendations favoring routine systemic antifungal therapy for most critically ill trauma patients. Such policies have led to a progressive shift toward resistant species of *Candida* in less than a decade. Further investigation into the roles of antibiotic ordering policies, use of surveillance cultures, alternatives to enteral nutritional support, and control of local immune systems needs to be done before such recommendations are generally put into effect.

The study was supported by a grant from Pfizer Roerig Inc, New York, NY.

Presented at the 106th Scientific Session of the Western Surgical Association, Indianapolis, Ind, November 17, 1998.

We thank George Burnstein, RN, for help in gathering data, Andrew Michaels, MD, for review and statistical assistance, and John Woon, PharmD, for support and encouragement.

Corresponding author: Anthony P. Borzotta, MD, 501 N Graham St, Suite 125, Portland, OR 97227.

REFERENCES

1. Beck-Sague C, Jarvis WR. Secular trends in the epidemiology of nosocomial fungal infections in the United States, 1980-1990: National Nosocomial Infections Surveillance System. *J Infect Dis.* 1993;167:1247-1251.
2. Dean DA, Burchard KW. Fungal infections in surgical patients. *Am J Surg.* 1996; 171:374-382.
3. Harvey RL, Myers JP. Nosocomial fungemia in a large community teaching hospital. *Arch Intern Med.* 1987;147:2117-2120.
4. Komshian SV, Uwaydah AK, Sobel JD, Crane LR. Fungemia caused by *Candida* species and *Torulopsis glabrata* in the hosptialized patient: frequency, characteristics, and evaluation of factors influencing outcome. *Rev Infect Dis.* 1989; 11:379-390.
5. Wey SB, Mori M, Pfaller MA, Woolson RF, Wenzel RP. Hosptial-acquired candidemia: the attributable mortality and excess length of stay. *Arch Intern Med.* 1988;148:2642-2645.
6. Wey SB, Mori M, Pfaller MA, Woolson RF, Wenzel RP. Risk factors for hospital-acquired candidemia. *Arch Intern Med.* 1989;149:2349-2353.
7. Fraser VJ, Jones M, Dunkel J, Storfer S, Medoff G, Dunagan WC. Candidemia in a tertiary care hospital: epidemiology, risk factors and predictors of mortality. *Clin Infect Dis.* 1992;15:414-421.
8. Smith DJ, Thomson PD. Changing flora in burn and trauma units: historical perspective experience in the United States. *J Burn Care Rehabil.* 1992;13:276-280.
9. Karabinis A, Hill C, Leclerq B, Tancrede C, Baume D, Andremont A. Risk factors for candidemia in cancer patients: a case-control study. *J Clin Microbiol.* 1988; 26:429-432.
10. Anaissie E, Bodey GP. Nosocomial fungal infections: old problems and new challenges. *Infect Dis Clin North Am.* 1989;3:867-882.
11. Mahr CC, Fildes JJ, Becker EJ, et al. The alarming rate of fungal recovery in critically ill trauma patients with unresolved sepsis. In press.
12. Safran DB, Dawson E. The effect of empiric and prophylactic treatment with fluconazole on yeast isolates in a surgical truama intensive care unit. *Arch Surg.* 1997;132:1184-1189.
13. Cornwell EE, Belzberg H, Berne TV, et al. The pattern of fungal infections in critically surgical patients. *Am Surg.* 1995;61:847-850.
14. Solomkin JS, Anaissie E. *Candida* infections and candidemia. In: Fry DE, ed. *Surgical Infections.* Boston, Mass; Little Brown & Co Inc; 1995:577-589.
15. Savino JA, Agarwal N, Wry P, Policastro AI, Cerabona T, Austria L. Routine prophylactic antifungal agents (clotrimazole, ketoconazole and nystatin) in nontransplant/nonburned critically ill surgical and trauma patients. *J Trauma.* 1994; 36:20-26.
16. Nassoura Z, Ivatury RR, Simon RJ, Jabbour N, Stahl WM. Candiduria as an early marker of disseminated infection in critically ill surgical patients: the role of fluconazole therapy. *J Trauma.* 1993;35:290-295.
17. Vincent JL, Anaissie E, Bruining H, et al. Epidemiology, diagnosis and treatment of systemic *Candida* infection in surgical patients under intensive care. *Intensive Care Med.* 1998;24:206-216.
18. Abi-Said D, Anaissie E, Uzun O, Raad I, Pizcowski H, Vartivarian S. The epidemilogy of hematogenous candidiasis caused by different *Candida* species. *Clin Infect Dis.* 1997;24:1122-1128.

19. *The Abbreviated Injury Scale: 1990 Revision.* Des Plaines, Ill: Association for the Advancement of Automotive Medicine; 1990.
20. Baker SP, O'Neill B, Haddon W, et al. The injury Severity Score: a method for describing patients with multiple injuries and evaluating emergency care. *J Trauma.* 1974;14:187-192.
21. Bodey GP, Anaissie EJ, Edwards JE. Appendix: definitions of *Candida* infections. In: Bodey GP, ed. *Candidiasis: Pathogenesis, Diagnosis and Treatment.* New York, NY; Raven Press; 1993.
22. Solomkin JS. Pathogenesis and management of *Candida* infection syndromes in non-neutropenic patients. *New Horiz.* 1993;1:202-213.
23. Klein JJ, Watanakunakorn C. Hospital-acquired fungemia: its natural course and clinical significance. *Am J Med.* 1979;67:51-58.
24. Pittet D, Monod M, Suter PM, Frenk E, Auckenthaler R. *Candida* colonization and subsequent infections in critically ill surgical patients. *Ann Surg.* 1994;220:751-758.
25. Marsh PK, Tally FP, Kellum J, et al. *Candida* infections in surgical patients. *Ann Surg.* 1983;198:42-47.
26. Conly JM, Grieves K, Peters B. A prospective, randomised study comparing transparent and dry gauze dressings for central venous catheters. *J Infect Dis.* 1989; 159:310-319.
27. Maki DG, Stolz SM, Wheeler S, Mermel LA. Prevention of central venous catheter–related bloodstream infection by use of an antiseptic impregnated catheter: a randomized, controlled trial. *Ann Intern Med.* 1997;127:257-266.
28. Maki DG, Cobb L, Garman JK, Shapiro JM, Ringer M, Helgerson RB. An attachable silver-impregnated cuff for prevention of infection with central venous catheters: a prospective randomized multicenter trial. *Am J Med.* 1988;85:307-314.
29. Raad I, Darouiche R. The broad-spectrum activity and efficacy of catheters coated with minocycline and rifampin. *J Infect Dis.* 1996;173:418-424.
30. Horowitz HW, Dworkin BM, Savino JA, Byrne DW, Pecora NA. Central catheter-related infections: comparison of pulmonary artery catheters and triple lumen catheters for the delivery of hyperalimentation in a critical care setting. *JPEN J Parenter Enteral Nutr.* 1990;14:588-592.
31. Yeung WITH, May J, Hughes R. Infection rate for single lumen v triple lumen subclavian catheters. *Infect Control Hosp Epidemiol.* 1988;9:154-158.
32. Wade JC. Epidemiology of *Candida* infections. In: Bodey GP, ed. *Candidiasis: Pathogenesis, Diagnosis and Treatment.* New York, NY: Raven Press; 1993:85-107.
33. Sherertz RJ, Gledhill KS, Hamptom KD, et al. Outbreak of *Candida* bloodstream infections associated with retrograde medication administration in a neonatal ICU. *J Pediatr.* 1992;120:455-461.
34. Tezabwala BU, Bennett M, Grundy SM. Immunotoxicity of polyunstaturated fatty acids in serum-free medium. *Immunopharmacol Immunotoxicol.* 1995;17:365-383.
35. Battistella FD, Widergren JT, Anderson JT, Siepler JK, Weber JC, MacColl K. A prospective, randomized trial of intravenous fat emulsion administration in trauma victims requiring total parenteral nutrition. *J Trauma.* 1997;43:52-60.
36. Gogos CA, Kalfarentzos F. Total parenteral nutrition and immune system activity: a review. *Nutrition.* 1995;11:339-344.
37. Palmblad J. Intravenous lipid emulsions and host defense: a critical review. *Clin Nutr.* 1991;10:303-308.
38. Hostetter MK. Handicap or host defence: effects of hyperglycemia on C3 and C. albicans. *Diabetes.* 1990;39:271-275.
39. Overett TK, Bistrian BR, Lowry SF, et al. Total parenteral nutrition in patients with insulin-requiring diabetes mellitus. *J Am Coll Nutr.* 1986;5:79-89.
40. Shou J, Lappin J, Minnard EA, Daly JM. Total parenteral nutrition, bacterial translocation, and host immune function. *Am J Surg.* 1994;167:145-150.
41. Shou J, Lappin J, Daly JM. Impairment of pulmonary macrophage function with total parenteral nutrition. *Ann Surg.* 1994;219:291-297.
42. Kudsk KA, Croce MA, Fabian TC, et al. Enteral versus pareneral feeding. *Ann Surg.* 1991;215:503-513.
43. Moore FA, Feliciano DV, Andrassy RJ, et al. Early enteral feeding, compared with parenteral, reduces postoperative septic complications: the results of a meta-analysis. *Ann Surg.* 1992;216:172-183.
44. Solomkin JS, Anaissie E. Care of the surgical patient: fungal infection: approach to the surgical patient at risk for candidiasis. *Sci Am.* 1994;10:1-12.
45. Stone HH, Kolb LD, Currie CA, Geheger CE, Cuzzell JZ. *Candida* sepsis: pathogenesis and principles of treatment. *Ann Surg.* 1974;179:697-710.
46. Walsh TJ, Merz WG. Pathologic features in the human alimentary tract associated with invasiveness of *Candida* tropicalis. *Am J Clin Pathol.* 1986;85:498-502.
47. Richet HM, Andremont A, Tancrede C, et al. Risk factors for candidemia in patients with acute lymphocytic leukemia. *Rev Infect Dis.* 1991;13:211-215.
48. Pfaller M, Cabezudo I, Koontz F, et al. Predicitive value of surveillance cultures for systemic infection due to *Candida* species. *Eur J Clin Microbiol.* 1987;6:628-633.
49. Rutledge R, Mandel SSR, Wild RE. *Candida* sepsis: insignificant contaminant or pathogenic species? *Am Surg.* 1986;52:299-302.
50. Burchard KW. Fungal sepsis. *Infect Dis Clin North Am.* 1992;6:677-692.
51. Solomkin JS, Flohr AB, Quie PG, Simmons RL. The role of *Candida* in intraperitoneal infections. *Surgery.* 1980;88:524-530.
52. Rosemurgy AS, Drost TF, Murphy CG, Kearney RE, Albrink MH. Treatment of candidosis in severely injured adults with short-course, low-dose amphoteracin. *B J Trauma.* 1990;30:1521-1523.
53. Klein HG. Allogeneic transfusion risks in the surgical patient. *Am J Surg.* 1995; 170(suppl):21-26.
54. Chaudry IH, Ayala A. Potential mechanism(s) of immunosuppression following hemorrhage. In: *Immunological Aspects of Hemorrhage.* Austin, Tex: RG Landes Co; 1992:83-102.
55. Botas CM, Kurlat I, Young SM, Sola A. Disseminated *Candida* infections and intravenous hydrocortisone in preterm infants. *Pediatrics.* 1995;95:883-887.
56. Flynn PM, Marina NM, Rivera GK, Hughs WT. *Candida tropicalis* infections in children with leukemia. *Leuk Lymphoma.* 1993:70:369-376.
57. Tang E, Tang G, Berne TV. Prognostic indicators in fungemia of the surgical patient. *Arch Surg.* 1993;128:759-763.
58. Vartivarian S, Smith CB. Pathogenesis, host resistance, and predisposing factors. In: Bodey GP, ed. *Candidiasis: Pathogenesis, Diagnosis and Treatment.* New York, NY: Raven Press; 1993:59-84.
59. Bodey GP. Fungal infections complicating acute leukemia. *J Chronic Dis.* 1966; 19:667-687.

DISCUSSION

John A. Weigelt, MD, St Paul, Minn: Dr Borzotta, one of our new members, has produced an analysis of fungal infection in a critically ill injured population. He and his coworker amassed a considerable amount of data on their index population that is represented in the article. Their purpose was to confirm risk factors for fungal infections in this patient population. They also had a secondary purpose in trying to identify whether fungal prophylaxis should be used. Their data suggest that many of the reported risk factors for fungal infections do not exist in the severely injured patient. Their statistical manipulations seem correct; however, their numbers are small and despite their adequate statistical methods, I have great concern for a type 2 error that must be acknowledged.

However, let's look at what we can learn from these data. Twenty cases of fungal infection occurred in 3 years—not very many. One third of all of the patients had fungal colonization, and colonization did not relate to fungal infection. Mortality was no different with or without fungal sepsis and, in fact, most patients with fungal sepsis also had severe bacterial infections. I realize the Centers for Disease Control and Prevention says that we are all in an epidemic of fungal infections, but I think analyses like these allow individual institutions to say, "Maybe we don't have as big a problem as people say we should."

I do have some questions that I would like Dr Borzotta to answer to better understand this article. First, was fungal prophylaxis used in any patient? What drug was used? What dosage was used? How was it given, if it was given? You had 2 resistant fungal infections that developed during fluconazole treatment. You quote your highest fluconazole dosage at 400 mg/d. Do you think this is drug failure or failure to use a proper use of fluconazole? We use at least 800 mg to treat fungal infections.

Do you believe your data show us a method to decrease the risk of fungal infections in critically ill patients other than good ICU care?

Finally, after doing this study and putting that last slide up, do you use fungal prophylaxis at all, and, once again, if so, what patients, what drug, what dose, what route?

Donald E. Fry, MD, Albuquerque, NM: I would like to commend Dr Borzotta on a very lucid presentation of a very, very difficult and actually very contentious subject depending upon one's personal perspective. The contentiousness really begins with defining what is *Candida* infection. The spectrum of opinions on that from this audience would span from those who don't believe that *Candida* causes infection at all and that presence of *Candida* even in the blood simply represents a collapse of host defense. Others would treat any positive culture for *Candida* and would be apt to treat all 109 patients that Dr Borzotta identified in his presentation who had the organism cultured from one anatomical site. The conventional definition would require that a blood culture be positive, or that 2 or more anatomical sites be culture positive. But even at that, we are dealing with a very difficult problem when Dr Borzotta included urinary tract infection. I would assume that all of those patients, even with greater than 100 000 colonies per milliliter, all had a urinary catheter in place. A catheter in place I think makes the sacred 100 000 organisms per milliliter suspicious at best in defining whether infection exists. So I am really curious as to whether you have reexamined the data in just looking at blood-borne infections. Obviously that is problematic for you because there are only 7 in the entire series.

Dr Borzotta has identified that the duration of antibiotics did not seem to be predictive of *Candida* infection. However, he hasn't really tried to detail the types of antibiotics. I am absolutely convinced that our continued practice of obliterating anaerobic colonization of the patient when they are in the ICU and experiencing nosocomial infections, which are never anaerobic, proves to be a liability for the host. Anaerobes are in fact man's best friend when they are colonizing the colon. They are not our best friend when they are in our soft tissues and in our peritoneal cavity. So one of the questions that arises is whether anaerobic antibiotic administration on an aggressive and long-term basis in the setting of the ICU patient may selectively be a negative issue. I would be interested in whether he has examined the presence or absence of anaerobic bacterial activity in the antibiotics as a variable in predicting *Candida* infection in his situation.

Everybody likes to bash on total parenteral nutrition (TPN). I am now old enough to remember when it was considered the saving grace of surgical science. I am curious as to whether we might take the flip side in this argument and say, not that TPN is bad, but rather that enteral feeding is good. Dr Borzotta noted in his comments that the TPN patients receiving TPN did so late in their course, and that patients receiving enteral feeding did so earlier in their course. The question then is whether *Candida* can be prevented by going to fewer antianaerobic antibiotics in our ICU and earlier applications of enteral feeding.

Michael A. West, MD, Minneapolis, Minn: I would also like to compliment Dr Borzotta on a very nice presentation and particularly compliment him on the relatively low use of antibiotics in the ICU where only a couple of patients in the ICU for the greater than 3 or 4 days were on more than one antibiotic. Several of the patients were not on any antibiotics at all.

My question relates to the very marked difference seen in the infected patients vs the control patients in the duration of time in the ICU. Is this because they developed infection, or did they develop infection with *Candida* because they were in the ICU for a long time? Was there a difference in the duration of ICU treatment prior to the development of the infection?

Basil A. Pruitt, Jr, MD, San Antonio, Tex: I think that you were wise to confine your conclusions to *Candida* and not generalize to all fungi since the true or filamentous fungi are quite different. *Candida* often colonize and seldom invade so I would ask whether you had occasion to look at other fungi in this population of patients since true fungi often invade and can be quite troublesome. Infections caused by true fungi have been found to be associated with acidosis, so I ask whether acidosis was a common risk factor in your ICU population. Since the length of stay in the ICU was more than twice as long in the candidemia patients or candidiasis patients, how could you control for antibiotics? In most critically ill populations, candidiasis is a perverse index of management success. In burn patients, candidemia, on the average, occurs 35 to 41 days after injury and candidal infections correlate with repetitive or prolonged antibiotic treatment. I am quite surprised that in your patients with candidal infections with over twice as long a stay in the ICU that there was no correlation with antibiotic therapy.

Katherine J-M Liu, MD, Chicago, Ill: I also thoroughly enjoyed this article regarding a very difficult problem that we see in some of the very ill patients. My question concerns the nutritional support of these patients. As you stated, parenteral nutritional support in the control group was initiated early during the course and later in the study patients. My question is whether there was any difference in nutritional status between the 2 groups, and when the study group was initiated later, could this lack of nutritional support actually have contributed to the fungal infection? Also, as you all know, the protocol for care for the parenteral nutritional support, the types of catheters, and many other factors involved influence the infection rate in patients receiving the parenteral nutrition. I wondered if you can comment on these aspects.

Dr Borzotta: There is very little I can do about a type 2 error. I think it is apparent that we had relatively few cases, and it is most obvious in terms of the use of steroids. If we had a few more cases, I suspect that would have shown statistical significance on a univariate basis.

None of the patients really had prophylaxis in the index group. Three patients did have prophylaxis in the control group for as long as 9 days, but there were no *Candida* isolates or there was simply 1 respiratory *Candida* isolate in 1 of the 3 cases.

Yes, our dosing tended to be low. There has been an evolution over the last 5 years of dosing recommendations from a minimum of 100 mg/d up to the very large 600 or 800 mg/d doses. Interestingly, in leukemics there is a nice article showing that low-dose amphotericin at half the usual dose is an excellent prophylaxis against candidiasis. I think it is not going to be the case with fluconazole. There is going to be selective pressure on the many *Candida* varieties in a given human being for potential overgrowth.

At this time we are not using any antifungal prophylaxis. We simply treat as we see an infection arises and I think we have backed away from putting fluconazole into patients just because we find *Candida* during an acute enteric spill.

Dr Fry's comments are interesting. There was one candiduria case really that occurred on the ward. He had an fever of unknown origin for 2 weeks. He had progressively increasing numbers of colonies of *Candida* in the urine and finally broke the 100 000 mark and so was put on a course of treatment which effectively resolved his septic state.

Among the 7 candidemia patients, there were 3 concurrent bacteremias. There was only 1 preceding bacteremia, which has been considered a risk factor. The date of onset of candidemia was 2 weeks after injury. The mean population onset was 13.5 days, but a significant number, to address one of the other questions, occurred 3 to 4 weeks into their hospital course. Wey and others have shown that candidemia, in particular, may not show itself for 4 weeks after the onset of illness, admission to the ICU, or date of injury.

The question regarding other fungi by Dr Pruitt: we actually set out to look for all fungal isolates, but all we found were *Candida*. We did not find any other zygomycoses or other kinds of nonyeast pathogens.

I don't have information about acidosis as a specific risk factor in this group.

The use of antibiotics, TPN, and mechanical ventilation were significantly longer throughout the entire ICU course in the infected patients than in the control patients. It's very hard to find a time to cut off use of central venous catheters in the control group for comparison purposes. In the infected group, it is obviously when the fungal isolate occurred, that being at about 10 days. There is roughly a 2-day difference between the infected group and the control group in terms of central venous catheter use. I suspect this is not significant but I have to look at that mathematically.

Dr Liu, I think TPN plays multiple roles here. It's partly a reflection that the gut won't allow enteral nutrition to be done. It's life-saving in that regard. It may increase risk itself, but it may also be a marker of a patient at increased risk because of multiple systems being dysfunctional. We use Arrowgard catheters, multilumen, to deliver our TPN. We also deliver it via a Swan-Ganz catheter, which is relatively safe early on, and then we switch over to enteral feeding as soon as feasible.

The Acute Inflammatory Response and Its Regulation

Peter A. Ward, MD; Alex B. Lentsch, PhD

The acute inflammatory response is composed of an elaborate cascade of both proinflammatory and anti-inflammatory mediators. The balance between these mediators often determines the outcome after injury. In clincal scenarios, such as trauma or sepsis, there is often unregulated production of proinflammatory mediators that can cause multiple organ failure. Further understanding of the endogenous mechanisms that control the inflammatory response is needed to facilitate development of therapeutic options. In this review, we discuss the current knowledge of the mechanisms leading to development of acute inflammatory injury as well as the factors that regulate this response. *Arch Surg. 1999;134:666-669*

The inflammatory process is a vital response to injury, infection, trauma, and many other insults. For a successful outcome after injury (including surgically induced trauma), the inflammatory response must be triggered to bring about recruitment of blood leukocytes, activation of tissue macrophages, and production of a series of mediators. The results of this may include ultimate resolution of the inflammatory process, triggering events that lead to cell regeneration and wound healing, or progression of the inflammatory response, which often leads to progressive organ dysfunction. Understanding how the inflammatory process is activated and how it is contained are key to developing strategies designed to block or reduce inflammatory responses, similar to immunosuppressive interventions when immune responses are unwanted (eg, allograft rejection) or exaggerated (eg, autoimmune responses). A good example of an undesirable inflammatory response occurs in the "systemic inflammatory response syndrome" during sepsis. In this situation, cytokines (eg, interleukin 1 [IL-1], IL-6, tumor necrosis factor α [TNF-α]) are detectable in the plasma, suggesting unregulated generation of these highly inflammatory peptides.[1] Under such conditions multiorgan failure often occurs. What remains to be determined is why, during sepsis, there is uncontrolled production of cytokines and how these cytokines may be involved in multiorgan failure.

From the Department of Pathology, University of Michigan Medical School, Ann Arbor (Dr Ward), and the Department of Surgery, University of Louisville, Louisville, Ky (Dr Lentsch).

THE INFLAMMATORY CASCADE AND NEUTROPHIL RECRUITMENT

Much of our work, which has provided information about mediation of the acute inflammatory process, has occurred in the context of acute inflammation in lungs of rats. For convenience, these reactions are triggered by distal airway deposition of IgG immune complexes, which trigger complement activation and macrophage activation that ultimately result in large accumulations of neutrophils, interstitial and intra-alveolar edema, and intra-alveolar hemorrhage, each of which can be precisely quantitated.[2] The general scheme of the inflammatory response is outlined in **Figure 1**. The inflammatory pathways in this particular model are very similar to events related to lung injury caused by ischemia,[3] by the presence of bacteria,[4] or by bacterial lipopolysaccharide.[5] These events trigger complement activation as well as activation of tissue macrophages. Activated macrophages generate the "early response cytokines," TNF-α and IL-1. A chief function of these cytokines is to stimulate vascular endothelial cells to express vascular adhesion molecules, such as intercellular adhesion molecule 1 (ICAM-1) and E-selectin.[6] Through a series of adhesion-promoting events, blood neutrophils adhere intermittently to endothelial cells (the "rolling" phenomenon), followed by firm attachment and transmigration into the

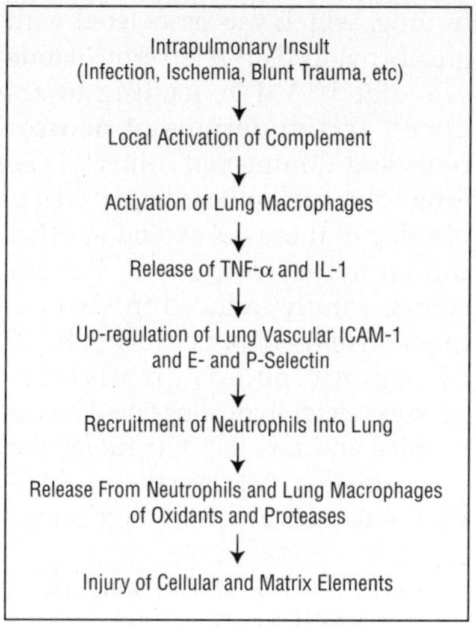

Figure 1. *Model of acute inflammatory lung injury induced by intrapulmonary deposition of IgG immune complexes. TNF-α indicates tumor necrosis factor α; IL-1, interleukin 1; and ICAM-1, intercellular adhesion molecule 1.*

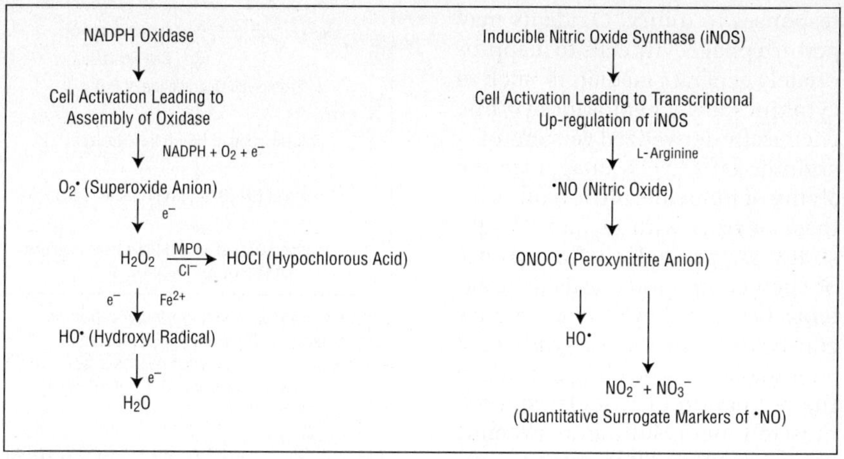

Figure 2. *Mechanisms of oxidant production by activated phagocytic cells. NADPH indicates nicotinamide adenine dinucleotide phosphate (reduced form).*

interstitial and alveolar compartments. The intermittent attachment phenomenon features endothelial selectin interactions with "counterreceptors" on neutrophils that contain oligosaccharides with the sialyl Lewis^x motif.[7] Firm attachment of neutrophils to the endothelium involves endothelial ICAM-1 interactions with neutrophil β2 integrins (CD11a/CD18 and CD11b/CD18).[8] Activated endothelial cells also express platelet-activating factor and IL-8, powerful neutrophil-stimulating agonists.[9] Accordingly, when neutrophils adhere to the activated endothelium, they also become activated or "primed," so that arrival at an extravascular site containing a neutrophil agonist such as TNF-α causes an exaggerated functional response in these neutrophils. The entry of neutrophils into the alveolar compartment together with tissue-activated macrophages sets the stage for injury of both lung cells and matrix glycoproteins (eg, collagens, elastin). Injury is related to generation of oxidants by phagocytic cells (described below) and the release of proteases (serine proteases and matrix metalloproteases).[10]

OXIDANT-GENERATING PATHWAYS

Most oxidants generated during the inflammatory response derive from phagocytic cells (neutrophils, macrophages, and monocytes) and are released into the extracellular environment, in part at least because one of the oxidants (nicotinamide adenine dinucleotide phosphate [NADPH] oxidase) is assembled in an enzymatically active form on surfaces of phagocytic cells. As shown in **Figure 2**, the 2 chief oxidant-generating pathways include NADPH oxidase and inducible nitric oxide synthase.[11,12] The former enzyme exists as inactive subunits that are located both on the cell membrane and in the cytosol. Cell activation causes translocation of cytosolic subunits to the cell membrane, resulting in a multimeric complex that exhibits oxidase activity. The pathway of oxidant generation by NADPH oxidase is described in Figure 2 and is characterized by an unusual series of single (rather than double) additions of electrons. In the presence of the oxidase, NADPH undergoes oxidation. The released electrons interact with molecular oxygen to cause its reduction, forming superoxide anion ($O_2^{\cdot}$). One function of $O2^{\cdot}$ is to reduce intracellular iron, converting Fe^{3+} to Fe^{2+}. A further electron addition to $O_2^{\cdot}$ converts it to hydrogen peroxide (H_2O_2), which can be further reduced to the most active of all oxygen-centered radicals, the hydroxyl radical ($HO^{\cdot}$). Generation of hydroxyl radical requires a heavy metal (such as iron) in its transition (unstable) state (Fe^{2+}). In giving up an electron to hydrogen peroxide, Fe^{2+} is reoxidized to Fe^{3+}. Hydroxyl radical is a highly reactive and damaging radical. If it is further reduced, the product is water. In the context of phagocytic cells, such as neutrophils, release of myeloperoxidase in the presence of a halide, such as chloride (Cl^-), will enzymatically convert hydrogen peroxide to hypochlorous acid, another potent oxidant.

A second major oxidant-generating pathway in phagocytic cells involves inducible nitric oxide synthase, which is typically not expressed in resting (nonstimulated) cells, especially macrophages. On cell activation, however, inducible nitric oxide synthase is transcriptionally up-regulated, reacting with L-arginine to generate nitric oxide (NO), which relaxes smooth muscle cells and is mildly reactive with aromatic amino acids to form stable adducts, such as nitrotyrosine. These modifications of tyrosine-containing proteins have often been found at sites of inflammation. Depending on the protein and the position of the tyrosine residue, nitrosylation may impair protein function. Nitric oxide is converted to peroxynitrite anion ($ONOO^{\cdot}$), which is highly reactive with thiol groups. Peroxynitrite anion can be further converted to hydroxyl radical in the absence of the requirement for a heavy metal cation. Finally, peroxynitrite anion is ultimately broken down into NO_2^- and NO_3^-, which serve as convenient quantitative surrogate markers of nitric oxide.

These 2 oxidant-generating pathways in phagocytic cells account for many tissue-damaging outcomes of inflammatory responses and may well impair physiological responses to injury. Oxidants may perturb phagocytic cells to inappropriately generate mediators, such as cytokines and chemokines. While chemically derivatized versions of L-arginine effectively antagonize the ability of inducible nitric oxide synthase to react with its natural substrate (L-arginine), the in vivo use of such compounds leads to problems, because they also antagonize constitutive nitric oxide synthase of endothelial cells, leading to a loss in the regulation of vascular smooth muscle tone, resulting in systemic hypertension. There are, to our knowledge, no reliable, specific, and effective inhibitors in vivo for either NADPH oxidase or inducible nitric oxide synthase.

MECHANISMS OF PHAGOCYTIC CELL ACTIVATION

Since phagocytic cells, especially macrophages, are key sources of inflammatory mediators (such as cytokines and chemokines), understanding their activation process is important if inhibition of their mediator generation is to be successful. When a macrophage is activated (eg, after contact with bacteria, bacterial lipopolysaccharide, TNF-α, or many other agonists), a series of intracellular events leads to transcriptional activation of the cell (**Figure 3**). A heterodimeric complex termed *nuclear factor* κ *B* (NF-κB) contains 2 subunits, most often p50 and p65.[13] This complex has the ability to bind with promoter sequences in DNA and to inaugurate transcription (generation of messanger RNA) for many inflammatory peptides. However, the NF-κB complex is held in check in the cytosol by inhibitors of the inhibitor κ B (IκB) family, which bind to the NF-κB complex and prevent its entry into the nucleus (translocation) and subsequent binding to DNA.[14] Typically, when the macrophages are activated, IκB undergoes phosphorylation and ubiquination. Those changes set the stage for the 26S proteosome to enzymatically cleave IκB. The liberated NF-κB complex can then translocate to the nucleus, engage DNA-promoter sequences, and cause transcriptional up-regulation of mediators such as

NF-κB (p50, p65) Complexed With IκB
↓ Cell Activation
Proteolytic Degradation of IκB
↓
Translocation of NF-κB Into Nucleus
↓
Binding of NF-κB to DNA Promotor Sites
↓
Transcriptional Activation and Ultimate Production of TNF-α, IL-1, ICAM-1, etc

Figure 3. *Pathways leading to activation of nuclear factor* κ *B (NF-κB). IκB indicates inhibitor* κ *B; TNF-α, tumor necrosis factor α; IL-1, interleukin 1; and ICAM-1, intercellular adhesion molecule 1.*

TNF-α, IL-1, and ICAM-1. Details of the NF-κB pathway are especially relevant to understanding how the inflammatory system is regulated by certain interleukins.

REGULATORY INTERLEUKINS

As described above, the experimental model of IgG immune complex–induced acute alveolitis is known to be self-regulated. After 4 hours, there is no further progression in the albumin leak, cessation in further neutrophil recruitment, and rapid disappearance of mediators such as TNF-α. There is evidence that these inflammatory reactions also initiate the appearance of a series of regulatory cytokines that prevent continuation of the inflammatory response.

Regulatory ILs were originally discovered by their ability to inhibit cytokine (TNF-α) generation in macrophages stimulated in vitro with agonists such as lipopolysaccharide. Several of these ILs also inhibit in vitro T-cell responses. Animals that are unable to express IL-10 ("IL-10 knockout" mice) develop a progressive chronic inflammatory bowel disease similar to that in found in ulcerative colitis.[15] Interleukin 10 knockout mice are also reported to be unable to contain a variety of other inflammatory responses (acute inflammation, delayed type hypersensitivity, etc). Using the model of immune complex–induced alveolitis in rats, several ILs were found to have a strong anti-inflammatory response, the rank (from most potent to least potent) being IL-10 = IL-13>IL-4>IL-6>IL-12.[16] The addition of exogenous ILs to rat lung caused reduced generation of TNF-α in lung, which was associated with greatly reduced up-regulation of lung vascular ICAM-1, leading to reduced accumulations of neutrophils and diminished injury of the lung. The anti-inflammatory effects of some of these ILs extend to other inflammatory responses. For instance, virally induced in vivo expression of IL-10 or delivery of IL-10 by osmotic pumps greatly suppresses rejection of allografted hearts in mice and rats.[17,18] The molecular mechanisms to explain these inhibitory outcomes are described below.

ROLES OF ENDOGENOUS REGULATORY ILs

The rat lung inflammatory model described above was used to assess the role of endogenous ILs. Complementary DNA for candidate ILs were cloned in the rat, the proteins were expressed, and blocking antibodies were developed. Assessing candidate endogenous regulatory ILs required the ability to demonstrate expression in lung of messenger RNA and protein for a given IL. In the most critical part of these studies, animals were treated with blocking antibody to the appropriate IL and the inflammatory response was quantitated. If a regulatory IL were blocked in vivo, then the expected outcome of the inflammatory response would be increased production in lung of TNF-α, increased expression of lung vascular ICAM-1, increased neutrophil accumulation in lung, and enhanced evidence of lung injury. Studies have identified the appearance of at least 3 regulatory ILs in the lung inflammatory response: IL-6, IL-10, and IL-13.[19-21] Blockade of any 1 of these 3 ILs increased TNF-α levels in lung and caused an increase of at least 50% in the number of neutrophils recruited into lung.

Another regulatory factor identified in these studies was the IL-1 receptor antagonist (IL-1ra). IL-1ra is known to be a product of stimulated macrophages. It is often released in vitro following macrophage production of TNF-α and IL-1 and functions as a receptor "decoy," binding to the IL-1 receptor without triggering a cell response, thus competing with the ability of IL-1 to bind to its natural receptor and to trigger signal transduction events. In the lung inflammatory model, both messenger RNA and protein for IL-1ra were found in lung tissues. Indeed, the protein could be detected both in macrophages and in neutrophils recruited into the lung. Antibody-induced blockade of endogenous IL-1ra, as with anti–IL-10, increased neutrophil accumulation by nearly 200%, notably increased the degree of extravascular albumin leak, and caused a nearly 2-fold increase in bronchoalveolar lavage levels of IL-1β (but did not affect bronchoalveolar lavage levels of TNF-α).[22] These data fairly convincingly indicate that endogenous IL-1ra is another regulator of the inflammatory response, at least in the lung.

MECHANISM OF REGULATION OF THE INFLAMMATORY RESPONSE

How regulatory ILs (eg, IL-10, IL-13) regulate the inflammatory response has been determined. As indicated in Figure 3, when the inflammatory response is triggered, there is in cytosolic extracts a rapid and profound loss of IκB because of its hydrolysis by the 26S proteasome. This allows translocation of NF-κB to the nucleus, where gene activation occurs. In the presence of IL-10 or IL-13, activation of NF-κB fails to take place and the generation of inflammatory mediators is accordingly suppressed.[23] The striking finding was that IL-10 or IL-13 prevented the loss of IκB in the inflamed tissue. In other words, breakdown of IκB failed to occur, for reasons that are not known. There was no evidence that either IL-10 or IL-13 cause transcriptional up-regulation (appearance of messenger RNA) of IκB. Retention of IκB prevented the translocation of NF-κB to the critical binding sites on DNA. The failure in breakdown of IκB may be related to the ability of IL-10 or IL-13 to interfere with the phosphorylation and ubiquination of IκB, or interference in the enzymatic activity of the 26S proteosome. Whatever the explanation, IL-10 and IL-13 seem to inhibit fundamental mechanisms leading to signal transduction and gene activation in pathways of the inflammatory response. It remains to be determined to what extent in vivo inhibition of NF-κB activation will represent a new approach for anti-inflammatory therapy.

CONCLUSIONS

The acute inflammatory response is an essential and protective response in injured tissues; when successful, it restores the tissues to their preinjury state. On the other hand, there are many diseases and syndromes in which the inflammatory response produces adverse and sometimes life-threatening outcomes. In sepsis, it seems that the inflammatory response is no longer regulated, causing the appearance systemically of a variety of proinflammatory cytokines. These mediators cause expression of vascular adhesion molecules that facilitate the recruitment of blood leukocytes, especially neutrophils. Injury resulting from the inflammatory response is due to phagocytic cell production of oxidants and proteases. Central to generation of inflammatory mediators is activation in phagocytic cells of NF-κB. The inflammatory response is naturally regulated by a variety of endogenous factors, including IL-10 and IL-13. These ILs suppress the inflammatory response by blocking activation of NF-κB. The data suggest that a novel approach to inhibition of the inflammatory response would be to suppress the activation of NF-κB in vivo.

Corresponding author: Alex B. Lentsch, PhD, Department of Surgery, University of Louisville School of Medicine, JGBBC 426, 529 S Jackson St, James Graham Brown Cancer Center, Louisville, KY 40202 (e-mail: ablent01@ulkyvm.louisville.edu).

REFERENCES

1. Casey LC, Balk RA, Bone RC. Plasma cytokine and endotoxin levels correlate with survival in patients with the sepsis syndrome. *Ann Intern Med.* 1993;119:771-778.
2. Johnson KJ, Ward PA. Acute immunologic pulmonary alveolitis. *J Clin Invest.* 1974;54:349-357.
3. Caty MG, Guice KS, Oldham KT, Remick DG, Kunkel SL. Evidence for tumor necrosis factor-induced pulmonary microvascular injury after intestinal ischemia-reperfusion injury. *Ann Surg.* 1990;212:694-700.
4. Lechner AJ, Ryerse JS, Matuschak GM. Acute lung injury during bacterial or fungal sepsis. *Microsc Res Tech.* 1993;26:444-456.
5. Simons RK, Junger WG, Loomis WH, Hoyt DB. Acute lung injury in endotoxemic rats is associated with sustained circulating IL-6 levels and intrapulmonary CINC activity and neutrophil recruitment. *Shock.* 1996;6:39-45.
6. Thorp KM, Southern C, Bird IN, Matthews N. Tumor necrosis factor induction of ELAM-1 and ICAM-1 on human umbilical vein endothelial cells. *Cytokine.* 1992;4:313-319.
7. Bevilacqua MP, Nelson RM. Selectins. *J Clin Invest.* 1993;91:379-387.
8. Albeda SM, Smith CW, Ward PA. Adhesion molecules and inflammatory injury. *FASEB J.* 1994;8:504-512.
9. Kuijpers TW, Hakkert BC, Hart MH, Roos D. Neutrophil migration across monolayers of cytokine-prestimulated endothelial cells. *J Cell Biol.* 1992;117:565-572.
10. Varani J, Ginsburg I, Schuger L, et al. Endothelial cell killing by neutrophils. *Am J Pathol.* 1989;135:435-438.
11. Rosen GM, Pou S, Ramos CL, Cohen MS, Britigan BE. Free radicals and phagocytic cells. *FASEB J.* 1995;9:200-209.
12. Royall JA, Kooy NW, Beckman JS. Nitric oxide-related oxidants in acute lung injury. *New Horiz.* 1995;3:113-122.
13. Liou HC, Baltimore D. Regulation of the NF-kappaB/rel transcription factor and I kappa B inhibitor system. *Curr Opin Cell Biol.* 1993;5:477-487.
14. Baldwin AS. The NF-kappa B and I kappa B proteins *Annu Rev Immunol.* 1996;14:649-683.
15. Kuhn R, Lohler J, Rennick D, Rajewsky K, Muller W. Interleukin-10-deficient mice develop chronic enterocolitis. *Cell.* 1993;75:263-274.
16. Mulligan MS, Warner RL, Foreback JL, Shanley TP, Ward PA. Protective effects of IL-4, IL-10, IL-12, and IL-13 in IgG immune complex-induced lung injury *J Immunol.* 1997;159:3483-3489.
17. Qin L, Chavin KD, Ding Y, et al. Retrovirus-mediated transfer of viral IL-10 gene prolongs murine cardiac allograft survival. *J Immunol.* 1996;156:2316-2323.
18. Mulligan MS, Warner RL, Bolling S, Ward PA. Protective role of IL-10 in cardiac allograft rejection [abstract]. *FASEB J.* 1996;10:A1279.
19. Shanley TP, Foreback JL, Remick DG, Ulich TR, Kunkel SL, Ward PA. Regulatory effects of interleukin-6 in immunoglobulin G immune complex-induced lung injury. *Am J Pathol.* 1997;151:193-203.
20. Shanley TP, Schmal H, Friedl HP, Jones ML, Ward PA. Regulatory effects of intrinsic IL-10 in IgG immune complex–induced lung injury. *J Immunol.* 1995;154:3454-3460.
21. Lentsch AB, Czermak BJ, Jordan J, Ward PA. Regulation of acute lung inflammatory injury by endogenous interleukin-13. *J Immunol.* 1999;162:1071-1076.
22. Shanley TP, Peters JL, Jones ML, Chensue SW, Kunkel SL, Ward PA. Regulatory effects of endogenous interleukin-1 receptor antagonist protein in immunoglobin G immune complex-induced lung injury. *J Clin Invest.* 1996;97:963-970.
23. Lentsch, AB, Shanley TP, Sarma V, Ward PA. In vivo suppression of NF-kappa B and preservation of I kappa B alpha by interleukin-10 and interleukin-13. *J Clin Invest.* 1997;100:2443-2448.

Proctectomy and Coloanal Anastomosis for Rectal Cancer

Thomas E. Read, MD; Ira J. Kodner, MD

Fueled by a greater understanding of pelvic physiology along with an improved comprehension of rectal cancer spread, we are now able to offer most patients restoration of intestinal continuity following oncologic proctectomy. Coloanal or ultralow colorectal anastomosis can be performed in most patients with midrectal cancers, provided that anal sphincter function is not impaired preoperatively. Functional results may be improved by construction of a colonic pouch with pouch-anal anastomosis. Temporary fecal diversion, usually with a diverting loop ileostomy, may be prudent, especially in patients undergoing neoadjuvant chemoradiation.

Arch Surg. 1999;134:670-677

The overwhelming majority of patients undergoing coloanal anastomosis have carcinoma of the rectum. Until recently, most patients with mid or distal rectal cancers underwent abdominoperineal resection. Technical issues notwithstanding, surgeons were loathe to consider preservation of the distal rectum or anal canal in these patients because of their concern of distal intramural spread of tumor. Careful pathologic studies have shown, however, that distal spread of rectal adenocarcinoma (either in the wall of the rectum or mesorectum) greater than 2 cm is rare, and is associated with advanced lesions and poor prognosis.[1-7] On the other hand, direct radial extension of tumor into the mesorectum or pelvic sidewall is of critical importance.[8] Cure and the avoidance of local recurrence after treatment of mid and distal rectal cancers depend on the adequacy of lateral pelvic clearance and the removal of all mesorectal tissue in its fascial envelope.[9,10] Preservation of anal sphincter function is possible following proctectomy for mid and distal cancers, provided that the distal margin of the tumor is several centimeters above the anorectal muscular ring.

Precise definition of coloanal anastomosis is lacking. Removal of the rectum to the level of the levators with anastomosis in, or just above, the anal canal is considered a coloanal anastomosis by some surgeons. Others have a more rigorous definition, requiring anastomosis at the dentate line, and refer to the former as an ultralow colorectal anastomosis. Technique of dissection and anastomosis also varies. The dissection can be performed from the abdomen with distal division of the rectum and anastomosis performed using surgical staplers. Alternatively, some surgeons advocate transanal dissection to define the distal margin for low tumors, with a handsewn anastomosis. Regardless of technique, the concept of removal of the rectum and mesorectum with restoration of intestinal continuity in the region of the anal sphincter complex remains constant.

Construction of a neorectum using a colonic pouch has received considerable attention recently. Stool frequency and urgency are reduced as compared with straight coloanal anastomosis, probably because of increased reservoir capacity.[11-18] The advantage of the pouch-anal anastomosis over a straight coloanal anastomosis seems to be most pronounced in the first 1 to 2 years following construction. The typical colonic pouch is constructed in a "J" fashion using a 6- to 10-cm limb length. Larger pouches may impair emptying, although the functional differences emphasized in some studies of pouch limb length may be negated by changes in pouch volume over time.[19,20]

From the Section of Colon and Rectal Surgery, Washington University School of Medicine, St Louis, Mo.

Many surgeons perform a temporary diverting stoma to minimize the consequences of anastomotic disruption should it occur. The low level of the anastomosis and the increased length of suture line at risk when a colonic pouch is constructed increase the risk of leak and pelvic sepsis. Anastomotic leak may cause pelvic fibrosis, rendering the neorectum stiff and noncompliant. Patients may thus suffer from tenesmus and fecal incontinence. The most commonly used diverting stoma is the loop ileostomy, because its construction and subsequent takedown are straightforward, and the colonic mesentery is not threatened by such manipulation. Temporary fecal diversion may also be prudent in cases where neoadjuvant chemoradiation is used. Although dramatic reductions in tumor size can be achieved with the use of preoperative chemoradiation, it may predispose to anastomotic problems in patients not undergoing temporary diversion at the time of proctectomy and coloanal anastomosis.[21]

PATIENT EVALUATION

Patients with rectal cancer undergo evaluation with digital rectal examination, rigid proctoscopy, and transrectal ultrasound. Invasion of the anorectal muscular ring precludes restoration of intestinal continuity. Surgeons should not be seduced into triumphs of technique over judgment in cases where the tumor is very low in the rectum. It is not advisable to jeopardize oncologic cure because of enthusiasm to perform low anastomosis. As Heister remarked in 1739, speaking of intestinal stomas: "... it is surely better to part with one of the conveniences of life than to part with life itself."[22]

Colonoscopy is performed to search for synchronous neoplasms. Abdominopelvic computed tomography and a chest radiograph are obtained to rule out distal metastases. Transrectal ultrasound and pelvic computed tomography can detect extensive mesorectal lymph node involvement and help guide decisions regarding neoadjuvant treatment. Patients undergoing neoadjuvant external beam radiation with or without chemotherapy are reexamined by the surgeon prior to operation to assess tumor response to therapy.

Before considering coloanal anastomosis, sphincter function must be assessed. A detailed continence history and physical examination by an experienced surgeon is probably the most predictive of postoperative function.[23] However, anal manometry may help in equivocal cases. Despite the enthusiasm of many patients to restore intestinal continuity at all costs, it should be remembered that an abdominal colostomy is preferable to a perineal colostomy in cases where sphincter function is impaired.

OPERATIVE PREPARATION

Consent for operation should include the possibility of temporary or permanent stoma construction. Stoma sites should be marked preoperatively by the surgeon or enterostomal therapist with the patient in the sitting, standing, and supine positions. A mechanical and antibiotic bowel preparation is used. Intravenous broad-spectrum antibiotics are given perioperatively for 24 hours. Deep venous thrombosis prophylaxis is indicated. Our policy has been to use heparin, 5000 U subcutaneously every 12 hours, and intermittent pneumatic compression stockings. Ureteral catheters should be considered in cases where invasion or impingement on the ureters or bladders is suspected. Although some authors have found that ureteral catheters are not useful in preventing injury, we have found them extremely helpful in facilitating difficult pelvic dissection. The patient is placed in the lithotomy position and a Foley catheter is inserted. Digital rectal examination and proctoscopy with the patient under anesthesia can be helpful in determining tumor level and degree of fixation. We routinely employ rectal irrigation with saline and dilute povidone-iodine prior to operation, and leave a rectal tube in place.

EXPLORATION

A midline incision is made and the abdomen explored. The presence of unresectable metastases makes coloanal anastomosis ill-advised. If a temporary diverting stoma is constructed, the patient may never be fit enough to have the stoma closed. Even if the patient does not require a diverting stoma, the initial 6 to 18 months following coloanal anastomosis are often marked by frequent loose stools and occasional incontinence. The patient may not survive long enough to benefit from the gradual improvement in function of the neorectum. If the patient is treated with chemotherapy postoperatively, the risk of diarrhea and fecal incontinence are increased further. Low anterior resection with Hartmann closure of the rectal stump is a more prudent option for these patients. Tumor mobility in the pelvis is then assessed. Apparent fixation to pelvic structures may not preclude cure, as inflammatory or fibrotic reaction may be responsible, especially in cases where preoperative radiation or chemoradiation has been used. However, if during the course of pelvic dissection it becomes obvious that tumor invasion of pelvic structures makes complete resection impossible, low anastomosis should be abandoned because of the high risk of persistent tumor growth in the pelvis.

MOBILIZATION

The left colon is mobilized from its retroperitoneal attachments (**Figure 1**, A and B). The bloodless plane lateral to the descending colon mesentery is developed first, initially avoiding the pelvic brim, where the ureter and iliac vessels are most prone to injury. The small bowel should be protected during this mobilization because of the risk of penetrating through the thin avascular area at the base of the descending colon mesentery. We routinely accomplish this by carefully placing a large laparotomy pad over the small bowel and retracting it medially. After the descending colon has been mobilized and the ureter identified, the sigmoid is mobilized from its lateral attachments.

Several maneuvers are then performed to allow the descending colon to reach into the deep pelvis. We use the descending colon to per-

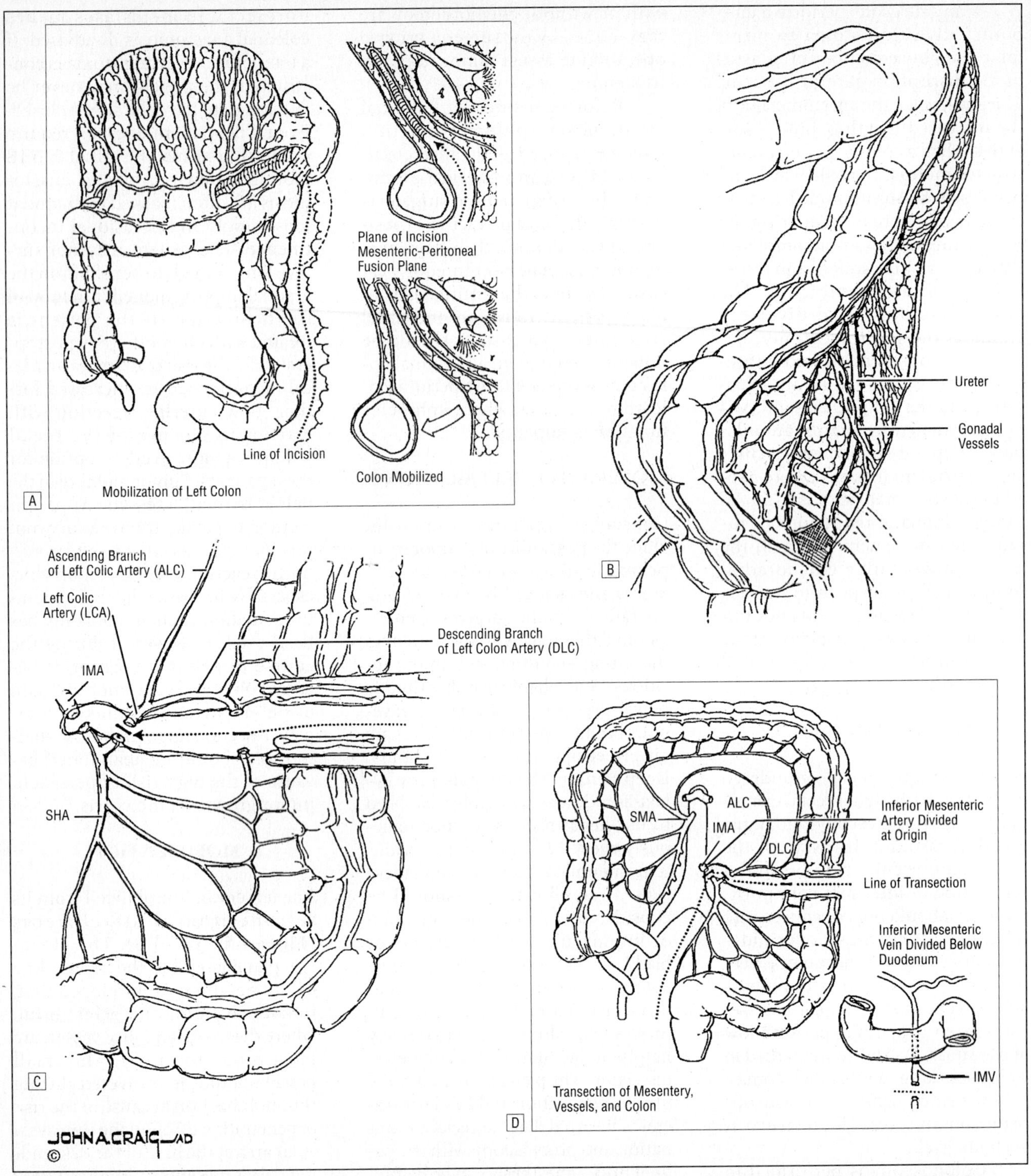

Figure 1. *Mobilization of the left colon. A, Line of incision in the avascular fusion plane between the left colon mesentery and retroperitoneum. B, Left colon reflected medially, exposing retroperitoneum. C, Inferior mesenteric artery divided close to aorta. The arcade of Riolan is preserved and the left colon and its mesentery are divided at the junction of the descending and sigmoid colon. D, Proximal ligation of inferior mesenteric vein for extra mobility.*

form all pelvic anastomoses because the sigmoid colon is narrow and has muscular hypertrophy in most patients. In addition, if preoperative external beam radiation has been used, the sigmoid may have been included in the radiation field and should not be used for the anastomosis. The splenic flexure is completely mobilized. The omentum is separated from the distal half of the transverse colon. An incision is made at the base of the sigmoid and descending colon mesentery on the right from the sacral promentory to the duodenum. It is frequently necessary to divide small filmy attachments of the distal duodenum and proximal jejeunum to the colonic mesentery to completely expose the origin of the inferior mesenteric artery (IMA) and the inferior mesenteric vein (IMV). The IMA is divided at its origin (Figure 1, C). Care should be taken to avoid the lumbar sympathetic plexus during IMA division. The IMV is divided adjacent to the ligament of Treitz (Figure 1, D). The blood supply to the proximal bowel is thus dependent on arcades originating from the middle colic artery.

Dissection then proceeds from the IMA origin toward the pelvis. Keeping the hypogastric nerves protected posteriorly, the plane just posterior to the superior hemorrhoidal artery is opened. This plane is used to gain entrance to the presacral space at the sacral promontory, and can be followed in the posterior midline to the anal canal without encountering a blood vessel.

Once the splenic flexure, descending colon, and sigmoid have been completely mobilized and the IMA and IMV divided, the proximal colon is divided. Although this step can be deferred until after pelvic dissection, division at this point in the operation allows the surgeon to retract on the rectosigmoid without danger of causing injury to the descending colon. The descending colon mesentery is divided between clamps beginning just proximal to the IMA. The line of mesenteric dissection extends perpendicular to the bowel to avoid jeopardizing proximal blood supply. We routinely divide the colon in an area of soft descending colon, leaving the sigmoid with the specimen. By performing the aforementioned mobilization, the descending colon should reach to the level of the anus. If additional length is needed, the omentum can be completely removed from the transverse colon and congenital attachments between the transverse mesocolon and retroperitoneum divided. It is rarely necessary to divide any of the arcade vessels originating from the middle colic artery, and great care should be exercised to ensure that pulsatile flow remains to the distal bowel. If a straight double-stapled anastomosis is planned, the bowel can be divided between clamps. A purse-string suture is placed and the proximal bowel sized to accommodate the anvil of the end-to-end stapler. If a colonic pouch or handsewn anastomosis is planned, the proximal bowel can be transected using a linear cutting stapler.

Pelvic dissection then proceeds (**Figure 2**). The goal is to remove the mesorectum intact within its fascial envelope and to achieve adequate radial and distal margins from the tumor. Sharp dissection under direct vision is required. Blunt tearing maneuvers should be avoided. A strong headlight and lighted retractors are invaluable in this phase of the operation. The peritoneum on either side of the mesorectum is divided. The line of incision should be just medial to the ureter on either side, and extend anteriorly to the seminal vesicles or rectovaginal septum. Posteriorly, the areolar tissue between the mesorectum and the presacral fascia is divided. Sharp dissection with electrocautery or scissors under direct vision can be accomplished with anterior retraction of the rectosigmoid. It is often helpful to use a curved malleable blade to retract the mesorectum as the dissection proceeds to the level of the coccyx. The risk of injury to the basivertebral veins on the anterior surface of the sacrum is minimized if the urge to perform this portion of the dissection bluntly with a hand behind the mesorectum is suppressed.

Anterior dissection is facilitated with a deep pelvic retractor placed between the anterior rectal wall and the posterior wall of the bladder. An assistant standing between the patient's legs places anterior retraction of these tissues. In a man, the plane posterior to the seminal vesicles is opened, the fascia of Denonvilliers incised, and the anterior rectal wall separated from the posterior capsule of the prostate. Palpation of the posterior surface of the pubis or palpation of the Foley catheter in the urethra distal to the prostate indicate that the distal aspect of the dissection is adequate. In a woman, the rectovaginal septum is separated to the level of the anal canal.

The lateral stalks are then divided. Most of this tissue can be divided using the electrocautery, working from the bloodless plane opened posterior to the mesorectum and proceeding in an anterior direction. In some cases it is prudent to divide the middle hemorrhoidal vessels between clamps and ligate the vessels. In other cases, these vessels can be controlled with cautery alone. Irrespective of the method of division, the lateral stalks should be divided as lateral as possible without jeopardizing the ureters. After completion of this maneuver, the rectum should rise out of the pelvis and the mesorectum should appear as a fatty bilobed structure posterolateral to the rectum encased in a glistening fascial envelope. It is now possible to divide any remaining tissue attachments to the distal rectum and proximal anal canal. The levators should be clearly visible, the mesorectum completely mobilized, and the anal canal exposed. In difficult cases where the exact level of distal dissection is uncertain, the surgeon may place a finger in the anal canal with the other hand palpating through the abdomen. The tumor should be well above the level of distal exposure of the muscular tube of anorectum, optimally 5 cm, although 2 cm has found to be adequate. If the tumor is found to be invading the levators or sphincter complex intraoperatively, abdominoperineal resection should be performed.

The pelvic autonomic nerves that innervate the genitalia and bladder are subject to injury during mobilization of the rectosigmoid. The preaortic sympathetic plexus can be drawn up into the resected specimen when the IMA is divided. The hypogastric plexus, located at the aortic bifurcation, and the hypogastric nerves, which are the condensation of those sympathetic fibers, are vulnerable to injury during mobilization of the mesorectum from the sacral promontory and lateral pelvic sidewalls. Sympathetic injury will result in retrograde ejaculation, or a "dry orgasm."

The pelvic plexus contains sympathetic fibers from the hypogastric nerves as well as parasympathetic fibers from the pelvic splanchnic nerves. This plexus is superior to the levators, anterior and lateral to the rectum, and between the peritoneum and the endopelvic fascia. Injury to the pelvic plexus can occur at the time of division of the lateral stalks or during the dissection of the rectum from the region of the seminal vesicles and prostate. Injury to both of the pelvic plexuses will result in complete impotence in the male.

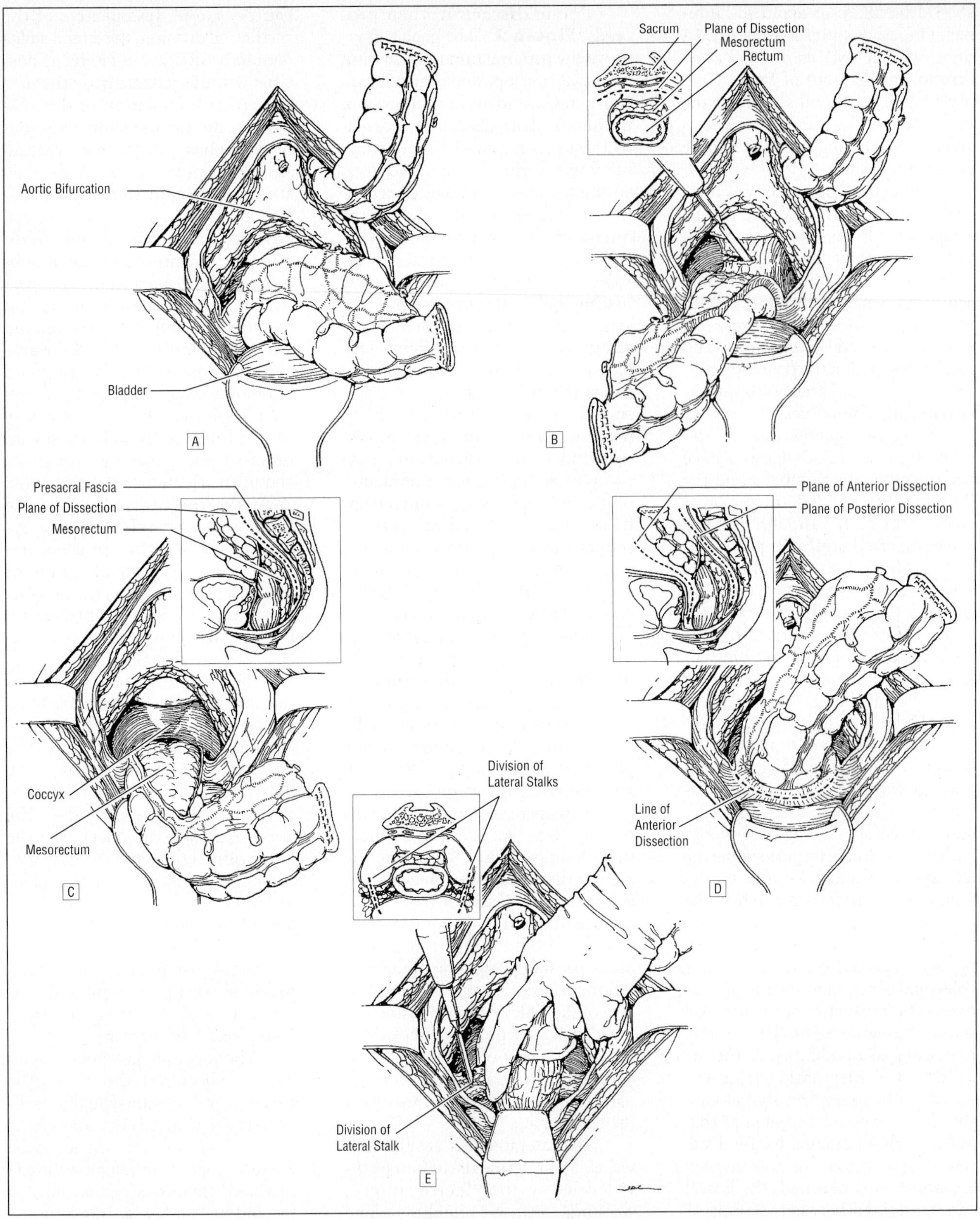

Figure 2. *Pelvic dissection. A, Incision of peritoneum at lateral borders of the mesorectum, just medial to the ureters. B, The areolar tissue plane posterior to the mesorectum is dissected sharply. C, The posterior aspect of the mesorectum appears as a bilobed structure when viewed from above, enclosed in a glistening fascial envelope. D, Anterior peritoneal incision. E, Division of lateral stalks.*

DISTAL TRANSECTION OF THE ANORECTUM

Division of the anal canal or very distal rectum can usually be accomplished through the abdomen using a linear stapler

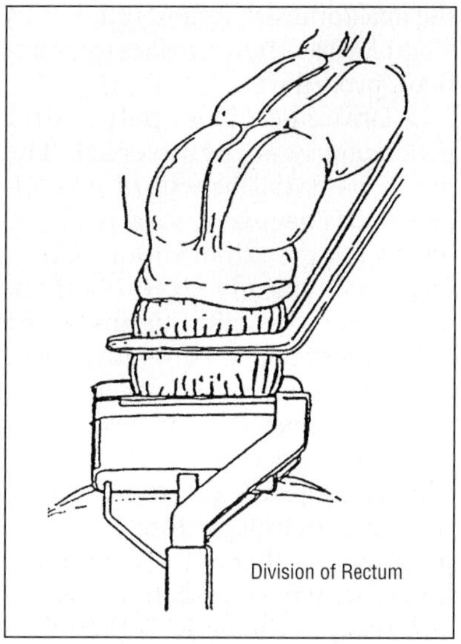

Figure 3. *Division of distal rectum using linear stapler distally and occlusive clamp proximally.*

(**Figure 3**). The site of division should be below the tail of mesorectum so that all mesorectal tissue accompanies the specimen. The rectum is retracted superiorly and posteriorly, with a deep pelvic retractor exposing the anterior surface of the rectum. We frequently use a "perineal pusher," an assistant standing between the patient's legs using folded towels enclosed in a sturdy clamp to manually elevate the perineum in a superior direction. After the stapler has been applied, a long occlusive clamp is placed on the rectum just proximal to the stapler and the bowel divided. It is crucial to have the specimen retrieved by the pathologist and have the radial margins inked prior to opening the specimen. Our pathologists now routinely report radial margin distance on all rectal cancer specimens.

Some surgeons are enthusiasts of the combined transanal-transabdominal resection procedure, where the distal margin is defined and the distal dissection is performed from a transanal approach. We have found very few indications for this technique. In most patients, the proximal anal canal can be exposed from the abdomen and a stapling instrument applied below the tumor. If the tumor is so low that division in the proximal anal canal would not provide an adequate distal margin, then perhaps an abdominoperineal procedure would be safer from an oncologic standpoint. There may be a few patients who, because of a narrow pelvis or other aspect of body habitus, might benefit from such a technique.

ANASTOMOSIS

Adequate mobilization of the proximal colon and lack of tension are reconfirmed. Blood supply to the proximal margin can be reassessed as the proximal bowel has now been dependent on unidirectional flow from the middle colic artery for the entire period of pelvic dissection. ("If

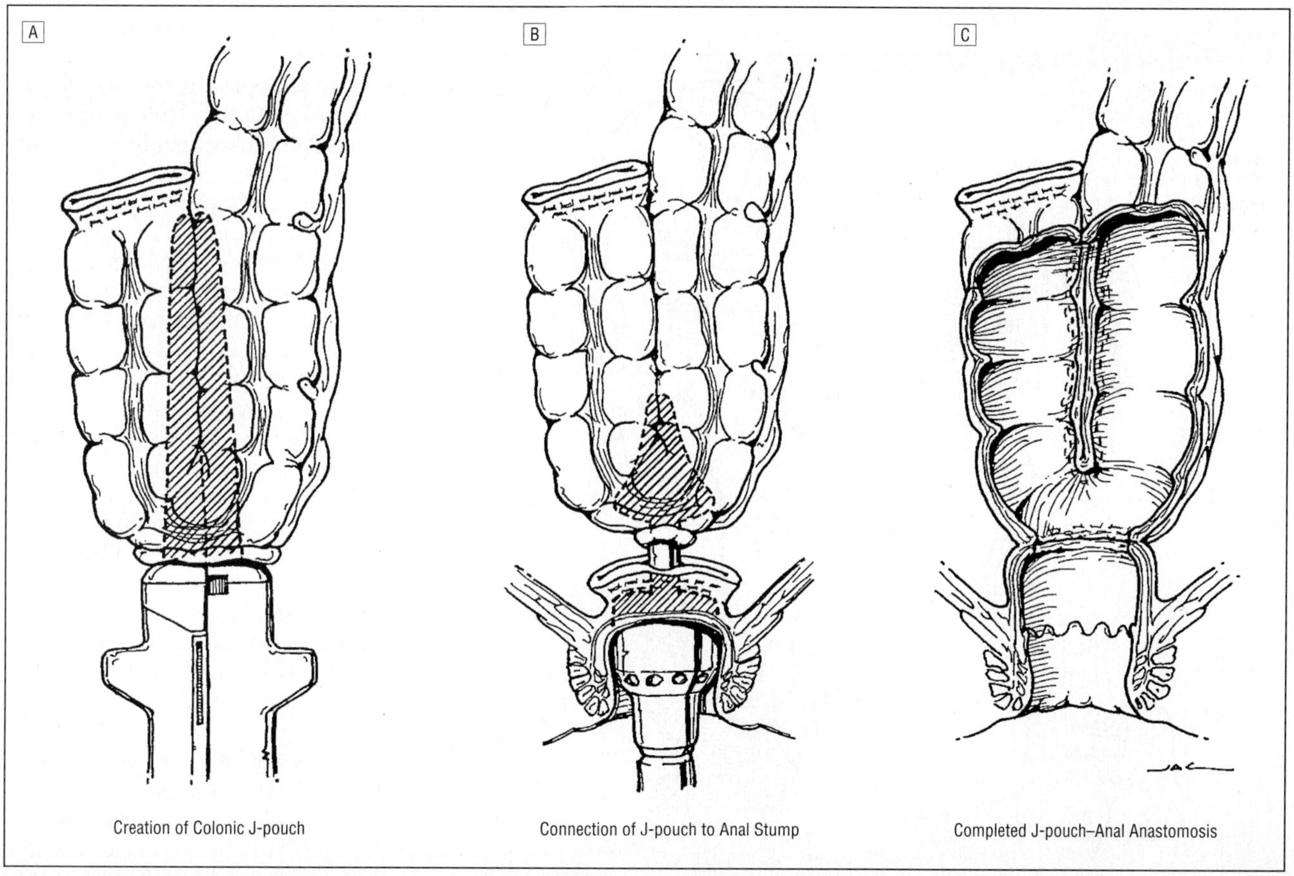

Figure 4. *Colonic J-pouch construction and pouch-anal anastomosis. A, The colon is folded in a J configuration and the stapler is passed through the apex of the pouch. B, The anvil of the stapler is secured at the apex of the pouch with a purse-string suture and the stapler passed through the anus. C, Completed anastomosis.*

it looks blue, it is blue.") Poor blood supply to the proximal margin must be corrected prior to anastomosis.

We routinely use a double-stapled technique to perform coloanal or ultralow colorectal anastomosis, and with increasing frequency we are constructing a colonic J-pouch (**Figure 4**). The colon is folded into a J-configuration with an approximately 8-cm limb length. The apex of the pouch is opened and a linear cutting stapler is used to create the pouch. Care must be taken to avoid incorporating the colonic mesentery into the staple line. Usually a single fire of a 75- or 90-mm stapler will create adequate pouch length. If there is a long blind end remaining, this can be corrected with a second fire of the linear cutting stapler. A purse-string suture is placed around the opening at the pouch apex and the anvil of the end-to-end stapler inserted. We usually use a 28- or 29-mm stapler in this situation.

Retractors are replaced and hemostasis in the pelvis confirmed. The stapler is placed gently in the anus with adequate lubrication. For low anastomosis, there is often not enough remaining length of the anorectum for the stapler head to slip above the sphincter complex and thus give the feeling of being properly positioned. Great care must be exercised in this situation to avoid forcing the stapler and bursting through the distal staple line. The staple head is aligned and the spike of the stapler is advanced through the distal staple line. Although it is tedious at times, we routinely place a purse-string suture in the distal bowel to make it fit snugly around the spike of the stapler. We feel this prevents extrusion of the distal bowel from the anastomosis during closure of the stapler.

Carefully retracting the vagina and any other tissue at risk, the anvil is attached to the spike and the stapler closed and fired. After removal of the stapler, the adequacy of the tissue doughnuts are assessed and the anastomosis inspected gently with a proctoscope. The integrity of the pouch and anastomosis are tested by instilling air via the proctoscope with the pelvis filled with warm saline. Bubbles are an indication of a leak and should be investigated and repaired. If there is a small separation at the anastomotic line low in the pelvis, it may be difficult to expose transabdominally and transanal repair with absorbable suture is indicated. Large leaks may require takedown and reconstruction of the anastomosis, although the short length of distal bowel makes this a difficult procedure.

Drainage of the pelvis after proctectomy is controversial. The major potential benefit of postoperative drainage is removal of blood, which is a growth medium for bacteria. We typically place 2 soft, Silastic, closed-suction drains in the pelvis after proctectomy with pouch-anal anastomosis. However, if hemostasis is excellent at the conclusion of the procedure, drains may be unnecessary. We do not routinely make an attempt to close the pelvic peritoneum. If the descending colon mesentery is loose, however, we will reapproximate it to the retroperitoneum. We have had a case of small bowel becoming entrapped posterior to the mesentery of the descending colon, necessitating reoperation.

In our opinion, the risk of anastomotic or pouch leak with pelvic sepsis and subsequent fibrosis of the neorectum outweighs the benefits of avoiding temporary fecal diversion in our patient population. In addition, most patients undergoing proctectomy and coloanal anastomosis for rectal cancer will have stage II or stage III lesions. We routinely treat these patients with postoperative chemotherapy. As mentioned above, chemotherapy-induced diarrhea in a patient first adapting to a neorectum will cause fecal incontinence. For these reasons, a temporary loop ileostomy is constructed (**Figure 5**). After chemotherapy is completed, the pouch and anastomosis are assessed endoscopically and radiographically and ileostomy takedown is performed.

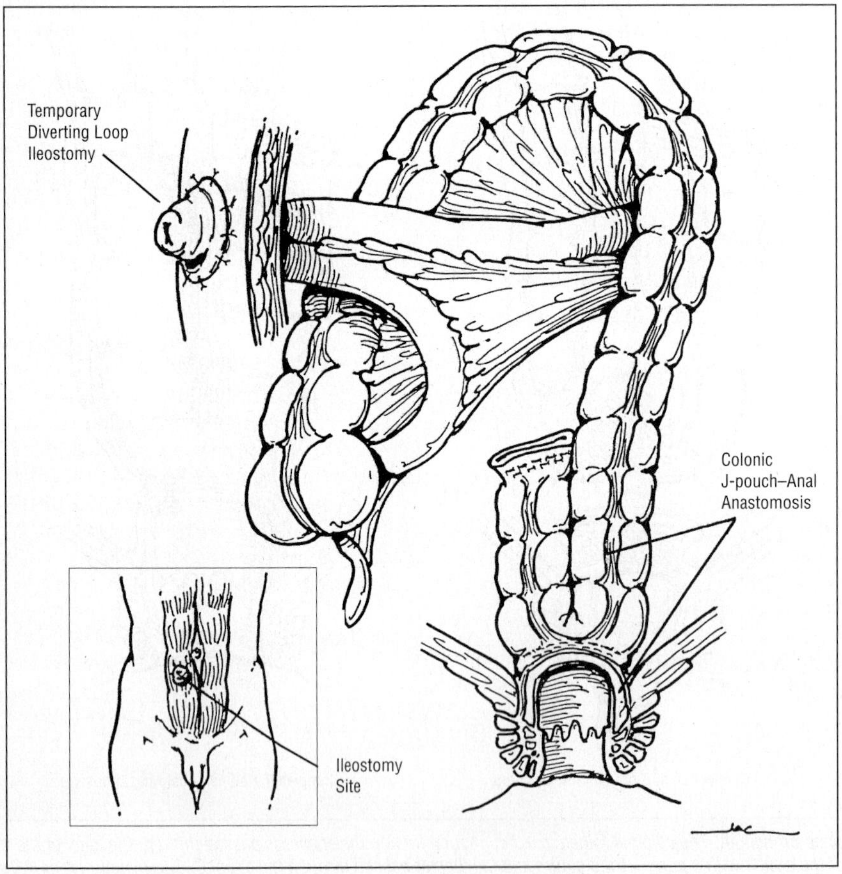

Figure 5. *Completed anastomosis with temporary diverting loop ileostomy.*

We thank John A. Craig, MD, for producing the illustrations.

Corresponding author: Thomas E. Read, MD, Section of Colon and Rectal Surgery, 216 S Kingshighway (North Campus), St Louis, MO 63110 (e-mail: readt@msnotes.wustl.edu).

REFERENCES

1. Quer E, Dahin D, Mayo C. Retrograde intramural spread of carcinoma of the rectum and rectosigmoid. *Surg Gynecol Obstet.* 1953;96:24-30.
2. Grinnell R. Distal intramural spread of rectal carcinoma. *Surg Gynecol Obstet.* 1954;99:421-430.
3. Black U, Waugh J. The intramural extension of carcinoma of the descending colon, sigmoid and rectosigmoid: a pathological study. *Surg Gynecol Obstet.* 1948;1948:457-464.
4. Scott N, Jackson P, al JT, Dixon MF, Quirke P, Finan PJ. Total mesorectal excision and local recurrence: a study of tumour spread in the mesorectum distal to rectal cancer. *Br J Surg.* 1995; 82:1031-1033.
5. Williams NS, Dixon MF, Johnston D. Reappraisal of the 5 centimetre rule of distal excision for carcinoma of the rectum: a study of distal intramural spread and of patients' survival. *Br J Surg.* 1983; 70:150-154.
6. Dukes C. The surgical pathology of rectal cancer. *Proc R Soc Med.* 1943;37:131.
7. Goligher J, Dukes C, Bussey H. Local recurences after sphincter-saving excisions for carcinoma of the rectum and rectosigmoid. *Br J Surg.* 1951; 39:199-211.
8. Quirke P, Durdey P, Dixon MF, Williams NS. Local recurrence of rectal adenocarcinoma due to inadequate surgical resection: histopathological study of lateral tumour spread and surgical excision. *Lancet.* 1986;2:996-999.
9. Heald RJ, Ryall RD. Recurrence and survival after total mesorectal excision for rectal cancer. *Lancet.* 1986;1:1479-1482.
10. Zaheer S, Pemberton JH, Farouk R, Dozois RR, Wolff BG, Ilstrup D. Surgical treatment of adenocarcinoma of the rectum. *Ann Surg.* 1998;227: 800-811.
11. Macmanus J. Perforations of the intestine by ingested foreign bodies. *Am J Surg.* 1941;111:393-402.
12. Mortensen NJ, Ramirez JM, Takeuchi N, Humphreys MM. Colonic J-pouch anal anastomosis after rectal excision for carcinoma: functional outcome. *Br J Surg.* 1995;82:611-613.
13. Lazorthes F, Chiotasso P, Gamagami RA, Istvan G, Chevreau P. Late clinical outcome in a randomized prospective comparison of colonic J-pouch and straight coloanal anastomosis. *Br J Surg.* 1997;84:1449-1451.
14. Hallbook O, Sjodahl R. Comparison between the colonic J-pouch anal anastomosis and healthy rectum: clinical and physiological function. *Br J Surg.* 1997;84:1437-1441.
15. Seow-Choen F, Goh HS. Prospective randomized trial comparing J colonic pouch-anal anastomosis and straight coloanal reconstruction. *Br J Surg.* 1995;82:608-610.
16. Ho YH, Tan M, Seow CF. Prospective randomized controlled study of clinical function and anorectal physiology after low anterior resection: comparison of straight and colonic J pouch anastomoses. *Br J Surg.* 1996;83:978-980.
17. Ortiz H, De MM, Armendariz P, Rodriguez J, Chocarro C. Coloanal anastomosis: are functional results better with a pouch? *Dis Colon Rectum.* 1995; 38:375-377.
18. Nicholls RJ, Lubowski DZ, Donaldson DR. Comparison of colonic reservoir and straight coloanal reconstruction after rectal excision. *Br J Surg.* 1988;75:318-320.
19. Lazorthes F, Gamagami R, Chiotasso P, Istvan G, Muhammad S. Prospective, randomized study comparing clinical results between small and large colonic J-pouch following coloanal anastomosis. *Dis Colon Rectum.* 1997;40: 1409-1413.
20. Hida J, Yasutomi M, Fujimoto K, et al. Functional outcome after low anterior resection with low anastomosis for rectal cancer using the colonic J-pouch: prospective randomized study for determination of optimum pouch size. *Dis Colon Rectum.* 1996;39:986-991.
21. Hyams DM, Mamounas EP, Petrelli N, et al. A clinical trial to evaluate the worth of preoperative multimodality therapy in patients with operable carcinoma of the rectum: a progress report of National Surgical Breast and Bowel Project Protocol R-03. *Dis Colon Rectum.* 1997;40:131-139.
22. Heister L. *A General System of Surgery.* London, England: W Innys; 1743.
23. Church JM, Saad R, Schroeder T, et al. Predicting the functional result of anastomoses to the anus: the paradox of preoperative anal resting pressure. *Dis Colon Rectum.* 1993;36:895-900.

IN OTHER AMA JOURNALS

JAMA

Market Forces and Unsponsored Research in Academic Health Centers

Joel S. Weissman, PhD; Demet Saglam, MS; Eric G. Campbell, PhD; Nancyanne Causino, EdD; David Blumenthal, MD, MPP

Context Increased competitive pressures on academic health centers may result in reduced discretionary funds from patient care revenues to support the performance of unsponsored research, including institutionally funded and faculty-supported activities.
Objective To measure the amount and distribution of unsponsored research activities and their outcomes.
Design and Setting Survey conducted in academic year 1996-1997 of 2336 research faculty in 117 medical schools. Responses were weighted to provide national estimates.
Main Outcome Measures Institutionally funded research as a proportion of total direct costs of research was compared across stages of market competition. Logistic regression was used to assess the relationship of performing unsponsored research to faculty characteristics and market stage.
Results Overall, 43% of faculty received institutional funding for research. Young faculty were more likely than others to receive institutional support (adjusted odds ratio [OR], 1.4; 95% confidence interval [CI], 1.1-1.9; $P = .004$). The amount of institutional support as a proportion of total funding was more than twice as high in less competitive markets (6.1%) compared with the most competitive markets (2.5%; $P = .05$). Most faculty (55%) performed faculty-supported research. Clinical researchers (OR, 1.6; 95% CI, 1.1-2.3), principal investigators (OR, 4.3; 95% CI, 2.8-7.0), faculty with high levels of research effort (OR, 6.2; 95% CI, 4.0-9.5) or institutional funding (OR, 1.9; 95% CI, 1.4-2.6), and faculty in the most competitive markets (OR, 1.9; 95% CI, 1.4-2.5) were more likely than others to conduct faculty-supported research. When undertaken by clinical researchers, these activities were supported by clinical income, extra hours worked, and discretionary funds, and often led to publications (76%) or grant awards (51%).
Conclusions Many academic health center faculty receive institutional support to conduct their research or fund the research themselves. Market pressures may be affecting the level of institutional funding available to faculty. (*1999;281:1093-1098*) www.jama.com

Corresponding author and reprints: Joel S. Weissman, PhD, Institute for Health Policy, Massachusetts General Hospital, 50 Staniford St, Ninth Floor, Boston, MA 02114 (e-mail: weissman@gem.mgh.harvard.edu).

George W. Stephenson, MD, FACS (1902-1998)

A Personal Remembrance

THE TELEPHONE would ring and I would answer it.

From the other end, "Are ya runnin' dry?" The voice was that of George Willoughby Stephenson, MD, FACS, archivist of the American College of Surgeons.

"Seems like it," I would say.

"Be right up!"

Then George and I would have a cup of coffee together in the small lounge provided by the college and together solve all but the stickiest problems of our world. For the stickiest problems, George's pronouncement would be, "It's a puzzlement."

This sequence, occurring late in the morning of most days, was not exactly a ritual, but it happened, whenever nothing else got in the way, for a decade.

When I joined the staff of the American College of Surgeons, late in 1987, George was in his late 80s and had been employed at the college since 1950, having been recruited from a private general surgery practice in Bloomington, Ill. He had directed the fellowship department of the college for many years and, in addition to overseeing the process by which surgeons become fellows of the college, had done the spadework for many of the collaborations of the college with other major medical organizations—the American Board of Medical Specialties and its various surgical boards, the Accreditation Council for Graduate Medical Education and its surgical residency review committees, and others.

It is not easy for me to say why George and I became close to each other very quickly, but I believe a lot of it had to do with the fact that George was a born instructor, and I needed a lot of instruction at that time. For my part, I thought George was a great guy, but he also had special knowledge that I thought would serve me extremely well in my own position at the college. I have said, since that time, that George knew everything that had been written about the college, but, more importantly, he knew everything that had not been written about it.

We were close friends for 10 years, during which he became progressively less able to walk the half mile from his apartment (he had voluntarily stopped driving years before), so whenever I was able, I would drive him home at the end of the day. He never got over having trouble getting his seat belt buckled, but we developed a reasonably efficient system of getting it done.

George was not, from his body language, a "hail fellow well met" type of individual; in fact, even in his later years, when he had mellowed considerably, George was perceived by some as severe. The perception was very different when you met and talked to him. He was anything but ebullient or effusive and was always very careful with his choice of words, lest he use too many or lose the precise meaning he wished to convey. He had spent many years scrutinizing the English language for the benefit of the college, and this was evident in conversing with him. He was called, by some members of the college staff who worked with him, the "king of the commas" because of his precision in writing with consummate brevity. But what made talking to George a memorable experience was his down-to-earth sophistication, his dry humor, his prodigious memory, and, even in his tenth decade of life, his broad and continuing interest in the world.

One of my favorite memories of talking to George is of one day when he was about 93. We were having another cup of coffee.

He said, "Rosey Clooney is coming to town."

I said, "I heard that."

George said, "She's gotten pretty big, but she still sings fine."

I said, "You know, George, I remember her first big hit in the summer of 1951."

"Yeah, 'Come on-a My House.'"

When he met someone new, he was always eminently courteous and almost always had something to say that would generate a smile. When he met someone new from the fellowship of the college, he almost always could strike up a conversation based on his experiences at the college, which would immediately kindle the curiosity of his new acquaintance.

He seldom talked about his family, but when he did, it was always with pride. His second wife, Martha, had died some years before I met him, and he certainly loved and was proud of his 2 children, Steve and Ann. Oddly enough, Ann's children had gone to school with mine in Darien, Conn, many years before my wife and I knew George.

George was a quiet patriot, loved his country deeply, and served during World War II. He saw active duty early in the war in the Aleutian Islands, and then later on in Africa and Italy. He was a member of one of the most famous medical units of any American war, the Second Auxiliary, which had been based on the medical team from Massachusetts General Hospital. During the last few years of his life, he was one of the 5 surviving surgeons who had served with the "Second Aux," and may have ultimately been the last. Certainly, all of those whom I knew or knew of had previously died.

He was not overly fond of foreigners and had very specific biases against some countries, most of them rooted in his experiences during the war. The exception was his great love and admiration for the British, and he had many surgical friends among the "Brits," Lord Smith being highly favored. He felt that, in many ways, if the United States could emulate the "tight little island," we would be much better off.

George used shopping bags for things he had to carry that would not fit in his ancient leather briefcase. A few months before his death, George gave me 2 shopping bags that contained the press clippings he had gathered during World War II. I was at first surprised at how few of the articles had anything personally to do with George, until I realized that George thought of himself as a small part of the system, doing his duty. That attitude was also pervasive in his thinking about his role within the college, and was reflected whenever he discussed it. On the other hand, he was very much aware that his own "personal war," as he referred to it, had been different from anybody else's experiences.

If he had not become a surgeon, George would have been an engineer. He was very proud of the shower facilities he had designed and had built for his army unit on the island of Kiska in the Aleutians. He was always fascinated by the way things worked and loved to tinker. He even built his television set from a kit.

Although he had not been much of an athlete, he was a great watcher of Chicago sports—the Cubs, Bears, and Bulls—and he knew in detail what was wrong with them. He always insisted that if the management of those teams would only listen to him . . .

George was very much an idealist, but he was also a genuine realist. I found it interesting that, in George, I could easily distinguish between realism and pragmatism. George bowed to undesirable reality only when he considered that the price for doing otherwise was clearly absurd. He never rationalized his ideals, and his ethics were anything but situational. I never sensed that George was likely to call on God for answers, but he seemed to believe strongly in what he considered a "Scottish" attitude: in the face of seemingly intolerable but unchangeable situations, one had to rely on the evolution of circumstances, over time, to solve the problem. He did not change his mind; he simply thought that waiting would bring beneficence. He was not religious in the sense of organized religion, but had great respect for aspects of some religions, particularly the Quaker faith.

He believed strongly in Swarthmore College, the University of Pennsylvania, and the Mayo Clinic. At Swarthmore, he obviously had a meaningful college experience that convinced him of the excellence of the Quakers. At the University of Pennsyvania and the Mayo Clinic, he engaged the medical training that made him what he most wanted to be, a "real 'get 'em well' doc." He regularly shared with me the publications from these worthy institutions, but was by no means incapable of critiquing some aspects of what he found in them. Most of what George was likely to criticize were signs of the times, which were certainly not unique to his own bastions of knowledge.

He retired in February 1998, having devoted half of his life to the work of the college. He did not get around very well because his legs refused to support him. On May 1, 1998, he fell and fractured his hip. To those of us who visited him in the next 2 months, it was difficult to see any silver lining to this cloud. George was stoic through the surgical and postoperative period, but, as we had frankly discussed on many occasions, he did not regard death as an enemy. When pneumonia struck 4 days before his death, he emphatically declined any aggressive attempts to reverse it or to support his life. Fortunately, his daughter and one of his closest friends from his days at the college were with him when he quietly died on the afternoon of June 23, 1998.

For me, George was a giant of the college, largely unheralded, by his own choosing, except when the American College of Surgeons' Distinguished Service Award, its highest honor for any surgeon, was bestowed on him in 1973. He was a special friend to both my wife and me, and the fellows of the college owe him much more than most of them know.

Gerald O. Strauch, MD, FACS
Chicago, Ill

Surgical Anatomy

The meandering **artery of Gonzalez** is a proximal collateral arterial arcade of the colon that shadows and is proximal and medial to the marginal artery. The **space of Riolan** is an avascular area in the mesentery to the left of the mid-colic artery. **Sudeck's Point** is a watershed between the superior hemorrhoidal artery and the middle hemorrhoidal artery.

1. Blackbourne LH, Fleischer KJ. *Advanced Surgical Recall*. Baltimore, Md: Williams & Wilkins; 1997:40-41.

Anesthesia During the Civil War

INITIALLY, THE GENERAL ignorance of the average Civil War "surgeon" regarding the use of chloroform and ether, combined with widely reported incidents of anesthetic mishaps, accounted for considerable controversy over whether anesthesia was appropriate in the military setting. This dispute led to romanticized tales of uncountable soldiers biting a bullet or getting rip-roaring drunk as a prelude to their confronting the surgeon's knife. Despite a tinge of truth, many of these surgical stories represent nothing more than imaginative folklore. The simple fact is that surgical anesthesia had been available for almost 15 years and was extensively applied early in the war, and by the end of the conflict it was universally used. With more than 80 000 known instances of anesthetic renderings, it would become apparent that few clinical lessons proved of greater value to the evolution of American surgery than this vast and positive experience with surgical anesthesia.

The actual anesthetic record of Civil War surgeons was quite remarkable. Of the 8900 cases where the anesthetic agent was definitely known (76% chloroform, 15% ether, and 9% mixed agents), a total of just 37 deaths from chloroform, 4 from ether, and 2 from a combination of both were reported. This is an extraordinary fact, largely attributable to the rapidity with which battlefield surgical procedures had to be carried out. Unfortunately, of the deaths, little can be learned about the actual cause of expiration, since autopsies were not always performed, and concepts of cellular pathology and physiology were not understood by the average physician/surgeon.

What can be speculated, however, is that by dispensing short-term doses of anesthetic agents, the surgeon inadvertently averted many complications, most notably sudden death from heart stoppage, which had plagued the worldwide use of inhalation anesthesia since its discovery. Chloroform rapidly became the anesthetic of choice because of its nonflammability and speed of action. The technique for administering it was a model of military efficiency, now colloquialized as the "open method." The sweet-smelling liquid was liberally sprinkled onto a sponge, handkerchief, or cotton cloth, which was held in place over the soldier's nose and mouth. Ingeniously designed inhalers were sometimes used to protect the hands of the person who administered the corrosive chloroform and also to help prevent excessive evaporation. The chloroform or ether was given until the patient became limp, which was a crude, but for that era fairly accurate way of determining adequate depth of surgical anesthesia. Since the actual procedure was usually so brief, inhalation of the agent was promptly suspended with little need to ever renew the dosage.

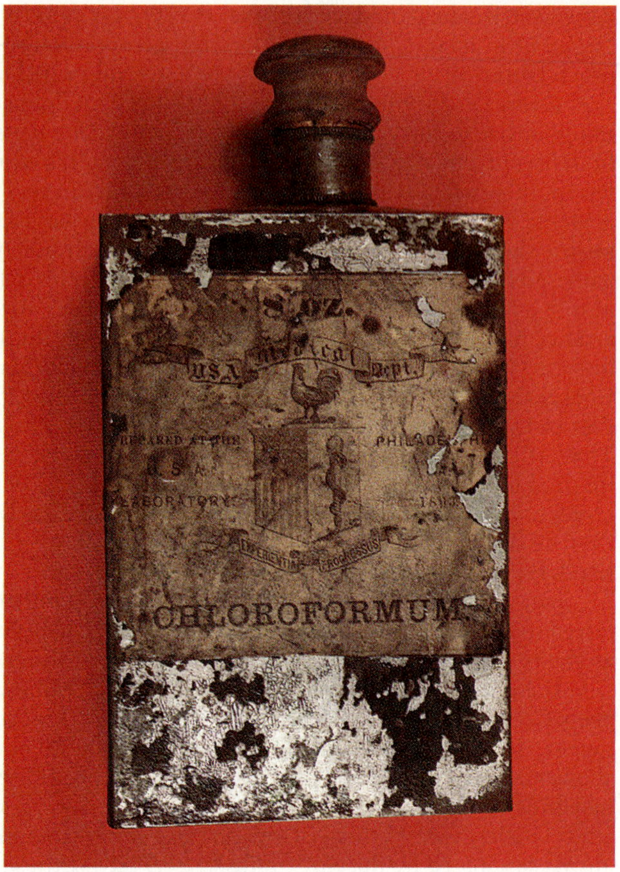

This rare extant example of bottled chloroform was prepared in 1863 at the US Army Laboratory in Philadelphia, Pa (Courtesy of Alex Peck, Antique Scientifica, Charlestown, Ill).

Cruel as it may seem, chloroform and ether were not invariably available, especially for Southern troops, who were often without important supplies. Nor, for that matter, did surgical anesthesia always appear necessary. Phoebe Pember, a matron at the renowned Chimborazo Hospital in Richmond, Va, observed that following the engagement at Crury's Bluff in May 1864, the men "were so exhausted by forced marches, lying in entrenchments and loss of sleep that few even awoke during the operations." Believable or not, that manner of behavior was similarly related by a Northern surgeon who told of how, during amputation, some of his patients "frequently lay and smoked their cigars, and kept up a conversation with their fellow sufferers."

Ira M. Rutkow, MD, MPH, DrPH

PRODUCTS & SERVICES

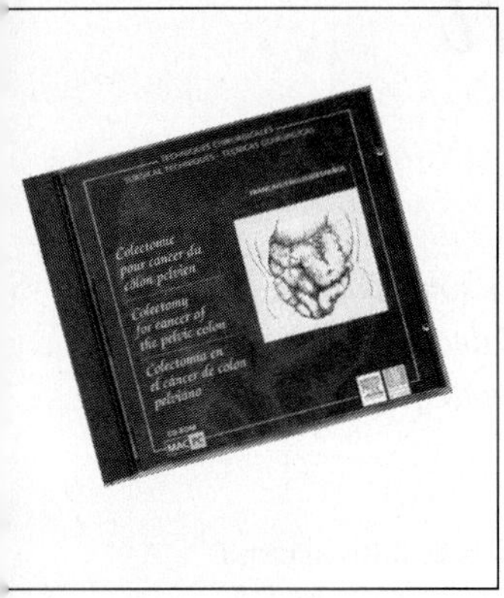

RGICAL CD-ROM —

MKAT, Inc, introduces a new urgical technique CD-Rom, Colectomy for cancer of the pelvic olon. It is available in English, panish and French on the same D-Rom. It is also available for oth Mac and PC platforms.

he CD-Rom on "Colectomy for ancer of the pelvic colon" is omposed of the basic operative teps for this operation. Each step s explicitly illustrated by the ideo sequence accompanied by exts and figures which can op-up at any time. More ever a ection called "additional nformation" in which the reader an find additional information oncerning technical variations, ossible difficulties or complica-ions is included.

he CD-Rom is based on ommented analysis on filmed operation illustrating the surgical echnique as performed in daily ractice.

or information write
AMKAT, Inc
12310 Riverfalls Ct
Boca Raton, FL 33428

all toll free
800-482-2386

-mail
amkat98@aol.com

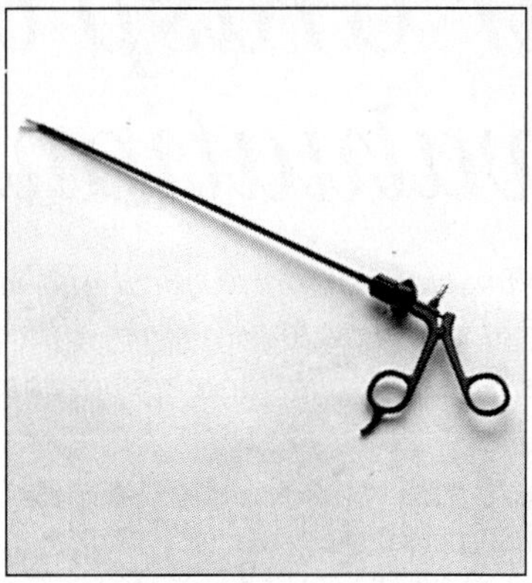

SURGICAL PRODUCT —

Aslan Medical Technologies has introduced a non-locking scissors-grip handle with the new VersaLap™ line of instruments for minimally invasive surgery. The conventional grip is offered as an alternative to the new Sensor™ handle, which made its debut with the VersaLap™ system of interchangeable instrument tips.

The non-locking, electrocautery-capable handle is made of surgical stainless steel with an autoclavable insulating coating. It can be sterilized and re-used with dozens of VersaLap™ tip styles.

For information write
ASLAN MEDICAL TECHNOLOGIES
Attn: Robert Sheldon
4110 South 9th Street
Kalamazoo, MI 49909

Call toll free
800-551-4561

Phone
612-338-5098

Fax
616-372-9639

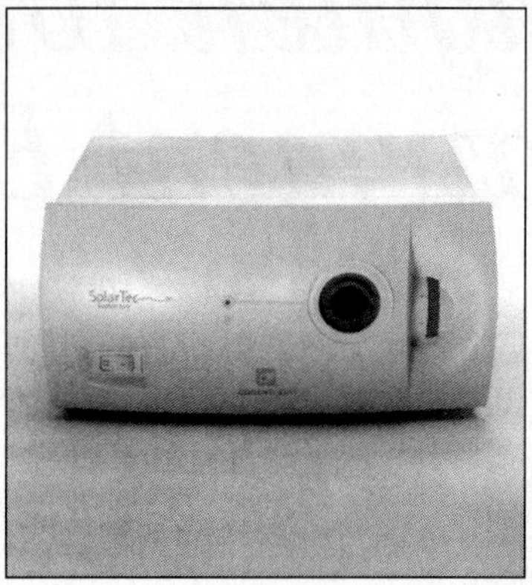

SURGICAL ANESTHETIC —

Cogent Light® Technologies introduces the SolarTec line of Micro Illumination™ light source platforms. SolarTec light sources outpace the competition by combining lower purchase and operating costs with enhanced performance. It powers surgical headlights, endoscopes, and lighted surgical instruments with sunlight quality illumination.

Equipped with the fully integrated Multi Link™ port, a SolarTec Source accepts traditional fiber bundles and the new line of low cost Micro Link® plastic single-fiber light guides.

SolarTec light source platforms are available in a variety of configurations, single fiber only, universal, or specially optimized to deliver higher power to fiber bundles and larger plastic fibers compared to conventional light sources. Lamp options include the xenon SolarTec 100, and the new SolarTec 270.

For information contact
Cogent Light Technologies, Inc
Att: Dennis Davis
26145 Technology Drive
Santa Clarita, CA 91355-1137

Call toll free
800-294-2989

Phone
805-294-2900

Fax
805-294-2904

Web site
www.cogentlight.com

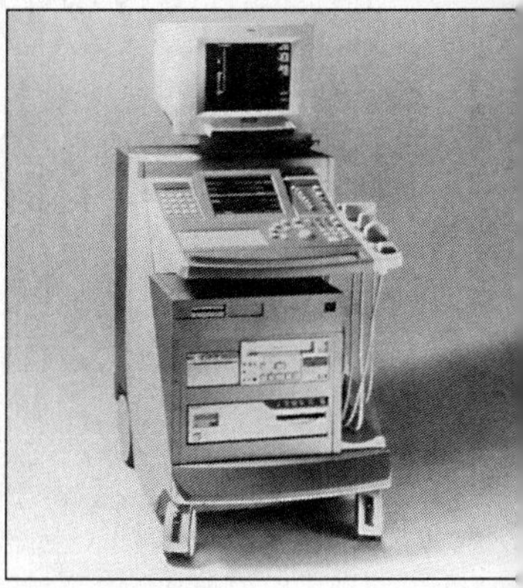

INFORMATIONAL CD-ROM

Siemens Medical Systems, Inc, Ultrasound Group has released an advanced ultrasound software that gives clinicians a new method for evaluating cancer and determining the health of vital organs. Siemens patented Ensemble™ Contrast Harmonic Imaging offers clinicians new views of blood flow within the body's tiniest capillaries.

Ultrasound contrast can be used to detect a lack of blood flow in organs, such as kidneys and the heart, and in transplants, providing clinicians an early warning of poor organ health.

Ultrasound contrast agents are administered through a simple intravenous line and the microbubbles dissolve harmlessly within the body, typically within a few minutes. Ensemble Imaging enhances these unique contrast agent signals to depict minute differences in blood flow information. This allows the SONOLINE® Elegra Ultrasound system to create precise images of complex blood vessel networks, including rare views of flow within microscopic feeder vessels.

For information write
SIEMENS MEDICAL SYSTEMS, INC
Attn: Sara Britton
22010 SE 51st St
Issaquah, WA 98029-7002

Call toll free
800-367-3569

Phone
206-448-1200

Web site
www.siemens-ultrasound.com

Classified Advertising

Academic/Faculty
Cardiovascular/Thoracic Surgery
CME Corner
Chiefs/Department Heads/ Directors
Courses/Symposia/Seminars
Facial Plastic Surgery
Graduate Training/ Residencies/Fellowships
Locum Tenens Wanted
Neurosurgery
Multiple Specialties/Group Practice
Notices
Othopedic Surgery
Pediatric Surgery
Plastic Surgery
Practices For Sale
Surgical Specialties
Thoracic Surgery
Vascular Surgery

Sales Information

1999 CLASSIFIED ADVERTISING RATES

Regular	1x 1.65/wd	*3x 1.55/wd
Bold	1x 1.85/wd	*3x 1.75/wd

*In order to receive the 3-time frequency price, the request must be made upon initial placement. The minimum charge is 20 words. A word consists of one or more letters surrounded by space on each side. For information on display advertising and our network buys contact an account representative.

POLICY

Orders for classified advertising must be submitted in writing. Although the American Medical Association believes the classified advertisements in these pages to be from reputable sources, the Association does not investigate the offers made and assumes no liability concerning them. Acceptance of advertising is restricted to professional opportunities, practices for sale, and medical office space available. The Association reserves the right to decline, withdraw, or edit advertisements at its discretion. Every care is taken to avoid mistakes but responsibility cannot be accepted by the Association for clerical or printer's errors.

REPLY BOX SERVICE

Confidential box numbers are available for an additional $25 per issue, plus the words: Box ________, c/o SUR. When responding to a box number, please send to Archives of Surgery, Box ________, c/o SUR, 515 N State St, Chicago, IL 60610.

CANCELLATIONS/CHANGES

Cancellations/changes must be received in writing at least 25 days prior to the date of the issue. In order to expedite, please fax to 312-464-5909 to the attention of your account representative.

GENERAL INFORMATION

To contact a Classified Advertising account representative, call 312-464-2475/2490/2491/4485 or 800-AMA-2260. Or fax your insertion order to 312-464-5909. Mail your materials to AMA Classified Advertising, 12th Floor, 515 N State St, Chicago, IL 60610.

ANNOUNCEMENT

Travel Grants for Research

The Burroughs Wellcome Fund (BWF) is accepting applications for 3 types of research travel grants, which enable US and Canadian scientists and medical historians to work for brief periods (2 weeks to 6 months) in the United Kingdom or the Republic of Ireland. The BWF annually makes approximately 50 research travel grants, including 10 grants in the history of medicine. The grants cover travel and subsistence expenses and range from $1000 to $15 000. Candidates must be citizens or permanent residents of the United States or Canada. Scientific investigators and medical historians must have a MD or PhD degree and hold an academic appointment at the assistant professor level or above at a degree-granting institution. Postdoctoral fellows must be early in their careers, and graduate students must be within a year of receiving their doctorates.

There are 3 application deadlines per year: March 1, July 1, and November 1. For information contact Rolly Simpson, Program Associate, telephone (919) 991-5110, e-mail: mailback@bwfund.org, or visit the Web site at http://www.bwfund.org.

CHIEFS/DEPARTMENT HEADS/ DIRECTORS

CHAIR, DEPARTMENT OF SURGERY: The Fallon Clinic, serving the community for 70 years, is seeking a dynamic B/C Surgeon with a subspecialty interest to lead the Surgery Department into the next century. We are a physician directed multi-specialty group practice, nationally recognized for quality and innovation. The Department of Surgery includes: General and Vascular Surgery, Urology, Otolaryngology, Orthopedics and Ophthalmology. Our ideal candidate should have demonstrated clinical and managerial experience, enjoy the rewards of clinical practice, and welcome the opportunity to make a significant impact on the delivery of surgical care in Central Massachusetts. We are seeking an individual with a vision for the future and the ability to plan and implement creative ideas for healthcare delivery. Research and teaching opportunities are available. We are also affiliated with a nationally acclaimed HMO. An excellent salary and benefits package is available. The Fallon Clinic is located in Worcester, New England's second largest city, located 45 minutes west of Boston. Enjoy New England at its best . . . beautiful landscapes, excellent schools, and quick access to mountains, the seashore, and major metropolitan areas. Please send CV and cover letter to Elizabeth Smiley or Mary Wright, Physician Services, 100 Central St, Worcester, MA 01608; Phone: 508-795-1157; Fax: 508-793-0909; E-mail: omd@fallon-clinic.com EOE.

ANNOUNCEMENT

Scholarships in Medical Science

The Charles E. Culpeper Foundation is accepting applications for its Year 2000 Scholarships in Medical Science Program designed to support the career development of academic physicians.

Up to 4 awards of $100 000 per year for 3 years will be made to US medical schools or equivalent US educational institutions on behalf of candidates who are US citizens or aliens who have been granted permanent US residence (proof required); who received their MD degree from a US medical school or the equivalent of an MD degree from an educational institution equivalent to a US medical school in 1991 or later; and who are judged worthy of support by virtue of the quality of their research proposals. All scientific research relevant to human health is eligible for consideration. No institution may nominate more than 1 candidate.

Deadline is August 16, 1999. Application forms and instructions may be obtained on the Web at www.culpeper.org or by contacting the Charles E. Culpeper Foundation at Financial Centre, 695 E Main St, Stamford, CT 06901-2155; telephone: (203) 975-1240; fax: (203) 975-1847.

ANNOUNCEMENT

Chronic Fatigue Registry of Physicians

The University of Washington is continuing to develop and enlarge its registry of more than 70 physicians with chronic fatigue syndrome, chronic fatigue, or fibromyalgia for research and other beneficial uses for patients and providers. Physicians with suggestive symptoms who have never been evaluated are welcome.

For information, contact Ellen Kleyman, Harborview Medical Center, 325 Ninth Ave, Box 359780, Seattle, WA 98104; phone: (206) 521-1929; fax: (206) 521-1930; e-mail: ekleyman@u.washington.edu.

ANNOUNCEMENT

Call for Abstracts: Cochrane Colloquium

The Cochrane Collaboration is accepting abstracts for oral and poster presentation at its Seventh Cochrane Colloquium. It will be held in Rome, Italy on October 5 through 9, 1999. Issues should pertain to the theme of the Best Evidence for Health Care: The Role of the Cochrane Collaboration. Topics covered include the history of evidence-based medicine and systematic reviews; systematic reviews and their effects on research planning; assessing clinical and public health relevance; individual vs statistical benefits and risks; and barriers to accepting systematic reviews as research.

For information, contact VII International Cochrane Colloquium, c/o Eurosymposia s.r.l., Via di Tor Fiorenza, 31, 0199 Rome, Italy; telephone: (39) 06-86328042; fax: (39) 06-86386644; e-mail: eurosy.congr@flashnet.it. The submission form can be downloaded at www.areas.it/roma99.

SOUTH TEXAS - GENERAL SURGERY: If you enjoy "Quality of Life" issues such as, low crime, excellent schools, no state income tax, clean air, and a low cost of living, then this practice opportunity is for you. A brand new hospital with a medical service area of 78,000 needs additional general surgery coverage. A generous income guarantee, no managed care, and an established referral system, are all excellent reasons why you should call to get additional information. This is a predominantly Hispanic community. If you're looking for unlimited income potential and a family oriented community, then please call for further details. For more information, call Robert Overfield, 800-839-4728. E-mail: overfield@beck-field.com Fax: 210-651-4338.

SURGERY: SURGICAL SPECIALTIES

CENTRAL, CA: 5 surgeon group seek MD for diverse General, Vascular, and Thoracic Surgery private practice. Family oriented rural commuity. Easy access to Yosemite, Sequoia, LA and SF. Early Partnership. BC/BE only. Fax CV to 559-585-2150, attn: Susan, or write to Kings Surgical Specialist, 470 N Greenfield, Suite 37, Hanford, CA 93230. Ph: 559-585-2100.

TWO-SURGEON PRACTICE, located in central New York, seeks general surgeon with laparoscopic, vascular, and/or thoracic capabilities. Recent fellowship training desirable. Based in the scenic and cosmopolitan home of Cornell University. The practice serves two progressive medical centers. Excellent lifestyle opportunities abound in housing, education, and recreation. Reply to Box 323, c/o SUR, 515 N State St, 12th Fl, Chicago, IL 60610.

ANNOUNCEMENT

Bupropion Pregnancy Registry

The Bupropion Pregnancy Registry is an ongoing national prenatal exposure registration and follow-up study established by Glaxo Wellcome in conjunction with the Centers for Disease Control and Prevention and experts in obstetrics and gynecology, teratology, clinical genetics, pediatrics, internal medicine, and epidemiology.

The purpose of the registry is to monitor for evidence of any major effect on developing fetuses when women have intentionally or inadvertently taken bupropion (Wellbutrin, Zyban) during any portion of their pregnancy. Patient confidentiality is strictly maintained.

If you have patients who have taken bupropion at any time during their pregnancy, you are encouraged to notify the registry, as early in the pregnancy as possible. To obtain a copy of the most recent interim report and/or to register patients, health care providers can contact the registry at (888) 825-5249, ext 39441 or call collect (919) 483-9441.

SURGERY: VASCULAR

MARYLAND: TWO VASCULAR SURGEONS sought to take over busy practice in suburb of DC. 240-bed hospital with certified vascular lab. Fellowship training in vascular preferred. Beautiful tree-lined community boasting wonderful schools and new golf course developments. Immediate need. Contact Todd Dillon at800-883-7345; Fax: 810-603-2942; E-mail: tdillon@cejka.com ID#6572AR. Visit our website at www.cejka.com

---

SALT LAKE CITY: BC/BE vascular trained surgeon for heart/lung group. Excellent compensation/ benefits/travel and relocation. PPS: 800-824-9275; Fax CV: 435-673-8423.

MacGregor Medical ASSOCIATION

Surgery Department Chair

Houston, Texas

Large multispecialty group practice in Houston is seeking a Board Certified General Surgeon to serve as Department Chair. Candidates should have five or more years of surgical experience, be familiar with contract negotiations and departmental productivity analysis as well as posses a record of demonstrated leadership. The incumbent can expect to spend 75% of time in patient care and 25% in completing administrative duties.

The surgeons operate in the prestigious Texas Medical Center and enjoy academic affiliation with local medical schools. The group serves over 160,000 patients and our diverse patient population is comprised of 90% managed care and 10% fee for service clients.

For an information packet, fax or mail your CV to:

MacGregor Medical Association
2550 Holly Hall
Houston, TX 77054

Fax: 713-746-5441

Check out our web site: http://medjobs.macgregor.com/

You can also call us at: 800-716-6060

The University of Medicine and Dentistry of New Jersey-New Jersey Medical School has the following Surgery positions available at the University Hospital, a level I Trauma Center for northern New Jersey.

EMERGENCY DEPARTMENT

BC/BE in Surgery required for our very busy ED, which has a total of 72,000 visits per year. Responsibilities include participating in the initial evaluation and resuscitation of trauma patients. Duties also include supervising residents, patient care, teaching medical students and clinical research. Positions offer faculty rank at the Instructor or Assistant Professor level.

Qualified candidate send resumes to: **Edwin A. Deitch, MD, Chairman, Department of Surgery, UMDNJ-New Jersey Medical School, 185 South Orange Ave., Room G506, Newark, NJ, 07103.** UMDNJ, New Jersey's University of the Health Sciences, is an Affirmative Action/Equal Opportunity Employer, m/f/d/v

UMD NEW JERSEY

Document Delivery Information

Copies of individual articles are available from the following:

UnCover
Tel: 800-787-7979
303-758-3030
Fax: 303-758-5946
URL: http://uncweb.carl.org
e-mail: uncover@carl.org

Institute for Scientific Information (ISI)
Tel: 800-336-4474
215-386-0100
Fax: 215-386-6362
URL: http://www.isinet.com

Index of Advertisers

CLASSIFIED ADVERTISING 683-688
http://www.ama-assn.org

ETHICON INC
Suture Assist .... Cover 2

GLAXO WELLCOME
Panorex 588

PFIZER, US PHARMACEUTICAL GROUP
http://www.pfizer.com
Trovan .... Cover 4

While every precaution is taken to ensure accuracy, we cannot guarantee against the possibility of an occasional change or omission in the preparation of this index.